Theory & Practice of Therapeutic Massage

FIFTH EDITION

Theory & Practice of Therapeutic Massage

Mark F. Beck

Photography by Yanik Chauvin

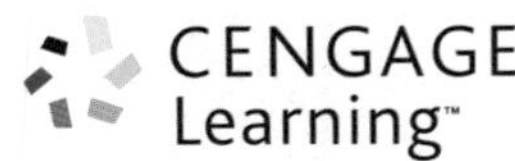

Australia • Brazil • Japan • Korea • Mexico • Singapore • Spain • United Kingdom • United States

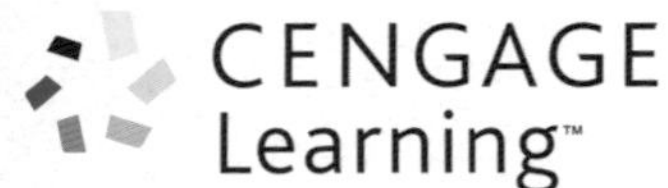

Theory & Practice of Therapeutic Massage
5th Edition
by Mark F. Beck

President, Milady: **Dawn Gerrain**

Publisher: **Erin O'Connor**

Acquisitions Editor: **Martine Edwards**

Senior Product Manager: **Philip Mandl**

Editorial Assistant: **Maria Hebert**

Director of Beauty Industry Relations: **Sandra Bruce**

Executive Marketing Manager: **Gerard McAvey**

Production Director: **Wendy Troeger**

Senior Content Project Manager: **Angela Sheehan**

Senior Art Director: **Joy Kocsis**

Library of Congress Control Number: 2009938144

Hard Cover – ISBN-13: 978-1-4354-8523-5
Hard Cover – ISBN-10: 1-4354-8523-8

Soft Cover – ISBN-13: 978-1-4354-8524-2
Soft Cover – ISBN-10: 1-4354-8524-6

Milady
5 Maxwell Drive
Clifton Park, NY 12065-2919
USA

Cengage Learning products are represented in Canada by Nelson Education, Ltd.

For your lifelong learning solutions, visit **milady.cengage.com**

Visit our corporate website at **www.cengage.com**

Notice to the Reader

Publisher does not warrant or guarantee any of the products described herein or perform any independent analysis in connection with any of the product information contained herein. Publisher does not assume, and expressly disclaims, any obligation to obtain and include information other than that provided to it by the manufacturer. The reader is expressly warned to consider and adopt all safety precautions that might be indicated by the activities described herein and to avoid all potential hazards. By following the instructions contained herein, the reader willingly assumes all risks in connection with such instructions. The publisher makes no representations or warranties of any kind, including but not limited to, the warranties of fitness for particular purpose or merchantability, nor are any such representations implied with respect to the material set forth herein, and the publisher takes no responsibility with respect to such material. The publisher shall not be liable for any special, consequential, or exemplary damages resulting, in whole or part, from the readers' use of, or reliance upon, this material.

Printed in the United States of America
2 3 4 5 XX 10

CONTENTS AT A GLANCE

CONTENTS

PART II Human Anatomy and Physiology

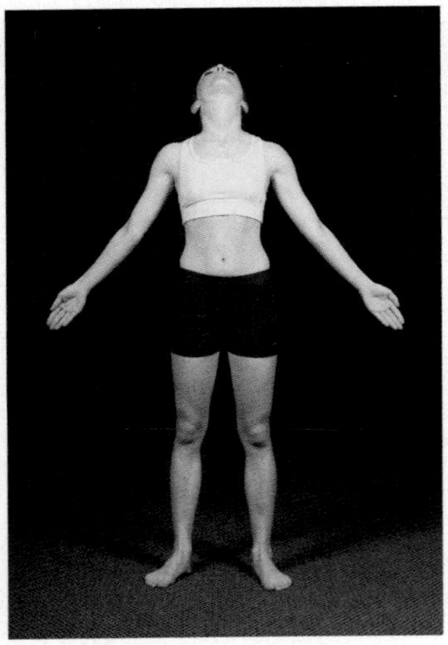

PART III Massage Practice

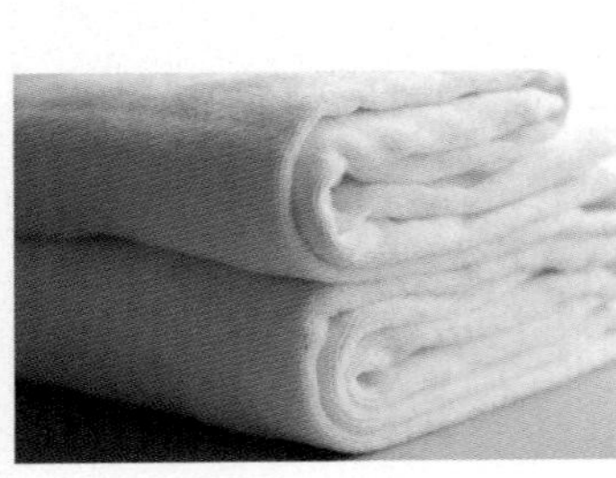

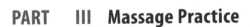

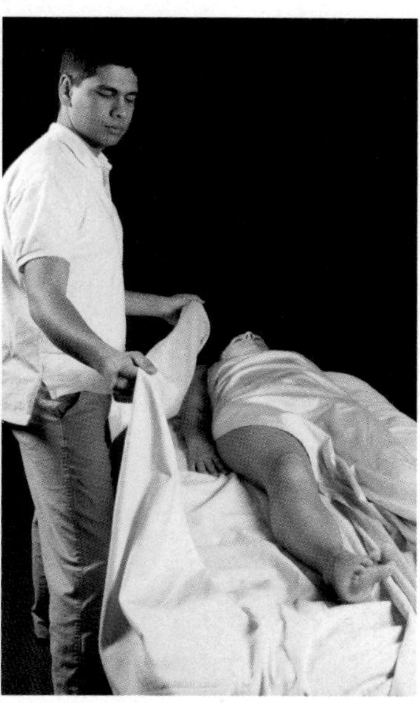

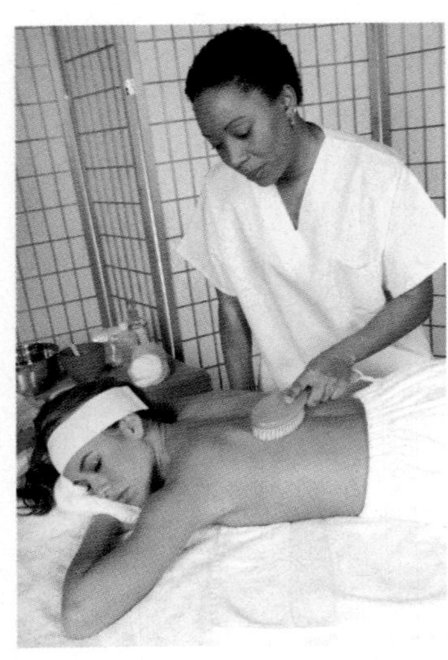

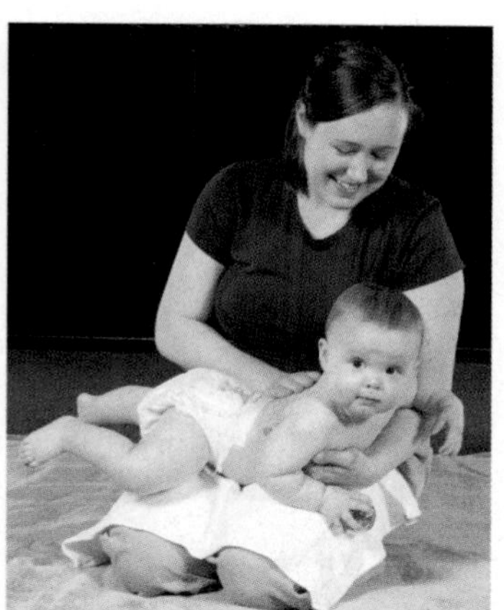

PART IV Massage Business Administration

PREFACE

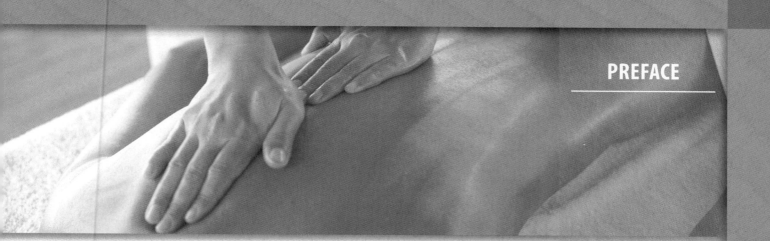

Welcome to the new *Theory & Practice of Therapeutic Massage*, Fifth Edition. It is very exciting to present the new edition of this classic text, containing all of the vital material of the past editions that you have come to trust, plus new information essential to today's student of massage. The text is primarily written for massage students in 500- to 1,200-hour massage programs and their instructors. This comprehensive text is also an important reference for massage therapists who want to refresh and expand their knowledge of the massage profession. *Theory & Practice of Therapeutic Massage*, Fifth Edition, is a basic textbook and starting point for students entering the massage profession. It contains the essential knowledge base for a massage therapist in an easily accessible form, as well as being a treasure trove of vital information for many possible career paths within the massage profession.

As more states regulate massage, massage education is becoming more standardized and organized, with a core body of knowledge reflected in licensing requirements, the National Certification Examination and the Federation of State Massage Board's Licensing Examination. Although most massage training takes place in one of many private massage schools, more massage programs are being offered in community colleges and business/career schools. All of these programs depend on solid core curriculum materials augmented with ancillary products. *Theory & Practice of Therapeutic Massage* and its ancillary products fit these programs perfectly, providing instructors and students with easily accessible materials that contain the fundamental knowledge base needed to become a successful massage practitioner.

Most massage education in the United States begins with a 500- to 1,000-hour program that lasts 6 months to 1 year. Programs include instruction in anatomy, physiology, kinesiology, ethics, sanitation, business practices, and the application of massage technique; most also include clinical practice. Many schools include instruction in some specialty techniques. Most of these programs provide a good foundation for a student to begin the journey as a massage professional. *Theory & Practice of Therapeutic Massage* is an excellent core textbook for these programs, because it contains all of the vital information about these basic subjects in one text.

Graduating from massage school is a first and important step in becoming a successful massage professional. The journey continues as the new professional therapist gains experience by performing massages and exchanging with other therapists while building and expanding a knowledge base through continuing education and personal study. In the massage profession, there are many paths and a wide variety of techniques. Although *Theory & Practice of Therapeutic Massage* provides the strong foundation that a student requires for entering the massage field, the text also provides introductions into several areas within the profession, with chapters devoted to spa massage, lymph massage, clinical massage techniques, therapeutic procedure, athletic massage, and massage in medicine. The somatic modalities chapter has been augmented with expanded discussions on chair massage, reflexology, Asian bodywork, and chakra balancing. Although entire books have been written on many of these subjects, this book provides enough of an overview of these modalities for the student to get a sense of whether he or she might want to pursue further study of a particular specialty. There is a lifetime of learning condensed into this text, and it is only the beginning of what is possible. There is always more to learn.

HISTORY OF THEORY & PRACTICE OF THERAPEUTIC MASSAGE

Frank Nichols was the author of the 1948 publication of *Theory & Practice of Body Massage* by Milady Publishing. Initiated in 1984, the first edition of *Theory & Practice of Therapeutic Massage* was a revision of the Nichols book and a collaborative effort of several writers under the editorial direction of Bobbi Ray Madry of Milady Publications, when Milady was a small, stand-alone publisher. It was not until the text was ready to go to the printer that I was asked for permission to use my name as the author because I was the largest contributor and they could not use Frank Nichols' name. Little did I know that I would become the author of *Theory & Practice of Therapeutic Massage* and would still be working on the project more than 25 years later.

I am honored to be involved in the continuing evolution of *Theory & Practice of Therapeutic Massage*. As an insatiable student of massage, my yearning to learn was only whetted by the 1,000-hour massage apprenticeship program I completed in 1974. Reading numerous books on topics such as anatomy and natural healing techniques and accumulating hundreds of hours of continuing education while working with a steadily growing clientele created more questions than answers. More schooling in a holistic practitioner program increased my skills. I started teaching massage in 1978 and became a massage school owner and director in 1980. As school director for over 15 years, I developed curricula, taught classes, and continued a part-time clinical practice. I served on the boards of state and national massage organizations in different capacities, including secretary of education, secretary of certification, and president. In 1992, I returned to school and earned a bachelor's degree in vocational education, with an emphasis on massage therapy. When Milady Publishing invited me to be a consultant for the revision of Frank Nichols' *Theory & Practice of Body Massage* in 1984, I saw it as an opportunity to participate in the creation of a much-needed textbook for the emerging massage therapy profession. In 1988, *Theory & Practice of Therapeutic Massage* was introduced as the first comprehensive massage therapy textbook on the market. Since then, each new edition has been expanded and updated in response to the emerging trends and needs of the fastest-growing profession in the United States, including this newest fifth edition.

The first edition provided the industry with a much-needed textbook for massage education. The second edition was updated to contain the vital knowledge and concepts needed by the student to enter the massage profession. The third edition added important features so that the instructor had all the elements to assist the student in gaining the skills and knowledge to become a massage practitioner. The fourth edition strengthened key subjects, including ethics and therapeutic application of massage, and added important chapters to help students to choose a career path as they move into the massage profession. Finally, the fifth edition expands and refocuses the clinical and therapeutic applications of classical, neuromuscular, and lymph massage techniques.

NEW TO THE FIFTH EDITION

The new fifth edition builds on the solid content of the former editions. The text maintains an easily readable style. Revisions have been made throughout the text to reflect the latest industry standards and research. In addition to the basic information for Western/Swedish massage and skills focusing on wellness and relaxation massage, there are several new chapters. Two new chapters have been added to the core of the text that provide important information about clinical skills, including neuromuscular and myofascial techniques as well as lymph massage. Another new chapter discusses special massage considerations for special populations, including prenatal massage, infant massage, massage for elderly clients, and massage for critically ill clients and people with cancer.

Theory & Practice of Therapeutic Massage is full of invaluable knowledge and fundamental concepts for learning massage. Although the text provides excellent information, instruction from a competent instructor and guided practice are required to become proficient at using the techniques described in the text. Hands-on classroom instruction and literally hundreds of hours of practice and application of skills in a clinical setting on real clientele are required to master the techniques.

ORGANIZATION

The text is organized into sections that can be studied sequentially, or better yet, simultaneously.

Part I, The History and Advancement of Therapeutic Massage (Chapters 1 through 3), gives a general introduction to therapeutic massage. Chapter 1 is an overview of the history of massage, which has been practiced in some form since prehistoric times. Chapter 2 discusses the legal and educational requirements to practice massage. Chapter 3 is concerned with professional standards and contains an expanded discussion of ethical considerations in the practice of therapeutic massage.

Part II, Human Anatomy and Physiology (Chapters 4 and 5), is a richly detailed presentation of anatomy, physiology, and pathology, the study of which is a foundation for the understanding and practice of therapeutic massage. Full-color illustrations enhance the descriptions in the text of structure and function, especially of the skeletal, muscular, circulatory, and nervous systems, as well as the other systems of the body.

Part III, Massage Practice (Chapters 6 through 21), combines theory with the practice of massage. Chapter 6 covers benefits, indications, and contraindications of massage. Chapter 7 discusses equipment and supplies, and Chapter 8 addresses hygiene, sanitation, and safety practices. Chapter 9 covers the preliminary consultation, communication skills, and charting for basic wellness massage. Chapters 10 through 12 define the classification of massage movements and describe the application of massage technique and the procedure for a general full-body relaxation massage.

Chapter 13 introduces the student to the therapeutic uses of water and hydrotherapy. Chapter 14 expands on the content of the hydrotherapy chapter and provides insight into the expectations and requirements of spa massage and working in the fast-growing spa industry.

Chapter 15 introduces the student to a variety of clinical massage techniques, including neuromuscular techniques to address trigger points, myofascial techniques, and craniosacral therapy. Chapter 16 is an introduction to lymph massage.

Chapter 17 takes the application of massage to the therapeutic level, in which each client is considered for the specific conditions that he or she brings to the session. Assessment techniques are introduced to determine the client's needs and the specific soft tissues involved, and modalities are indicated to address soft tissue dysfunction.

The remaining chapters in Part III provide fundamental information to enhance and expand the student's skills in several specialty areas. Chapter 18, "Athletic/Sports Massage," introduces students to the fundamentals of sports massage, working with athletes, and the various applications of specialized massage in the sports world. Chapter 19 is a new chapter that discusses massage applications for special populations, including prenatal and infant massage, elderly clients, and critically ill people or those with cancer. Chapter 20 explores medical massage historically and reviews the current use of therapeutic massage as it integrates with modern medicine. Chapter 21 discusses other somatic modalities, including chair massage, reflexology, Asian bodywork techniques, and chakra balancing.

Part IV, Massage Business Administration, is devoted to the business side of a massage practice. Which type of workplace setting appeals to you—sports clinic, day spa, chiropractor's office, your home? Should you start your own business or work for someone else? Learn about licensing, setup costs, bookkeeping, advertising, and other aspects of running a successful business.

The instructor might design the curriculum so that the student is studying several different sections of the text at the same time. For example, early in the program, the student could study the history of massage, begin the study of anatomy and physiology, and begin learning the classification of massage movements all at the same time. As the program continues, the curriculum might cover legal requirements and ethics at the same time as benefits, indications, and contraindications, while the study of anatomy and massage techniques continues. When the student has progressed to the point of doing full-body massages, the consultation is covered as the study of anatomy and kinesiology continues. Advanced and specialty applications of massage follow at the same time as business practices and more anatomy, physiology, and pathology.

SPECIAL FEATURES

The textbook is organized and designed to make retention easier and learning more enjoyable.

- *Clear, step-by-step instructions* augmented by hundreds of dynamic full-color photos guide the student through basic and advanced massage techniques.
- *Learning Objectives* at the beginning of each chapter focus student learning and are excellent tools for study and review.
- *Margin glossary terms.* Important terms are highlighted, with definitions conveniently displayed in the page margin for easy referral and study. A comprehensive glossary at the back of the book gives students immediate access to definitions.
- *Charts and tables* emphasize crucial concepts. An extensive table in Chapter 5 illustrates the insertion, origin, and action of skeletal muscles, knowledge essential to the effective practice of therapeutic massage. More than 40 full-color illustrations help the student to identify and locate all the major muscle groups.
- *Informational text boxes and bulleted lists* throughout the text highlight important content for easy reading and enhanced review.
- *Review of specialized massage applications.* In addition to a strong foundation in basic massage, explore the therapeutic application of massage, clinical massage, sports massage, spa massage, massage in a medical setting, lymph massage, soft tissue interventions, chair massage, reflexology, and more.
- *Questions for discussion and review.* At the end of each chapter, test your comprehension and identify which areas need to be reviewed by answering questions covering material in the chapter. The answers are located in Appendix II of the textbook.

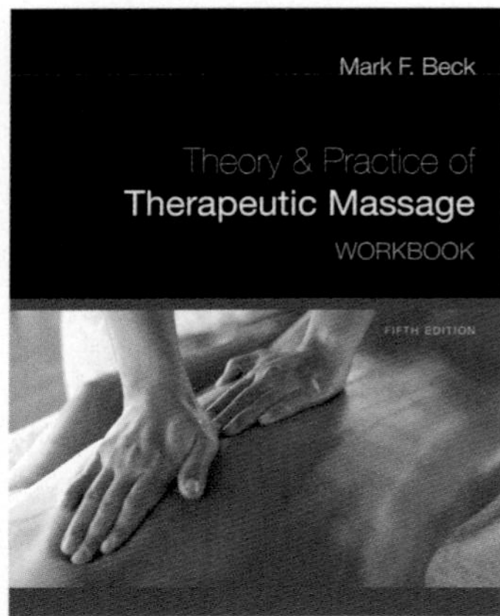

EXTENSIVE TEACHING AND LEARNING PACKAGE

Several ancillary materials accompany *Theory & Practice of Therapeutic Massage*, Fifth Edition. These materials are designed to support student learning and to provide massage instructors with everything they need to teach the concepts in the core textbook successfully.

Theory & Practice of Therapeutic Massage, Fifth Edition Workbook

The Workbook is made up of questions that directly correspond to each chapter of the textbook. Questions are in the form of fill-in-the-blank, matching, multiple choice, word reviews, and labeling illustrations. The workbook questions help the student to prepare for certification and licensing examinations.

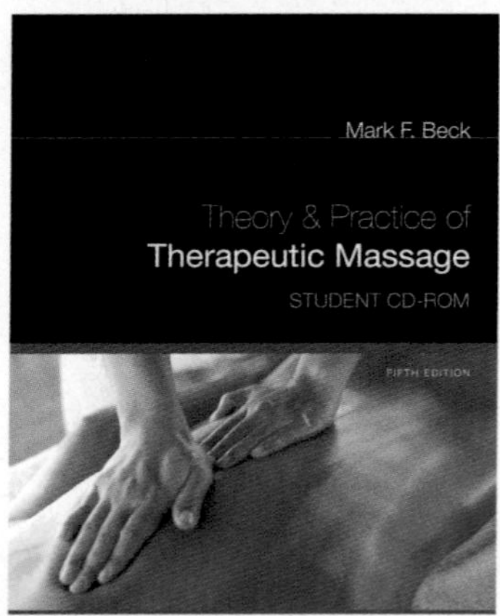

Theory & Practice of Therapeutic Massage, Fifth Edition Student CD-ROM

This interactive student product was designed to reinforce classroom learning, stimulate the imagination, and aid in preparation for board examinations. Featuring video clips and graphical animations to demonstrate practices and procedures, this exciting educational tool also contains a test bank, learning games, and an audio glossary that pronounces and defines each term. The student CD-ROM is available in two versions: an individual user version and a networkable school version.

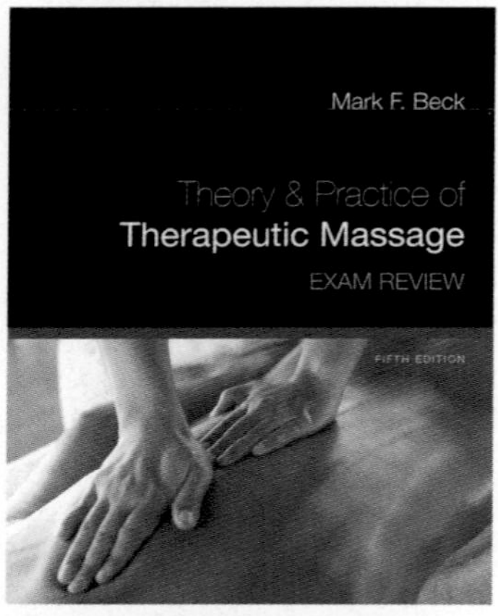

Theory & Practice of Therapeutic Massage, Fifth Edition Exam Review

This review book contains questions similar to those found on state licensing examinations for massage therapists. It employs the multiple-choice type question, which has been widely adopted and approved by most state licensing boards. Groups of questions are arranged under major subject areas. Like the core textbook, the Exam Review is also available in Spanish.

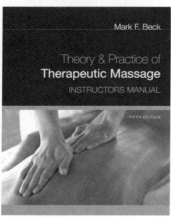

Theory & Practice of Therapeutic Massage, Fifth Edition Instructor's Manual

The Instructor's Manual is a comprehensive teaching aid that contains

- lesson plans, each keyed to a section of the text
- an outline of topics to cover in both the theory and practical sessions of each class
- time allotments for each activity
- suggested projects, resources, and assignments
- teaching tips to help instructors engage and instruct students successfully
- skills checklists that can be used to gauge and track students' mastery of specific massage skills
- additional resources and sources for information

- answer key for the student workbook included on the CD-ROM provided with the Instructor's Manual

The *Instructor's Manual* is designed to help massage educators by simplifying and organizing classroom preparation and presentation. Teaching becomes more efficient, more effective, and more enjoyable.

Theory & Practice of Therapeutic Massage, Fifth Edition Course Management Guide CD-ROM

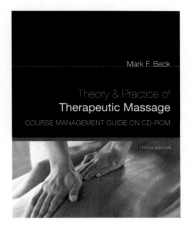

The Course Management Guide CD-ROM is an innovative instructor resource to support customized instruction. This CD-ROM for instructors contains excellent tools, including

- a detailed lesson plan for each chapter in the book.
- learning reinforcement ideas or activities that can be implemented in the massage therapy classroom.
- the answer key to the review questions from the *Theory & Practice of Therapeutic Massage,* Fifth Edition Workbook
- *a Computerized Test Bank* of over 1,100 questions in multiple-choice, matching, and short-answer format, as well as the accompanying answers, organized by chapter, which can be used to generate quizzes and tests.
- a searchable *Image Library* containing all of the color drawings and figures from *Theory & Practice of Therapeutic Massage*, Fifth Edition, to incorporate into lectures, electronic presentations, assignments, testing, and handouts.
- *student Skills Proficiency Checklists* in both ready-to-use PDF and customizable MS Word formats.
- *a Customizable Syllabus* that instructors can tailor to meet individual teaching styles and course objectives, complete with course schedules, assignments, grading options, paper topics, and more.

The Course Management Guide CD-ROM is an incredibly powerful resource that instructors can customize to fit their individual instructional goals.

Theory & Practice of Therapeutic Massage, Fifth Edition Instructor Support Slides

(Microsoft PowerPoint Presentation)

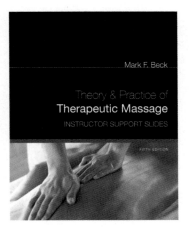

The PowerPoint® presentation created to accompany *Theory & Practice of Therapeutic Massage*, Fifth Edition, makes lesson plans simple yet incredibly effective. Complete with photos and art, this chapter-by-chapter CD-ROM has ready-to-use presentations that will help to engage students' attention and keep their interest through its varied color schemes and styles. Instructors can use it as is or adapt it to their own classrooms by importing photos they have taken, changing the graphics, or adding slides.

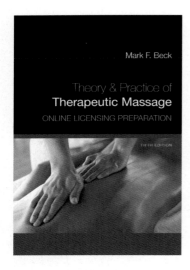

Online Licensing Preparation: Theory & Practice of Therapeutic Massage, Fifth Edition

Online Licensing Preparation: Theory & Practice of Therapeutic Massage, Fifth Edition, provides students with an online alternative for additional preparation for state board examinations. One thousand multiple-choice questions, different from those in the Exam Review, appear with rationales for correct and incorrect choices. Students have the flexibility to study from any computer, whether at home or at school. Because examination review preparation is available to students at any time of day or night, class time can be used for other activities, and students gain familiarity with a computerized test environment as they prepare for licensure.

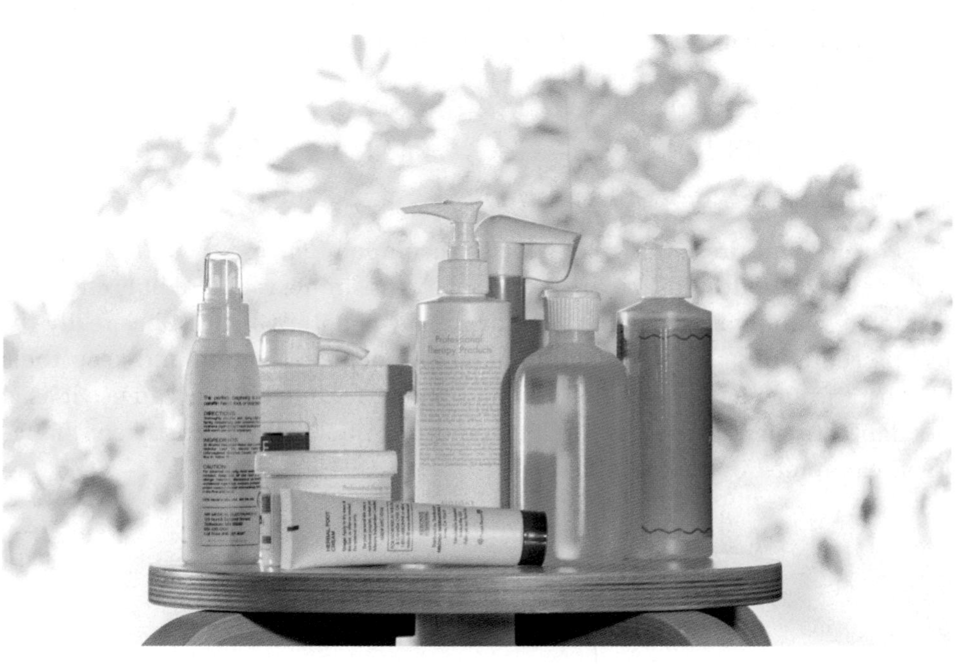

ACKNOWLEDGMENTS

The author and Cengage Learning wish to express our deep appreciation to the many professional people who have contributed their valuable time and counsel during the preparation of this text. Massage therapy has developed over hundreds of years. There is actually very little information that is unique, original, or new in this text, although each edition has been refined and expanded to contain the fundamental and vital concepts needed for today's serious student of therapeutic massage. Literally hundreds of people have been involved in both the production and the content of this text throughout its history and development. The fifth edition would not be possible without the four editions that preceded it and all of the work and talent of the many individuals that went into those editions. We are indebted to and appreciative of every contributor.

We especially want to thank the following people for their contributions in their special areas of expertise:

Richard Van Why and Judy Calvert for their unceasing research into the history of massage and the information provided in the history chapter.

Jack Meagher, Pat Archer, and Gay Koopman for the material that they provided in the athletic massage chapter.

David Palmer, founder and director of TouchPro Institute in San Francisco, for contributions in the section on chair massage.

Cherie Sohnen-Moe for her valuable contributions to the massage profession and especially to the business and ethics chapters of this text.

Steve Capellini for the valuable addition of the spa chapter and his expert help during the photo shoot for the fourth edition.

Maria K. Hebert, LMT, LE for her expert help during the photo shoot for this new fifth edition.

Susan Beck for the Infant Massage portion of the Special Populations chapter in this edition and her continuous support through the development of the first two editions of the text.

Steve Schenkman for his valuable contributions about Asian bodywork.

Richard Eidson for his contributions to the Hydrotherapy chapter.

Yanik Chauvin for the incredible photography in the fourth and fifth editions.

Dan Cronin of the Center for Natural Wellness School of Massage Therapy, Albany, New York, for inviting us to hold the photo shoot at his beautiful facility and providing us unlimited access to the school's resources.

All of the models in the photos, each one a licensed massage therapist or a student on the road to a massage career, with special thanks to Dale Perry, LMT, CLT, NSMT, for sharing his expertise in lymph massage and Lou Alpy for sharing his expertise in neuromuscular therapy and craniosacral therapy.

Faye Schenkman for lending her expertise on pharmacology, herbology, and nutritional supplements as they relate to the practice of massage therapy in Appendix I.

The author also expresses a special appreciation to the following people:

Bobbi Ray Madry, editor of the original *Theory & Practice of Therapeutic Massage*, for her encouragement of my involvement in this project and her gift of the authorship of the text.

Bob Rogers for the training that began my journey into the marvelous and rewarding profession of massage.

My mentors, teachers, students, and many clients who have provided me with the knowledge and skills that were the foundation of my own practice and the curriculum at the massage schools at which I directed and taught.

My wife, Kiri Saftler, for her continuous support and encouragement as I spend countless hours tucked away in my office revising the text.

The creation of this magnificent fifth edition would not have been possible without the expertise and dedication of the entire production team and Cengage Learning, including:

Martine Edwards, Acquisitions Editor
Philip Mandl, Senior Product Manager
Maria K. Hebert, Editorial Assistant
Angela Sheehan, Senior Content Project Manager
Joy Kocsis, Senior Art Director

To the many reviewers, for their assistance, comments, and expertise in reviewing the developing text.

REVIEWERS OF *THEORY & PRACTICE OF THERAPEUTIC MASSAGE, 5TH EDITION*

Garfield Lee Adkins
Institute of Beauty and Massage
Lurana Bain, LMT
Elgin Community College
Susan Beck, BS, NCTMB
Idaho State University
Bernice Bicknase, BS, ACMT
Ivy Tech Community College-Northeast
Monique Blake, LMT, MS
Keiser Career College
Felicia Brown, LMBT Spalutions
Christine Clinton
ITEC-USA
Christopher Cude
United Education Institute College
Sheila Decora. DC, CMT
Chase College
Jennifer DiBlasio, AST, CHT, ACMT
Career Training Academy, Inc.
Betty Echols, LMT
Instructor, NAME OF SCHOOL TK
Brooke Galo LMT
Apollo College
Shari Golightly, EDS
Entanglements Training Center
Jamie Graham, LAc, LMT, MTI
McLennan Community College
Belinda Green, LMT
Mildred Elley
Laura Hash
Kathleen Hunt, LMT
Elizabeth Grady School of Esthetics and Massage Therapy
Michael Konsor
Glendale Career College
Dawn Langnes, BS, LMT, CNMT
Barral Institute-Upledger Institute
Scott LaSalle, MSW, LMT, CNMT
Florida Career College
Todd Lorentz, MA, LMT
Natural Health Practitioners of Canada Association
Dave MacDougall, MA, LMT
North Country Community College
Gloria Mathiesen, MA, LMT, NCTMB
Pima Community College
Beverly May, BA, NCTMB, AMTA
Rewood Massage & Sauna
Dale Perry, LMT, CLT
CNW School of Massage Therapy

Susan Pomfret, MA, LMT
Central Arizona College
Donna Redman-Bentley, PT, PhD
Western University of Health Sciences
Teressa Sloan, PhD, DD, NCMT, LMT
Bluegrass Professional School of Massage Therapy
Deborah Valentine Smith, BA, LMT, AOBTA(R)CI, Dipl. ABT (NCCAOM)
Massage Arts Center of Philadelphia
Heather H. Smith, BS, LMT, SET
Education Affiliates/Florida Career Institute
Anna Stookey, MA, MFT, CHt, CMT
Bodymind Psychotherapist & Massage Therapist
Carolyn Talley-Porter, LMT
Greenville Technical College
Deborah Taylor, LMT, BS
East West College of the Healing Arts
Maureen C. Thacker, BS, LMT, NCBTMB, NCEA
Academy of Career Training
Dawn Turner, RN, LMT, Reiki Master
Mildred Elley
Denise Van Nostran, MM, BM, LMT
Technical College of the Lowcountry
Tamela Voorhees, NCTMB, LMT, AMTA
High Tech Institute
Blayne Wiley, BA, LMT
Eagle Gate College
Tracy Wright, LMT, NCBTMB
Educating Hands School of Massage

I want to acknowledge Frank Nichols, author of the original *Theory & Practice of Body Massage* (1948), for the original work from which *Theory & Practice of Therapeutic Massage* evolved.

Finally, Natasha, wherever you are, thank you for my first real massage and the advice, "Whenever your back hurts like that, find someone who knows how to do massage."

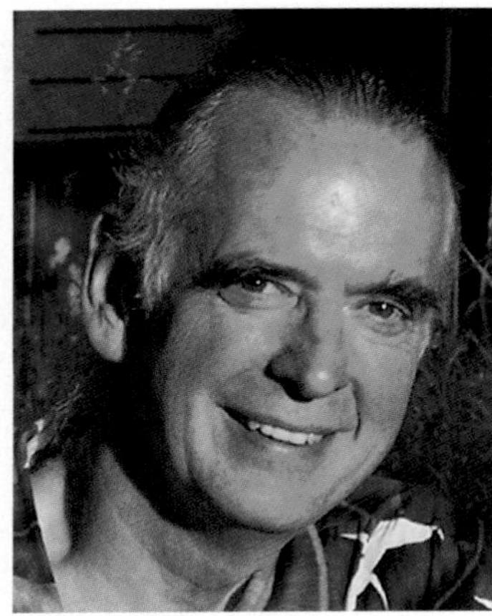

ABOUT THE AUTHOR

Mark Beck began his massage career in 1974 (more than 35 years ago) after completing a massage apprenticeship under the guidance of Bob Rogers. One of the main things that he gained in his training was the knowledge of how expansive the world of massage is and an insatiable appetite to learn more. He completed a program to become a holistic practitioner in 1979 and has taken hundreds of hours of continuing education classes. He has been the owner and director of two massage schools and has been active in state and national professional massage organizations. He holds a bachelor's degree in vocational education with an emphasis in massage therapy from the University of Idaho. Mark developed the Structural Muscular Balancing Seminars and is coauthor of the *Structural Muscular Balancing Manual.*

Because of a spinal cord injury in 1990, Mark retired from the practice of massage therapy but continues to be an advocate for excellence in massage education. He has also become an ambassador for disability advocacy.

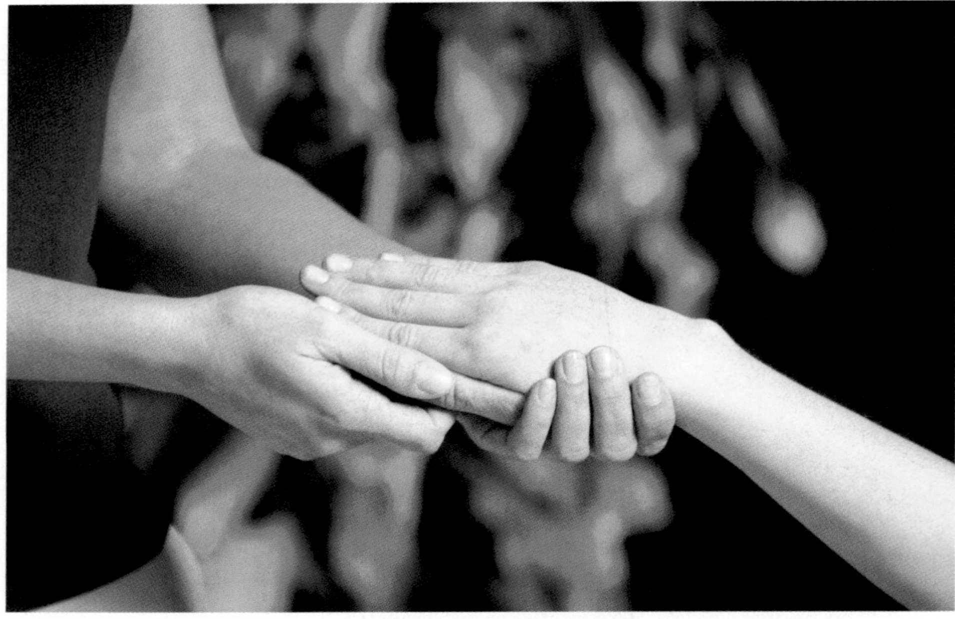

CONTRIBUTORS TO *THEORY & PRACTICE OF THERAPEUTIC MASSAGE*, FIFTH EDITION

Susan Beck

Susan Beck BS, NCTMB, is the program coordinator and lead instructor for the Massage Therapy Program, Department of Health Occupations, College of Technology at Idaho State University and is obtaining a Masters in Human Resource Training and Development. Susan was the owner/operator of the Massage Clinic in Twin Falls, Idaho from 1979–1996. Susan is an instructor-trainer for the International Loving Touch Foundation where she travels and teaches a 3-day seminar for Certification for Infant Massage Instructors. From 1982–1990, she was co-owner with Mark Beck of the Magic Valley Massotherapy Institute, a 500-hour program in massage therapy. She has been actively academically involved in the development of *The Theory and Practice of Therapeutic Massage* 1st & 2nd, and 5th edition by Mark Beck, as well as reviewing other new texts. Susan Beck is a long standing member of the American Massage Therapist Association (AMTA) and a member of the Alliance for Massage Therapy Education (AFMTE).

Steve Capellini

Steve Capellini has been a licensed massage therapist since 1984. He has worked in the spa industry for over 25 years as a therapist, supervisor, trainer, manager, and consultant. He has written many articles for industry publications and was a spa columnist for Massage Today for 9 years. His books include the new textbook entitled *The Complete Spa Book for Massage Therapists, The Royal Treatment, Massage Career Guide for Hands-On Success,* and *Massage for Dummies.* He teaches workshops for therapists who plan to integrate spa services into their practices and is currently writing a textbook to complement spa training curricula in massage schools.

Yanik Chauvin

Yanik Chauvin is a former administrative director of a leading massage therapy school in Gatineau, Quebec, Canada. He is also a professional photographer selling massage therapy images through his Web site (www.touchphotography.com) and offering his photography services to various organizations through another site (www.yanikchauvin.com). He specializes in corporate and health-oriented imagery and has been working closely with Cengage Learning since early 2005 as the designer and photographer of the book covers for the complete massage therapy line.

Faye N. Schenkman

Faye Schenkman is a licensed massage therapist in New York and holds a master's degree in Chinese history. She is a diplomate of Asian bodywork therapy and Chinese herbal medicine and the National Certification Commission for Acupuncture and Oriental Medicine (NCCAOM). She is a charter member and certified instructor of the American Organization of Bodywork Therapies of

Asia (AOBTA). She is a former faculty member of The University of Illinois Oriental Studies Department and a teacher of Chinese in several New York City high schools. Faye is currently an instructor of Integrative Therapies, Graduate School of Nursing at Columbia University. She is a former Board of Trustees member of the New York College for Wholistic Health Education and Research, and she was director of the Wholistic Health Center at the college for more than 10 years. Faye was also the chair of the Massage Therapy School at New York College, as well as the dean of the Advanced *Amma* program, where she taught Advanced *Amma* Therapeutic Massage, Chinese and Western herbal medicine, Eastern nutrition, and Oriental sciences. Faye has been an advanced practitioner of *Amma* Therapeutic Massage for more than 20 years. She is a cofounder, with her partner Kim Rosado, of Wholistic Healing Arts, LLC, in Huntington, New York, where patients are treated for a wide range of physical illnesses using *amma*, acupuncture, herbal medicine, holistic nutrition, craniosacral therapy, uterine massage, and Qi Gong. Faye and Kim conduct workshops throughout the United States.

Steven Schenkman

Steven Schenkman, a licensed New York State Massage Therapist since 1984, is an established leader in the field of Complementary and Integrative Medicine. He served as President of The New York College for Holistic Health, Education, and Research (now known as the New York College of Health Professions) from 1989 through 2001. The college offers associates and bachelor's degree programs in massage and bodywork therapy, master's degrees in acupuncture and Oriental medicine, certificate programs in holistic nursing and physical arts. There he developed the first associate's degree program in massage therapy in the United States in 1996. Since 2001 Mr. has been a consultant and curriculum specialist to career colleges, allied health and business Schenkman schools and schools of massage therapy specializing in assistance with accreditation, administration, licensing, reorganization, curriculum, new program and business development and marketing & advertising. Steven was also a founding member of the National Certification Board for Therapeutic Massage and Bodywork (NCBTMB). He served as Chairman of the New York State Massage Therapy Board and was also founding member and the first President of the American Organization for Bodywork Therapies of Asia (AOBTA). Most recently, Mr. Schenkman completed a one year project as a member of the Massage Therapy Body of Knowledge (MTBOK) Task Force with the release of the MTBOK document at the Massage Therapy Foundation's 2010 Highlighting Research Conference in Seattle, Washington. The Task Force was responsible for defining, developing and articulating a massage therapy body of knowledge for the profession. Steven is a member of the Cengage Learning Massage Therapy Advisory Board and Books of Discovery Advisory Council. He practices Advanced Amma Therapeutic Massage, a form of Asian Bodywork Therapy. Mr. Schenkman is a master tai chi practitioner and instructor. To contact Steven, call 1-631-659-3090 or visit his website, http://www.schenkmanconsulting.com.

HOW TO USE *THEORY AND PRACTICE OF THERAPEUTIC MASSAGE, 5TH EDITION*

Learning Objectives

Before beginning a chapter, review the Learning Objectives for a "road map" of what the chapter will cover. These Learning Objectives cover the main points of each chapter and are also an excellent tool for review and study.

LEARNING OBJECTIVES

After you have mastered this chapter, you will be able to:

1. **Explain why massage is known as one of the earliest remedial practices for the relief of pain and discomfort.**
2. **Explain why massage is a natural and instinctive remedy for some illnesses and injuries.**
3. **Identify three historic Greeks who professed the benefits of exercise and massage.**
4. **Explain how developments in the nineteenth century influenced modern massage therapy.**
5. **Describe the basic differences in massage systems.**
6. **Explain why massage practitioners should understand massage history.**

Key Terms and Margin Definitions

The amount of new terminology faced by the massage therapy student can be overwhelming. To help the reader quickly and easily master important terms, new words are bolded in color in the text on their first use. This key term is then defined in the margin, providing immediate access to the definition. All terms bolded and defined in the margin are also included in the text's main glossary, found at the back of the book. Readers are encouraged to use the margin glossary terms while studying and reviewing.

shiatsu

is a massage technique from Japan in which points of stimulation are pressed to affect the circulation of fluids and ki (life force energy).

tschanpua

is a Hindu technique of massage in the bath.

Questions for Discussion and Review

At the conclusion of each chapter are questions to help focus learning and spark thoughtful discussion. These are an excellent review tool and can be done independently or as part of an organized assignment. While the answers to all the questions can be found in the chapter itself, they are also provided at the back of the book for easy reference.

QUESTIONS FOR DISCUSSION AND REVIEW

1. Define *massage*.
2. How do we know that ancient civilizations used therapeutic massage and exercise in their social, personal, or religious practices?
3. Why is massage said to be the most natural and instinctive means of relieving pain and discomfort?
4. What did the Chinese call their early massage system?
5. Why did the Greeks and Romans place so much emphasis on exercise and massage?
6. Which Greek physician became known as the father of medicine?
7. Why were the Middle Ages also called the Dark Ages?
8. How did the Arabic Empire and the rise of Islam help to preserve the practice of massage?
9. Why was the Renaissance an important turning point for the arts and sciences?
10. How did the invention of the printing press in the fifteenth century help to further the practice of massage and therapeutic exercise?
11. What is the basis of Per Henrik Ling's Swedish Movement Cure?
12. Who introduced the Swedish Movement Cure to the United States?
13. What are some of the reasons for the decline of massage at the turn of the twentieth century?
14. Why did the acceptance of massage and therapeutic exercise increase during World Wars I and II?
15. Why did manual massage become a secondary treatment following World War II?
16. How has more awareness of health and personal wellness in recent years caused a renewed interest in massage?
17. What is the difference between passive and active exercise?
18. Describe the theory on which the Japanese shiatsu system of massage is based.
19. What is the role of proper exercise and use of massage in athletics?
20. Of what benefit is the history of therapeutic massage to the student who wishes to pursue a career in the field?
21. Which massage system is the most widely used in general massage?
22. In what way are the Chinese and Japanese systems similar?
23. Why is massage used as a treatment in sports or athletic medicine?

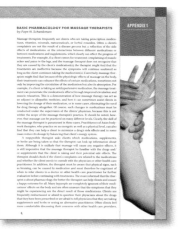

Appendix I: Basic Pharmacology for Massage Therapists

Increasingly, massage therapists are expected to have a basic understanding of pharmacology for certification and licensure. This new appendix on Basic Pharmacology for Massage Therapists is a general introduction to this important information. Covering basics of pharmacology as well as drugs, vitamins and minerals, and herbs, this is an excellent resource.

APPENDIX 1

BASIC PHARMACOLOGY FOR MASSAGE THERAPISTS

by Faye R. Schenkman

PHOTO CREDITS

Unless otherwise noted in the photo captions throughout the text, all images in this text fall under the copyright of Milady, a part of Cengage Learning. Photography by Yanik Chauvin. Athletic Sports Massage photos in Chapter 18 by Dino Petrocelli.

PART 1

THE HISTORY AND ADVANCEMENT OF THERAPEUTIC MASSAGE

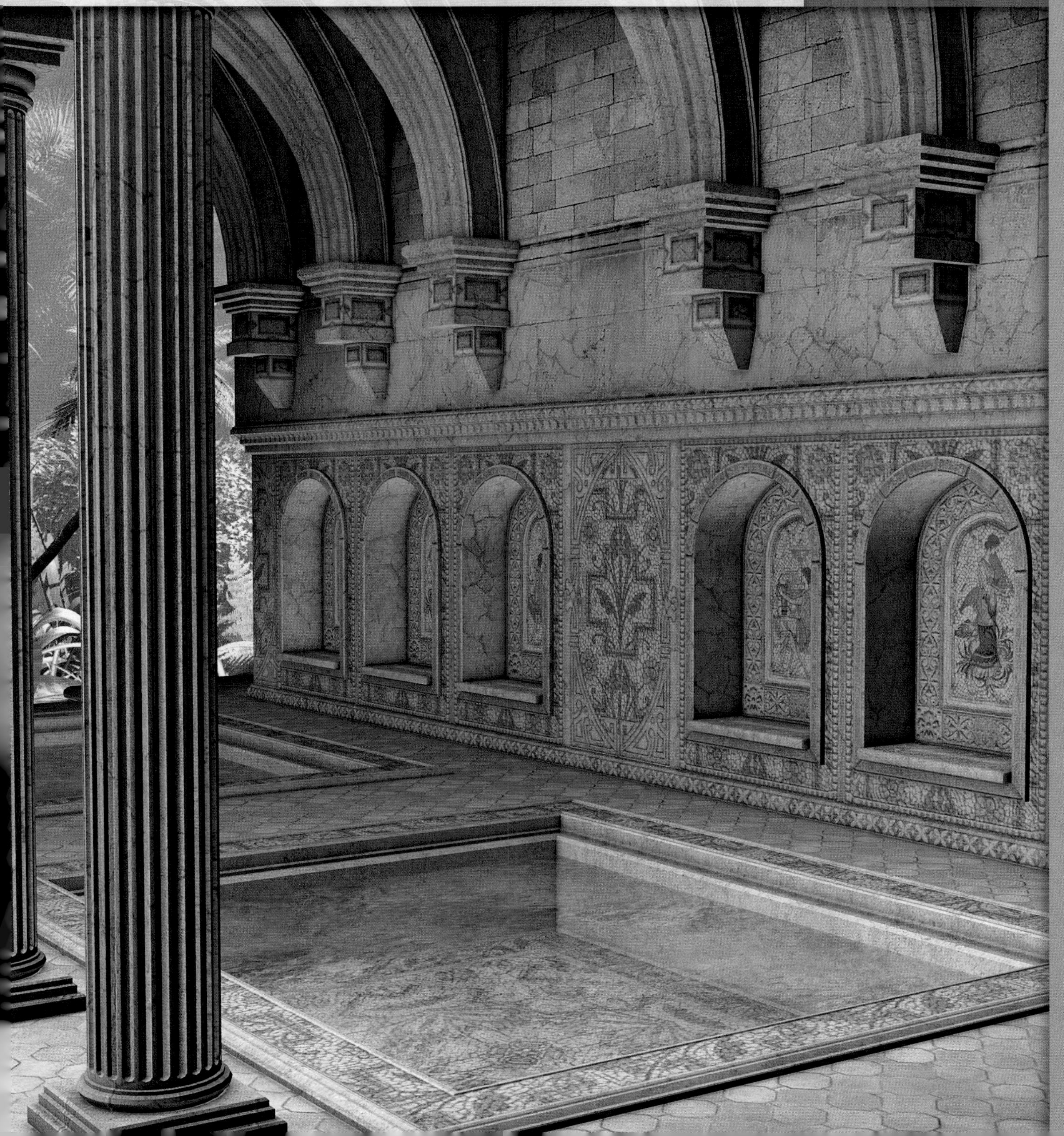

CHAPTER

1

Historical Overview of Massage

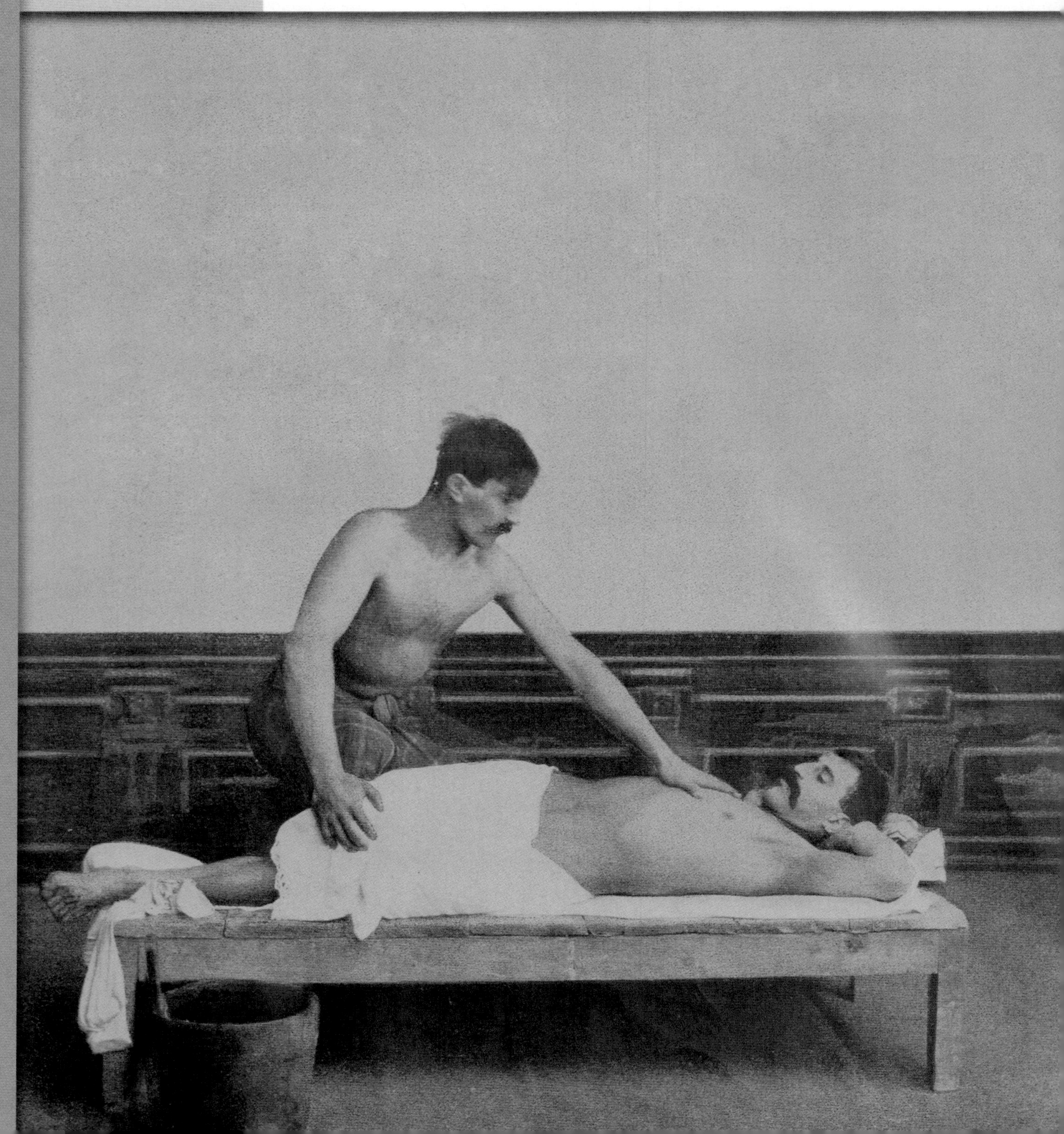

LEARNING OBJECTIVES

After you have mastered this chapter, you will be able to:

1. **Explain why massage is known as one of the earliest remedial practices for the relief of pain and discomfort.**
2. **Explain why massage is a natural and instinctive remedy for some illnesses and injuries.**
3. **Identify three historic Greeks who professed the benefits of exercise and massage.**
4. **Explain how developments in the nineteenth century influenced modern massage therapy.**
5. **Describe the basic differences in massage systems.**
6. **Explain why massage practitioners should understand massage history.**

INTRODUCTION

Massage (muh-SAHZH) is defined as the systematic manual manipulations of the soft tissues of the body by movements such as rubbing, kneading, pressing, rolling, slapping, and tapping for therapeutic purposes such as promoting circulation of the blood and lymph, relaxation of muscles, relief from pain, restoration of metabolic balance, and other benefits both physical and mental. (*Note*: The definition of massage varies according to jurisdiction or source.)

massage
is the systematic manual or mechanical manipulations of the soft tissues of the body for therapeutic purposes.

The massage practitioner has been referred to as a *massage technician* or *massotherapist*. In the past, a male massage practitioner might have been called a *masseur* (ma-**SUR**), and a female practitioner a *masseuse* (ma-**SOOS**). Today, most professionally trained men and women prefer to be called *massage practitioners* or *massage therapists*. For practical purposes, *massage practitioner* or *massage therapist* are the terms used throughout this book.

The origin of the word ***massage*** can be traced to at least five sources:

- The Greek root ***masso***, or ***massein***, which means to touch or to handle but also to knead or to squeeze.
- The Latin root ***massa*** comes directly from the Greek ***masso*** and has the same meaning.
- The Arabic root ***mass'h***, or ***mass***, means to press softly.
- The Sanskrit word ***makeh*** also means to press softly.

The modern use of the term *massage* to denote using the hands to manipulate the soft tissues is of fairly recent origin. The term was first used in American and European literature in approximately 1875. In America, near the end of the nineteenth century, Douglas Graham from Massachusetts first popularized the use of the word *massage*. The term *massage*, as well as the common names for the strokes (e.g., *effleurage, petrissage, tapotement*) and frictions, is generally attributed to a Dutch man, Johann Georg Mezger (1817–1893).

MASSAGE IN ANCIENT TIMES

Although the term *massage* is fairly new, the practice of several of its techniques can be traced back to antiquity. Massage is one of the earliest remedial practices of humankind and is the most natural and instinctive means of relieving pain and discomfort. When a person has sore, aching muscles, abdominal pains, or a bruise or wound, a natural and instinctive impulse is to touch, press, and rub that part of the body to obtain relief.

Artifacts have been found in many parts of the world to support the belief that prehistoric men and women massaged their muscles and rubbed herbs, oils, and various substances on their bodies as healing and protective agents. Many ancient cultures practiced some form of touch or massage. In many groups, a special person such as a healer, spiritual leader, or doctor was selected to administer healing power. Some ancient civilizations used therapeutic massage not only as a pain reliever but also to improve their sense of well-being and physical appearance.

Massage has been a major part of medicine for at least 5,000 years and an important part of Western medical traditions for at least 3,000 years. Massage was the first and most important of the medical arts and was practiced, developed, and taught primarily by physicians. Since 500 B.C., authors have written extensively about massage in medical books. Massage was also a major topic in the first medical texts printed after the invention of the printing press.

Chinese Anmo Techniques

In the British Museum, records reveal that the Chinese practiced massage as early as 3000 B.C. *The Cong Fou* of Tao-Tse is one of the ancient Chinese books that describes the use of medicinal plants, exercises, and a system of massage for the treatment of disease and the maintenance of health. The Chinese continued to improve their massage techniques through a special procedure they called *anmo* or *amma*. This massage technique was developed through many years of experience in finding the points on the body where various movements such as rubbing, pressing, or manipulations were most effective. Today, massage is an integral part of the Chinese health system and is practiced in China's medical clinics and hospitals. A more modern term for Chinese medical massage is **tui-na** (TOOY-nah), which literally means "push-pull." Traditional Chinese Medical practice also includes acupuncture, a method of assessing and treating the physical and energetic body that employs various methods of stimulating acupuncture points, including needles, heat, and pressure. *Acupressure* is derived from acupuncture and is the use of finger pressure and touch on specified points to promote balance.

Japanese Tsubo and Shiatsu

tsubo

are points on the body that are sensitive to pressure applied during shiatsu.

The practice of the *anmo* method of massage entered Japan around the sixth century A.D. (Figure 1-1). The points of stimulation remained much the same as the Chinese pressure points but were called **tsubo** (TSOO-boh). These points are pressed to affect the circulation of fluids and *Ki* (i.e., life force energy also called chi) and stimulate nerves in a finger pressure technique that the Japanese called **shiatsu** (**shee-AHT-soo**). This massage method has become quite popular in recent years. Early records show that the Japanese published a book on massage, *The San-Tsai-Tou-Hoei*, in the sixteenth century that described both passive and active massage procedures. The art of massage or *amma* in Japan was practiced almost exclusively by blind persons as a way of providing them with a means of income, and this employment was sanctioned and supported by the government.

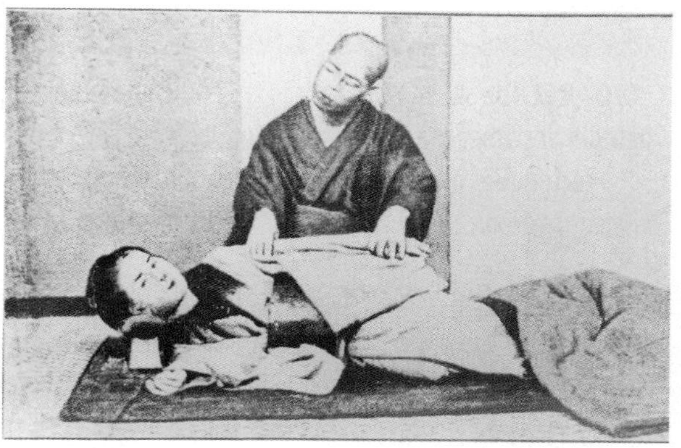

FIGURE 1–1 A blind practitioner in Japan (ca. 1880).

Indian and Hindu Practices

Massage has been practiced on the Indian subcontinent for more than 3,000 years. Knowledge of massage came to India from the Chinese and was an important part of the Hindu tradition. The *Ayur-Veda* (*Art of Life*), a sacred book of the Hindus written approximately 1800 B.C., included massage treatments among its hygienic principles. In writings dating back to 300 B.C., *The Laws of Manu* (*The Laws of Man*) defined the duties of everyday life. These duties included diet, bathing, exercise, and **tschanpua,** or massage at the bath. *Tschanpua* included kneading the extremities, tapotement, frictioning, anointing with perfumes, and cracking the joints of the fingers, toes, and neck.

shiatsu

is a massage technique from Japan in which points of stimulation are pressed to affect the circulation of fluids and ki (life force energy).

tschanpua

is a Hindu technique of massage in the bath.

Greek Massage and Gymnastics

From the East, the practice of massage spread to Europe and is thought to have flourished well before 300 B.C. The Greeks made gymnastics and the regular use of massage a part of their physical fitness rituals. The Greek priest-physician Asclepius, who lived in the seventh century B.C., was the first in a long line of Greek physicians. He was later worshipped as the god of medicine. He is said to have combined exercise and massage to create gymnastics and founded the first **gymnasium** to treat disease and promote health. The gymnasium and baths became important centers where philosophers and athletes gathered to exercise and discuss ideas. These were places where the young were educated, soldiers trained, and the sick healed. Asclepius's staff, with its entwined serpents, remains today as the symbol of medicine and pharmacy.

The Greek physician Herodicus of the fifth century B.C. prolonged the lives of many of his patients with diet, exercise, and massage by using beneficial herbs and oils. Herodotus, the Greek historian of the time, wrote of the benefits of massage. Hippocrates (460–380 B.C.), a pupil of Herodicus and a descendant in the lineage of Ascelpius, later became known as the father of medicine. His famous code of ethics for physicians, the **Hippocratic Oath**, is still in use today. This oath, which incorporates a code of ethics for physicians and those about to receive medical degrees, binds physicians to honor their teachers, do their

gymnasium

is a center where exercise and massage are combined to treat disease and promote health.

Hippocratic Oath

is a code of ethics for physicians.

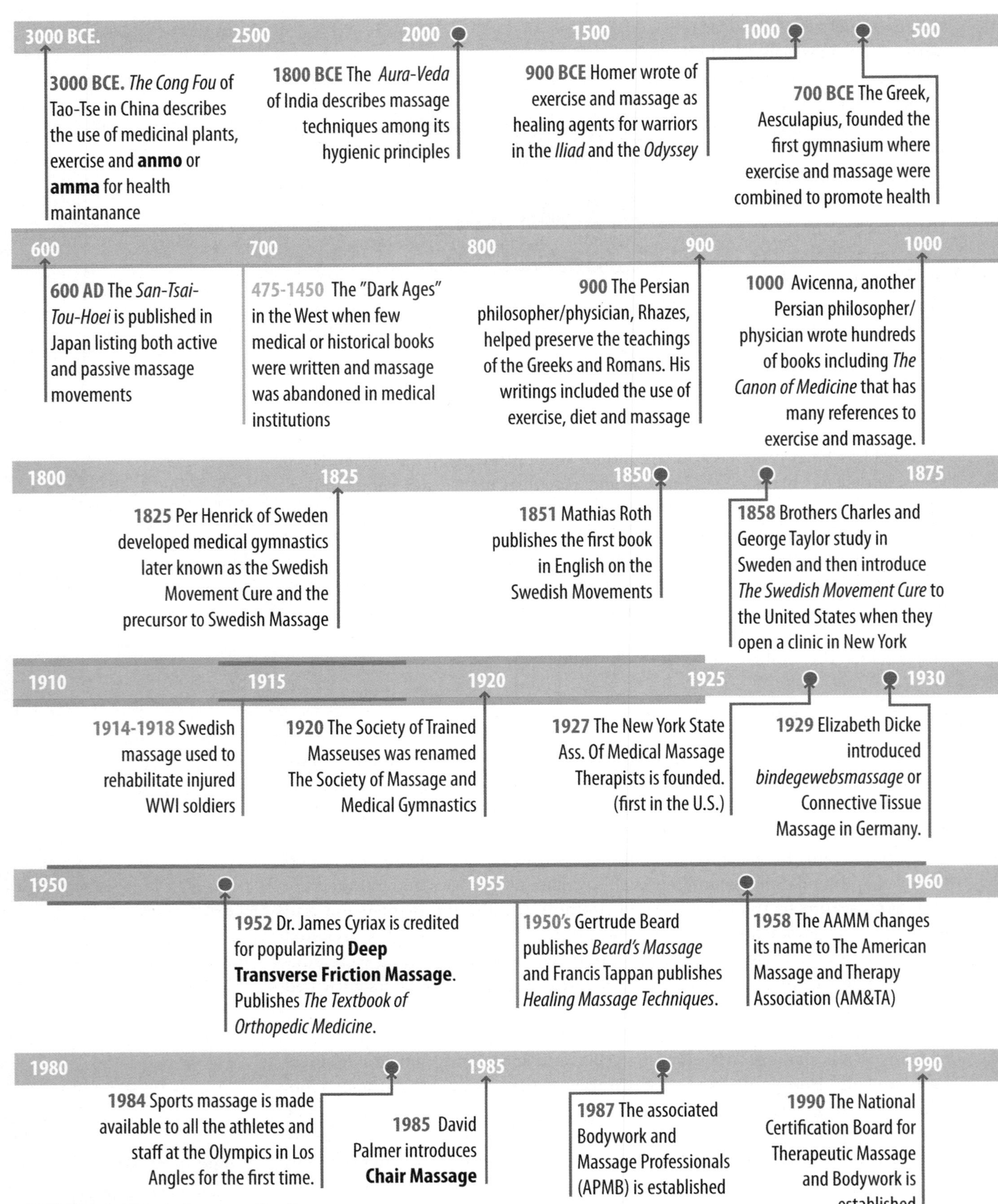

3000 BCE.
2500
2000
1500
1000
500
3000 BCE. The Cong Fou of Tao-Tse in China describes the use of medicinal plants, exercise and anmo or amma for health maintanance
1800 BCE The Aura-Veda of India describes massage techniques among its hygienic principles
900 BCE Homer wrote of exercise and massage as healing agents for warriors in the Iliad and the Odyssey
700 BCE The Greek, Aesculapius, founded the first gymnasium where exercise and massage were combined to promote health
600
700
800
900
1000
600 AD The San-Tsai-Tou-Hoei is published in Japan listing both active and passive massage movements
475-1450 The "Dark Ages" in the West when few medical or historical books were written and massage was abandoned in medical institutions
900 The Persian philosopher/physician, Rhazes, helped preserve the teachings of the Greeks and Romans. His writings included the use of exercise, diet and massage
1000 Avicenna, another Persian philosopher/physician wrote hundreds of books including The Canon of Medicine that has many references to exercise and massage.
1800
1825
1850
1875
1825 Per Henrick of Sweden developed medical gymnastics later known as the Swedish Movement Cure and the precursor to Swedish Massage
1851 Mathias Roth publishes the first book in English on the Swedish Movements
1858 Brothers Charles and George Taylor study in Sweden and then introduce The Swedish Movement Cure to the United States when they open a clinic in New York
1910
1915
1920
1925
1930
1914-1918 Swedish massage used to rehabilitate injured WWI soldiers
1920 The Society of Trained Masseuses was renamed The Society of Massage and Medical Gymnastics
1927 The New York State Ass. Of Medical Massage Therapists is founded. (first in the U.S.)
1929 Elizabeth Dicke introduced bindegewebsmassage or Connective Tissue Massage in Germany.
1950
1955
1960
1952 Dr. James Cyriax is credited for popularizing Deep Transverse Friction Massage. Publishes The Textbook of Orthopedic Medicine.
1950's Gertrude Beard publishes Beard's Massage and Francis Tappan publishes Healing Massage Techniques.
1958 The AAMM changes its name to The American Massage and Therapy Association (AM&TA)
1980
1985
1990
1984 Sports massage is made available to all the athletes and staff at the Olympics in Los Angles for the first time.
1985 David Palmer introduces Chair Massage
1987 The associated Bodywork and Massage Professionals (APMB) is established
1990 The National Certification Board for Therapeutic Massage and Bodywork is established

FIGURE 1–2 Historical massage timeline.

400 | 300 | 200 | 100 | 0 | 100 AD | 200

400 BCE Hippocrates, the father of modern medicine, described the effects of various massage movements

300 BCE In India, the *Laws of Manu* defined **tschanpua**, a Hindu technique of massage in the bath

20-30 AD Celsus, a Roman, wrote **de Medi** includes descriptions of exercise, bathing and massage

220-237 AD Roman Emporer Constantine, who converted to Christianity, destroyed the baths and gymnasium because of widespread "abuses" of a sexual nature

1400 | 1500 | 1600 | 1700 | 1800 | 1900

1450-1600 The Renaissance

1569 Italian, Mercurialis, wrote *De Arte Gymnastica* on gymnastics and the benefits of massage

1570 French barber/surgeon, Ambroise Pare, wrote about the positive effects and employed gentle, medium and vigorous friction and joint movements

1800 English surgeon and practitioner of **chirurgy** (healing with the hands) John Grosvenor wrote about the value of frictions for the relief of gout, stiff joints and rheumatism

1875 | 1880 | 1885 | 1890 | 1900

1874-1925 Dr. Douglas Graham of Boston wrote extensively about the benefits of "massage" (first in U.S to use the term). Founding member of The American Physical Education Assn. in 1885

1880-1909 Dr. Johan of Holland establishes scientific massage as a basis of rehabilitation preferring the French terminology **effleurage, petrisage** and **tapotement** still in use today

1894 The Society of Trained Masseuses was formed in England

1900 German Dr. Albert Hoffa published *Technic Der Massage*

1935 | 1940 | 1945

1936 Drs. Emil and Estrid Vodder introduce Lymphatic Drainage massage in Paris

1940 Elizabeth Dicke introduces *Bindegewebsmassage* or Conective Tissue Massage in Germany. Boris Chaitow and Dr. Stanley Lief establish Neuromuscular Therapy in Europe

1943 The American Association of Massures and Massuses (AAMM) is established in Chicago. Later to become the AMTA

1960 | 1965 | 1970 | 1975

1962 Esalen Institute, a center for the development of the Human Potential Movement develops Esalen Massage

1970's John Barnes introduced Myofascial Release, Milton Trager introduces Trager, Moshe Feldenkrais introduces Feldenkrais, Fredrick Alexander introduces the Alexander Technique and Paul St. John develops the St. John Method of Neuromuscular Therapy

1971 Ida Rolf opens the Rolf Institute in Boulder, CO

1990 | 1995 | 2000 | 2005

1992 The NCBMTB administers the first National Certification exam

1992 The Touch Research Institute is founded

1998 The National Institute of Health established the Center for Complementary and Alternative Medicine

2005 The Federation of State Massage Licensing Boards was established.

best to maintain the health of their patients, honor their patients' secrets, and prescribe no harmful treatment or drug. The Hippocratic Oath can be found in its entirety in most medical dictionaries.

anatripsis is the art of rubbing a body part upward.

That Hippocrates understood the effects of massage is revealed in one of his descriptions of massage movements. He said, "Hard rubbing binds, much rubbing causes parts to waste, and moderate rubbing makes them grow." Scholars have interpreted this to mean that rubbing can help to bind a joint that is too loose or loosen a joint that is too tight. Vigorous rubbing can tighten and firm; moderate rubbing tends to build muscle. In his writings, Hippocrates used the word **anatripsis**, which means the art of rubbing a part upward, not downward. He stated that it is necessary to rub the shoulder after reduction of a dislocation. This advice can still serve as a valuable guideline for modern practitioners. Hippocrates thought that all physicians should be trained in massage as a method of healing.

Roman Art of Massage and Therapeutic Bathing

The Romans acquired the practice of therapeutic bathing and massage from the Greeks. The Romans built public baths that were available to rich and poor

Box 1.1

The Hippocratic Oath (A classical translation)

I swear by Apollo Physician and Asclepius and Hygieia and Panaceia and all the gods and goddesses, making them my witnesses, that I will fulfill according to my ability and judgment this oath and this covenant:

To hold him who has taught me this art as equal to my parents and to live my life in partnership with him, and if he is in need of money to give him a share of mine, and to regard his offspring as equal to my brothers in male lineage and to teach them this art—if they desire to learn it—without fee and covenant; to give a share of precepts and oral instruction and all the other learning to my sons and to the sons of him who has instructed me and to pupils who have signed the covenant and have taken an oath according to the medical law, but no one else.

I will apply dietetic measures for the benefit of the sick according to my ability and judgment; I will keep them from harm and injustice.

I will neither give a deadly drug to anybody who asked for it, nor will I make a suggestion to this effect. Similarly I will not give to a woman an abortive remedy. In purity and holiness I will guard my life and my art.

I will not use the knife, not even on sufferers from stone, but will withdraw in favor of such men as are engaged in this work.

Whatever houses I may visit, I will come for the benefit of the sick, remaining free of all intentional injustice, of all mischief and in particular of sexual relations with both female and male persons, be they free or slaves.

What I may see or hear in the course of the treatment or even outside of the treatment in regard to the life of men, which on no account one must spread abroad, I will keep to myself, holding such things shameful to be spoken about.

If I fulfill this oath and do not violate it, may it be granted to me to enjoy life and art, being honored with fame among all men for all time to come; if I transgress it and swear falsely, may the opposite of all this be my lot.

Translation from the Greek by Ludwig Edelstein. From The Hippocratic Oath: Text, Translation, and Interpretation, by Ludwig Edelstein. Baltimore: Johns Hopkins Press, 1943.

alike. A brisk rubdown with fragrant oils could be enjoyed after the bath. The art of massage was also highly respected as a treatment for weak and diseased patients and as an aid to remove stiffness and soreness from muscles.

The Romans, similar to the Greeks before them, used massage as part of their gymnastics. Celsus, who lived during the reign of Emperor Tiberius (about 42 B.C.–A.D. 37), was considered to be one of the most eminent Roman physicians. He wrote extensively on many subjects, including medicine. *De Medicina* discusses prevention and therapeutics extensively and advises using massage, exercise, and bathing. Celsus recommended rubbing the head to relieve headaches and rubbing the limbs to strengthen muscles and to combat paralysis. Massage was used to improve sluggish circulation and internal disorders and to reduce edema. Although circulation of the blood was not completely understood, physicians of the time followed the teaching of Hippocrates and thought that rubbing upward was more effective than rubbing downward.

The Greek physician Claudius Galen (A.D. 130–200), who became physician to the Roman emperor Marcus Aurelius, is said to have discovered that arteries and veins contain blood. William Harvey (1578–1657), an English physician, is credited with discovering the circulation of the blood in 1628, however. Galen was a prolific writer, and his medical texts were the principal sources used for more than 1,000 years. As a physician to the gladiators, Galen gained great knowledge of anatomy. His books on hygienic health, exercise, and massage stressed specific exercises for various physical disorders. Greek and Roman philosophers, statesmen, and historians such as Cicero, Pliny, Plutarch, and Plato wrote of the importance of massage and passive and active exercise to the maintenance of a healthy body and mind. Even Julius Gaius Caesar, Roman general and Emperor of Rome (100–44 B.C.), is said to have demanded his daily massage for the relief of neuralgia and prevention of epileptic attacks.

The Decline of Arts and Sciences in the West

With the decline of the Roman Empire, beginning approximately A.D. 180, the popularity of bathing and massage also declined. According to Richard van Why, "The Roman emperor Constantine (A.D. 228–337) who converted to Christianity, abolished and destroyed the baths and gymnasiums because of widespread abuses of a sexual nature." Oribasius, Antyllus, Caelius Aurelianus, Aetius of Amida, and Paul of Aegina are some of the medical writers and physicians who lived during the decline of the Roman Empire. They all wrote favorably about the use of massage, exercise, and bathing as therapeutic and conditioning agents.

Little recorded history of health practices during the Middle Ages (also known as the Dark Ages) has survived. This period, between classical antiquity and the European Renaissance, extends from the downfall of Rome in approximately A.D. 476 to about 1450. Both the sciences and the arts suffered severe setbacks during the Dark Ages. Few medical or historical books were written during this time, and much recorded history was lost. This decline was partly because of wars but also because of religious superstitions that made people fear placing too much importance on the physical self. During the Middle Ages in Europe, medical institutions abandoned massage in favor of other remedies.

Laypeople, folk healers, and midwives still practiced massage sporadically, but practitioners were occasionally the objects of persecution.

The Arabic Empire and the Rise of Islam

Beginning in the seventh century, the spread of Islam throughout North Africa, Asia Minor, Mesopotamia, and Persia actually served to preserve much of the Greco-Roman culture. As the Greco-Roman culture fell into decay in the Middle Ages, the Persians continued many of the important teachings of the great physicians and philosophers from the classical era. The Islamic Persian philosopher/physician *Rhazes*, or *Razi* (A.D. 860–932), was a follower of Hippocrates and Galen and a prolific writer. He wrote several books, the most important of which was an encyclopedia of Arabic, Roman, and Greek medical practices that esteemed the use of exercise, diet, and massage in the treatment of disease and the preservation of health. Another prominent Persian philosopher/physician, Avicenna (A.D. 980–1037), authored the *Canon of Medicine*, which is considered to be the most important single book in medical history. Avicenna was an ardent follower of Galen, and his text made numerous references to the use of massage, exercise, and bathing. Eventually these volumes paved the way for the Renaissance as these writings returned to the West through trade and conquest.

The Renaissance Revives Interest in Health Practices

The Renaissance (1450–1600) revived interest in the arts and sciences. After a long intellectual slumber, the classical writings of the ancient Greek, Roman, and Persian masters were rediscovered and studied as a basis from which to develop new ideas. Once again, people became interested in the maintenance and improvement of physical health and appearance. By the second half of the fifteenth century, the printing press had been invented, which led to the publication of many scholarly writings in the arts and sciences. The greater availability and distribution of printed materials also helped to stimulate interest in better health practices.

The Growth and Acceptance of Massage as a Healing Aid

By the sixteenth century, medical practitioners began to reinvent and employ massage as part of their healing treatments. Ambroise Paré (1517–1590), a French barber-surgeon, one of the founders of modern surgery and inventor of the ligation of arteries, described the positive effects of massage in the healing process in one of his publications. He classified massage movements as gentle, medium, and vigorous frictions and employed flexion, extension, and circumduction of joints. His concepts were passed down to other French physicians who believed in the value of physical therapeutics. During his lifetime, Paré served as personal physician to four of France's kings. He is credited with restoring the health of Mary, Queen of Scots (1542–1587) by use of massage. In 1569, Mercurialis (1530–1606), a professor of medicine at the University of Padua, Italy, published a book, *De Arte Gymnastica*, on gymnastics and the benefits of massage when integrated with other therapies for the body and mind.

The sixteenth, seventeenth, and eighteenth centuries witnessed an expansion in all fields of knowledge. Emerging literature from English, French, German, and Italian authors reestablished massage as a preferred scientific practice for the maintenance of health and the treatment of disease.

Frictions, manipulations, anointing, bathing, and exercise were regarded as important tools in the medical armamentarium. These subjects were taught in institutions of higher learning to physicians and other practitioners of the healing practices and were based in the sciences of anatomy, physiology, and pathology, as these specialties were known in that day and age.

Throughout history, a variety of massage or hands-on healing has been practiced by laypeople or commoners. Because it was often practiced by folk healers and midwives, it was passed on as an art and a gift. A body of knowledge was never established and codified, however, so that techniques were lost and rediscovered through the ages.

THE DEVELOPMENT OF MODERN MASSAGE TECHNIQUES

In the early part of the nineteenth century, John Grosvenor (1742–1823), a well-respected English surgeon and a practitioner of **chirurgy** (healing with the hands), emphasized to his colleagues the value of friction in the relief of stiff joints, gout, and rheumatism. His efforts helped to further the belief in massage as an aid to healing.

Per Henrik Ling (1776–1839) of Smaaland, Sweden, a physiologist and fencing master, is known as the father of physical therapy (Figure 1-3). Ling systematized and developed movements that he found to be beneficial in improving his own physical condition, calling the system of movements **medical gymnastics**. He based this system on the developing science of physiology. The Ling System's primary focus was on gymnastics as applied to the treatment of disease and consisted of movements classified as active, duplicated, and passive. *Active movements* were performed by the patient and could be referred to as exercise. *Duplicated movements* were performed by the patient in cooperation with the therapist. These correspond to modern resistive or assistive exercises. *Passive movements* were performed by the therapist to the patient and would be considered range-of-motion therapy and massage. In 1813, Ling established the Royal Swedish Central Institute of Gymnastics, which was chartered and financed by the Swedish government. Ling died in 1839, but his students published his works posthumously. The Ling System, more commonly called *Swedish Movements* or the *Movement Cure*, spread throughout Europe and Russia. By 1851, there were 38 institutions for education in the Swedish Movements in Europe, most of them located in Germany. These schools were generally open to learned men. The programs were as long as three years, with classes lasting six to eight hours a day.

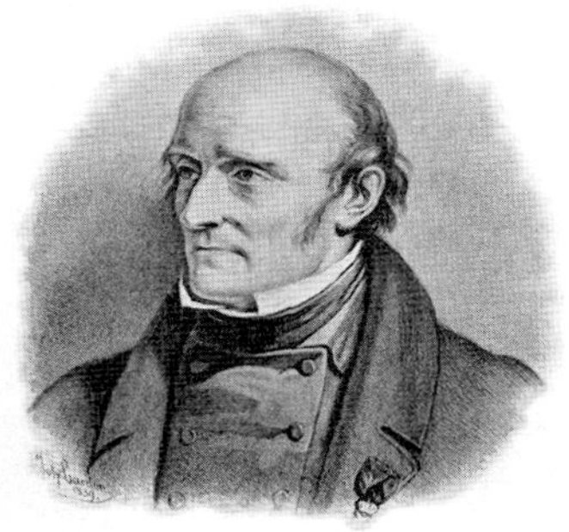

FIGURE 1-3 Per Henrick Ling (1776–1839), known as the father of physical therapy.

chirugy

is healing with the hands.

medical gymnastics

gymnastics applied to the treatment of disease consisting of active, duplicated, and passive movements.

Mathias Roth, an English physician, studied under Ling at the Royal Central Institute and in 1851 published the first book in English on the Swedish Movements. He established the first institute in England to teach Swedish Movement Gymnastics and gave private instruction to Charles Fayette Taylor, a New York physician, who in 1858 introduced the methods to the United States. In the United States, the technique became known as the *Swedish Movement Cure*. Charles's brother, George Henry Taylor, attended the Dr. Sotherberg Institute in Stockholm and completed full training in the Swedish Movements. The brothers returned to the United States and started an orthopedic practice in New York, where they specialized in the Swedish Movements. Within a year they had dissolved their joint practice, but both continued to practice and write about the Swedish Movement Cure. In 1860, George Henry published the first American textbook on the Swedish Movement Cure and established the Improved Movement Cure Institute in New York City. Charles Fayette wrote many articles and published a textbook introducing the Swedish Movements in 1861. Both brothers practiced and taught the cure until their deaths in 1899. Thus it was the competitive Taylor brothers who introduced the Swedish Movement Cure to the United States and brought massage more into public and medical acceptance.

Modern Massage Terminology

effleurage

is a succession of strokes applied by gliding the hand over an extended portion of the body.

petrissage

lifts, squeezes, and presses the tissues.

tapotement

movements include tapping, slapping, hacking, cupping, and beating.

Modern massage terminology is credited to Dr. Johann Mezger (1839–1909) of Amsterdam, Holland, who established the practice and art of massage as a scientific subject for physicians in the remedial treatment of disease. He was acknowledged by many of the authors of his day as the founder of scientific massage. Through Mezger's efforts, massage became recognized as fundamental to rehabilitation in physical therapy. Mezger's preference for the French terminology has remained an influence to this day (thus the use of the terms **effleurage, petrissage, tapotement,** and even *massage* itself). The word *massage* was not used in the United States until 1874, when Douglas Graham from Boston and Benjamin Lee and Charles Mills from Philadelphia published articles using Mezger's terminology. Dr. Douglas O. Graham was a practitioner and a historian of massage who wrote extensively about the subject from 1874 to 1925, more than 50 years. He was a founding member of the American Physical Education Association. Dr. John Harvey Kellogg (1852–1943) ran the Battle Creek Sanitarium in Battle Creek Michigan and wrote extensively on the benefits of massage and hydrotherapy (Figure 1-4). In 1929, Kellogg published The *Art of Massage: A Practical Manual for the Nurse, the Student and the Practitioner*. He was the author of numerous magazine articles and the editor of the popular magazine *Good Health*.

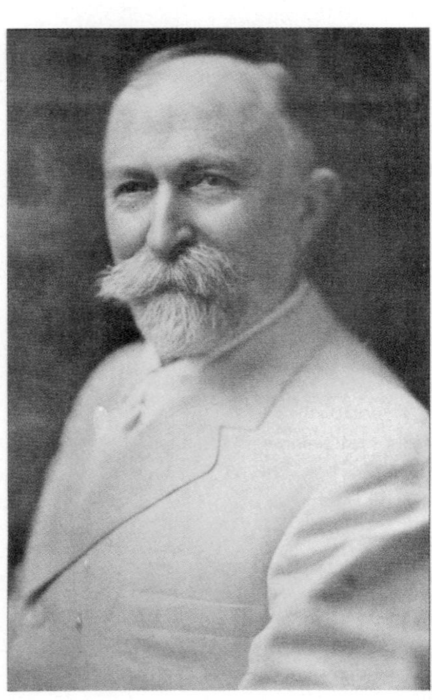

FIGURE 1-4 Dr. John Harvey Kellogg (1852–1943).

By the early part of the twentieth century, physicians in medical schools in Germany and Scandinavia were including massage in their teachings as a dignified and beneficial asset in the medical field. In 1900, the distinguished German physician Albert J. Hoffa published *Technik Der Massage*. The publication remains one of the most basic books in the field and contains many of the techniques used in Swedish massage.

Throughout Germany, Denmark, Norway, and Sweden, physicians recommended therapeutic exercises, massage, and baths for the restoration and maintenance of health. These physicians thought that massage helped the body to rid itself of toxins, relieved ailments such as rheumatism, and promoted the healthy functioning of all body systems.

In 1894, a group of women formed the Society of Trained Masseuses in England. By 1920, this society had grown in members and prestige. Later, the society became known as the Chartered Society of Massage and Medical Gymnastics; it was registered in 1964 as the Chartered Society of Physiotherapy.

THE DECLINE OF MASSAGE IN THE TWENTIETH CENTURY

The beginning of the twentieth century brought with it a decline in the scientific and medical use of massage. There were several reasons for this decline. The increasing popularity of massage in the nineteenth century precipitated an increase in not only qualified practitioners and schools but also lay practitioners and unscrupulous schools.

A special inquiry by the British Medical Association in 1894 revealed numerous abuses in the education and practice of massage practitioners, which dealt a severe blow to the profession's reputation. The inquiry found many schools using unscrupulous recruitment practices and offering inadequate training. As a result, graduates were unqualified or incompetent and in debt to the school. To repay that debt, students and graduates were required to work in clinics that offered poor massage and often were no more than houses of prostitution. Other abuses included false certification and deceptive advertising, in which exorbitant claims were made that were totally unfounded and untrue. The reputation of massage was damaged among physicians and the general public alike.

Technical innovations also had a detrimental affect on massage. The invention of electricity and various electrical apparatuses (e.g., the vibrator) greatly diminished the use of hands-on therapy in favor of these new electrical modalities (Figures 1-5a and b and Figure 1-6). This trend continues to this day.

Technical and intellectual advances in medicine resulted in new treatment strategies based more on pharmacology and surgical procedures. The old ideas of treating disease through diet, exercise, and bathing gave way to the more sophisticated practices of modern medicine. Physicians no longer learned massage as a part of their training, nor did they employ trained therapists. The place of massage in nursing was reduced to no more than the administering of a back rub.

CONTEMPORARY DEVELOPMENTS IN MASSAGE

Several important developments during the second quarter of the twentieth century continue to influence modern massage.

An Austrian named Emil Vodder (1897–1986) and his wife Astrid developed a method of gentle rhythmic massage along the superficial lymphatics that accelerates the functioning of the lymphatic system and effectively treats chronic lymphedema (limf-e-**DEE**-muh) and other diseases of venous or lymph circulation. Today this system is widely known and taught as **Dr. Vodder's Manual Lymph Drainage.**

Dr. Vodder's Manual Lymph Drainage

is a method of gentle, rhythmic massage along the superficial lymphatics that aids in lymphatic system functioning and treats chronic lymphedema..

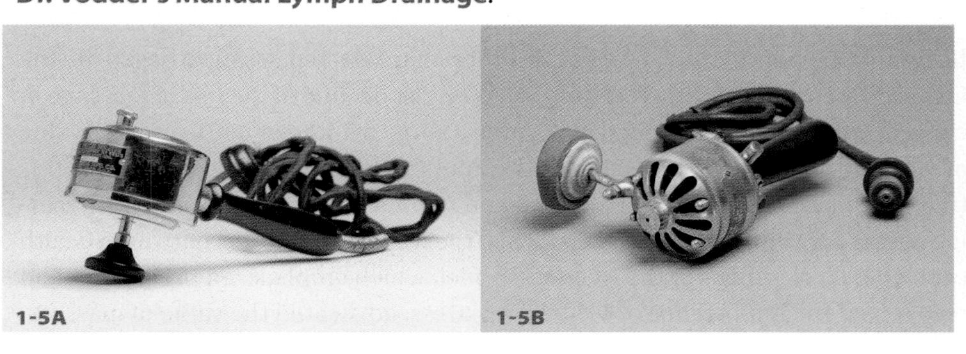

FIGURES 1-5A, B Electric vibrators from the early twentieth century. A. The Star Electric Vibrator (ca.1918). B. The New Lite vibrator by Hamilton Beach (*ca.*) 1902.

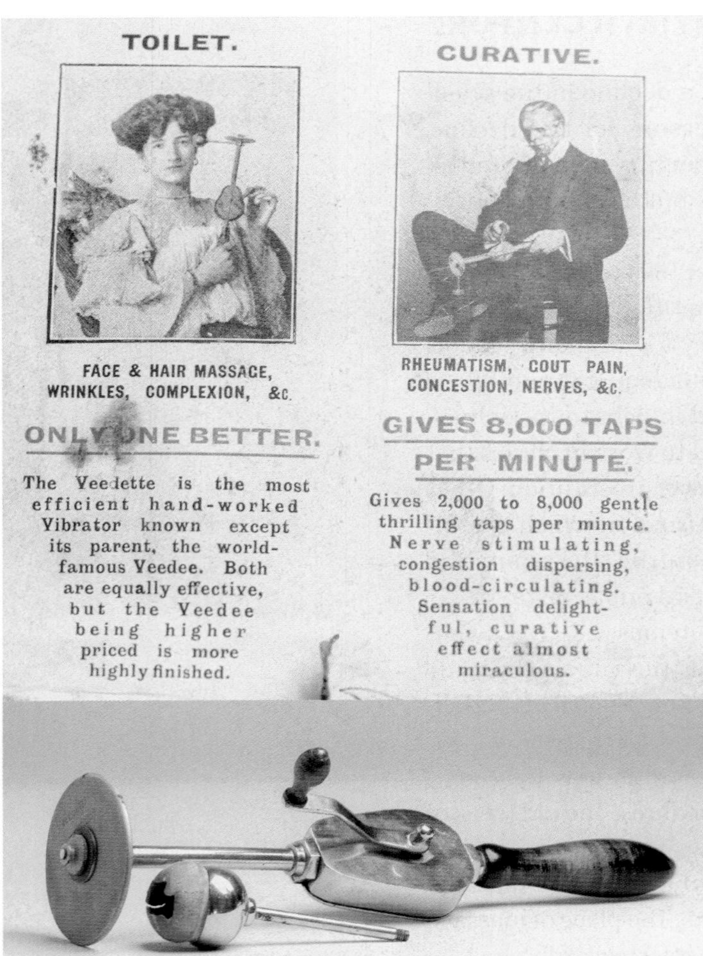

TOILET.
FACE & HAIR MASSAGE,
WRINKLES, COMPLEXION, &c.
The Veedette is the most efficient hand-worked Vibrator known except its parent, the world-famous Veedee. Both are equally effective, but the Veedee being higher priced is more highly finished.
CURATIVE.
RHEUMATISM, GOUT PAIN,
CONGESTION, NERVES, &c.
GIVES 8,000 TAPS
PER MINUTE.
Gives 2,000 to 8,000 gentle thrilling taps per minute. Nerve stimulating, congestion dispersing, blood-circulating. Sensation delightful, curative effect almost miraculous.

FIGURE 1-6 Mechanical vibrator with advertisements demonstrating its use

In the 1940s, a German, Elizabeth Dicke (1884–1952), developed *Bindegewebsmassage*, or **Connective Tissue Massage**, which was later popularized in England by Maria Ebner. *Bindegewebsmassage* is directed toward the subcutaneous connective tissue and is thought to affect vascular and visceral reflexes related to a variety of pathologies and disabilities. This method continues to be widely employed in many countries for pathologic conditions of circulation or visceral disease.

Dr. James H. Cyriax (1905–1985), an English orthopedic physician, is credited with popularizing **Deep Transverse Friction Massage**. This method broadens the fibrous tissues of muscles, tendons, or ligaments, breaking down unwanted fibrous adhesions and thereby restoring mobility to muscles in a way that cannot be achieved by passive stretching or active exercise. Transverse friction massage retains its popularity today in physical therapy and massage therapy regimes as an effective treatment in the restoration and rehabilitation of muscle and soft tissue injuries.

Two American physical therapists who have had a major impact on massage therapy in the United States are Gertrude Beard and Frances Tappan. Both devoted much of their lives to promoting massage as an important part of the health care system. Tappan's book, Healing Massage Techniques, and Beard's Massage remain as standards in the massage industry.

Massage played an important role immediately after World War I (1914–1918), when it proved beneficial as a restorative treatment in the rehabilitation of injuries. In World War II (1939–1945), massage was again employed on an even larger scale in the hospitals of the Armed Forces. In the years after World War II, however, manual massage played a secondary role in physical therapy as more mechanical and electrical means of stimulation and rehabilitation gained popularity. During the postwar recovery, massage was directed more toward relaxation and athletic activities and less toward rehabilitation. Most practitioners were employed in athletic clubs, YMCAs, or as trainers for athletic teams.

Connective Tissue Massage

is massage directed toward the subcutaneous connective tissue, thought to affect vascular and visceral reflexes related to a variety of pathologies and disabilities.

Deep Transverse Friction Massage

is massage that broadens the fibrous tissues of muscles, tendons, or ligaments, breaking down unwanted adhesions and restoring mobility to muscles.

A MASSAGE RENAISSANCE IN THE UNITED STATES

Beginning in approximately 1960, another massage renaissance began in the United States and continues to this day. With the decline of the use of massage in conventional or allopathic medicine came a surge of interest in the use and value of massage in the paraprofessional and lay public. Several factors precipitated this trend. Increased awareness of physical and mental fitness, as well as the increasing cost of conventional medicine, opened the way for viable alternatives in health care. The development of the wellness model, which emphasized prevention and recognized the importance of controlling stress, advocated the value of massage.

The psychological benefits of touch and its proven use in the treatment of pain returned massage to a place of prominence in the health care system.

In 1962, Esalen Institute in Big Sur, California, was founded and soon became a popular center for the burgeoning human potential movement. Some of the early leaders included Aldous Huxley, Alan Watts, Abraham Maslow, and Fritz Pearls (father of Gestalt). Esalen was one of the first places where contemporary massage and bodywork were taught. Moshe Feldenkrais, Milton Trager, and Ida Rolf taught at Esalen as well as many others. Esalen massage was developed at the Institute. Esalen massage is a deeply relaxing experience based on Swedish massage, with influences of meditation, gestalt, Oriental techniques, polarity, Trager, and yoga. Today, Esalen Institute continues to offer hundreds of seminars a year, and Esalen massage is always available to participants and guests.

The human potential movement and interest in Eastern practices, preventive health, and wellness led to the publication of numerous books and the development of a wide variety of bodywork modalities. During the 1970s and 1980s, a significant rise in the popularity of massage as well as several other forms of bodywork occurred in the United States. Several professional associations and numerous schools emerged to teach and promote a variety of massage disciplines.

In 1943, the American Massage Therapy Association (AMTA), the oldest national professional massage association in the United States, was established in Chicago by graduates of the College of Swedish Massage. The original name of the organization was the American Association of Masseurs and Masseuses (AAMM). In 1958, the AAMM changed its name to the American Massage and Therapy Association and then in 1983 simplified the name to the American Massage Therapy Association. The association's popular publication, *The Massage Therapy Journal*, carries a variety of articles that are of interest to the massage professional. The Association of Bodywork Professionals (ABMP) and the International Massage Association (IMA) were both created in the 1980s to offer an alternative for massage professionals to obtain professional liability insurance. The ABMP also publishes *Massage and Bodywork Magazine* and offers several membership benefits, including networking, marketing, and business tools to practitioners of all the diverse bodywork modalities. The American Organization for Bodywork Therapies of Asia (AOBTA) also originated in the 1980s as a professional membership organization for practitioners of Asian body therapies. In 1985, *Massage Magazine* began publication as an independent trade magazine to bring the science, art, and business of massage to the general public. In 2000, *Massage Today* began publication as a no-cost subscription available to anyone in the massage industry, with news of current events as well as articles from industry leaders.

Articles about massage have appeared in a wide variety of news magazines, including *Time*, *Life*, and *Newsweek*. Newspapers ran common interest stories about massage or massage practitioners. Most of these articles were about the practitioners and the positive effects and benefits of massage. Massage therapists in communities gave presentations at club meetings and gatherings about the positive aspects of massage. As the public became more aware of the effects and benefits of therapeutic massage, the unfortunate association between massage and prostitution dissipated.

During the 1970s and 1980s, the growing popularity of massage continued, with more people receiving massage and more people choosing to learn massage, either for personal satisfaction or to become massage practitioners. Massage training programs varied widely in content and length, with classic Swedish or Western massage being at the core of most of the curriculums. Early programs were as short as 100 hours for an introductory course. Adult education programs at community colleges or universities sometimes had "Friends and Family" massage classes that were as short as a weekend or a few evening classes. Training for those wishing to practice massage tended to be somewhat longer, with the length and content often determined by local or state licensing requirements. In 1990, the establishment of the *National Certification Board for Therapeutic Massage and Bodywork* required an applicant to have a minimum of 500 hours of training from a state-recognized school to take the *National Certification Examination*. Massage school curriculums tended to be between 500 and 600 class hours, with courses consisting of anatomy, physiology, business practices, and massage techniques. A few schools offered longer, more comprehensive programs of up to 1,000 to 1,200 class hours. Massage training was done mostly at private massage schools or through apprenticeships. Many private massage schools were established after 1970, with more than 1,000 schools in the United States by the year 2000. With the growing popularity of massage and massage education, and the increase in states regulating massage, private business schools and public community colleges began offering accredited massage training programs.

Massage was consistently becoming more visible, accessible, and popular with the American public. Massage of athletes became more commonplace. Athletes at organized runs, marathons, and triathlons lined up after their events to receive their postevent massage at the **sports massage** tent. At the 1984 Summer Olympics, sports massage services were made available to the athletes for the first time. Since that time, athletic massage has been part of every Summer and Winter Olympics. Many professional and even semiprofessional athletic teams, including baseball, football, basketball, hockey, and tennis, either employed or provided for the services of sport massage therapists. Serious athletes from a variety of sports would seek out the services of a skilled massage therapist to help maintain the highest level of performance while addressing the myriad physical and sometimes emotional conditions that accompany the sport.

sports massage

is a method of massage designed to enhance an athlete's performance.

Whereas sports massage teams at athletic events provided relief to athletes from the rigors of competition, another type of massage team began appearing at the sites of disasters. Specially trained emergency response massage teams coordinated with the Red Cross to provide the relief of massage to firefighters, emergency workers, and sometimes the victims of disasters such as floods, wildfires, or earthquakes. Team members set up massage tables or chairs in relief areas where emergency workers could take much-needed breaks from the long, intense hours at the scene and enjoy a few minutes of caring and rejuvenating massage before heading back to the front lines.

Seated massage, or **chair massage**, was a great innovation that helped to demystify massage and make it more accessible to a wider audience. Introduced in 1985 by David Palmer, chair massage is performed with the client clothed and seated on a special massage chair. This innovative massage application brought massage out of the studio and into the public arena. Massage no longer required a table, sheets, lubricants, or the removal of clothing. Suddenly, massage could be practiced in corporate offices, teacher's lounges, shopping malls, airports, health fairs, state legislatures, and on the street. Massage was less of a mystery and therefore less threatening and safer. In the 1990s, corporate massage became more popular, and therapists started taking massage chairs into

chair massage

takes place in a chair, which is a better choice for people unable to or not amenable to receiving full-body massage on a table.

offices, schools, hospitals, or other workplace settings to offer 15-minute massage breaks. Finally, massage was coming out!

In the late 1980s, efforts to return massage and bodywork to the mainstream of health and wellness care prompted members from the various disciplines to come together and share ideas. In 1988, Robert Calvert (1946–2006), editor of *Massage Magazine*, created a forum called Head, Heart and Hands that had three gatherings, one in the center of the country, one on the East Coast, and one on the West Coast, in an attempt to discuss common issues and organize massage on a national level. In 1991, a Federation of Bodywork Organizations was formed to ensure equitable recognition of the different forms of bodywork in the development of standards and legislation.

The trend toward massage regulation steadily progressed during the final quarter of the twentieth century. Most massage regulation from the 1950s through the 1970s consisted of local ordinances initiated to control prostitution. Since the 1980s, most massage legislation has been practitioner based, focusing on educational standards, scope of practice, title protection, and protecting the public from harm. The AMTA, in cooperation with individual state organizations, actively pursued state legislatures to enact state licensing for massage therapists. In 1985, only ten states regulated massage. By 2009, 42 states and the District of Columbia had state-wide massage licensing.

In 1988, the AMTA provided funding for the development of a National Certification for Massage Therapists. In 1990, the National Certification Board for Therapeutic Massage and Bodywork (NCBTMB) became an independent certifying entity, and the first examinations were administered in 1992. The National Certification Examination (NCE) was originally designed to be a voluntary examination that a practitioner could take to become recognized as being nationally certified in therapeutic massage and bodywork. Since its inception, however, several states that license massage have adopted the NCE as part of their licensing requirements. As of the publication of this text, 35 of the 42 states requiring massage licensing use the successful completion of the National Certification Examination as a qualification for licensing. As a result, many massage schools' curricula are guided by the requirements and content of the exam.

In 2005, the Federation of State Massage Therapy Boards (FSMTB) was established when members from 22 state massage therapy licensing agencies convened in Albuquerque, New Mexico, where bylaws were unanimously adopted and the first board was elected and installed. Among the most significant concerns were the need for a valid and reliable licensing examination and the desire to bring commonality to licensing requirements, to assist with reciprocity and professional mobility of massage practitioners between licensed states. The federation promotes networking and communication between state massage licensing boards and has developed a comprehensive licensing examination (MBLEx) for use among the member states. The MBLEx is a 125-item multiple-choice test with 13 percent of its content devoted to the topic of ethics, reflecting the Federation's commitment to professionalism and client safety. As of 2009, 30 of the 42 regulated states are members of the FSMTB, and 18 states use the MBLEx.

The recognition, acceptance, and growth of massage continued through the 1990s. In 1990 and 1997, surveys by David Eisenberg, MD, published in the

New England Journal of Medicine and the *Journal of the American Medical Association* respectively, indicated that an increasing number of Americans were using complementary and alternative medicine (CAM) therapies and paying for them at a rate estimated at $27 billion in 1997, which exceeded the out-of-pocket expenditures for all U.S. hospitalizations. The same studies showed that massage was the third most common CAM modality used after chiropractic and relaxation practices such as deep breathing and meditation.

Another phenomenon that began in the 1990s and has continued into the new century is the proliferation of massage research. Research, which is funded by various sources, validates the effects and benefits of massage and helps to legitimize massage in the eyes of the medical community and the public. Some of the leaders in promoting massage research include the Touch Research Institute (TRI), the Massage Therapy Foundation, and the National Institutes of Health (NIH) Center for Complementary and Alternative Medicine.

TRI was founded in 1992 under the direction of Tiffany M. Fields, in collaboration with the University of Miami Medical School expressly to study the effect of touch therapy on human well-being. Studies at TRI have shown that massage can induce weight gain in premature infants, alleviates depressive symptoms, reduces stress hormones, alleviates pain, and positively alters the immune system in children and adults with various medical conditions.

In 1990, the AMTA Foundation was formed as an independently governed public charity to advance the knowledge and practice of massage by supporting scientific research, education, and community service. The foundation accepts and solicits donations, then grants funds for research, community service, and

Box 1.2

The Federation of Therapeutic Massage, Bodywork, and Somatic Practice Organizations

In 1991, the Federation of Therapeutic Massage, Bodywork and Somatic Practice Organizations was formed to ensure equitable recognition of all forms of bodywork in the formation of public wellness policy and practice. The federation's vision is to promote networking, share expertise, and create programs that advance the fields of touch and movement, and to encourage coalitions in the development of appropriate legislation. Members of the federation include these organizations:

- American Massage Therapy Association (AMTA)
- American Organization for Bodywork Therapies of Asia (AOBTA)
- American Polarity Therapy Association (APTA)
- American Society for the Alexander Technique (AmSAT)
- Feldenkrais Guild of North America (FGNA)
- International Somatic Movement Education and Therapy Association (ISMETA)
- The Rolf Institute
- United States Trager Association

educational scholarships. The foundation also provides direct consultation to the medical and research community and educates massage therapists about research methods. In September 2004, the AMTA Foundation was renamed the Massage Therapy Foundation.

In 1998, the NIH established the National Center for Complementary and Alternative Medicine (NCCAM; http://nccam.nih.gov). The NIH started providing grants for the research of complementary medicine modalities to verify the effectiveness of their use. Massage research also continues to advance through other funding sources.

With the continuing research, the growing number of states requiring massage licensing, and the development of more sophisticated educational standards, massage continues to emerge as a recognized and respected allied health profession.

MASSAGE SYSTEMS

The methods of massage generally in use today descend directly from the Swedish, German, French, English, Chinese, and Japanese systems.

1. The Swedish system is based on the Western concepts of anatomy and physiology and employs the traditional manipulative techniques of *effleurage, petrissage,* vibration, friction, and *tapotement.* The Swedish system also employs movements that can be slow and gentle, or vigorous and bracing, according to the results that the practitioner wishes to achieve.
2. The German method combines many of the Swedish movements and emphasizes the use of various kinds of therapeutic baths.
3. The French and English systems also employ many of the Swedish massage movements for body massage.
4. Acupressure stems from the Chinese medical practice of acupuncture. It is based on the traditional Oriental medical principles for assessing and treating the physical and energetic body and employs various methods of stimulating acupuncture points to regulate *Qi* (the life force energy). The aim of this method is to achieve therapeutic changes in the person being treated as well as to relieve pain, discomfort, or other physiologic imbalances.
5. The Japanese system, called *shiatsu,* a finger pressure method, is based on the Oriental concept that the body has a series of energy points (*tsubo*). When pressure is properly applied to these points, circulation is improved and nerves are stimulated. This system is said to improve body metabolism and to relieve a number of physical disorders.

At the time of publication of this text, there are more than 70 styles or modalities of massage therapy being practiced in the United States, most of which have developed since the 1960s. It is not practical to describe or list all of them; however, the following is a small sample of systems that have gained recognition as beneficial forms of massage.

Sports massage refers to a method of massage especially designed to prepare an athlete for an upcoming event and to aid in the body's regenerative and restorative capacities following a rigorous workout or competition. This effect is achieved through specialized manipulations that stimulate circulation of the blood and lymph. Some sports massage movements are designed to break down lesions and adhesions or reduce fatigue. Sports massage generally follows the Swedish system, with variations of movements applied according to the judgment of the practitioner and the results desired. Sports teams, especially those in professional baseball, football, basketball, hockey, ice skating, and swimming, often retain a professionally trained massage practitioner. Athletes, dancers, and others who must keep muscles strong and supple are often instructed in automassage (i.e., how to massage one's own muscles) and in basic massage on a partner. (See Chapter 18)

polarity therapy
uses massage manipulations derived from Eastern and Western practices.

Polarity therapy is a method developed by Randolph Stone (1890–1971) using massage manipulations derived from both Eastern and Western practices. Exercises and thinking practices are included to balance the body both physically and energetically.

Dr. Milton Trager developed the Trager method, which uses movement exercises called mentastics and a massage-like, gentle shaking of different parts of the body to eliminate and prevent pent-up tensions.

rolfing
aligns the major body segments through manipulation of the fascia or the connective tissue.

Rolfing is a systematic program developed from the technique of structural integration by Dr. Ida Rolf. Rolfing aligns the major body segments through manipulation of the fascia (**FAH**-shuh) or the connective tissue.

reflexology
stimulates particular points on the surface of the body, which in turn affects other areas or organs of the body.

The **reflexology** method originated with the Chinese and is based on the idea that stimulation of particular points on the surface of the body has an effect on other areas or organs of the body. Dr. William Fitzgerald is credited with first demonstrating the effects of reflexology in the early 1900s. Eunice Ingham worked for Fitzgerald, and in the 1930s, she systemized the technique (popular today) that focuses mainly on the hands and feet. (See Chapter 21)

Box 1.3

Valuable Massage Therapy Websites

American Massage Therapy Association	www.amtamassage.org
Association of Massage and Bodywork Professionals	www.abmp.com
American Organization of Body Therapies of Asia	www.aobta.org
International Massage Association	www.imagroup.com
National Certification Board for Therapeutic Massage and Bodywork	www.ncbtmb.org
Federation of State Massage Therapy Boards	www.fsmtb.org
Federation of Therapeutic Massage, Bodywork and Somatic Practice Organizations	www.federationmbs.org
The Massage Therapy Foundation	www.massagetherapyfoundation.org
Touch Research Institute	www6.miami.edu (in the search field enter "touch research" and select the Touch Research Institute link)
National Center for Complementary and Alternative Therapies	nccam.nih.gov

Touch for Health is a simplified form of applied kinesiology (ki-nee-see-**AHL**-o-jee; principles of anatomy in relation to human movement) developed by Dr. John Thie. This method involves techniques with both Eastern and Western origins. Its purpose is to relieve stress on muscles and internal organs. There are also several styles of bodywork and alternative health-related practices that use specialized kinesiology (a form of muscle testing) to derive information about the conditions of the body or how a particular substance or type of treatment might affect it.

Touch for Health

is a simplified form of applied kinesiology that involves techniques having both Eastern and Western origins.

Neuromuscular techniques originated in Europe around 1940 with the work of osteopaths Drs. Stanley Lief and Boris Chaitow. Western approaches have been developed or advanced by Paul St. John, Bonnie Prudden, Janet Travell, Lawrence Jones, Judith DeLany, and Dr. Leon Chaitow, among others. Varieties include Neuromuscular Therapy, Myotherapy, trigger point therapy, muscle energy technique, Orthobionomy, and Strain/counterstrain. Neuromuscular techniques use manipulations common to Swedish massage to systematically activate or sedate neuroreceptors usually located in contractile tissue. Reflex activity tends to normalize contractile tissue and brings the body more toward balance.(See Chapter 15)

neuromusculartechniques

a group of techniques that assess and address soft tissue dysfunction by affecting the neurologic mechanisms that control the muscle.

Craniosacral therapy has been developed by Dr. John Upledger and researchers at the Upledger Institute in Palm Beach Gardens, Florida. Craniosacral therapy is a gentle, hands-on method of evaluating and enhancing the functioning of a physiologic body system called the craniosacral system. During craniosacral therapy, trained practitioners use a light touch (i.e., equivalent to a nickel's weight) to feel the rhythmic motion theoretically created by the movement of the cerebrospinal fluid within the craniosacral system. Craniosacral therapy treatment techniques are noninvasive and usually indirect approaches, intended to resolve restrictive barriers and restore symmetric, smooth craniosacral motion. Craniosacral therapy is effective for a wide range of physiologic conditions associated with pain and dysfunction and is used as a preventive health practice because of its ability to improve the function of the central nervous system and bolster the body's resistance to disease.(See Chapter 15)

craniosacral therapy

lis a gentle, hands-on method of evaluating and enhancing the functioning of the craniosacral system.

The foregoing is a brief list and does not include the many and varied types of massage and bodywork being practiced today. Although there are many excellent massage methods, the Swedish system is still the most widely used and has been incorporated into many other procedures. Whichever method a practitioner prefers, it is essential to have a thorough knowledge of all technical movements and their effects on the various systems of the body. Practitioners must be thoroughly trained in anatomy, physiology, pathology, medical communication, and technique in schools that are licensed or have credentials meeting the professional standards required by state boards and ethical associations. The objectives of all professional practitioners are generally the same: to provide a service that enhances the client's physical health and sense of well-being.

(For a more concise history of massage, the author recommends *The Bodywork Knowledgebase, Lectures on History of Massage* by Richard P. van Why and *The History of Massage* by Robert Calvert, from which a good portion of this chapter was adapted.)

This chapter is dedicated to the memory of Robert Noah Calvert (1946–2006), massage therapist, educator, author and collector. The artwork in this chapter comes from his expansive collection of massage artifacts with permission of his widow, Judi Calvert.

QUESTIONS FOR DISCUSSION AND REVIEW

1. Define *massage.*
2. How do we know that ancient civilizations used therapeutic massage and exercise in their social, personal, or religious practices?
3. Why is massage said to be the most natural and instinctive means of relieving pain and discomfort?
4. What did the Chinese call their early massage system?
5. Why did the Greeks and Romans place so much emphasis on exercise and massage?
6. Which Greek physician became known as the father of medicine?
7. Why were the Middle Ages also called the Dark Ages?
8. How did the Arabic Empire and the rise of Islam help to preserve the practice of massage?
9. Why was the Renaissance an important turning point for the arts and sciences?
10. How did the invention of the printing press in the fifteenth century help to further the practice of massage and therapeutic exercise?
11. What is the basis of Per Henrik Ling's Swedish Movement Cure?
12. Who introduced the Swedish Movement Cure to the United States?
13. What are some of the reasons for the decline of massage at the turn of the twentieth century?
14. Why did the acceptance of massage and therapeutic exercise increase during World Wars I and II?
15. Why did manual massage become a secondary treatment following World War II?
16. How has more awareness of health and personal wellness in recent years caused a renewed interest in massage?
17. What is the difference between passive and active exercise?
18. Describe the theory on which the Japanese shiatsu system of massage is based.
19. What is the role of proper exercise and use of massage in athletics?
20. Of what benefit is the history of therapeutic massage to the student who wishes to pursue a career in the field?
21. Which massage system is the most widely used in general massage?
22. In what way are the Chinese and Japanese systems similar?
23. Why is massage used as a treatment in sports or athletic medicine?

CHAPTER

2

Requirements for the Practice of Therapeutic Massage

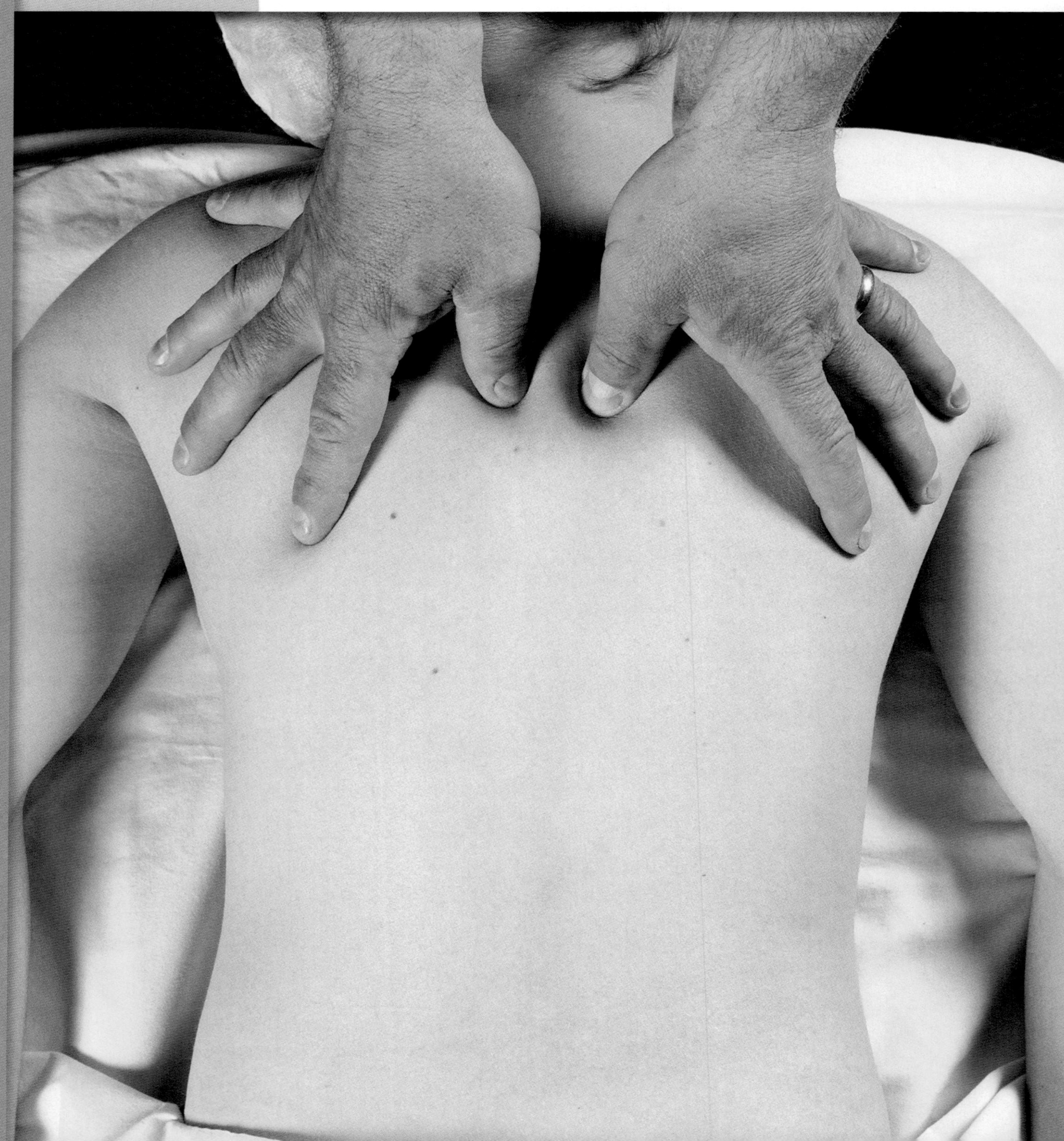

LEARNING OBJECTIVES

After you have mastered this chapter, you will be able to

1. **Explain the educational and legal aspects of scope of practice.**
2. **Explain how state legislation defines the scope of practice of therapeutic massage.**
3. **Explain why the massage practitioner must be aware of the laws, rules, regulations, restrictions, and obligations governing the practice of therapeutic massage.**
4. **Explain why it is necessary to obtain a license to practice therapeutic body massage.**
5. **Explain the difference between certifications and licenses.**
6. **Give reasons why a license to practice massage might be revoked, canceled, or suspended.**

INTRODUCTION

Therapeutic massage is a personal health service employing various soft tissue manipulations for the improvement of the client's health and well-being; therefore, the massage practitioner has an ethical responsibility to the public and to individual clients. In addition to being technically well trained, the practitioner must understand the laws, rules, regulations, limitations, and obligations concerning the practice of massage, especially in the area where he or she chooses to practice.

SCOPE OF PRACTICE

In the world of health care, practitioners can perform certain duties as prescribed by their occupation, their license, and their level of training. For instance, in a health care facility, a nurse's aide can attend to a patient's comfort and care but cannot distribute medications. In some instances, a licensed practical nurse may distribute specified medications except for narcotics, injections, and intravenous (IV) drugs. A registered nurse must oversee these distributions and handle the dangerous drugs and injections, and the orders for any of these agents must come from a physician. According to law, only doctors and nurse practitioners can diagnose illness and other medical conditions and prescribe the medications and course of treatment for those conditions. Each of these practitioners is operating within his or her scope of practice.

Scope of practice defines the rights and activities that are legally acceptable according to the licenses of a particular occupation or profession. The scope of practice of any licensed occupation is described in the legal description and definitions contained in the licensing regulation. The scope is determined in part by the educational focus of the professional training. A professional person's scope of practice is directly related to the skills he or she has gained and the training received. Massage and bodywork encompass a wide range of styles and techniques. Each professional chooses particular specialties or interests within the broader profession and directs the training and practice toward those specialties. A person's scope of practice is also influenced by personal limitations such as belief systems, personal bias, choice of preferred clientele,

scope of practice

defines the rights and activities legally acceptable according to the licenses of a particular occupation or profession.

and physical stature or endurance. By honoring personal scope of practice and respecting other professionals' scope of practice, professional people better serve their clients by providing quality service in what they do best or by referring clients to other professionals when appropriate.

Many occupations and professions have national or state regulatory boards that help to define and enforce adherence to a scope of practice. National or state boards develop and upgrade professional standards and oversee testing and licensing procedures.

At the time of publication of this text, 43 of the 50 states, the District of Columbia in the United States, and 4 Canadian provinces have adopted licensing regulations governing the practice of massage. The definition of massage and the educational requirements contained in those regulations define the scope of practice of massage in those states (See Box 2.1). Whereas there is some basic agreement among those states regarding the need to license massage, there is great diversity in defining the purpose, object, procedure, or educational requirements. With more than 3/4 of the states requiring licenses for massage, there is not a clearly defined scope of practice for massage therapy. Regardless of this fact, massage practitioners must recognize and practice within their legal and professional boundaries and refer clients to appropriately trained and licensed professionals when indicated.

Box 2.1

Legislative Definitions of Massage Therapy

This box contains excerpts from legislative documents from selected states that license massage and define the term *massage therapy*. The educational requirements for licensing and continuing education requirements for license renewal are also listed. These states were selected to show the diversity of the definition of massage therapy and the educational requirements to practice. Become familiar with the laws of the state or municipality where you choose to practice.

Maine

Educational requirement:	500 hours from an accredited school
Continuing education requirement:	None

"Massage therapist" or "massage practitioner" means a person who provides or offers to provide massage therapy for a fee, monetary or otherwise.

"Massage therapy" means a scientific or skillful manipulation of soft tissue for therapeutic or remedial purposes, specifically for improving muscle tone and circulation and promoting health and physical well-being. The term includes, but is not limited to, manual and mechanical procedures for the purpose of treating soft tissue only, the use of supplementary aids such as rubbing alcohol, liniments, oils, antiseptics, powders, herbal preparations, creams or lotions; procedures such as oil rubs, salt glows, and hot or cold packs; or other similar procedures or preparations commonly used in this practice. This term specifically excludes manipulation of the spine or articulations and excludes sexual contact of any kind.

New Mexico

Educational requirement:	650 hours
Continuing education requirement:	16 hours biennial

"Massage therapy" means the assessment and treatment of soft tissues and their dysfunctions for therapeutic purposes primarily for comfort and relief of pain. It is a health care service that includes gliding, kneading, percussion, compression,

Box 2.1 cont'd

vibration, friction, nerve strokes, stretching the tissue and exercising the range of motion, and may include the use of oils, salt glows, hot or cold packs, or hydrotherapy. Synonymous terms for massage therapy include massage, therapeutic massage, body massage, myomassage, bodywork, body rub, or any derivation of those terms. Massage therapy is the deformation of soft tissues from more than one anatomical point by manual or mechanical means to accomplish homeostasis and/or pain relief in the tissues being deformed, as defined in the Massage Therapy Practice Act, NMSA 1978, Section 61-12C-3.E.

Nebraska

Educational requirement:	1,000 hours from an accredited massage school
Continuing education requirement:	24 hours biennial

"Massage Therapist" means a person licensed to practice massage therapy.

"Massage Therapy" means the physical, mechanical, or electrical manipulation of soft tissue for the therapeutic purposes of enhancing muscle relaxation, reducing stress, improving circulation, or instilling a greater sense of well-being and may include the use of oil, salt glows, heat lamps, and hydrotherapy. It does not include diagnosis or treatment or use of procedures for which a license to practice medicine or surgery, chiropractic, or podiatry is required nor the use of microwave diathermy, shortwave diathermy, ultrasound, transcutaneous electrical nerve stimulation, electrical stimulation of >35 volts, neurologic hyperstimulation, or spinal and joint adjustments.

The definitions above were attained from the Internet Web site of the various states. Those sites as of July 2009 are
Maine—http://www.state.me.us, search for "professional licensing".
New Mexico—http://www.rld.state.nm.us
Nebraska—http://www.hhs.state.ne.us

LICENSES: THEY ARE THE LAW

In the United States, laws and regulations for massage can fall under the auspices of the state, the county, or the municipality, or they might not exist at all. Where massage laws are in effect, massage practitioners must register with the proper authorities, satisfy certain requirements to obtain a license to practice, and operate their practice in accordance to those regulations. These requirements vary depending on the licensing agency and the original motives for instituting the legislation. Many municipalities adopt ordinances to curb unethical practices, misleading advertising, and the use of the term *massage* to conceal questionable or illegal activities, especially prostitution or illicit drug sales and distribution. This type of licensing often requires mug shots, fingerprinting, and criminal record searches and has little regard for massage proficiency. As massage becomes more recognized as a reputable and respected health care practice, most of these ordinances are being replaced with licensing laws that contain educational, technical, ethical, and sanitation requirements.

Laws and regulations vary greatly from state to state and city to city. Being licensed in one state does not guarantee that the same license is valid or recognized in another state. If your license is from a city, it is almost guaranteed that the only place where that license is valid is in the city where the license was issued. A practitioner who has a license and wishes to practice in another city or state should contact the proper agency in the area where he or she wishes to practice. Usually the county commissioner's office, the city attorney, city clerk, or the mayor's office can provide information about massage regulations. If there is reciprocity between the two licensing agencies, the valid license will be honored; if not, the practitioner should provide proof of ability to meet any requirements and make applications as required.

In the United States, a growing number of states are adopting legislation that requires all massage practitioners to obtain and maintain a license or registration. These state laws usually take precedence over city and county laws and are professional licenses wherein the applicant must apply and satisfy certain requirements before being issued a license to practice massage. As of the publication of this text, in the United States 43 states and the District of Columbia license massage therapists. Each of these states has an agency or board that oversees the licensing process. The requirements for licensure vary somewhat from state to state, but most require the applicant to be at least 18 years of age, be a high school graduate, complete massage therapy training from a school or program of a minimum specified length that is recognized by the board, and successfully complete a written examination. Of the 43 regulated states (including the District of Columbia), 35 use the National Certification Examination for Therapeutic Massage and Bodywork as a requirement for licensing. In 2007, the Federation of State Massage Therapy Licensing Boards (FSMTB) created the Massage and Bodywork Licensing Examination (MBLEx) as a valid, reliable licensing examination to determine entry-level competence. A growing number of states are joining the Federation and adopting the MBLEx as an alternative to the National Certification Examination. Both the NCE and the MBLEx use a multiple choice format and cover subjects such as anatomy, physiology, kinesiology, pathology, contraindications, assessment, benefits, treatment planning, business practices, and ethics.

Both the NCE and the MBLEx charge a fee to administer the examination. All states that license massage therapists require a fee for the initial license and for either an annual or biennial renewal. The amount of these fees varies according to the state. States that regulate massage require licenses or registrations to be renewed either every year or every other year, and there is a fee to renew the license. It is not necessary to retake the licensing examination; however, many states do require a specified number of continuing education hours. **Continuing education** is any class or workshop that practitioners attend that is related to their profession or practice. The term *continuing education hours* refers to the length of these classes in hours. The massage practitioner's responsibility is to know the licensing requirements where they live and practice according to his or her state and local regulations.

continuing education

any class or workshop that a professional attends that relates to his or her profession or practice after graduation from the initial training.

Licensed physical therapists, physicians, registered nurses, osteopaths, chiropractors, athletic trainers, and podiatrists may practice massage as part of their therapeutic treatments. These professionals, however, usually obtain a license specifically for the practice of massage when they wish to be known as massage practitioners. It is outside a massage therapist's scope of practice to perform services that require a professional license to practice, such as chiropractic, acupuncture, and psychotherapy. A massage therapist cannot diagnose illness or prescribe medication or medical intervention. A massage therapist can perform a variety of assessments to determine which therapeutic modalities are most appropriate for soft tissue conditions that a client might have or if a prospective client would be better served by being referred to another professional, however.

Massage establishments must abide by local laws, rules, and regulations. Where it is required, they must be licensed and employ only licensed practitioners.

In addition to massage ordinances and licenses, local business and zoning laws must be followed when one is setting up a massage business. Most states require massage practitioners to display their licenses at their place of business.

STUDENT ACTIVITY

1. Determine the massage licensing requirements to practice massage where you currently reside.
2. Choose a neighboring state or a state to which you would like to move and determine the licensing requirements to practice massage in that location. (*Hint*: the AMTA maintains a website of all states that regulate massage. (http://amtamassage.org, select "Legislation/ Regulation")

EDUCATIONAL REQUIREMENTS

The educational requirements to practice massage or bodywork vary depending on the discipline or techniques and the licensing requirements of the city or state where the practice is located. There are many disciplines or styles of hands-on therapies in practice, and few of these have clearly defined educational requirements. Professional organizations affiliated with these various disciplines often set educational guidelines that include the length and content of training programs and recognize schools that comply with those guidelines. The American Massage Therapy Association (AMTA) Council of Schools, for example, requires member schools to have a curriculum of at least 500 in-class hours, whereas the Commission for Massage Therapy Accreditation (COMTA) requires that schools have a minimum of 600 classroom hours of training before they can be considered for accreditation. Required subjects include the following:

- Anatomy, physiology, and pathology of the human body
- Knowledge of the effects of massage and bodywork techniques
- Indications, contraindications, and precautions for massage
- Application of massage therapy, including assessment, planning, and performance
- Ethics and development of successful therapeutic relationships with clients

If a license is required to practice massage, an educational requirement is usually included in the licensing legislation. Without a national standard for massage therapy, educational requirements contained in licensing laws vary widely. City or municipal licenses can contain no educational requirement or can require as many as 1,000 hours of training. Of the states that license massage at the time of publication of this text, the educational requirements vary from 500 to 1,000 hours of training; some Canadian provinces require as many as 2,200 hours of schooling.

The National Certification for Therapeutic Massage and Bodywork recommends a minimum standard educational requirement, which has been established as the equivalent of 500 hours of training and includes the subjects of anatomy, physiology, pathology, business practices, massage technique, and ethics.

Educational requirements for licensure and national certification reflect an entry-level knowledge base and are often the basis on which many massage schools build their core curriculum. Although this provides a solid foundation to begin a professional career, it is only the beginning of what is possible. Massage education does not end with graduation and licensure or certification. There is an extensive variety of massage and bodywork modalities available through classes and continuing education seminars to enhance therapists' skills to better serve their clients. Continuing education programs vary in length from a few hours to hundreds of hours or even several years. Modalities introduced in massage school, such as sports massage, orthopedic massage, neuromuscular therapy, myofascial release, and craniosacral therapy, can be enhanced with more extensive training after graduation. Most state massage boards, the National Certification Board, the ABMP, and the AMTA include continuing education among requirements for license or membership renewal. Dedicated massage professionals expand their technical skills, refresh their interest, improve their businesses, and become better therapists by regularly participating in continuing education courses.

HEALTH REQUIREMENTS FOR PRACTITIONERS

Because massage is a hands-on profession, one involving touch, the massage practitioner should be physically and mentally fit and be free of any communicable diseases. Some state licensing requirements or employers request a health certificate or written confirmation of this fitness from a physician. It is the practitioner's duty to keep him- or herself in top physical condition. Massage is hard work and requires the therapist to stand for extended periods, especially when performing multiple massages. The practitioner must have physical stamina and the ability to concentrate on giving a therapeutic massage.

REASONS WHY LICENSES CAN BE REVOKED, SUSPENDED, OR CANCELED

Because the practice of massage concerns the health and welfare of the public and specifically that of individual clients, the profession must be regulated by the issuance of licenses only to people who have met the requirements to practice. The professional massage practitioner must have integrity, the necessary technical skills, and a willingness to comply with rigid health standards.

The following are grounds on which the practitioner's license can be revoked, canceled, or suspended:

1. Being guilty of fraud or deceit in obtaining a license
2. Having been convicted of a felony
3. Being engaged currently or previously in any act of prostitution
4. Practicing under a false or assumed name
5. Being addicted to narcotics, alcohol, or similar substances that interfere with the performance of duties
6. Being willfully negligent in the practice of massage so as to endanger the health of a client
7. Prescribing drugs or medicines (unless you are a licensed physician)
8. Being guilty of fraudulent or deceptive advertising
9. Ethical or sexual misconduct with a client
10. Practicing beyond the scope permitted by law or performing professional responsibilities that the licensee knows he or she is not competent to perform

LICENSE VERSUS CERTIFICATION

A *license* is issued from a state or municipal regulating agency as a requirement for conducting a business or practicing a trade or profession. A *certification*, on the other hand, is a document that is awarded in recognition of an accomplishment or achieving or maintaining some kind of standard. A certification can be given for successfully completing a course of study or passing an examination

Box 2.2

Licensing versus Certification

Licensing	Certification
Issued by a governmental agency	Issued by a nongovernmental agency
Required to practice a trade or profession in a regulated jurisdiction	Voluntary to show proficiency or accomplishment
Specifies a scope of practice	Some licenses require certification
Determines minimum requirements for compliance	May show levels of competence beyond what is required for licensure
Must be renewed at predetermined intervals	May indicate membership in an organization

to show a level of proficiency or ability. Certificates are awarded by schools and institutions to show the successful completion of a course of study. Professional organizations have certificates of membership to indicate that the recipient has met the qualifications to become a member. Many professions (the massage profession included) have a national certification program whereby proficiency toward a national standard can be achieved and certified. Since 1992, the National Certification Board for Therapeutic Massage and Bodywork (NCBTMB) has administered the National Certification Examination for Therapeutic Massage and Bodywork (NCETMB). Participation in national certification is voluntary; however, several states that license massage require successful completion of the National Certification Examination to be licensed. Successful completion of the National Certification Examination earns the one taking the test the designation of being nationally certified in therapeutic massage and bodywork. In 2005, the National Certification Board added another credentialing examination, the National Certification Examination for Therapeutic Massage (NCETM), which focuses on classic Western massage without the Asian bodywork component. These certifications do lend an air of credibility to a practitioner but do not take the place of a license in locales where a license is required to practice.

QUESTIONS FOR DISCUSSION AND REVIEW

1. Why must the massage practitioner be concerned about the laws, rules, regulations, and obligations pertaining to the practice of therapeutic body massage?
2. What are the legal and educational aspects of scope of practice?
3. Why do laws governing the practice of massage often differ from one state to another?
4. Does having a license in one locale permit a practitioner to practice anywhere? Why or why not?
5. What is the general educational requirement for a license to practice massage?
6. What are the reasons for which a person would receive a certificate?
7. What are the specific grounds on which a practitioner's license may be revoked, canceled, or suspended?

CHAPTER

3

Professional Ethics for Massage Practitioners

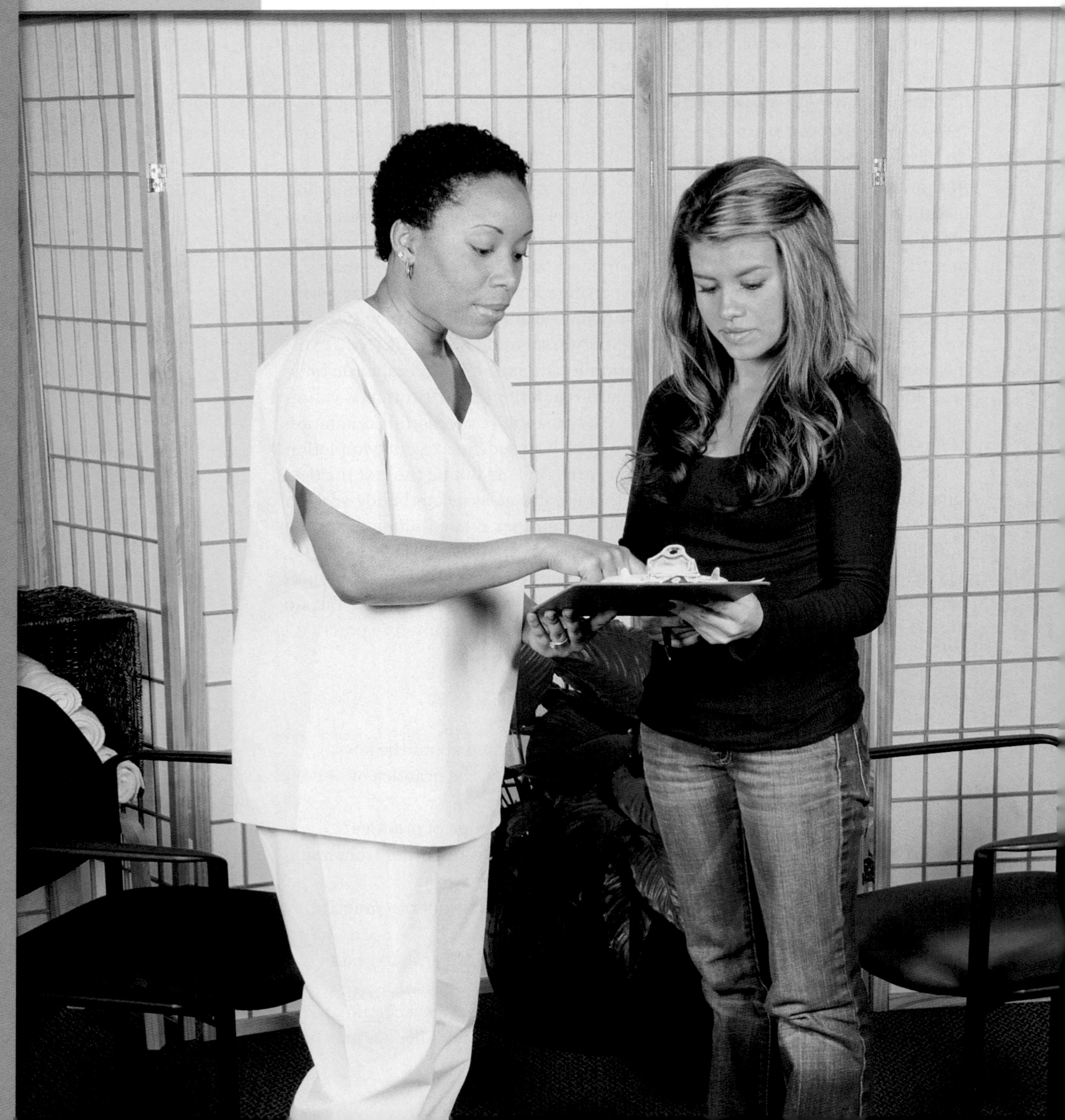

LEARNING OBJECTIVES

After you have mastered this chapter, you will be able to

1. **Define the meaning of professional ethics.**
2. **Explain how the practice of good ethics helps to build a successful massage practice.**
3. **Differentiate between personal and professional boundaries.**
4. **Designate at least eight areas to consider when establishing professional boundaries.**
5. **Define a therapeutic relationship and a client-centered relationship.**
6. **Explain the effects of a power differential in the therapeutic relationship.**
7. **Explain the effects of transference, countertransference, and dual relationships in the therapeutic setting.**
8. **Discuss why sexual arousal can occur during a massage session and what to do if it does.**
9. **Discuss why and how to desexualize the massage experience.**
10. **Define supervision and its importance to the massage professional.**
11. **Discuss the importance of good health habits and professional projection.**
12. **Discuss the importance of human relations and success attitudes.**
13. **Discuss ways to build a sound business reputation.**

INTRODUCTION

When a massage therapy student completes the initial course of study and graduates from massage school, you enter the profession of massage. You become a professional therapist. Being a professional is more than simply having a job. A professional has completed a course of study to gain knowledge in a specific field of practice, usually to provide a service. A profession is usually regulated, is represented by a professional association, and adheres to a **code of ethics**.

code of ethics

a set of guiding moral principles that governs a person's choice of action.

Professionalism in massage not only encompasses the application of massage technique to a client but also involves clear communication, managing boundaries, and ethical business practices. Professional standards include educational requirements, scope of practice, state and local regulations, codes of ethics, and standards of practice.

Massage professionals engage in therapeutic relationships with clients. A healthy therapeutic relationship requires an understanding and respect for personal and professional **boundaries**. Personal boundaries provide protection and a sense of self. Each person's set of boundaries is unique depending on life experiences. Professional boundaries are the foundation of an ethical practice. Honoring personal boundaries and maintaining professional boundaries ensure that the therapeutic relationship benefits the client and avoids ethical problems.

boundaries

are personal comfort zones that help a person to maintain a sense of comfort and safety. They can be professional, personal, physical, emotional, intellectual, and sexual.

Ethics is the study of the standards and philosophy of human conduct and is defined as a system or code of morals of an individual person, a group, or a profession. To practice good ethics is to be concerned about the public welfare, the welfare of individual clients, your reputation, and the reputation of the profession you represent. *Ethics* are moral guidelines that are established by experienced professionals to reduce the incidence and risk of harm or injury in the professional relationship because of an abuse of a position of power. A professional person is one who is engaged in an avocation or occupation requiring some advanced training to gain knowledge and skills. Without ethics there can be no true professionalism.

Ethical conduct on the part of the practitioner gives the client confidence in the place of business, the services rendered, and the entire industry. A satisfied client is your best means of advertising, because that person's good recommendation helps you to maintain public confidence and build a sound business following. The business establishment that becomes known for its professional ethics will stay in business longer than one that makes extravagant claims and false promises or one that is involved in questionable practices. (See Box 3.1 for two examples of ethics codes.)

Box 3.1

Codes of Ethics

Codes of ethics are adopted by professions, professional organizations, and sometimes by state regulatory agencies. This box presents the Code of Ethics of the American Massage Therapy Association and the National Certification Board for Therapeutic Massage and Bodywork.

AMTA Code of Ethics

This Code of Ethics is a summary statement of the standards by which massage therapists agree to conduct their practices and is a declaration of the general principles of acceptable, ethical, professional behavior.

Massage therapists shall:

1. Demonstrate commitment to provide the highest quality massage therapy/bodywork to those who seek their professional service.
2. Acknowledge the inherent worth and individuality of each person by not discriminating or behaving in any prejudicial manner with clients and/or colleagues.
3. Demonstrate professional excellence through regular self-assessment of strengths, limitations, and effectiveness by continued education and training.
4. Acknowledge the confidential nature of the professional relationship with clients and respect each client's right to privacy.
5. Conduct all business and professional activities within their scope of practice, the law of the land, and project a professional image.
6. Refrain from engaging in any sexual conduct or sexual activities involving their clients.
7. Accept responsibility to do no harm to the physical, mental, and emotional well-being of self, clients, and associates.

Box 3.1 (cont'd)

Codes of Ethics

National Certification Board for Therapeutic Massage and Bodywork

Code of Ethics

revised 6/23/2007

Massage and bodywork therapists shall act in a manner that justifies public trust and confidence, enhances the reputation of the profession, and safeguards the interest of individual clients. To this end, massage and bodywork therapists in the exercise of accountability will:

1. Have a sincere commitment to provide the highest quality of care to those who seek their professional services.
2. Represent their qualifications honestly, including education and professional affiliations, and provide only those services that they are qualified to perform.
3. Accurately inform clients, other healthcare practitioners, and the public of the scope and limitations of their discipline.
4. Acknowledge the limitations of and contraindications for massage and bodywork and refer clients to appropriate health professionals.
5. Provide treatment only where there is reasonable expectation that it will be advantageous to the client.
6. Consistently maintain and improve professional knowledge and competence, striving for professional excellence through regular assessment of personal and professional strengths and weaknesses and through continued education training.
7. Conduct their business and professional activities with honesty and integrity, and respect the inherent worth of all persons.
8. Refuse to unjustly discriminate against clients or health professionals.
9. Safeguard the confidentiality of all client information, unless disclosure is requested by the client in writing, is medically necessary, required by law, or necessary for the protection of the public.
10. Respect the client's right to treatment with informed and voluntary consent. The certified practitioner will obtain and record the informed consent of the client, or client's advocate, before providing treatment. This consent may be written or verbal.
11. Respect the client's right to refuse, modify, or terminate treatment regardless of prior consent given.
12. Provide draping and treatment in a way that ensures the safety, comfort, and privacy of the client.
13. Exercise the right to refuse to treat any person or part of the body for just and reasonable cause.
14. Refrain, under all circumstances, from initiating or engaging in any sexual conduct, sexual activities or sexualizing behavior involving a client, even if the client attempts to sexualize the relationship.
15. Avoid any interest, activity, or influence which might be in conflict with the practitioner's obligation to act in the best interests of the client or the profession.
16. Respect the client's boundaries with regard to privacy, disclosure, exposure, emotional expression, beliefs, and the client's reasonable expectations of professional behavior. Practitioners will respect the client's autonomy.
17. Refuse any gifts or benefits that are intended to influence a referral, decision, or treatment, or that are purely for personal gain and not for the good of the client.
18. Follow all policies, procedures, guidelines, regulations, codes and requirements promulgated by the National Certification Board for Therapeutic Massage and Bodywork.

BOUNDARIES

Any discussion of ethical professional practices must include an understanding of boundaries, both personal and professional. Boundaries delineate personal comfort zones, the realm in which people operate with a sense of safety and control. Boundaries also help to screen input about what is appropriate for our personal comfort. Everyone has boundaries that dictate how they act and interact with the world and other people.

Boundaries are individual, personal, and usually intangible. There are many kinds of boundaries that we establish and maintain in order to keep a sense of comfort and safety. Some of those boundaries may be classified as physical, emotional, intellectual, and sexual. They act as personal protection. A boundary is like a safety net or force field that surrounds every person. Boundaries are contextual depending on circumstances and relationships. The field shifts depending on the situation.

Personal boundaries help to define who we are emotionally, intellectually, and spiritually. They help to determine how and with whom we choose to share our lives and beliefs. Boundaries are defined by our experiences, beliefs and expectations. They separate us as individual persons and provide a framework to safely function in the world. People with a good sense of boundaries are able to claim their own space, embrace their own emotions, be spontaneous, take in information easily, make clear decisions, and be responsive and sensitive to the needs of others.

Some determining factors in the formation of personal boundaries include family, school, or religious upbringing. Cultural and ethnic influences also shape attitudes about relationships, privacy, and touch. Boundaries are flexible, permeable, and constantly changing according to new information. Although many boundaries are established early in our lives, relationships, both good and bad, continue to influence our boundaries and comfort zones in the way that we relate to others.

Personal boundaries vary widely among individual people. Relationships involve the interaction between the boundaries of individual persons. Often, one person in the relationship gives in to the other's wishes or needs, thereby shifting the boundaries. People with whom we interact have different boundaries, and so we must be sensitive and able to respond with understanding. In some situations, we must hold strong boundaries, and at other appropriate times we must be flexible to merge or expand our experience. Many minor boundary fluctuations occur with very little impact, depending on the level of trust in the relationship. When a boundary is severely invaded or violated, this might constitute a situation of neglect or even abuse. Even in the case of minor boundary infractions, there can be a sense of discomfort or confusion.

When we move outside of our own boundaries or push beyond another's, we find ourselves in dangerous territory that can easily lead to disappointment, questionable behavior, emotional turmoil, or abuse.

Professional Boundaries

Professional boundaries are predetermined practices that protect the safety of the client and the therapist. An important aspect of a professional practice is to recognize, respect, and honor the client's personal boundaries. A new client seeking massage is asked to stretch one's personal boundaries in several ways. The client enters an unfamiliar facility and discloses personal information relative to a physical condition to a practitioner who is a stranger. The client disrobes and lies down on a table under a sheet, rather passively, while the practitioner applies touch and manipulations that sometimes approach levels of discomfort. In each of these activities, the client might move beyond the normal comfort boundary. What allows the client to do this is trust that the massage practitioner will maintain certain professional boundaries.

Professional boundaries are preliminarily outlined in policy and procedure statements that are presented to the client very early in the therapeutic relationship. These boundaries create a stable framework and a safe environment from which to practice.

Cherie Sohnen-Moe and Ben Benjamin, in their exceptional book *The Ethics of Touch*, list eight major areas to consider in establishing professional boundaries: location of service, interpersonal space, appearance, self-disclosure, language, touch, time, and money.

Location

The *location* refers to the therapeutic setting where the massage takes place; it should be professional, safe, and comfortable. Therapeutic massage can be performed in a wide variety of settings, ranging from a medical office, to a cabana on the beach, to an outdoor tent at a marathon, to a client's home, to a cruise ship or a home office. Seated massage can take place just about anywhere a massage chair can be set up. Regardless of the setting, consideration must be taken to ensure safety, comfort, and security for the client and a sense of professionalism from the practitioner that inspires confidence and respect.

Interpersonal Space

Interpersonal space refers to the actual space maintained between the client and practitioner during interactions before and after the actual massage. Creating an appropriate space means maintaining a physical space between the client and practitioner that makes both parties comfortable. Height variation is also considered. Carry on conversations at eye level whenever possible. Sit or stand so neither party must look up or down when discussing topics relevant to the session. Try to complete most of the important conversation before the client lies down on the table. Discussions that take place when both persons are at the same height minimize the power differential.

Appearance

Appearance refers to the way the practitioner looks and dresses when providing or promoting massage. Professional appearance includes appropriate clothing and good personal hygiene (Figure 3-1). The goal is to foster a sense of comfort, trust, and safety in the client. Avoid clothing that is too casual, revealing, or sexually provocative, or that focuses attention on the practitioner instead of the client.

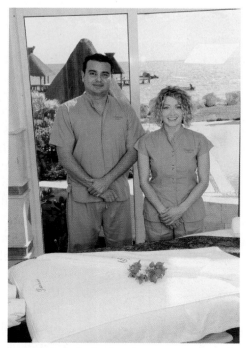

FIGURE 3-1 Professional appearance includes appropriate clothing and good personal hygiene.

Self-disclosure

Seek and provide self-disclosure appropriate to the therapeutic relationship. During the pre-session interview, the client discloses personal information at the request of the practitioner. The extent and depth of that information should cover only what is relevant to the conditions presented for treatment. Avoid probing for personal information that does not pertain to the session.

In an effort to impress or get closer to the therapist, clients sometimes expound on personal and sensitive information. The client might be unclear as to the client's own or the therapist's boundaries and give information in an attempt to gain psychological support or to leverage the practitioner to somehow act on the client's behalf beyond the scope of the therapy session.

The practitioner must also be aware of appropriate self-disclosure practices. Pertinent information regarding training, experience, modalities practiced, treatment plan, appointment policies, and fees are necessary to gain informed consent and confidence from the client. Beyond this, the practitioner must exercise caution that any personal information he or you choose to share somehow benefits the client and the therapeutic goals of the session. Some level of sharing personal experience can actually strengthen the therapeutic relationship, whereas certain personal information tends to direct the focus toward the practitioner rather than the client. This should be discouraged and avoided.

Language

According to Sohnen-Moe and Benjamin, "language is one of the most potent means for creating and maintaining healthy boundaries" (p. 55). Choice of words, voice intonation, and overall skills as a communicator are vital aspects of creating effective boundaries.

Touch

Touch and how it is applied can create a feeling of comfort and safety, or it can be threatening and uncomfortable. Touch is directly related to physical boundaries both on and off the table. Be aware of appropriate touch when greeting and saying good-bye to a client. Is a hug or a hand on the shoulder called for, or is a handshake more appropriate?

On the treatment table, touch boundaries include which parts of the practitioner's body touch the client, which parts of the client's body are and are not touched, and the depth and quality of touch. In the treatment setting, the practitioner uses the body in a nonsexual manner to perform the massage. Predominantly, the hands, forearms and elbows are used. In some modalities such as Thai massage and shiatsu, the practitioner can also use the feet and knees. Care is taken that other body parts do not inadvertently touch the client. Only areas of the client's body that are being therapeutically treated are included in the treatments. The genitals and anus are not included in a therapeutic massage treatment. Women's breasts are included as a part of a massage only when therapeutically indicated and only after obtaining written informed consent from the client before the massage begins. Therapeutic massage does not include any kind of sexually oriented touch.

Quality and depth of touch should be discussed before the session begins and included in the informed consent. Touch that is too light or too deep can cause discomfort, violate boundaries, and be inappropriate. Avoid inflicting excessive pain on a client. Some types of deep tissue work can be quite intense; however, when the pain threshold is crossed, trust is broken and it is difficult or impossible to restore. Whenever any aspect of touch goes beyond or deviates from what was discussed in the original informed consent, there must be clear and complete disclosure with the client so that the client can once again give informed consent. This greatly reduces the possibility of crossing boundaries.

Time

A defining aspect of a professional relationship is time. The client comes for a massage at an appointed time and expects a treatment that lasts a predetermined amount of time. The way in which a practitioner manages time sets clear boundaries. Beginning and finishing sessions on time honors professional and personal boundaries. Adequate time should be scheduled to accommodate a preliminary interview, assessments, undressing, dressing, and closure. Schedule enough time between appointments to complete records, return phone calls, take a break, or accommodate an unexpected late or long appointment. The client should expect to be able to come for, receive, and complete a massage within a certain time frame and can schedule a day around those activities. Establishing and maintaining policies regarding session length, late arrivals, no shows, and missed appointments define boundaries, letting clients know what to expect.

Money

In a therapeutic relationship, the practitioner provides a service that is of benefit in exchange for a set fee. The fee is predetermined and adds value to the client's experience. The amount of the fee is determined based on the service provided and should directly reflect the value of the service. When establishing a fee structure, the practitioner establishes boundaries, further defining a professional practice. Fees that are too low or exorbitantly high for the services rendered are professional boundary infractions. Charging different fees to different populations for the same service should be avoided or done with extreme scrutiny. Clients challenge boundaries by not bringing money or a check to pay for a session, by writing a check with insufficient funds, by being late paying, or by not paying a bill at all.

Be aware of and honor a client's personal boundaries. Respect a client's comfort levels with respect to room temperature, level of dress or undress, amount of pressure used during the massage, and parts of the body to omit or give extra attention. Early in the therapeutic relationship, the practitioner can help the client to become more aware and responsive to boundary issues and at the same time reduce the chance of inadvertently invading or violating those boundaries with a statement like: "At any time while we are together, if I ask, say, or do anything that causes any discomfort at all, please let me know what it is." This empowers the client and provides the opportunity to discuss and clarify the reason for whatever might be the cause of the discomfort so that the session can be adjusted to better serve the needs of the client.

When applying any technique that might be in any way intrusive, such as ischemic compression on a trigger point or approaching a sensitive area on the body, a similar statement informs and empowers the client with more control over the session.

Recognizing and honoring a client's boundaries and maintaining clear professional boundaries are the cornerstones for building and maintaining an ethical professional practice.

THE THERAPEUTIC RELATIONSHIP

The *therapeutic relationship* is a practitioner/client relationship that is client centered, in which all activities benefit and enhance the client's well-being and maintain or promote individual welfare. Therapeutic relationships directly influence people's mental, emotional, and physical well-being. Inherent in the therapeutic relationship is an implicit contract between the therapist and the client. The client comes by appointment to a prearranged location, receives an agreed-on treatment, for a specified length of time and an agreed-on fee. The client expects to receive treatment to address certain conditions or otherwise enhance the state of wellness in accordance with the knowledge of the therapist and dependent on the therapist's skills and education. It is the responsibility of the practitioner to provide an environment that is secure and safe. Clients put trust in the practitioner to always act in the client's best interests.

A client enters a therapeutic relationship expecting to gain from the skills of the practitioner. A central goal in developing a therapeutic relationship is to create a safe environment, a place where any client is secure enough to allow healing to occur; a place that is safe enough to be vulnerable, to be open, to release, to relax, be nonthreatened; a place of trust or a safe haven in which to unwind. The client assumes there is safety from physical, emotional, or sexual impropriety.

Confidentiality in the practitioner/client relationship is the foundation of safety, protection, trust, and respect. It helps to provide an environment for the client to relax, open, release, transform, and heal. To uphold confidentiality, the practitioner keeps all personal information regarding any client, including the fact of being a client, private except with permission of the client or in certain circumstances required by law. The client should sign a release of medical information before the practitioner confers with other health care providers concerning the client. (This is discussed on pages 51 and 633.) There is a legal requirement that the practitioner report to authorities situations of imminent or life-threatening danger by or to a client or situations of child abuse. This requirement is known as *the duty to warn and protect.* Clients must be informed about the limits of confidentiality near the beginning of the initial interview or assessment.

In a client-based relationship, a good litmus test to determine whether an activity or procedure is appropriate is to ask "To whose benefit is the questioned activity?" If the answer is not "the client's," the decision should be not to proceed.

In the therapeutic relationship, being sensitive to, respecting, and maintaining both personal and professional boundaries is critical to avoiding potential ethical dilemmas.

Power Differential

Throughout their lifetimes, people experience many kinds of relationships. Relationships include those with friends, schoolmates, siblings, parent/child, romantic partner, spouse, employer/employee, and therapist/client. Each kind of relationship involves various levels of intimacy, commitment, and responsibility, and in each there is a balance or imbalance of power. In some relationships, such as friendships or romantic couplings, the balance of power is fairly even or shifts back and forth according to what is happening at any given moment. In relationships such as parent/child, teacher/student, or employer/employee, there is an evident power differential in which more authority is held by the person on one side of the relationship, whereas the other person is in a more vulnerable or submissive role. With that power comes responsibility.

Practitioner/client relationships by their very nature exhibit a power differential. The client seeks out the services of the practitioner because of the practitioner's knowledge, skill, and authority. The practitioner is in a place of power to provide actions or services to enhance the well-being of the more vulnerable client. Owing to the nature of the massage session, the practitioner stands over the client who is lying unclothed (although draped) on a massage table. The client literally looks up to and submits to the ministrations of the practitioner. The client is often passive while the practitioner actively uses the hands to manipulate the client's body. There is an inherent power differential favoring the practitioner, whereas the client is in a more vulnerable position. Because of the power differential, the client might quietly succumb to the actions of the practitioner rather than articulate any discomfort. If the client thinks that the practitioner is "all knowing," the client might not speak up when needs are not being met or when the practitioner does or does not do something that crosses or violates the client's boundaries.

Because we are human, it is inevitable that boundaries are crossed or even violated. When subtle boundary crossings occur, they can be experienced as a feeling of discomfort or unease on the part of either party owing to the action usually of the other. These small discomforts should be noted and articulated. When the practitioner notices signs of discomfort such as withdrawal or fidgeting during the interview or grimacing during the session, you should encourage the client to articulate those feelings. The practitioner can help to balance the power differential by discussing treatment options with the client and giving a choice on how to proceed at the beginning of the session. Establishing a policy early in the therapeutic relationship that encourages the client to speak up anytime there is discomfort of any kind during the course of treatment empowers the client to better direct the experience and reduces the likelihood of personal boundaries being severely crossed. Clear communication is the most effective tool to both prevent and clarify boundary issues.

In the therapeutic relationship, the practitioner holds the advantage in the power differential and therefore has the responsibility to establish and maintain a safe and healthy therapeutic environment where the client's well-being, safety, and comfort are the focus of all activities. It is the role of the practitioner to ensure that the power differential is not abused to the client's detriment.

The practitioner has the responsibility to be sensitive to, to respect, and to maintain both personal and professional boundaries, even if the client initiates the questionable activity.

Transference

When a client seeks the services of a professional, an authority figure, someone to whom the client can defer judgment, that client enters a relationship in which it is comfortable to respond as done with other authority figures in the past. There is sometimes an unconscious tendency for the client to project onto the practitioner attributes of someone from a former relationship. The client might also seek more out of the relationship than is therapeutically appropriate. Psychotherapists have been aware of this type of phenomenon since the time of Freud. When a client tries to personalize the therapeutic relationship, it is known as **transference**. Transference involves misperceptions that the client might have toward the practitioner or therapist. Those misperceptions can be positive or negative. Transference can surface in any relationship in which there is a power differential. This occurs quite unconsciously. Transference usually tends to diminish the effectiveness of the therapeutic relationship.

transference

happens when a client personalizes, either negatively or positively, a therapeutic relationship by unconsciously projecting characteristics of someone from a former relationship onto a therapist or practitioner.

The therapist should be aware of the signs of transference and take necessary measures to reduce its occurrence.

Transference usually happens at an unconscious level. Some signs of transference include the following:

- The client attempts to become more personally involved with the practitioner.
- The client asks personal questions not related to the reason for the visit.
- The client might vie for extra time during or at the end of the session.
- The client might invite the practitioner to social activities, or try to get closer physically, socially, or emotionally.
- The client brings or offers gifts or favors.
- The client proposes friendships or sexual involvement.
- The client might become more demanding of the practitioner's time and attention or even become angry, disappointed, or rejected if the practitioner does not respond.
- The client might want to adore, befriend, and please the practitioner or berate and mistrust the practitioner.

All of these behaviors are signs of transference. They are not necessarily about the practitioner but are related to the power differential and the attempts of the client to personalize the therapeutic relationship.

Ultimately, it is the responsibility of the practitioner to maintain clear professional boundaries when transference occurs to uphold a healthy therapeutic relationship.

Countertransference

Occasionally, transference works in the other direction—the practitioner begins to personalize or take the relationship with the client personally. When the practitioner tends to personalize the relationship, it is known as

countertransference. Countertransference involves misperceptions of the practitioner toward the client. It is usually unconscious and always detrimental to the therapeutic process.

countertransference

happens when a therapist or practitioner personalizes a therapeutic relationship by unconsciously projecting characteristics of someone from a former relationship onto a client. This is almost always detrimental to a therapeutic relationship.

Signs of countertransference include the following:

- Strong emotional feelings toward the client, either positive or negative.
- Thinking excessively about a client between sessions.
- Dressing in a special manner when a certain client is coming.
- Making special provisions or spending extra time with a client.
- Fantasizing or having sexual feelings toward a client.
- Yawning excessively during an appointment.
- Dreading an upcoming appointment with a client.
- Negative reactions to a client, such as:
  - Feeling guilty, frustrated, or angry if a client does not respond to treatment.
  - Feeling anger or disappointment if a client is late or cancels.
  - Experiencing fatigue, disappointment, depression, or even infatuation after a session.

Any strong feelings toward a client can signal countertransference. Feelings range from love, sexual attraction, and a need to rescue, to avoidance, aggravation, and anger.

Many times a client's transference, when unrecognized, will spawn countertransference on the part of the unwitting practitioner. This is nearly always a recipe for disappointment and possible disaster for the practitioner.

Transference and countertransference are natural, unconscious phenomena that occur in therapeutic relationships in which there is a power differential. If not recognized and effectively defused, the result has a negative impact on the relationship, possibly emotionally harming the client and potentially devastating the professional's practice.

Maintaining healthy professional boundaries is the best defense against transference and countertransference. When boundaries are stretched or when a professional is tempted to move beyond those boundaries, it is a warning sign to assess motivations and how one is operating as a professional and seek supervision.

In a relationship in which there is a power differential, it is ultimately the responsibility of the person in the more powerful role to provide a safe, secure environment. The practitioner is therefore responsible for recognizing and ensuring that transference and countertransference issues are not acted out in a manner that is in any way harmful to the client or the therapeutic relationship. In some circumstances, this requires discontinuing the relationship and referring the client to another practitioner.

Dual Relationships

The therapeutic relationship is a practitioner/client relationship that is client centered, which means every activity of the relationship is directed to the benefit of the client in exchange for the predetermined fee for service.

A *dual relationship* is any situation that combines the therapeutic relationship with a secondary relationship that extends beyond the massage practitioner/client relationship. Dual relationships span a broad spectrum.

Dual relationships usually involve various dynamics with complicated tendencies that affect both sides of the relationship. There is increased potential that evolving circumstances in one relationship can adversely affect the other. Because the numerous risks of dual relationships are generally not favorable to a healthy therapeutic relationship, Dual or multiple relationships are preferably avoided.

Awareness of dual relationships and potential pitfalls originated in the field of psychology, in which strong standards now exist that discourage or even prohibit dual relationships. Numerous cases of sexual impropriety stemming from dual relationships between therapists and clients in the 1960s and 1970s were documented, prompting authorities and regulators in the mental health professions to establish regulations that dissuade practitioners and therapists from engaging in dual relationships with patients.

Dual relationships can arise when someone whom the practitioner knows becomes a client, such as a family member, a friend, a work associate, or someone from the practitioner's club, organization, or church. This situation is especially common for students who are eager for bodies to practice on or for new practitioners in the beginning stages of building a practice.

In smaller communities, the chance of a client and practitioner interacting socially increases. When encountering a client in a social setting, to uphold and honor confidentiality, it is professionally and ethically proper to engage the client only if the client initiates the contact. If the client initiates the conversation, limit the interaction to social discussion and steer clear of therapy-related topics unless the client introduces them.

In rare cases, if not exploitive or sexual, and when well managed, the dual relationship can benefit or at least not interfere with the therapeutic relationship. The fact that someone already knows the practitioner might influence the decision to call for a massage appointment. In some cases, knowing someone's personal life circumstances can help when designing a personal care plan.

There are several factors to consider concerning dual relationships. Which came first, the therapeutic relationship or the social relationship? Who initiated the secondary relationship? What is the nature of the nontherapeutic relationship? Relationships of a sexual or romantic nature are never appropriate. What is the reason for or nature of the therapeutic relationship? What is the frequency or how intimate is the nontherapeutic relationship? Can the relationships be separate and independent? Remember, the best interest of the client must always be served in the therapeutic relationship.

Another type of dual relationship develops when we barter either work or services for our services. When we barter health services, for instance, we switch from the role of therapist to the role of client, while the other party does the same. This has the potential to become complicated if one party does not feel to be receiving or giving equally. Work barters can become difficult if the quality of work does not meet the expectations of the therapist or hard feelings arise over the seemingly inequitable number of hours of work in exchange for a one-hour massage.

The classic dual relationship, however, and the one of more concern, is when a client and practitioner take on another relationship role. The relationship begins when a prospective client makes an appointment and comes in for a session.

An attraction, one for the other or mutual, results in a social or romantic relationship outside or beyond the therapeutic relationship.

If the feelings or attractions are on the part of the client, the practitioner must clearly state professional boundaries and the responsibility to uphold them. If the feelings are on the part of the practitioner, then you should seek out supervision to clarify the origin of the feelings and strengthen your boundaries, or refer the client to another practitioner for the sake of the safety of both parties.

Because of the power differential in the therapeutic relationship, it is the practitioner's responsibility to act ethically. The practitioner can pose questions such as: how will the client-centered therapeutic relationship be affected? Will the dual relationship improve or enhance the client's well-being? Choices must be made that maintain and enhance the well-being of the client. The professional is ultimately responsible for maintaining boundaries even when the client initiates the activities. It is the practitioner's responsibility to inform the client of the possible positive and negative implications of pursuing the relationship. If there is a strong mutual attraction, both parties should openly discuss the ramifications and complexities before proceeding. It is important to carefully examine the motives of entering the nontherapeutic relationship. Mutual and equal consent is essential. Without good communication, feelings are hurt, which leads to all aspects of the relationship suffering. Before becoming involved or pursuing any social relationship, the client/practitioner relationship should end. The practitioner should seek supervision with peers or a supervisor to explore the source of the feelings. If the feelings persist and the client seeks the practitioner outside of the therapeutic setting, the practitioner should use extreme caution before establishing any social relationship. It is usually a good idea to wait a period of time after the professional relationship is discontinued before continuing a personal or romantic relationship. Dual relationships are a normal part of human interaction but are nearly always detrimental to the therapeutic relationship.

ETHICAL TOUCH

The massage practitioner is a professional who is engaged in the business of giving appropriate, nurturing, and ethical touch. The massage or bodywork profession is unique in that human touch is the primary vehicle whereby services are performed. Whether it is relaxation, wellness massage, sports massage, Therapeutic Touch, or the specifically applied soft tissue manipulation of clinical massage, it is the beneficial human response to skillfully applied touch that is the basis for the success of the massage profession.

In *Touching: The Human Significance of the Skin*, Ashley Montague presents compelling anthropologic evidence that touch is an essential element for healthy growth and development. He illustrates the importance of how, from a very early age, positive touch affects human physical and emotional health throughout our lives. This book is highly recommended for anyone entering any touch or health profession.

Multiple studies by Tiffany Fields and her colleagues at the Touch Research Institute in Miami, Florida, show that the positive touch of massage reduces stress and lowers blood levels of cortisol and norepinepherine, while increasing levels of serotonin and dopamine. Low levels of serotonin and dopamine are evident in people who suffer from depression, whereas significantly higher levels are associated with elevated moods.

The United States, however, is mostly a low-touch society. Usually infants and young children are the only ones who receive a significant amount of positive touch. By the time that they enter school, children are taught to "keep their hands to themselves." Beyond the adolescent years, positive touch primarily occurs with a handshake, an occasional pat on the back or hug, in contact sports, in romantic relationships, or in touch-related therapies. For many adults, the only experience of caring touch is related to romantic relationships, happens only in the most intimate settings, and is often associated with sexual activity.

In the therapeutic setting, the practitioner is the giver, and the client is the recipient of touch. The massage professional's business is to provide caring, compassionate touch to the client. Massage therapists practice it every day and are comfortable administering touch as therapy. The client's experience of touch is personal, individual, and dependent on a multitude of factors. The way in which the client perceives and responds to touch not only depends on which techniques are applied but also on who the client is, personal history, and the individual circumstances that the client brings to the table. Perceptions are also influenced by ethnic, cultural, familial, or religious backgrounds, as well as previous experiences involving touch, both good and bad. Every client comes with a personal reason for seeking massage. It is the practitioner's responsibility to be sensitive to the individual client's needs and boundaries.

The touch professional is unique in that the primary means in which services are rendered is through caring touch. The practitioner applies skilled touch to assess and treat the client in exchange for some kind of remuneration. Although there is some verbal communication, usually at the beginning of a therapy session, touch is the primary means of communication between the client's body and the practitioner's hands. The practitioner feels the conditions of the soft tissues of the client and applies appropriate touch to soothe and normalize the tissues. How that touch is perceived depends on the intention of the giver, which body part does the touching, the quality of touch (including pressure and movement), which part of the body is touched or the sequence in which parts of the body are touched, verbal communication that accompanies the touch, previous experience of the recipient with the giver, or similar touch modalities. The client might have different reactions to touch applied to different areas of the body. Some areas of the body, such as the anterior torso or face, are more vulnerable and must be approached with caution and sensitivity. Certain areas can trigger an emotional response because of a previous experience such as trauma, surgery, or abuse. During a full-body massage, the practitioner applies massage to nearly every skin surface of the client's body, except the genitals and other sensitive areas. This gives the client the opportunity to literally get in touch with or become conscious of the entire body.

Generally, reactions to therapeutically applied touch are positive unless the touch is perceived as threatening or is more intimate than expected. Physical and sexual abuse is common in our society. People who have been victims of abuse at one extreme perceive a touch as threatening or, on the other hand, might have great difficulty setting appropriate boundaries. Some types of therapeutic touch can be perceived as invasive, like the touch experienced in some medical procedures or settings.

Touch can be classified as hostile, aggressive, casual, pleasurable, sensual, erotic, and therapeutic. Touch is considered hostile or aggressive when it is applied to do harm to or dominate the receiver. That is not appropriate in the therapeutic setting. If a practitioner harbors any ill will toward or is angry or upset with a client, it is wise to refer that client to another practitioner or at least postpone any therapy session until the difficulties are resolved. Even though the practitioner does not employ any aggressive or harmful manipulations, the intention with which touch is applied might carry elements of the hostility.

Professional massage does not include touch that is intentionally sexual or erotic, although sometimes a client might perceive touch to be erotic that is not applied with that intention. Clients might bring sexual issues into the session in the way of a history of abuse, a sexual disorder, or poor sexual boundaries. The client might project sexual issues onto the therapist, or the practitioner might have sexual feelings toward the client. Sexual feelings are normal, healthy, and pleasurable. In a therapeutic relationship, however, acting out those feelings is always inappropriate and detrimental to the relationship. Sexual intimacy, including seductive behavior or language, is never appropriate in a therapeutic relationship. In a therapeutic setting, touching the genitals, erotic touch, or touch with the intention of sexual arousal is never appropriate. Touch is never used with the intent of sexually stimulating a client. As a practitioner, you are responsible to maintain clear sexual boundaries regarding your own actions and to monitor and prohibit any sexual behavior on the part of the client.

Clear communication with a client, stating how, where, and which forms of touch will be used, informing the client of any changes in the treatment plan, and getting consent from the client help to create a safe environment. Always impress on clients that there is always the option to say no to any portion of the session.

Touch and Arousal: The Sexual Response

Massage is a sensual experience. A possible effect of touch during the massage session is sexual arousal. Sexual arousal is a natural physiologic and cognitive response to a stimulation that is perceived as erotic by the body. Sexual arousal does not necessarily correspond to sexual desire or attraction. It is not usually an overt sign or a request to respond sexually to the arousal.

Conditions that can initiate sexual arousal vary. It is possible that the only previous touch experiences of the client have been sexual. The type of touch, the position of the client, the degree of undress, or the way in which draping is done can play a role. The same nerve plexus that controls the genitals also serves the lower abdomen, buttocks, and thighs. Slow, rhythmic massage of those areas can initiate an arousal response.

Sexual arousal is quite obvious in men in the form of a penile erection. Arousal is more difficult to recognize in women. Proper draping conceals most signs of a woman's arousal. Visual signs include a slight flushing in the face or fidgeting. During a massage, a spontaneous erection or arousal might become uncomfortable or even fearful for the practitioner, the client, or both.

The appropriate response to sexual arousal depends on the circumstance. If there is apparent discomfort or embarrassment on the part of the client or practitioner, take immediate steps to defuse the situation. If the practitioner has been massaging an area adjacent to the genitals, usually discontinuing the massage, re-draping the area, and moving to a less vulnerable and sensitive area of the body remedies the situation. Usually sexual arousal passes quickly when the initiating stimulus is removed. The practitioner can open a dialogue with the client acknowledging the reaction. Reassure the client that it can be a natural response to touch stimulation and give the client the opportunity to respond. It might be helpful to simply have the client turn face down and continue the massage. If there are no other signs of discomfort by either party, the session can continue and the arousal might simply dissipate.

It is the practitioner's responsibility to act in a nonsexual manner, clarify to the client that there is no sexual intent or involvement in the relationship, and maintain appropriate boundaries.

In the case that the client indicates—verbally or nonverbally—persistent sexual intent, it is the practitioner's responsibility to stop the session and reestablish clear professional boundaries, wherein sexual activity is not part of the relationship. If the client agrees, the session can continue if the practitioner feels comfortable enough to resume. If the client persists with any sort of sexual intent, the session is terminated. The practitioner can state, "I no longer feel comfortable with this massage, and the session is now over." At this point, the practitioner tells the client to get dressed and leaves the room.

Desexualizing Massage

In today's society, touch is often sexualized. The media predominantly portrays touch as either sexual or violent. Even touch involving massage in the media often has a sexual context. For many years, massage was related to sexual activities in massage parlors. Therapeutic massage has made great strides in shedding the massage parlor persona; nevertheless, there are still those who use massage as a front for erotic and sexual endeavors. The massage profession has worked hard to separate itself from these practices; however, there is still the occasion when a new prospective client calls for an appointment seeking services that include sexual massage. It is usually easy to recognize these callers. Use a simple question such as "What type of massage services are you seeking?" or "What conditions would you like to address during the massage?" Responses to this type of question usually reveal the caller's intentions. If the caller is seeking sexual services, a simple statement such as "I am a health professional and do not provide any kind of sexual services," or "I practice only therapeutic massage and do not engage in sexual practices of any kind" either ends the conversation or clarifies your policy. If and when such people do come in for an appointment, they know what to expect.

Clarity in advertising and communication greatly reduces the incidence of callers wanting illicit or sexual massage. A clear statement of your policies is usually sufficient to deter sexual advances in the office.

Occasionally, a client attempts to sexualize the therapy session. Sexual comments, overt advances, or requests for sexual favors can be prompted by physical attraction, by former experiences, or because sexual abuse has blurred the client's perception of appropriate boundaries. Because such acts can cause confusion, anger, or other emotional response, it is the responsibility of the practitioner not to succumb to the client's suggestive behavior and to redirect the therapeutic process, reestablish boundaries, and educate the client about appropriate behavior and the limits of the relationship. Remind them that professional therapeutic massage does not include any kind of sexual practice or intentional erotic stimulation. The firm statement "I am a professional massage practitioner, and I do not offer any type of sexual activity" might be all that has to be said. If the client persists, the practitioner must end the session and the relationship. The practitioner can state discomfort with the client's comments and intentions and therefore has terminated the session. The practitioner then instructs the client to dress and leave, and then promptly leaves the treatment room. The practitioner should document in the session notes what took place and which actions were taken.

Supervision

When a therapist finds oneself involved in instances of transference, countertransference, or dual relationships, a common and helpful activity to pursue is supervision. Supervision means meeting with a professional or peer group to discuss questionable or uncomfortable situations that can occur during professional interactions. Supervision also helps when dealing with issues of confidentiality, prejudice, guilt, intimacy, sexuality, and with many other difficulties that surface when working with clients. Supervision has been practiced in the mental health professions for decades. It has more recently become an important aspect of the wellness professions, especially for those who practice body therapy.

Supervision can take place with a counselor who is familiar with supervision, the massage profession, and with issues involving transference and countertransference; with a mentor, who is more experienced, who is trusted, and who understands supervision and the pitfalls of transference and countertransference; or with a peer group, made up of other practitioners with similar backgrounds and experiences. Supervision is an opportunity to explore why transference or countertransference happens in certain situations and to gain insight into how to respond to feelings positively when they surface.

Mental health professionals often include supervision as one of many services. Psychotherapists, psychologists, and mental health counselors practice supervision within their professions and might be available as supervisors to other health care providers. A good supervisor is trained in issues of transference and countertransference, is familiar with the massage therapy profession, and is an invaluable model and support in helping to establish and maintain healthy personal and professional boundaries.

Massage practitioners new to the profession often find a more experienced therapist who becomes a mentor. A mentor can be very helpful, providing insight into many aspects of developing a successful massage business or practice. A trusted mentor can also be a great asset in handling difficult clients, with special circumstances, or with issues of transference and countertransference.

Supervision in a peer group is done with a small group of practitioners and offers the possibility of sharing stories and scenarios with colleagues who might have similar experiences and have ideas on how to work with difficult situations. It offers a chance to explore problematic situations in a supportive atmosphere. Supervision through a small group of practitioners who practice similar styles of therapy creates a support system in which one can learn from another's experience and, in doing so, not feel as isolated and alone when handling difficult situations.

Peer group supervision consists of several people practicing similar forms of therapy who agree to meet regularly and consistently, using an agreed-on format in an atmosphere of honesty, warmth, respect, openness, and confidentiality. Some advantages of peer supervision are that it offers multiple perspectives on any situation, decreases professional isolation while increasing professional support and networking opportunities, and is generally free.

A professional clinical supervisor initially might help to start the peer group and establish a format to examine issues. After that, the supervisor might be called in to rejoin the group occasionally to delve more deeply into issues or concerns of the group.

Regular supervision offers a way to improve therapeutic relationships with clients. Seeking supervision is not looking for someone to tell the practitioner what to do. A good supervisor points out strong points and helps to shore up mistakes or pitfalls that a practitioner might stumble into when handling issues of transference and countertransference in the practice of massage therapy. Rather than dictate which action a practitioner should take, a good supervisor helps the practitioner to explore the internal underlying issues related to the problem; defines appropriate boundaries related to the client and practitioner, and helps to devise appropriate actions to maintain healthy therapeutic relationships (see Box 3.2).

Box 3.2

Reasons for Supervision

Some reasons to seek supervision include the following:

- You have a client or clients who are difficult or controlling.
- Difficult or confusing situations arise in your practice.
- Clients challenge professional or personal boundaries.
- You experience feelings of exhaustion or burnout at the end of a session or day.
- You sense disappointment, depression, agitation, or ill will related to a client.
- You are working with clients who have been sexually or physically abused.
- You stretched or crossed a professional boundary with a client.
- You are attracted to a client or a client is attracted to you.
- Sexual or romantic feelings enter into a therapeutic relationship.
- You have strong feelings toward a client, either positive or negative.
- You have feelings for a client that alter the way in which you work with that client.
- You have feelings of infatuation, intimidation, powerlessness, anger, or frustration toward any client.
- You change your regular care protocol for a particular client.
- You have feelings for any client that come up outside of the therapy session.

A practitioner who uses supervision must have permission from the client to specifically discuss the client's case with a supervisor, or the practitioner must not identify the client specifically when discussing issues relating to that person. Supervisors are sworn to the same or even more rigid rules of confidentiality as are practitioners.

When working with clients who have been sexually abused or are mentally ill (e.g., depressed, bipolar, or schizophrenic), supervision with someone familiar with these conditions is invaluable to help the practitioner to understand possible reactions these clients might have to bodywork.

Supervision should offer a trusted, shame-free environment in which to sort out emotional or boundary issues that arise in the professional arena. Proper supervision is self-care for the practitioner.

ETHICAL BUSINESS PRACTICES

Ethics are the basis for standards of acceptable and professional behavior by which a person or business conducts business. The following are ethical standards of practice to which you as a massage professional should adhere:

1. Treat all clients with the same fairness, courtesy, respect, and dignity.
2. Provide the highest quality care for those who seek your professional services.
3. Have knowledge of and always stay within the limitations of your scope of practice.
4. Respect and protect client confidentiality. Solicit only that information from the client that is relevant to the therapeutic relationship. Never share a client's name, condition, or any information from conversation or written forms with anyone outside the therapy session without the client's written approval. Obtain a "Release of Medical Information" form, signed and dated by the client, before conferring with any other health care provider for the purpose of aiding the quality of service to the client.
5. Set an example of professionalism by your conduct at all times.
6. Be respectful of the therapeutic relationship, and maintain appropriate boundaries.
7. Be aware of the effects of transference and countertransference and avoid dual relationships that might adversely affect the therapeutic relationship.
8. In no way allow or encourage any kind of sexual activity in your practice. Do not participate in any sexual relationship with a client at any time during the term of the therapeutic relationship.
9. Do not participate in the practice of massage when under the influence of drugs or alcohol.
10. Retain the right to refuse or terminate service to any client who is sexually inappropriate, abusive, or under the influence of drugs or alcohol.
11. Disclose to clients adequate information regarding your qualifications, the massage procedures, and the expected outcome, and obtain an informed consent from the client or an advocate (in the case that the client is under the age of 18 or is not competent) before providing treatment.

Respect the client's right to refuse, terminate, or modify treatment regardless of prior consent.

12. Provide massage services only when there is a reasonable expectation that it will be advantageous to the client.
13. Represent your education, professional affiliations, certifications, and qualifications honestly and provide only those services that you are qualified to perform.
14. Respect and cooperate with other ethical health care providers to promote health and wellness, and refer to appropriate medical personnel when indicated.
15. Maintain accurate and truthful client records and make them available to review with the client.
16. Provide adequate draping procedures so that the client feels safe, secure, comfortable, and warm at all times (Figure 3-2).

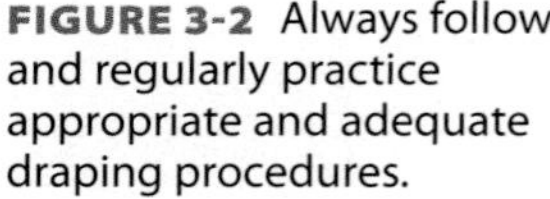

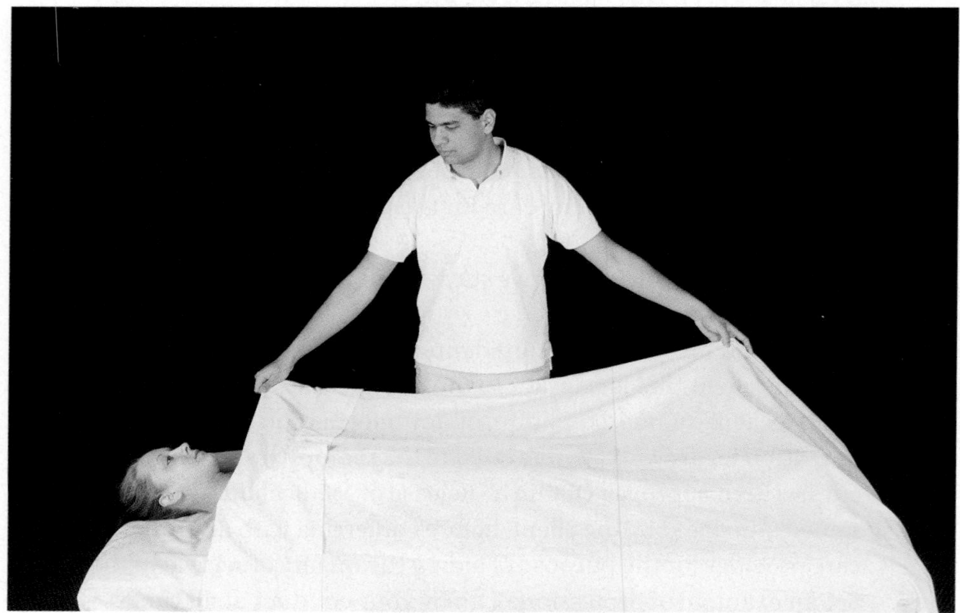

FIGURE 3-2 Always follow and regularly practice appropriate and adequate draping procedures.

17. Provide a safe environment, employ hygienic practices, and use universal precautions.
18. Charge fair prices for all services. Disclose fee schedules and discuss any financial arrangements in advance of the session.
19. Know and obey all laws, rules, and regulations of your city, county, and state pertaining to your work.
20. Strive to improve the credibility of massage as a valuable health service by educating the public and medical community as to its benefits.
21. Be fair and honest in all advertising of services.
22. Communicate professionally on the telephone, in personal conversations, and in letters.
23. Refrain from the use of improper language and any form of gossip.
24. Eliminate prejudice in the profession and do not discriminate against colleagues or clients.

25. Be well organized so that you make the most of your time.
26. Maintain your physical, mental, and emotional well-being so that you are looked on as a credit to your profession. Seek out and use supervision when indicated and appropriate.
27. Dress in a manner that is professional, modest, and clean.
28. Continue to learn about new developments in your profession by participating in local and national professional associations and pursuing continuing education and training.
29. Keep foremost in your mind that you are a professional person engaged in giving an important and beneficial personal service. Operate all aspects of your business with honesty and integrity.
30. Do your utmost to keep your place of business clean, safe, comfortable, and according to all legal requirements.

Remember that people judge you by first impressions (see Box 3.3).

Box 3.3

Personal Hygiene and Health Habits

To inspire confidence and trust in your clients, you should project a well-groomed, professional appearance at all times. In a personal service business, personal health and good grooming are assets that clients admire and are essential for your protection and that of the client.

Your personal health and grooming habits should include the following:

1. Bathe or shower daily and use deodorant as necessary.
2. Keep your teeth and gums healthy. Visit your dentist regularly.
3. Use mouthwash and avoid foods that contribute to offensive breath odor.
4. Keep your hair fresh and clean, and wear an appropriate hairstyle. Hair should be worn in a style that you do not have to touch during a massage session. In addition, your hair must not touch the client during the session.
5. Avoid strong fragrances such as perfumes, colognes, and lotions.
6. Keep your hands free of blemishes and calluses. Use lotion to keep your hands soft and smooth.
7. Keep your nails clean and filed so that they do not extend to the tips of the fingers. Sharp nails should never come in contact with the client's skin. Do not wear nail polish.
8. Wear appropriate makeup in appropriate colors for your skin tone. Be sure makeup is applied neatly.
9. Keep facial hair neat and well groomed. If you prefer the clean-shaven look, be sure to shave as often as necessary.
10. Avoid gum chewing in the presence of clients.
11. Do not smoke before doing massage. The odor that lingers on hands and breath can be offensive to the client.
12. Keep your face clean and free of blemishes.
13. Practice all rules of sanitation for the client's and for your own protection.
14. Have a complete physical examination by a physician before beginning work as a massage practitioner. Continue to have checkups, follow your physician's advice, and do all that is possible to maintain optimum health.
15. If you perspire heavily, take precautions so that your perspiration does not drop on your client.
16. Take time for relaxation and physical fitness. Receive massages regularly. A regimen of daily exercise is recommended. This may be accomplished by participation in active sports of your choice (e.g., swimming, tennis), working out at the gym, or by devising a set of beneficial exercises that you can do at home.

Box 3.3 (cont'd)

Personal Hygiene and Health Habits

17. Eat a well-balanced, nutritious diet. Maintain your normal weight for your height and bone structure.
18. Be aware of good posture and proper body mechanics when walking, standing, sitting, and working. Poor posture habits such as slouching contribute to fatigue, foot problems, and strain to your back and neck.
19. Wear the appropriate clothing for your profession. Refrain from low-cut necklines and tight or sexually provocative clothing. Clothing should be loose enough to allow for optimal movement. It should be free of accessories that might catch on the massage table or touch the client when you are performing the massage (e.g., long chains, necklace or tie, a wide belt, or long sleeves). Consider clothing that allows your body heat to escape. Clothing made of natural fibers such as cotton is good. Some synthetic fabrics hold the heat of your body and can be uncomfortable for the physical exertion of this profession.

COMMUNICATION SKILLS

In addition to gaining the necessary technical skills as a professional massage practitioner, you must be able to understand your client's needs. This is the basis of all good human relations. A pleasant voice, good manners, cheerfulness, patience, tact, loyalty, empathy, and interest in the client's welfare are some of the desirable traits that help to build the client's confidence in you and your place of business (Figure 3-3).

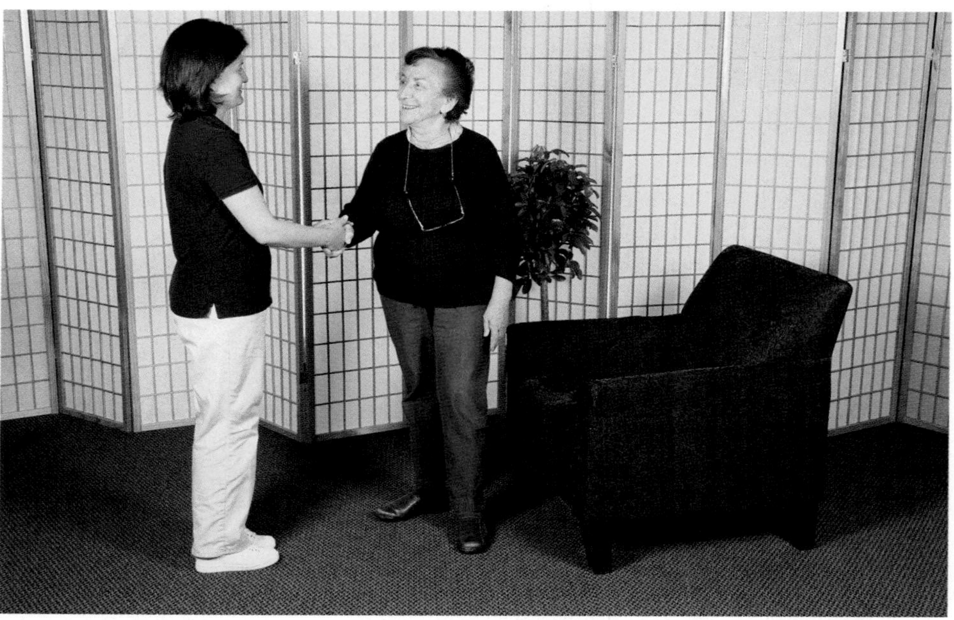

FIGURE 3-3 Communication is the basis of all good human relations.

It is important to be able to interact with people without becoming too familiar. Often, clients will confide personal feelings and trust you not to betray the confidence put in your hands. This is where the art of listening is an invaluable asset. Listen with empathy, tactfully change the subject when necessary, and never betray the client's confidence in you.

The following rules for good human relations will help you interact successfully with people from all walks of life:

Tact: Tact is required with a client who is overly critical, finds fault, and is hard to please. It might be that the client simply wants attention. Tact helps you to deal with this client in an impersonal but understanding manner. To be tactful is to avoid what is offensive or disturbing and to do what is most considerate for all concerned. For example, you might discover that a client needs medical care and you feel you should suggest that he see a physician. You must approach this problem with the utmost tact and diplomacy.

Cheerfulness: A cheerful attitude and a pleasant facial expression go a long way toward putting a client at ease.

Patience: Patience is the ability to be tolerant under stressful or undesirable conditions. Your patience and understanding will be the best medicine when you work with people who are ill, agitated, or in pain. Patience helps you to change negative situations to more positive ones.

Honesty: To be honest does not mean that you must be brutally frank with a client. You can answer questions factually but tactfully. For example, if a client has unrealistic expectations about the benefits of a treatment, you can discuss what can or cannot be accomplished in a sincerely but conscientiously.

Intuition: Intuition is your ability to have insight into people's feelings. When you genuinely like people, it is easier to show sympathy and understanding for their problems. People often confide in you when their intuition tells them you are trustworthy. In turn, your own intuition will help you to avoid embarrassing situations and involving yourself in problems that you cannot solve. Remember, one of the primary reasons why your clients come to you is for relaxation. Keep conversations to a minimum to allow the client's maximum relaxation.

Sense of humor: It is important to have a sense of humor, especially when dealing with difficult people or situations. A good sense of humor helps you to remain optimistic, courteous, and in control.

Maturity: Maturity is not so much a matter of how old you are, but what you have gained from your life experience. Maturity is the quality of being reliable, responsible, self-disciplined, and well adjusted.

Self-esteem: Self-esteem is projected by your attitudes about yourself and your profession. If you respect yourself and your profession, you will be respected by others.

Self-motivation: Self-motivation is your ability to set positive goals and put forth the energy and effort required to achieve those goals. It means making sacrifices when necessary to save time and money and to achieve your goals.

BUILDING A PROFESSIONAL IMAGE

If you want to be successful in business, you must prepare for success. Preparation, planning, and performance are the assets that help you to do your job in the most professional manner. You should take every opportunity to pursue new avenues of knowledge. Attend professional seminars, read trade journals and other publications relating to your business, and become active in associations where you can exchange ideas with other dedicated people.

Your business image is important and should be built on good service and truth in advertising. A reliable reputation is particularly important in the personal service business because you are dealing with the health and well-being of people. Consistently high standards and good service are the foundations on which successful businesses are built. (Refer to Chapter 22 Business Practices, for more ideas on massage business management.)

YOUR BUSINESS NAME

Using appropriate wording in your business name in advertising helps you to establish a good reputation. You can see how the name "Smitty's Massage Parlour" or "Smith Massage Clinic" can totally change how your business is perceived by potential clients.

Some massage professionals, especially those entering a new community, might think that advertising should state that only therapeutic and nonsexual massage is given. Keeping regular business hours, rather than late-night hours, also stresses your professional reputation.

Another point to remember is that using proper draping techniques to ensure your client's privacy is very important in building a good reputation. Word of mouth is the massage professional's best advertising. Satisfied clients will spread the message that you work in a professional manner.

QUESTIONS FOR DISCUSSION AND REVIEW

1. Why is it important to have a code of ethics for your business?
2. Why is a satisfied client your best means of advertising?
3. Why do successful business managers prefer employees who are concerned with personal and professional ethics?
4. What is the connection between boundaries and ethics?
5. Differentiate between personal and professional boundaries.
6. What are major areas to consider when establishing professional boundaries?
7. Who does the power differential favor in the therapeutic relationship?
8. What is the effect of a boundary's being crossed?
9. What can a practitioner do to reduce the risk of crossing a client's boundary?
10. Define transference and countertransference.
11. Whose responsibility is it to manage boundary issues and instances of transference or countertransference?
12. What constitutes a dual relationship in a therapeutic setting?
13. How should a practitioner respond if a client becomes sexually aroused?
14. What is supervision?
15. Why is it necessary for the massage practitioner to have strict personal hygiene and health habits?
16. What is meant by professional projection in attitude and appearance?

17. How do you define human relations as applied to working with or serving others?
18. Why is the practice of human relations so important to the massage practitioner?
19. When building your business (practice) image, how can you be sure that the public gets the right message?

PART 2

HUMAN ANATOMY AND PHYSIOLOGY

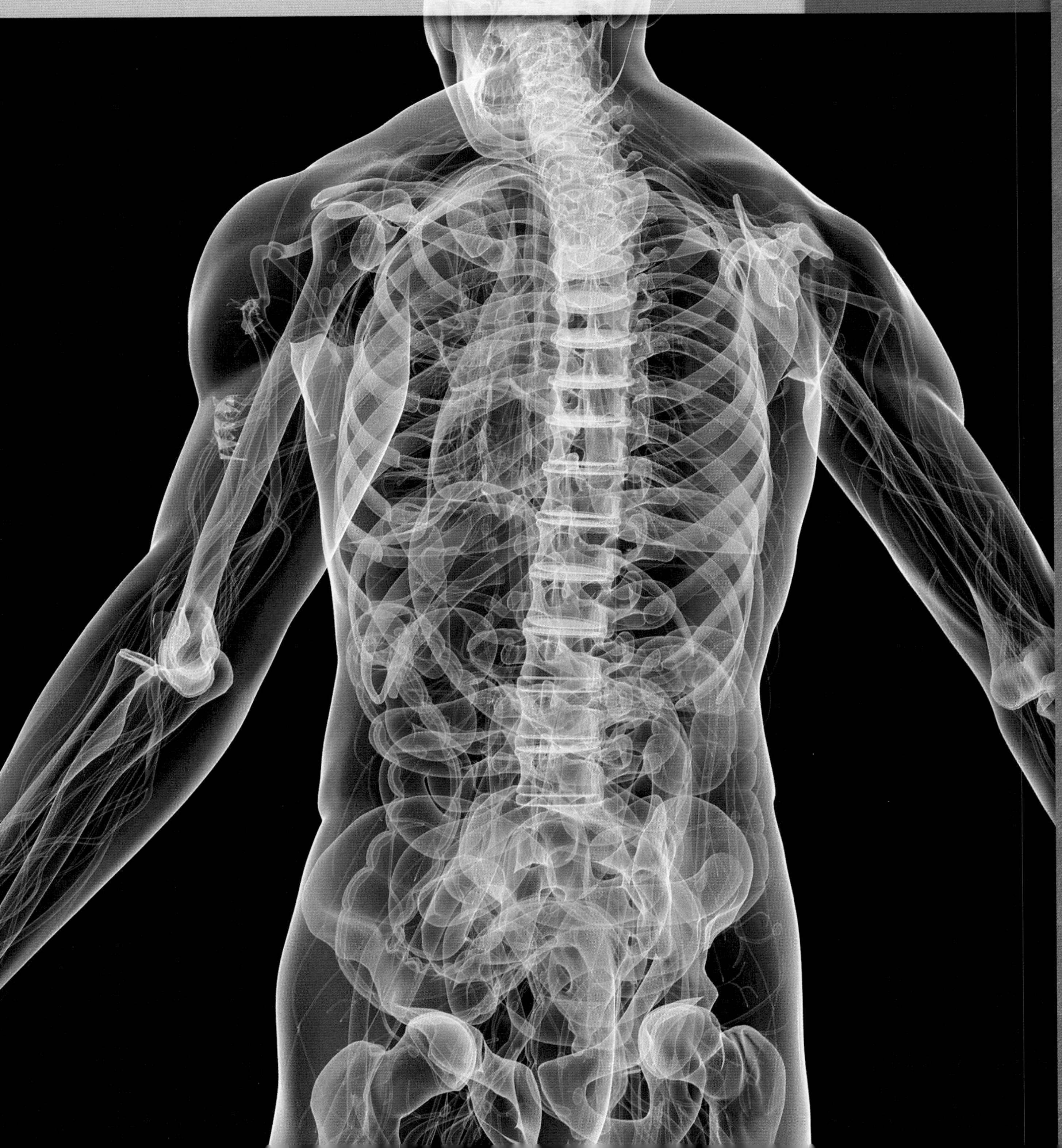

CHAPTER 4

Overview

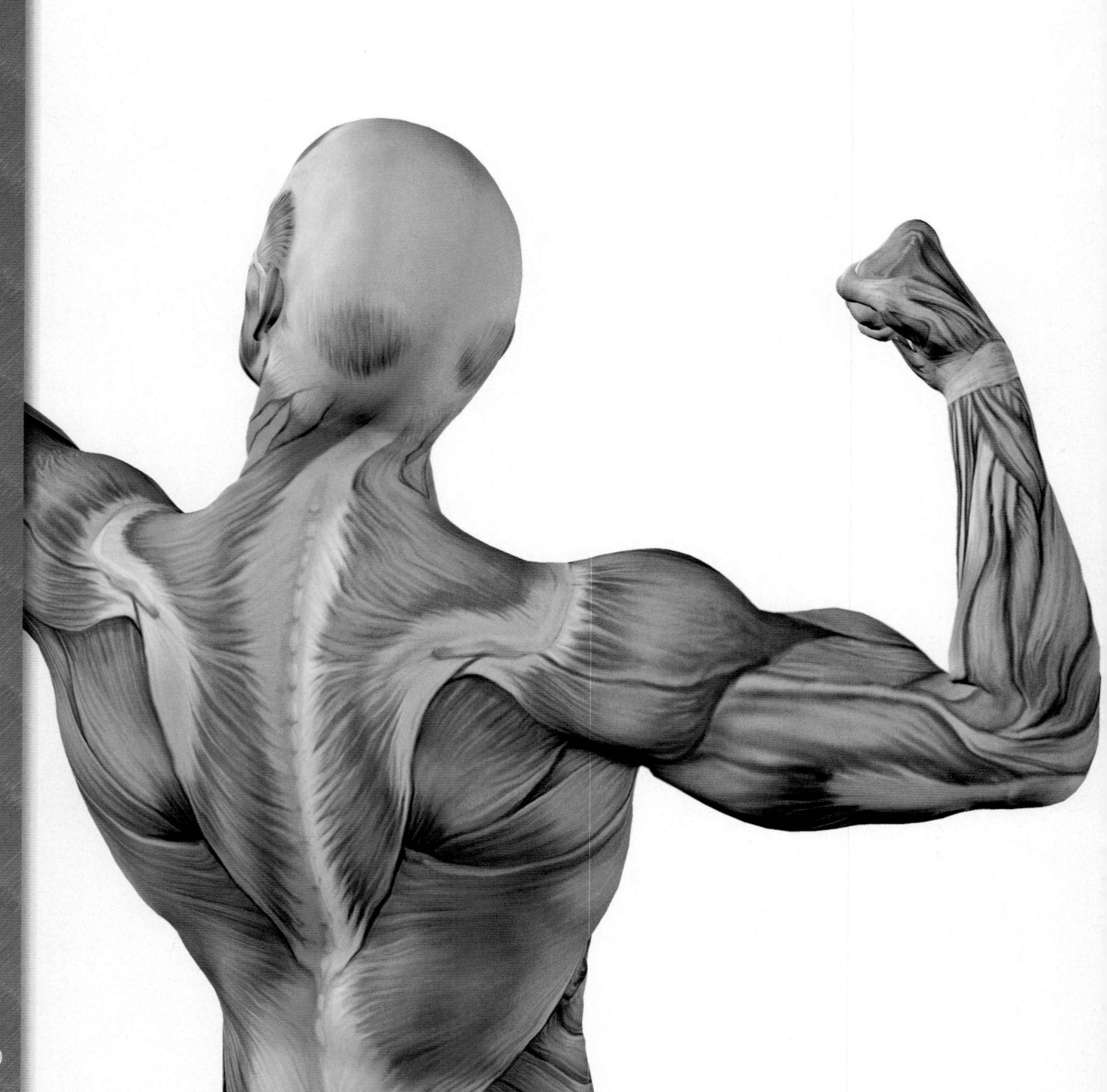

LEARNING OBJECTIVES

After you have mastered this chapter, you will be able to

1. **Explain the meanings of the important terms in boldface listed in this chapter.**
2. **Explain why a massage therapist should have a good understanding of anatomy, physiology, and pathology.**
3. **Explain the physiologic and psychological effects of stress and pain and the role of massage therapy in the management of stress and pain.**
4. **Describe the healing functions of the body in terms of inflammation and tissue repair.**
5. **Describe the wellness model and how massage can be a part of that model.**
6. **Be able to derive the meaning of medical terms by breaking the terms into their parts and defining those parts.**

INTRODUCTION

A basic knowledge of **anatomy, physiology, kinesiology,** and **pathology** is necessary in mastering the theory and practice of therapeutic massage. The massage practitioner should study the structures and functions of the human body to know when, where, and how to apply massage movements for the most beneficial results. This knowledge enables the practitioner to adjust the massage treatment to the needs of the individual client and to anticipate results.

anatomy

is the study of the gross structure of the body and the interrelations of its parts.

physiology

is the science and study of the vital processes, mechanisms, and functions of an organ or system.

kinesiology

is the scientific study of muscular activity and the anatomy, physiology, and mechanics of body movement.

pathology

is the study of the structural and functional changes caused by disease.

DEFINITION OF ANATOMY AND PHYSIOLOGY

Anatomy is the science of structure of an organism or body. *Physiology* concerns the normal functions performed by the various systems of the body. Anatomy and physiology are interrelated in that the structures are associated with their functions. Structure and function depend on the interaction of the organism's parts, and each part has a role in the operation of the whole.

Anatomy (uh-**NAT**-o-mee) is defined as the study of the gross structure of the body or the study of an organism and the interrelations of its parts. For example, when describing the skeleton or other anatomic parts of the body, naming the parts and how they relate to one another, we are describing anatomy.

Physiology (fiz-ee-**AH**-lo-jee) is the science and study of the vital processes, mechanisms, and functions of an organ, system of organs, or the entire organism. When we describe how the organs or parts of the body function and how their functions relate to one another, we are speaking about physiology.

Kinesiology (kin-ee-see-**AH**-lo-jee) is the scientific study of muscular activity and the anatomy, physiology, and mechanics of body movement. It is the functional study of the interaction of the bones, joints and muscles.

Pathology (pa-**THAL**-o-jee) is the study of the structural and functional changes caused by disease. Anatomy, physiology, and kinesiology provide an understanding of how the healthy body works. Pathology examines what happens when the body or body part is in a state of dysfunction or disease.

RELATIONSHIP OF ANATOMY AND PHYSIOLOGY TO MASSAGE AND BODYWORK

Therapeutic massage is applied to and directly affects the structures and the functions of the human organism. It has direct effects such as increased local circulation of venous (**VEE**-nuhs) blood and lymph (**LIMF**), stretching of muscle tissue, and loosening of adhesions and scar tissue. Massage has indirect effects of increased circulation to the muscles and internal organs, reduced blood pressure, and general relaxation of tense muscles. Massage also has reflex effects, such as reduced heart rate and slower, deeper breathing.

An important purpose of massage and bodywork is to promote functional improvement in the recipient's body. The more understanding that therapists have of the human body and how it functions, the better they can direct their treatment to produce desired effects. A working knowledge of anatomy, physiology, kinesiology, and pathology gives therapists a basis on which they can plan effective treatments and discuss those applications with other health care professionals. As the popularity of massage increases and research continues to verify the positive benefits of massage, more people are using massage for the relief of discomfort or as a part of an integrated health plan. Many of these clients have conditions that preclude massage or at least would influence the decision of what and how massage is applied for the maximal benefit and minimal risk. A basic knowledge of pathology provides massage therapists with an understanding of disease processes so that they can make decisions as to which massage services they can safely provide or refer clients to appropriate medical professionals. Through clear understanding of kinesiology and the structures involved in body movement, the massage therapist can better identify which specific structures are involved in the areas of pain or dysfunction when working with clients. As therapists continue to develop therapeutic skills by learning more effective methods of bodywork, a thorough knowledge and understanding of anatomy, physiology, kinesiology, and pathology become essential.

The study of these sciences helps the therapist to understand more of how the body functions; however, it is important to remember that a person's body functions as an integrated organism. When studying these subjects, the student has the opportunity to closely examine various aspects of the structure and function of the body's systems and parts. This is helpful to begin to understand the body, but these systems all working together are what determines the well-being of the individual person.

PHYSIOLOGIC CHANGES DURING DISEASE

Physiologically, the body strives to maintain the delicate balance in its internal environment. Changes in the stresses posed by the external environment constantly force the body to compensate to maintain that delicate internal balance called **homeostasis** (ho-mee-o-**STAY**-sis). When the body's homeostasis is disturbed, the person can experience symptoms of disease.

homeostasis

is the internal balance of the body.

Signs and Symptoms of Disease

Disease is an abnormal and unhealthy state of all or part of the body wherein it is incapable of carrying on its normal function. Diseases generally have **symptoms** and **signs**. A *symptom* is caused by the disease and is perceived by the subject, such as dizziness, chills, nausea, or pain. A symptom is a clear message to the organism that something is wrong. Signs of a disease are observable indications such as abnormal pulse rate, fever, abnormal skin color, or physical irregularities. When signs and symptoms of disease appear, it is advisable to seek help from proper medical authorities. A therapist can recognize some signs or symptoms when a client comes for a session, but it is beyond their scope of practice to diagnose the condition, and they should refer the client to the appropriate medical professional. Symptoms and signs, along with medical examinations, medical histories, and laboratory tests, are the bases for proper diagnosis and treatment of most disease conditions.

disease

is an abnormal and unhealthy state of all or part of the body wherein it is incapable of carrying on its normal function.

symptom

is subjective evidence of disease or bodily disorder.

sign (of disease)

is an observable indication of disease or bodily disorder.

There are many possible direct causes for disease, including disease-producing organisms, trauma, environmental agents, malnutrition, degenerative processes, and stress. Other conditions that can be predisposing factors include age, working or living conditions, gender, and heredity.

Stress

Stress is any psychological or physical situation or condition that causes tension or strain. Stress can be any element or situation that requires our body or mind to compensate to maintain the body's delicate internal balance and harmony. Stress can affect individual persons differently. What is extremely stressful to one person might not affect another at all. If too many stressful conditions occur without an effective method to manage or cope with them, however, the health of the person suffers. Regardless of the source or nature of the stress, the physiologic reaction of the body is essentially the same.

stress

is any psychological or physical situation or condition that causes tension or strain.

Stress is most notably associated with the **adrenal glands** and their secretion of the "fight-or-flight" hormones. The principal and most understood adrenal hormones are *adrenaline* (uh-**DREN**-uh-lin) and *cortisol* (**KAUR**-ti-zol). When we encounter high levels of stress, the adrenal secretions give us a physical and mental boost that heightens our senses, sharpens our reflexes, and prepares our muscles for maximum exertion. The adrenal glands by no means work alone, however. In conjunction with the *pituitary* (pi-**TOO**-i-tar-ee) and the *hypothalamus* (high-po-**THAL**-uh-muhs), they affect the function of most of the internal systems. Muscle tone increases, blood pressure rises, and breathing deepens. Blood is directed toward the skeletal muscles and nervous system and away from the digestive organs; in fact, digestion virtually stops. Glycogen, glucose, and oxygen-carrying red blood cells are mobilized. Blood-coagulating chemicals are added to the blood, and the kidneys retain fluids in case of injury and bleeding. Cortisol promotes the breakdown of the body's proteins to form glucose, which is a quick energy source and acts as an anti-inflammatory and antiallergenic.

adrenal glands

situated on the top of each kidney, produce epinephrine, norepinephrine, and corticosteroids.

These biochemical effects are essential in emergency, fight-or-flight situations; however, if the dosage of these hormones is sustained over a long period, as it would be with long-term stress, the consequences can be devastating. The ongoing anti-inflammatory effect of cortisol, for example, would inhibit the natural inflammatory response to injury. The body's healing process of flooding the injured area with wound-healing leukocytes, nutrients, fibroblasts, and oxygen would be interfered with, and eventually the body's ability to resist infection of all kinds is decreased. Continued secretion of adrenaline would eventually exhaust not only the adrenal glands but, because of its effect on the sympathetic nervous system, would have the same effect on the organs as severe loss of sleep—exhaustion! Other effects of sustained levels of these hormones include gastric ulcers, high blood pressure, depressed immune system function, **atherosclerosis** (ath-eer-o-skler-**O**-sis), and finally, death.

atherosclerosis

is characterized by an accumulation of fatty deposits on the inner walls of the arteries.

Stress in and of itself is not the problem. Life is inherently stressful. When effectively worked with, stress tends to strengthen our physical, mental, and emotional resolve. When we load ourselves with unrelenting, inescapable, and overburdening stress, however, it becomes unhealthy and even deadly.

Pain

pain

is the result of stimulation of specialized nerve endings called nociceptors. It has a primarily protective function in that it warns of tissue damage or destruction somewhere in the body.

Pain is one of the body's primary sensations, along with touch, pressure, heat, and cold. Its function is primarily protective in that it warns of tissue damage or destruction somewhere in the body. Pain is the result of stimulation to specialized nerve endings called nociceptors located near the surface of the body, in the periosteum of the bones, in the arterial and intestinal walls, and, to a lesser extent, in the deeper organs, muscles, and viscera (**VIS**-er-uh).

There are two responses to pain: psychological and physical. The physical response to pain is very similar to the body's response to stress. Blood pressure and pulse increase, and blood flow is shifted from the intestines and brain to the muscles as mental alertness intensifies, readying the body for fight or flight. The physical experience of pain also tells the location, intensity, and duration of the affliction.

The person's psychological and emotional reaction to pain varies depending on many factors, such as previous experience with pain, training in coping with pain, anxiety, tension, and fatigue. The fear and anxiety associated with pain can be more debilitating than the actual pain.

Pain-Spasm-Pain Cycle

A painful syndrome of interest to the massage therapist is the *pain-spasm-pain cycle* associated with muscle spasms. The cycle can start with a rather minor injury such as a bruise or muscle strain that in itself has little effect on the function of the organism. The natural reflex reaction to the tissue damage and pain is a contraction of the muscles that surround the injury, which acts to support and protect the damaged tissue. The contracted muscles constrict the blood vessels and capillaries in the muscles, inhibiting blood flow to the area (a condition known as **ischemia** [is-**KEE**-mee-uh]). At the same time,

ischemia

is localized tissue anemia caused by obstruction of the inflow of blood.

the metabolic activity of the contracting muscles increases, consuming more energy. Oxygen and nutrients are burned, producing increased amounts of metabolic waste. The available oxygen is quickly burned, and the amounts of lactic acid and other toxins collect in the tissues. Soon, *ischemic pain* appears, which is often more intense than the pain from the original injury. The reflex reaction to the ischemic pain is identical to the response to the original injury. Pain causes muscle contraction and ischemia, thereby causing a spasm that causes more pain. It is easy to see how this can become a vicious cycle that can perpetuate itself and continue long after the original injury heals.

THE ROLE OF THERAPEUTIC MASSAGE IN STRESS, PAIN, AND THE PAIN-SPASM-PAIN CYCLE

Therapeutic massage combines the power of sensitive touch with the knowledge of anatomy, physiology, and kinesiology to become a valuable tool in relieving the psychological and physical suffering of stress and pain. Skillfully applied massage provides pleasurable stimulation that is carried to the brain on thicker, faster, more numerous nerve fibers that actually override or drown out the pain signals. Even though the diversion is temporary, it gives the person a chance to relax and disassociate from the noxious stimulus, possibly long enough to shut down the fight-or-flight reaction. Psychologically, the reassuring touch of the therapist helps to relieve anxiety and fear. The person in many cases is able to regain some sense of control over the situation. Physically, as soothing, pleasant sensations flood the brain, adrenal secretions subside, breathing slows and deepens, blood pressure lowers, pulse rate slows, and the body relaxes and begins to recuperate.

In the case of the pain-spasm-pain cycle, in which pain is intensified because of ischemia, skillfully applied massage therapy is very effective in breaking the cycle, relieving the pain, and restoring mobility. Sensitive touch can divert some attention away from the acute intensity of the pain. By gentle palpation, the actual source of the pain can be isolated and differentiated from the contracted and ischemic areas around it. By massaging the contracted ischemic tissues, chronic spasms can be relieved and circulation restored. As oxygen and nutrients flood the area, and lactic acid and other irritants are removed, the pain disappears and mobility is restored.

Even though massage is an effective tool in controlling pain, remember that pain is an indication of tissue damage or nerve irritation. Generally, the more severe the pain, the more severe the tissue damage. Acute or severe pain is a warning that something is physically wrong and should be checked by a physician. If massage is used as an aid for controlling pain, the attending physician should be advised. If massage increases the overall level of pain, it should be discontinued. Please note that some massage techniques can be uncomfortable as they are being applied; however, the discomfort should not be so intense that it hurts the client or lingers beyond the direct application of the manipulation.

HEALING MECHANISMS OF THE BODY

Infection

bacteria

are minute, unicellular organisms exhibiting both plant and animal characteristics and are classified as either harmless or harmful.

virus

is any class of submicroscopic pathogenic agents that transmit disease.

fungus

(pl. *fungi*) is a diverse group of organisms potentially capable of causing disease that thrive or grow in wet or damp areas and live by absorbing nutrients from organic matter.

parasite

is an organism that can potentially cause disease that exists and functions at the expense of a host organism without contributing to the survival of the host.

local infection

is invading organisms confined to a small area of the body.

systemic infection

is invading organisms that have spread throughout the body.

inflammation

is a protective tissue response characterized by swelling, redness, heat, and pain.

fever

is an elevated body temperature.

The most common cause of disease in humans is the invasion of the body by disease-producing *microorganisms* such as **bacteria, viruses, fungi,** or **parasites.** If microorganisms enter the body in sufficient numbers to multiply and become harmful and are capable of destroying healthy tissue, the body reacts by developing an infection. If the invading organisms are confined to a small area, the condition is considered a **local infection.** If, however, the organisms spread throughout the body, the condition is termed a **systemic infection.**

Massage should not be applied in cases of systemic infection or to the site of local infection.

Inflammation

If invading microorganisms cause any destruction of tissue, inflammation occurs. Inflammation also results from physical injury such as a sprain or blow; excessive heat, cold, or radiation; or physical irritants such as splinters, stings, and chemical exposure in which tissue is damaged.

When tissue is damaged, substances are released that cause dramatic secondary reactions that are collectively called **inflammation**. Inflammation is a protective tissue response that is characterized by swelling, redness, heat, and pain. Blood vessels in the area of the damaged tissues dilate, increasing blood flow to the area and causing redness and heat. Capillary walls become more permeable, allowing large quantities of blood plasma and white blood cells to enter the tissue spaces, resulting in swelling. The swelling puts pressure on local nerve endings, causing pain. Increased numbers of white blood cells, called *leukocytes* and *phagocytes*, flood the area to engulf and digest the invading organisms and the damaged tissue debris (*phagocytosis*).

Sometimes, toxic bacteria or the reaction between the invading organisms and the white blood cells releases a substance into the bloodstream that affects the body's heat-regulating system. The resulting elevated body temperature is called a **fever**. Fever is a warning sign that usually accompanies infectious diseases or infected burns and cuts. In cases of sudden-onset or high fever (>102° F), a physician should be consulted. In some ways, fever, if it is not extremely high, is a natural protective device. Fever increases the metabolic rate and the production of the immune substances that battle the invading organisms. The increased temperature itself destroys certain organisms. At the same time, the discomfort and weakness that accompany fever causes the patient to rest, thereby conserving energy to battle the infection. Prolonged fever causes dehydration, and therefore fluids must be replaced. Extreme or prolonged fever can be dangerous or even fatal. Fevers >106° to 108° F can cause damage to the tissues of the kidneys, liver, or other organs or can cause irreparable brain damage, possibly resulting in death.

Massage of inflamed tissue or while fever is present is contraindicated.

Tissue Repair

The degree of tissue repair varies depending on the location and type of tissue and the nature of the damage or injury. Skin and surface tissues undergo a great deal of wear and tear and are easily and quickly repaired. Bone and ligaments repair much more slowly and can require immobilization. Muscle and tendons repair with noticeable scarring and weakness. Neurons of the central nervous system that are injured by trauma or infection repair very slowly or not at all.

Injury or wound healing and repair take place only when infection-causing pathogens have been destroyed. Escaping fluid from the damaged tissues and capillaries fill the wound and coagulate, forming a clot to seal the wound. Connective tissue cells called *fibroblasts* migrate to the area and produce connective tissue fibers that begin to span the wound, providing a structure for regenerating vascular and epithelial tissue. When the wound is healed, this formation of fibrous connective tissue is called **scar tissue.** If the wound is small, the damage is completely and quickly restored to normal. If the wound is large, however, measures must be taken to bring the wound surfaces close together to prevent the formation of excessive scar tissue.

scar

a dense fibrous tissue that forms as an injury, wound, burn, or sore heals.

Properly applied tissue stretching and friction massage will minimize the formation of scar tissue and adhesions resulting from tissue trauma.

THE WELLNESS MODEL

Wellness is a concept in which people take personal responsibility for their own state of health. It is a preventive plan wherein a person makes an effort to recognize conditions, situations, and practices that can be threatening or detrimental to health and takes steps to change or eliminate them to live a more healthful life. Wellness involves taking a personal and active role in being healthy, and adopting practices that enhance health such as a low-fat, high-fiber diet, exercise, a balance between work and play, and a positive mental and spiritual attitude. Wellness also means reducing health risks and eliminating practices that add stressful dangers to our lifestyles.

wellness

is a concept where people take personal responsibility for their own physical, emotional, mental and spiritual state of health.

Wellness takes into consideration more than the state of physical health. Wellness is often represented as an equilateral triangle with the sides depicting body, mind, and spirit or physical, psychological/mental, and attitude/emotional. When all three aspects are healthy and in balance, optimal wellness is experienced. A wellness-oriented person strives to attain a healthy balance among these three (Figure 4-1).

Health might be gauged on a scale that ranges from –5 to 0 to 5. Minus five equates with severe illness combined with a poor attitude. Zero is okay (that is, there is no perceivable sickness). Five equates with optimal health and vitality. Most of our society hovers between –3 and 2. A wellness-oriented person would strive to maintain a health rating >3 on the scale (Figure 4-2).

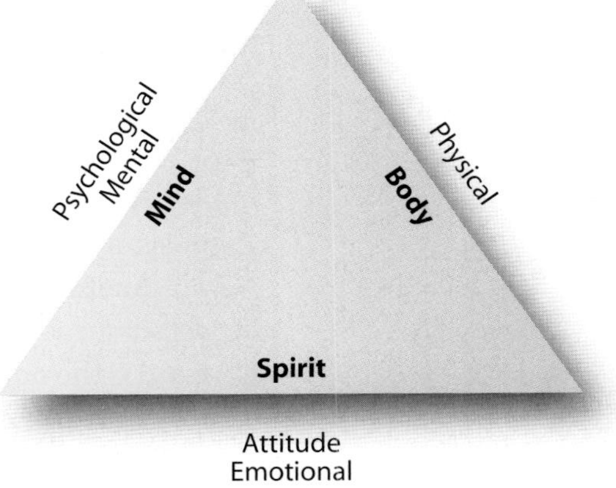

FIGURE 4-1 Wellness model.

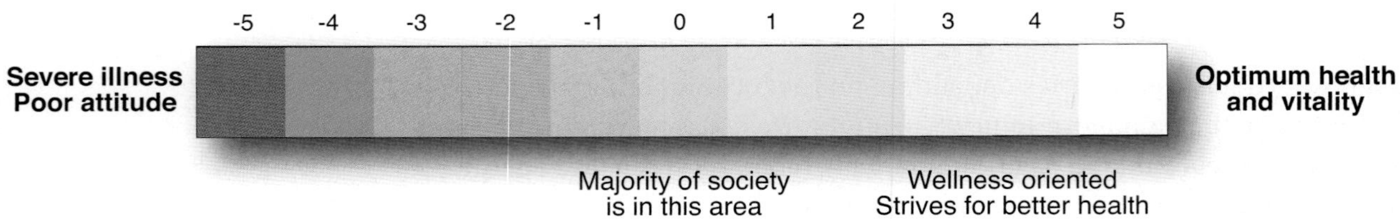

FIGURE 4-2 Scale of health.

MEDICAL AND ANATOMIC TERMINOLOGY

Any profession or trade uses a language or vocabulary that is specific or peculiar to the practices, equipment, and processes of that system. The field of massage and bodywork is no different. Most of the terminology related to massage is derived from the health care and medical field.

Anatomic and medical terminology refers to the vocabulary or jargon commonly used by health professionals when communicating to one another concerning conditions of patients, descriptions of procedures, and anatomic structures. Massage therapists must have an understanding of the body's structure and function, and therefore, becoming familiar with the related terminology is essential. By having an understanding of how medical terms are constructed, the massage therapist will be less intimidated by the long words, be better able to communicate with other health care professionals, and (by speaking their language) be better respected and accepted by the medical community.

The history of medical terminology goes back nearly 2,000 years, to the time when Western civilization first began systematically studying the human body. Because the languages of these first researchers were Greek and Latin, these became and remain the source languages for medical terminology.

Composition of Medical Terminology

In medical terminology, long words are compound words constructed of root words (or stems), prefixes, and suffixes. There are many terms that are constructed from relatively few word parts.

The *stem*, or *root word*, generally indicates the body part or structure involved. Occasionally, two or more stems are combined to show relation or position (e.g., cardiopulmonary pertaining to heart and lung). When stems are combined, a single-letter syllable is often used to create what is called a combining form. This is a word root plus a vowel that is used with another word root to form a compound word. A combining form is usually an "o" or an "i."

A *prefix* is one or more syllables added in front of the stem to further its meaning. A *suffix* likewise is added to the end of the word. Suffixes often denote a diagnosis, symptom, or surgical procedure or identify a word as a noun or adjective.

Anatomic terms often include more than one word. Generally, the first word acts as an adjective and indicates the region or location of the structure. The second word is the noun and names the structure (e.g., femoral artery, thoracic duct).

By breaking the terms into their parts, one can derive the logical meaning. Table 4.1 provides a list of prefixes, suffixes, and stem words and their meanings. As you study the following chapters, be aware of anatomic and medical terms and decipher their meanings by examining the parts. During discussions with peers and other health care practitioners, use proper terminology and make note of unfamiliar terms. Examine them and determine their meaning by breaking them apart and defining their parts. Practice and become familiar with the language. When in doubt, always keep a medical dictionary available. When an unfamiliar term is used, check the dictionary.

TABLE 4.1.

ALPHABETICAL LISTING OF COMMON WORD ELEMENTS USED TO CONSTRUCT MEDICAL TERMS

PREFIXES			PREFIXES, cont'd		
WORD PART	DEFINITION	EXAMPLE	WORD PART	DEFINITION	EXAMPLE
a-	absent, without, away from	abacterial	infra-	beneath	infraspinatus
ab-	away from	abduction	inter	between	intercellular
ad-	to, toward	adduction	intra-	inside	intravenous
ambi-	both	ambidextrous	leuk-(o)	white	leukocyte
a-; an-	without	atypical	macr-(o)	large, long	macrophage
anti-	against	antibody, antidote	mal-	abnormal, bad	malpractice
ante-	before	anterior	medi-	middle, midline	medial
auto	self	autoimmune	mega-	large, extreme	megadose
bi-	two	biceps	micr-(o)	small	microscope
bio-	life	biology	mon-(o)	one, single	monolith
carcin-(o)	cancer	carcinogenic	multi-	many, multiple	multiply
circum-	around	circumvent	narc-	stupor, numbness	narcotine
co-	with, together	cooperate	ne-(o)	new	neophyte, neonatal
contra-	against, counter to	contraindicate	necr-(o)	dead	necrosis
de-	down, from	descend	nutri-	nourish	nutrition
di-	two	dissect	para-	next to, resembling, beside	paralysis, paraplegic
dis-	apart, away from	dislocate	path-	pertaining to disease	pathology
dors-	back	dorsal	per-	through	perforate
dys-	abnormal, impaired	dysfunction	peri-	around	periosteum
e-	out, from	emetic	poly-	many, much	polyunsaturated
ect-	outside, without	ectoplasm	post-	after, later in time	posthumous
end-(o)	inside, within	endoderm	pre-, pro-	before in time	previous
epi-	upon, over, in addition	epimysium	pseud-(o)	false	pseudonym
ex-	out of	exit, excrete	quad-	four	quadriplegic
extra-	beyond, outside of, in addition	extracellular	re-	back, again	repeat, review
flex-	bent	flexion	retro-	backward	retrofit
front-	front, forehead	frontalis	semi	half	semicircle
hemi-	half	hemiplegic	sub-	under, below	subscapularis
hetero-	the other	heterosexual	super-	above, in addition	superior
hom-	common, same	homogenous	supra-	over, above, upper	supraspinatus
hydro-	denoting water	hydrotherapy	syn-	together, along with	synergist
hyper-	above, extreme	hypertensive	tri-	three	triceps
hypo-	under, below	hypodermic	trans	across	transcutaneous
in-	within, into, not, negative	internal, inept	uni-	single, one	unilateral

TABLE 4.1, (cont'd)

ALPHABETICAL LISTING OF COMMON WORD ELEMENTS USED TO CONSTRUCT MEDICAL TERMS

SUFFIXES		
WORD PART	DEFINITION	EXAMPLE
-al; -ar	pertaining to an area	femoral, clavicular
-algia	painful condition	neuralgia
-ase	denoting an enzyme	lactase
-cyte	cell	lymphocyte
-desis	a binding	tenodesis
-ectomy	surgical removal of body part	tonsillectomy
-emia	blood condition	anemia
-genic	producing or causing	autogenic
-gram	a record	sonogram
-graph	write, draw, record	electrocardio-graph
-ia	a noun ending of a condition	leukemia
-ic	a noun/adjective ending	pelvic, hypo-dermic
-ism	condition	autism
-ist	one who does	artist, antagonist
-itis	inflammation	arthritis
-meter	a devise for measuring	cytophotometer
-oid	resembling	styloid, lipoid
-ology	study of, science of	biology
-oma	tumor	carcinoma
-osis	abnormal condition	lymphocytosis
-ostomy	forming an opening	colostomy
-otomy	incision, cutting into	lobotomy
-pathic	diseased	psychopathic
-plegia	paralysis	quadriplegia
-phobia	morbid fear of	claustrophobia
-rrhea	profuse flow	dysmenorrhea
-scope	examination instrument	cystoscope
-scopy	a procedure using a scope	cystoscopy
-tomy	surgical procedure	colostomy

COMMON WORD ROOTS OF STEMS

Many root words add an "o" or an "i" at the end when combined with other words.

WORD PART	DEFINITION	EXAMPLE
abdomin	abdomen	abdominal
adren	adrenal	adrenaline
arteri	artery	arteriosclerosis
aur	ear	auricular
arth(ro)	joint	arthritis
brachi	arm	brachialis
bronch	bronchial	bronchitis
cardi	heart	cardiac
cephal	head	brachiocephalic

COMMON WORD ROOTS OF STEMS, cont'd

WORD PART	DEFINITION	EXAMPLE
cerebr(o)	brain	cerebrospinal
cervic	neck	cervix, cervical
chondr(o)	cartilage	osteochondritis
cost	rib	intercostal
crani	skull	cranial
cyst	bladder, cyst	cystoscopy
cyt	cell	leukocyte
dent	teeth	dentin, dental
derm	skin	subdermal
encephal	brain	encephalitis
entero	intestine	enterocolitis
fibr	fiber	fibrositis
gastr(o)	stomach	gastritis
gyn	woman	gynecology
hem	blood	hematoma
hepat	liver	hepatitis
hist	tissue	histology
hydr	water	hydrotherapy
labi	lip	quadratus labii
mamm	breast	mammogram
my(o)	muscle	myology
nephr(o)	kidney	nephritis
neur(o)	nerve	neurology
ocul	eye	ocular
oss, ost(e)	bone	osteoblast
ot	ear	otology
ped	child, foot	pediatric, pedicure
phleb	vein	phlebitis
pneum	lung	pneumonia
pod	foot	podiatrist
psych	mind	psychologist
pulmo	lung	cardiopulmonary
rhin	nose	rhinovirus
therm	heat	thermometer
thorac	chest	thoracic cavity
throm	clot	thrombosis
thyr	thyroid	thyroxine, thyrotropin
toxic	poison	toxicologist
ur	urine	urogenital
uter	uterus	uterine cancer
vas	vessel	vascular
ven	vein	venous
vertebr	spine	vertebral

QUESTIONS FOR DISCUSSION AND REVIEW

1. What is anatomy?
2. What is physiology?
3. What is kinesiology?
4. What is pathology?
5. Define disease.
6. Differentiate between a sign and a symptom of a disease.
7. What is the physiologic reaction to stress?
8. What is the physical reaction of the body to pain?
9. Describe what is meant by the pain-spasm-pain cycle.
10. Describe the role of the massage therapist in breaking the pain-spasm-pain cycle.
11. Explain the difference between infection and inflammation.
12. What are the four principal signs and symptoms of inflammation?
13. What is fever?
14. When does fever become dangerous?
15. How are medical terms constructed?
16. What do the parts of a medical term generally indicate?

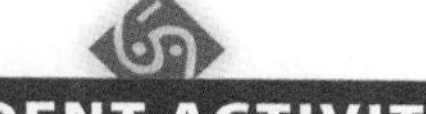

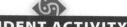

STUDENT ACTIVITY

Separate the following medical terms into roots, prefixes and suffixes and determine their meaning. Check with a medical dictionary to confirm your results.

Electrocardiograph

Cerebral thrombosis

Antispasmodic

Cystosarcoma

Cytology

Intracellular

Polymyositis

Microcephaly

Neurofibroma

Subcutaneous

CHAPTER

5

Human Anatomy and Physiology

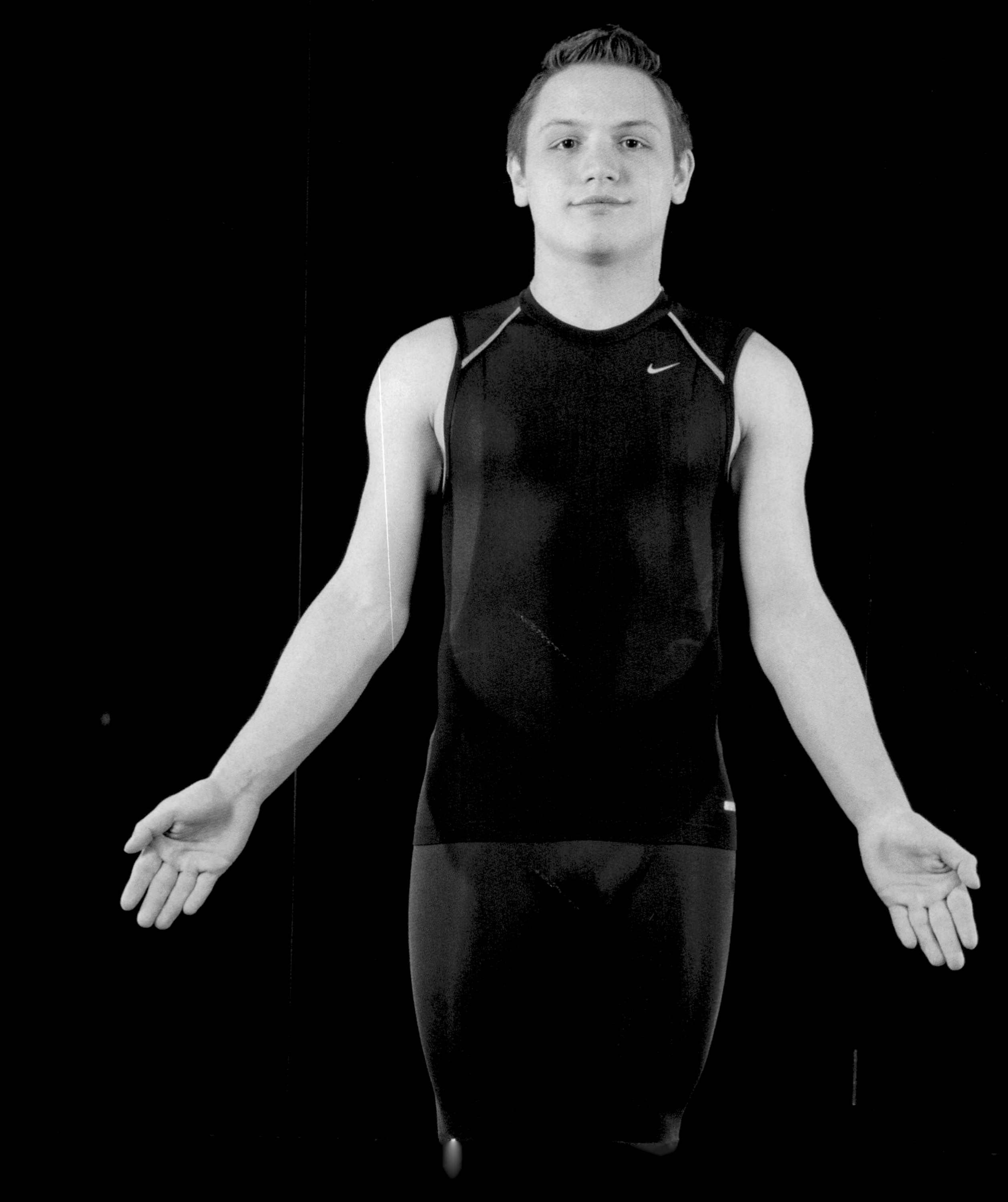

LEARNING OBJECTIVES

After you have mastered this chapter, you will be able to:

1. **Demonstrate knowledge of basic human anatomy and physiology as a requisite in mastering the theory and practice of therapeutic massage.**
2. **Name the anatomic planes, regions, cavities, and parts of the body.**
3. **Name the ten most important body systems.**
4. **Explain the structures and functions of the various body systems.**

INTRODUCTION

An elementary knowledge of anatomy, physiology, kinesiology, and pathology is necessary in mastering the theory and practice of therapeutic massage. To obtain the most beneficial results, the practitioner who knows the principles of anatomy, physiology, and kinesiology is better able to adjust the massage treatment to the needs of the client and to maximize desired results. An understanding of pathology is important so that the practitioner can recognize certain irregularities or conditions and make appropriate decisions either to work on a client or refer that client to a doctor for further diagnosis and treatment.

Anatomy (a-**NAT**-o-mee) is the science of **morphology** (morf-**AL**-o-jee), or structure of an organism or body. *Physiology* (fiz-ee-**OL**-o-jee) concerns the normal functions performed by the various systems of the body. *Pathology* (path-**OL**-o-jee) is the study of disease and disease processes. *Kinesiology* (kin-ee-see-**OL**-o-jee) is the scientific study of muscular activity and the mechanics of body movement. Through clear understanding of the structures involved in body movement, the massage therapist can better identify the areas of pain and/or dysfunction when working with clients.

morphology

is the science or study of the structure of an organism or body.

atoms

consist of subatomic particles that all substances are composed of.

cells

are basic functional units of all living matter.

tissues

are collections of similar cells that carry out specific bodily functions.

LEVELS OF COMPLEXITY OF LIVING MATTER

All substances are made of subatomic particles that form **atoms**. Atoms are arranged in specific patterns and structures called **molecules**. Molecules are arranged in such a way as to produce compounds and matter. Within the human organism, the basic unit of structure and function is the **cell**. Cells are organized into layers or groups called **tissues**. Groups of tissues form complex structures that perform certain functions. These structures, called **organs**, are arranged in **organ systems**. Organ systems are arranged to form an organism. The human body is the organism we study in relation to therapeutic massage (Figure 5-1).

organs

a combination of tissues and cells that form a complex structure to perform a certain function within the system.

organ system

is several organs working together to perform a bodily function.

CELLS

All living matter is composed of **protoplasm** (**PRO**-to-plazm), a colorless, jelly-like substance in which food elements, such as protein, fats, carbohydrates, mineral salts, and water, are present. Cells are the basic functional units of all living

protoplasm

is a colorless, jelly-like substance in which food elements, such as protein, fats, carbohydrates, mineral salts, and water, are present.

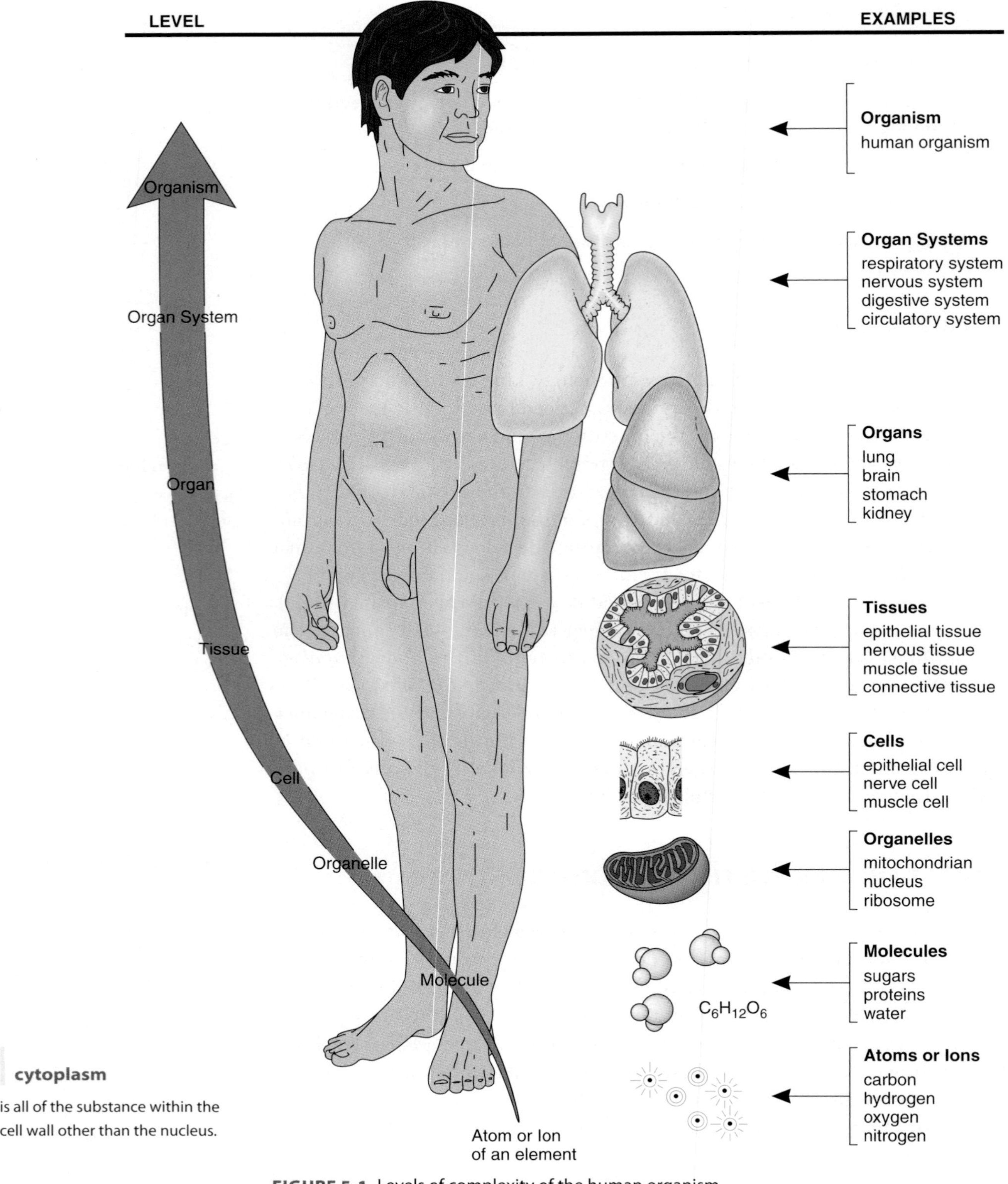

FIGURE 5-1 Levels of complexity of the human organism.

cytoplasm

is all of the substance within the cell wall other than the nucleus.

nucleus

the main central body of living cells that contains the genetic information for continuing life.

matter of animals, plants, and bacteria. Living cells differ from one another in size, shape, structure, and function. In the human body, cells are highly specialized to perform such vital functions as movement, digestion, thought, and reproduction.

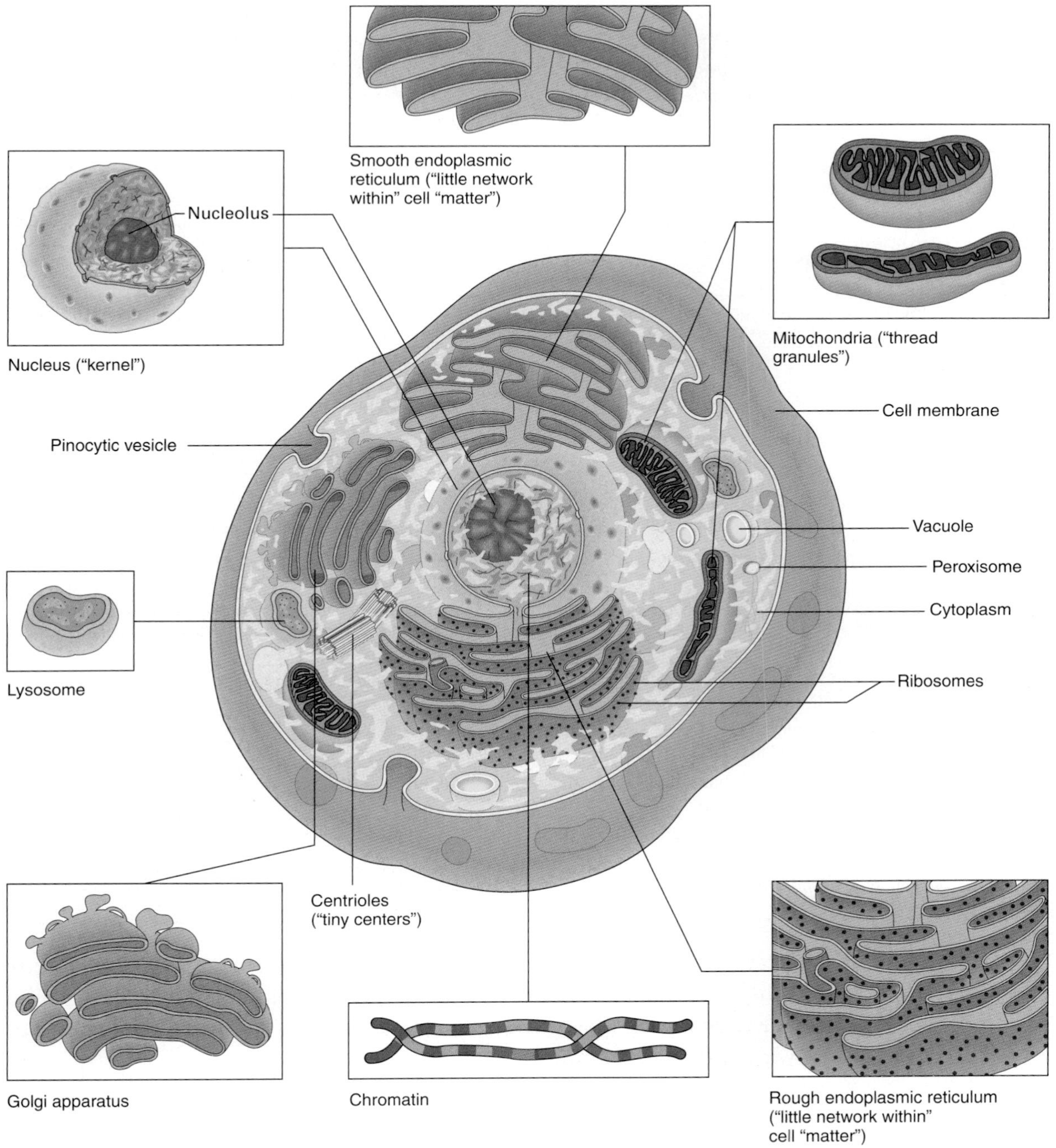

FIGURE 5-2 Structure of a typical animal cell.

The principal parts of a cell are the **cytoplasm** (**SIGH**-to-plazm), **nucleus**, and **cell membrane**. A thin cell membrane or wall separates one cell from another and permits soluble substances such as nutrients and waste products to enter and leave the cytoplasm. Near the center of the cell is a nucleus (dense protoplasm). Outside the nucleus is the cytoplasm (less dense protoplasm).

The cytoplasm contains a network of various membranes that mark off several distinct parts called **cytoplasmic organelles** (Figure 5-2). Organelles perform specific functions necessary for cell survival (Table 5.1.) As long as the cell receives an adequate supply of food, oxygen, and water, eliminates waste

cell membrane

permits soluble substances to enter and leave the protoplasm.

cytoplasmic organelles

discrete structures within a cell, having specialized functions, identifying molecular structures, and a distinctive chemical composition.

TABLE 5.1

STRUCTURE AND FUNCTION OF CELLULAR ORGANELLES		
ORGANELLE	**STRUCTURE**	**FUNCTION**
An *organelle* is a discrete structure within a cell, having specialized functions, identifying molecular structures, and a distinctive chemical composition.		
Cell membrane	A thin covering of the outer surface of the cytoplasm composed of protein and lipid molecules	Transports materials between the outside and inside of the cell, helps to control cell activity, and contains cellular material
Centrosome	A nonmembranous structure near the nucleus composed of two rod-shaped centrioles	Divides into two parts during mitosis and moves to the opposite poles of the dividing cell; helps to distribute the chromosomes into the daughter cells
Chromatin	Network of fibers composed of protein and DNA that form the chromosomes	Contains the genes by which hereditary characteristics are transmitted and determined
Endoplasmic reticulum	Network of sacs and canals connected to the cell membrane, the nuclear membrane, and other organelles	There are two varieties: a smooth type that produce lipid and a rough type that has ribosomes attached to its surface; provides for the transportation of materials within the cell
Fibrils and microtubules	Minute rods and tubules	Support the cytoplasm and contribute to movement of substances within the cytoplasm
Golgi apparatus	Composed of flattened membranes and small vesicles	Collects the products of cell synthesis, synthesizes carbohydrates, holds protein molecules for secretion
Lysosome	Membranous structure containing hydrolytic enzymes	Digests proteins, carbohydrates, and other foreign substances that enter the cell
Mitochondria	Shape varies according to function, but all exhibit a double membrane with the inner membrane, lifted into folds	Contains enzymes for releasing energy and converting it to useful forms for cell operation in the form of adenosine triphosphate (ATP)
Nuclear membrane	The covering structure of the nucleus that separates the nucleus and the cytoplasm	Controls passage of substances between the nucleus and the cytoplasm
Nucleolus	A dense body composed mainly of protein with some RNA molecules, found in the nucleus of most cells	Forms ribosomes
Nucleus	Protein-coated heredity material (DNA) containing chromosomes that transmit heredity	Supervises all cell activity
Ribosome	Minute particle or granule composed of RNA and protein molecules	Synthesizes proteins
Vacuole	Membrane-lined containers	Involved in rapid ejection of fluids or introduction of substances

products, and is surrounded by a favorable environment (proper temperature and the absence of waste products, toxins, and pressure), it will continue to grow and function. When these requirements are not provided, the cell stops growing and eventually dies.

Cell Division

The human body is composed of more than 70 trillion cells, which develop from a single cell, the fertilized ovum (egg). During the early developmental stages, the repeated division of the ovum results in many specialized cells that differ from one another in composition and function. The cells specialize into epithelial, muscle, nerve, and connective tissue cells. This process is termed **differentiation** (dif-er-en-shee-**A**-shun).

differentiation

is the repeated division of the ovum during early developmental stages, resulting in specialized cells that differ from one another.

After the tissues and organs of the organism have developed, growth and maintenance of the various tissues are carried on through cell division. As a cell matures and is nourished, it grows in size and eventually divides into two smaller (daughter-like) cells that are genetically and functionally identical to the original cell. This form of cell division, called **mitosis** (migh-**TO**-sis), produces new cells.

mitosis

is the process of cell division in which a cell divides into two cells identical to the parent cell.

In the human body, some cells reproduce continually, some occasionally, and some not at all. For example, skin and intestinal lining cells are exposed to continuous wear and tear and reproduce continually throughout life. Most body cells are capable of growth and self-repair during their life cycle; however, delicate nerve cells in the central nervous system are incapable of self-repair after injury or destruction and disease.

The *life cycle* of a cell begins at the time the cell forms and continues until it reproduces and divides into two duplicate daughter cells. In the human body, when a cell reaches maturity, reproduction takes place by indirect division or *mitosis,* in which a series of changes occurs in the nucleus before the entire cell divides into two identical daughter cells.

Mitosis is accomplished in five stages: interphase, prophase, metaphase, anaphase, and telophase (Figure 5-3).

1. ***Interphase:*** This is a normal state of the cell during which most of the cellular work and growth are done. This is the time when the cell is maturing, metabolizing, and functioning according to its design. Interphase means between phases and is not actually a part of cell division. During interphase, chromosomes exist in thin threads within the nucleus called *chromatin.* It is during mitosis that the chromosomes assume the twin helical (rodlike) structure.
2. ***Prophase:*** Prophase occurs when the chromosomes, composed of deoxyribonucleic acid (DNA), which house the genes, become larger and more defined. They can be seen within the cell duplicated as two coiled strands called ***chromatids*** (**KRO**-muh-tids). The centrioles begin to migrate to opposite sides of the cell and form a system of microtubules between them. During the last part of prophase, the nuclear membrane disappears.
3. ***Metaphase:*** During metaphase, the chromosomes arrange themselves around the center of the cell in a plane called the *equatorial plane* and are held in place by the microtubules. The nuclear membrane and the nucleolus are absent.
4. ***Anaphase:*** During anaphase, the duplicated chromatids are separated and pulled toward the centrioles by the shortening microtubules. As the chromatids are separated, they are again called chromosomes.
5. ***Telophase:*** This is the stage when the chromosomes reach the centrioles (small bodies) and begin to uncoil. The microtubules break down and a new nuclear membrane forms around the new chromosomes as they defuse back into chromatin. In animal cells, the centrioles duplicate (plant cells do not have centrioles). The cytoplasm continues to divide into two parts or two cells in a process called *cytokinesis*

Meiosis

Meiosis is a special kind of cell division that, in animals, takes place only in the sex glands and produces the egg and sperm required for reproduction. In the male this takes place in the testes; in the female, in the ovary. Meiosis is a reduction cell division in which the resultant cells, called *gametes,* have only one half the number of hereditary chromosomes as the parent cell. A human has 46

meiosis

is cell division that takes place in the sex organs of animals to produce the egg and sperm required for fertilization, and in which the resultant cells have only one half the number of hereditary chromosomes as the parent cell.

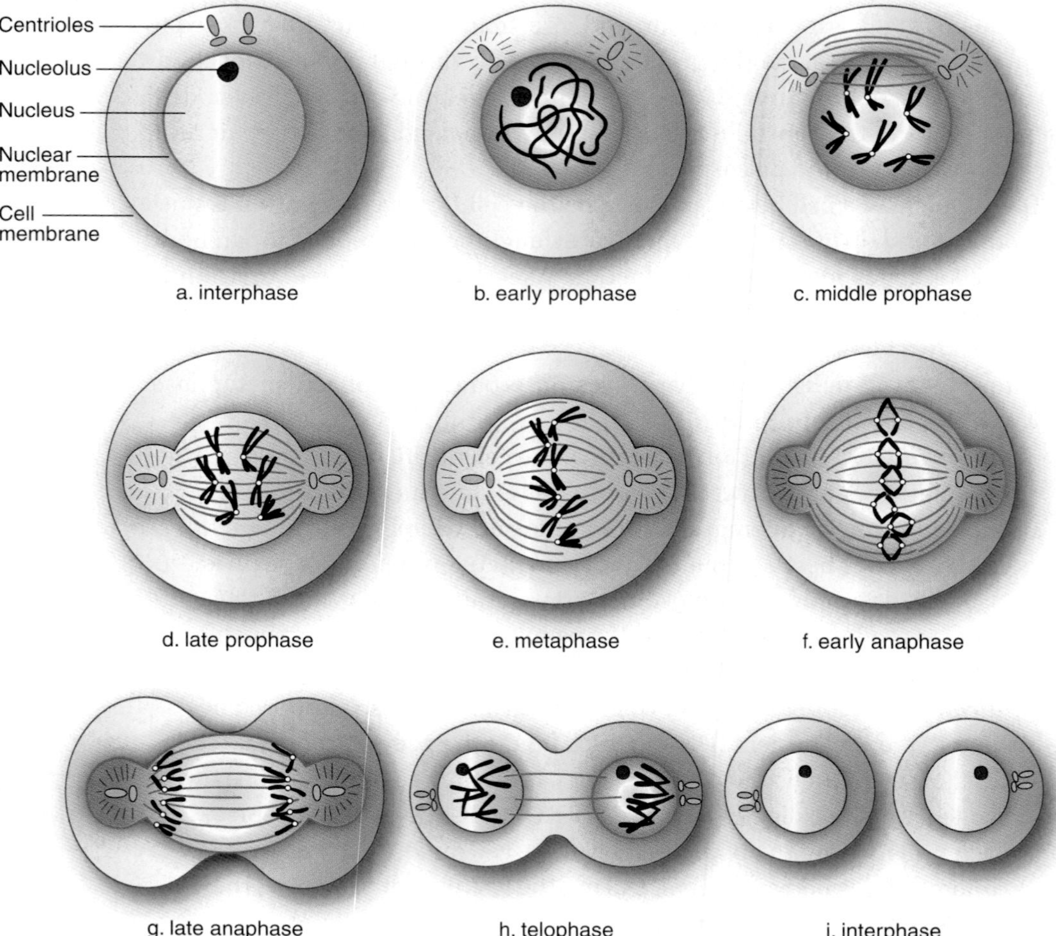

FIGURE 5-3 Stages of mitosis in animal cells.
a. interphase
b. early prophase
c. middle prophase
d. late prophase
e. metaphase
f. early anaphase
g. late anaphase
h. telophase
i. interphase

chromosomes in the nucleus of the body's cells. Through the process of meiosis, the sperm and egg each have 23 chromosomes. When the two cells unite, the resulting zygote again has 46 chromosomes, uniting the hereditary material from two different organisms, thereby increasing the genetic variability. The result is a being that is similar to, but not identical to, either parent.

Cellular Activity

The activity of cells can be divided into three categories: vegetative, growth and reproduction, and specialized.

1. ***Vegetative:*** Vegetative activities include maintenance of the cell such as absorption, assimilation, and excretion of waste products.
2. ***Growth and reproduction:*** Growth involves the development of additional structural materials. Reproduction is the process of mitosis or indirect division of cells. The centriole and nucleus play important roles in this process.

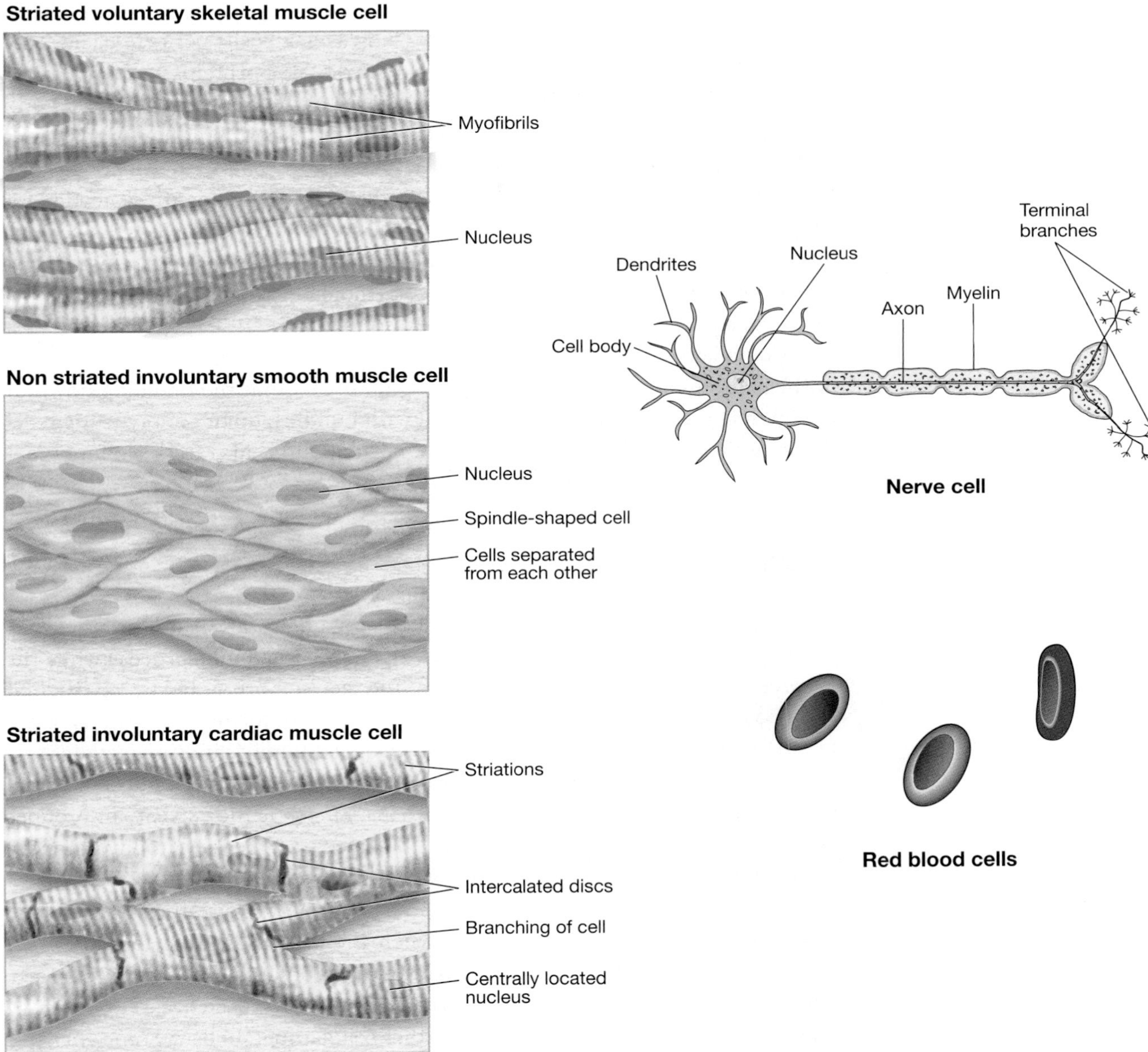

FIGURE 5-4 Variations in specialized cells.

3. ***Specialized activities:*** Because of cell differentiation (Figure 5-4), different cells perform different functions. For example, muscle cells exhibit contractility. Epithelial cells secrete and absorb. Nerve cells transmit nerve impulses. The cell is usually in the vegetative state, and then as time passes it either grows and reproduces or undergoes regression (atrophy) and finally dies.

Metabolism

As the basic units of life, cells perform individually much like small factories. All chemical reactions within a cell that transform food for cell growth and operation are broadly termed *cellular metabolism*. **Metabolism** is the complex chemical and physical process that takes place in living organisms whereby the

metabolism

is the process taking place in living organisms whereby the cells are nourished and carry out their activities.

cells are nourished and carry out their various activities. Different kinds of cells perform specialized metabolic processes; however, all cells perform basic reactions that include the building up or breaking down of proteins, carbohydrates, fats, and other nutrients. There are two phases of metabolism: *anabolism* and *catabolism*. **Anabolism** (a-**NAB**-o-lizm) is the process of building up of larger molecules from smaller ones. This process requires energy because it is the constructive phase of cellular metabolism during which substances needed for cell growth and repair are manufactured. **Catabolism** (ka-**TAB**-o-lizm) is the breaking down of larger substances or molecules into smaller ones. This process releases energy that can be stored by special molecules to be used for other reactions, such as muscle contraction or heat production.

anabolism

is the process of building up of larger molecules from smaller ones.

catabolism

is the breaking down of larger substances into smaller ones.

Anabolism and catabolism are carried out simultaneously and continuously in the cells. Their activities are closely regulated so that the breaking-down or energy-releasing reactions are balanced with building-up or energy-using reactions. Homeostasis (the maintenance of normal, internal stability in an organism) therefore is maintained.

ENZYMES

Enzymes are protein substances that act as organic catalysts to initiate, accelerate, or control specific chemical reactions in the metabolic process while the enzymes themselves remain unchanged. The reaction promoted by a particular enzyme is very specific. Because cellular metabolism includes hundreds of different chemical reactions, there are hundreds of different kinds of enzymes.

enzymes

are proteins that act as catalysts for chemical reactions in metabolism while remaining unchanged themselves.

Enzymes are involved in the process of releasing energy from nutrients, principally from carbohydrates, fats, and proteins. Energy is the capacity to produce change in matter or to do work. During the digestive process, carbohydrates are broken down into simple sugars (glucose), fats are split into fatty acids, and proteins are converted into amino acids. These materials are absorbed by the blood and transported to the cells of the body, where they become the fuel for cell metabolism. As they are further broken down into other compounds, energy is released. Some of this energy is in the form of heat, whereas some is used to carry on the various cellular functions or to promote further cellular metabolism. Some energy is stored in a special molecule called **adenosine** (a-**DEN**-o-seen) **triphosphate (ATP).** ATP stores the energy until it is needed for muscular and other cellular activity.

adenosine triphosphate(ATP)

a molecule that stores energy in the body and releases it when it breaks down into adenosine diphosphate (ADP).

TISSUES

The basic unit of tissue is the cell. Tissues are collections of similar cells that carry out specific functions of the body. Tissues compose all body organs and are subdivided into four main categories:

1. Epithelial tissue
2. Muscle tissue
3. Nerve tissue
4. Connective tissue

The human body develops from a single cell. By the second week of growth of a human fetus (the embryonic stage), distinct layers of cells develop.

The innermost layer of cells is called the **endoderm**, the middle layer is the **mesoderm**, and the outermost layer is called the **ectoderm**. These layers form the primary germ layer, which in turn forms all tissues and organs of the body.

The *endodermal* (inner layer) cells produce the epithelial linings of the respiratory and digestive tracts as well as the linings of the urethra and urinary bladder. The *mesodermal* (middle layer) cells develop into all types of muscle, bone, blood, blood vessel tissues, various connective tissues, lymph, and the linings of all body cavities, as well as the kidneys and the reproductive organs. The *ectodermal* (outer layer) cells form the glands of the skin, linings of the mouth, the anal canal, the epidermis, hair, nails, and the nervous system.

endoderm

is the innermost layer of cells of the zygote.

mesoderm

is the middle layer of cells of the zygote.

ectoderm

is the outermost layer of cells of the zygote.

Epithelial Tissue

Epithelial tissue is a thin protective layer or covering that functions in the process of absorption, excretion, secretion, and protection. There are various classifications of epithelial tissue, named according to the shape or number of layers of cells. Epithelial cells are classified by shape as *squamous* (**SKWA**-muhs; flat), *cuboidal* (small cube shape), and *columnar* (tall or rectangular). These cells are also classified according to arrangement. For example, a simple squamous arrangement is one cell thick, the stratified squamous arrangement is several cells thick, and the transitional squamous is an arrangement of several layers of cells that are flat and closely packed (Figure 5-5).

epithelial tissue

is a protective layer that functions in the processes of absorption, excretion, secretion, and protection.

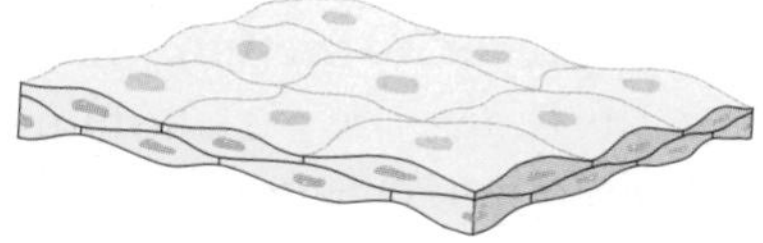

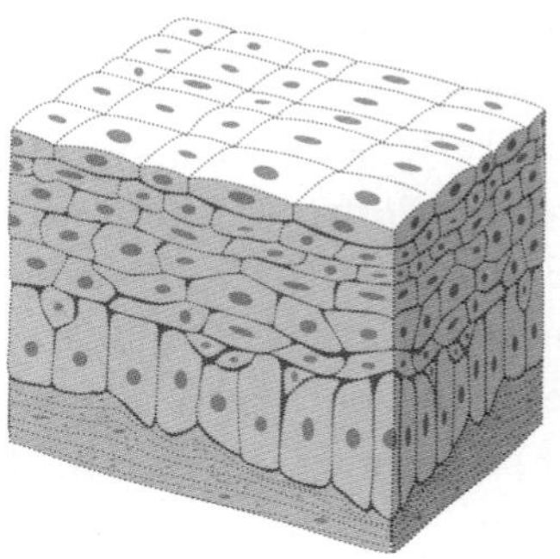

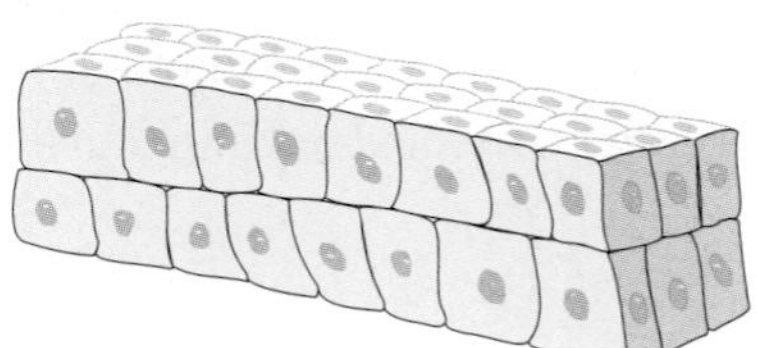

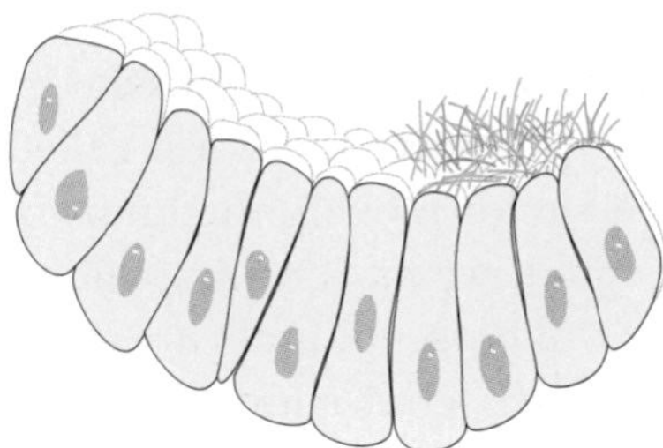

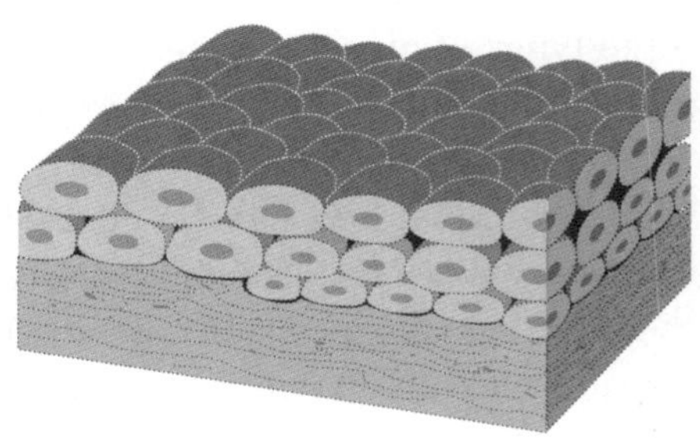

FIGURE 5-5 Types of epithelial tissue.

Epithelial tissue covers all the surfaces of the body both inside and out. It forms the skin, the covering of the organs, and the inner lining of all the hollow organs. These cells also make up the major tissue of the glands. Because epithelial tissue acts as a surface covering or a lining, it always has a free surface that is exposed to outside influences, whereas the other surface is well anchored in the connective tissue from which it derives nourishment.

Membranes

Membranes are structures closely associated with epithelial tissue. There are two main categories of membranes: epithelial membranes and fibrous connective tissue membranes. *Epithelial membranes* have their outer surface faced with epithelium. They are further divided into two main subgroups: mucous membranes and serous membranes. *Mucous membranes* produce mucus, a thick, sticky substance that acts as a protectant and lubricant. Mucous membranes line the surfaces of body cavities and canals that lead to the outside of the body such as the digestive and upper respiratory tracts. In some instances their secretions contain a high number of enzymes that perform specific actions, such as digestion.

Serous membranes produce serous fluid, a watery substance that also acts as a lubricant. Serous membranes line the closed body cavities and sometimes form the outermost surface of the organs contained in those cavities. The covering of the serous membranes in the body cavities is a special epithelial tissue called the ***mesothelium*** (mez-o-**THEE**-lee-um). This is a smooth covering that allows the movements of the organs to take place with little or no friction. Three major serous membranes are the pleura that encase the lungs, the pericardium around the heart, and the peritoneum that lines the abdominal cavity.

Skeletal membrane covers bones and cartilage. The membrane covering bone is the **periosteum** (per-ee-**OS**-tee-um). The membrane covering cartilage is the **perichondrium** (per-i-**KON**-dree-um). Cavities and capsules in and around joints are lined with a connective tissue membrane called **synovial membrane**, which secretes *synovium*, or synovial fluid, an agent that acts as a lubricant between the ends of bones in the joint cavity and in spaces of great activity and friction. There are many other membranes in the body. All can be classified as either epithelial or connective.

skeletal membrane

covers bone and cartilage.

periosteum

is a fibrous membrane that functions to protect the bone and serves as an attachment of tendons and ligaments.

perichondrium

is the membrane covering cartilage.

synovial membrane

is a connective tissue membrane lining cavities and capsules in and around joints.

Muscle Tissue

The main function of muscle tissue fibers is to contract their elongated cells, which pulls attached ends closer together, causing a body part to move. The three types of muscle tissue are skeletal muscle tissue, smooth muscle tissue, and cardiac muscle tissue (Figure 5-6).

Skeletal muscles are usually attached to bone or other muscle by way of tendons and can be controlled by conscious effort. These are called **voluntary muscles**. Skeletal muscles are responsible for moving the limbs of the body, facial expression, speaking, and other voluntary movements. Voluntary muscle cells appear long and threadlike under a microscope and have alternating light and dark cross-markings called *striations* (strigh-**A**-shuns). Muscles containing striations are called *striated muscles.*

Smooth muscle tissue lacks striations (i.e., is non-striated) and cannot usually be stimulated to contract by conscious effort. Smooth muscle

skeletal muscles

are attached to bone by tendons and are responsible for moving the limbs, facial expression, speaking, and other voluntary movements.

voluntary muscles

are skeletal muscles that can be activated by conscious effort.

smooth muscle tissue

lacks striations and cannot be stimulated to contract by conscious effort.

contractions generally result from involuntary nerve impulses from the autonomic nervous system or from glandular activity. Smooth muscle tissue is found in the hollow organs of the stomach, small intestine, colon, bladder, and the blood vessels. Non-striated muscle is responsible for the movement of food through the digestive tract, the constriction of blood vessels, and the emptying of the bladder.

Cardiac muscle tissue occurs only in the heart. Cardiac muscle cells are striated, cylindrical, and connected end to end with other cardiac cells at junctions called *intercalated* (in-**TER**-kah-**lay**-ted) disks. It is controlled involuntarily and can continue to function without being directly stimulated by nerve impulses. Cardiac tissue causes the beating of the heart and is responsible for pumping blood through the heart into the blood vessels.

cardiac muscle tissue

occurs only in the heart and is responsible for pumping blood through the heart into the blood vessels.

nervous tissue

is composed of neurons; it initiates, controls, and coordinates the body's adaptation to its surroundings.

neuron

is the structural unit of the nervous system.

Nerve Tissue

Nervous or nerve tissue is composed of **neurons** (**NOOR**-ons; nerve cells) and is found in the brain, spinal cord, and associated nerves. Nerves are sensitive to specific types of stimuli from their environment and are able to transmit impulses through specialized extensions of their cell bodies to other nerves, the brain, and muscles. Nerves act as channels for the transmission of messages to and from the brain and various parts of the body, such as sensory nerves in the skin and organs of hearing, taste, smell, and sight. Nervous tissue initiates, controls, and coordinates the body's adaptation to its surroundings. Neurons (nerve cells) are linked together to form nerve pathways.

Connective Tissue

Connective tissue binds structures together, provides support and protection, and serves as a framework. Connective tissue cells produce a variety of structural substances into the intercellular spaces, including collagen, elastin and reticulin fibers, and a matrix of ground substance. The various proportions of the matrix and fibrous content differentiate the type of connective tissue. Connective tissue can be categorized as loose connective tissue, dense connective tissue, and specialized connective tissue.

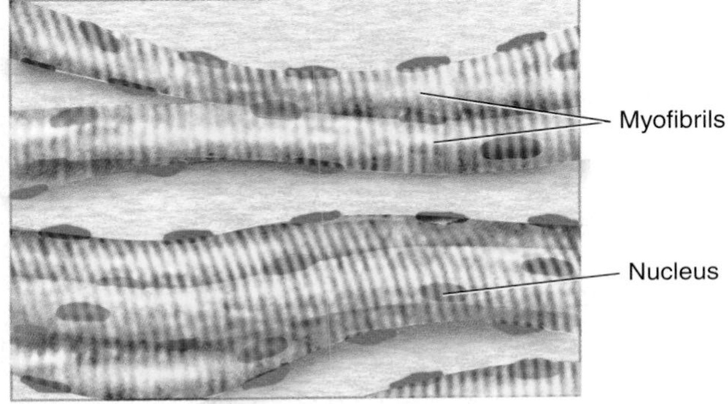

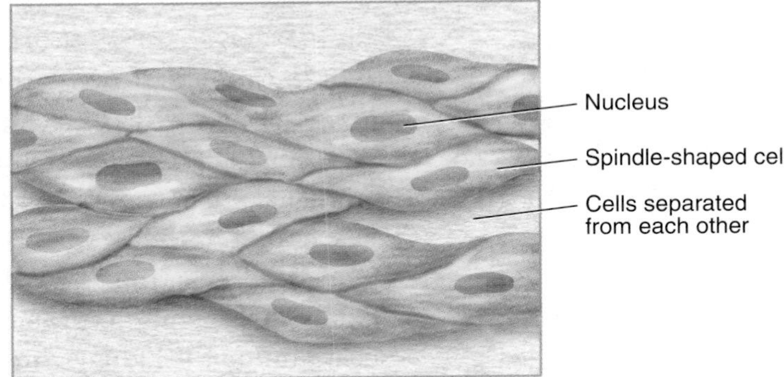

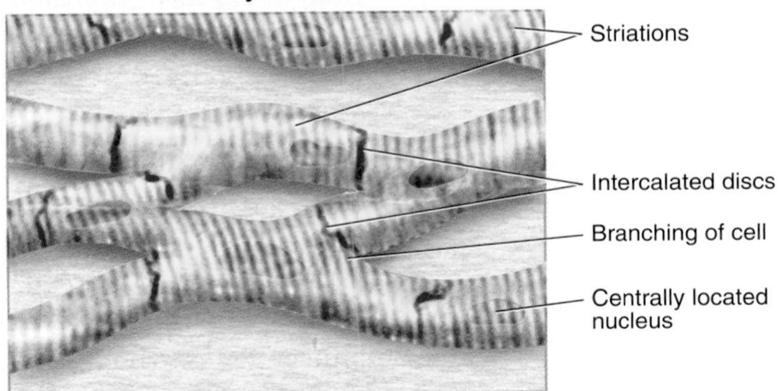

FIGURE 5-6 Types of muscle tissue.

Classifications of Connective Tissue

Loose Connective Tissue (Figure 5-7)

Areolar – Abundance of collagen and elastic fibers

Adipose – Tissue containing fat cells

Reticular – Provides framework of liver and other lymphoid organs

Dense Connective Tissue

Regular – Tendons, ligaments and aponeuroses

Irregular – Muscle sheaths and joint capsules

Cartilage

Fibrocartilage – Characterized by collagenous fiber in the matrix

Hyaline – Fundamental type of cartilage consisting of fine white fibers

Elastic – Characterized by elastic fibers in the matrix

Specialized Connective Tissue

Bone – Skeletal structure

Liquid – Represented by blood, lymph, and interstitial fluid

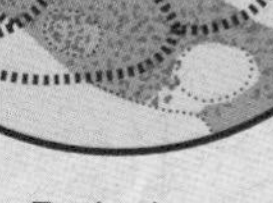

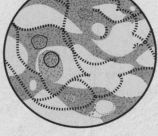

FIGURE 5-7 Loose connective tissue.

areolar tissue

is loose connective tissue that binds the skin to the underlying tissues and fills the spaces between the muscles.

superficial fascia

refers to the connective tissue layer between the skin and those structures underlying the skin.

adipose tissue

is areolar tissue with an abundance of fat cells.

reticular tissue

is composed of fibers that form the framework of the liver and lymphoid organs.

The loose connective tissue, or **areolar** (a-**REE**-o-lar) **tissue**, binds the skin to the underlying tissues and fills the spaces between the muscles. This is the tissue that lies beneath most layers of epithelium and is also known as **superficial fascia**. It is rich in blood vessels and provides nourishment to the epithelial tissues. **Adipose tissue** is areolar tissue that has an abundance of fat-containing cells. Adipose tissue acts as a protection against heat loss and stores energy in the form of fat molecules. It is found in abundance in certain abdominal membranes, and around the surface of the heart, between the muscles, around the kidneys, and just beneath the skin.

Reticular tissue resembles fine fibers when viewed under a microscope. These fibers form the framework of the liver and lymphoid organs. Reticular tissue is abundant in embryos and is eventually replaced by more mature collagen fibers. **Dense connective tissue** is composed of collagen (albuminoid substance) and elastic fibers that are more closely packed and can be divided into two subgroups, depending on how the fibers are arranged. Regular dense connective tissues include tendons, ligaments, and aponeuroses. **Tendons** or *sinews* are white, glistening cords or bands that serve to attach muscle to bone and consist of mostly tough collagen fibers aligned parallel to each other. Aponeuroses are wide flat tendons. **Ligaments** are tough, fibrous bands that connect bones to bones or support viscera and contain a combination of closely arranged collagen and elastin fibers. Irregular dense connective tissue is characterized by dense muscle sheaths surrounding muscles and the capsules surrounding synovial joints.

dense connective tissue

is composed of collagen and elastin fibers that are closely arranged to form tendons and ligaments.

Fascia

Fascia is a term denoting the areolar connective tissue that forms a fibrous network that is continuous from the top of the skull to the tips of the toes and throughout the body. It is a continuous membranous envelope that glistens with a sticky, lubricating fluid, surrounding every organ, blood vessel, nerve, bone, and muscle. Fascia is composed of collagen and elastin fibers in viscous, gel-like ground substance. It envelops, supports, separates, and gives shape to the body and its component parts. Fascia provides form and cohesiveness and at the same time allows movement between different structures without irritation. Fascia has different names according to its location. Around the brain and spinal cord it is the meninges. Around the heart, it is the pericardium. In the abdominal cavity, it is the peritoneum. The layer just under the skin is the superficial fascia, whereas **deep fascia** envelops and permeates the skeletal muscles. Deep fascia covers each muscle fiber (endomysium), the muscle fascicles (perimysium), the whole muscle (epimysium), and groups of muscles (investing fascia). Each layer of deep fascia is invested into the next. The fasciae in muscles organize and separate the muscle fibers, allowing them to move independently while at the same time directing the muscle contraction into the muscle attachments, thereby creating movement. Muscles and fascia are anatomically inseparable. Without fascia, muscle would be without form or functionality. Fascia also provides support and pathways for nerves, blood, and lymph vessels. All fascia throughout the body is continuous (Figure 5-8).

tendons

are bands that attach muscle to bone.

ligaments

are bands of fibrous tissue that connect bones to bones.

fascia

fibrous connective tissue that forms a network throughout the body, surrounding every structure to support, separate, and give shape to the body.

deep fascia

envelops and permeates the skeletal muscles.
refers to fibrous tissue sheaths that penetrate deep into the body, separating muscle groups

Cartilage

Fibrocartilage is found between the vertebrae and in the pubic symphysis, where strong support and minimal range of movement are required. In dense fibrous connective tissue, repair to damaged tissue is slow because of low vascularity.

Hyaline (**HIGH**-a-lin) is a type of cartilage that contains little fibrous tissue and is made up of cells embedded in a somewhat translucent matrix, as is found in the nose and trachea and on the end of bones and in movable joints.

Elastic cartilage is the most resilient of cartilages and is found in the external ear, the larynx, and similar structures (Figure 5-9).

fibrocartilage

is found between the vertebrae and pubic symphysis.

Bone Tissue

Bone or osseous (bonelike) tissue is connective tissue in which the intercellular substance is rendered hard by being impregnated with mineral salts, chiefly calcium phosphate and calcium carbonate. Compact, dense material forms the dense, outer layer of a long bone; cancellous (porous) material forms the bone's inner tissue. *Dentne*, the substance beneath the enamel of the teeth, closely resembles bone but is harder and denser. Unlike bone, dentne contains no distinct cells or blood vessels.

bone tissue

is connective tissue in which the intercellular substance is rendered hard by mineral salts, chiefly calcium carbonate and calcium phosphate.

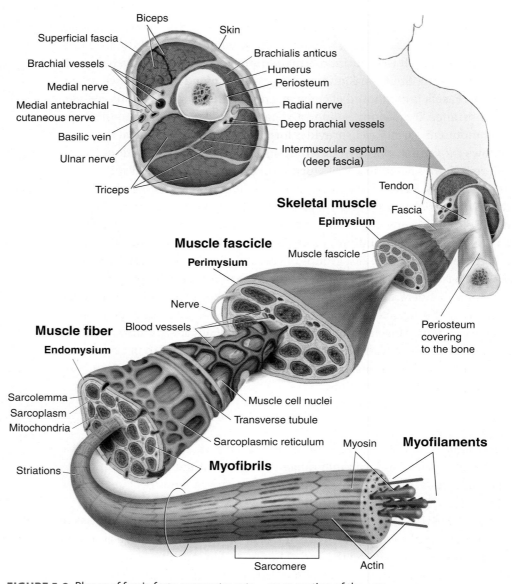

Biceps
Skin
Superficial fascia
Brachialis anticus
Brachial vessels
Humerus
Periosteum
Medial nerve
Radial nerve
Medial antebrachial cutaneous nerve
Deep brachial vessels
Basilic vein
Intermuscular septum (deep fascia)
Ulnar nerve
Triceps
Tendon
Skeletal muscle
Fascia
Epimysium
Muscle fascicle
Muscle fascicle
Perimysium
Nerve
Blood vessels
Periosteum covering to the bone
Muscle fiber
Endomysium
Sarcolemma
Sarcoplasm
Mitochondria
Muscle cell nuclei
Transverse tubule
Sarcoplasmic reticulum
Myosin
Myofilaments
Striations
Myofibrils
Sarcomere
Actin

FIGURE 5-8 Planes of fascia form compartments—cross-section of the arm.

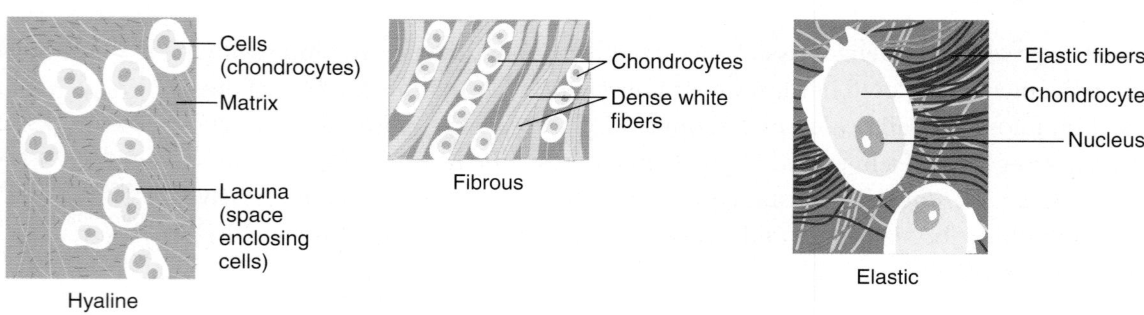

FIGURE 5-9 Cartilage.

Liquid Connective Tissue

Liquid connective tissue is represented by blood, lymph, and interstitial fluid. Blood is a fluid tissue that circulates throughout the body and from which the body cells obtain nutrients and by which waste products are removed. Lymph is derived from the blood and tissue fluid and is collected into the lymphatic vessels along with metabolic waste and toxins. Lymphoid tissue, found in the lymph nodes (small, compact, knotlike structures) and in the adenoids, thymus, tonsils, and spleen, is important in the production of antibodies. Interstitial fluid is the liqudy substance found outside the cell walls and between the cells of the body that bathes the cells and is the means of transport of nutrients and cellular wastes between the cells and the circulatory system.

SECTION QUESTIONS FOR DISCUSSION AND REVIEW

1. Why is the cell called the basic unit of all living matter?
2. Name the three principal parts of a cell.
3. Which parts of the cell control reproduction?
4 Which conditions are required for a cell to grow and function?
5. By which process does cell reproduction occur in human tissue?
6. Name the five phases of cell mitosis.
7. Name the two phases of metabolism.
8. Explain anabolism.
9. Explain catabolism.
10. What are enzymes and what is their function?
11. Of which substances are tissues composed?
12. Name the four main categories of tissues.
13. What do the terms *endoderm, mesoderm,* and *ectoderm* refer to?
14. Where is epithelial tissue found and what is its function?
15. Name the two main types of membranes
16. Name the three types of muscle tissue.
17. What is the difference between striated and smooth muscle tissue?
18. In which part of the body is cardiac muscle tissue found?
19. What is the main function of nervous tissue?
20. Where is liquid tissue found?
21. What is the main function of connective tissue?
22. What is the main function of areolar (loose) tissue?
23. What is adipose tissue?
24. Name the three types of cartilage.
25. What makes bone tissue hard?

THE ANATOMAL POSITION OF THE BODY

anatomic position

standing with feet shoulder-width apart, arms at the side, with the palms of the hands facing forward.

sagittal plane

divides the body into left and right parts.

coronal plane

divides the body into the front and back.

transverse plane

divides the body horizontally into an upper and lower portion.

When studying anatomy, you will find it helpful to know the anatomal terms that designate specific regions of the body. These terms refer to the body as seen in the **anatomic position**, which shows a figure standing upright with the palms of the hands facing forward.

Anatomists divide the body with three imaginary planes called the *sagittal* (vertical), the *coronal* (frontal), and the *transverse* (horizontal) planes (Figure 5-10).

1. The **sagittal** (**SAJ**-i-tal) **plane** divides the body into left and right parts by an imaginary line running vertically down the body. *Midsagittal* refers to the plane that divides the body or an organ into right and left halves.
2. The **coronal** (**KOR**-on-al) **plane**, sometimes referred to as the *frontal plane*, is an imaginary line that divides the body into the anterior (front) or ventral half of the body and the posterior (back) or dorsal half of the body.
3. The **transverse plane** is an imaginary line that divides the body horizontally into upper and lower portions. A *transverse section* cuts through a body part perpendicular to the long axis of the body part.

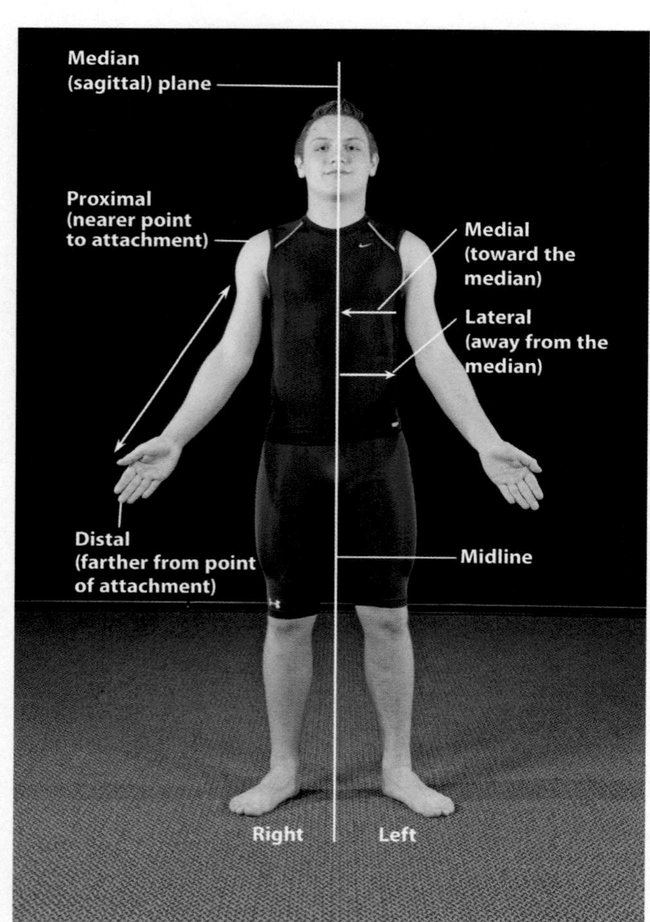

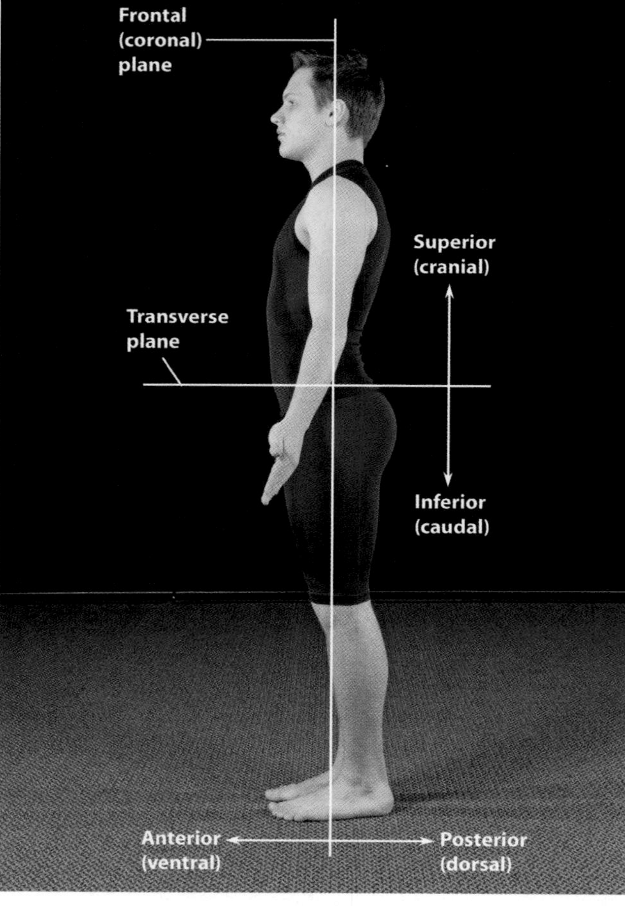

FIGURE 5-10 Planes of the body in terms of location and position.

ANATOMIC TERMS AND MEANINGS

The following chart presents anatomic terms and their meaning:

	TERM	MEANING
1.	Cranial or superior aspect	Situated toward the crown of the head
2.	Caudal or inferior aspect	Situated toward the feet
3.	Anterior or ventral aspect	Situated before or in front of
4.	Posterior or dorsal aspect	Situated behind or in back of
5.	Transverse plane	Division of the body into an upper and lower parts. Transverse section refers to a plane through a body part perpendicular to the axis, which is the vertical centerline around which the body part is arranged.
6.	Sagittal plane	Pertaining to the sagittal suture of the cranium (vertical plane or section dividing the body into right and left sides). A midsagittal section divides the body into equal left and right halves.
7.	Coronal plane	Pertaining to the coronal suture of the cranium. The coronal plane, which is also referred to as the frontal plane or section, passes through the long axis of the body, dividing it into front and back halves.
8.	Medial aspect	Pertaining to the middle or center, nearer to the midline
9.	Lateral aspect	On the side, farther from the midline or center
10.	Distal aspect	Farthest point from the origin of a structure or point of attachment. Relatively farther from the median, trunk, or center.
11.	Proximal	Nearest the origin of a structure or point of attachment. Relatively nearer to the trunk or median.

BODY CAVITIES AND ORGANS

Knowing the body plane makes is easier to remember where body cavities and organs are located. There are two groups of body cavities: the dorsal or posterior cavities and the ventral or anterior cavities. The *dorsal cavities* contain the brain and spinal cord, with the skull forming the *cranial cavity* and the vertebrae forming the *vertebral* or *spinal cavity.* The *ventral cavities* are the *thoracic cavity* and *abdominopelvic cavities.* The thoracic cavity is subdivided into the pericardial cavity, which contains the heart, and the pleural cavities, which contain the lungs. The abdominal cavity is situated below the diaphragm and contains the liver, stomach, spleen, pancreas, small and large intestines. The *pelvic cavity* is the lower third of the abdominopelvic cavity and contains the bladder, rectum, and some of the reproductive organs (Figure 5-11).

Body Cavities

1. Cranial cavity (dorsal)
2. Spinal cavity (dorsal)
3. Thoracic cavity (ventral)
4. Abdominal cavity (ventral)
5. Pelvic cavity (ventral)

FIGURE 5-11 Body cavities.

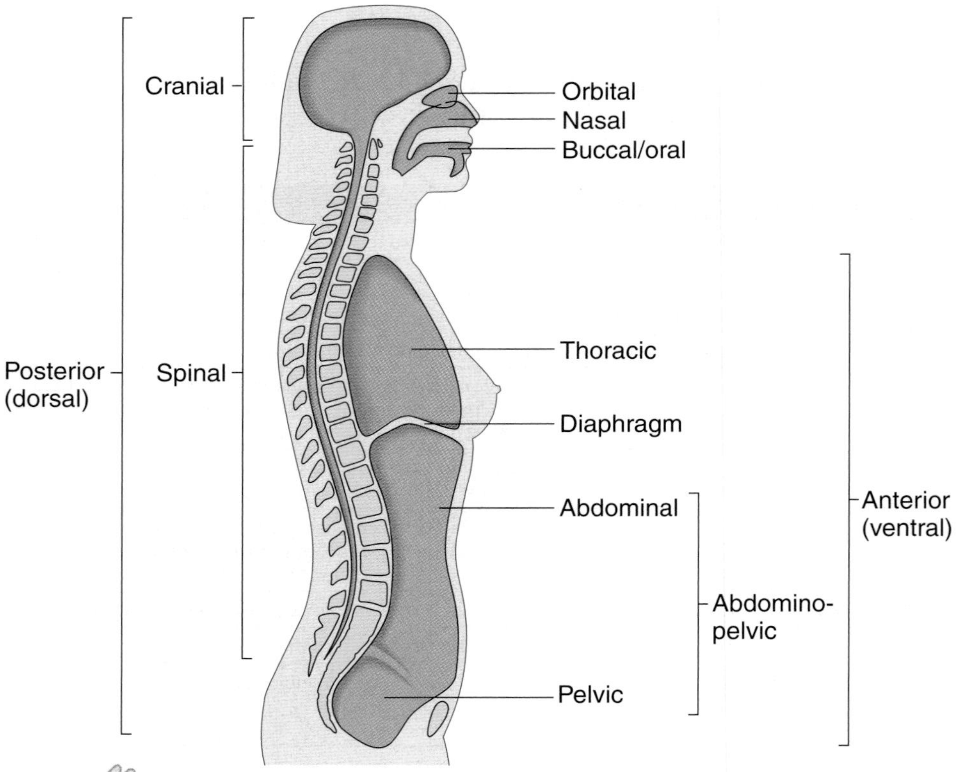

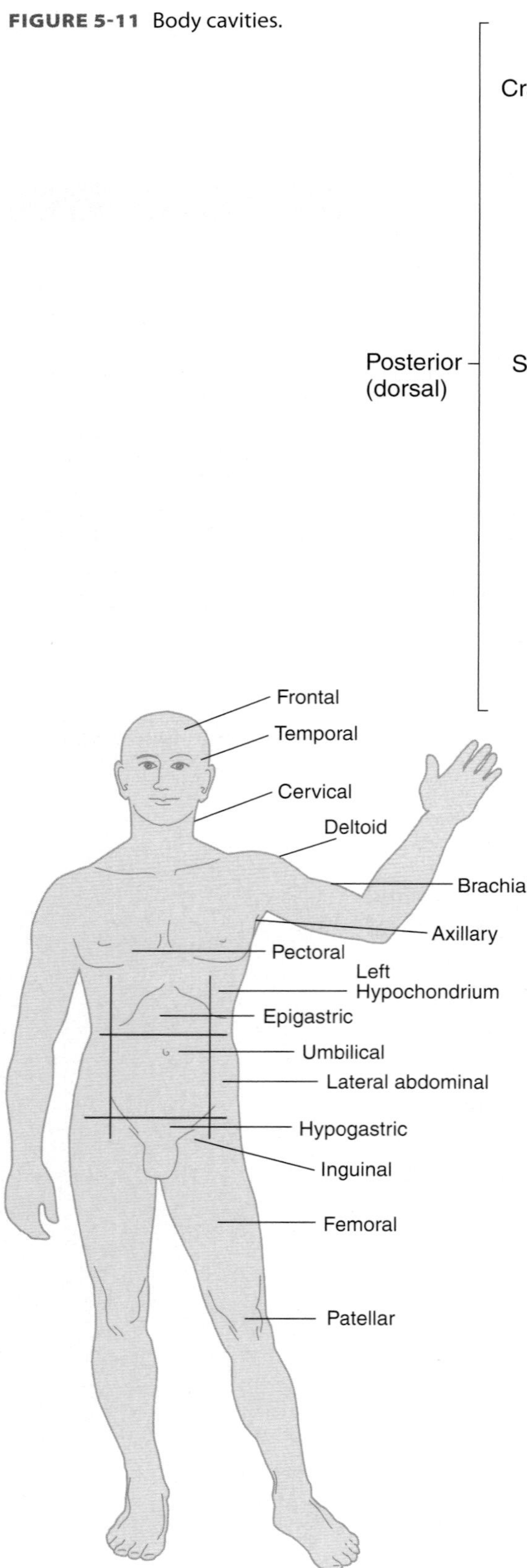

FIGURE 5-12 Regions of the body (anterior view). Areas or regions of the body have been identified and named to aid in locating and describing the location of anatomic structures and conditions.

THE REGIONS OF THE HUMAN BODY

Knowing the regions of the body helps to pinpoint a particular area of the body. For example, the pectoral muscle is located in the pectoral or chest region. The brachial nerve is located in the brachial region. The lower back is the lumbar region. Study the illustrations of the regions of the body until you can locate each region and name the parts of the body associated with each region.

Anterior View of the Human Body Regions

1. ***Frontal:*** Region of the head
2. ***Temporal:*** Region of the temples
3. ***Cervical:*** Region of the neck
4. ***Deltoid:*** Region of the shoulder joint and deltoid muscle
5. ***Axillary:*** Region of the armpit
6. ***Brachial:*** Region between the elbow and shoulder
7. ***Hypochondrium:*** Region of the abdomen lateral to the epigastric region
8. ***Umbilical:*** Region of the navel (umbilicus); the middle of the three median abdominal regions, below the epigastric region and above the pubic region
9. ***Hypogastric:*** Region under the stomach and inferior to the umbilical region
10. ***Patellar:*** Region of the knees and kneecap
11. ***Femoral:*** Region of the femur or thigh

12. ***Inguinal:*** Region of the groin
13. ***Epigastric:*** Region of the abdomen
14. ***Pectoral:*** Region of the breast and chest (Figure 5-12)

Posterior View of the Human Body Regions

1. ***Occipital:*** Region of the back of the head
2. ***Parietal:*** Region of the head, posterior to the frontal region and anterior to the occipital region
3. ***Mastoid:*** Region of the temporal bone behind the ear
4. ***Cervical:*** Region of the neck
5. ***Scapular:*** Region of the back of the shoulder or shoulder blade
6. ***Thoracic:*** The upper trunk surrounded by the rib cage, containing the lungs, heart, esophagus and part of the trachea. The thoracic portion of the spine includes vertebrae T-1 through T-12
7. ***Lumbar:*** Region of the lower back
8. ***Sacral:*** Region over the sacrum, below the low back and between the gluteal
9. ***Gluteal:*** Region of muscles of the buttocks
10. ***Popliteal:*** A diamond-shaped area behind the knee joint (Figure 5-13)

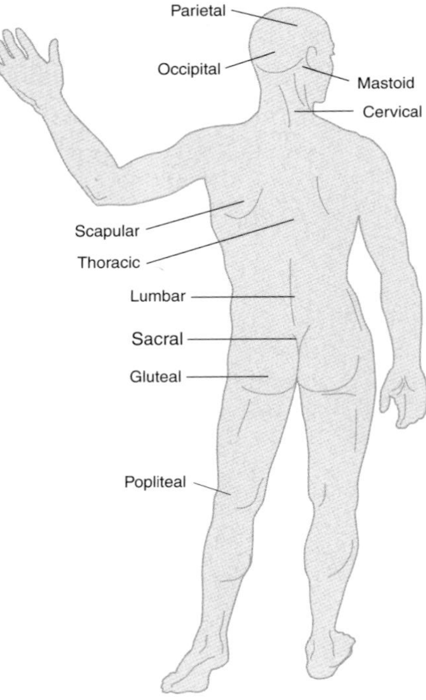

FIGURE 5-13 Regions of the body (posterior view). Regions of the body are generally named for underlying bones, joints, muscles, or other anatomic structures in the immediate area.

THE STRUCTURE OF THE HUMAN BODY

The main anatomic parts of the body are the following:

1. The head
2. The spine
3. The trunk
4. The extremities

The head is subdivided into:

- The cranium: The upper portion of the head, housing the brain.
- The face: The front and lower part of the skull, including the eyes, nose, and mouth.

The spine is a column of bones that supports the head and trunk of the body and protects the spinal cord.

The trunk is subdivided into:

- The thorax or chest: The upper part of the trunk containing the ribs, lungs, heart, esophagus (food tube), and part of the trachea or windpipe.
- The abdomen: Situated below the diaphragm, containing the stomach, intestines, liver, and kidneys. The diaphragm is a muscular partition located between the *thoracic cavity* and the *abdominal cavity*. It is the main muscle associated with breathing. The *pelvic cavity* is located below the abdomen and contains the bladder, some of the reproductive organs, the lower bowel, and the rectum.

The extremities include:

- The upper limbs: The shoulder, arm, wrist, and hand.
- The lower limbs: The hip, thigh, leg, ankle, and foot.

STUDENT ACTIVITY

Pair up with a classmate (or ask a friend or family member), and locate the major anatomic regions on the anterior and posterior aspects of the body.

Body Organs

Body organs are structures containing two or more major different tissues that combine to accomplish a definite function. Among the major organs of the body are the brain, heart, lungs, kidneys, liver, sense organs, organs of digestion, and the organs of reproduction.

Organ Systems

When several organs work together to perform a bodily function, they constitute an organ system. Systems carry on specific functions but are not independent units. All of the body organ systems cooperate for a common purpose, namely, the maintenance or function of the entire organism.

The human body is composed of the following ten important organ systems (Table 5.2):

1. Integumentary system (skin)
2. Skeletal system
3. Muscular system
4. Circulatory system (blood-vascular and lymph-vascular)
5. Nervous system
6. Endocrine system
7. Digestive system
8. Respiratory system
9. Excretory system (including the urinary system)
10. Reproductive system

The Integumentary System

integumentary system is composed of the skin, hair, and nails. (See also Skin.)

The skin is the largest organ of the body. It is often referred to as the outer covering or the **integumentary** (in-teg-you-**MEN**-ta-ree) **system**. The skin's functions include protection, heat regulation, secretion and excretion, sensation, absorption, and respiration.

The Skeletal System

The skeletal system is the structure and hard framework on which the other body systems depend for support and protection. The skeletal system is the physical foundation of the body. It is composed of differently shaped bones united by movable and immovable joints. The main function of the skeletal system is to serve as a means of protection, support, and attachment for muscles of locomotion.

The Muscular System

The muscular system is made up of voluntary and involuntary muscles that are necessary for movement of the parts of the body. The muscular system covers and shapes the skeleton. Practically every contraction and movement of the body is due to the action of the muscles. The obvious movements of the arms and hands, the contraction of the heart and stomach, and the changes in facial expression are the direct result of muscular activity.

The Circulatory System (Blood-Vascular and Lymph-Vascular)

The circulatory (vascular) system controls the circulation of blood and lymph throughout the body. This system consists of two divisions: the blood-vascular system and the lymph-vascular system. The blood-vascular system includes the heart and blood vessels (i.e., arteries, veins, and capillaries). The pumping action of the heart distributes the vital fluids through the blood vessels to all parts of the body. The blood acts as a two-way carrier of supplies, bringing oxygen and nutritional materials to the cells and taking away waste products and secretions from the tissues.

The lymph (a clear, yellow fluid) bathes all cells and assists in the exchange of supplies required by the cells and carries waste and impurities away from the cells. The lymph-vascular system consists of lymph, lymph nodes, and lymph vessels (lymphatics) through which the lymph circulates. The lymph system also includes the spleen, thymus, tonsils, adenoids, and Peyer's patches, lymphoid tissue located on the walls of the small intestines.

The Nervous System

The nervous or neurologic system controls and coordinates all of the body systems, helping them to work efficiently and harmoniously. The neurologic system includes all of the nerves of the body, spinal cord, and brain. It is a highly developed and sensitive organization of nerve tissues. Through the nervous system, the person is made aware of his existence and relationship to the outside world. Nerves, branching out from the brain and spinal cord, coordinate all of the voluntary and involuntary functions of the body.

The Endocrine System

The endocrine system represents a group of specialized organs or glands capable of manufacturing secretions called *hormones* that affect many functions of the body, including growth, reproduction, and health. The endocrine glands, such as the pituitary and thyroid, secrete hormones into the blood to regulate the processes of growth and metabolism. Reproduction is made possible by the sex glands and their secretions.

The Digestive System

The digestive system consists of all of the structures involved in the process of digestion, including the mouth, stomach, intestines, and salivary and gastric glands. The intestines are part of a continuous tube about 30 feet in length. The function of digestion is to break down complex food substances into simple materials fit to be absorbed and used by the body cells. Various digestive glands, including the salivary glands, pancreas, and liver, and the glands in the stomach and small intestine, form and discharge enzymes that act on food in the process of digestion.

The Respiratory System

The respiratory system includes the lungs, air passages, nose, mouth, pharynx, trachea, and bronchial tubes, which lead to the lungs. The blood, as it passes through the lungs, is purified by the removal of carbon dioxide and the intake of oxygen.

The Excretory System

The excretory system includes the skin, kidneys, bladder, liver, lungs, and large intestines, which eliminate waste products from the body. The skin (integumentary system) gives off perspiration. The lungs exhale carbon dioxide gas. The kidneys excrete urine by way of the bladder. The large intestine discharges digestive refuse from the body. The liver produces bile and urea, which contains certain waste products.

The Reproductive System

The function of the reproductive system is the system is to ensure continuance of the species by the reproduction of other human beings. In women, the ovaries discharge an ovum or egg cell that appears prior to menstruation. The testes in men manufacture sperm cells. The union of the ovum with sperm results in fertilization and conception.

In the following sections of this chapter, each organ system is discussed in more detail.

TABLE 5.2

ORGAN SYSTEMS		
SYSTEM	**ORGANS IN THE SYSTEM**	**FUNCTIONS**
Integumentary System	Epidermis, dermis, hair, sudoriferous and sebaceous glands	Protects, regulates temperature, secretion, excretion, sensation, absorption, respiration
Skeletal System	Approximately 206 bones united by movable and immovable joints attached by ligaments	Protects organs, supports body structure, and serves as attachments for the muscles of locomotion
Muscular System	Voluntary and involuntary muscles	Supports body structure; produces heat and motion, contractions of the heart, peristalsis of digestion, facial expression, locomotion, and other body movements
Circulatory System	Heart, blood vessels, capillaries, blood, lymph vessels and nodes, and lymph	Controls the movement of blood and lymph throughout the body
Nervous System	Brain, spinal cord, and nerves	Controls and coordinates all of the voluntary and involuntary functions of the body's systems
Endocrine System	Pituitary, pineal, thyroid, parathyroid, thymus, adrenals, pancreas, ovaries, testes	Manufactures and secretes various hormones that regulate or affect numerous body functions
Digestive System	Mouth, stomach, intestines, gastric and salivary glands, plus the accessory organs: the liver, gallbladder, and pancreas	Breaks down complex food substances to be absorbed into the lymph and blood to be used by body cells
Respiratory System	Lungs and the air passages that lead to the lungs, including the nose, mouth, pharynx, trachea, and bronchial tubes	Absorbs oxygen into and releases carbon dioxide from the blood
Excretory System (including the Urinary System)	Kidneys, bladder, ureters, urethra, liver, large intestines, skin and lungs	Eliminates waste products from the body
Reproductive System	Female: ovaries, fallopian tubes, uterus, vagina, vulva Male: testes, vas deferens, seminal vesicles, prostate, penis	Provides for reproduction, thereby ensuring the continuation of the species

SECTION QUESTIONS FOR DISCUSSION AND REVIEW

1. What is anatomic position?
2. What are three anatomic planes of the body?
3. Why is it important to know the anatomic position and the planes and regions of the human body?
4. Name the subdivisions of the ventral and dorsal cavities and the major organs found in each.
5. What are the four main anatomic parts of the body and the structures found in each?
6. Name the ten important organ systems of the body.

REVIEW

I. Match each term in the left column with the correct definition in the right column.

______	1.	superior	a.	farthest from center
______	2.	inferior	b.	pertaining to the middle
______	3.	anterior	c.	dividing front and back
______	4.	posterior	d.	toward the side
______	5.	transverse plane	e.	dividing left and right
______	6.	sagittal plane	f.	closer to the origin
______	7.	coronal plane	g.	toward the top
______	8.	medial	h.	dividing upper and lower
______	9.	lateral	i.	toward the front
______	10.	distal	j.	toward the feet
______	11.	proximal	k.	toward the back

II. Match each term in the left column with the correct definition in the right column.

________	1.	cervical	a.	region of the groin
________	2.	axillary	b.	side of the cranium
________	3.	femoral	c.	region of the armpit
________	4.	lumbar	d.	behind the knee
________	5.	inguinal	e.	inferior to the umbilical region
________	6.	popliteal	f.	region of the neck
________	7.	gluteal	g.	region of the lower back
________	8.	parietal	h.	between the shoulder and elbow
________	9.	hypogastric	i.	region of the thigh
________	10.	brachial	j.	region of the buttocks

SYSTEM 1 THE INTEGUMENTARY SYSTEM—THE SKIN

The word *integument* means covering or skin. The skin is the largest organ of the body and serves as an interface with the environment and protection for the body.

The principal functions of the skin are the following:

1. Protection: The skin protects the body from injury and bacterial invasion.
2. Heat regulation: The healthy body maintains a constant internal temperature of approximately 98.6°F (37°C). As changes occur in the outside temperature, the blood and sweat glands of the skin make the necessary adjustments in their functions.

3. Secretion and excretion: By means of its sweat (sudoriferous) and oil (sebaceous) glands, the skin acts both as a secretory and an excretory organ. The sudoriferous (sweat) glands excrete (eliminate) perspiration, which is mostly water with a small amount of waste matter. The sebaceous (oil) glands secrete (produce and release) sebum, which is a lubricant. The skin is about 50 to 70 percent moisture. Sebum (oil) coats the surface of the skin and helps to maintain its moisture level. The sebum level slows down evaporation of moisture and keeps excess water from penetrating the skin.
4. Sensation: The papillary layer of the dermis provides the body with a sense of touch. Nerves supplying the skin register basic types of sensations, such as heat, cold, pain, pressure, and touch. Nerve endings are most abundant in the fingertips. Complex sensations, such as the feelings of vibration, seem to depend on a combination of these nerve endings.
5. Absorption: The skin has limited powers of absorption through its pores. Some cosmetics, chemicals, and drugs can be absorbed in small amounts.
6. Respiration: The skin breathes through its pores much as the body breathes through its lungs, but on a much smaller scale. Oxygen is taken in, and carbon dioxide is discharged.

The Structure of the Skin

epidermis

is the outermost layer of the skin.

dermis

is the deeper layer of the skin that extends to form the subcutaneous tissue.

The structure of the skin contains two clearly defined divisions: the **epidermis** (cuticle, or scarf), which is the outermost layer, and the **dermis** (corium, or true skin), which is the deeper layer that extends to form the subcutaneous tissue.

Although the epidermis comprises almost a solid sheet of cells, the dermis is a more semisolid mixture of fibers, water, and a gel-like material called *ground substance*. There are three kinds of fibers that intermingle with the cells of the dermis: collagen, reticulum, and elastin. Collagen makes up about 70 percent of the dry weight of the skin and gives it strength, form, and flexibility. Reticulum fibers form a fine branching pattern in connective tissue that helps to link the bundles of collagen fibers. The dermis also contains a protein called *elastin* that has elastic properties and helps to give the skin its resiliency. The dermis is a connective tissue network of cells through which are distributed nerves, blood and lymph vessels, and sweat and oil glands (Figures 5-14 and 5-15).

The Epidermis

The epidermis is the outermost layer of the body and forms a protective layer covering every part of the body; it varies in thickness, being thickest on the palms of the hands and soles of the feet and thinnest on the inner sides of the limbs. It consists of several variable layers of cells.

The *stratum corneum* is the outermost layer. The protoplasm of the cells changes into a protein substance called *keratin*, forming a waterproof covering. Next is a very thin, nearly invisible layer of clear cells called the *stratum lucidum*.

The *stratum granulosum* (gran-you-**LO**-sum; granular layer of the skin) consists of cells that look like granules. These cells are almost dead and undergo a change into cells of the more superficial layers.

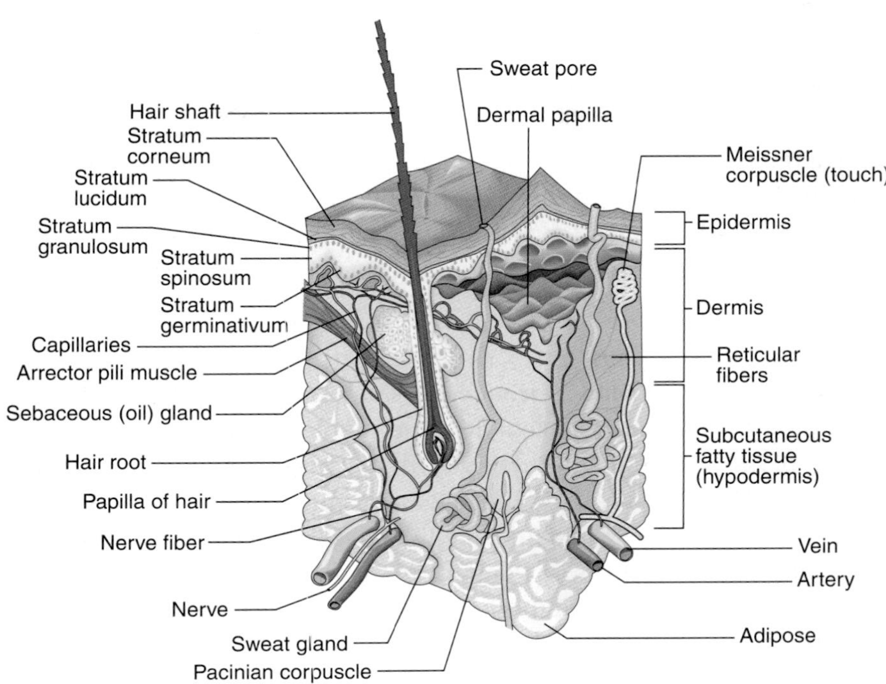

FIGURE 5-14 The integumentary system (showing skin and hair).

The *stratum spinosum* (also called *stratum mucosum*) varies in thickness and consists of irregularly shaped cells containing *melanin* (**MEL**-a-nin) (coloring matter) of the skin. Melanin helps to protect the sensitive cells from the action of strong solar rays.

The *stratum germinativum* (jer-mi-na-**TEE**-vum) is the deepest layer of the epidermis, comprising a single layer of cells that are well nourished by the dermis. These are the only cells in the skin that undergo mitosis, pushing other cells closer to the body surface. This layer also contains the melanocytes that produce the pigment melanin.

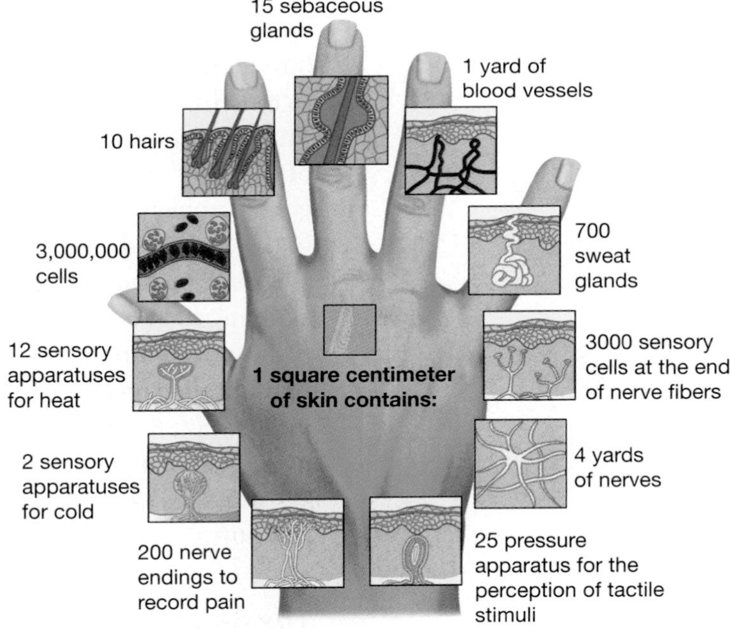

FIGURE 5-15 Structures in the skin.

The Dermis

The *papillary layer* of the skin (directly beneath the epidermis) contains the papillae, the conelike projections made of fine strands of elastic tissue that extend upward into the epidermis. Some of the papillae contain looped capillaries; others contain terminations of nerve fibers called *tactile corpuscles.*

The *reticular layer* of the skin contains fat cells, blood and lymph vessels, sweat and oil glands, hair follicles, and nerve endings.

The **subcutaneous** (sub-kyou-**TAY**-nee-us) **tissue** (subcutis) is regarded as a continuation of the dermis. The subcutaneous tissue is continuous with the superficial fascia, which connects the skin with the underlying structures. It varies in thickness according to the age, sex, and general health of the person. Fatty (adipose) tissue gives smoothness and contour to the body, provides a reservoir for fuel and energy, and serves as a protective cushion for the upper skin layers.

subcutaneous tissue is regarded as a continuation of the dermis.

Nutrition and the Skin

Blood and lymph supply nutrients to the skin. As much as one half of the total blood supply of the body is distributed to the skin. Blood and lymph, as they circulate through the skin, contribute certain materials for growth, nourishment, and repair of skin, hair, and nails. In the subcutaneous tissue are found networks of arteries and lymphatics, which send their smaller branches to hair papillae, hair follicles, and the glands of the skin. Capillaries are quite numerous in the skin.

Aging Skin

As people age, the collagen and elastin network of the skin tends to lose its elasticity, causing the skin to become less firm and supple. With age, the deeper or dermal layer of the skin undergoes changes. The sebaceous glands produce less sebum to moisturize the skin. The skin becomes thinner, drier, and more prone to growths. It can become lined and crepe-like. Swelling (edema) of tissues can appear around and under the eyes. Pliability of the skin depends on elasticity of the fibers of the dermis. For example, after expansion, healthy skin regains its former shape almost immediately.

Structural Changes of the Skin

Because the skin is the covering for the entire body, its condition must be taken into consideration before massage treatment is given. The skin can be sensitive to touch, or it can show signs of damage owing to disease or injury. The massage practitioner must be aware of any skin condition that might require the attention of the client's physician. Freckles, birthmarks (port-wine stains), and the like present no problem; however, a lesion or any discontinuity of tissue should be reported to the client and referred to a physician before the client receives a massage.

Healthy skin is slightly moist, soft, flexible, and slightly acidic. The texture of skin, revealed by feel and appearance, should be smooth and fine grained. The color of the skin depends partly on the blood supply but more on the coloring matter called melanin. Skin pigment varies in different people and is determined by genetics. Regardless of native pigmentation, healthy skin is of good color. An overly pale, ashy, reddish, or yellow cast to the skin can indicate health problems.

Massage benefits the skin by improving circulation of the blood, which carries nutrients to the cells.

The Appendages Associated with the Skin

Glands of the Skin

The skin contains two types of duct glands (exocrine glands) that extract materials from the blood to form new substances. These are the *sudoriferous* (soo-du-**RIF**-er-us; sweat) glands and *sebaceous* (see-**BAY**-shus; oil) glands. Sebaceous glands connect to the hair follicles and produce sebum, which, when secreted, lubricates and moisturizes the skin. Sweat glands are under the control of the autonomic nervous system and are located in the dermis. They consist of a coiled base or fundus and a tubelike duct that terminates at the surface of the skin to form a sweat pore. Practically all parts of the body are supplied with sweat glands, but they are more abundant in the armpits, soles of the feet, palms of the hands, and forehead. The activity of the sweat glands is greatly increased by heat, exercise, and mental excitement (Figure 5-16).

The sudoriferous glands respond to elevated body temperatures resulting from environmental conditions or physical activity. Sweating is an important physiologic process. As the moisture evaporates, it has a cooling effect on the body. The tubular extensions of these glands open at the body surface as a pore. Fluid secreted by the *eccrine* glands is mostly water and contains some bodily wastes, such as lactic acid, ammonia, urea, and uric acid; therefore, the skin acts in some degree as an organ of excretion.

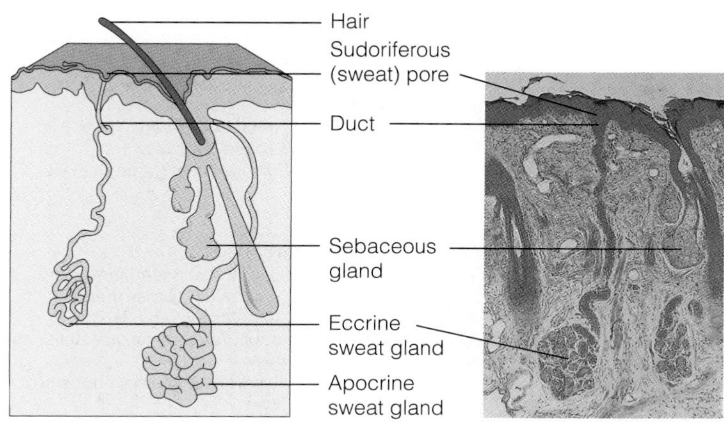

FIGURE 5-16 Sebaceous and sudoriferous glands.

The Hair and Nails

Hair and nails are appendages of the skin. They are composed of hard keratin, a protein that, in its soft form, is found in skin. Hard keratin, as found in hair, has a sulfur content of 4 to 8 percent and a lower moisture and fat content than soft keratin and is a particularly tough, elastic material. It forms continuous sheets (fingernails) or long fibers (hair). Soft keratin contains about 2 percent sulfur, 50 percent moisture, and a small percentage of fats. In the epidermis, keratin occurs as flattened cells or dry scales (Figures 5-17 and 5-18).

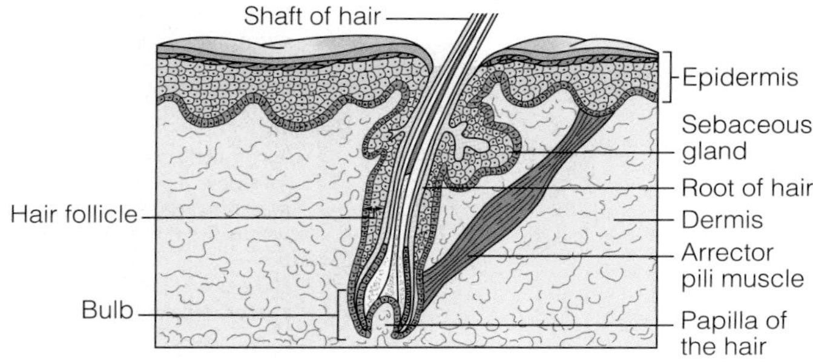

FIGURE 5-17 Hair follicle.

Hair grows over the entire body, with the exception of the palms of the hands, soles of the feet, some areas of the genitalia, the mucous membranes of the lips, the nipples, the navel, and the eyelids. The heavier concentration of hair is on the head, under the armpits, on and around the genitals, and on the arms and legs. A person's genes strongly influence the distribution of hair, its thickness, quality, color, and rate of growth, and whether it is curly or straight.

Each hair develops from a tubelike depression (hair follicle) that extends through the epidermis, into and through the dermis, and into the subcutaneous layer. As epidermal cells at the base of the follicle are nourished by the blood supply, they divide and push up through the hair follicle, die, and keratinize, becoming a shaft of hair.

Associated with hair follicles are sebaceous (oil) glands and arrector pili (a-**REK**-tor **PIGH**-ligh) muscles. The arrector pili muscles are fanlike muscles connected to the base of the follicle and positioned in such a way that they contract in reaction to cold or emotional stimuli. This reaction often results in a condition called *goose bumps* because the skin appears bumpy, like that of a plucked goose.

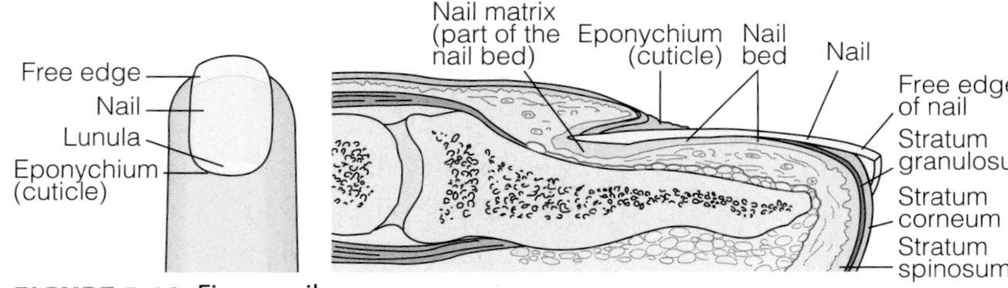

FIGURE 5-18 Fingernail.

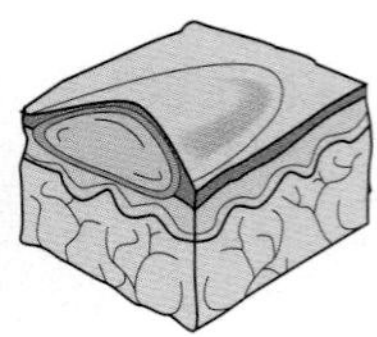

Bulla:
Same as a vesicle only greater than 0.5 cm
Example:
Contact dermatitis, large second-degree burns, bulbous impetigo, pemphigus

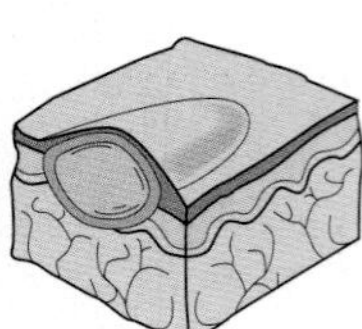

Tubercle:
Solid and elevated; however, it extends deeper than papules into the dermis or subcutaneous tissues, 0.5-2 cm
Example:
Lipoma, erythema, nodosum, cyst

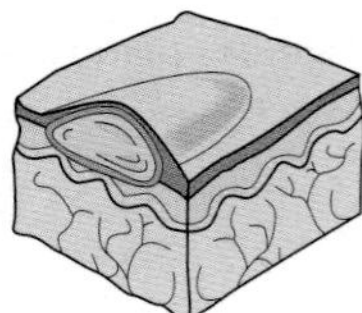

Pustule:
Vesicles or bullae that become filled with pus, usually described as less than 0.5 cm in diameter
Example:
Acne, impetigo, furuncles, carbuncles, folliculitis

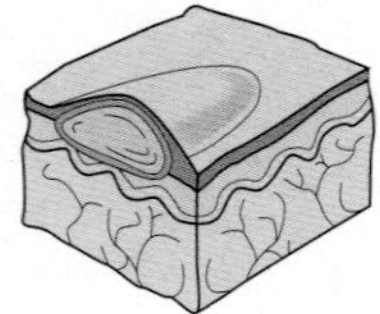

Vesicle:
Accumulation of fluid between the upper layers of the skin; elevated mass containing serous fluid; less than 0.5 cm
Example:
Herpes simplex, herpes zoster, chickenpox

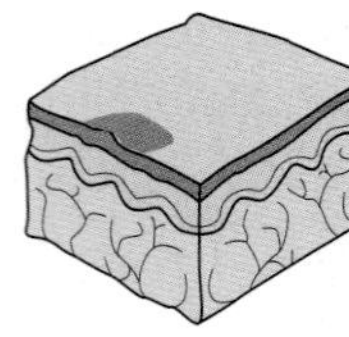

Macule:
Localized changes in skin color of less than 1 cm in diameter
Example:
Freckle

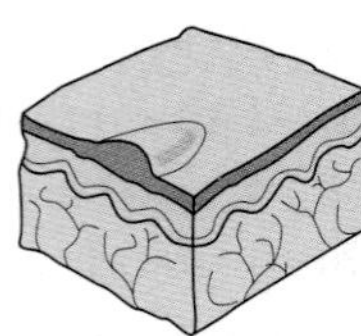

Papule:
Solid, elevated lesion less than 0.5 cm in diameter
Example:
Warts, elevated nevi

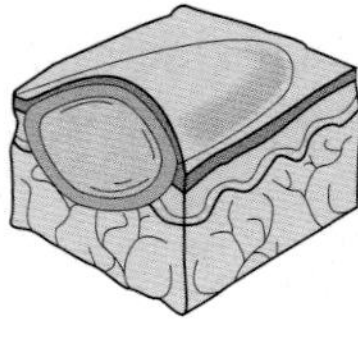

Tumor:
The same as a nodule only greater than 2 cm
Example:
Carcinoma (such as advanced breast carcinoma); **not** basal cell or squamous cell of the skin

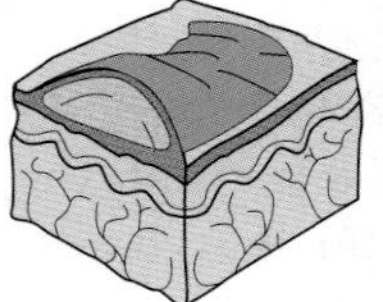

Wheal:
Localized edema in the epidermis causing irregular elevation that may be red or pale
Example:
Insect bite or a hive

FIGURE 5-19A Skin lesions (primary).

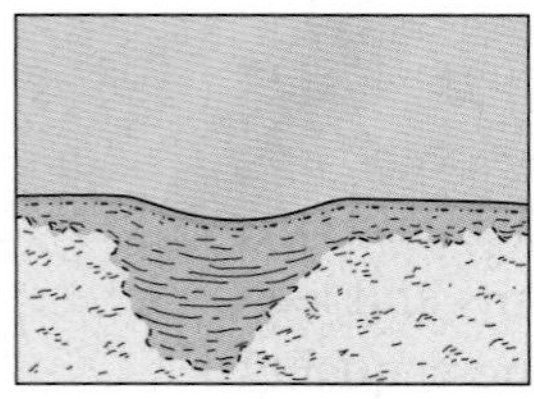

Scar

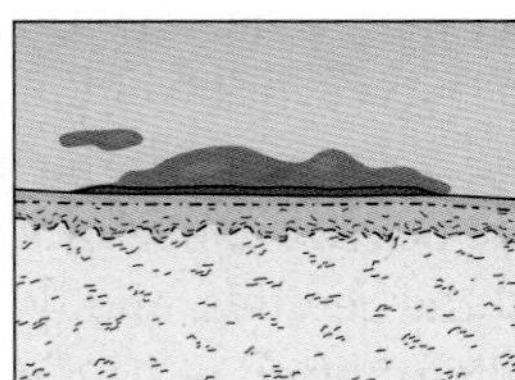

Crust

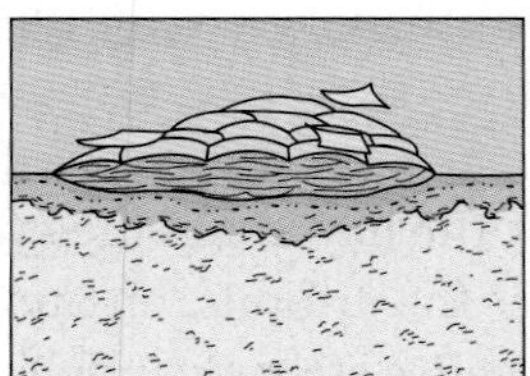

Scale

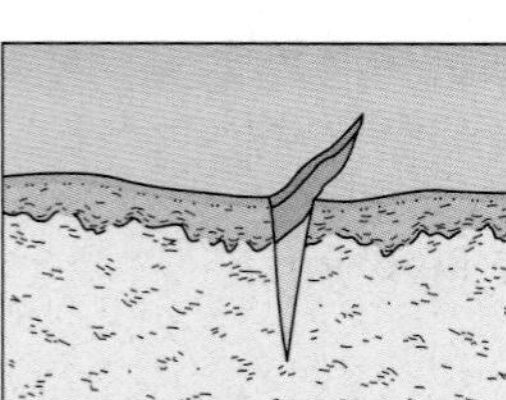

Fissure

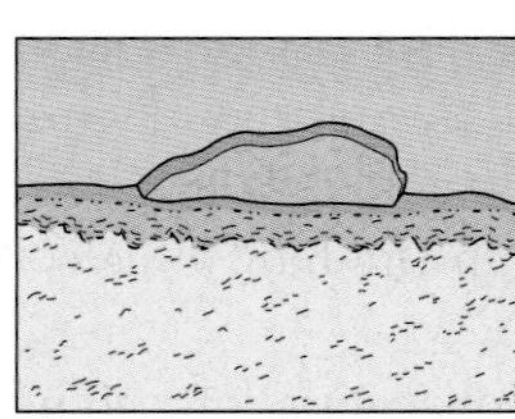

Excoriation

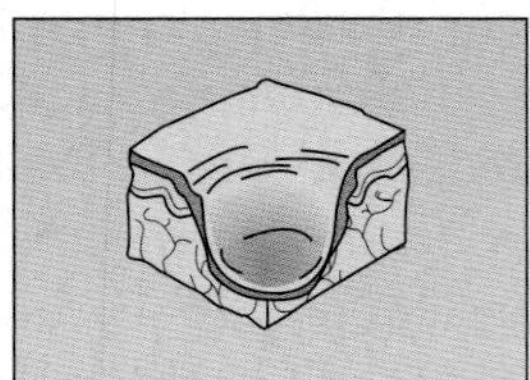

Ulcer

FIGURE 5-19B Skin lesions (secondary).

Lesions of the Skin

A *lesion* is a structural change in the tissues caused by injury or disease. There are three types: primary, secondary, and tertiary. Knowing how to identify the principal skin lesions helps the practitioner to avoid affected areas. The client should be advised to seek medical attention for any suspicious lesions.

Definitions Pertaining to Primary Lesions (Figure 5-19a)

Bulla: A blister containing a watery fluid, similar to a vesicle, but larger (example: contact dermititis, large second-degree burns, bulbous impetigo, or pemphigus)

Macule: A small, discolored spot or patch on the surface of the skin, neither raised nor sunken, such as freckles

Papule: A small, elevated pimple in the skin, containing fluid, but which can develop pus (examples: warts or elevated nevi)

Pustule: An elevation of the skin having an inflamed base, containing pus (examples: acne, impetigo, furuncles, carbuncles, or folliculitis)

Tubercle: A solid lump larger than a papule. It projects above the surface or lies within or under the skin. It varies in size from a pea to a hickory nut (examples: lipoma, erythema nodosum, or cyst).

Tumor: An external swelling, varying in size, shape, and color, such as carcinoma

Vesicle: A blister with clear fluid in it, vesicles lie within or just beneath the epidermis (example: poison ivy, herpes, or chickenpox)

Wheal: An itchy, swollen lesion that lasts only a few hours (examples: hives, or the bite of an insect, such as a mosquito)

Definitions Pertaining to Secondary Lesions

The secondary skin lesions are those in the skin that develop as a result of injury, from external conditions or in the later stages of disease (Figure 5-19b).

Crust: An accumulation of serum and pus, mixed perhaps with epidermal material (example: the scab on a sore)

Excoriation: A skin sore or abrasion produced by scratching or scraping (example: a raw surface due to the loss of the superficial skin after an injury)

Fissure: A crack in the skin penetrating into the derma, as in the case of chapped hands or lips

Scale: An accumulation of epidermal flakes, dry or greasy (example: abnormal or excessive dandruff)

Scar (cicatrix; **SICK**-ay-trix): Likely to form after the healing of an injury or skin condition that has penetrated the dermal layer

Stain: An abnormal discoloration remaining after the disappearance of moles, freckles, or liver spots, sometimes apparent after certain diseases

Ulcer: An open lesion on the skin or mucous membrane of the body, accompanied by pus and loss of skin depth

Disorders of the Skin

Problem, Blemished Skin

It is outside the scope of practice of massage therapists to diagnose or treat skin disorders, but they should be able to recognize some of the more common conditions to explain to the client why massage should or should not be given. The practitioner can suggest or recommend that the client see a dermatologist for skin conditions that are contraindications for massage.

Blackheads (comedones) are small masses of hardened, discolored sebum that appear most frequently on the face, shoulders, chest, and back. Blackheads are often accompanied by pimples during adolescence and are primarily caused by overstimulated sebaceous glands. Proper cleansing of the skin helps to reduce the skin's oiliness. Any case of excessive pimples or blackheads should be treated by a dermatologist.

Massage can be given to someone who has blackheads; however, massage should not be given over areas where these skin conditions are more severe. Stimulation of blood circulation is beneficial, and massage, exercise, and proper diet will, in most cases, improve these conditions.

A client can have a condition of the skin known as *staphylodermatitis,* an inflammation caused by staphylococci, bacteria that are generally found in milk and other dairy products. Massage should not be given when the skin is inflamed. The client should have the condition diagnosed by a physician.

A *bruise* is a superficial injury (contusion) generally caused by a blow or impact with some object; although the skin is not broken, the blow causes a reddish-blue or purple discoloration. Massage can be done above and below a bruise or contusion but not directly over the injured area.

Acne is a chronic inflammatory disorder of the skin, usually related to hormonal changes and overactive sebaceous glands during adolescence. Common acne is also known as *acne simplex* or *acne vulgaris.* Although acne generally starts at the onset of puberty, it also afflicts adult men and women.

Modern studies show that acne is often due to heredity, but the condition can be aggravated by emotional stress and environmental factors. A well-balanced diet, drinking plenty of water, and developing healthful personal hygiene are recommended. Acne can be present on the back, chest, and shoulders. Acne can be accompanied by blackheads, pustules, and pimples that are red, swollen, and contain pus. In more advanced cases of acne, cysts (which are red, swollen lumps beneath the surface of the skin) appear. Massage should be avoided when severe acne is present.

Seborrhea (seb-o-**REE**-uh) is a skin condition caused by overactivity and excessive secretion of the sebaceous glands. An oily or shiny condition of the nose, forehead, or scalp indicates the presence of seborrhea. It is readily detected on the scalp by the unusual amount of oil on the hair. Seborrhea is often the basis of an acne condition. Massage should not be given over infected areas.

Rosacea (ro-**ZAY**-shee-uh) is associated with excessive oiliness of the skin and a chronic inflammatory condition of the cheeks and nose. It is characterized by redness owing to dilation of blood vessels and the formation of papules and pustules. The skin becomes coarse, and the pores enlarged. Rosacea is usually caused by an inability to digest certain foods and an intolerance to strong beverages. It can also be caused by overexposure to extreme climate, faulty elimination, and hyperacidity. Massage is not given over affected areas.

A *steatoma* (stee-uh-**TOE**-muh) or *sebaceous cyst* is a subcutaneous tumor of the sebaceous glands that contains sebum. It usually appears as a small growth on the scalp, neck, or back. A steatoma is sometimes called a *wen.* Massage is not given over the affected area.

Asteatosis (as-tee-uh-**TOE**-sis) is a condition of dry, scaly skin, characterized by absolute or partial deficiency of sebum, usually due to aging or bodily disorders. In local conditions, such as scaling of the hands, it can be caused by alkalis in soaps and similar products. If the skin is unbroken, a mild lubricant can be massaged into the skin.

Impetigo is an acute, highly contagious, bacterial skin infection that is most common in children. It begins as an itchy, reddish discoloration that develops into pustules that form into a yellowish crust. Massage is contraindicated, and the client should be referred to a doctor for treatment.

A *furuncle* (**FYOU**-rung-kl), or *boil*, is caused by bacteria that enter the skin through the hair follicles. It is a subcutaneous abscess that fills with pus. A boil can be painful if neglected and should be treated by a physician.

A *carbuncle* is a mass of connected boils. Massage on the area is avoided, and the client should be referred to a doctor.

Warts are caused by the papillomavirus and are classified as common, plantar, and venereal. *Common warts* have a raised, rough surface and are generally found on the hands. *Plantar warts,* generally found on the soles of the feet, grow inward and are often painful and hard to remove. All warts are contagious. Avoid touching them, and wash your hands after making any contact.

Corns are cone-shaped areas on or between the toes caused by pressure or friction. They are not contagious but are sometimes painful to touch or pressure.

A *keratoma* (ker-a-**TOE**-muh), or callus, is a superficial, thickened patch of epidermis caused by friction on the hands and feet. This condition is usually treated by a podiatrist.

Fungal conditions such as *ringworm* and *athlete's foot* thrive in moist environments but respond well to antifungal preparations. Avoid using lubricants near the infected area, and wash hands thoroughly, because the fungus can be transmitted by contact.

Decubitus ulcers (pressure sores or bedsores) are caused by a persistent pressure against the skin, usually in the area of a bony projection. The pressure causes a lack of circulation to the skin and underlying tissues. The lack of blood supply, oxygen, and nutrition causes tissue necrosis. The cells die, and an ulcer forms. Pressure sores are a concern for people who are bedridden who do not turn enough, people who use wheelchairs and do not shift their weight enough, and people who must wear casts or braces that do not fit properly. Degrees of pressure sores vary from a persistent red spot to crusted or broken skin to an open wound that can penetrate clear to the bone. Massage is contraindicated over open decubitus ulcers; however, massage to increase circulation over areas that are prone to pressure sores can help to prevent them from ever forming.

decubitus ulcers are bedsores.

Skin Cancers and Tumors

The massage practitioner should not attempt to diagnose any kind of bump, lesion, ulceration, or discoloration as skin cancer but should be able to recognize serious skin disorders and suggest that the client seek medical attention without delay. A massage therapist has the best opportunity for a close-up inspection of a client's skin. If you notice a change in appearance or behavior of an existing skin blemish or suspect the appearance of a new one, bring it to the attention of the client or refer the client to a doctor.

There are three kinds of skin cancer. The least malignant and most common is called **basal cell carcinoma.** This type of cancer begins as a small raised nodule that develops a crusty plaque with a slightly elevated, whitish border. Another

basal cell carcinoma is a type of skin cancer.

Box 5.1

A-B-C-D-E Warning for Malignant Melanoma

Asymmetry of any pigmented lesion

Borders that are irregular, notched, or indistinct

Color that is widely variable (black, brown, red, blue, or white)

Diameter larger than a pencil eraser

Elevation or partial elevation from the skin level

variety of basal cell carcinoma appears on the body as a flat sore that does not heal properly. The sore can then develop a crust, shed that crust, and then form another. It is most common in light-skinned people over age 40 who have had excessive exposure to the sun. Basal cell carcinoma develops slowly and can be treated successfully with minor surgery or local applications of freezing. Massage is locally contraindicated on or near the lesion. If the lesions are located on the client's body, the massage therapist might be the first to notice them. The client should be referred to a dermatologist or other physician for diagnosis and treatment before any other massage is performed.

Squamous cell carcinoma is different in appearance from the basal type; it consists of scaly, red papules. Blood vessels are not visible. This cancer is more serious than the basal cell carcinoma because it can metastasize into deeper tissues and the lymph system and tends to spread more quickly than basal cell carcinomas. It can occur anywhere on the skin but is more common on the lips, ears, hands, and sun-exposed areas where the skin has had to repair irritated tissue repeatedly. As with basal cell carcinoma, squamous cell carcinoma is characterized by a sore or lesion that repeatedly crusts over but does not heal. Squamous cell carcinoma is usually successfully treated by freezing the lesions or with local surgical removal.

Massage is contraindicated for persons with squamous cell carcinoma. If a massage practitioner discovers a suspicious lesion, the client must be referred to a dermatologist immediately. A client who has been recently treated for squamous cell carcinoma should obtain an approval or release from his physician before receiving massage.

malignant melanoma is the most serious form of skin cancer.

The most serious but least common skin cancer is the **malignant melanoma**. This cancer is characterized by dark (brown, black, or discolored) patches on the skin. Early diagnosis of malignant melanoma is essential because it can metastasize quickly and can be fatal. Malignant melanoma often arises from an existing mole and can appear on any part of the body, so that it is important to recognize the signs or the A-B-C-D-E warning of this disease (see Box 5.1).

Malignant melanoma is a result of cumulative damage to melanocytes in the dermis from repeated exposure to the UV rays of the sun. Because melanoma tends to be so aggressive, the treatment is usually radical, including surgery, radiation, and removal of local lymph nodes. Survival depends on the successful removal of all cancerous cells before they spread to other organs or tissues through the lymph system. Because melanoma metastasizes through the lymph system, massage is contraindicated except in cases in which the patient is terminally ill and chooses to have massage for comfort and palliative care.

A **tumor** is an abnormal growth of swollen tissue that can be located on any part of the body. Some tumors are benign (mild in character) and are not likely to recur after removal, which means they are not harmful. These include moles, skin tags, and sebaceous cysts. Unless these begin to change shape or color, they are harmless. If they seem irritated, change color, or begin to grow they should be checked by a doctor. Some tumors are malignant and are more serious, as they can recur after removal. Tumors are removed by surgery, radiation therapy, or chemotherapy.

tumor

is an abnormal growth of swollen tissue that can be located on any part of the body.

Sexually Transmitted Diseases

Sexually transmitted diseases *(STDs),* also known as *venereal diseases*, or sexually transmitted infections, are those diseases associated with the sexual organs and are characterized by sores and rashes on the skin. STDs can become latent and appear at a later time. This can be dangerous because the affected person might not seek treatment. STDs can also affect unborn children.

sexually transmitted diseases

are associated with the sexual organs and are characterized by sores and rashes on the skin.

Syphilis (**SIF**-i-lis) is a serious disease that is transmitted by sexual contact with an infected person. When a sore first appears, especially one that is hard and ulcerated (with a hole in the center), a physician should be consulted. Without treatment, the sore might go away only to appear later in the form of a rash. This is called *secondary syphilis,* which can cause degeneration of various parts of the body and ultimately cause death. *Tertiary syphilis* can occur 1 to 50 years after the initial infection as tumor-like balls of infection that affect nearly any part of the anatomy, including the skeleton, heart, or brain.

syphilis

is a serious disease that is transmitted by sexual contact with an infected person.

Gonorrhea (gon-o-**REE**-uh) is a more common disease than syphilis and is characterized by a discharge and burning sensation when urinating. Women sometimes show no symptoms. If gonorrhea is left untreated, harmful bacteria can enter the bloodstream.

gonorrhea

is a venereal disease characterized by a discharge and burning sensation when urinating.

Herpes

Herpes simplex is a recurrent viral infection that is highly contagious and tends to lie dormant in its carrier until stress or a depressed immune system creates an outbreak. The acute phase of the infection is usually a tingling or burning sensation, followed by an outbreak of an oozing blister or blisters that scab over after a few days. An outbreak can last two to three weeks between the first signs and healing of the blisters. There are several strains of the herpes virus. *Type I* generally affects the face, around and sometimes inside the mouth with what are commonly called *cold sores* or *fever blisters.*

herpes

is a virus that affects the mouth, skin, and other facial parts, commonly called cold sores and fever blisters.

Herpes simplex Type II or genital herpes outbreaks generally occur on the genitals, buttocks, or inner thigh. *Herpes whitlow* is a rarer variety, with the outbreaks occurring around the nail beds of the fingers. The virus is transmitted from the site of the outbreak by skin-to-skin contact. Each of these forms of herpes is very contagious in its acute phase and is at least a local contraindication for massage. Because the virus is quite virulent and can exist outside of its host, linens used with clients who have an acute outbreak of herpes should be isolated and washed in hot water with a cup of bleach added to the wash and dried in a hot dryer. Face rests must be sanitized between clients if there is any sign of herpes, to prevent infecting other clients. Practitioners with active fever blisters must take extra precaution to ensure that no client is at risk. This might mean refraining from practicing massage during the acute phase of the outbreak, and thorough hand washing and not touching the infected area during the subacute phase. When herpes is in its latent state, with no symptoms, massage is not contraindicated.

shingles

is an acute inflammation of a nerve trunk by the herpes varicella-zoster virus.

Herpes zoster, or **shingles**, is a very painful viral infection of the nervous system that is caused by the chickenpox virus. Shingles is characterized by pain in a particular dermatome, usually of the intercostal nerves, followed and accompanied by watery blisters. The pain and blisters are usually isolated to a portion of the affected dermatome and only on one side of the body. Unlike herpes simplex, herpes zoster does not seem to be particularly contagious. Generally, a person with this painful condition will not seek massage. In milder cases, massage is locally contraindicated, depending on the tolerance of the client. When the pain has subsided and the blisters have healed, massage is appropriate.

Allergies

An *allergy* is a sensitivity that certain persons develop to normally harmless substances. Contact with certain types of cosmetics, medicines, and hair preparations or consumption of certain foods can result in an itching skin eruption, accompanied by redness, swelling, blisters, oozing, and scaling. Many allergies are accompanied by headaches, congestion, or emotional inconsistency.

Millions of people suffer from various forms of allergies. Allergic dermatitis (eczema), one of the more common allergies, can be caused by several different factors: food, substances in the air, or materials that the person uses. Many objects, including necklaces, rings, hairpins, and bracelets, contain metals (e.g., nickel) that cause dermatitis. Hair dyes, makeup, and chemicals are a few of the substances to which some people are allergic.

Dermatitis (der-ma-**TIE**-tis) is an inflammatory condition of the skin. The lesions come in various forms, such as scales, vesicles, or papules.

Eczema (**EG**-ze-muh), an inflammation of the skin, either acute or chronic in nature, can appear in many forms of dry or moist lesions. The term *eczema* is applied to any number of surface lesions. It is usually a red, blistered, oozing area that itches painfully. Eczema can be the result of some type of allergy or internal disorder, and the client should be referred to a physician for treatment.

Contact dermatitis refers to abnormal conditions resulting from contact with chemicals or other exterior agents. Some people develop allergies to ingredients in some substances with which they work—for instance, when a cosmetologist becomes allergic to hair tints.

The appropriateness of massage in cases of dermatitis and eczema is dependent on the causes and extent of the inflammation. If blisters or other skin lesions are present, massage is locally contraindicated. Skin that is irritated, hot, red, and puffy contraindicates massage until the inflammation has subsided. If the irritation is minor and isolated, however, questioning the client might indicate the cause, and general massage might be appropriate.

Psoriasis (so-**RYE**-a-sis) is a common chronic inflammatory skin disease, the cause of which is unknown. It is usually found on the scalp, elbows, knees, chest, and lower back, but rarely on the face. The lesions are round dry patches covered with coarse, silvery scales. If the lesions become irritated, bleeding points can occur. Although not contagious, psoriasis can be spread by irritation. Massage over such a condition should be avoided.

Urticaria (hives) are red, raised lesions or wheals accompanied by severe itching, caused by an allergic or emotional reaction. The condition is not contagious, but the area should be avoided when doing massage.

Pigmentations of the Skin

Changes in skin color are observed in various skin disorders and in many systemic disorders. Certain drugs taken internally can affect pigmentation. Foods eaten in excess can affect the skin; the carotene in carrots is an example. A suntan is an example of external changes in the pigmentation of the skin. The fairer the skin, the easier it is to sunburn and the more difficult it is to acquire an even suntan.

Generally, a skin that tans easily is not sensitive to massage. Skin that has been overexposed can become sensitive, however. When there is sunburn or peeling from sunburn, massage can be painful.

Lentigines (len-**TIJ**-i-neez), or freckles, are small yellowish to brownish color spots on parts exposed to sunlight and air.

Stains are abnormal brown skin patches, having circular or irregular shapes. Their permanent color is due to the presence of blood pigment. They occur during aging, after certain diseases, and after the disappearance of moles, freckles, and liver spots. The cause of these stains is unknown.

Chloasma (klo-**AZ**-muh) is characterized by increased deposits of pigment in the skin. It is found mainly on the forehead, nose, and cheeks. Chloasma is also called *moth patches* or *liver spots.*

A *nevus,* commonly known as a birthmark, is a small or large discoloration of the skin from pigmentation or dilated capillaries and is present on the skin at birth. Generally, such colored spots or areas are not affected by massage.

Leukoderma (loo-ko-**DER**-muh) are abnormal light patches of skin, caused by congenital defective pigmentations. *Vitiligo* (vit-i-**LYE**-go) is an acquired condition of leukoderma that affects skin or hair.

Albinism (**AL**-bin-izm) is a congenital absence of melanin pigment in the body that affects the color of the skin, hair, and eyes. In albinos the hair is silky and white, and the skin is pinkish white and does not tan.

Changes of the skin, such as a crack on the skin, a type of thickening, or any discoloration, ranging from shades of red to brown and purple to almost black, can be danger signals, and should be examined by a dermatologist.

SECTION QUESTIONS FOR DISCUSSION AND REVIEW

1. What is the integumentary system?
2. Name the major functions of the skin.
3. Name the two main layers of the skin.
4. Name the layers of the epidermis.
5. Name two forms of keratin and where they are found in most abundance.
6. What is subcutaneous tissue?

7. How does the skin receive its color?
8. Name the layers of the dermis.
9. What is a gland?
10. Name the two major glands found in the skin and give the function of each.
11. Define the following: sebum, duct.
12. Name the appendages of the skin.
13. What is a lesion?
14. Which kind of skin condition is contact dermatitis?
15. Why is it important for the massage practitioner to observe a client's skin condition?

epiphysis

is an enlarged area on the ends of long bones that articulates with other bones.

articular cartilage

is a layer of hyaline cartilage covering the end surface of the epiphysis.

diaphysis

is the bone shaft between the epiphyses.

periosteum

is a fibrous membrane that functions to protect the bone and serves as an attachment of tendons and ligaments.

SYSTEM 2 THE SKELETAL SYSTEM

The skeletal system is the bony framework of the body. It is composed of bones, cartilage, and ligaments. The skeletal system has five main functions:

1. To offer a framework that supports body structures and gives shape to the body
2. To protect delicate internal organs and tissues
3. To provide attachments for muscles and act as levers in conjunction with muscles to produce movement
4. To manufacture blood cells in the red bone marrow
5. To store minerals such as calcium phosphate, calcium carbonate, magnesium, and sodium

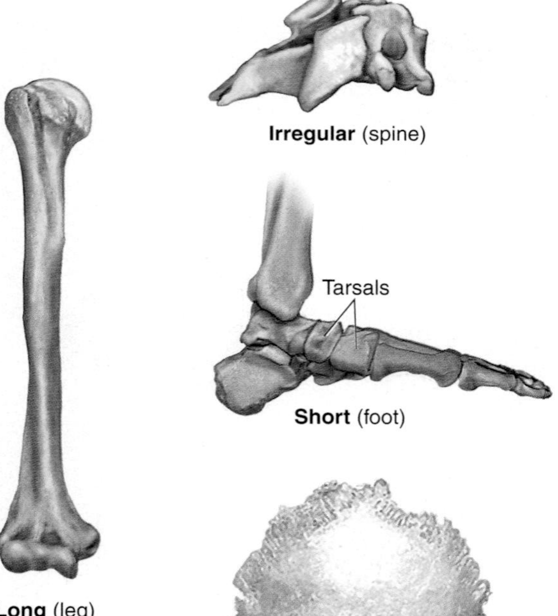

FIGURE 5-20 Bone shapes.

Composition of Bones

Other than dentin—the dense hard tissue that forms the body of a tooth—bone is the hardest structure of the body. Despite its solid and inert appearance, bone is a complex and ever-changing organ. Bone is composed of approximately one-third animal matter and two-thirds mineral or earthy matter. The animal (organic) matter consists of bone cells (osteocytes), blood vessels, connective tissues, and marrow. The mineral (inorganic) matter consists mainly of calcium phosphate and calcium carbonate.

Bone Forms or Shapes

There are several forms or shapes of bones found in the human body (Figure 5-20), namely:

- Flat bones, such as those in the skull, pelvis, and ribs (costals)
- Long bones, such as those in the legs, arms, fingers, and toes
- Short bones, such as those in the carpals and tarsals
- Irregular bones, such as the vertebrae (spine)
- Sesamoid bones, such as the patella

Characteristics of Long Bones

A typical long bone (Figure 5-21) has enlarged areas on the ends, called the **epiphysis** (e-**PIF**-i-sis), which articulate with other bones. The end surface of the epiphysis is covered with a layer of hyaline cartilage called **articular cartilage**. The articular cartilage provides a smooth, shock-absorbing surface where two bones meet to form a joint. The shaft of the bone between the epiphysis is the **diaphysis** (die-**AF**-i-sis).

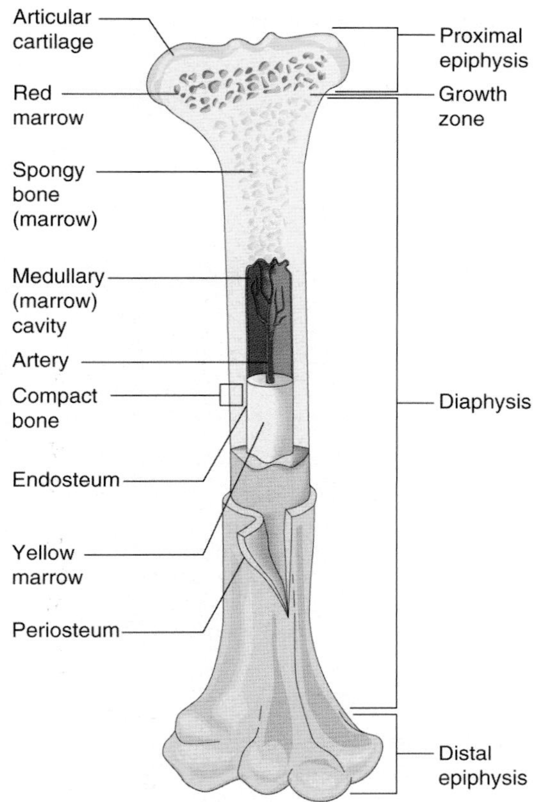

FIGURE 5-21 Structure of a long bone.

Except for articular cartilage, the bone is covered by the **periosteum** (per-ee-**OS**-tee-um). The periosteum is a fibrous membrane, the function of which is to protect the bone and serve as an attachment for tendons and ligaments. It contains an abundance of nerves, blood, and lymph vessels and is essential to bone nutrition and repair. Beneath the periosteum, the walls of the diaphysis are composed of **compact bone tissue**. Compact bone tissue forms the hard bone found in the shafts of long bones and along the outside of flat bones. This bone tissue is strong and rigid.

The inner portion of the bone is made up mostly of **cancellous bone**, also called *spongy bone*, which consists of irregularly shaped spaces defined by thin, bony plates called trabeculae. This provides a lightweight yet surprisingly strong interior structure to the bones. The cancellous bone tissue in the flat bones and at the ends of the long bones is filled with red bone marrow and is the site of production for blood cells. The **medullary cavity** is a hollow chamber formed in the shaft of long bones that is filled with yellow bone marrow.

Marrow is the connective tissue filling the cavities of bones. Its function is largely concerned with the formation of red and white blood cells. There are two types of bone marrow, *red* and *yellow* marrow. Red bone marrow functions in the production of red and white blood cells and platelets. It occupies nearly all of the bone cavities of the newborn; however, in the adult it is found in the bone spaces of the skull, ribs, sternum, vertebrae, and pelvis. Yellow marrow is the result of inactive blood-producing cells filling with fatty material and is located in the medullary cavity of the long bones. In some cases of severe blood loss, yellow marrow converts back to red marrow to increase the production of red blood cells.

compact bone tissue
forms the hard bone found in the shafts of long bones and along the outside of flat bones.

cancellous bone
located inside long bones and flat bones, consists of irregularly shaped spaces defined by thin, bony plates.

medullary cavity
is a hollow chamber formed in the shaft of long bones that is filled with yellow bone marrow.

marrow
is the connective tissue filling in the cavities of bones that forms red and white blood cells.

Bone Nutrition

Bone receives its nourishment through a highly organized system of blood vessels (capillaries) that make their way through the periosteum into the interior of bones. Bone marrow also aids in the nutrition of bone. For proper growth and hardening of bony structures, the diet should contain an adequate amount of calcium, phosphorus, and vitamin D.

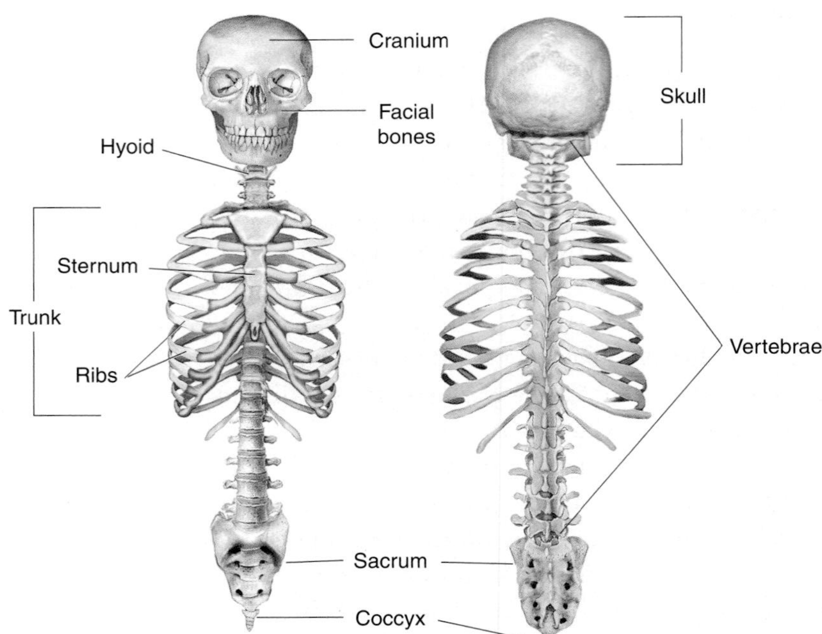

FIGURE 5-22 Axial skeleton.

axial skeleton

is made up of bones of the skull, thorax, vertebral column, and the hyoid bone.

appendicular skeleton

is made up of bones of the shoulder, upper extremities, hips, and lower extremities.

THE SKELETON AS A WHOLE

The skeleton is divided into two main parts: the **axial skeleton** and the **appendicular skeleton.** The cranial and facial bones of the skull, thorax, vertebral column, and the hyoid bone compose the axial skeleton (Figure 5-22). The appendicular skeleton is made up of bones of the shoulder, upper extremities, hips, and lower extremities. The name *appendicular* identifies these parts as appendages or extensions of the axis or axial skeleton.

In the human adult, the skeleton consists of 206 bones, distributed as follows (numbers in parentheses indicate the number of bones):

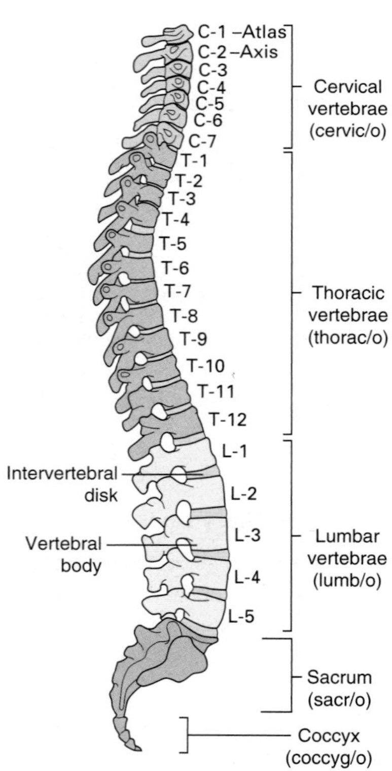

FIGURE 5-23 Vertebral column.

The Axial Skeleton

- **Cranium** (8)—forms a protective structure for the brain: frontal (1), parietal (2), occipital (1), temporal (2), sphenoid (1), ethmoid (1)
- **Face** (14)—forms the structure of the eyes, nose, cheeks, mouth, and jaws: maxilla (2), palatine (2), zygomatic (2), lacrimal (2), nasal (2), vomer (1), inferior nasal concha (2), mandible (1)
- **Ear** (6)—forms the internal structure of the ears: malleus (2), incus (2), stapes (2)
- **Hyoid bone** (1)—supports the base of the tongue
- **Vertebral column** (26)—forms the spinal column, which supports the head and the trunk, protects the spinal cord, and provides attachment for the ribs: cervical vertebrae (7), thoracic vertebrae (12), lumbar vertebrae (5), sacrum (1), coccyx (1)
- **Thoracic cage** (25):
  ribs (costals; 24)—forms a protective cage for the lungs and heart
  sternum (1)—serves as an attachment for the ribs at the front of the chest

The Appendicular Skeleton

- **Upper extremities** (64):
  clavicle (2), scapula (2), humerus (2), ulna (2), radius (2), carpals (16), metacarpals (10), phalanges (28)
- **Lower extremities** (66):
  pelvis (fusion of three bones: the ischium, pubis, and ilium) (6), femur (2), patella (2), tibia (2), fibula (2), tarsals (14), metatarsals (10), phalanges (28)

The form or outline of the bones must be carefully followed and the limitations of the range of movements considered when practicing massage therapy. Knowing the names of bones serves as a guide in recalling the names of related structures connected with the body part being massaged (Figures 5-23 to 5-27).

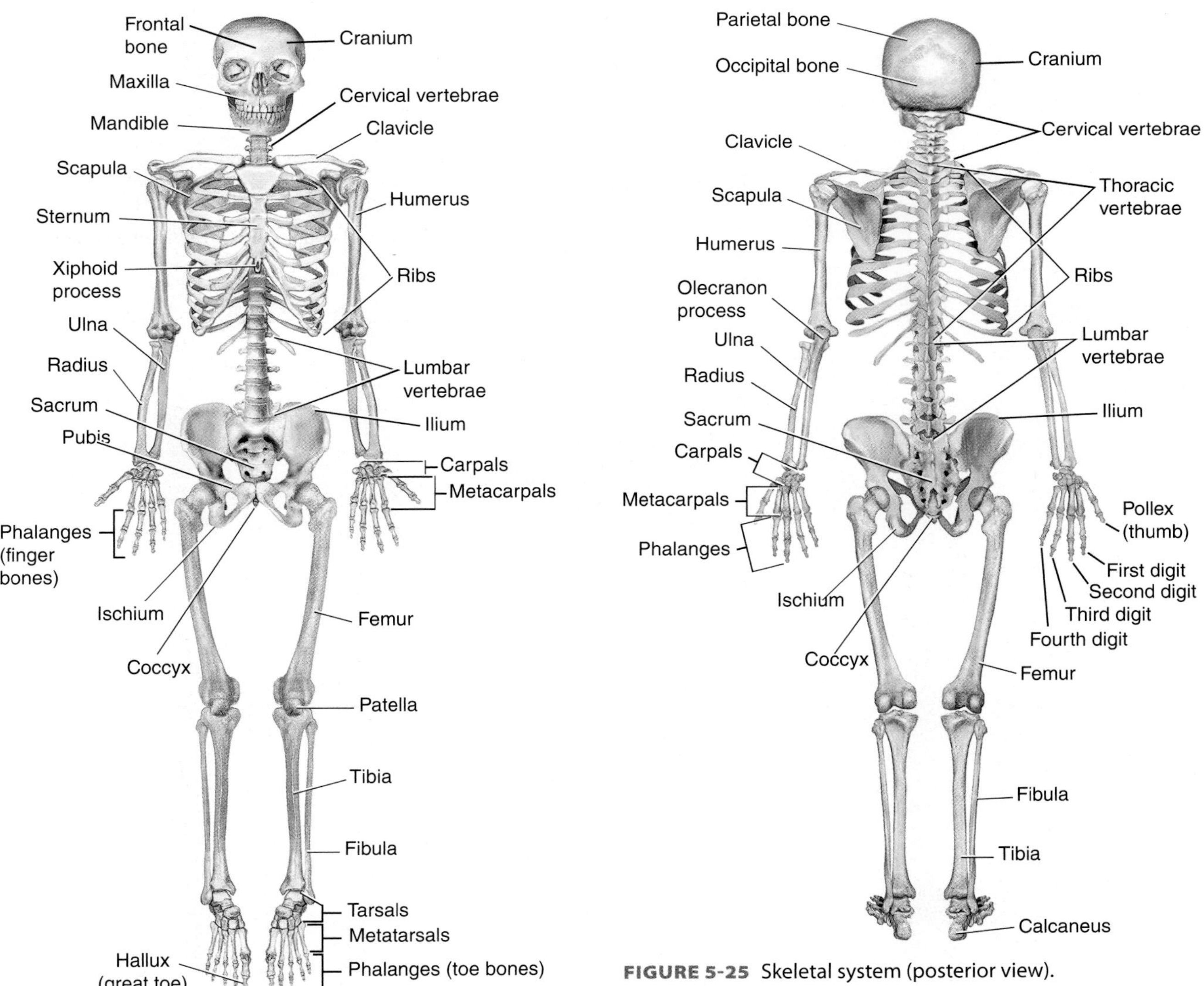

FIGURE 5-24 Skeletal system (anterior view).

FIGURE 5-25 Skeletal system (posterior view).

Labels for Bony Landmarks (Figure 5-26)

1. Medial malleolus; inside or medial "ankle bone."
2. Shaft of the tibia; "shin bone."
3. Tuberosity of the tibia; prominent bump inferior to the patella.
4. Patella; "kneecap."
5. Pubic arch; the middle is the pubic symphysis, the lateral portion (about one and one-half inch to each side of the symphysis) is the ramus of the pubic bone.
6. Styloid process of the ulna; small bump at the distal end of the ulna just proximal to the wrist.
7. Anterior superior iliac spine (ASIS); pointed bone at the front of the hip.
8. Styloid process of the radius; lateral process at the distal end of the radius.
9. Lateral epicondyle of the humerus; bump on outside of the elbow at the end of the humerus. Attachment of many of the wrist extensor muscles.

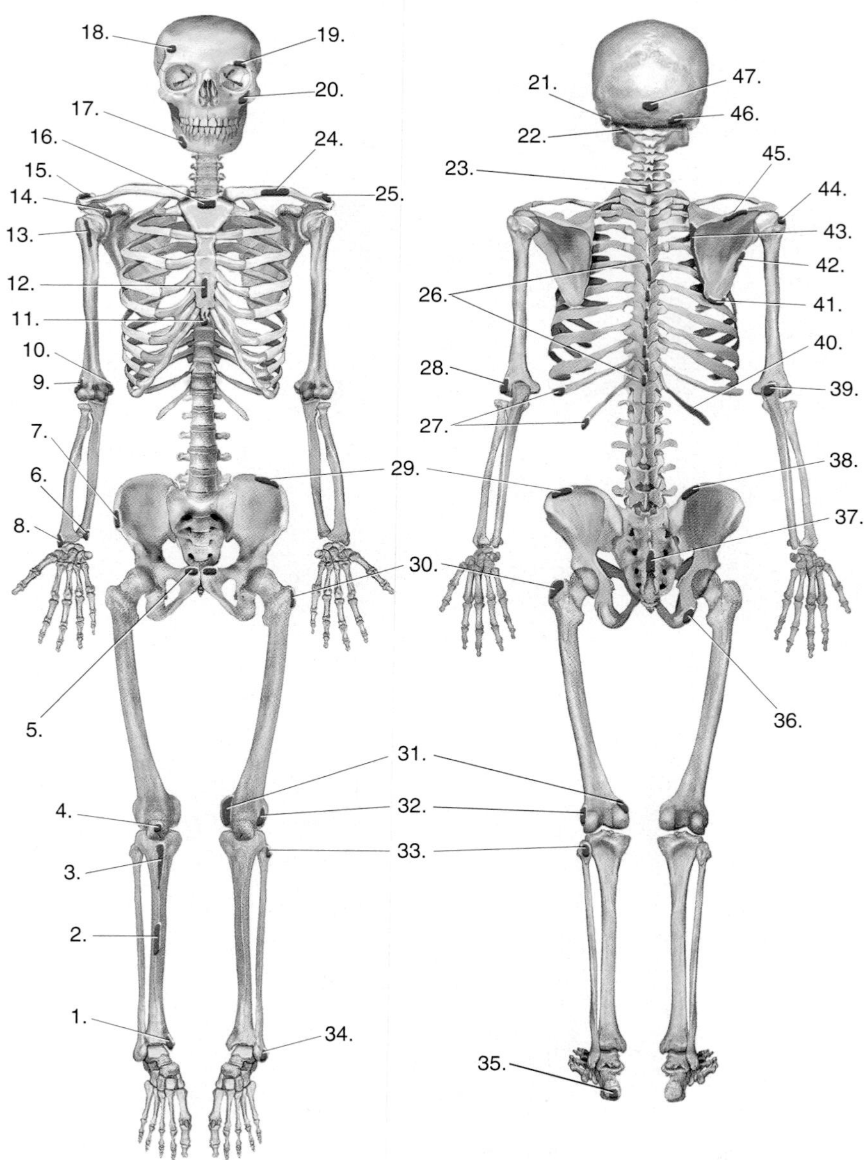

FIGURE 5-26 Major bony landmarks on the body.

10. Medial epicondyle of the humerus; bump on inside of elbow at the end of the humerus. Attachment of many of the wrist flexor muscles.
11. Xiphoid process; point at the inferior end of the sternum.
12. Sternum; breastbone, between ribs on the front of the chest.
13. Bicipital groove; groove between the greater and lesser tuberosity of the humerus, location of the tendon of the long head of the biceps muscle.
14. Coracoid process.
15. Cromioclavicular (AC)joint; joint between the acromion process of the scapula and the clavicle.
16. Sternal notch; hollow just superior to the sternum and between the heads of the clavicles.
17. Ramus of the mandible; point at the angle of the jawbone.
18. Frontal eminence; slight rise between the eyebrow and hairline.
19. Supraorbital ridge; upper part of eye socket, under the eyebrow.
20. Zygomatic bone; "cheekbone."
21. Mastoid process; bony point behind lower portion of the ear.
22. Transverse process of first cervical vertebra; just below and deeper than mastoid process.
23. Spinous process of the seventh cervical vertebra; topmost of the palpable spinous processes.
24. Clavicle; collarbone.
25. Acromion process; lateral point of the spine of the scapula.
26. Spinous processes of the vertebra.
27. Ends of the floating ribs.
28. Lateral epicondyle of the humerus; refer to #9.
29. Crest of the ilium; the "hip bone," also called the iliac crest.
30. Greater trochanter of the femur; bony knob at the top of the leg bone.
31. Medial epicondyle of the femur; bony enlargement on the inside of the knee.
32. Lateral epicondyle of the femur; bony enlargement on the outside of the knee.
33. Head of the fibula; bump on the outside of the leg just below the knee.
34. Lateral malleolus; outside or lateral ankle bone, distal end of the fibula.
35. Calcaneus; "heel bone."
36. Ischial tuberosity; "sit bone."
37. Distal end of sacrum; prominent bone at upper end of gluteal crease. (The coccyx or tailbone is located deep between the buttocks.)
38. Posterior superior iliac spine (PSIS); bony prominence of the low back at the posterior end of the iliac crest.
39. Olecranon process; point of the elbow at the proximal end of the ulna.
40. Twelfth rib; last rib.
41. Inferior angle of the scapula; lower tip of the scapula.
42. Axillary border of the scapula; lateral edge of the scapula from the interior angle to the "armpit."
43. Vertebral border of the scapula; medial edge of the scapula nearest the spine.
44. Greater tuberosity of the humerus; proximal prominence of the humerus.
45. Spine of the scapula; bony ridge on the posterior scapula.
46. Occipital ridge; lowest palpable bony ridge on the posterior skull.
47. Occipital protuberance; small bump on the posterior skull.

FIGURE 5-27 Cranium, neck, and face bones.

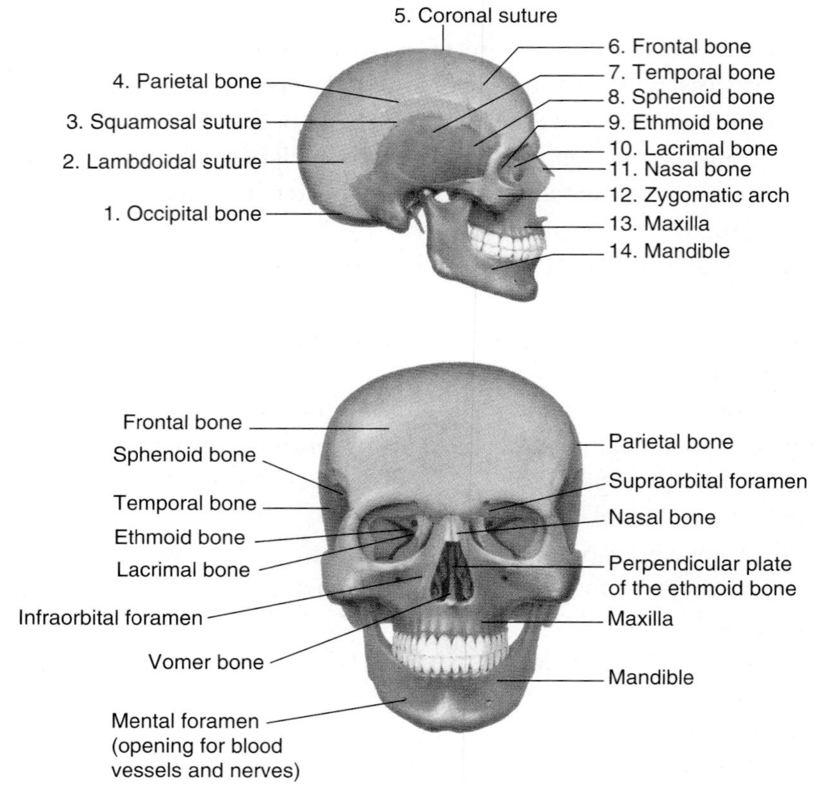

STUDENT ACTIVITY

Pair up with another student (or ask a friend) and palpate the major bony landmarks on his or her body. Name the landmarks as they are found. Exchanges places so your partner can locate the bony landmarks.

synovial membrane

is a connective tissue membrane lining cavities and capsules in and around joints that produce synovial fluid.

fibrous joints

have no space and are held together by fibrous connective tissue.

cartilaginous joints

are joints held together with cartilage with no joint cavity.

synovial joints

are freely movable joints with a joint cavity surrounded by an articular capsule.

Joints

The bones of the skeleton are connected at different parts of their surfaces. Such connections are called *joints* or *articulations.*

Joints are classified according to the amount of motion that they permit.

Synarthrotic (**SIN**-ar-thro-tic) *joints,* such as those in the skull, are essentially immovable.

Amphiarthrotic (**AM**-fee-ar-thro-tic) *joints* have limited motion. Examples are the symphysis pubis and sacroiliac joints.

Diarthrotic (**DIE**-ar-thro-tic) *joints* are freely movable. The articulating ends of the bones that meet at these joints are covered with hyaline cartilage called *articular cartilage.* A strong fibrous joint capsule surrounds the joint and is firmly attached to both bones. The outside of the capsule is constructed of ligaments that attach the bones; the inner surface or the lining of the capsule consists of **synovial membrane**, which secretes *synovial fluid* that lubricates the joint surfaces. Diarthrotic joints have a variety of shapes and are capable of several kinds of movements: pivot movement, as in turning the head; saddle movement, as in the thumb; ball and socket movement, as in the hip; and hinge movement, as in the knees (Figure 5-28).

Besides the functional classification of joints as discussed, joints are also classified according to their structure (Table 5.3). The structural classification of joints is based on the type of fibrous tissue that holds the joint together and the amount and quality of space between the articulating bones. Joints with no space that are held together by fibrous connective tissue are classified as **fibrous joints**. Joints held together with cartilage with no joint cavity are **cartilaginous joints**. **Synovial joints** do have a joint cavity that is surrounded by an articular capsule.

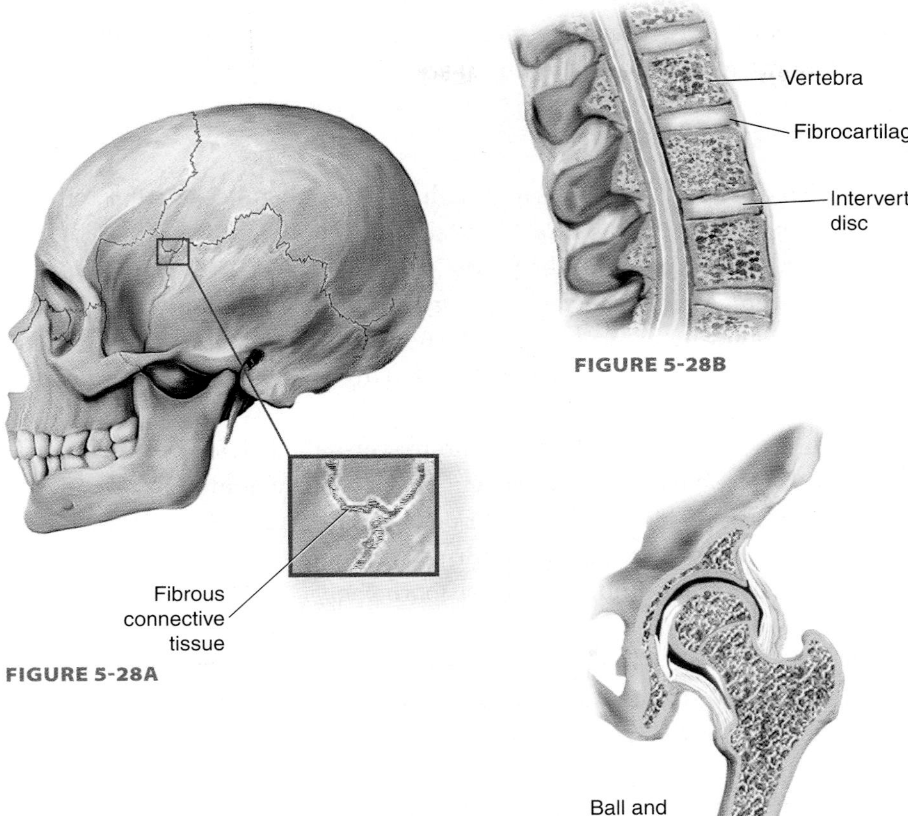

FIGURE 5-28A

FIGURE 5-28B

FIGURE 5-28C

FIGURE 5-28 Classification of joints: a. synarthrosis or immovable joint; b. amphiarthrosis or slightly movable joint; c. diarthrosis or freely movable joint.

TABLE 5.3

TYPES OF JOINTS BASED ON FUNCTIONAL AND STRUCTURAL CLASSIFICATION			
TYPE	CLASSIFICATION	DESCRIPTION	EXAMPLE
Suture	Immovable Fibrous	Bones separated by a thin fibrous layer	Found only in the sutures of the skull
Gomphosis	Immovable Fibrous	Cone-shaped peg fits in socket connecting bones with periodontal ligament	Roots of teeth in mandible and maxilla
Synchondrosis	Immovable Cartilaginous	Connecting material is hyaline cartilage	The junction between the epiphysis and the diaphysis of growing long bones
Syndesmosis	Slightly movable Fibrous	Bones held together with dense fibrous tissue	Distal ends of fibula and tibia
Symphysis	Slightly movable Cartilaginous	Connected by flat disc of fibrocartilage	Symphysis pubis and intervertebral joints
Pivot	Freely movable Synovial	Rounded bone rotates in a ring made of bone and ligament	Joint at proximal ends of radius and ulna and the joint between axis and atlas
Hinge	Freely movable Synovial	Allows movement only in one plane (i.e., flexion/extension)	Elbow, knee, interphalangeal joints
Ball and socket	Freely movable Synovial	Ball-like surface fits into cuplike socket	Hip and shoulder joint
Gliding	Freely movable Synovial	Flat articulating surfaces	Intertarsal and intercarpal joints
Saddle	Freely movable Synovial	Two saddle-shaped bones fit together	Joint between thumb metacarpal and wrist carpal (trapezium)
Condyloid Ellipsoid	Freely movable Synovial	Oval-shaped condyle fits into ellipsoidal socket	Joint between carpals and radius

Immovable joints (synarthroses) and slightly movable joints (amphiarthroses) are *fibrous* or *cartilaginous joints.* A distinguishing factor in freely movable joints (diarthroses) is that they are *synovial joints.*

Cartilage and Ligaments

Cartilage (also called *gristle*) is a firm, tough, elastic substance, similar to bone but without its mineral content. Cartilage serves the following purposes:

1. To cushion the bones at the joints
2. To prevent jarring between bones in motion, as in walking
3. To give shape to external features, such as the nose and ears

There are three types of cartilage, each having a slightly different makeup depending on their structural role:

- Hyaline cartilage, the most common, often called *articular cartilage,* caps the articulating surfaces of bones in synovial joints.
- Fibrocartilage contains a greater density of collagen fibers, is the toughest form of cartilage and forms amphiarthrotic, cartilaginous joints such as the pubic symphysis of the pelvis and the intervetebral disks of the spine.
- Elastic cartilage has a higher proportion of elastin fibers; this makes it more flexible. It is found in the structure of the external ear.

ligaments

are bands of fibrous tissue that connect bones to bones.

bursae

are fibrous sacks lined with synovial membrane and lubricated with synovial fluid, functioning as a cushion in areas of pressure.

Ligaments are bands or sheets of fibrous tissue that connect bone to bone and help to support the bones at the joints, as in the wrist and ankle.

Bursae (**BER**-suh) are fibrous sacks lined with synovial membrane and lubricated with synovial fluid. The purpose of the bursae is to function as a slippery cushion in areas where pressure is exerted, such as between bones and overlying muscle, tendons, or skin. Injury to bursae can cause inflammation and swelling and is called bursitis (ber-**SIGH**-tis). The *synovial fluid* is the lubricating fluid produced by the synovial membrane, the function of which is to prevent friction within the bursa and joint capsules.

Types of Movable Joints

The various types of movable joints found in the human body (Figure 5-29) are classified as follows:

- Pivot joints have an extension on one bone that rotates in relation to the bone it articulates with, such as in the neck between the atlas and the axis, or between the radius and ulna just distal to the elbow.
- Hinge joints move through one plane only, such as in the elbow, knees, and two distal joints of the fingers.
- Ball-and-socket joints permit the greatest range of movement. A bone with a ball-shaped head articulates in a socket-shaped depression, such as in the hips and shoulders.
- Gliding joints have nearly flat surfaces that glide across one another, such as in the spine or carpal and tarsal.
- Saddle joints involve bones with concave articulating surfaces, such as in the thumb.

Condyloid or ellipsoid joints have an oval-shaped end of one bone that articulates with an ellipsoid basin of another such as between the distal end of the radius and the trapezium at the wrist.

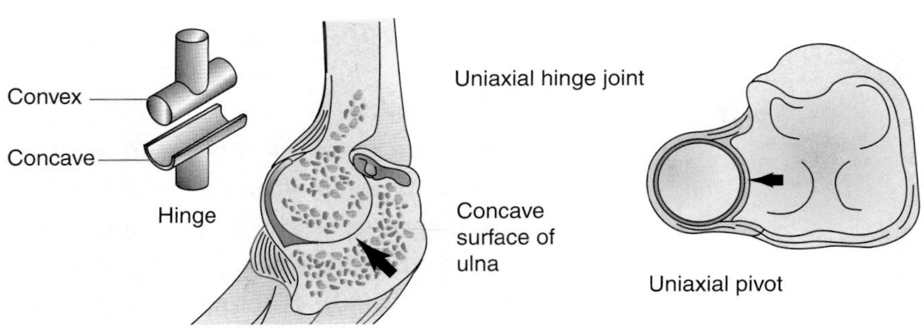

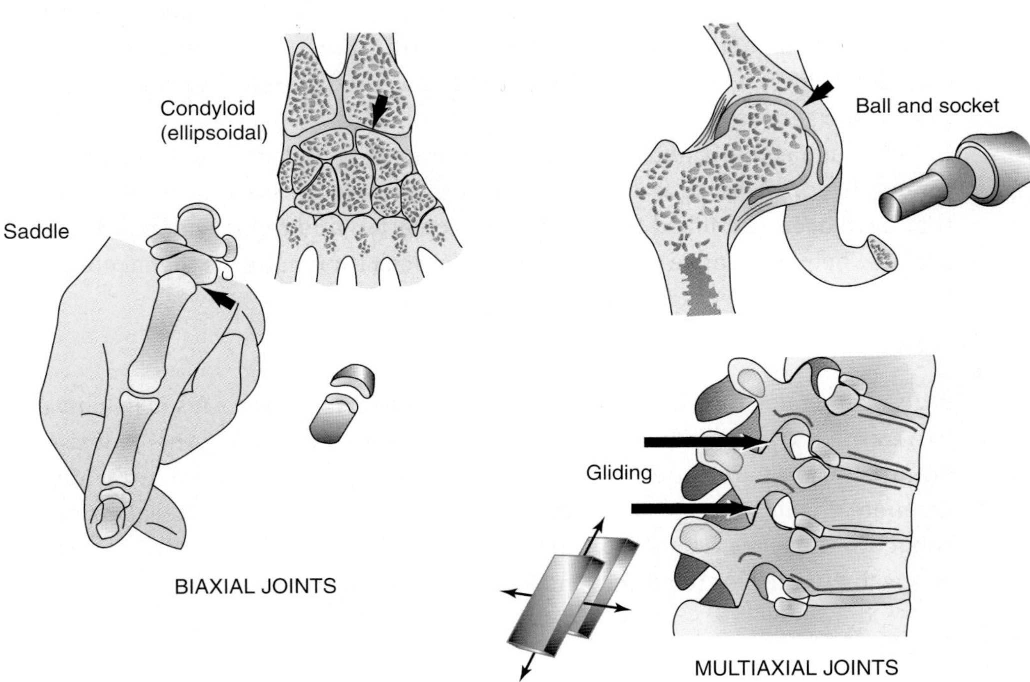

FIGURE 5-29 Types of movable joints.

Words That Describe Bone Structures

Condyle (**KON**-dil)	A rounded, knuckle-like prominence, usually at a point of articulation
Crest	A ridge
Foramen (fo-**RAY**-mun)	A hole
Fossa (**FOS**-uh)	A depression or hollow
Head	A rounded articulating process at the end of a bone
Line	A less prominent ridge of a bone than a crest
Meatus (**MEE**-ay-tus)	A tubelike passage
Process	A bony prominence or projection
Sinus or antrum	A cavity within a bone
Spine	A sharp, slender projection
Trochanter (**TRO**-kan-tur)	A large process for muscle attachment
Tubercle (**TEW**-bur-kul)	A small, rounded process
Tuberosity	A large, rounded process

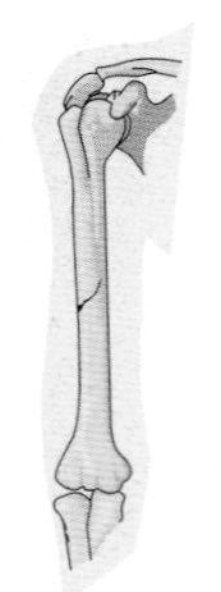
Incomplete (greenstick)

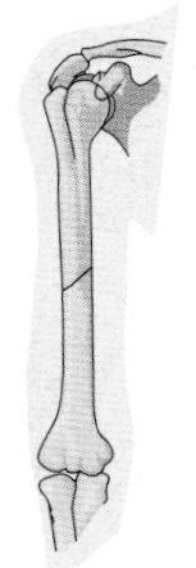
Closed or simple

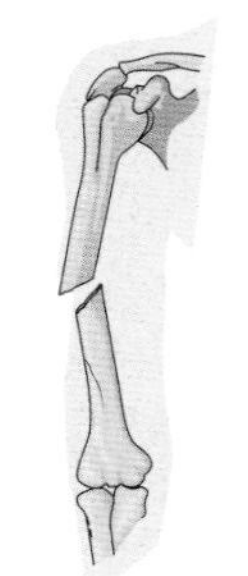
Open or compound

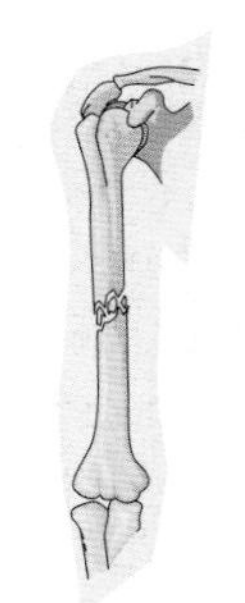
Comminuted

FIGURE 5-30 Types of fractures.

Skeletal and Joint Disorders

Fractures

A *fracture* is a break or rupture in a bone. There are several types of fractures classified according to the severity of the injury: simple or closed, compound or open, greenstick, comminuted, and spiral (Figure 5-30). Fractures are relatively easy to identify. Usually the result of a traumatic event, fractures are painful and limit the function of the associated joint. A decisive diagnosis is verified by x-ray or magnetic resonance imaging (MRI). Fractured bones usually heal completely after being immobilized by either a cast or surgically implanted pins, plates, and screws.

Massage is contraindicated for acute fractures that have not been set and immobilized. Massage is appropriate in the subacute stage around fractures that have been stabilized to encourage circulation and reduce edema. Massage can also help to balance the developing compensation patterns that accompany the restricted movement caused by the fracture.

Dislocation

A *dislocation* occurs when a bone is displaced within a joint. This is usually due to a traumatic injury that stretches or tears the ligaments and other soft tissues around the joint and requires reduction (realigning the bones) and rest while the ligaments heal. Massage is contraindicated during the acute phase. During the subacute stage, massage can be used to reduce scar tissue and address splinting or spasmed muscles related to the formerly dislocated joint.

Herniated Disk

herniated disk

is a weakening of the intervertebral disc resulting in a protrusion into the vertebral canal, potentially compressing the spinal cord.

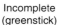

A **herniated disk** is a weakening of the intervertebral disk that results in a protrusion of the nucleus pulposis or the annulus fibrosis of the disk into the vertebral canal, potentially compressing the spinal nerve root or the spinal cord. Herniated disks usually occur in the lumbar or cervical spine. Symptoms include neck or back pain, numbness, and tingling or pain down the limb of the impinged nerves.

A client with a suspected herniated disk should be referred to a physician for a definitive diagnosis by x-ray, myelogram, or MRI, because similar symptoms can be caused by other conditions such as ligament damage, spondylosis, or bone cancer, all of which require very different treatments.

Successful treatment for herniated disks involves reducing the protrusion, preferably by reabsorption of the nucleus pulposis into the disk and healing of the annulus fibrosis. This can be accomplished with therapies such as chiropractic or osteopathic manipulations, traction, strict bedrest, physical therapy, or special exercises done with the intention of strengthening the core muscles and creating more space for the disk to heal. If these are unsuccessful, or if the disk is putting severe pressure on the spinal cord or spinal nerve, surgical intervention might be required.

Massage is not recommended during an acute episode of a herniated disk. After a definitive diagnosis and initial treatment, as part of a team approach, massage may be helpful to address the muscle spasms, referred pain, and compensation patterns that accompany the condition.

Sprain

A **sprain** is an injury to a joint that results in the stretching or tearing of the ligaments but is not severe enough to cause a dislocation. Sprains are classified according to their severity.

sprain
is an injury to a joint resulting in stretching or tearing of the ligaments.

Class I sprain: There is a stretch in the ligament, some discomfort, and minimal loss of function.

Class II sprain: The ligament is torn with some loss of function. Discoloration from tissue damage and bleeding might be present.

Class III sprain: This is the most severe sprain, in which the ligaments are torn and there is internal bleeding and severe loss of function.

All classes of sprain cause swelling and require rest and support while the tissues heal.

Sprains cause inflammation (i.e., pain, heat, redness, and swelling) as a result of tissue damage plus a painful loss of function in the associated joint. Passive movement of the joint that stretches the sprained ligament causes pain. Massage is contraindicated during the acute stage of a sprain, when signs of inflammation are present. Massage is appropriate during the subacute and healing stages to help to reduce adhesions, edema, and stiffness while enhancing circulation and flexibility.

Arthritis

Arthritis is an inflammatory condition of the joints often accompanied by pain and changes of bone structure. There are many kinds of arthritis; the most common are rheumatoid arthritis, osteoarthritis, and gouty arthritis.

Rheumatoid arthritis is a chronic, systemic, autoimmune inflammatory disease and is the most serious and crippling form of arthritis. It is a systemic disease, often involving several joints, that first affects the synovial membrane that lines the joints. The joints become swollen, hot, and red. The inflammation causes the articular cartilage to erode and the joints to calcify and eventually become immovable. Its cause is unknown, but treatments are available to slow the progress and reduce the discomfort. Massage is contraindicated in the acute stage because it aggravates the condition. In the remission stage, gentle massage and joint movement well within pain tolerance can be beneficial.

Osteoarthritis is a chronic disease that accompanies aging. It usually affects synovial joints that have experienced much wear and tear or trauma. The knees, hips, and spine are common sites for this degenerative disease, which erodes the articular cartilage and results in abnormal bone thickening and progressive joint immobility. Arthritic pain can come and go and ranges from mild to unbearable. In the acute, inflammatory stage, the affected joint can be swollen, hot, and painful. In the subacute stage, the pain in the joint subsides somewhat, but there is noticeable stiffness. There is no cure for osteoarthritis, but medication, exercise, and massage help to relieve pain and maintain mobility. Surgery is sometimes indicated to remove *spurs* or replace affected joints. Massage is contraindicated during the inflammatory, acute stages of osteoarthritis, but it is indicated during the subacute stages to help to relax related muscle tension, reduce pain, and maintain flexibility.

spondylosis

a degenerative arthritic condition affecting the vertebrae.

Spondylosis is osteoarthritis of the spine that can affect the cervical, lumbar, or thoracic vertebrae. It is characterized by the degeneration of the intervertebral disks and the formation of bony growths on the vertebra called *osteophytes* or *bone spurs*. Spondylosis is a slow-progressing, degenerative condition that affects middle-aged to elderly people. There might be no symptoms until the osteophytes grow enough to put pressure on a spinal nerve, the spinal cord, or begin to limit movement between vertebrae. Gentle exercise and movement help to slow the progression of the disease. Massage may be appropriate with caution and in cooperation with the primary care provider.

Acute gouty arthritis, also referred to as *gout,* is caused by a high concentration of uric acid in the blood that precipitates out into the interstitial and synovial spaces in the form of sharp, needlelike crystals. Uric acid is a metabolic by-product of purine and is normally excreted from the body by the kidneys. High blood levels of uric acid (*hyperuremia*) can result from eating foods high in purine such as shellfish, red meat, organ meats, and lentils, or from consuming high amounts of alcohol, which interferes with the kidney's ability to eliminate uric acid, or because of low-functioning kidneys. The most common place for the crystals to settle is in the metaphalangeal joint of the large toe, where an immune system response to the presence of the uric acid crystals causes the classic inflammatory symptoms of pain, swelling, heat, and redness. Other joints that can be affected by gout include the ankle, knee, fingers, wrist, and elbow. Attacks usually last a few days and subside on their own. Over time, attacks can become more frequent and severe. Uric acid crystals can also cause kidney stones. Gout can be an indicator of other medical conditions. Before proceeding with massage, a client with symptoms of gout should receive medical clearance. In the acute stage, gout is a systemic contraindication for massage; in a subacute stage or remission, it is a local contraindication.

Ankylosing spondylitis is a type of inflammatory arthritis that targets the sacroiliac joint and the spinal articulations, including the ribs, although it can also affect other areas of the body such as the shoulders, hips, and small joints of the hands and feet. Sometimes the eyes become involved, and—rarely—the lungs and heart can be affected. It is a genetic autoimmune disease that primarily affects men between the ages of 15 and 35. Chronic ankylosing spondylitis begins with stiffness and pain in the low back and hips, then progresses up the back and neck. In severe cases, bone formation leads to spinal and vertebrocostal fusion, leaving the body in a forward-stooping posture and the rib cage frozen, which compromises breathing. Currently there is no cure, but medications and proper treatment help to slow the progression and reduce symptoms. Anti-inflammatory drugs and proper exercise are essential to reduce pain and maintain posture and flexibility.

As with other inflammatory conditions, massage is contraindicated during the acute stages of ankylosing spondylitis. The appropriateness of massage during the subacute and remission stages has not been determined and must be decided on a case-by-case basis in close cooperation with the client's physician.

Bursitis

Bursitis is an inflammation of the small fluid-filled sacs (bursae) located near the joints that reduce the friction of overlying structures during movement.

There are more than 150 bursae in the body located between moving structures such as bones, muscles, skin, and tendons. The bursae act as a cushion to allow smooth gliding between these structures. Bursitis is a painful condition that results from repeated irritation or trauma. The most common site of bursitis is the subdeltoid bursae of the shoulder, but it can develop at any joint. Pain from an acute case of bursitis drastically limits joint mobility. After the inflammation subsides, mobility remains limited because of pain and contracted muscles. Massage is locally contraindicated during the acute stage of bursitis; however, in the subacute stage, mild exercise, range of motion, and massage are very effective for restoring mobility.

Osteoporosis

Osteoporosis (**OS**-tee-o-pour-**O**-sis) literally means increased porosity of the bones. Osteoporosis affects four times as many women as men, and its prevalence increases with age. Until around the age of 35, the body builds bone density by storing various minerals, mostly calcium. After that, it begins to slowly demineralize, increasing the risk of osteoporosis. Besides aging, other risk factors that play a part in the development of osteoporosis are genetics, having a small bone structure, smoking, alcohol abuse, and a sedentary lifestyle.

Osteoporosis is a silent disease because there are no apparent symptoms. Often, the first indicator is a fracture after a minor accident. A definitive diagnosis is done with a bone mineral density test and x-ray studies. The best treatment for osteoporosis is prevention through good nutrition with ample amounts of calcium and vitamin D and regular weight-bearing exercise throughout life. Increased reabsorption of calcium into the bloodstream causes a thinning of bone tissue, leaving it more fragile and prone to fracture (especially where bones are weight bearing, such as in the spine and pelvis). When severe osteoporosis is present, the massage therapist must be very cautious and avoid any deep pressure or forceful joint movements that could lead to the possibility of fractures of the delicate bones.

Spinal Curvature

The healthy adult spine has a double S curve when viewed from the side. The cervical and lumbar portions of the spine are concave and have a normal lordotic (lor-DOT-ick) curve. The thoracic portion of the spine is convex and has a normal kyphotic (kye-FAH-tick) curve. These curvatures help to position the head over the pelvis and provide flexibility, strength, shock absorption, and balance. Sometimes, abnormal curvatures develop in the spine.

In some instances, abnormal curvatures of the spine (Figure 5-31) begin as functional conditions of posture or soft tissues pulling the spine out of alignment. If left untreated, the constant pull of the soft tissues or gravity cause the vertebrae and other skeletal structures to change shape and become more of a structural dysfunction.

Scoliosis is a lateral curvature of the spine that involves a rotation of the vertebrae.

Lordosis is an exaggerated lordotic or concave curve most commonly found in the lumbar spine, creating a condition commonly known as *swayback*.

Kyphosis is an abnormally exaggerated kyphotic or convex curve of the thoracic spine. This condition is also termed *hyperkyphosis*. *Postural kyphosis* usually

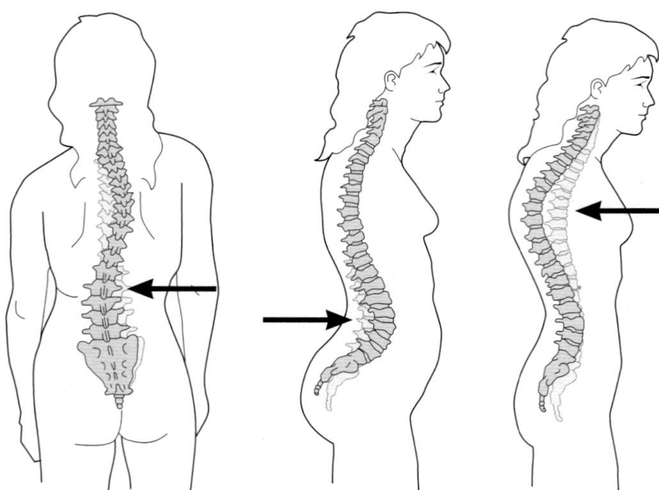

FIGURE 5-31 Abnormal curvature of the spine: (a) scoliosis, b) lordosis, (c) kyphosis.

becomes apparent during adolescence and is associated with slouching. *Scheuermann's kyphosis* is a genetic condition that also becomes apparent during the early teenage years but tends to be more severe, with irregularly formed vertebrae and disks.

These abnormal curves can develop because of a congenital defect, habitually poor body mechanics, aging, or other reasons that are not easily discernable. Regardless of their origin, these abnormal conditions cause tremendous biomechanical stress on the body. Massage and exercise, although not offering a cure for these conditions, are very effective in counteracting the stress and pain associated with these abnormalities.

SECTION QUESTIONS FOR DISCUSSION AND REVIEW

1. Which structures make up the skeletal system?
2. Name five functions of bones.
3. Name the organic and inorganic matter found in bones.
4. Name two types of bone tissue and indicate where they are found.
5. Which covering protects the bone?
6. How are the bones nourished?
7. Name the various shapes of bones found in the body. Give an example of each.
8. Name two kinds of marrow and where each is found.
9. What is the function of red bone marrow?
10. What are the two main parts of the skeleton?
11. Name three classifications of joints and differentiate between them.
12. Which structure cushions the bones at the joints?
13. Which structure connects and supports the bones at the joints?
14. Which fluid lubricates the joints?
15. Approximately how many bones are found in the human body?
16. Why must the skeletal system be considered in the practice of massage therapy?
17. List five types of movable joints and give an example of each.
18. What is a fracture?
19. What is a sprain? Describe the difference between the three classes of sprains.
20. What is arthritis? What are the three most common types of arthritis?
21. What is osteoporosis? Which precautions must be observed when massaging a person with osteoporosis?
22. Describe three abnormal curves of the spine.

REVIEW

Matching Test I

Insert the letter of the proper term in front of each definition.

________	1.	upper arm	a.	femur
________	2.	wrist bones	b.	tarsus
________	3.	ankle bones	c.	scapula
________	4.	toe or finger bones	d.	tibia
________	5.	palm bones	e.	phalanges
________	6.	spinal column	f.	vertebrae
________	7.	collarbone	g.	carpals
________	8.	shoulder blade	h.	metacarpals
________	9.	thigh bone	i.	humerus
________	10.	shin bone	j.	clavicle

True or False Test

Carefully read each statement and decide if it is true or false; draw a circle around the letter T or F.

1. T F The hyoid bone supports the base of the ear.
2. T F The metatarsals and metacarpals are different bones.
3. T F The patella forms the front of the knee joint.
4. T F The upper limbs are attached to the pelvis.
5. T F The clavicle and scapula serve as an attachment for the lower limbs.
6. T F The femur is found in the thigh.
7. T F The ulna and radius are found in the forearm.
8. T F The lungs and heart are found in the thorax.
9. T F The vertebrae provide an attachment for the ribs.
10. T F The pelvis is known as the kneecap.

Matching II

Match the definition in the right column with the correct word in the left column.

________	1.	crest	a.	rounded prominence at a joint
________	2.	head	b.	a hole
________	3.	spine	c.	a ridge
________	4.	tuberosity	d.	a hollow or depression
________	5.	foramen	e.	articulating end of a bone
________	6.	condyle	f.	less prominent ridge on a bone
________	7.	fossa	g.	bony prominence
________	8.	trochanter	h.	sharp, slender projection
________	9.	line	i.	larger process for muscle attachment
________	10.	process	j.	large rounded process

SYSTEM 3 THE MUSCULAR SYSTEM

Muscle is the main organ of the muscular system. Muscle is made of specialized cells or fibers that have the unique ability to change their length. The action of muscle cells produces nearly all the movement of the body. Muscle movement is responsible for locomotion and all motor functions. It is responsible for breathing, moving fluids such as blood and urine, and transporting food through the digestive system. By their action on the fascia, tendons, ligaments, and bones, muscles also provide the stability to support the body in an erect and weight-bearing posture.

The muscular system shapes and supports the skeleton. Depending on a person's physical development, muscles comprise approximately 40 to 60 percent of the total body weight. The skeletal muscular system consists of over 600 muscles, large and small.

Metabolically, muscles use most of the food and oxygen that we consume to produce energy for movement and heat that the body uses for heat regulation. The muscular system relies on the skeletal, nervous, vascular, digestive, and respiratory systems for its activities.

Stiff, sore, achy, tired, tense, injured, and overworked muscles benefit immensely from massage. Massage has a profound effect not only on the common soft tissue dysfunctions of muscles such as strains and spasms, but also on the activity of the blood, lymph, and nerves associated with the muscles of the body. The effects and benefits of massage on muscles and other systems is addressed in Chapter 6.

Types of Muscles

There are three types of muscular tissue (Figure 5-32):

1. Voluntary, striated, or skeletal muscles are controlled by the will.
2. Involuntary, nonstriated or smooth muscles function without the action of the will.
3. Heart or cardiac muscle is found only in the heart, and it is not duplicated anywhere else in the body.

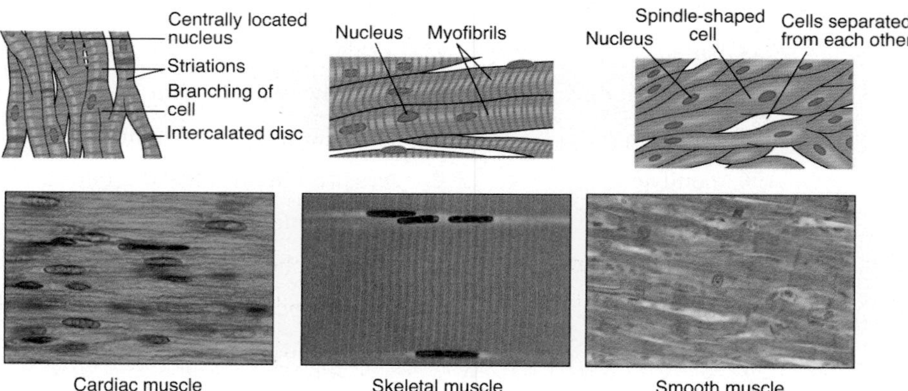

FIGURE 5-32 Types of muscle.

Skeletal (striated) muscles or *voluntary* muscles are put into action by conscious will. They are governed by the central nervous system (CNS) and appear striated or striped under the microscope. They make up the fleshy areas of the body, are attached to the skeleton, and are in turn fastened to the bones, skin, or other muscles.

Smooth (visceral or involuntary) muscles function without the action of the will. They are controlled by the autonomic nervous system. Smooth muscle consists of spindle-shaped, nonstriated cells that overlap at the ends, often forming fibrous bands, such as those found in the walls of the stomach, intestines, and blood vessels. Smooth muscle does not attach to bone, is rather slow acting, can maintain a contraction for a long time, and does not fatigue easily.

Cardiac (heart) muscle is only found in the heart. It is composed of cells that are as distinctly striated as the cells of skeletal muscle. Cardiac muscle cells are quadrangular, joined end to end, and grouped in bundles supported by a framework of connective tissue.

Characteristics of Muscles

The characteristics that enable muscles to perform their functions of contraction and movement are irritability, contractility, and elasticity. **Irritability** or excitability is the capacity of muscles to receive and react to stimuli, whether mechanical (massage), electrical (currents), thermal (heat), chemical (acid or salt), or impulses of nervous origin.

Muscle also has **contractility**, which is the ability to contract or shorten and thereby exert force. When cardiac muscle contracts, it reduces the area in the chambers of the heart, causing a pumping action. Likewise, when smooth muscle contracts, the diameter of the related organ decreases. If a skeletal muscle is attached to a pair of articulating bones, when the muscle contracts the attachments are drawn closer together, resulting in movement of the bones.

Muscle has **elasticity**, which is the ability to return to its original shape after being stretched. **Extensibility** is the ability of the muscle to stretch.

irritability

or excitability, is the capacity of muscles to receive and react to stimuli.

contractility

is the ability of a muscle to contract or shorten and thereby exert force.

elasticity

refers to the tissue's ability to return to normal resting length when a stress that has been placed on it is removed.

extensibility

is the ability of a muscle to stretch.

Structure of Skeletal Muscles

Massage primarily is performed on and affects the skeletal muscles; therefore, the rest of this chapter focuses on skeletal muscles.

Skeletal muscles contain several tissues, including muscle tissue, blood and other fluids, nerve tissue, and a variety of connective tissues. The structure of skeletal muscle is unique, with its arrangement of contractile fibers aligned and supported in such a way that by contracting, they exert a force on the bony levers of the skeleton, producing movement.

Muscle Tissue

Muscle tissue consists of contractile fibrous tissue arranged in separate parallel bundles (*fascicles*), which in turn consist of several parallel muscle fibers that are held in place by an extensive and intricate connective tissue system. The connective tissue supports the muscle fibers in such a way that when the fibers contract, a force is exerted on whichever structure the muscle is attached to, causing movement.

Muscle tissue is also supplied with a vast network of blood and lymph vessels, capillaries, and nerve fibers. The blood supplies the oxygen and nutrients that are essential to carry on the intense metabolic activity as well as carry away the wastes and by-products of muscle activity. The nerves not only provide the motor impulses to the muscles from the CNS but also supply the CNS with a variety of sensory information from sensory nerve ends and proprioceptors located in the skin, muscles, tendons, and joints.

Connective Tissue and Fascia

Connective tissues form a continuous netlike framework throughout the body. Connective tissue consists largely of a fluid matrix (ground substance) and collagen fibers that support, bind, and connect the wide range of body structures. Depending on its consistency and the varying proportions of fluid to fibers, a wide array of connective tissues are formed. Some examples are the fluid intercellular environment, the superficial fascia just below the skin, the fascia of the muscles, the tendons and ligaments, the tough cartilage, and even bone.

The muscular system is a highly organized system of compartmentalized contractile fibrous tissues that work together to produce movement. The contractile tissue is organized and supported by an intricate network of connective tissue commonly called *fascia. Fascia* organizes muscles into functional groups, surrounds each individual muscle, extends inward throughout the muscle creating muscle bundles, and eventually surrounds each muscle fiber. Connective tissue also creates a supporting structure for the intricate network of blood vessels and nerves. The fascia projects beyond the ends of the muscle to become tendons or flat tendinous sheaths (aponeuroses) that connect the muscles to other structures. Aponeuroses can attach muscles to bones, to other muscles, or to the skin; tendons intertwine with the fibrous coverings of bones (periosteum). Other connective tissue binds and supports the organs and structures in their proper place and forms anchors for lymph and blood vessels and nerves, holding them in their proper place among the organs, muscles, and bones.

The *superficial fascia* is situated just below the skin and covers the entire muscular system. The fascia penetrates to the bone (deep fascia), separating muscle groups and covering individual muscles, holding them in their relative positions and at the same time allowing them to move somewhat independently. The layer of fascia that closely covers an individual muscle is the *epimysium* (ep-i-**MI**-see-um). The *perimysium* (**PAR**-a-**MI**-see-um) extends inward from the epimysium and separates the muscle into bundles of muscle fibers or *fascicles* (**FAS**-i-kls). Within the fascicle, each muscle fiber has a delicate connective tissue covering called the *endomysium.* Indeed, muscle tissue and fascia are structurally and functionally inseparable. The term **myofascial** has been coined to describe the combined muscle and fascial tissues.

myofascial

the combination of muscle tissue and its related connective tissue or fascia.

The connective tissue organizes the muscle fibers and connects the muscle to tendons, tendons to bones, and even bones to bones. Without this complicated system of connecting sheets, hinges, and ropes that transfers the action of the muscle fibers to the levers of the skeleton, motion and postural stability would not be possible (Figure 5-33).

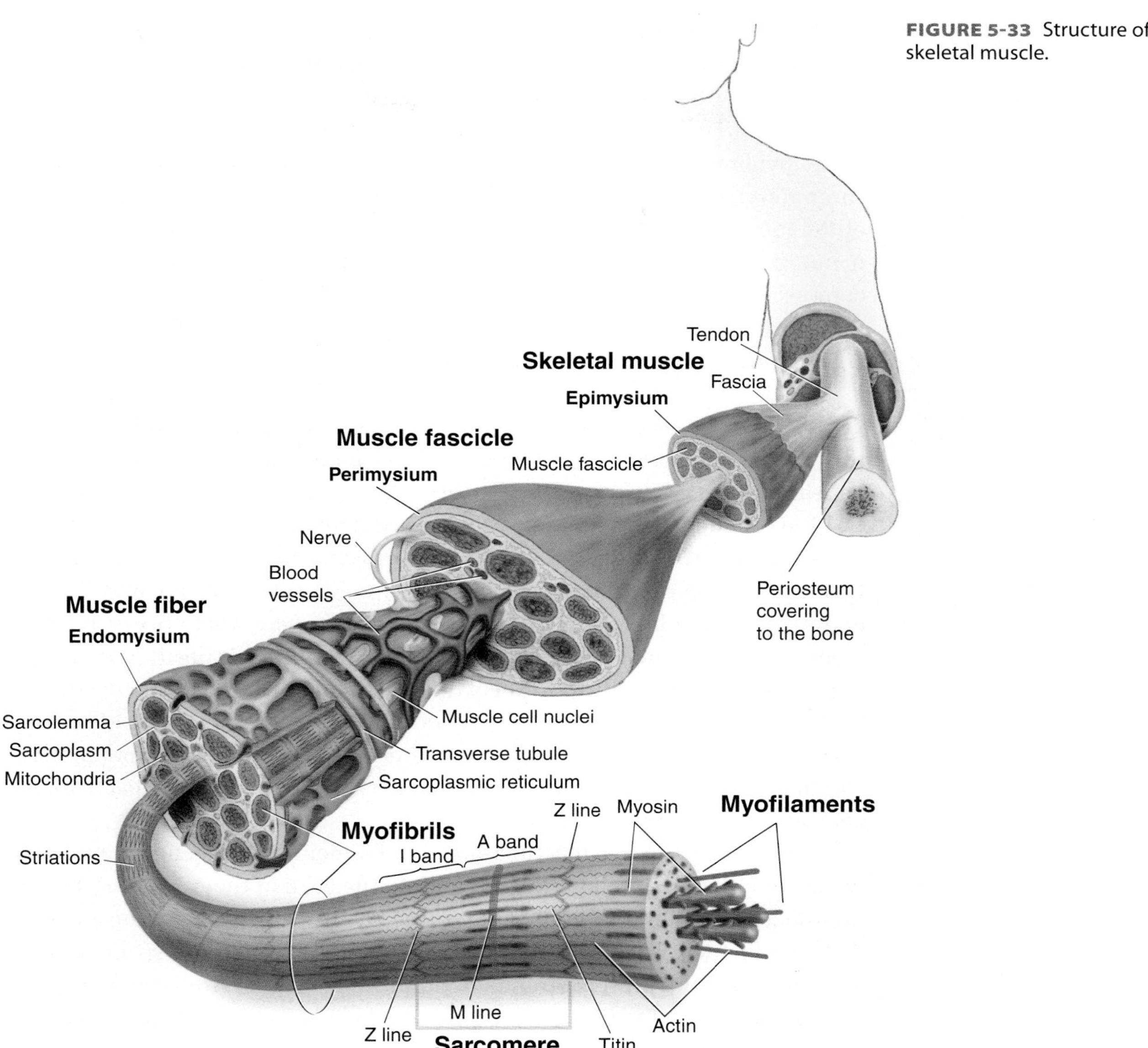

FIGURE 5-33 Structure of skeletal muscle.

Muscle Cells or Fibers

The *muscle fiber* or muscle cell is the functional contractile unit of muscle tissue. The muscle cells are long, cylindrical, wormlike structures that can extend the entire length of the muscle. Muscle fibers vary in length from 1 to 50 mm. Muscle cells are multinucleated. A single muscle cell can have hundreds of nuclei distributed just beneath the cell membrane. These nuclei produce the enzymes and proteins necessary in muscle contractions. Multiple nuclei all along the cell speed up the process. The muscle cell has a connective tissue covering (endomysium [**EN**-do-**MI**-see-um]) that maintains its parallel position with other cells. Toward the end of the muscle fiber, the collagen fibers of the endomysium combine with the fibers of the perimysium and the epimysium to become tendons or the broad sheath of the aponeurosis. The tendon fibers in turn attach usually to bone, where the fibers mesh into the periosteum and the bone matrix, providing a firm connection. As a result, the contraction of the muscle fiber is translated into a pull on the tendon and a movement of the bone.

sarcolemma

is the cell wall of the muscle cell.

sarcomere

the smallest functional unit of the muscle cell containing the actin and myosin filaments.

myosin

a protein that forms filaments that make up nearly 50 percent of muscle tissue and are involved in muscle contraction.

actin

a protein in muscle tissue that forms filaments that interact with myosin filaments to cause muscle contractions.

transverse tubules

a system of channels within the muscle cell containing extracellular fluid that helps transmit nerve impulses throughout the cell.

sarcoplasmic reticulum

is a network of membranous channels within the muscle cell that release calcium ions, causing muscle contraction.

Beneath the layer of connective tissue is a cell membrane (*sarcolemma*). Within the **sarcolemma** (**SAR**-ko-**LEM**-uh) the muscle cell is highly organized. Each muscle fiber can contain from several hundred to several thousand parallel *myofibrils* (my-o-**FYE**-brils), depending on the size of the muscle fiber.

A myofibril is as long as its muscle fiber and can consist of as many as 10,000 **sarcomeres** arranged end to end. The sarcomere is the smallest functional unit of the muscle fiber. Within every sarcomere is an arrangement of protein filaments that are made up largely of **myosin** or **actin**. The thicker filaments are composed of mostly myosin, and the thinner filaments of mostly actin. The manner in which the actin and myosin filaments are arranged in the sarcomeres gives the skeletal muscle the striped or striated appearance for which it is named. Under magnification, myofibrils appear to have darker A bands and lighter I bands. All the myofibrils in a muscle cell are aligned side by side so that the A and I bands appear consistent across the fiber, creating the striated appearance of skeletal muscles (Figure 5-34).

The A band is in the middle of the sarcomere and is caused by the thicker myosin filament. The width of the A band is equal to the length of the myosin filament. Within the A band are the M line, the H zone or band, and the zone of overlap. The M line is the midpoint of the sarcomere where the myosin filaments seem to connect with one another to stabilize their position in the cell. The H zone represents the portion of the myosin filament that is not overlapped by the thinner actin filament. The H zone is wider in a sarcomere at rest and narrower in a cell that is in a contracted position. The zone of overlap, which contains both myosin and actin filaments, is the area where the activities of contraction take place.

The I band contains only the thin actin filaments. The I band extends from the edge of the A band in one sarcomere to the edge of the A band in the next sarcomere. In the middle of the I band is the Z line, which acts as the anchor of the actin filaments and is the boundary between sarcomeres. Also anchored to the Z lines are the protein strands of titan, which extend from the ends of the myosin filaments. The titan strands seem to help keep the actin and myosin in proper alignment.

The interaction between the actin and myosin filaments in the sarcomere give muscle its unique contractile ability. When a muscle contracts, the zone of overlap becomes wider, the I band becomes narrower, and the Z lines come closer together. The contraction continues until the I band is nearly eliminated, indicating that the actin filaments slide across the thicker myosin filaments toward the M line as the end of the myosin filaments are drawn toward the Z line. This is known as the *sliding filament theory.*

Extending inward from the cell membrane in the area of the transverse Z lines that anchor the actin filaments is an intricate system of **transverse tubules** that encircle each myofibril and contain extracellular fluid. These tubules play an important role in the transmission of the stimulus of muscle contraction. The **sarcoplasmic reticulum** is a network of membranous channels within the muscle cell that surrounds each myofibril and is closely associated with the transverse tubules. When an impulse is transmitted through the cell membrane and transverse tubules, the sarcoplasmic reticulum releases calcium ions. In the high concentrations of calcium ions in the sarcoplasm (intercellular fluid of the

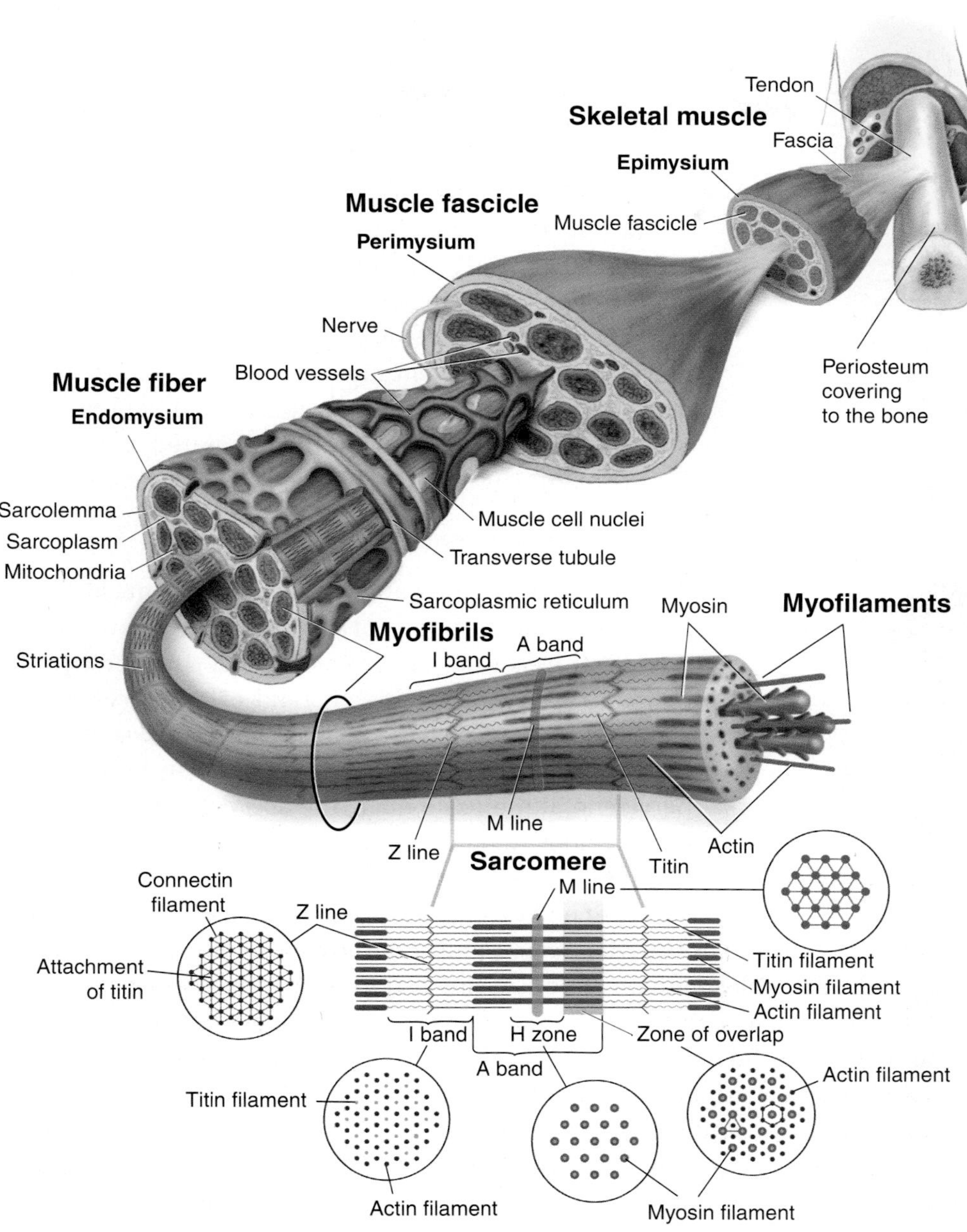

FIGURE 5-34 Structure of muscle fibers.

muscle cells), the actin filaments are drawn across the myosin filaments, resulting in the shortening of the cell and contraction of the muscle (Figures 5-34 and 5-35).

Neuromuscular Connection

Every skeletal muscle fiber is connected to a branch of a motor neuron. The site where the muscle fiber and nerve fiber meet is called the *neuromuscular junction* or **myoneural junction.** There are a few specialized muscle cells called **spindle cells** that have both sensory and motor functions and are essential for muscle control and coordination (more about these later in this chapter). Although a muscle fiber has only one nerve fiber connection, a motor nerve can have many branches and therefore connect to several muscle fibers. A motor

myoneural junction

the connection point of the motor nerve and the muscle cell.

spindle cells

located in the belly of muscle, alert the CNS as to the length, stretch, and speed of the muscle.

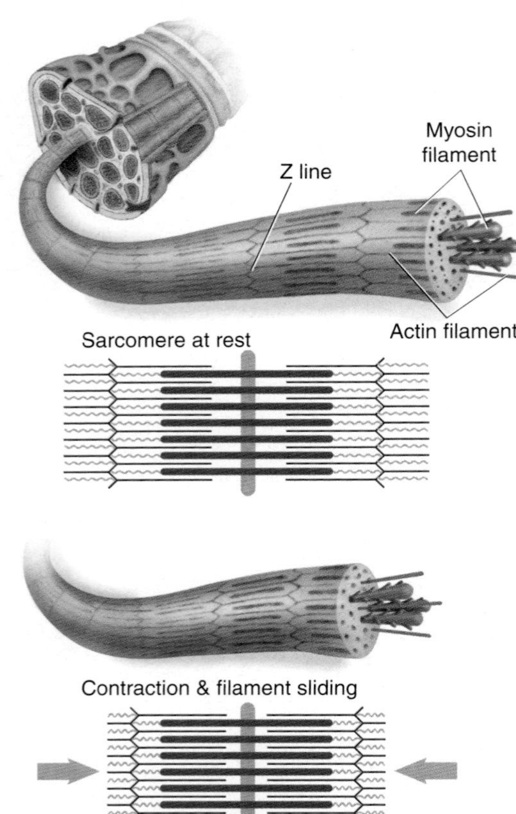

FIGURE 5-35 Model of muscle contraction. As actin filaments are pulled across myosin filaments, the Z lines are pulled closer together, and the overall length of the cell shortens.

neuron and all the muscle fibers that it controls constitute a **motor unit**. When a motor nerve transmits a stimulus, *all* of the muscle fibers connected by its many branches contract simultaneously. Generally, in small muscles that provide intricate movements (e.g., muscles that control speech or eye movement) the motor units can include as few as 6 to 12 muscle fibers, whereas larger muscles that provide less intricate movements (e.g., the vastus muscles or gastrocnemius) can have several hundred muscle fibers in a single motor unit. Motor units tend to overlap with the muscle fibers of adjacent motor units interspersed among one another. This allows muscle units to support each other and provides for smooth, integrated movements (Figure 5-36).

Skeletal Muscle Contraction

Muscle has the unique ability to change chemical energy into mechanical energy or movement. When a nerve impulse travels from the brain or spinal cord through the motor neuron and reaches the end of the nerve fiber, a chemical *neurotransmitter* called *acetylcholine* (as-e-til-**KOE**-leen) is released and bridges the gap between the nerve end and muscle fiber. The acetylcholine affects the muscle fiber membrane and causes an action potential much like a nerve impulse that immediately travels the length of and throughout the muscle fiber. The impulse is transmitted through the transverse tubules of the muscle fiber, where it contacts the sarcoplasmic reticulum, causing it to release a flood of calcium ions. The calcium ions bond to the actin filaments, which opens active sites on the actin where heads of the myosin molecules attach, pivot, detach, and repeat the process as long as calcium ions and ATP are available. This bridging action causes the actin and myosin filaments to merge, shortening the fiber and contracting the muscle. The sliding mechanism between the actin and myosin filaments involves complex chemical, mechanical, and molecular activity that is beyond the scope of this text. All of this mechanical activity requires energy.

The Energy Source for Muscle Activity

The energy for muscle contraction comes from the breakdown of the ATP molecule. When a muscle contracts, an enzyme causes one of the phosphates to split from the ATP molecule, releasing energy and forming *adenosine diphosphate (ADP).* There is only enough ATP stored in the muscle cells to sustain a contraction for a few seconds. Fortunately, within a fraction of a second, ADP is reconstituted into ATP in one of several ways.

Another cellular substance that has a high-energy phosphate bond is *creatine phosphate.* Even though the energy stored in creatine phosphate cannot be used directly by the muscle, when it contacts ADP, the energy causes the rebonding of the phosphate ion, producing ATP. Unfortunately, the combined amounts

motor unit

consists of a motor neuron and all of the muscle fibers it controls.

of creatine phosphate and ATP available in the cell are still sufficient to sustain a contraction for only a few seconds.

Most of the energy to reconstitute ADP is the result of cellular respiration. **Aerobic cellular respiration** takes place in the cells' mitochondria. Aerobic respiration is responsible for most of the sustained energy supply for the constant replenishing of ATP. By the time it goes through the digestive process and is transported to the cells, most of the food that we eat has been converted to glucose. As the glucose is transported through the cell to the mitochondria, it is converted to pyruvic acid. In the mitochondria, a complex metabolic process known as the *Krebs cycle* (or the citric acid cycle) takes place, resulting in the production of carbon dioxide, water, and energy in the form of heat and the synthesis of ATP.

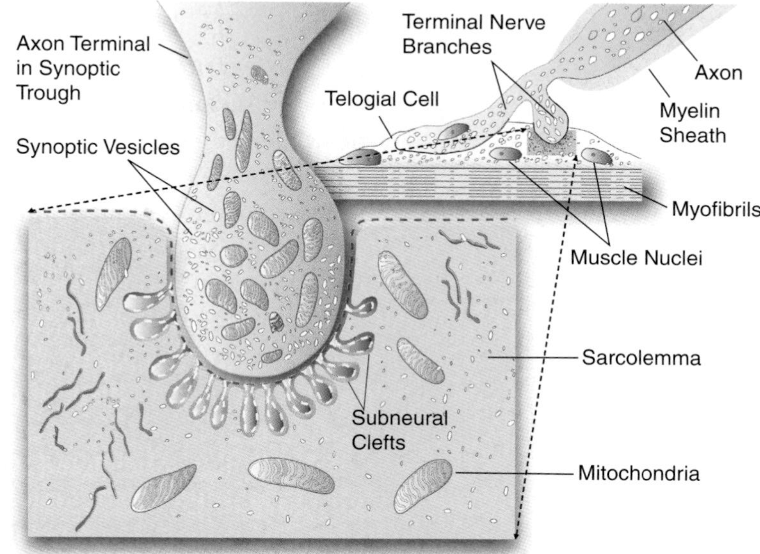

FIGURE 5-36 Myoneural junction.

aerobic cellular respiration makes energy for reconstituting ADP in cell mitochondrion.

The oxygen required to carry on aerobic respiration is carried to the cells from the lungs in the blood by the red blood cells. The amount of oxygen taken in and the rate at which it can be delivered to the mitochondria of the cells determines how much ATP can be reconstituted and therefore how much a muscle can do.

When the oxygen available for aerobic respiration is depleted, anaerobic respiration takes place. In **anaerobic respiration** (in the absence of oxygen), glucose is broken down, releasing enough energy to synthesize some ATP and produce pyruvic acid, which is converted to lactic acid. The lactic acid is carried by the bloodstream to the liver, where it is converted back to glucose (ATP is required for this conversion).

anaerobic respiration is a process in which glucose is broken down in the absence of oxygen.

During light or moderate activity, the lungs and circulatory system are able to supply the skeletal muscles with adequate amounts of oxygen to carry on aerobic respiration. After just a few minutes of strenuous output, however, the pulse and respiration rate increase. As the strenuous activity continues, the circulatory and respiratory systems cannot supply enough oxygen to the muscles, which forces them to rely on the less efficient anaerobic respiration. Anaerobic respiration produces pyruvic and then lactic acid. As lactic acid accumulates, the person develops *oxygen debt.* After the strenuous activity ceases, the heavy breathing and accelerated heart rate continue until the oxygen debt is paid off, and then normal breathing and pulse resume.

Muscle Fatigue

If rapid or prolonged muscle contractions continue to the point that oxygen debt becomes extreme, the muscle ceases to respond. This condition is **muscle fatigue.** Muscle fatigue results either because the circulation of blood cannot keep pace with the demand for oxygen or because the waste products accumulate faster than they can be removed, affecting the muscle's ability to respond to nerve impulses.

muscle fatigue is a condition in which the muscle ceases to respond because of oxygen debt from rapid or prolonged muscle contractions.

Muscle Fiber Types

Muscle fiber structure varies according to function. There are two distinctive types of muscle fibers: Type I, slow twitch fibers, and Type II, fast twitch fibers. Type II fibers are subdivided into Type IIa and Type IIb.

Type I, slow twitch fibers, have a relatively slower contraction time and a high resistance to fatigue. They contain a high number of mitochondria, large amounts of myoglobin, and have an ample capillary supply. Myoglobin is a form of hemoglobin in the muscle tissue that stores oxygen and gives muscle its red color. The rich blood supply and numerous mitochondria give the fibers a high capacity to generate ATP and sustain low-level contractions for a long time while resisting fatigue. Type I fibers are found in large quantities in postural muscles.

Type IIb, fast twitch fibers, produce powerful, high-velocity contractions for short periods. The contraction velocity is five to ten times faster than Type I fibers. They contain few mitochondria, low myoglobin content, and few capillaries, which give them a lighter, whitish color. They depend on glycogen and creatine phosphate for ATP generation, and they fatigue easily. Type II fibers are more prevalent in the arms, shoulders, and legs.

Type IIa fibers are rarely found in humans. It seems that through extensive endurance training, Type IIb fibers take on characteristics of Type I fibers, with better blood supply, higher concentrations of mitochondria, and more myoglobin to give muscle more endurance while maintaining explosive speed and strength. Table 5.4 presents an overview of muscle fiber characteristics.

Chicken provides a graphic example of muscle types. The white breast meat is made of Type II fibers; the darker leg and thigh is Type I muscle. The legs are continuously used for walking and consist of high-endurance Type I fibers. The breast muscles are used for very occasional short bursts of flying and therefore consist of Type II fibers.

Type I muscle is slow to fatigue because of an ample blood supply and numerous mitochondria available to generate adequate amounts of ATP by aerobic respiration to sustain low to moderate muscle activity. Ninety-five percent of the muscle's ATP production takes place in the cell's mitochondria. The aerobic respiration of Type I fibers uses oxygen and glucose supplied from the blood to produce ATP to energize the muscle contraction with byproducts of carbon dioxide and water, which are carried away by the bloodstream.

TABLE 5.4

MUSCLE FIBER CHARACTERISTICS			
MUSCLE FIBER TYPE	**TYPE I**	**TYPE IIA**	**TYPE IIB**
Contraction velocity	Slow	Fast	Fast
Fiber color	Red	Red	White
Fatigue time	Slow	Intermediate	Fast
Myoglobin content	High	High	Low
Capillary density	High	High	Low
Mitochondria density	High	High	Low

Type IIb muscle fibers provide on-demand, powerful, explosive contractions. These fibers tend to be larger, with more actin/myosin filaments but fewer mitochondria and less blood supply. Without the rich supply of blood and oxygen, ATP generation for Type IIb muscle contraction is supplied more by creatine phosphate and the anaerobic metabolism of glycogen, both of which are stored in the muscle. The muscle converts glycogen to glucose and then, in the absence of oxygen (anaerobic state), metabolizes ATP with lactic acid as a by-product. The depletion of stored creatine phosphate and glycogen and the buildup of lactic acid cause the Type IIb cell to fatigue rather quickly. Rest periods between bursts of activity allow circulation to remove lactic acid and restore the oxygen debt in fast twitch muscle fibers.

Most muscles contain both fiber types. The proportion of fast and slow twitch fibers depends on the primary function of the muscle and on genetics. Postural muscles contain a higher proportion of Type I fibers. Phasic muscles—those used for quick, infrequent, powerful movement—contain a higher proportion of Type II fibers. Postural muscles are stabilizers, and phasic muscles are movers. Different muscle fibers in a particular muscle might be called on for different functions. For example, if only slight muscle contractions are needed for a task, such as a gentle stroll down a lane, only Type I fibers in the legs are active. If stronger contractions are needed, say to chase after a dog that has stolen your favorite hat, Type IIb fibers would be activated. Each type of muscle fiber is energized by separate motor neurons. A single motor neuron can activate as few as 2 and as many as 2,000 muscle fibers. A single muscle can have hundreds of thousands of muscle fibers. A motor unit contains fibers of only one type and activates with a frequency conducive to those fibers. If the demand is light, slow twitch fibers are stimulated. When more intense movement is called for, Type IIb fibers activate. Type I fibers have a lower activation threshold than Type IIb fibers. The activation of the various motor units is controlled in the spinal cord and brain (Box 5.2).

Postural muscles support the body against gravity and are made up of a higher proportion of Type I fibers. They are slower to respond to stimulation but slower to fatigue. They respond to undue or sustained stress and strain by shortening, becoming hypertonic, and developing trigger points and fibrosis. Under continuous strain, the connective tissue of postural muscle thickens to support the structure.

Phasic muscles move the body by responding quickly and forcefully when stimulated. They consist of a higher proportion of Type IIb fibers. As postural muscles tend to tighten and shorten when stressed, associated phasic muscles tend to be inhibited and weaken. This is important to note when working with clients with postural concerns. Because phasic muscles contract quickly and forcefully, common problems include muscle strains, tendonitis, and microtrauma at the musculotendinous and tendinoperiosteal junctions.

Muscle Insertion and Origin

As explained earlier, the connective tissue surrounding the muscle fibers extends beyond the ends of the fibers to become the fibrous and rather inelastic tendons that anchor the ends of the muscle to the bones. The arrangement of muscle fibers and tendons varies according to muscle function and location. Some

Box 5.2

MAJOR PHASIC AND POSTURAL MUSCLES

- Phasic Muscles
- Respond to dysfunction and stress by hypotonicity and weakening
- Anterior neck flexors
- Scalenii
- Deltoid
- Lower pectorals
- Middle and lower trapezius
- Rhomboids
- Serratus anterior
- Rectus abdominis
- Gluteals
- Hamstrings
- Vastus muscles
- Peroneals
- Arm extensors

- Postural Muscles
- Respond to dysfunction and stress with hypertonicity and shortening
- Upper trapezius
- Levator scapulae
- Sternocleidomastoid
- Upper pectoralis major
- Pectoralis minor
- Latissimus dorsi
- Sacrospinalis
- Lumbar erector spinae
- Quadratus lumborum
- Iliopsoas
- Piriformis
- Oblique abdominals
- Adductor longus and magnus
- Tensor fascia lata
- Rectus femoris
- Medial hamstrings
- Soleus
- Gastrocnemius
- Tibialis posterior

origin of a muscle
is the point where the end of a muscle is anchored to an immovable section of the skeleton.

insertion of a muscle
is the more mobile attachment of a muscle to bone.

isometric contraction
occurs when a muscle contracts and the ends of the muscle do not move.

isotonic contraction
occurs when a muscle contracts and the distance between the ends of the muscle changes.

eccentric contraction
occurs when a muscle contracts while the ends of the muscle move farther apart.

muscles, such as the biceps, form cordlike tendons at either end of the muscle belly. Other muscles, such as the deltoid and trapezius, have their attachments spread over a broad area.

The structures to which the tendons attach determine the action that the contracting muscles produce. Skeletal muscles, as their name implies, have at least one end of the muscle that is attached to bone. The end of the muscle is anchored to a relatively immovable section of the skeleton called the **origin of the muscle**. The *origin* of a muscle is generally located more proximal to or nearer the center of the body.

The other end of the muscle attaches either to a bone, the deeper structures of the skin, or other muscles, and creates the action of the structure. The term applied to the more mobile attachment is the **insertion of the muscle**. The *insertion* of a muscle is generally attached to the more distal aspect of an appendage. In some movements, the roles of insertion and origin of a muscle can be reversed. The action of a muscle contraction can be derived from the knowledge of its insertion and origin (Figure 5-37).

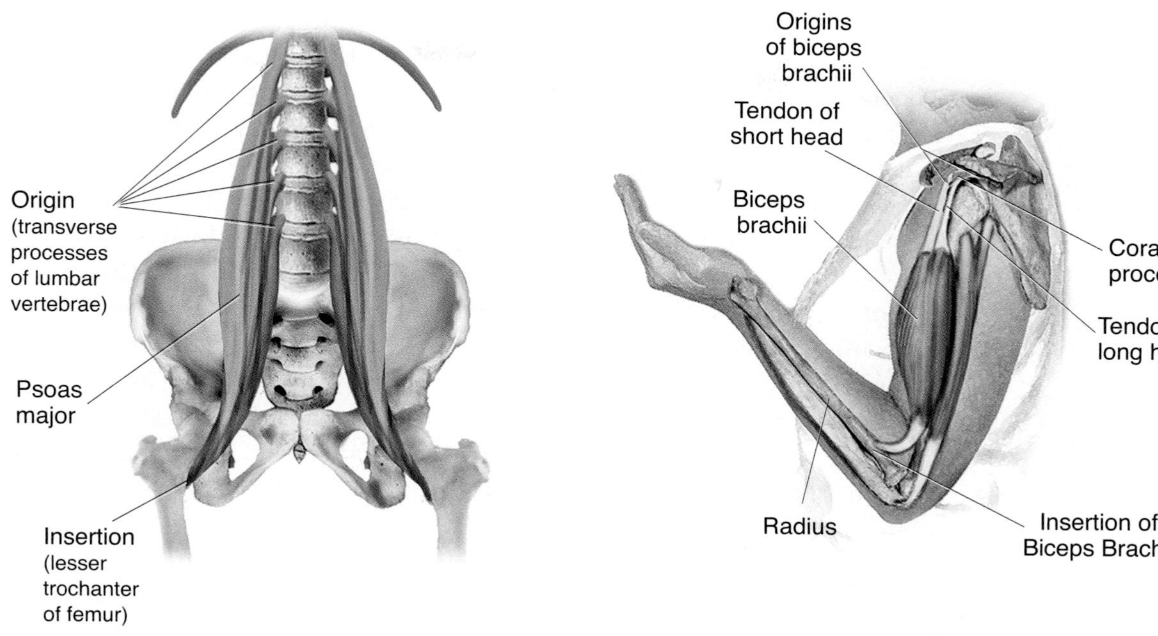

FIGURE 5-37 Muscle insertion and origin.

Isometric and Isotonic Contractions

When a muscle contracts and the ends of the muscle do not move or the body part that the muscle affects does not move, the contraction is an **isometric contraction.** When a person strains to move a heavy object that does not budge, the muscle effort is isometric. In the muscles that stabilize our bodies in an upright posture, most contractions are continuous and isometric.

When a muscle contracts and the distance between the ends of the muscle changes, it is an **isotonic contraction.** When the distance between the ends of a contracting muscle decreases, the isotonic contraction is said to be *concentric.* When the distance between the ends of a contracting muscle increases, the isotonic contraction is said to be **eccentric.** When you do a push-up, as you push up, the loaded muscles shorten, and the contraction is concentric. As you lower yourself to the floor, the loaded muscles are getting longer and the contraction is eccentric. In both directions, the contractions are isotonic.

Muscle Interaction

In some ways, the muscular system could be considered one continuous muscle that covers the entire body and is divided into various chambers by an intricate system of connective tissue. This muscle is controlled by a vast network of neuromuscular units that coordinate their activities through the CNS to produce smooth, coordinated, graceful movements.

The classic approach has been to study the effect of the individual muscles on joint action, but this is not physiologic. Normal muscle action is the patterned response of groups of muscles. Muscles have anatomic individuality, but they do not have functional individuality.

STUDENT ACTIVITY

Demonstrate and identify an eccentric, concentric, and an isometric contraction.

Begin by standing. Slowly squat down. Which type of contraction is occurring in the front of the legs (quadriceps)?

Now slowly, stand up again. Which type of contraction is occurring in the front of the legs (quadriceps)?

Begin to squat again, but stop part way down and hold that position. Which type of contraction is occurring in the front of the legs (quadriceps)?

Demonstrate at least one other example of each type of contraction.

prime mover

the primary muscle responsible for a specific movement.

agonist

a prime mover.

antagonist

the muscle that performs the opposite movement of the agonist.

synergists

muscles that assist the agonist.

fixator

muscles that act to stabilize a body part so that another muscle can act on an adjacent limb or body part.

Individual muscles, because of their specific attachments when contracted, generate a specific action; however, muscles never work alone. When an isolated and specific action occurs, the muscle responsible for that action is the **prime mover** (sometimes referred to as the **agonist**). When the prime mover contracts, there is a muscle that causes the opposite action. That opposing muscle is referred to as the **antagonist**. For instance, when the elbow is flexed with the hand in the supine position, the prime mover is the biceps. The opposite action would be to extend the arm. The muscle responsible for arm extension is the triceps, so the antagonist of the biceps is the triceps. It is clear from this example that when the prime mover contracts and shortens, the antagonist must extend. Most movement, however, is not that simple, and even when only one joint is considered, several muscles can be involved. Muscles that assist the prime mover are called **synergists** (**SIN**-er-jists). **Fixator** or stabilizer muscles stabilize more proximal joints so that more distal limbs can perform weight-bearing functions.

In observing the dynamics of movement, there are three components of motion: flexion/extension, abduction/adduction, and rotation. Most joints in the body function in at least two of these components, and many articulations involve all three. A muscle that acts across a joint has a primary function in one of the three components of motion, but the same muscle can have a secondary or even a tertiary action, depending on the mobility of the joint. For instance, in Figure 5-38, the primary function of the biceps is to flex the elbow; however, a secondary function of the biceps is to assist in supination of the forearm, and a minor, tertiary function of the short head of the biceps is to flex the shoulder (Figures 5-38 to 5-42). Table 5.5 gives a comprehensive presentation of the location and action of muscles.

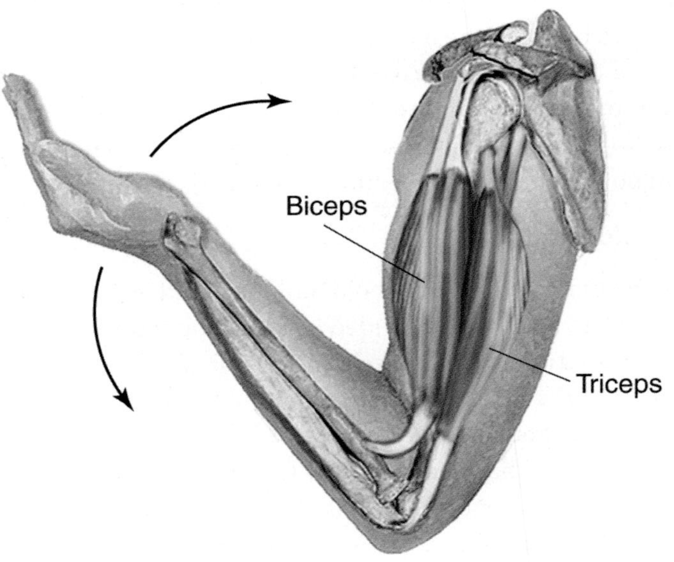

FIGURE 5-38 Muscle interaction.

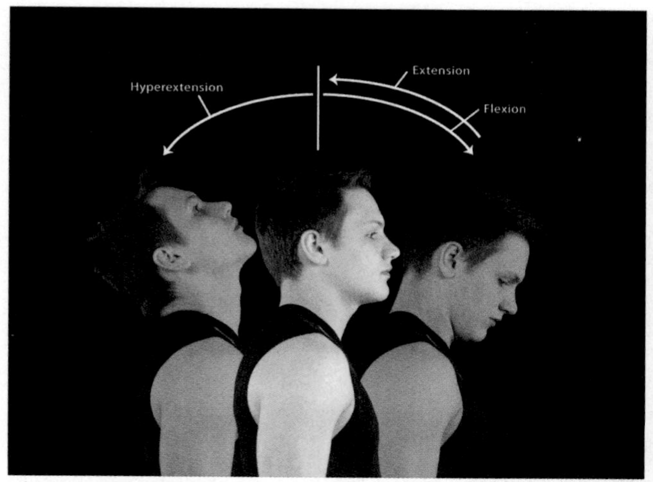

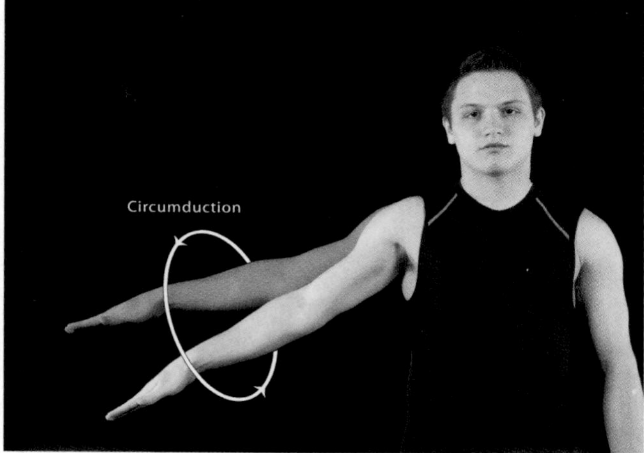

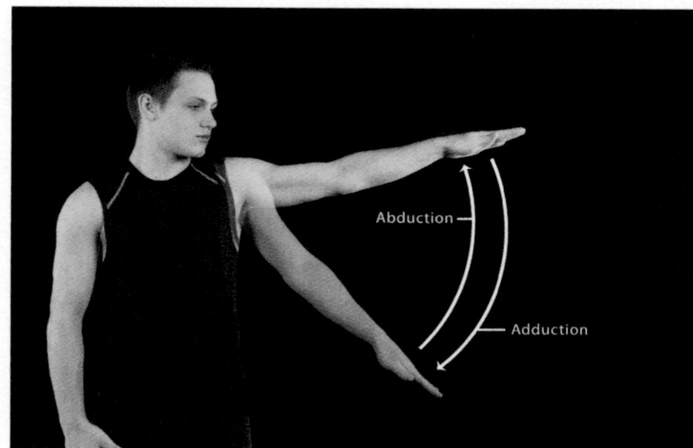

FIGURE 5-39A–C Motion in diarthrotic joints.

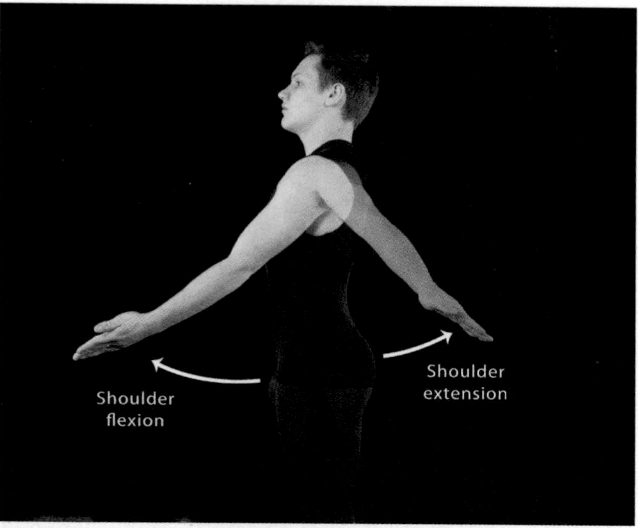

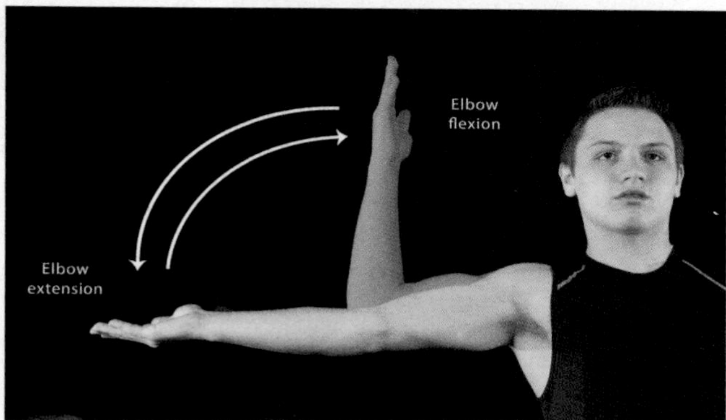

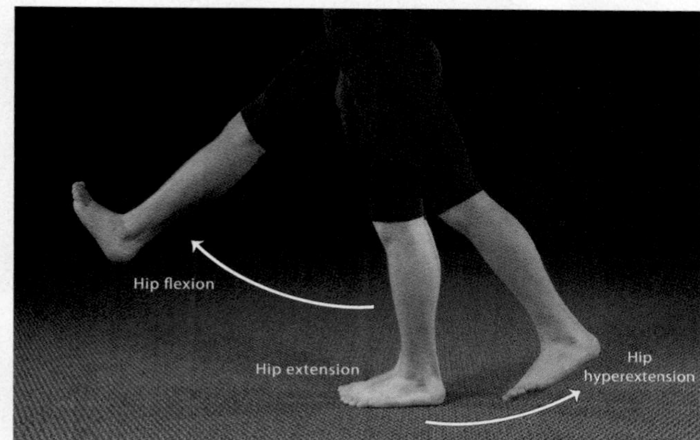

FIGURE 5-39D–F Motion in diarthrotic joints.

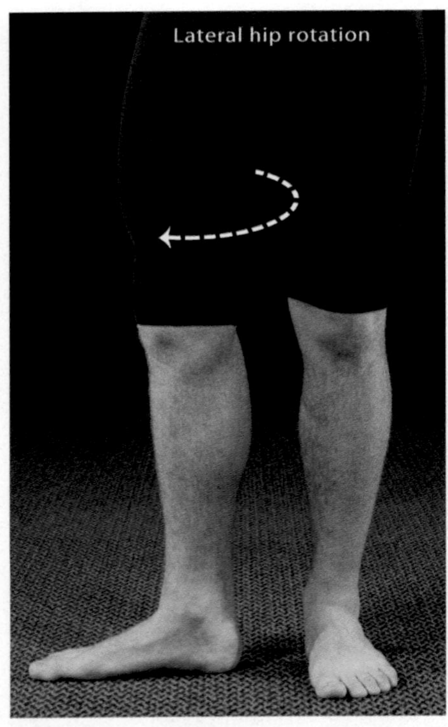

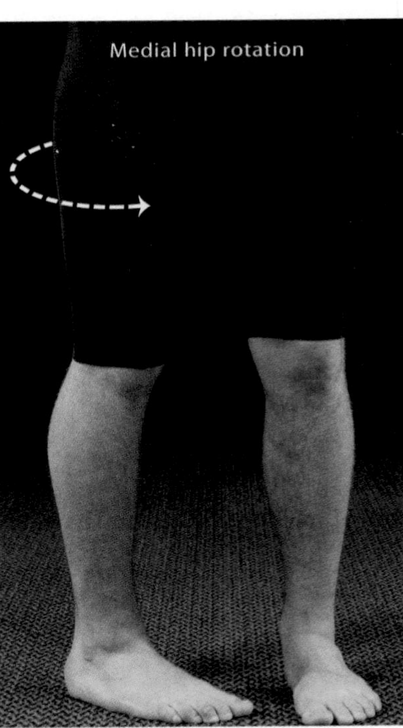

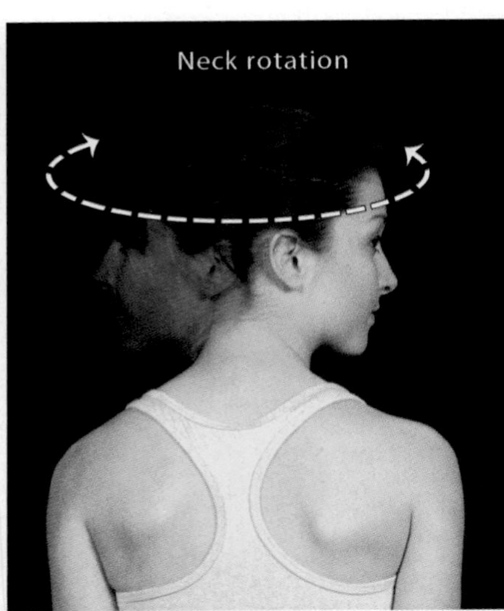

FIGURE 5-40A–C Motion in diarthrotic joints, continued.

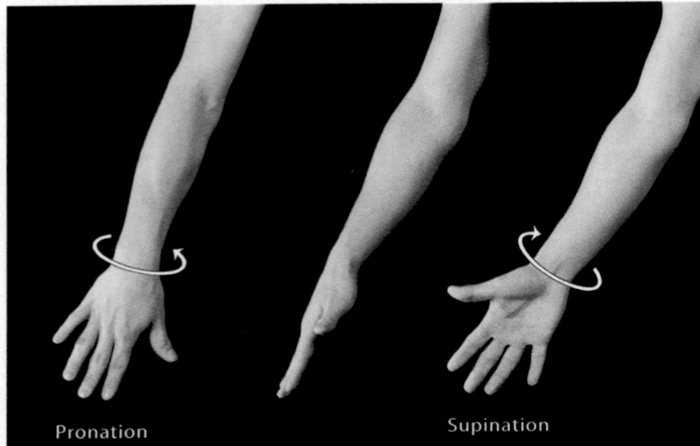

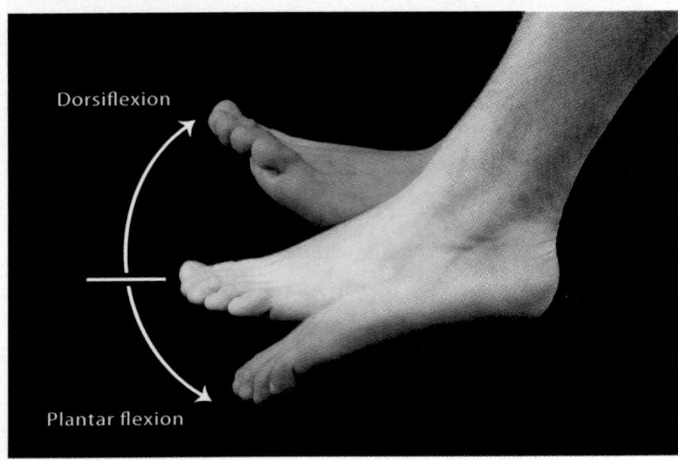

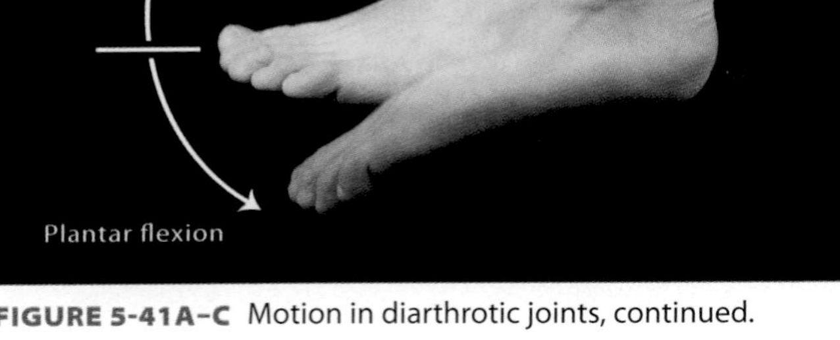

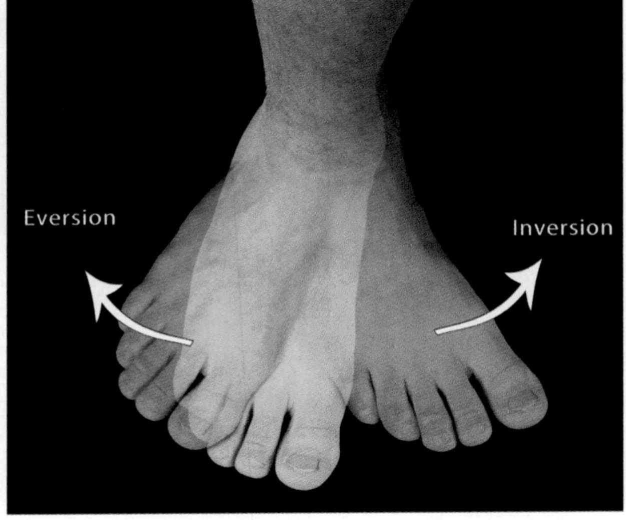

FIGURE 5-41A–C Motion in diarthrotic joints, continued.

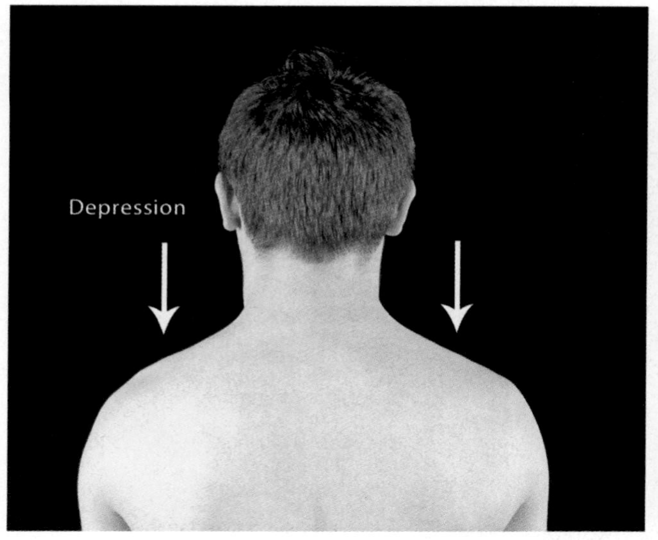

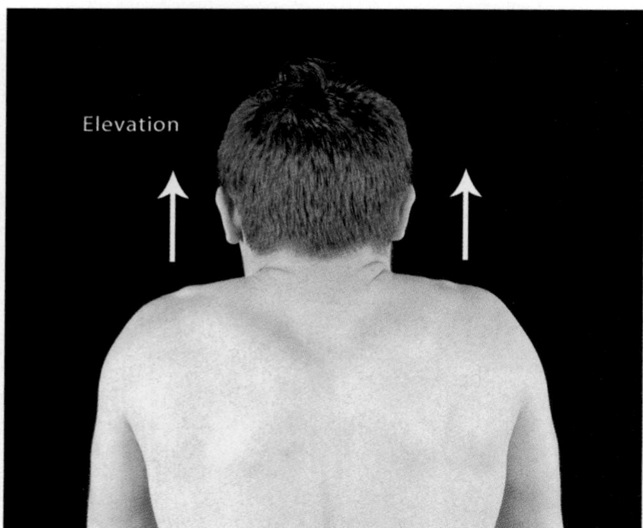

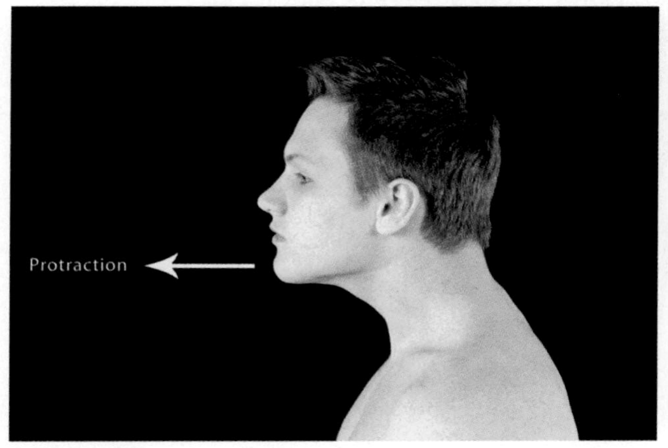

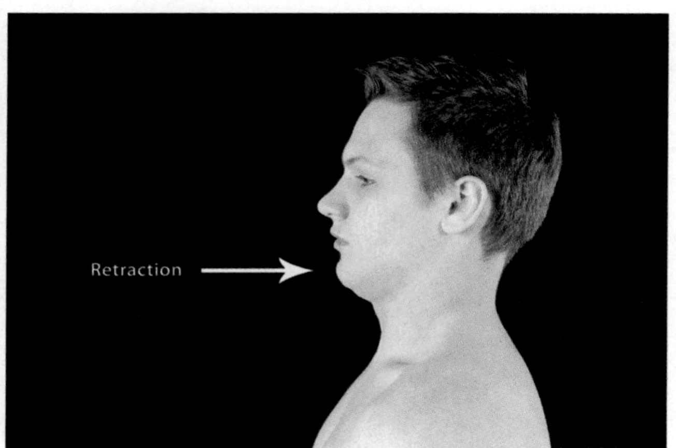

FIGURE 5-42A–D Motion in diarthrotic joints, continued.

Terms to Remember

A review of the words shown below will be helpful in understanding the meaning of technical terms when studying the muscular system (Figures 5-43 and 5-44).

Anterior: before, or in front of
Posterior: behind, or in back of
Superior: situated above
Inferior: situated lower
Oblique or anguli: at an angle
Levator: that which lifts
Dorsal: behind, or in back of
Medial: pertaining to the middle or center
Dilator: that which expands or enlarges
Depressor: that which presses or draws down
Proximal: nearer to the center or medial line
Distal: farther from the center or medial lines

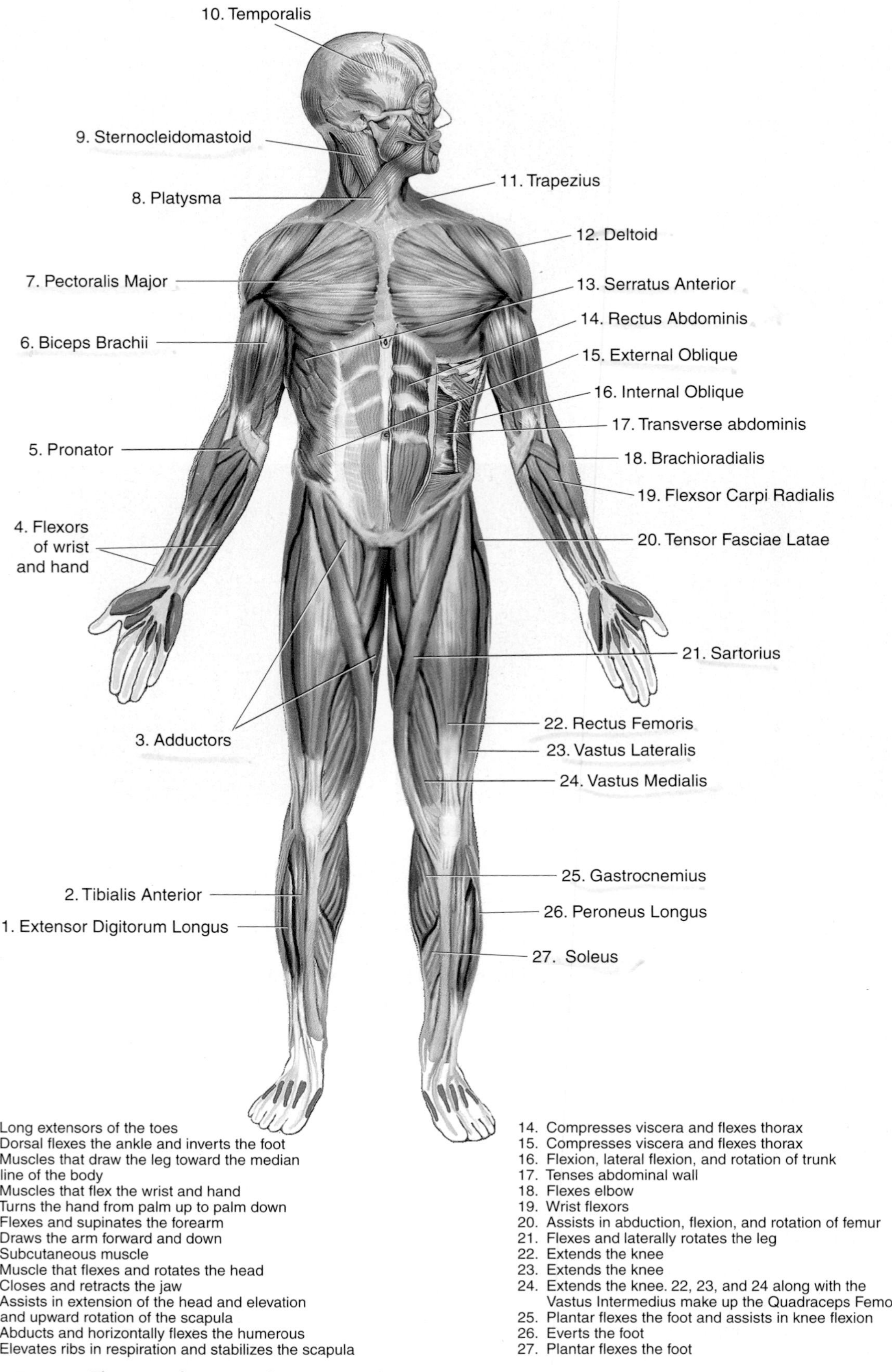
10. Temporalis
9. Sternocleidomastoid
11. Trapezius
8. Platysma
12. Deltoid
7. Pectoralis Major
13. Serratus Anterior
14. Rectus Abdominis
6. Biceps Brachii
15. External Oblique
16. Internal Oblique
17. Transverse abdominis
5. Pronator
18. Brachioradialis
19. Flexsor Carpi Radialis
4. Flexors of wrist and hand
20. Tensor Fasciae Latae
21. Sartorius
22. Rectus Femoris
3. Adductors
23. Vastus Lateralis
24. Vastus Medialis
25. Gastrocnemius
2. Tibialis Anterior
26. Peroneus Longus
1. Extensor Digitorum Longus
27. Soleus
1. Long extensors of the toes
2. Dorsal flexes the ankle and inverts the foot
3. Muscles that draw the leg toward the median line of the body
4. Muscles that flex the wrist and hand
5. Turns the hand from palm up to palm down
6. Flexes and supinates the forearm
7. Draws the arm forward and down
8. Subcutaneous muscle
9. Muscle that flexes and rotates the head
10. Closes and retracts the jaw
11. Assists in extension of the head and elevation and upward rotation of the scapula
12. Abducts and horizontally flexes the humerous
13. Elevates ribs in respiration and stabilizes the scapula
14. Compresses viscera and flexes thorax
15. Compresses viscera and flexes thorax
16. Flexion, lateral flexion, and rotation of trunk
17. Tenses abdominal wall
18. Flexes elbow
19. Wrist flexors
20. Assists in abduction, flexion, and rotation of femur
21. Flexes and laterally rotates the leg
22. Extends the knee
23. Extends the knee
24. Extends the knee. 22, 23, and 24 along with the Vastus Intermedius make up the Quadraceps Femoris
25. Plantar flexes the foot and assists in knee flexion
26. Everts the foot
27. Plantar flexes the foot

FIGURE 5-43 The muscular system (anterior view).

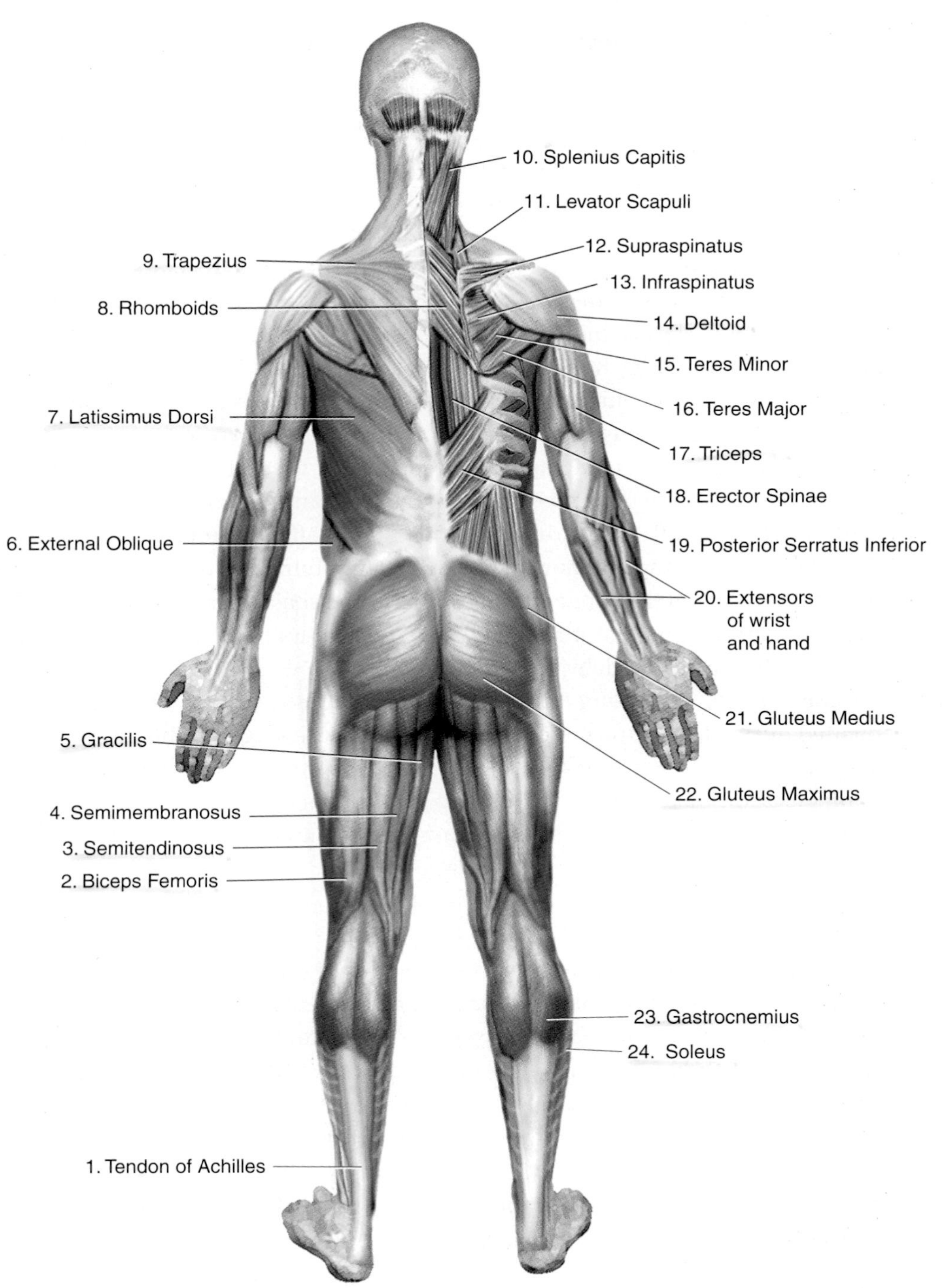

1. Attaches calf muscle to heel bone
2, 3, 4. Make up the hamstrings that flex the knee and assist in extension of the hip
5. Draws leg toward the mid-line
6. Supports abdominal viscera; flexes vertebral column
7. Draws arm backward and downward: rotates arm inward
8. Draws scapula toward the spine
9. Draws scapula toward the spine; rotates scapula either upward or downward; draws head backward
10. Draws head back or rotates the head
11. Elevation and/or downward rotation of scapula
12. Abducts the arm
13. Outward rotation and extension of arm
14. Abducts and rotates humerus
15. Lateral rotation of humerus
16. Inward rotation, abduction, and extension of humerus
17. Extends the forearm
18. Extension of the spine
19. Pulls ribs outward and down; opposes diaphragm
20. Extends the wrist and hand
21. Abducts and rotates the thigh
22. Extends, abducts, and rotates the thigh outward
23. Flexes the knee and plantar flexes the foot
24. Plantar flexes the foot

FIGURE 5-44 The muscular system (posterior view).

Common Dysfunctions and Diseases of the Muscular System

Muscle Spasms

Muscle spasms are the most common muscle dysfunction. A *spasm* is a sudden involuntary contraction of a muscle or a group of muscles. Spasms vary both in duration and intensity and can affect any muscle tissue (i.e., voluntary, involuntary, or cardiac). Spasms are considered *tonic* when they are sustained or *clonic* when they alternate between contraction and relaxation. Intense, short-lived, painful spasms are often designated as *cramps*. Some common examples of muscle spasms are hiccups, tics and twitches in the face, torticollis (**TOR**-ti-koll-is), charley horses, convulsions, and muscle "splinting" associated with injuries. Spasms can occur as a result of injury, disease, or emotional stress (stuttering). Usually, spasms cease when their cause is corrected.

The appropriateness for massage depends on the nature of the spasm or cramp. Massage directly on the site of an acute cramp or charley horse is contraindicated. Compressing from the ends of the affected muscle or resisting the contraction of the antagonist, however, can inhibit and quiet the spasming muscle. Massage in the subacute stage or after the spasm has subsided can help to restore circulation and nutrients to the muscle tissue while clearing the tissues of toxic waste and debris.

Massage on a splinting muscle that is protecting an injury site is contraindicated during the acute and even into the subacute stages of the injury. Occasionally, splinting continues well after the injured tissue has healed, causing compensation or restricted movement. This is when massage and soft tissue interventions are appropriate to release tension and restore circulation and flexibility.

Contractures

Contractures are shortened, contracted muscles or muscle groups in which the muscle atrophies and shrinks while the connective tissue thickens. Contractures are usually related to immobility or severe nerve damage and usually result in flexion rather than extension of the affected limb. Contractures are common in conditions such as cerebral palsy and spinal cord injury. Although massage is of little or no benefit when addressing contractures in an advanced or chronic state, massage and consistent stretching exercises can help to prevent or reduce the extent of a contracture if employed during the early stages of the condition, before the connective tissue thickens and the muscles atrophy.

Muscle Strains

Muscle strains (also called *torn* or *pulled* muscles) are the most common injury to muscle. There are three degrees or grades of muscle strain:

Grade I is an overstretching of a few of the muscle fibers with a minimal tearing of the fibers. There is some pain but no loss of function and no palpable or visual indications.

Grade II involves a partial tear of between 10 and 50 percent of the muscle fibers. There is considerable pain and some loss of function. There is a palpable thickening of the muscle tissue, and perhaps some tissue bleeding.

Grade III is the most severe injury, with between 50 and 100 percent muscle tearing. There is a palpable depression and/or bunching of the muscle, with severe pain and total or near total loss of muscle function.

Muscle strains can occur in different sites in the muscle. Most strains (80 percent) occur in the muscle belly or at the junction between the muscle and the tendon (musculotendinous junction). Other less common sites are at the insertion or the origin, or in the tendon of the muscle.

Torn fibers of a muscle strain initiate an inflammatory response, flooding the area with fluid containing white blood cells to carry away damaged debris and fibroblasts to create collagen fibers to begin to mend the injured tissues. The influx of fluid causes swelling and pain, which helps to limit movement. The preferred intervention during the acute stage of a muscle strain, which can last from 24 to 72 hours depending on the severity, is described by the acronym PRICE (protect, rest, ice, compression, and elevation). Massage is contraindicated during the acute stage of a muscle strain.

Specialized massage procedures are invaluable during the subacute stages (as the injury heals) to ensure that the newly forming scar tissue is strong and pliable, to limit the formation of adhesions between fascial sheaths, to promote circulation, and to restore range of motion. Certain massage procedures are helpful at the site of old muscle strains to reduce adhesions, improve mobility, and reduce the chance of reinjury.

Hypertrophy

Muscle hypertrophy is an enlargement of the breadth of a muscle as a result of repeated forceful muscle activity. Most of the hypertrophy is due to the increase in the size of the muscle fibers rather than an increase in the number of muscle fibers. As a result of the increased size, the power of the muscle increases as well as the metabolic support system (i.e., increased blood supply, sarcoplasm, ATP, mitochondria). It is also likely that the number of actin/myosin filaments and number of fibrils in the muscle fiber increase; however, this has not been substantiated.

Atrophy

Muscle *atrophy* is the reverse of hypertrophy and is the result of muscle disuse. If a muscle cannot be contracted or is contracted only very weakly, the muscle tissue rapidly degenerates and begins to waste away. The number and size of the capillaries supplying the muscle decrease as well as the sarcoplasm and its constituents (i.e., mitochondria, sarcoplasmic reticulum, glycogen, ATP). The size of the fibrils and the actin/myosin filaments is reduced, as is the power of the muscle. If the nerve supply to the muscle is interfered with, paralysis results and muscle atrophy progresses rapidly. If atrophy continues over an extended period, the contractile tissue will continue to degenerate until it is replaced with connective tissue, and rehabilitation becomes all but impossible.

Tendonitis and Tenosynovitis

Tendonitis is an inflammation of the tendon, often occurring at the musculotendinous or tenoperiosteal junction. Tenosynovitis is an inflammation of the tendon sheath. Both are accompanied by pain, stiffness, and often swelling.

Many times, they occur simultaneously. Massage is indicated to relieve muscle tension and to assist healing in the subacute stage but should be avoided on the lesion during the acute stages of inflammation.

Tendonosis

Tendonosis is a degenerative condition of a tendon that does not involve any inflammation. Tendonosis is characterized by degeneration of the collagen fibers in the tendon, tendon weakness, and abnormal growth of unhealthy blood vessels through the tendon. It is not an inflammatory condition. Many times the painful condition of tendonosis is mistaken and misdiagnosed for tendonitis. Tendonosis tends to be a more chronic condition that responds to proper rehabilitative exercise and massage.

Lupus Erythematosus

Lupus is a chronic inflammatory disease of the connective tissue that can affect many body tissues and organs. It is an autoimmune disorder that causes blood vessel inflammation (especially in the face), organ dysfunction, and arthritis. Massage may be given only under the supervision of a physician.

Fibromyalgia Syndrome

Fibromyalgia is characterized by pain, fatigue, and stiffness in the connective tissue of the muscles, tendons, and ligaments. It is associated with stress, poor sleep habits, and occupational or recreational strain, and is more prevalent in women. Systemic viral or bacterial infections can be a precursor, as well as cold, damp conditions. It is often related to chronic fatigue syndrome. There are identifiable trigger points. Massage to desensitize trigger points and range-of-motion exercises are beneficial. All massage should be gentle and done with great consideration of the condition. Each person's symptoms vary, as does tolerance to the modalities and pressure applied by the practitioner. Refer to and work in conjunction with a physician with these clients.

Dystrophy

Muscular dystrophy refers to a group of related diseases that seem to be genetically inherited and that cause a progressive degeneration of the voluntary muscular system. With muscular dystrophy, the contractile fibers of the muscles are gradually replaced by fat and connective tissue until those muscles become virtually useless. All of the visible effects of muscular dystrophy seem to be in the muscles. It rarely causes pain, and the intellect is not affected. Exercise and massage are helpful in prolonging muscular ability and maintaining flexibility.

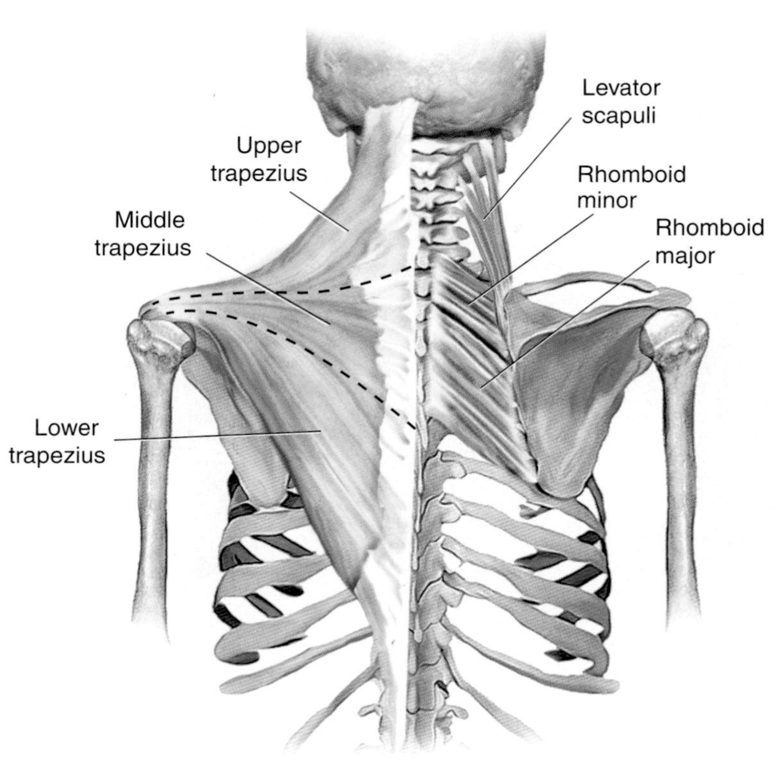

FIGURE T5-5-1 Posterior upper thorax: Trapezius. One side is cut away to show rhomboids and levator.

TABLE 5.5

MUSCLES OF THE UPPER EXTREMITIES Muscles That Act on and Support the Scapula						
MUSCLE	ORIGIN	INSERTION	ACTION	INNERVATION	PALPATION	FIGURE
Trapezius						T5-5-1
Upper	Occiput and ligamentum nuchae of cervical spine	Lateral one third of clavicle and acromion	Elevation and upward rotation of scapula	Cranial XI, Spinal Accessory	From below occiput to acromion	T5-5-1
Middle	Spinous process C7–T5	Spine of the scapula	Pulls scapula medially	C3–4	From spinous process T1–5 to acromion	T5-5-1
Lower	Spinous process T5–T12	Spine of the scapula	Depression and upward rotation of scapula	C3–4	From spinous process T5–12 to spine of scapula	T5-5-1
Rhomboid						
Major	Spinous process T2–5	Lower two thirds of vertebral border of scapula	Retracts and rotates scapula downward	C5 Dorsal scapular	Under Trapezius along vertebral border of scapula	T5-5-1
Minor	Spinous process C7–T1	Vertebral border at root of the spine of the scapula	Same as Rhomboid major	C5 Dorsal scapular	Just superior to Rhomboid major, hard to palpate	T5-5-1
Levator Scapulae	Transverse process C1–4	Superior one third of vertebral border of scapula	Elevation of scapula and moves neck laterally	C3–5	Anterior to upper Trapezius, hard to palpate	T5-5-1
Pectoralis Minor	Anterior ribs 3, 4, 5	Coracoid process	Forward rotation and depression of scapula	C8–T1 Medial pectoral	Under Pectoralis major in axillary space, hard to palpate	T5-5-2
Serratus Anterior	Anterior ribs 1–8	Anterior aspect of vertebral border of scapula	Stabilization, upward rotation and protraction of the scapula	C5, 6, 7 Posterior thoracic	Lateral ribs below axilla	T5-5-2

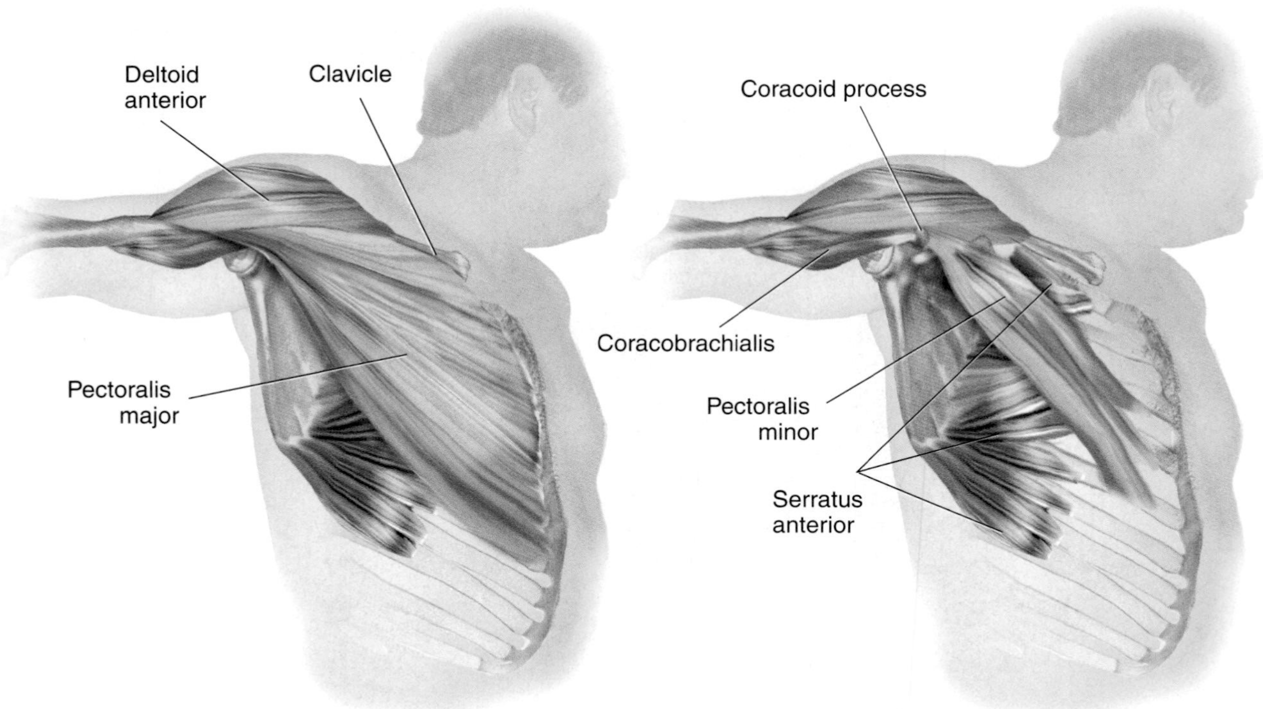

FIGURE T5-5-2 Anterior lateral upper thorax (pectoralis major cut away): serratus anterior and pectoralis minor.

TABLE 5.5 (continued)

MUSCLES OF THE UPPER EXTREMITIES (Continued) — Muscles That Act on the Upper Arm						
MUSCLE	**ORIGIN**	**INSERTION**	**ACTION**	**INNERVATION**	**PALPATION**	**FIGURE**
Pectoralis Major						
Clavicular	Medial half of clavicle, clavicular head	Lateral ridge of bicipital groove distal to pectoralis major sternal insertion	Adduction, horizontal adduction, medial rotation and flexion of humerus	C5, 6, 7 Lateral pectoral Accessory	Anterior of axilla to acromion	T5-5-3
Sternal	Sternum, costal cartilage of ribs 1–6	Lateral ridge of bicipital groove proximal to pectoralis major clavicular insertion	Same as clavicular plus extension of humerus from flexed position	C8, T1 Lateral and medial pectoral	Anterior of axilla	T5-5-3
Coracobrachialis	Coracoid process of scapula	Middle of medial humerus	Flexion and adduction of humerus	C6, 7 Musculocutaneous	Hard to palpate	T5-5-3
Deltoid						
Anterior	Lateral one third of clavicle	Deltoid tuberosity of humerus	Flexion, horizontal rotation	C5, 6 Axillary nerve adduction, medial	This is the rounded shoulder muscle; the anterior in front, the middle lateral to and the posterior in the back of the shoulder joint.	T5-5-2
Middle	Acromion and lateral spine of the scapula	Deltoid tuberosity of humerus	Abduction to 90 degrees	C5, 6 Axillary nerve		T5-5-3

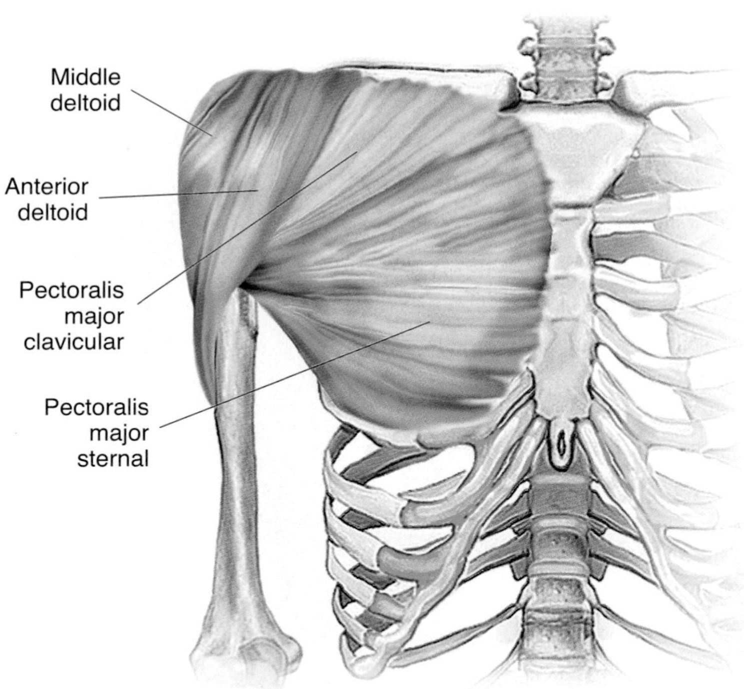

FIGURE T5-5-3 Anterior shoulder; pectoralis major, anterior and middle deltoid, overlay cut away to show coracobrachialis.

TABLE 5.5 (continued)

MUSCLES OF THE UPPER EXTREMITIES (Continued) Muscles That Act on the Upper Arm (continued)						
MUSCLE	ORIGIN	INSERTION	ACTION	INNERVATION	PALPATION	FIGURE
Deltoid, cont'd						
Posterior	Lower lip of the spine of the scapula	Deltoid tuberosity of humerus	Extension, horizontal abduction, lateral rotation	C5, 6 Axillary nerve		T5-5-4
Supraspinatus	Supraspinous fossa of scapula	Top of greater tubercle of the humerus	Initiates abduction of the humerus	C5 Suprascapular nerve	Above spine of scapula near acromion	T5-5-4
Infraspinatus	Infraspinous fossa of scapula	Greater tubercle of humerus	Lateral rotation of humerus	C5, 6 Suprascapular nerve	Below the spine of the scapula	T5-5-4
Subscapularis	Anterior surface of the scapula	Lesser tubercle of the humerus	Medial rotation of humerus	C6, 7 Subscapular nerve	Hard to palpate	T5-5-5
Teres Minor	Upper axillary border of scapula	Greater tubercle of humerus	Lateral rotation of of humerus	C5 Axillary nerve	Below posterior deltoid and above teres major	T5-5-4
Teres Major	Lateral border, inferior angle of scapula	Medial ridge of bicipital groove of humerus	Extension, adduction, medial rotation of humerus	C6, 7 Subscapular nerve	With latissimus dorsi forms posterior border of axilla	T5-5-4 T5-5-5
Latissimus Dorsi	Thoracolumbar aponeurosis from T7 to iliac crest, lower ribs, inferior angle of scapula	Bicipital groove of humerus	Extension, adduction, medial rotation of humerus	C6, 7, 8 Thoracodorsal nerve	Large muscle forming posterior axilla and extending down toward posterior ribs	T5-5-4

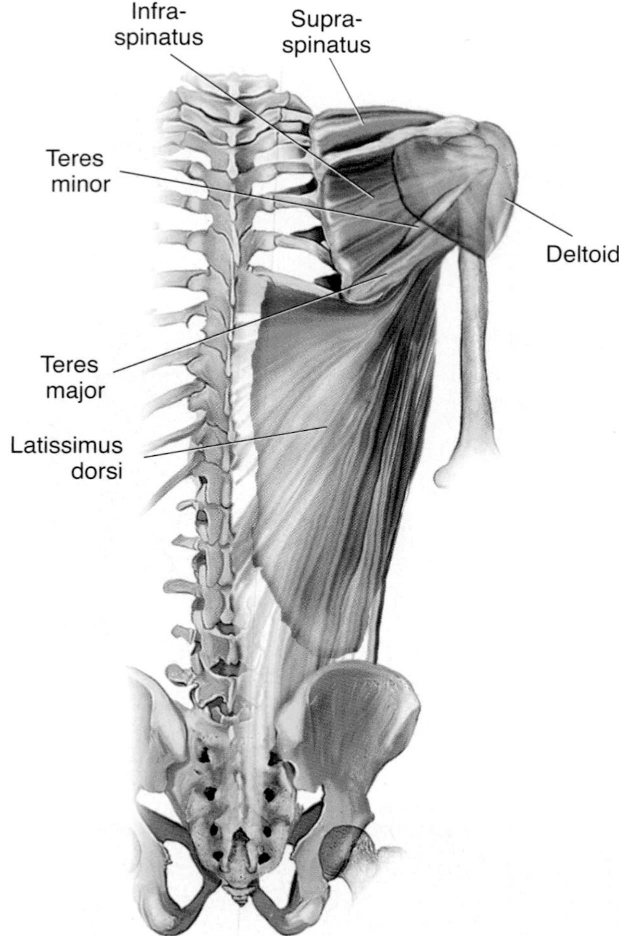

FIGURE T5-5-4 Posterior shoulder; supraspinatus and infraspinatus, posterior deltoid, teres major and minor, latissimus dorsi.

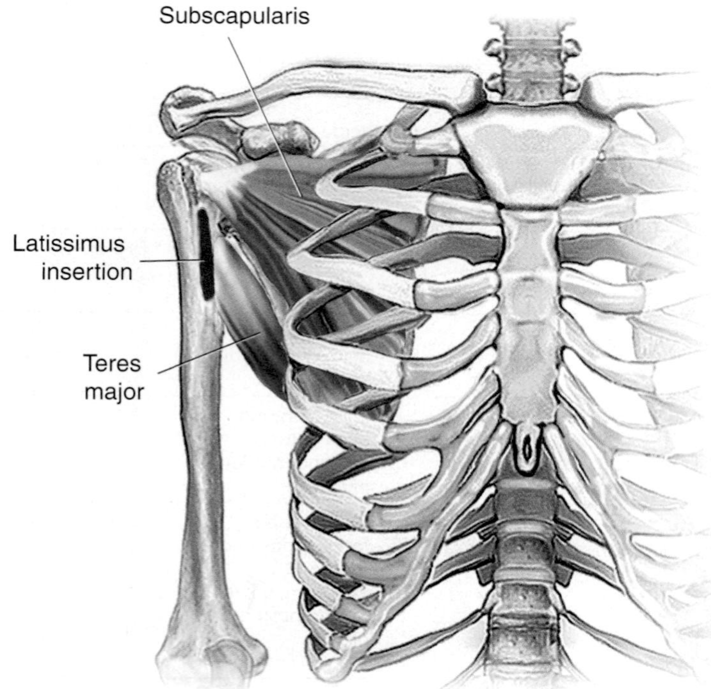

FIGURE T5-5-5 Anterior shoulder cutaway shows subscapularis muscle and teres major and latissimus dorsi insertion.

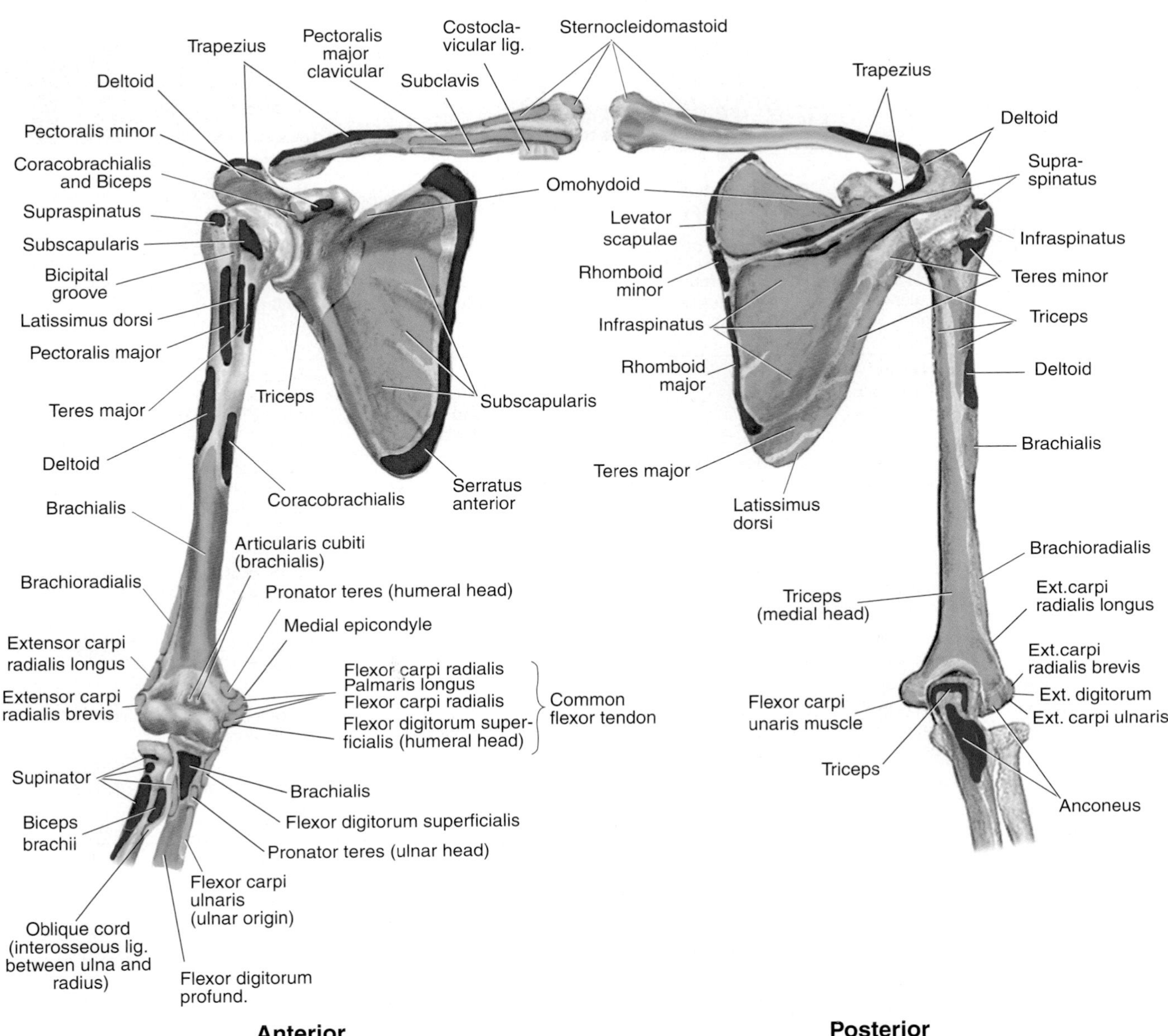

FIGURE T5-5-6 Muscle attachments for shoulder and upper arm.

TABLE 5.5 (continued)

MUSCLES OF THE UPPER EXTREMITIES (Continued) Muscles That Act on the Forearm						
MUSCLE	ORIGIN	INSERTION	ACTION	INNERVATION	PALPATION	FIGURE
Biceps Brachii						
Short Head	Coracoid process of the scapula	Posterior portion of the tuberosity of the radius	Flexion of arm, and forearm, supinates forearm	C5, 6 Musculocutaneous	Anterior surface of humerus	T5-5-7
Long Head	Tubercle at top of the glenoid fossa on scapula	Posterior portion of the tuberosity of the radius	Flexion of arm and forearm, supinates forearm	C5, 6 Musculocutaneous	Anterior surface of humerus	T5-5-7
Brachialis	Distal half of anterior aspect of the humerus	Tuberosity of the ulna	Flexion of the elbow	C5, 6 Musculocutaneous and C7, 8 Radial nerve	Medial to Biceps on distal anterior humerus	T5-5-7
Brachioradialis	Lateral supra-condylar ridge of humerus	Styloid process of radius	Flexion of the elbow	C5, 6 Radial nerve	Top of upper forearm when elbow is flexed	T5-5-7
Triceps Brachii						
Long Head	Infraglenoid tuberosity of the scapula	Olecranon process of ulna	Extension of the elbow	C7, 8 Radial nerve	Posterior aspect of humerus	T5-5-8
Lateral Head	Proximal half of posterior humerus	Olecranon process of ulna	Extension of the elbow	C7, 8 Radial nerve	Posterior aspect of humerus	T5-5-8
Medial Head	Distal two thirds of posterior humerus	Olecranon process of ulna	Extension of the elbow	C7, 8 Radial nerve	Posterior aspect of humerus	T5-5-8
Anconeus	Lateral epicondyle of humerus	Olecranon process of ulna	Extension of the elbow	C7, 8 Radial nerve	Hard to palpate	T5-5-8
Pronator Teres	Just proximal to medial epicondyle of humerus	Midlateral surface of radius	Pronates the hand, assists in elbow flexion	C6, 7 Median nerve	In resisted pronation, medial anterior proximal forearm	T5-5-7
Pronator Quadratus	Distal one fourth of anterior ulna radius	Distal one fourth of lateroanterior radius	Pronates the hand	C8, T1 Median nerve	Cannot palpate	T5-5-7
Supinator	Lateral epicondyle, radial collateral and annular ligament and the ridge of the ulna just below the radial notch	Lateral surface of the proximal one third of radius	Assists biceps to supinate hand and forearm	C6 Deep Radial nerve	Deep to brachioradialis on proximal forearm; hard to palpate	T5-5-7

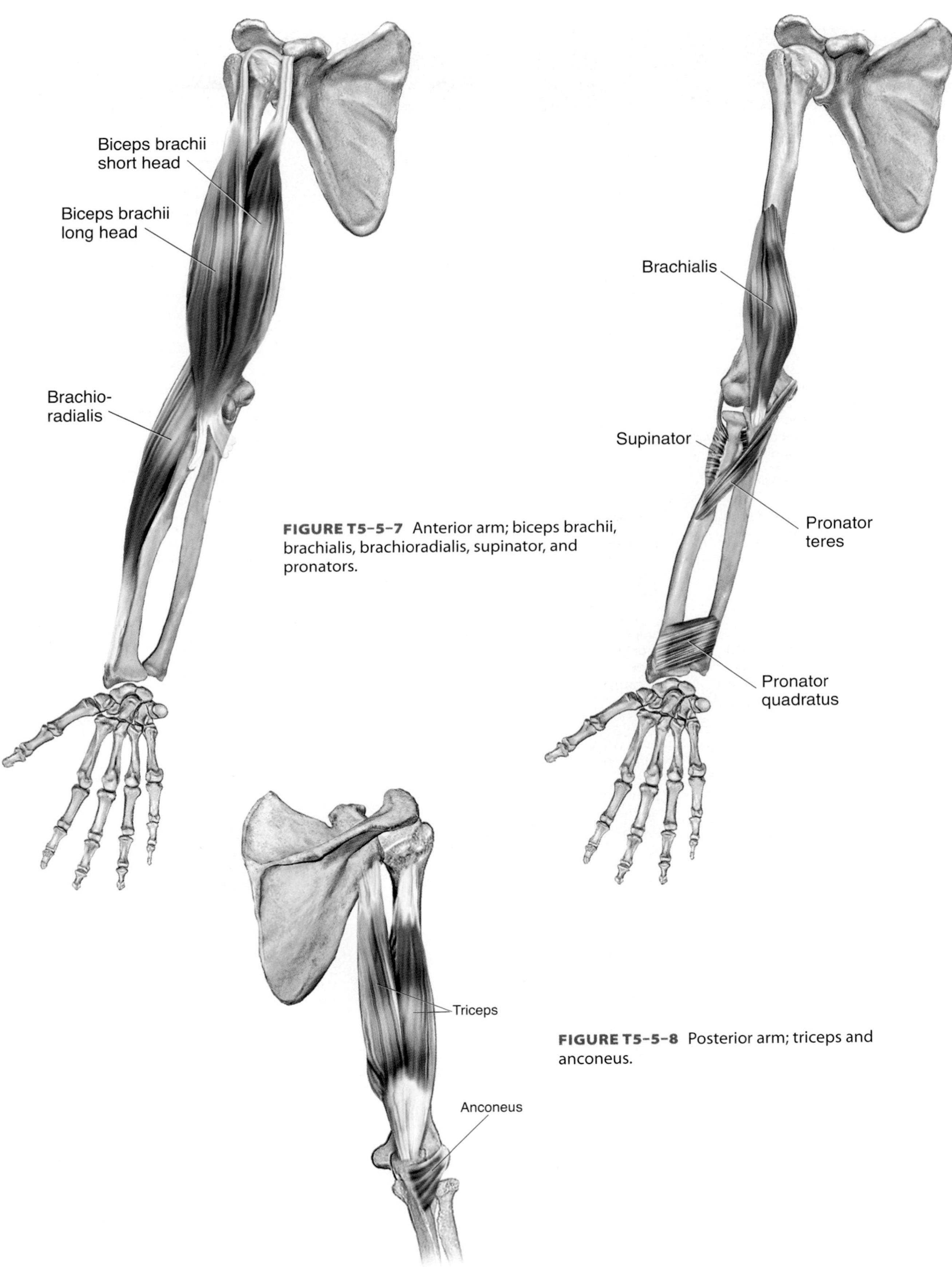

FIGURE T5-5-7 Anterior arm; biceps brachii, brachialis, brachioradialis, supinator, and pronators.

FIGURE T5-5-8 Posterior arm; triceps and anconeus.

TABLE 5.5 (continued)

MUSCLES OF THE UPPER EXTREMITIES (Continued) Muscles That Act on the Wrist and Hand						
MUSCLE	**ORIGIN**	**INSERTION**	**ACTION**	**INNERVATION**	**PALPATION**	**FIGURE**
Flexor Carpi Radialis	Medial epicondyle of the humerus	Base of the second and third metacarpals	Flexion, abduction of wrist	C6, 7 Median	Anterior surface of forearm; tendon prominent on radial side of Palmaris longus tendon at the wrist	T5-5-9
Flexor Carpi Ulnaris						T5-5-9
Humeral head	Medial epicondyle of humerus	Pisiform, hamate and base of fifth metacarpal	Flexion, abduction of wrist	C7, 8, T1 Ulnar	Muscle on proximal half of medial forearm tendon on medial anterior wrist proximal to pisiform bone	
Ulnar head	Proximal two thirds of posterior ulna and olecranon	Common insertion with Humeral head	Flexion, abduction of wrist	C7, 8, T1 Ulnar		
Palmaris Longus	Medial epicondyle of humerus	Palmar aponeurosis	Flexion of wrist	C7, 8 Median	Tendon palpated in middle of anterior wrist	T5-5-9
Extensor Carpi Radialis Longus	Distal one third of supra-condylar ridge of humerus	Dorsal surface of base of second metacarpal	Extension, abduction of wrist	C6, 7 Radial	Next to brachioradialis on dorsal surface of forearm	T5-5-10
Extensor Carpi Radialis Brevis	Lateral epicondyle of humerus	Dorsal surface of base of third metacarpal	Extension of wrist	C6, 7, 8 Radial	Next to Extensor carpi radialis longus, hard to differentiate	T5-5-10
Extensor Carpi Ulnaris	Lateral epicondyle of humerus and by aponeurosis from proximal posterior ulna	Lateral dorsal side of base of fifth metacarpal	Extension and abduction of wrist	C6, 7, 8 Deep radial	Ulnar border of dorsal forearm; tendon on dorsal wrist near ulnar styloid	T5-5-10
Flexor Digitorum Superficialis		By four tendons to the sides of the middle phalanges of digits 2–5	Initial action flexes middle phalanx digits 2–5; continued action flexes proximal phalanx of digits 2–5 and wrist	C7, 8, T1 Median	Muscle is hard to palpate; tendon is prominent on ulnar side of wrist between Palmaris longus and Flexor carpi ulnaris tendons	T5-5-11
Humeral head	Medial epicondyle of humerus and ulnar collateral ligament					
Ulnar head	Medial side of coronoid process of ulna					
Radial head	Oblique line of the radius					

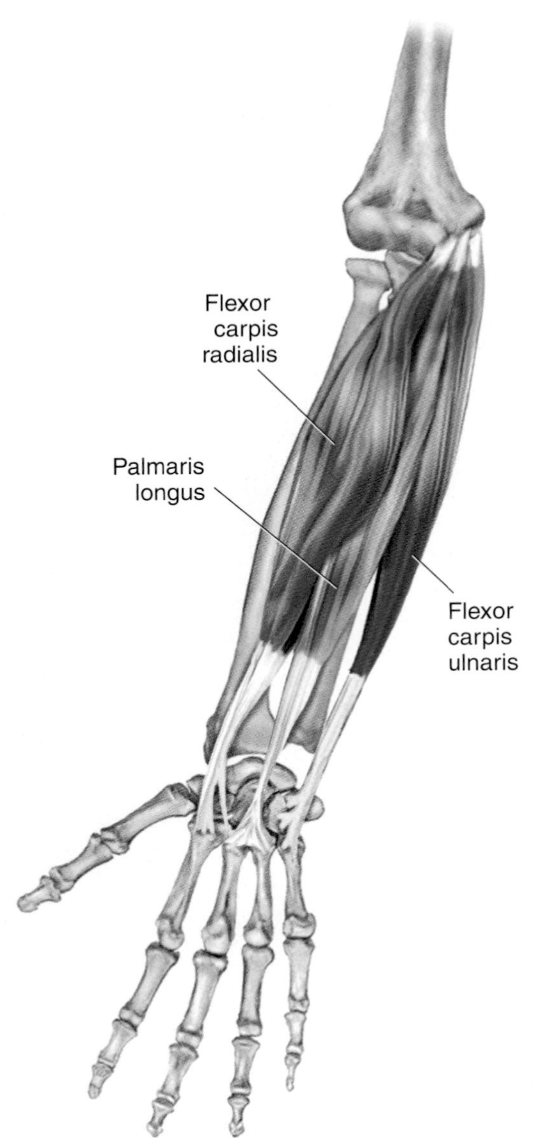

FIGURE T5-5-9 Anterior forearm; flexor carpi radialis and ulnaris and palmaris longus.

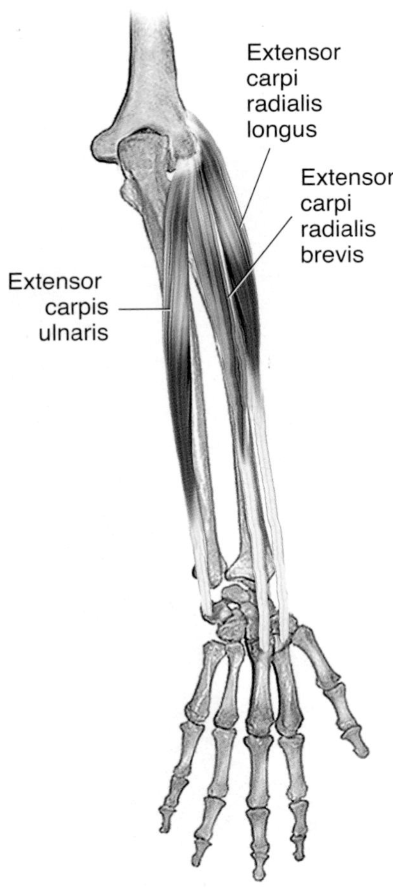

FIGURE T5-5-10 Posterior forearm; extensor carpi radialis longus and brevis, extensor carpi ulnaris.

TABLE 5.5 (continued)

MUSCLES OF THE UPPER EXTREMITIES (Continued) Muscles That Act on the Wrist and Hand (continued)						
MUSCLE	ORIGIN	INSERTION	ACTION	INNERVATION	PALPATION	FIGURE
Flexor Digitorum Profundus	Proximal three fourths of anterior and medial ulna and interosseus	By tendons to anterior bases of dist phalan 2–5	Initially flexes distal phalanges 2–5; continued action assists flexion of and wrist	Digit 2–3; C8, TI Median Digit 4–5; C7, 8 Ulnar	Muscle lies deep and is hard pass through split tendons of Superficialis tendons and can be palpated on anterior surface of middle phalanges	T5-5-11
Flexor Digiti Minimi	Hamate bone and flexor retinaculum	Base of proximal phalanx of little finger	Flexes metacarpophalangeal joint of little finger	C8, T1 Ulnar	Palmar surface of fifth metacarpal	T5-5-14

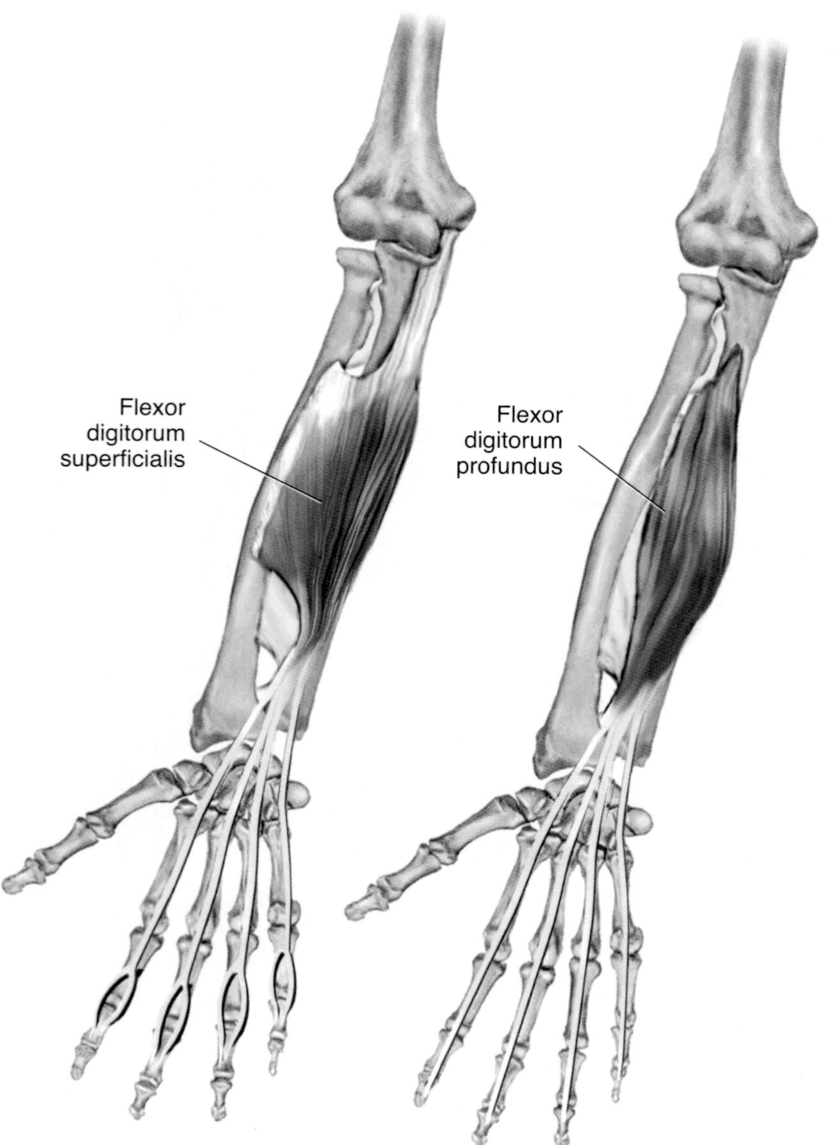

FIGURE T5-5-11 Anterior forearm and hand; flexor digitorum profundus and superficialis longus.

TABLE 5.5 (continued)

MUSCLES OF THE UPPER EXTREMITIES (Continued)						
Muscles That Act on the Wrist and Hand (continued)						
MUSCLE	ORIGIN	INSERTION	ACTION	INNERVATION	PALPATION	FIGURE
Extensor Digitorum	Lateral epicondyle of humerus	By four tendons to digits 2–5. To the dorsal base of the middle and distal phalanges	Extension of MP joints and with Lumbricalis and interossei extends PIP* and DIP** joints	C6, 7, 8 Radial	Prominent tendons on back of hand	T5-5-12
Extensor Indicis	Distal third of posterior ulna and interosseus membrane	Extensor expansion of index finger with Extensor digito-rum tendon	Extension of index finger at PIP* and DIP** joints with Lumbricalis and interosseous and extends MP† joint	C6, 7, 8 Radial	Dorsal surface of distal forearm. Tendon prominent on dorsal hand when pointing index finger	

TABLE 5.5 (continued)

MUSCLES OF THE UPPER EXTREMITIES (Continued) Muscles That Act on and Support the Scapula						
MUSCLE	**ORIGIN**	**INSERTION**	**ACTION**	**INNERVATION**	**PALPATION**	**FIGURE**
Extensor Digiti Minimi	Lateral epicondyle of humerus	Extensor expansion of little finger with Extensor digitorum tendon	Extension of MP† joint and with Lumbricalis and interosseous extends PIP* and DIP** joints	C6, 7, 8 Radial	Adjacent to Extensor digitorum; hard to palpate	T5-5-12
Abductor Digiti Minimi	Tendon of Flexor carpi ulnaris and pisiform	Ulnar side of proximal phalanx of little finger	Abduction of little finger at MP† joint	C8, T1 Ulnar	Ulnar border of fifth metacarpal	T5-5-14
Opponens Digiti Minimi	Hook of the Hamate and flexor retinaculum	Ulnar side of fourth metacarpal	Opposition of the fifth metacarpal	C8, T1 Ulnar	Hard to palpate	T5-5-14
Palmar interosseous						T5-5-14
First	Ulnar side of first metacarpal	Ulnar side of proximal phalanx of first digit	Adducts thumb, index finger, ring finger, and little finger toward axial line of hand through third finger; assists Lumbricalis in MP† flexion and DIP** and PIP* extension	C8, T1 Ulnar	Cannot palpate	
Second	Ulnar side of second metacarpal	Ulnar side of proximal phalanx of second digit				
Third	Radial side of fourth metacarpal	Radial side of proximal phalanx of fourth digit				
Fourth	Radial side of fifth metacarpal	Radial side of proximal phalanx of fifth digit				
Dorsal interosseous	Adjacent surfaces of all metacarpal bones	Extensor expansion and proximal bases of digits 2, 3, and 4	Abduction of index, middle, and ring fingers. Assists Lumbricalis in MP† flexion and DIP** and PIP* extension	C8, T1 Ulnar	Between metacarpals of dorsal surface of hand	T5-5-15
Lumbricals	Flexor digitorum tendons at level of metacarpals	Radial side of extensor expansion at proximal phalanx of digits 2, 3, 4, and 5	Flexion of MP† joints and extension of DIP** and PIP* joints	Digits 2 and 3, C6, 7, Median. Digits 4 and 5, 7 and 8, Ulnar	Hard to palpate	T5-5-14

- * proximal interphalangal joint
- ** distal interphalangal joint
- † metacarpalphalangal joint

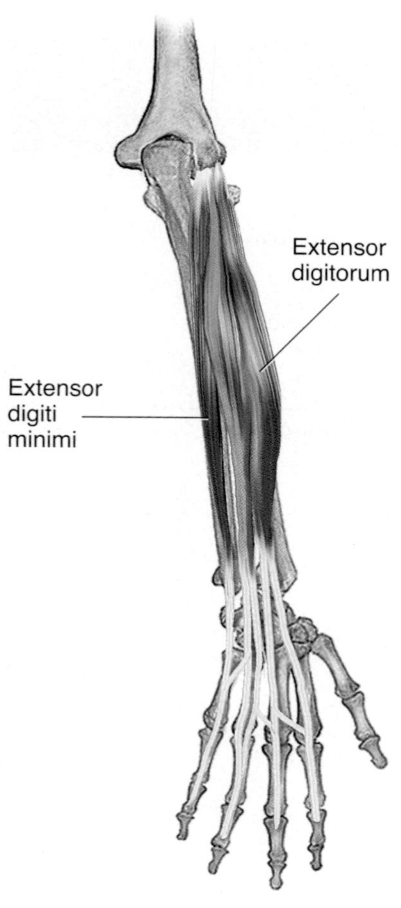

FIGURE T5-5-12 Posterior forearm and hand; extensor digitorum communis, extensor indicis, and extensor digiti minimi.

TABLE 5.5 (continued)

MUSCLES OF THE UPPER EXTREMITIES (Continued) — Muscles That Act on the Thumb						
MUSCLE	ORIGIN	INSERTION	ACTION	INNERVATION	PALPATION	FIGURE
Abductor Pollicis Longus	Middle third of posterior surface of ulna, radius, and interosseus	Base of radial side of first metacarpal	Abduction and extension of carpometa-carpal joint of thumb	C7, 8 Radial	Tendon palpated just anterior to Extensor pollicis longus on radial side of wrist	T5-5-16 T5-5-17
Abductor Pollicis Brevis	Flexor retinaculum, trapezium, and scaphoid	Radial side of proximal phalanx of thumb	Abduction of the thumb	C8, T1 Median	Radial side of palmar surface of first metacarpal	T5-5-17
Adductor Pollicis		Ulnar side of base of the first phalanx of the thumb	Adduction of the thumb	C8, T1 Deep branch of ulnar	Palmar surface of thumb web space	T5-5-17
Transverse Head	Palmar surface of third metacarpal					
Oblique Head	Capitate bone and base of second and third metacarpals					
Flexor Pollicis Longus	Anterior surface of middle radius and adjacent interosseus membrane	Base of palmar surface of distal phalanx of thumb	Initial action flexes distal joint of thumb; continued action assists flexion of two proximal joints	C8, T1 Palmar interosseus branch of Median nerve	Tendon palpated of radial side of anterior wrist	T5-5-17

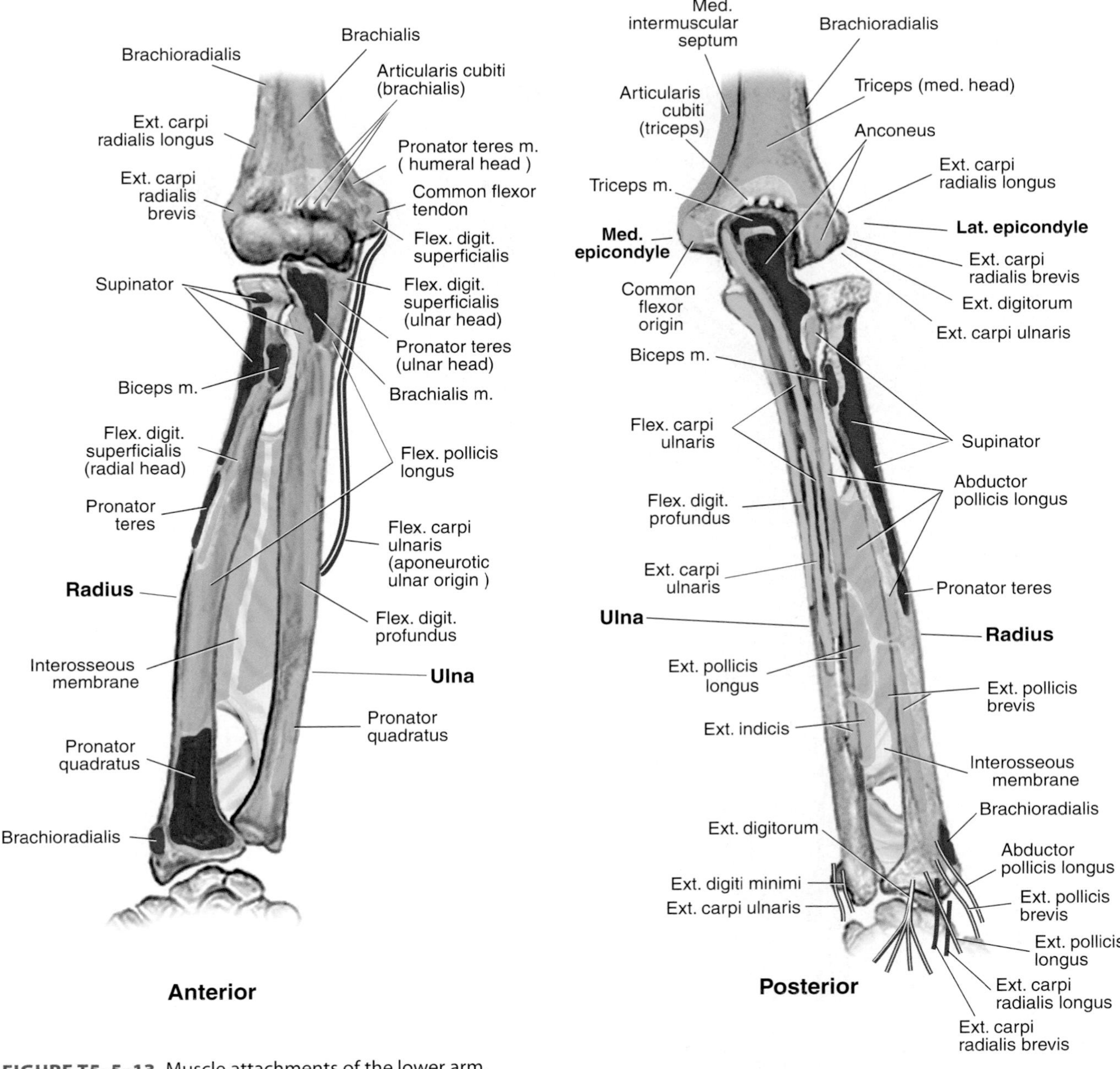

FIGURE T5-5-13 Muscle attachments of the lower arm.

TABLE 5.5 (continued)

MUSCLES OF THE UPPER EXTREMITIES (Continued)						
Muscles That Act on the Thumb (continued)						
MUSCLE	ORIGIN	INSERTION	ACTION	INNERVATION	PALPATION	FIGURE
Flexor Pollicis Brevis		Radial side of proximal phalanx of thumb and extensor expansion	Flexion of proximal phalanx and assists with opposition of thumb	C6, 7, 8 Median	Considered to be No. 1 Palmar interossei muscle with Abductor pollicis brevis and Opponens pollicis, makes up the thenar eminence	T5-5-17
Superficial Head	Flexor Retinaculum and trapezium bone					
Deep Head	Trapezoid and capitate bones			C8, T1 Ulnar		

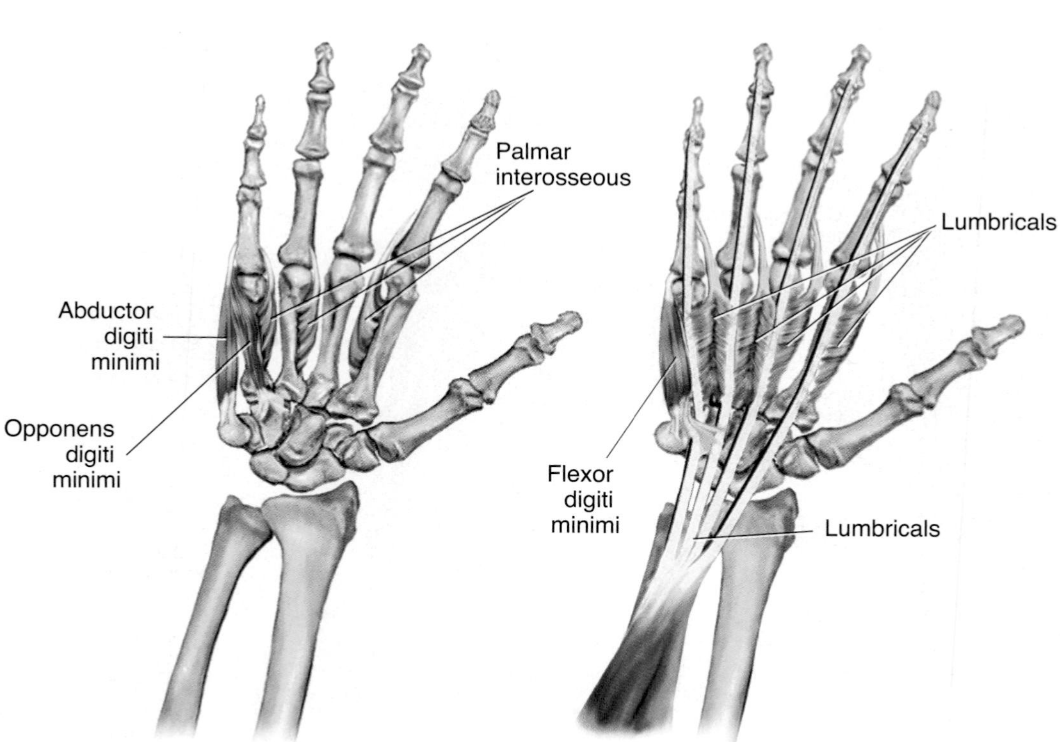

FIGURE T5-5-14 Anterior hand; flexor digiti minimi, abductor digiti minimi, opponens digiti minimi, palmar interosseous, and lumbricales.

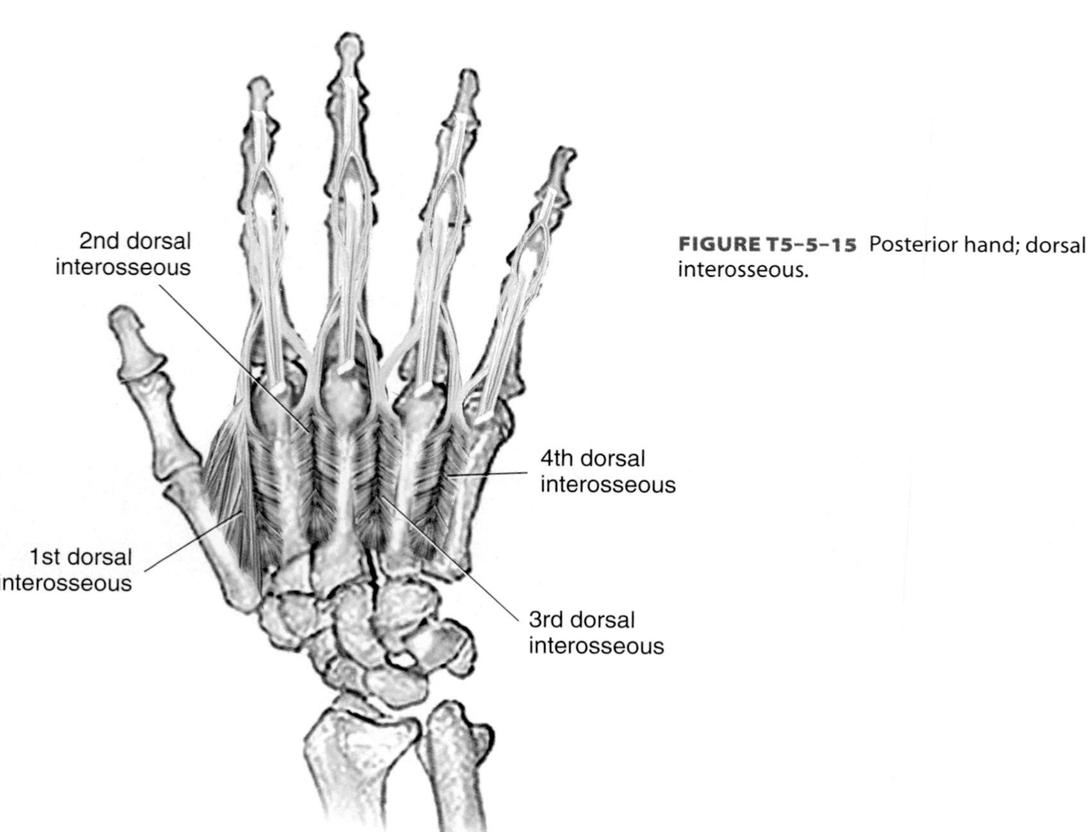

FIGURE T5-5-15 Posterior hand; dorsal interosseous.

TABLE 5.5 (continued)

MUSCLES OF THE UPPER EXTREMITIES (Continued) Muscles That Act on the Thumb (continued)						
MUSCLE	ORIGIN	INSERTION	ACTION	INNERVATION	PALPATION	FIGURE
Extensor Pollicis Longus	Middle third of posterior surface of ulna and interosseus membrane	Base of dorsal surface of distal phalanx of thumb	Extends distal phalanx of thumb; assists extension of proximal phalanx of thumb and wrist and abduction of wrist	C7, 8 Deep radial	Tendon palpated on radial side of first metacarpa on resisted extension just posterior to Extensor pollicis brevis tendon	T5-5-16
Extensor Pollicis Brevis	Posterior surface of radius and membrane distal to origin of Abductor pollicis longus	Dorsal surface of proximal phalanx interosseous	Extends proximal phalanx of thumb; assists in abduction of first metacarpal and wrist	C7, 8 Deep radial	Tendon palpated on radial side of first metacarpal on resisted extension just anterior to Extensor pollici longus tendon	T5-5-16
Opponens Pollicis	Flexor retinaculum and trapezium bone	Entire radial side of first metacarpal	Opposition of thumb	C6, 7, 8, T1 Median and Ulna	Part of thenar eminence. Along first metacarpal	T5-5-17

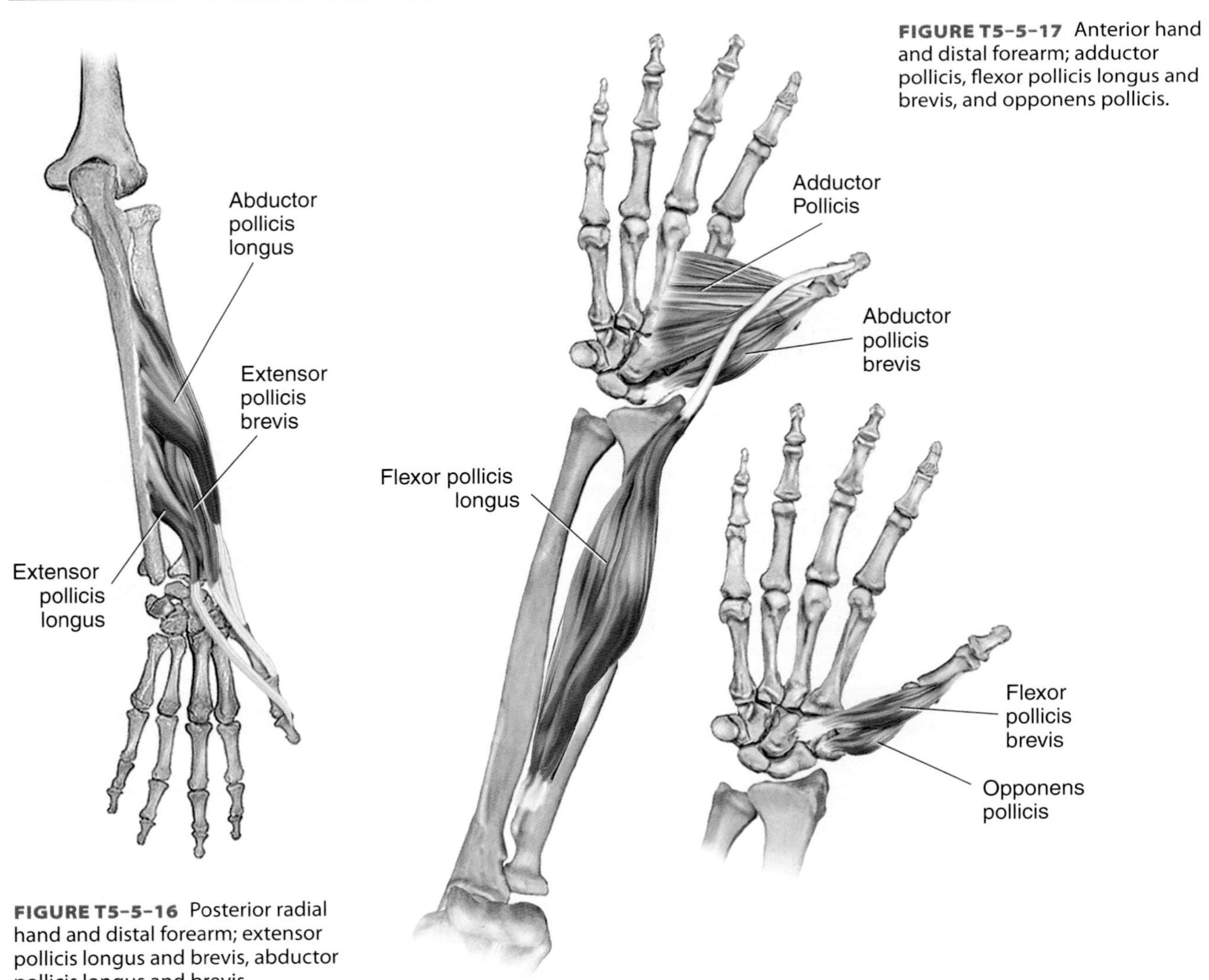

FIGURE T5-5-16 Posterior radial hand and distal forearm; extensor pollicis longus and brevis, abductor pollicis longus and brevis.

FIGURE T5-5-17 Anterior hand and distal forearm; adductor pollicis, flexor pollicis longus and brevis, and opponens pollicis.

TABLE 5.5 (continued)

MUSCLES OF THE LOWER EXTREMITIES Muscles That Act on the Thigh						
MUSCLE	**ORIGIN**	**INSERTION**	**ACTION**	**INNERVATION**	**PALPATION**	**FIGURE**
Psoas Major	Anterior Posterior surfaces of transverse processes and sides of bodies and disks of all lumbar vertebrae	Lesser trochanter of the femur	With fixed origin: Flexes thigh; with fixed insertion, bilaterally flexes hip, unilaterally assists lateral flexion of spine	L2, 3 Lumbar plexus	Deep in abdomen and just above inguinal crease; hard to palpate	T5-5-18 T5-5-31
Iliacus	Superior two thirds of iliac fossa and iliac crest	With Psoas major at lesser trochanter of the femur	Same as Psoas major; assists in abduction and lateral rotation of hip	L2, 3, 4 Femoral	Difficult to palpate	T5-5-18 T5-5-31
Gluteus Maximus	Posterior gluteal line of ilium and adjacent iliac crest, the posterior inferior surface of the sacrum and lateral surface of coccyx	Iliotibial tract of Fascia lata and gluteal tuberosity of femur	Extends and laterally rotates thigh; support extended knee	L5, S1, 2 Inferior gluteal	Posterior surface of buttock	T5-5-19
Gluteus Medius	Iliac crest and external surface of ilium	Lateral surface of greater trochanter of the femur	Abducts thigh. Anterior fibers rotate hip medially	L4, 5, S1 Superior gluteal	Lateral surface of hip between greater trochanter and iliac crest	T5-5-19
Gluteus Minimus	External surface of ilium inferior to gluteus medius muscle and margin of greater sciatic notch	Anterior border of the greater trochanter of femur	Abducts and medially rotates hip	L4, 5, S1 Superior gluteal	Under Gluteus medius	T5-5-19
Tensor Fascia Latae	Anterior portion of iliac spine and ASIS	Iliotibial tract of fascia lata	Abducts and rotates thigh medially; main tains extension of knee	L4, 5, S1 Superior gluteal	Below anterior iliac spine	
Pectineus	Superior ramus of anterior pubis	Between lesser tochanter and linea aspera on posterior femur	Adducts, flexes, and medially rotates thigh	L2,3,4 Femoral and obturator	Uppermost of medial thigh muscles, just superior to Adductor longus	T5-5-20
Adductor Brevis	Outer surface of the inferior ramus of the pubis	Proximal half of the linea aspera to the lesser trochanter on posterior femur	Adduction, flexion, and medial rotation of thigh	L3, 4 Obturator	Deep to Pectineus and Adductor longus; hard to palpate	T5-5-20
Adductor Longus	At the crest of pubis adjacent to pubic symphysis	Middle one third of medial lip of linea aspera	Adduction, flexion, and medial rotation of thigh	L3, 4 Obturator	Groin muscle just below pubis	T5-5-20

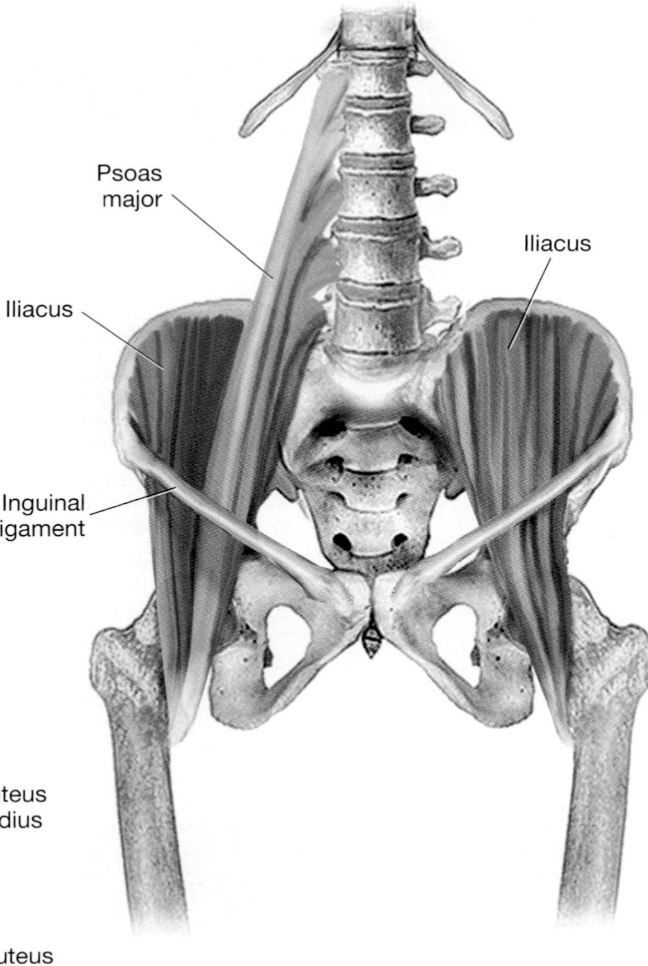

FIGURE T5-5-18 The iliacus and psoas muscles combined are known as the iliopsoas and considered to be the strongest hip flexor.

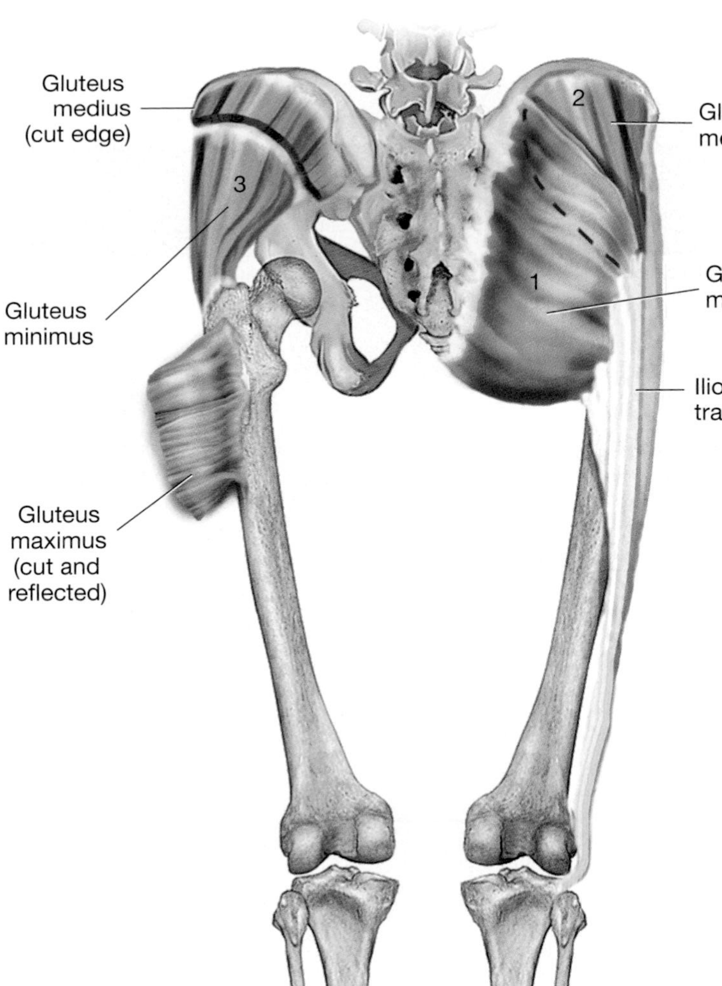

FIGURE T5-5-19 Gluteus maximus, gluteus medius, and gluteus minimus.

TABLE 5.5 (continued)

MUSCLES OF THE LOWER EXTREMITIES (Continued) Muscles That Act on the Thigh (continued)						
MUSCLE	**ORIGIN**	**INSERTION**	**ACTION**	**INNERVATION**	**PALPATION**	**FIGURE**
Adductor Magnus	Inferior pubic ramus, ischial ramus, and ischial tuberosity	The linea aspera, medial epicondylic ridge, and adductor tubercle of the medial femoral condyle	Powerful adduction; anterior fibers flexion and medial rotation posterior fibers extension and lateral rotation	L2, 3, 4 Obturator, L4, 5, S1 Sciatic	Medial surface of thigh	T5-5-20
Gracilis	Inferior half of symphysis pubis and inferior ramus of pubis	The pes anserine; medial surface of tibia inferior to medial tibial condyle	Adducts thigh, flexion and medial rotation of knee	L3, 4 Obturator	Medial thigh below pubis	T5-5-20
Sartorius	Anterior superior iliac spine and iliac notch just inferior to spine	Proximal medial surface of tibia; pes anserine	Flexes, laterally rotates and abducts thigh; assists with flexion and medial rotation of knee	L2, 3 Femoral	Just below ASIS and diagonally across thigh	T5-5-20

TABLE 5.5 (continued)

MUSCLES OF THE LOWER EXTREMITIES (Continued) Muscles That Act on the Thigh and Lateral Rotaters						
MUSCLE	**ORIGIN**	**INSERTION**	**ACTION**	**INNERVATION**	**PALPATION**	**FIGURE**
Piriformis	Anterior sacrum, greater sciatic notch, and anterior portion of the sacrotuberous ligament	Superior edge of greater trochanter of the femur	Lateral rotation of the thigh	L5, S1 Sacral plexus	Cannot palpate	T5-5-21
Gemellus Superior	Outer surface of ischial spine	Medial surface of the posterior greater trochanter of the femur	Lateral rotation of the thigh	L5, S1 Sacral plexus	Cannot palpate	T5-5-21
Obturator Internus	Ramus of the ischium, inner surface of the ilium, and superior and inferior ramus of pubis	Medial surface of the posterior greater trochanter of the femur	Lateral rotation of the thigh	L5, S1 Sacral plexus	Cannot palpate	T5-5-21
Gemellus Inferior	Ischial tuberosity	Medial surface of the posterior greater trochanter of the femur	Lateral rotation of the thigh	L5, S1 Sacral plexus	Cannot palpate	T5-5-21
Obturator Externus	Pubis and ischium around medial side of obturator foramen	The fossa of the greater trochanter of the femur	Lateral rotation of the thigh	L3, 4 Obturator	Cannot palpate	T5-5-21
Quadratus Femoris	Ischial tuberosity	Just distal to the greater trochantic crest	Lateral rotation of the thigh	L5, S1 Sacral plexus	Cannot palpate	T5-5-21

FIGURE T5-5-20 Pectineus, adductor magnus, adductor longus, adductor brevis, gracilis, sartorius.

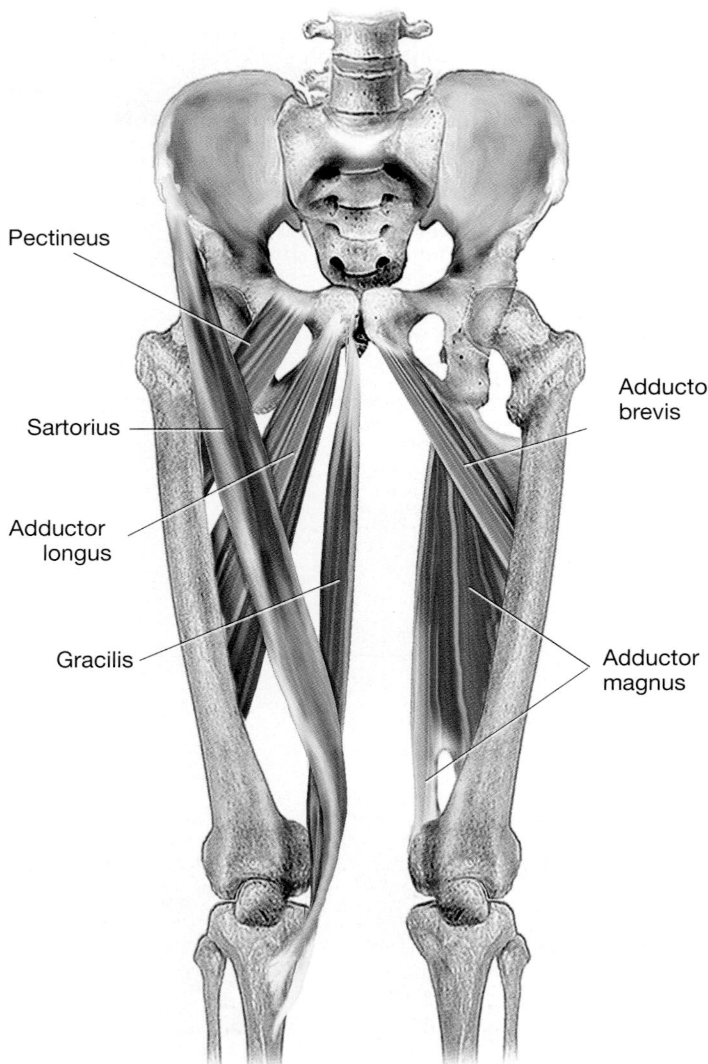

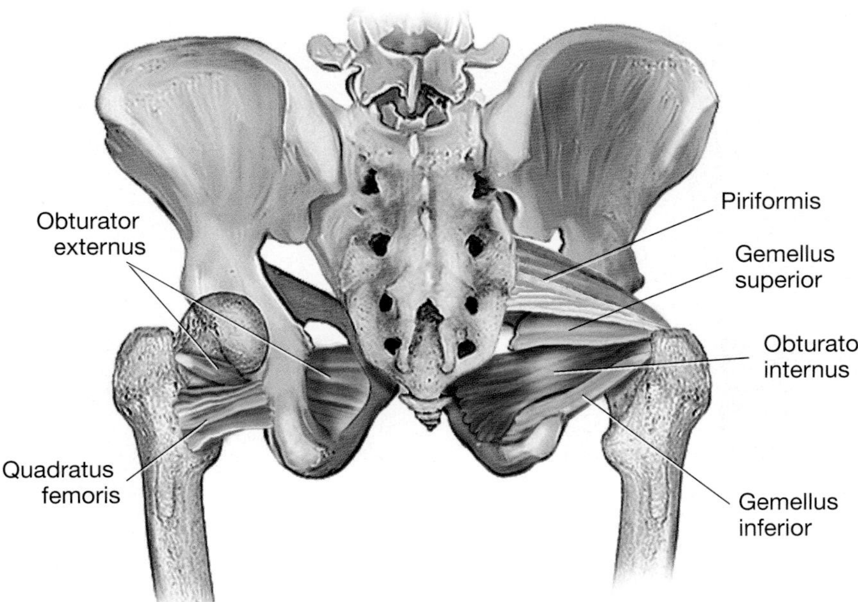

FIGURE T5-5-21 Deep rotators; piriformis, gemellus superior, obturator internus, gemellus inferior, obturator externus, and quadratus femoris.

TABLE 5.5 (continued)

MUSCLES OF THE LOWER EXTREMITIES (Continued) Muscles That Act on the Lower Leg						
MUSCLE	ORIGIN	INSERTION	ACTION	INNERVATION	PALPATION	FIGURE
Hamstrings						T5-5-22
Biceps Femoris Long Head	Ischial tuberosity and sacrotuberous ligament	Lateral side of the head of the fibula and the lateral condyle of the tibia	Both heads; flex and laterally rotate the leg	L5, SI, 2 Sciatic, tibial division	Muscle on posterior surface of thigh; tendon on lateral side of posterior knee	
Short Head	Lateral lip of the linea aspera		Long head; extends and assists in lateral rotation of the hip	L5, S1, 2 Sciatic, peroneal division		
Semi-tendinosus	Ischial tuberosity	Proximal part of medial surface of the tibia; pes anserine	Extends the thigh; flexes and medially rotates the knee	L5, S1, 2 Sciatic, tibial division	Muscle on posterior surface of thigh; tendon on medial side of posterior knee	T5-5-22
Semi-membranosus	Ischial tuberosity	Posteromedial aspect of medial condyle of the tibia	Extends the thigh; flexes and medially rotates the knee	L5, S1, 2 Sciatic, tibia division	Muscle on posterior surface of thigh; tendon deep and hard to palpate	T5-5-22

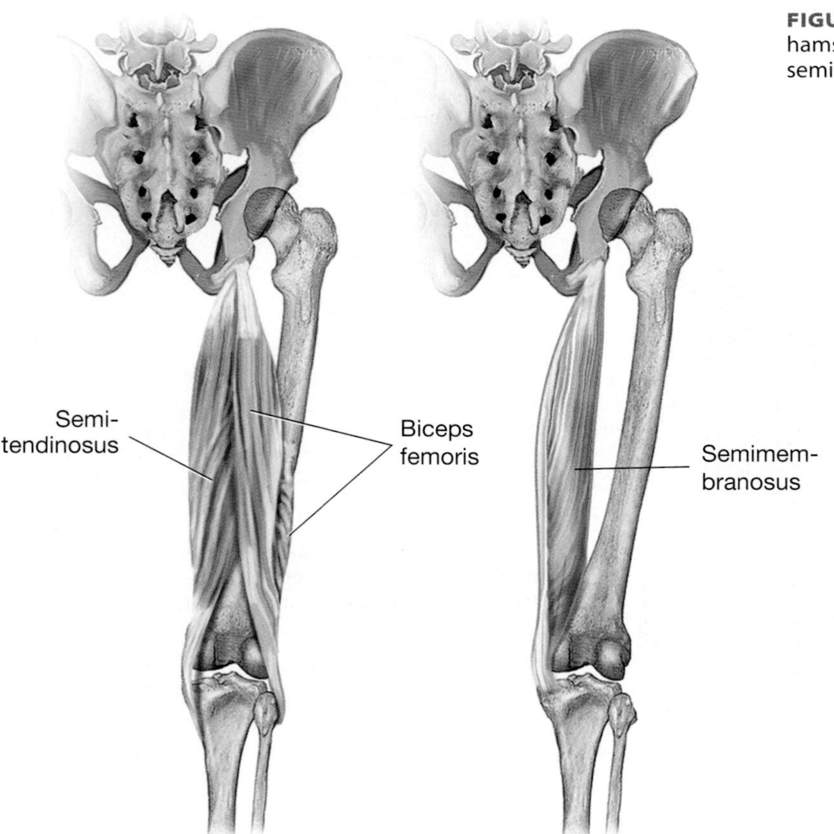

FIGURE T5-5-22 Posterior thigh; hamstrings; biceps femoris, semitendinosus, semimembranosus.

TABLE 5.5 (continued)

MUSCLES OF THE LOWER EXTREMITIES (Continued) Muscles That Act on the Lower Leg (continued)						
MUSCLE	ORIGIN	INSERTION	ACTION	INNERVATION	PALPATION	FIGURE
Quadriceps Femoris						T5-5-23
Rectus Femoris	Anterior inferior iliac spine and the groove above the acetabulum	Via quadriceps expansion and patella through patellar ligament to tuberosity of tibia	Extends the leg at the knee	L2, 3, 4 Femoral	Anterior surface of thigh	T5-5-23
Vastus Lateralis	Anterior and inferior border of greater tro-chanter, proximal one half of lateral linea aspera	Via quadriceps expansion and patella through patellar ligament to tuberosity of tibia	Extends the leg at the knee	L2, 3, 4 Femoral	Anterolateral surface of thigh	T5-5-23
Vastus Intermedius	Anterior and lateral surfaces of proximal two thirds of femur	Via quadriceps expansion and patella through patellar ligament to tuberosity of tibia	Extends the leg at the knee	L2, 3, 4 Femoral	Deep to rectus femoris; hard to palpate	T5-5-23
Vastus Medialis	Medial lip of linea aspera and posterior femur	Via quadriceps expansion and patella through patellar ligament to tuberosity of tibia	Extends the leg at the knee	L2, 3, 4 Femoral	Medial surface of distal two thirds of anterior thigh	T5-5-23

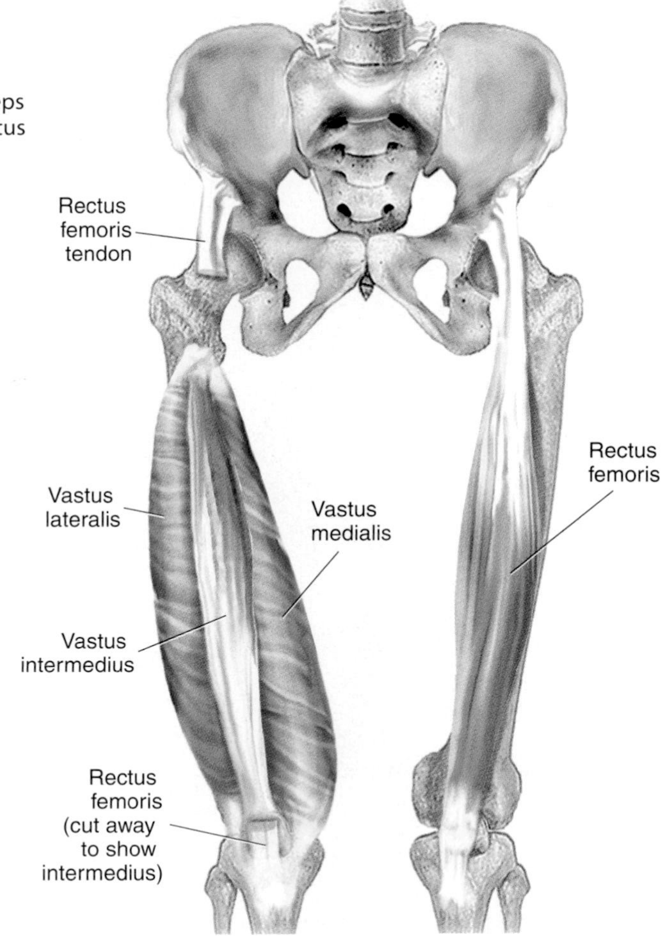

FIGURE T5-5-23 Anterior thigh; quadriceps femoris: rectus femoris, vastus lateralis, vastus intermedius, vastus medialis.

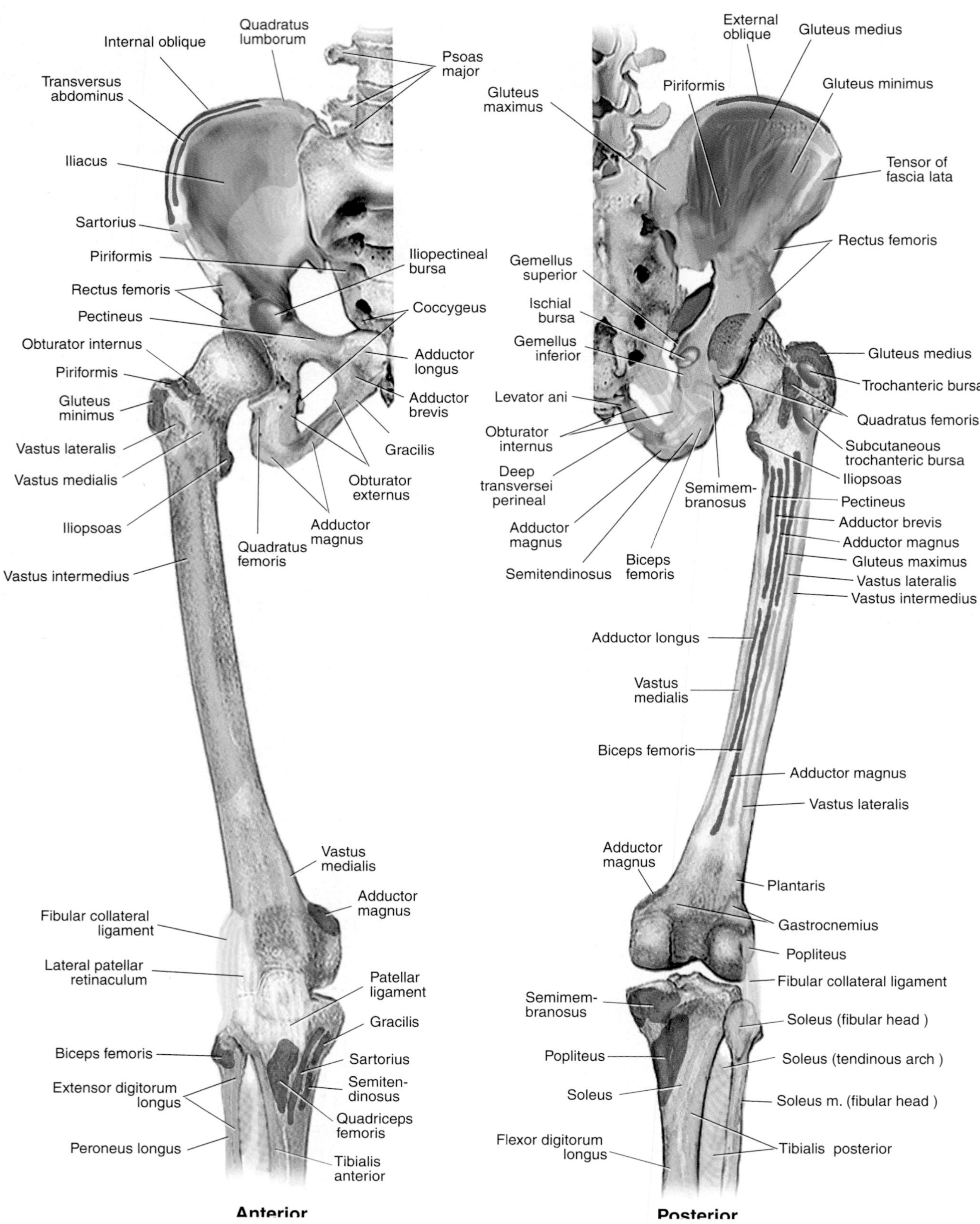

FIGURE T5-5-24 Muscle attachments for the hip and thigh.

TABLE 5.5 (continued)

MUSCLES OF THE LOWER EXTREMITIES (Continued) Muscles That Act on the Foot						
MUSCLE	**ORIGIN**	**INSERTION**	**ACTION**	**INNERVATION**	**PALPATION**	**FIGURE**
Popliteus	Lateral condyle of femur	Posterior surface of proximal tibia	Initiates leg flexion by unlocking the knee	L4, 5, S1 Tibial	Cannot palpate	T5-5-26
Tibialis Anterior	Lateral condyle and proximal one half of tibia, interosseous membrane	Medial and plantar surface of medial cuneiform and base of first metatarsal	Dorsal flexion of ankle and inversion of foot	L4, 5 Deep Peroneal	Lateroanterior surface of tibia; tendon palpated anterior ankle medial to Extensor hallucis longus	T5-5-27
Peroneus Tertius	Distal one third of anterior fibula	Base of fifth metatarsal	Dorsal flexion of the ankle, eversion of foot	L4, 5, S1 Deep Peroneal	Tendon just lateral to tendon of Extensor digitorum	T5-5-28
Extensor Digitorum Longus	Lateral condyle of tibia and proximal three fourths of the anterior fibula	By four tendons to the dorsal surfaces of the second and third phalanges of the four lateral toes	Extension of four lateral toes and dorsal flexion of ankle	L4, 5, S1 Deep Peroneal	Four tendons on dorsum of foot	T5-5-27
Extensor Hallucis Longus	Middle two quarters of anterior fibula and interosseous membrane	Base of distal phalanx of large toe	Extends large toe, dorsal flexes ankle and inversion of foot	L4, 5, S1 Deep Peroneal	Tendon on anterior ankle and dorsum of large toe	T5-5-27
Gastrocnemius						T5-5-25
Medial Head	Posterior surface of medial condyle of the femur	Middle of posterior surface of the calcaneus via Achilles tendon	Plantar flexes the ankle or assists the flexion of the knee	S1, 2 Tibial	Major muscle of posterior calf	
Lateral Head	Posterior surface of the lateral condyle of femur					
Plantaris	Distal lateral supracondylar line of the femur	Posterior surface of the calcaneus via the Achilles tendon	Plantar flexes the ankle or assists flexion of the knee	L4, 5, S1 Tibial	Hard to palpate	T5-5-25
Soleus	Head and proximal one third of posterior fibula and middle border and soleal line of tibia	Middle of posterior surface of the calcaneus via the Achilles tendon	Plantar flexes the ankle	L5, S1, 2 Tibial	Lateral surface of lower leg below gastrocnemius	T5-5-25
Flexor Digitorum Longus	Middle one third of posterior surface of tibia	By four tendons to the plantar surface of the distal phalanges of the four lateral toes	Flexes the four lateral toes; assists in plantar flexion and inversion of the foot	L5, S1, 2 Tibial	Tendon palpated posterior and inferior to media malleolus with Posterior tibialis and Flexor digitorum longus	T5-5-26
Flexor Hallucis Longus	Distal two thirds of posterior fibula and adjacent interosseous membrane	Base of plantar surface distal phalanx of large toes	Flexes large toe; assists plantar flexion and inversion of foot	L5, S1, 2 Tibial	Tendon palpated posterior and inferior to medial malleolus with Posterior tibialis and Flexor digitorum longus	T5-5-26

TABLE 5.5 (continued)

MUSCLES OF THE LOWER EXTREMITIES (Continued) Muscles That Act on the Foot (continued)						
MUSCLE	ORIGIN	INSERTION	ACTION	INNERVATION	PALPATION	FIGURE
Tibialis Posterior	Middle third of posterior tibia, proximal two thirds of medial fibula and interosseus membrane	Plantar surfaces of navicular, cuboid, second and third and fourth metatarsals	Inversion of foot; assists in plantar flexion of ankle	L5, S1, 2 Tibial	Tendon palpated posterior and inferior to medial malleolus with Flexor hallucis longus and Flexor digitorum longus	T5-5-26

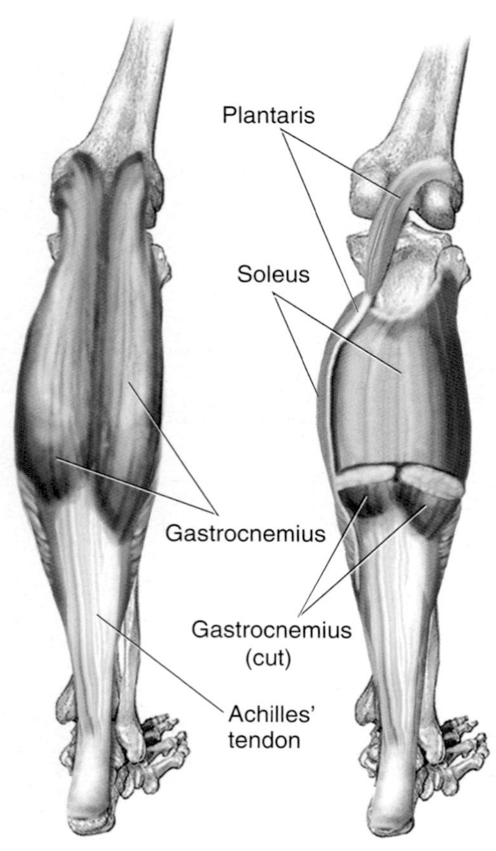

FIGURE T5-5-25 Posterior leg; gastrocnemius, soleus, plantaris.

TABLE 5.5 (continued)

MUSCLES OF THE LOWER EXTREMITIES (Continued) Muscles That Act on the Foot (continued)						
MUSCLE	ORIGIN	INSERTION	ACTION	INNERVATION	PALPATION	FIGURE
Peroneus Longus	Head and proximal two thirds of lateral surface of fibula and lateral condyle of tibia	Plantar surface of medial cuneiform and base of first metatarsal	Eversion of foot; assists plantar flexion of ankle	L4, 5, S1 Superficial Peroneal	Proximal half of lateral surface of lower leg	T5-5-28
Peroneus Brevis	Distal two thirds of lateral surface of fibula	Lateral surface of base of fifth metatarsal	Eversion of foot; assists plantar flexion of ankle	L4, 5, S1 Superficial Peroneal	Posterior and inferior to lateral malleolus with tendon of Peroneus longus	T5-5-28

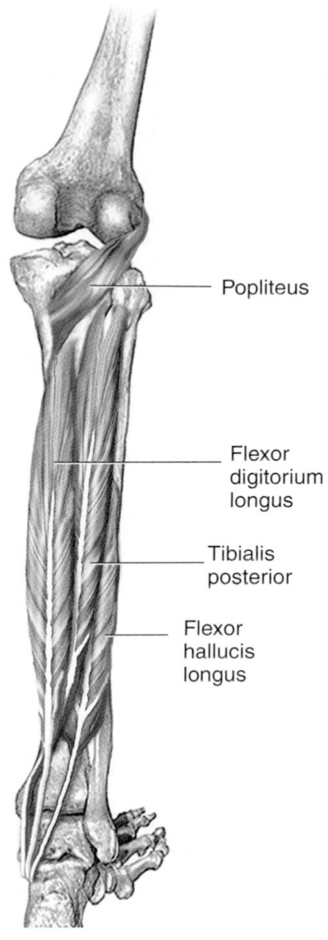

FIGURE T5-5-26 Posterior leg (deep); tibialis posterior, flexor digitorum, flexor hallucis, popliteus.

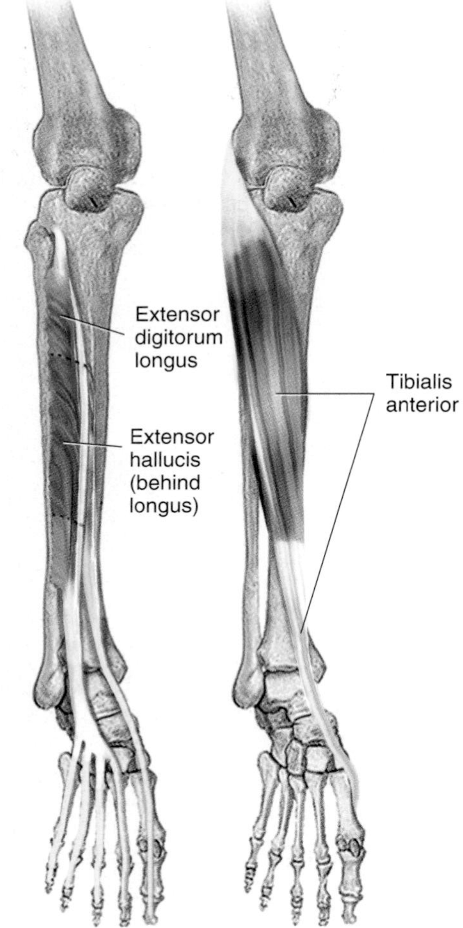

FIGURE T5-5-27 Anterior leg; tibialis anterior, extensor digitorum, extensor hallucis.

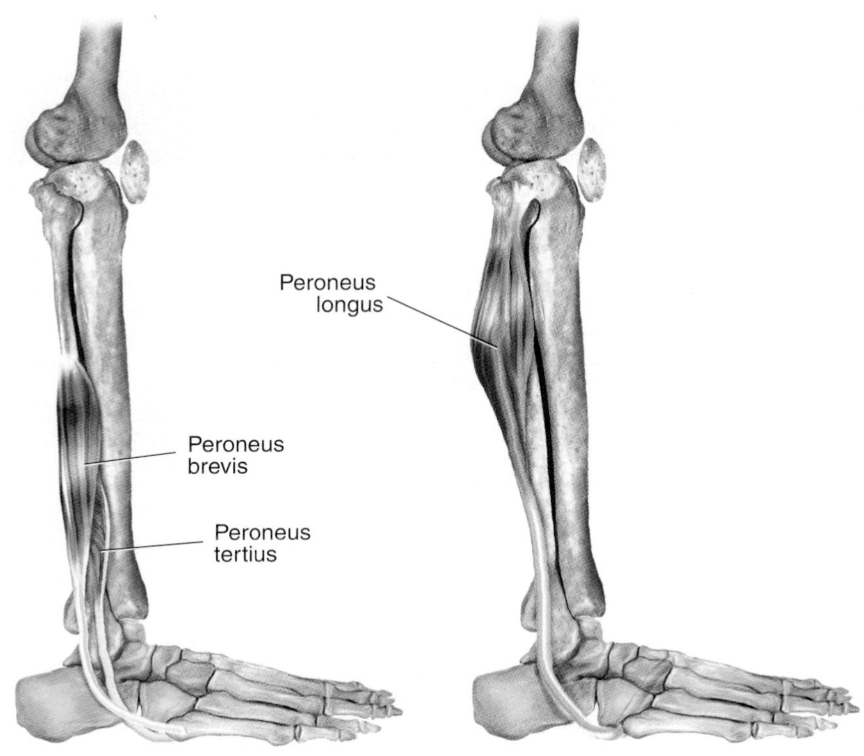

FIGURE T5-5-28 Lateral leg; peroneus tertius, peroneus longus, peroneus brevis.

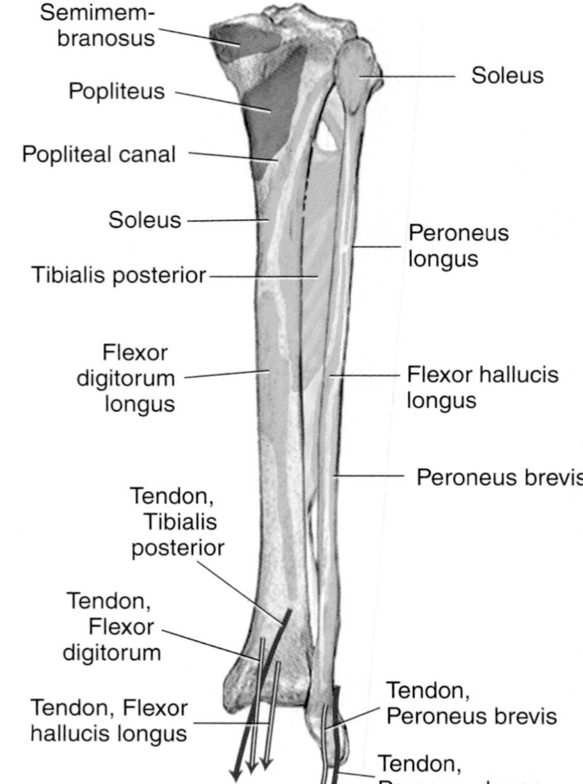

FIGURE T5-5-29 Muscle attachments for the posterior lower leg.

TABLE 5.5 (continued)

MUSCLES OF THE LOWER EXTREMITIES (Continued) Muscles That Act on the Abdomen						
MUSCLE	ORIGIN	INSERTION	ACTION	INNERVATION	PALPATION	FIGURE
Rectus Abdominis	Crest of the pubis and pubic symphysis	Xiphoid process and costal cartilage of fifth, sixth, and seventh ribs	Flexion of trunk; tenses abdominal wall and compresses contents	T5–12 Intercostal, Iliohypogastric, Ilioinguinal	Anterior abdomen from pubis to sternum	T5-5-30
External Oblique	External surface of eight lower ribs	Abdominal aponeurosis to linea alba and iliac crest	Bilaterally, same as above; unilaterally, Lateral flexion and rotation to opposite side	T8–12 Intercostal, Iliohypogastric, Ilioinguinal	Lateral surfaces of abdomen	T5-5-30
Internal Oblique	Inguinal ligament, Iliac crest and Thoracolumbar fascia	Abdominal aponeurosis, linea alba, and costal cartilages of four lower ribs	Bilaterally, same as above; unilaterally, Lateral flexion and rotation to same side	T8–12 Intercostal, Iliohypogastric, Ilioinguinal	Deep to External Oblique, cannot palpate	T5-5-30
Transverse Abdominis	Inguinal ligament, Iliac crest and Thoracolumbar fascia, and lower six ribs	Abdominal aponeurosis to linea alba and iliac crest	Tenses abdominal wall and compresses contents	T7–12 Intercostal, Iliohypogastric, Ilioinguinal	Cannot palpate	T5-5-30

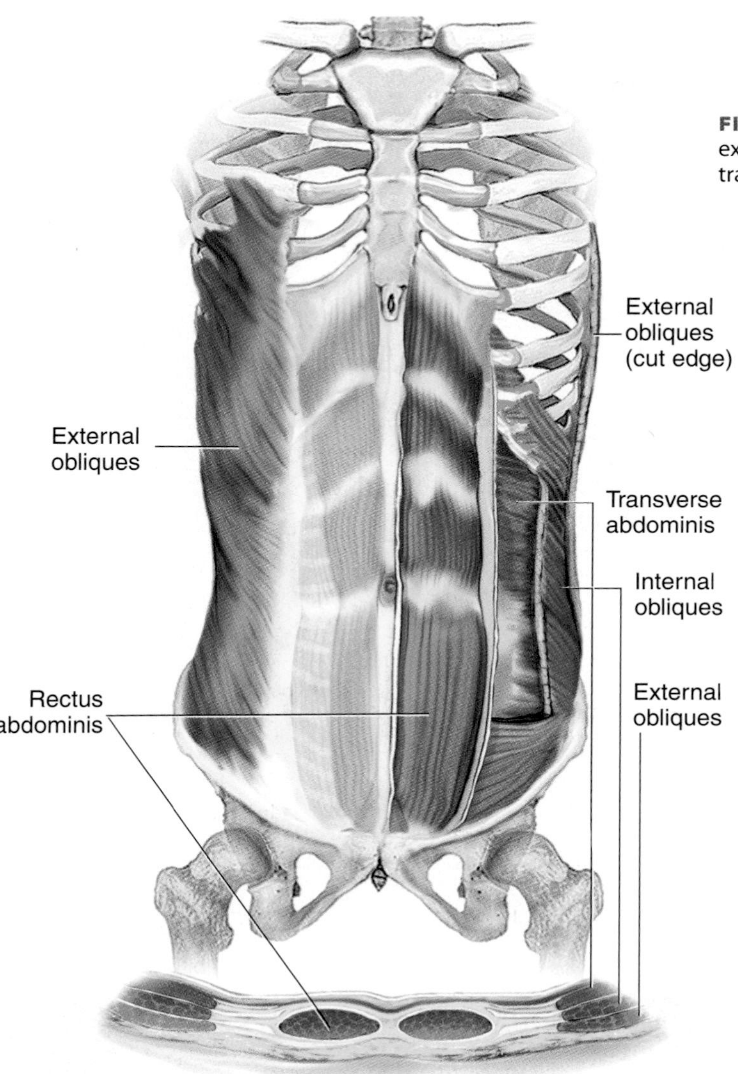

FIGURE T5-5-30 Abdominal area: external obliques, internal obliques, transverse abdominis, rectus abdominis.

TABLE 5.5 (continued)

MUSCLES OF THE TORSO (Continued)						
Muscles of Respiration						
MUSCLE	ORIGIN	INSERTION	ACTION	INNERVATION	PALPATION	FIGURE
Diaphragm	The xiphoid process, six lower ribs and costal cartilages, ligaments, bodies and transverse processes of upper lumbar vertebrae	Central tendon of the Diaphragm, a strong aponeurosis with no bony attachment	Main muscle of respiration, contracts during inspiration increasing thoracic volume; separates abdominal and thoracic cavities	C3, 4, 5 Phrenic	Cannot palpate; action can be observed on abdomen during respiration	T5-5-31

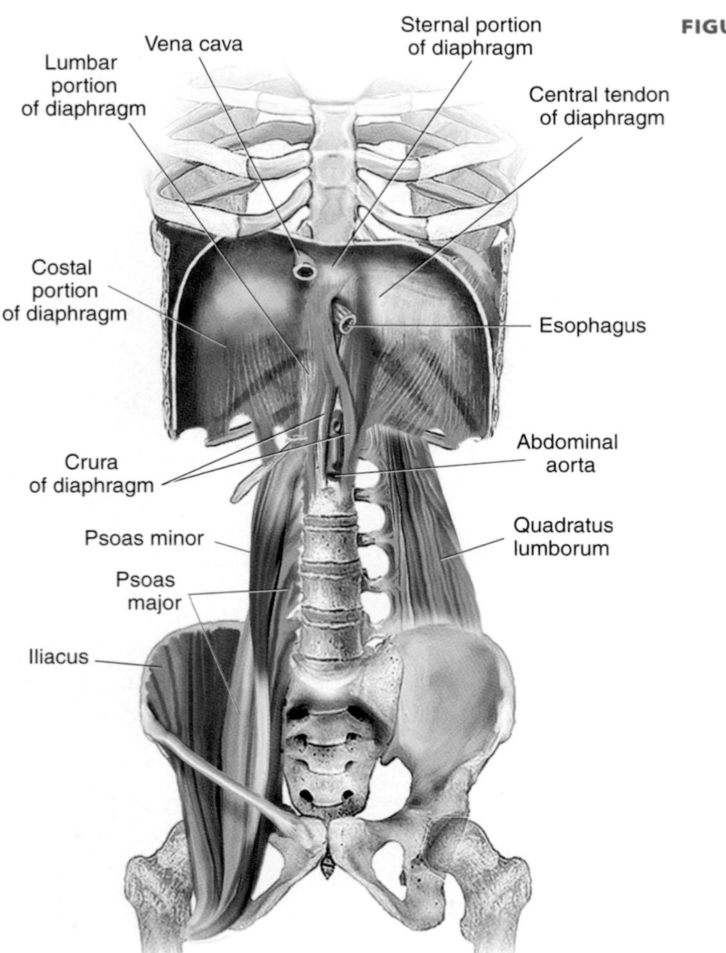

FIGURE T5-5-31 Diaphragm.

TABLE 5.5 (continued)

MUSCLES OF THE TORSO (Continued) — Muscles of Respiration (continued)						
MUSCLE	ORIGIN	INSERTION	ACTION	INNERVATION	PALPATION	FIGURE
Intercostals						T5-5-32
External	Inferior margin of the rib above	Superior margin of the rib below. Fibers angle 45 percent lateral to medial.	Pull ribs together and elevate ribs during inhalation	T1–12 Intercostal	External palpated between ribs	
Internal	Inferior margin of the rib above	Superior margin of the rib below. Fibers angle 45 percent medial to lateral.	Depress ribs during forced exhalation		External and internal intercostal situated perpendicular to each other, and innermost intercostals are too deep to palpate	
Innermost	Sternum and inferior margin of lower ribs	Inner surface of the ventral ribs				
Serratus Posterior Superior	Spinous process C7–T2, ligamentum nuchae C6–T1 supraspinous ligament	Posterior superior surfaces of ribs 2–5	Raises ribs during deep inhalation	T1–4 Intercostal	Cannot palpate	T5-5-33
Serratus Posterior Inferior	Spinous process T11–L3, supraspinous ligament	Inferior borders of ribs 8–12	Pulls ribs outward and down, opposes diaphragm	T9–12 Intercostal	Cannot palpate	T5-5-33

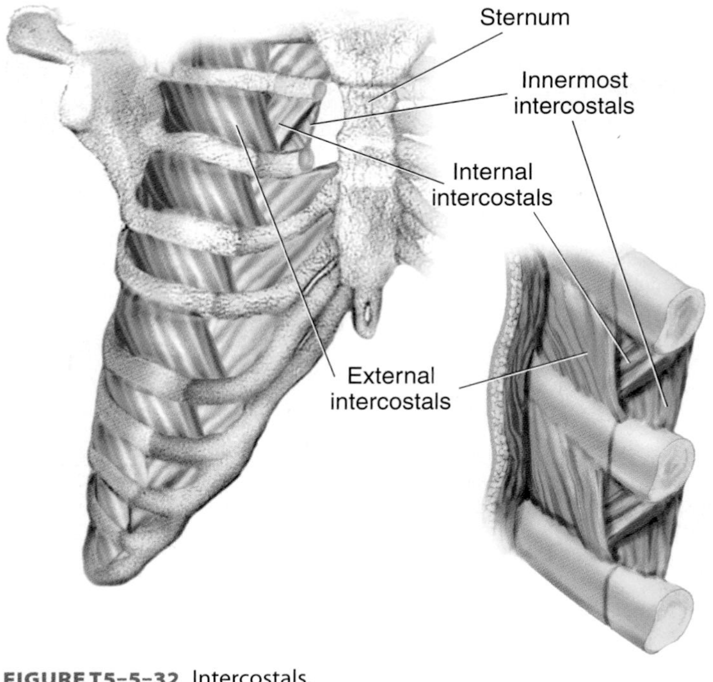

FIGURE T5-5-32 Intercostals.

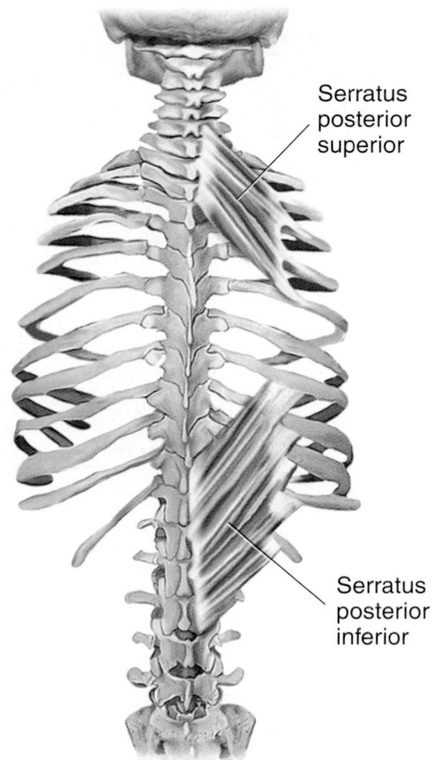

FIGURE T5-5-33 Serratus posterior superior, serratus posterior inferior.

TABLE 5.5 (continued)

MUSCLES OF THE TORSO (Continued) Muscles That Act On The Spine						
MUSCLE	ORIGIN	INSERTION	ACTION	INNERVATION	PALPATION	FIGURE
Quadratus Lumborum	Posterior iliac crest	Transverse process of L1–4 and inferior border of 12th rib	Lateral flexion of spine or raises hip	T12, L1, 2, 3 Lumbar plexus	Deep to Thoracolumbar sheath; hard to palpate	T5-5-31
Intertransversarii	Transverse processes of cervical, lumbar, and T10–12 vertebrae	Transverse process of vertebra directly above origin	Lateral flexion and stabilization of spine	Posterior branches of adjacent spinal nerves	Cannot palpate	T5-5-35a
Interspinales	In pairs between spinous process of cervical lumbar and T1–2 and T11–12 vertebrae	Spinous process of vertebra directly above origin	Extension and stabilization of spine	Posterior branches of adjacent spinal nerves	Cannot palpate	
Rotatores	Transverse process of each vertebra	Lamina of vertebra directly above	Extension, rotation to opposite side, and stabilization of spine	Posterior branches of adjacent spinal nerves	Cannot palpate	T5-5-35a
Multifidus	Transverse processes of C4–L5 PSIS, and posterior sacrum	Spans 2–4 vertebrae Inserts on spinous process	Extension, rotation to opposite side, and stabilization of spine	Posterior branches of adjacent spinal nerves	Cannot palpate	T5-5-35a

TABLE 5.5 (continued)

MUSCLES OF THE TORSO (Continued) Muscles That Act On The Spine (continued)						
MUSCLE	ORIGIN	INSERTION	ACTION	INNERVATION	PALPATION	FIGURE
Semispinalis			Bilaterally, Extension			T5-5-35a
Capitis	Transverse processes C4–T7	Occipital bone between inferior and superior nuchal lines	Unilaterally, Rotation to opposite side; stabilization of spine	Posterior branches of adjacent spinal nerves	Cannot palpate	
Cervicis	Transverse processes of T1–6	Spinous processes C2–5				
Thoracis	Transverse processes T6–12	Spinous processes C6–T8				
Spinalis			Bilaterally, Extension of spine	Posterior branches of adjacent spina nerves	Cannot palpate	T5-5-35a
Capitis	Inseparable from Semispinalis	Same as Semispinalis	Unilaterally, Lateral flexion of the spine			
Cervicis	Ligamentum nuchae	Spinous processes C2–4				
Thoracis	Spinous processes T10–L2	Spinous processes T4–8	Stabilization of spine			T5-5-34
Longissimus			Bilaterally, Extension of spine	Posterior branches of adjacent spina nerves	Deep to Thoracolumbar fascial latissimus dorsi and trapezius muscles on either side of spine; hard to palpate	T5-5-34
Capitis	Articular processes C4–7, Transverse processes T1–4	Posterior surface of mastoid process	Unilaterally, Lateral flexion of the spine			
Cervicis	Transverse processes T1–5	Transverse processes C2–6	Stabilization of spine			
Thoracis	Thoracolumbar fascia, transverse processes of lumbar vertebra	Transverse processes T1–12 and posterior surface of lower ten ribs				

TABLE 5.5 (continued)

MUSCLES OF THE UPPER EXTREMITIES (Continued) Muscles That Act On The Neck						
MUSCLE	ORIGIN	INSERTION	ACTION	INNERVATION	PALPATION	FIGURE
Iliocostalis Lumborum	Common origin by broad tendon arising from spinous process T12–L5, medial lip of iliac crest, and medial and lateral crest of the sacrum	Inferior borders of posterior angle of ribs 7–12	Bilaterally, extension of spine; unilaterally, Lateral flexion of the spine; stabilization of spine	Posterior branches of adjacent spinal nerves	Deep to thoracolumbar fascia, Latissimus dorsi, and Trapezius muscles on either side of spine; hard to palpate	T5-5-34
Thoracis	Upper borders of posterior angles of ribs 7–12	Transverse process of C7 and angles of ribs 1–6.				T5-5-34
Cervicis	Posterior angles of ribs 3–6	Transverse processes C4–6				

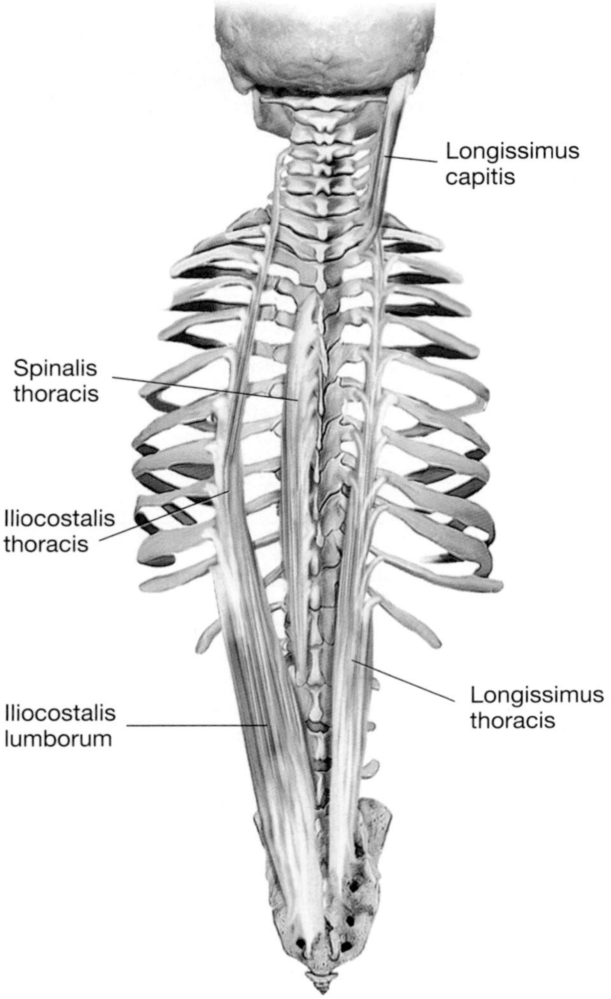

FIGURE T5-5-34 Iliocostalis group.

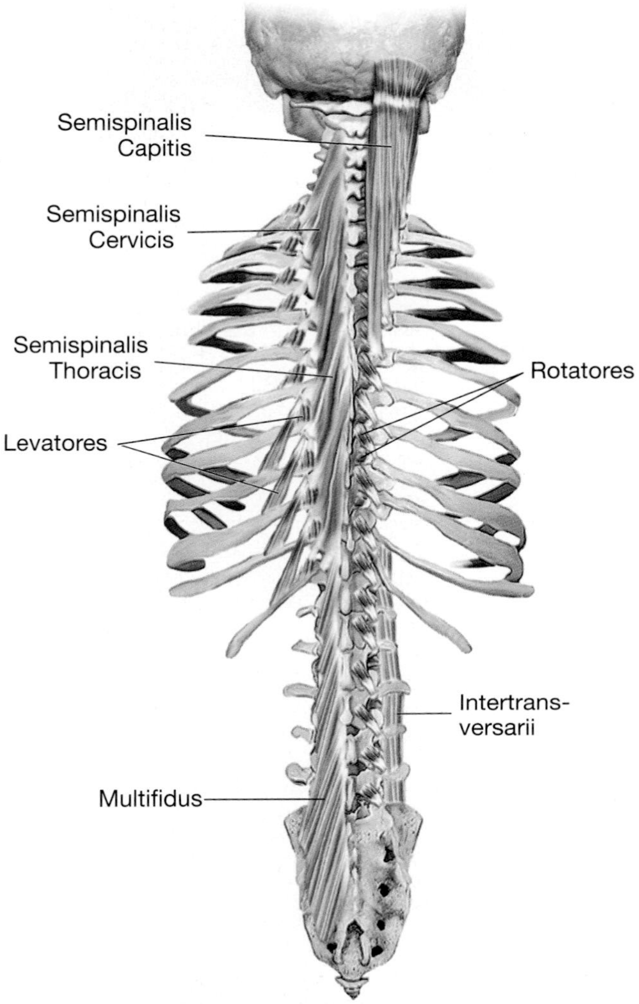

FIGURE T5-5-35A Semispinalis group.

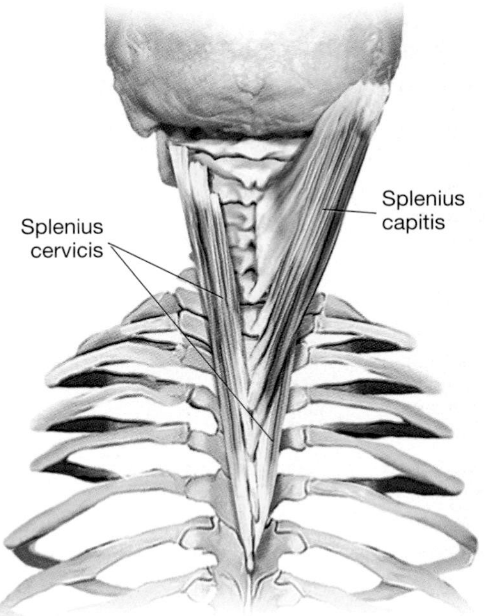

FIGURE T5-5-35B Splenius group.

TABLE 5.5 (continued)

MUSCLES OF THE NECK AND HEAD						
Muscles That Act On The Neck						
MUSCLE	**ORIGIN**	**INSERTION**	**ACTION**	**INNERVATION**	**PALPATION**	**FIGURE**
Splenius Capitis	Lower one half of ligamentum nuchae, spinous processes C7–T4	Mastoid process and lateral one third of occiput	Bilaterally, extension of neck; unilaterally, Rotation of head to same side	Posterior braches of cervical nerves	On posterior neck between Trapezius and Sternocleido-mastoid; hard to to palpate	T5-5-35b
Cervicis	Spinous processes T3–6	Transverse processes C1–3				
Sternocleido-mastoid	Sternal head: Superior aspect of manubrium. Clavicular head: Medial one third of clavicle	Mastoid process	Bilaterally, flexion of neck; unilaterally, Rotation of head to opposite side, lateral flexion	Accessory nerve and C2, 3	Anterolateral aspect of neck, diagonally from origin to insertion	T5-5-36
Scalenus						T5-5-38
Anterior	Anterior tubercles of transverse processes C3–6	Anterior superior aspect of first rib	Bilaterally, raise rib cage in deep inhalation, neck flexion;	C6, 7, 8	Lateral aspect of lower neck posterior to Sternocleido mastoid muscle from anterior	
Medial	Posterior tubercles of transverse processes C2–7	Lateral anterior aspect of first rib	unilaterally, Lateral flexion of neck, assists in neck rotation to opposite side		aspect of first rib to transverse process of cervical vertebra; hard to palpate	
Posterior	Posterior tubercles of transverse processes C5–7	Lateral anterior aspect of second rib				
Rectus Capitis						
Anterior	Anterior surface and transverse process of C1	Basal surface of occiput anterior to foramen magnum	Neck flexion, rotation to same side	Suboccipital	Cannot palapte	T5-5-39
Lateralis	Transverse process of C1	Basil surface of occiput lateral to foramen magnum	Lateral flexion of head	C1	Cannot palpate	T5-5-39
Posterior Minor	Posterior arch of C1spinous process of C2	Medial segment of inferior nuchal line of occiput	Neck, head extension	Occipital	Deep to Trapezius and Semispinalis; hard to palpate	T5-5-38
Posterior Major	Spinous process of C2	Inferior nuchal line of occiput lateral to RCP minor attachment	Head extension, and lateral flexion	Occipital	Cannot palpate	T5-5-38
Obliquus Capitis						
Superior	Superior aspect of transverse process of C1	Between inferior and superior nuchal lines of occiput	Head extension, rotation to same side	Occipital	Cannot palpate	T5--5-38
Inferior	Spinous process C2	Posterior aspect of transverse process of C1	Rotation to same side	Occipital	Cannot palpate	T5-5-38

TABLE 5.5 (continued)

MUSCLES OF THE NECK AND HEAD (Continued) Muscles That Act On The Neck (continued)						
MUSCLE	ORIGIN	INSERTION	ACTION	INNERVATION	PALPATION	FIGURE
Longus Colli	Anterior tubercles C3–5, Anterior vertebral bodies C5–T3	Anterior surface of vertebral bodies of C1–4, Anterior tubercles C5–6	Head flexion, lateral flexion and rotation to same side	C1–4	Cannot palpate	T5-5-39
Longus Capitis	Anterior tubercles of transverse processes C3–6	Inferior surface of occiput	Flexion of head	C1–3	Cannot palpate	T5-5-39

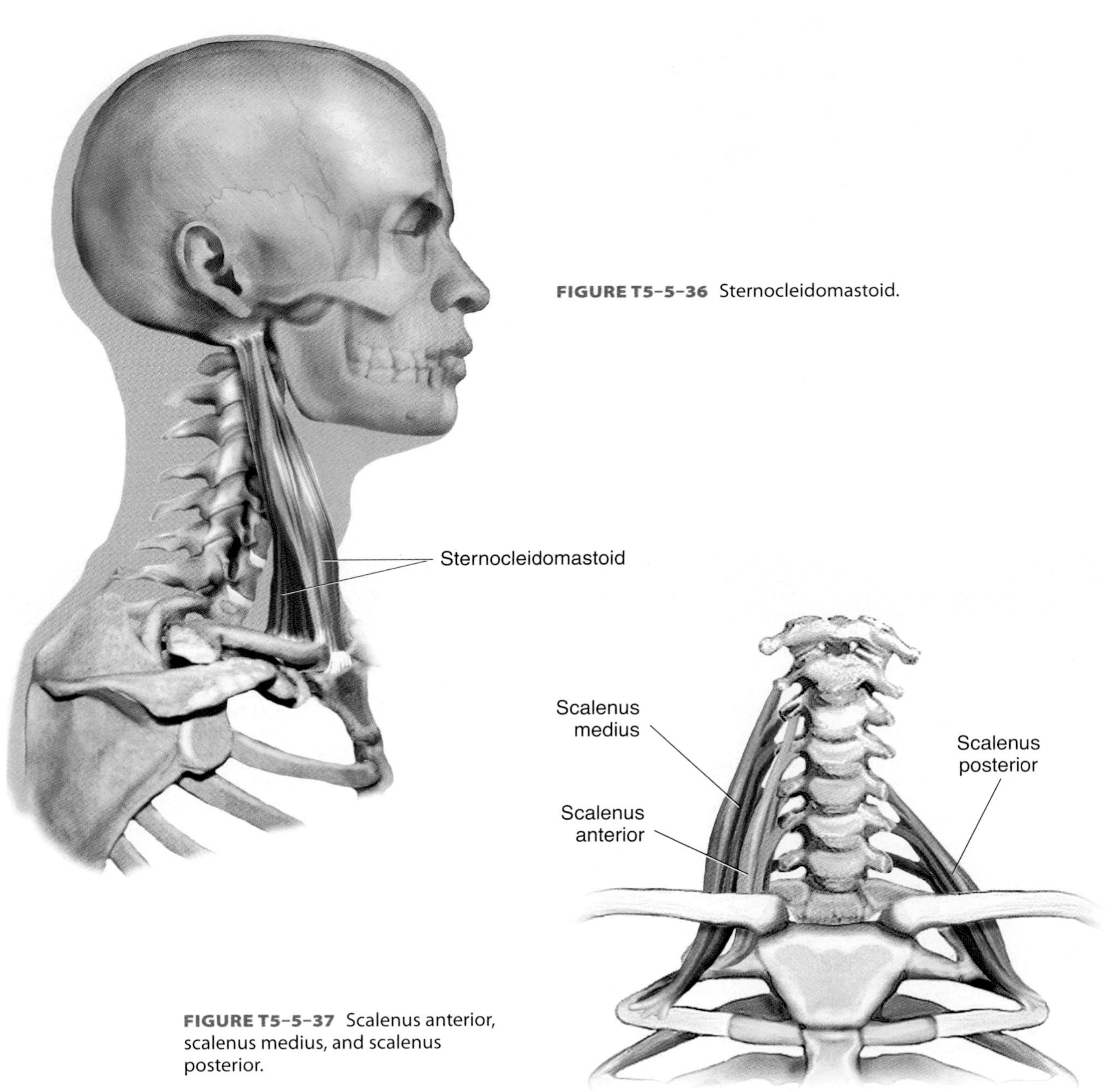

FIGURE T5-5-36 Sternocleidomastoid.

FIGURE T5-5-37 Scalenus anterior, scalenus medius, and scalenus posterior.

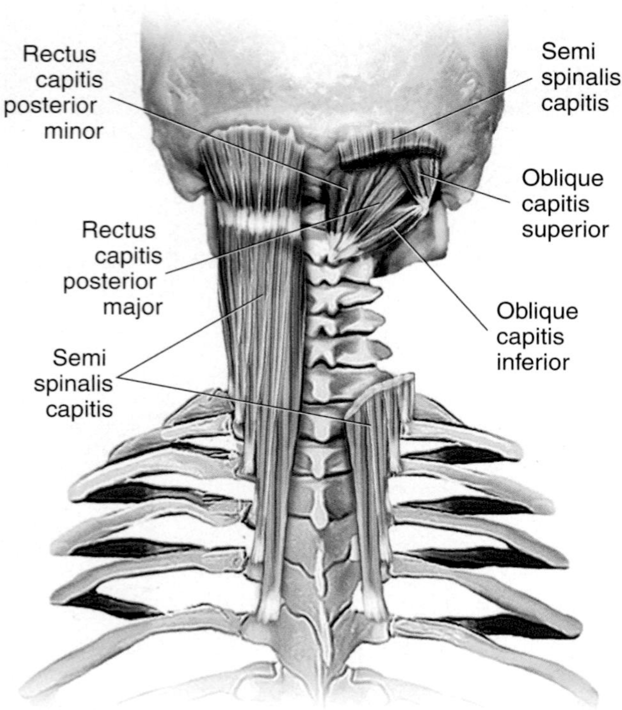

FIGURE T5-5-38 Posterior neck; rectus capitis posterior major and minor, obliques capitis superior and inferior.

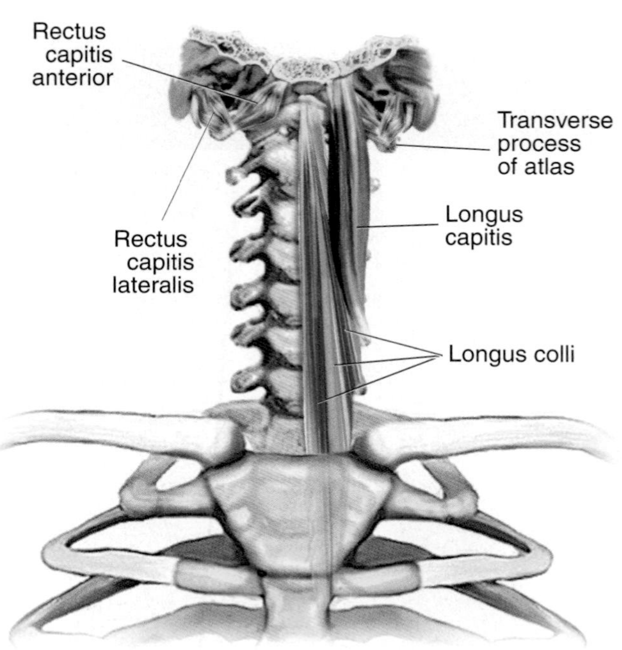

FIGURE T5-5-39 Anterior neck (deep): rectus capitis anterior and rectus capitis lateralis, longus colli and longus capitis.

TABLE 5.5 (continued)

MUSCLES OF THE NECK AND HEAD						
MUSCLE	ORIGIN	INSERTION	ACTION	INNERVATION	PALPATION	FIGURE
Infrahyoid Muscles						
Sternohyoid	Top of sternum and medial end of clavicle	Inferior body of hyoid	Depresses hyoid	C1, 2, 3	Lower anterior neck between SCM and trachea	T5-5-40
Sternothyroid	Top of sternum and costal cartilage of first rib	Thyroid cartilage	Depresses thyroid cartilage	C1, 2, 3	Lower anterior neck between SCM and trachea	T5-5-40
Thyrohyoid	Thyroid cartilage	Inferior body of hyoid	Depresses hyoid or raises thyroid cartilage	C1, 2, 3	Below hyoid, lateral to Sternohyoid; hard to differentiate and palpate	T5-5-40
Omohyoid	Superior border of scapula and by tendon to clavicle	Inferior body of hyoid	Depresses hyoid			T5-5-40

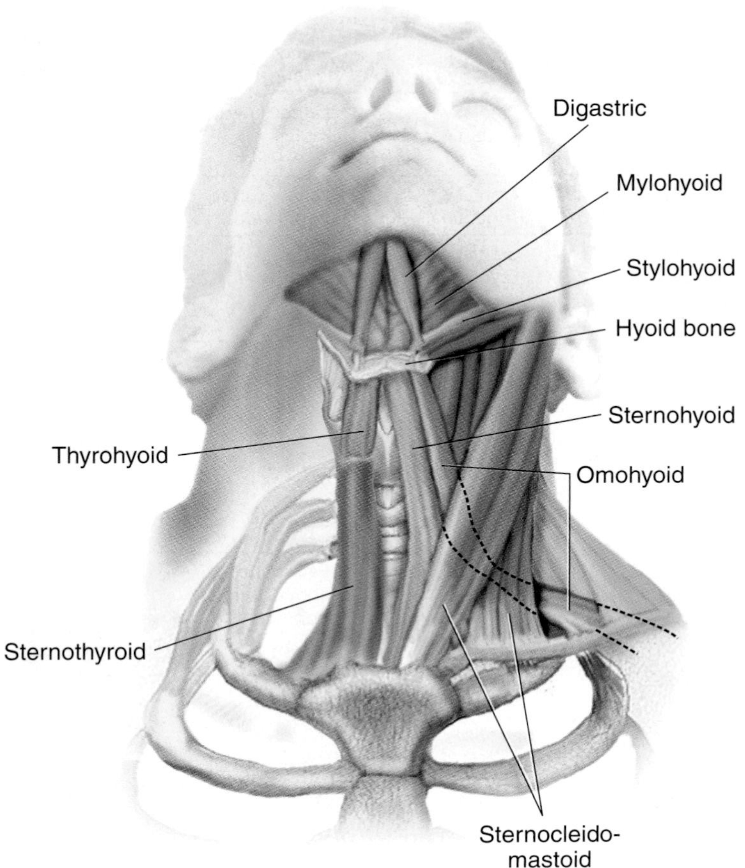

FIGURE T5-5-40 Anterior neck; hyoid muscles.

TABLE 5.5 (continued)

MUSCLES OF THE NECK AND HEAD (Continued)						
MUSCLE	ORIGIN	INSERTION	ACTION	INNERVATION	PALPATION	FIGURE
Suprahyoid Muscles						
Geniohyoid	Mandible under chin	Body of hyoid, superior aspect	Elevates hyoid or depresses mandible	C1, 2	Deep to Mylohyoid, cannot palpate	
Myohyoid	Mandible from ramus to under chin	Body of hyoid, superior aspect	Elevates hyoid or depresses mandible	Cranial V, Trigeminal	Deep muscle sheath under chin	T5-5-40
Stylohyoid	Styloid process of temporal bone	Body of hyoid, superior aspect	Elevates hyoid or moves hyoid posteriorly	Cranial VII, Facial	Between hyoid and ramus along with Posterior digastric	T5-5-40
Digastric Anterior belly	Mandible under chin	By tendon to body chin of hyoid, superior aspect	Elevates hyoid or depresses mandible	Cranial V, Trigeminal	From hyoid the point of chin between hyoid to ramus of mandible along with Stylohyoid muscle	T5-5-40
Posterior belly	Mastoid process			Cranial VII facial		

TABLE 5.5 (continued)

MUSCLES OF THE FACE						
MUSCLE	ORIGIN	INSERTION	ACTION	INNERVATION	PALPATION	FIGURE
Masseter	Zygomatic arch	Lateral surface of ramus of the mandible	Closes jaw	Cranial V, Trigeminal	Lateral jaw, over molars	T5-5-41
Temporalis	Temporal bone	Coronoid process and ramus	Closes and retracts jaw of mandible	Cranial V, Trigeminal	Lateral surface of temple area	T5-5-41
Buccinator	Maxilla and mandible	Angle of mouth, blending with Obicularis oris	Holds cheeks near teeth, positioning food for chewing	Cranial VII, Facial	Cheeks	T5-5-41
Internal Pterygoid	Medial surface of pterygoid plate of sphenoid	Medial surface of ramus of the mandible	Closes jaw; unilaterally, moves jaw to opposite side	Cranial V, Trigeminal	Hard to palpate	
External Pterygoid	Lateral surface of pterygoid plate of sphenoid	Anterior surface of condyle of mandible and TMJ capsule	Protrudes lower jaw	Cranial V, Trigeminal	Cannot palpate	
Epicranius Occipitalis	Posterior occiput above occipital ridge	Epicranial aponeurosis or the Galea aponeurotica	Draws Epicranius towards posterior	Posterior auricular and small occipital	Back of head above occipital ridge	
Frontalis	Blended into Procerus, corrugator, and Obicularis oculi	Epicranial aponeurosis or the Galea aponeurotica	Raises eyebrow and wrinkles the forehead	Cranial VII, Facial	Forehead, above eyebrows	T5-5-41
Corrugator	Medial aspect of supraorbital ridge	Deep surface of skin in middle of supraorbita arch	Draws eyebrows	Cranial VII,	Under medial	T5-5-41
Procerus	Fascia over upper nasal cartilage and lower nasal bone	Deep surface of skin between eyebrows	Draws nose up, causing wrinkles across nose	Cranial VII, Facial	Bridge of nose	T5-5-41
Orbicularis Oculi	Medial palpebral ligament to maxilla, nasal bone, nasal part of frontal bone	Fibers surround eye and blend with adjacent muscles	Closes the eye	Cranial VII, Facial	Eyelid and surrounding eye	T5-5-41
Nasalis	Maxilla above incisors	Blends into procerus	Compresses nostrils	Cranial VII, Facial	Side of nose	T5-5-41
Dilator Naris	Greater alar cartilage	Point of the nose	Expands opening of nostril	Cranial VII, Facial	Cannot palpate	
Quadratus Labii Superioris	Lower margin of orbit, frontal process of maxilla	Blends into Obicularis oris on upper lip	Raises upper lip	Cranial VII, Facial	Above upper lip, next to nose	
Zygomaticus Major	Zygomatic bone	Blends into Obicularis oris muscle at upper angle of mouth	Draws angle of mouth back and up	Cranial VII, Facial	Below zygomatic arch when smiling	T5-5-41
Minor	Continuous from inferior border of Obicularis oculi	Blends into Obicularis oris on upper lip	Raises upper lip	Cranial VII, Facial	Hard to differentiate from Quadratus labii	

TABLE 5.5 (continued)

MUSCLES OF THE FACE (Continued)						
MUSCLE	ORIGIN	INSERTION	ACTION	INNERVATION	PALPATION	FIGURE
Obicularis Oris	From numerous adjacent muscles surrounding mouth	Lips, external skin around mouth, and mucous membrane adjacent to the lips inside of mouth	Closes and protrudes lips	Cranial VII, Facial	The lips	T5-5-41
Risorius	Fascia over Masseter	Blends into Obicularis oris and skin at corner of the mouth	Draws angle of mouth back	Cranial VII, Facial	On cheek near corner of mouth; hard to palpate	T5-5-41
Depressor Anguli Oris	Anterior inferior surface of mandible	Blends into Obicularis oris and skin at corner of the mouth	Draws angle of mouth down	Cranial VII, Facial	On chin below corner of mouth	T5-5-41
Depressor Labii Inferioris	Anterior inferior surface of mandible	Blends into Obicularis oris and skin on lower lip ofthe mouth	Depresses lower lip	Cranial VII, Facial	On chin below lower lip	T5-5-41
Mentalis	Mandible below incisors	Deep skin at point of chin	Raises chin and protrudes lower lip as if pouting	Cranial VII, Facial	The chin	T5-5-41
Platysma	Superficial fascia of upper thorax and anterolateral aspect of neck	Blends into muscles of angle of mouth and chin	Depresses angle of mouth and wrinkles skin of neck	Cranial VII, Facial	Anterolateral aspect of neck; thin muscle and hard to palpate	T5-5-41
Auricularis Anterior Superior Posterior	Temporal bone	Deep skin around ear	Raises and moves ear	Cranial VII, Facial	In front, above, and behind ear; small muscles, hard to palpate	

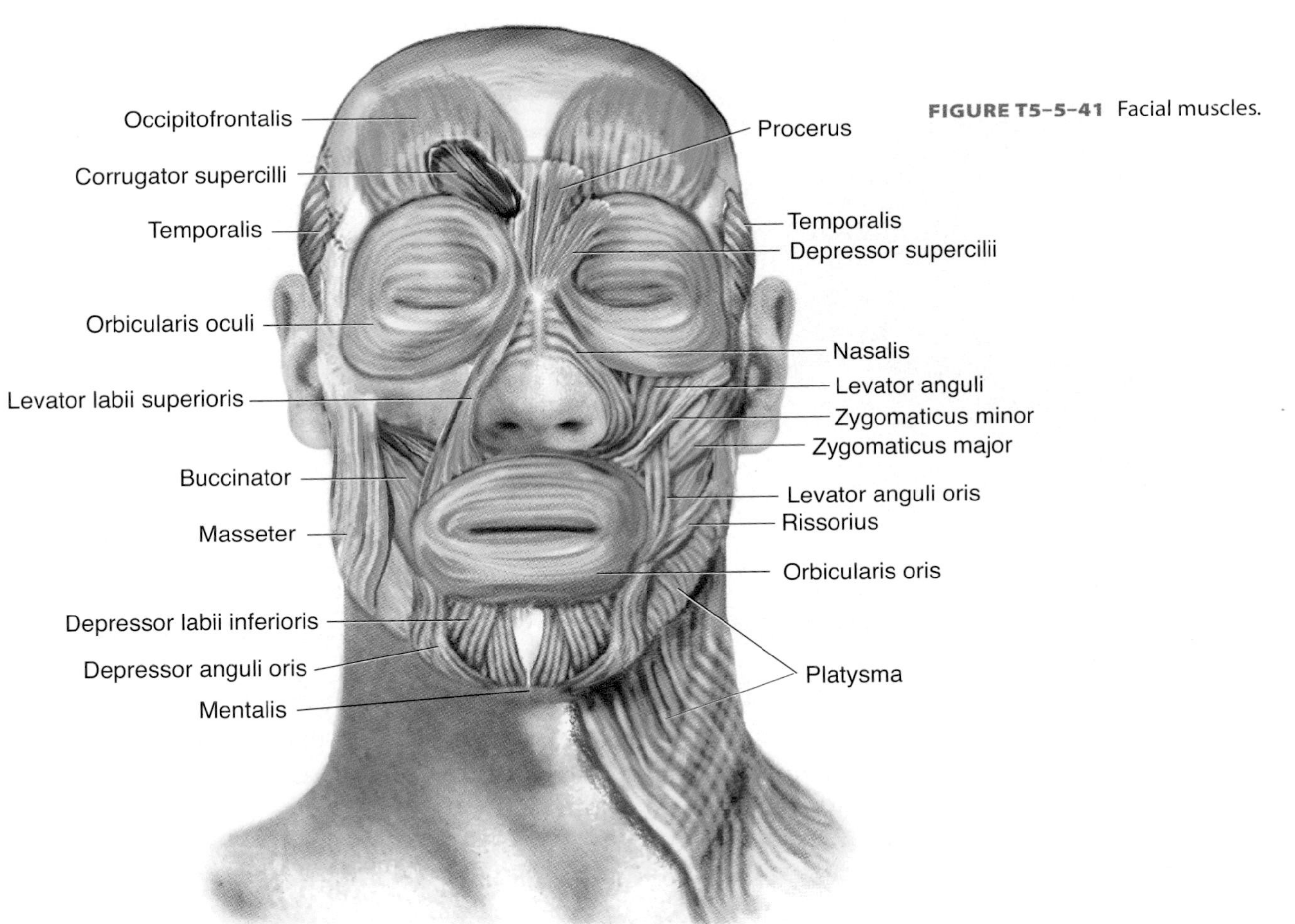

FIGURE T5-5-41 Facial muscles.

TABLE 5.5 (continued)

MUSCLES THAT ACT ON THE EYE (Continued)						
MUSCLE	**ORIGIN**	**INSERTION**	**ACTION**	**INNERVATION**	**PALPATION**	**FIGURE**
Levator Palpebrae Superioris	Common tendinous ring surrounding optic nerve near	Upper eyelid	Opens the eye	Cranial III, Oculomotor	Cannot palpate	T5-5-42
Superior Oblique	Common tendinous ring surrounding optic nerve by a tendon in superior orbit	Posterior lateral aspect of eyeball	Turns eye out and down	Cranial IV, Trochlear	Cannot palpate	T5-5-42
Supetior Rectus	Common tendinous ring surrounding optic nerve near optic foramen	Anterior superior aspect of eyeball	Rotates eye up	Cranial III, Oculomotor	Cannot palpate	T5-5-42
Lateral Rectus	Common tendinous ring surrounding optic nerve near optic foramen	Anterior lateral aspect of eyeball	Rotates eye laterally	Cranial VI, Abducens	Cannot palpate	T5-5-42
Inferior Rectus	Common tendinous ring surrounding optic nerve near optic foramen	Anterior inferior aspect of eyeball	Rotates eye down	Cranial III, Oculomotor	Cannot palpate	T5-5-42
Medial Rectus	Common tendinous ring surrounding optic nerve near optic foramen	Anterior medial aspect of eye	Rotates eye medially	Cranial III, Oculomotor	Cannot palpate	T5-5-42
Inferior Oblique	Orbital surface of maxilla	Posterior lateral aspect of eyeball	Rotates eye up and out	Cranial III, Oculomotor	Cannot palpate	T5-5-42

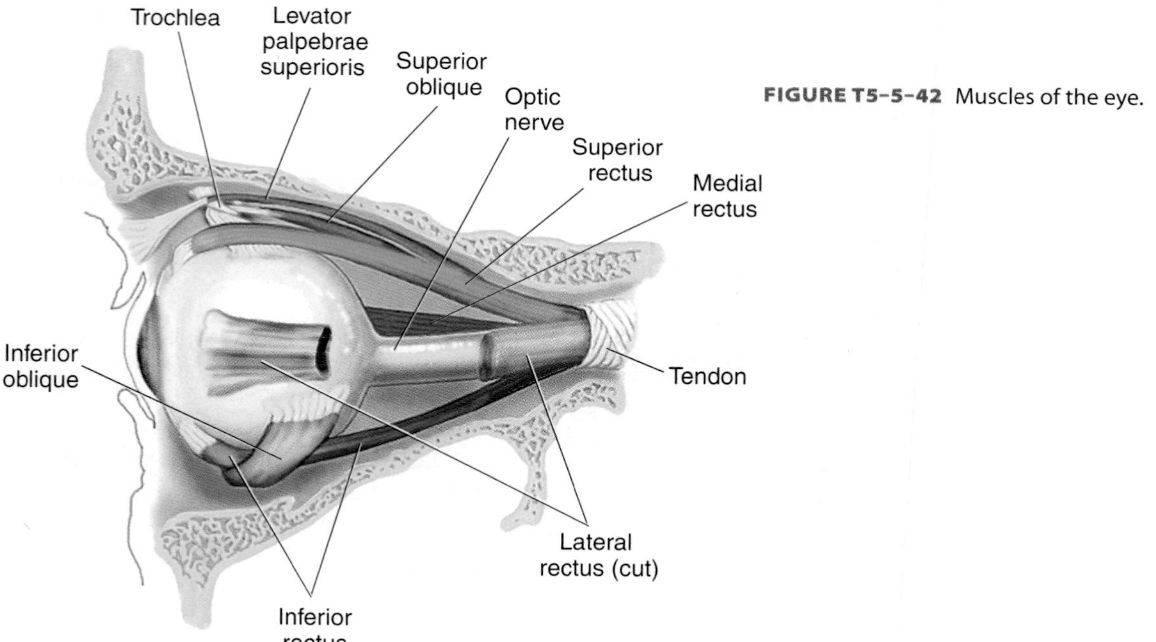

FIGURE T5-5-42 Muscles of the eye.

SECTION QUESTIONS FOR DISCUSSION AND REVIEW

1. What is the structure and function of muscles?
2. Approximately how many muscles are there in the human body?
3. Name three types of muscular tissue and give examples of where they are found.
4. What is the difference between voluntary and involuntary muscles?
5. Which characteristics enable muscles to produce movements?

6. What are skeletal muscles?
7. What is the functional unit of skeletal muscle?
8. What structures cause the striated appearance of skeletal muscles?
9. Which tissues are found in muscle?
10. To which structures are skeletal muscles attached?
11. What is the origin of a muscle? Give an example.
12. What is the insertion of a muscle? Give an example.
13. Which structure attaches the muscle to the bone?
14. What is the function of fibrous connective tissue in muscle?
15. What is fascia?
16. Name and locate the three connective tissue layers of muscle.
17. What is meant by the term *motor unit?*
18. What is acetylcholine? Where is it found, and what does it do?
19. Which molecular structure provides the energy for muscle contraction?
20. What is the relationship between oxygen debt and muscle fatigue?
21. What does the term *myofascial* refer to?
22. Name three things that differentiate Type I and Type II muscle fibers.
23. Why is it important for the massage practitioner to understand how muscles function?
24. What is meant by extensibility of muscle?
25. Explain the difference between isometric and isotonic muscle contractions.
26. Explain the difference between eccentric and concentric contractions. What do they have in common?
27. To what does the term *agonist* (or *prime mover*) refer?
28. When the elbow is flexed, is the triceps the prime mover or the antagonist?
29. What are the three components of motion?
30. Do diarthrotic joints remain motionless or are they capable of free movement?
31. Describe three degrees of muscle strain.
32. What is muscle atrophy?
33. Which joints have limited motion?
34. Are synarthrotic joints movable or immovable?

Matching Test I

Insert the letter of the proper term in front of each definition.

______	1.	move ears	a.	orbicularis oculi
______	2.	move scalp	b.	orbicularis oris
______	3.	opens eye	c.	auricularis
______	4.	presses lips together	d.	masseter
______	5.	raises lower jaw	e.	epicranius

True or False Test I

Carefully read each statement and decide whether it is true or false; draw a circle around the letter T or F.

1. T F Inferior oblique and superior oblique muscles do not rotate the eyeball.
2. T F Only the temporalis muscle moves the lower jaw.
3. T F The superior levator palpebrae muscle opens the eye.
4. T F The epicranius is also known as the occipitofrontalis muscle.
5. T F The corrugator muscle controls the movement of the mouth.

Muscles of the Neck and Chest

Matching Test II

Insert the letter of the proper term in front of each definition.

______	1.	rotates cranium	a.	intercostals
______	2.	draws head backward	b.	longus colli
______	3.	flexes cervical spine	c.	obliquus capitis inferior
______	4.	muscle of respiration	d.	obliquus capitis superior
______	5.	raises ribs in breathing	e.	diaphragm

True or False Test II

Carefully read each statement and decide whether it is true or false; draw a circle around the letter T or F.

1. T F Several muscles depress the jaw and raise the hyoid bone.
2. T F The sternocleidomastoid is the only muscle that bends the head forward and sideways.
3. T F The platysma muscle does not draw down the corners of the mouth.
4. T F The pectoralis major and minor muscles control the movement of the arm and shoulder.
5. T F Several groups of muscles raise the ribs in breathing.

Muscles of the Abdomen and Back

Matching Test III

Insert the letter of the proper term in front of each definition.

______	1.	flexes trunk	a.	rectus abdominis
______	2.	keeps spine erect	b.	quadratus lumborum
______	3.	draws head backward	c.	sacrospinalis
______	4.	draws arm backward	d.	trapezius
______	5.	compresses abdomen	e.	latissimus dorsi

True or False Test III

Carefully read each statement and decide whether it is true or false; draw a circle around the letter T or F.

1. T F The external oblique is an external muscle of the abdomen and back.
2. T F Only one muscle compresses the abdomen and bends the chest.
3. T F The infraspinatus and supraspinatus muscles control the movement of the arm.
4. T F The gluteus medius muscle extends the hip joint.
5. T F The spine is kept erect with the aid of the sacrospinalis and multifidus muscles.

Muscles of the Arms and Hands

Matching Test IV

Insert the letter of the proper term in front of each definition.

______	1.	flexes hand	a.	brachialis
______	2.	flexes forearm	b.	triceps brachii
______	3.	flexes arm	c.	interossei

______	4. separates fingers	d.	deltoid
______	5. extends forearm	e.	palmaris longus

True or False Test IV

Carefully read each statement and decide whether it is true or false; draw a circle around the letter T or F.

1. T F The movement of the thumb is controlled by one muscle.
2. T F The biceps brachii muscle draws the palm downward.
3. T F The brachioradialis muscle draws the palm upward.
4. T F Quick, short movements of the fingers are produced by the lumbricales muscles.
5. T F The subscapularis muscle rotates the humerus inward.

Muscles of the Legs and Feet

Matching Test V

Insert the letter of the proper term in front of each definition.

______	1. flexes leg	a.	flexor digitorum
______	2. extends leg	b.	biceps femoris
______	3. flexes hip	c.	rectus femoris
______	4. extends foot	d.	pectineus
______	5. flexes toes	e.	soleus

True or False Test V

Carefully read each statement and decide whether it is true or false; draw a circle around the letter T or F.

1. T F The sartorius muscle bends the thigh and leg.
2. T F The movement of the big toe is controlled by the extensor hallucis longus muscle.
3. T F The extensor digitorum brevis muscle does not extend the toes.
4. T F The soleus and gastrocnemius muscles both plantar flex the foot.
5. T F The gracilis adducts the femur and flexes the knee joint.

SYSTEM 4 THE CIRCULATORY SYSTEM

The vascular or circulatory system controls the circulation of the blood and lymph throughout the body by means of the heart, blood, and lymph vessels. The primary function of the circulatory system is to supply body cells with nutrient materials and carry away waste products.

There are two divisions to the vascular system:

1. The *blood-vascular system* or **cardiovascular system** includes the blood, heart, and blood vessels (i.e., arteries, capillaries, and veins).
2. The *lymph-vascular system*, or *lymphatic system*, consists of lymph, lymph nodes, and lymphatics through which the lymph circulates.

These two systems are intimately linked with each other.

cardiovascular system

cardiovascular system a network of structures including the heart, blood vessels, and blood that pumps and carries blood throughout the body

The Blood-Vascular System or Cardiovascular System

The *blood-vascular system* is a closed-circuit system that consists of the heart, the arteries, capillaries, veins, and the blood. This system continuously circulates the blood throughout the body. Even though the blood-vascular system is considered to be a closed system, in which the blood normally does not leave the blood vessels, in the capillaries there is a constant and extensive interchange of fluids and the substances that they contain.

The Heart

The *heart* is an efficient pump that keeps the blood circulating in a steady stream through a closed system of arteries, capillaries, and veins. The heart is a muscular, conical-shaped organ, about the size of a closed fist, located in the chest cavity between the lungs and behind the sternum. It is enclosed in a double-layered membrane, the **pericardium** (per-i-**KAR**-dee-um). The inner layer of the pericardium is a thin serous covering of the heart; the outer layer is a protective fibrous connective tissue sac that is attached to the diaphragm, the vertebral column, the back of the sternum, and the large blood vessels that emerge from the heart. Between these two layers is a space called the *pericardial cavity* that contains a serous fluid so that the heart is supported in position and at the same time allowed to move frictionlessly as it continually pulsates.

pericardium

is a double-layered membrane that encloses the heart.

The walls of the heart consist of three distinct layers. The **epicardium** is the protective outer layer that includes the inner pericardium. This layer includes and supports the nerves, blood and lymph capillaries, and the fat that surrounds the heart. The next thick layer is the cardiac muscle, or the **myocardium,** and is responsible for the muscular pumping action of the heart. The thin innermost layer is the **endocardium,** which provides a smooth protective covering that lines the inner chambers of the heart and heart valves and is continuous with the linings of the blood vessels (endothelium; Figure 5-45).

epicardium

is the protective outer layer of the heart.

myocardium

is the cardiac muscle.

endocardium

is the thin, innermost layer of the heart.

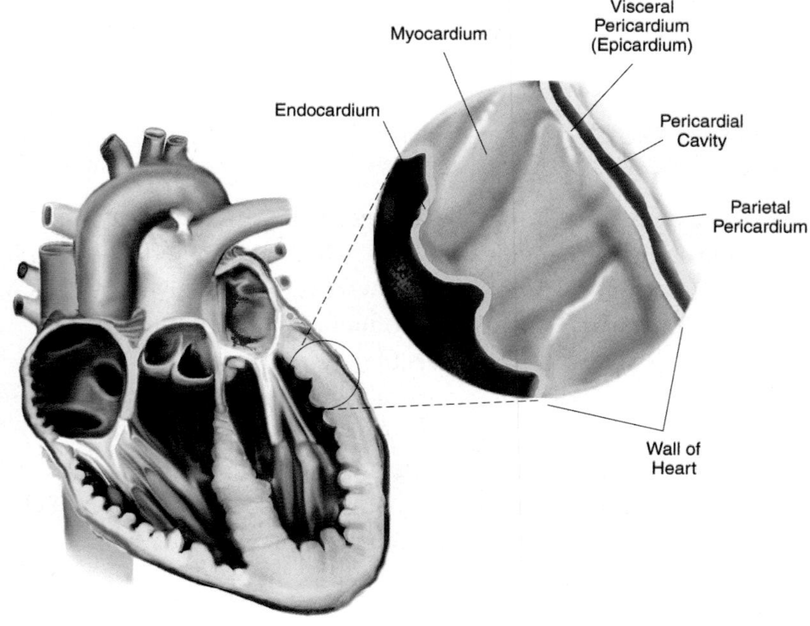

FIGURE 5-45 Wall of the heart, including the pericardium.

The interior of the heart contains four chambers, two on each side of a muscular wall called the **septum** (**SEP**-tum). The upper thin-walled cavities, the right and left atria (sometimes called the *auricles*), receive blood into the heart from the veins. The lower thick-walled chambers, the right and left ventricles, pump the blood out of the heart into the arteries. Four valves allow the blood to flow in only one direction. The **tricuspid valve**, located between the right atrium and right ventricle, allows blood to flow from the right atrium into the right ventricle and not the opposite direction. The **pulmonary semilunar valve**, positioned between the right ventricle and pulmonary artery, directs the blood from the right ventricle into the pulmonary arteries as blood travels to the lungs. The **bicuspid (or mitral) valve**, located between the left atrium and ventricle, allows blood to flow only from the left atrium into the left ventricle. The **aortic semilunar valve**, situated in the orifice of the aorta, permits the blood to be pumped from the left ventricle into the aorta but not the reverse. With each contraction and relaxation of the heart, the blood flows in, travels from the atria to the ventricles, and is then driven out to be distributed all over the body (Figure 5-46).

The impulses that generate the rhythmic heartbeat originate within the heart muscle. A system of specialized cardiac tissue initiates rhythmic impulses that transmit throughout the cardiac muscle and stimulate it to contract. This occurs without stimulation by outside nerve fibers or other agents. Even though the rhythmic heart contractions are initiated within the heart muscle, there is a complicated neurologic heart monitoring system that regulates the heart rate. Impulses from the *vagus* (**VAY**-gus) *nerve* and the *sympathetic nervous system* help to regulate the force of contraction and the heart rate. In a normal human adult, the heart beats about 60 to 80 times a minute.

The Blood Vessels

The **arteries, arterioles, capillaries, venules,** and **veins** transport blood from the heart to the various tissues of the body and back again to the heart. The

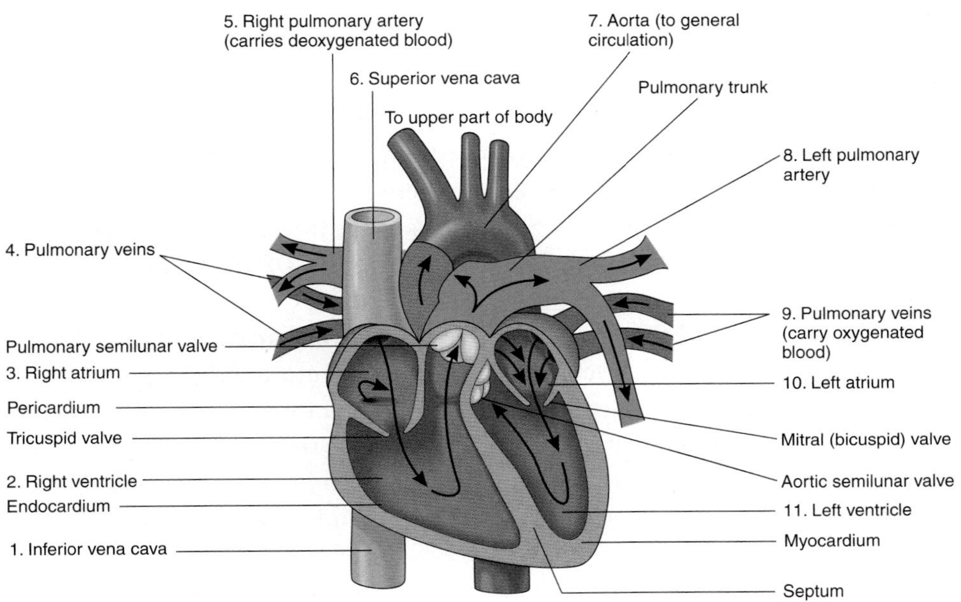

FIGURE 5-46 Anatomy of the heart.

septum
is the wall that separates the heart's chambers.

tricuspid valve
of the heart allows blood to flow from the right atrium into the right ventricle.

pulmonary semilunar valve
of the heart directs blood from the right ventricle into the pulmonary arteries.

bicuspid or mitral valve
of the heart allows blood to flow from the left atrium into the left ventricle.

aortic semilunar valve
of the heart permits the blood to be pumped from the left ventricle into the aorta.

arteries
are thick-walled muscular and elastic vessels that transport oxygenated blood from the heart.

arterioles
small blood vessels between the arteries and the capillaries.

capillaries
are the smallest blood vessels and connect arterioles with the venules.

venules
are microscopic vessels that continue from the capillaries and merge to form veins.

veins
are thinner-walled blood vessels that carry deoxygenated blood and waste-laden blood from capillaries back to the heart.

construction of all blood vessels, except the capillaries, is similar. The innermost layer is made up of endothelium, the middle layer is smooth muscle, and the outer layer is tough, protective connective tissue. The arteries and arterioles have thicker walls than those of the veins and venules. The farther from the heart, the finer and more delicate the vessels become. The capillary walls are made up of only a single layer of simple squamous epithelium to allow the passage of nutrients and wastes from and into the bloodstream. There are as many as 60,000 miles of continuous blood vessels that make up the circulatory system of an adult human.

Arteries and Arterioles

aorta

is the main artery of the body.

Arteries are thick-walled muscular and elastic vessels that transport oxygenated blood (except for the pulmonary artery) under relatively high pressure from the heart. The main artery of the body is the **aorta** (ay-**OR**-tuh), which arches up from the left ventricle of the heart, extending over and down along the vertebral column. Arteries branch into smaller and smaller vessels until eventually they become microscopic arterioles that control the rate of flow of blood into the capillaries. Arteries vary in size from the aorta, which is about an inch in diameter, to the microscopic capillaries, the walls of which are just a single cell in thickness and are only large enough to pass one blood cell at a time (Figure 5-47).

vasoconstriction

is the contraction of the arterial walls.

vasodilation

is the relaxation and enlargement of the arterial walls.

The smooth muscle tissue in the walls of the arteries and arterioles is richly supplied with nerves from the sympathetic portion of the autonomic nervous system. Impulses from these *vasomotor nerves* cause the smooth muscles of the arterial walls to contract, reducing the diameter of the vessel. This action is called **vasoconstriction.** When the nerve impulses are inhibited, the muscles relax and the diameter of the vessel enlarges or undergoes **vasodilation.** Changes in the diameter of the vessels affect the blood pressure and flow. The nerve response and control of the small arteries and arterioles regulate the flow of blood to the tissues in direct proportion to the tissue's specific needs.

Capillaries

Capillaries are the smallest microscopic, thin-walled blood vessels; their networks connect the small arterioles with the venules. The walls of the capillaries are extremely thin and permeable. The most important function of the capillaries is the two-way transport of substances between the flowing blood and the tissue fluids surrounding the cells. Substances move through the capillary walls either by the process of diffusion, filtration, or osmosis. Of these, diffusion is the most prevalent.

diffusion

is a process in which substances move from an area of higher concentration to an area of lower concentration.

In the process of **diffusion,** substances move from an area of higher concentration to an area of lower concentration. Blood entering the capillaries has a higher concentration of nutrients and oxygen than the fluid surrounding the cells, so that the oxygen and nutrients diffuse into the tissue spaces. By the same account, the concentrations of metabolic waste products and carbon dioxide are more highly concentrated in the tissue fluid and therefore tend to diffuse into the bloodstream.

The pressure of the blood, especially at the junction of the arteriole and the capillary, tends to push fluids and substances through the capillary wall and into the tissue spaces through a process called **filtration**. Because of a high concentration of proteins and other substances retained in the plasma, there is an osmotic pressure created that tends to draw water into the capillaries from the tissue spaces at almost the same rate as the blood pressure forces fluid out. Through these processes, substances can move back and forth between the bloodstream and tissues to support the needs of the cells and at the same time maintain the volume of the blood at a normal level.

filtration

is a process in which blood pressure pushes fluids and substances through the capillary wall and into the tissue spaces.

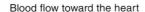

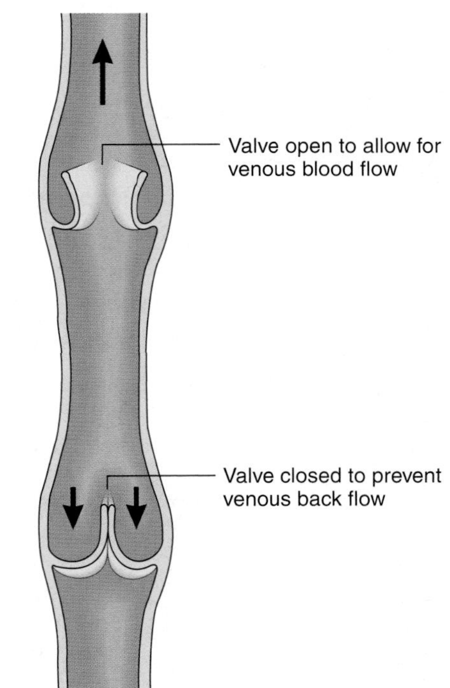

FIGURE 5–47 Valves in the veins.

Veins and Venules

Venules (**VEN**-yools) are the microscopic vessels that continue from the capillaries and merge to form veins. Veins are thinner-walled blood vessels that carry deoxygenated and waste-laden blood from the various capillaries back to the heart. Many veins, especially those in the arms and legs, have a system of valves that prevent blood from flowing backward in the vein and act as a *venous pump* to move the blood toward the heart. These valves are flaplike structures that protrude from the inside walls of the vein in such a way that blood moving toward the heart pushes past the valve, but if the blood attempts to move in the reverse direction, pressure against the valve forces it closed and blood cannot pass (Figure 5-48). The *venous pump* is a phenomenon that results when muscles contract and exert external pressure on the veins, which tends to collapse them. As the vein is repeatedly collapsed, the blood is forced along through the system of valves toward the heart. Massage strokes are very effective at encouraging the blood to move through the veins and therefore should always be directed to follow the venous blood flow toward the heart (Figure 5-49).

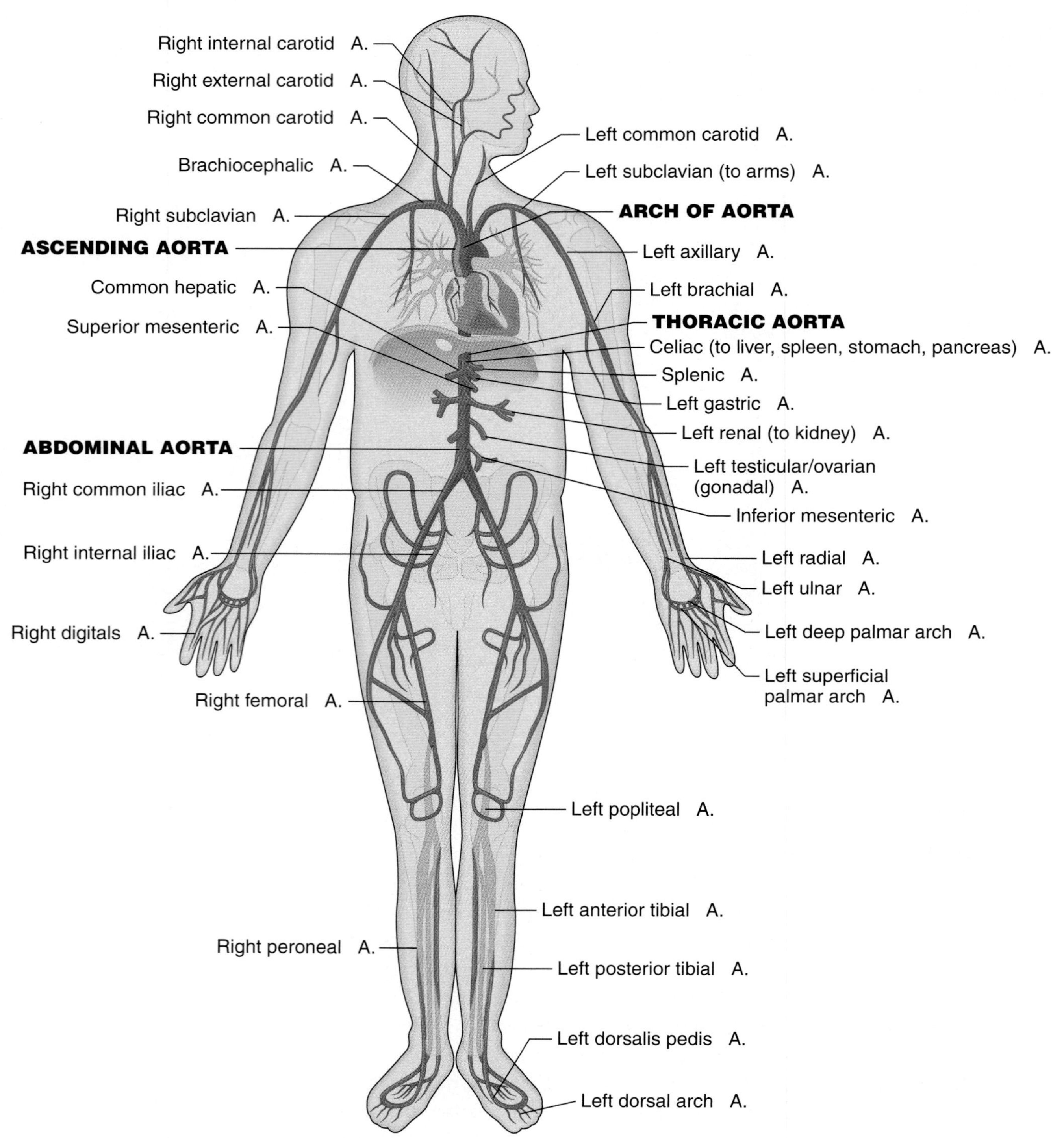
Right internal carotid A.
Right external carotid A.
Right common carotid A.
Brachiocephalic A.
Right subclavian A.
ASCENDING AORTA
Common hepatic A.
Superior mesenteric A.
ABDOMINAL AORTA
Right common iliac A.
Right internal iliac A.
Right digitals A.
Right femoral A.
Right peroneal A.
Left common carotid A.
Left subclavian (to arms) A.
ARCH OF AORTA
Left axillary A.
Left brachial A.
THORACIC AORTA
Celiac (to liver, spleen, stomach, pancreas) A.
Splenic A.
Left gastric A.
Left renal (to kidney) A.
Left testicular/ovarian
(gonadal) A.
Inferior mesenteric A.
Left radial A.
Left ulnar A.
Left deep palmar arch A.
Left superficial
palmar arch A.
Left popliteal A.
Left anterior tibial A.
Left posterior tibial A.
Left dorsalis pedis A.
Left dorsal arch A.

FIGURE 5-48 Major arteries of the circulatory system.

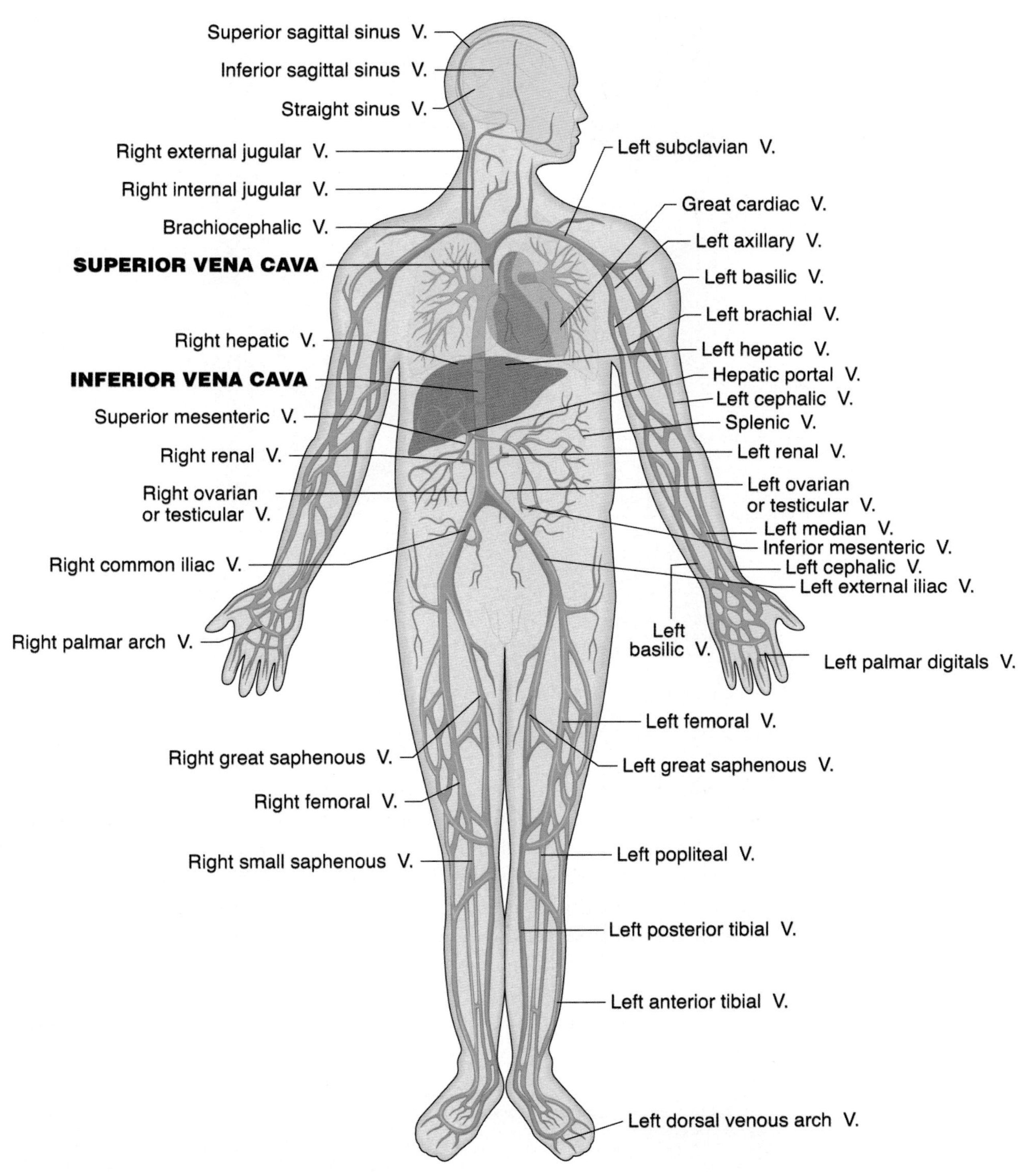
Superior sagittal sinus V.
Inferior sagittal sinus V.
Straight sinus V.
Right external jugular V.
Right internal jugular V.
Brachiocephalic V.
SUPERIOR VENA CAVA
Right hepatic V.
INFERIOR VENA CAVA
Superior mesenteric V.
Right renal V.
Right ovarian
or testicular V.
Right common iliac V.
Right palmar arch V.
Right great saphenous V.
Right femoral V.
Right small saphenous V.
Left subclavian V.
Great cardiac V.
Left axillary V.
Left basilic V.
Left brachial V.
Left hepatic V.
Hepatic portal V.
Left cephalic V.
Splenic V.
Left renal V.
Left ovarian
or testicular V.
Left median V.
Inferior mesenteric V.
Left cephalic V.
Left external iliac V.
Left
basilic V.
Left palmar digitals V.
Left femoral V.
Left great saphenous V.
Left popliteal V.
Left posterior tibial V.
Left anterior tibial V.
Left dorsal venous arch V.

FIGURE 5-49 Major veins of the circulatory system.

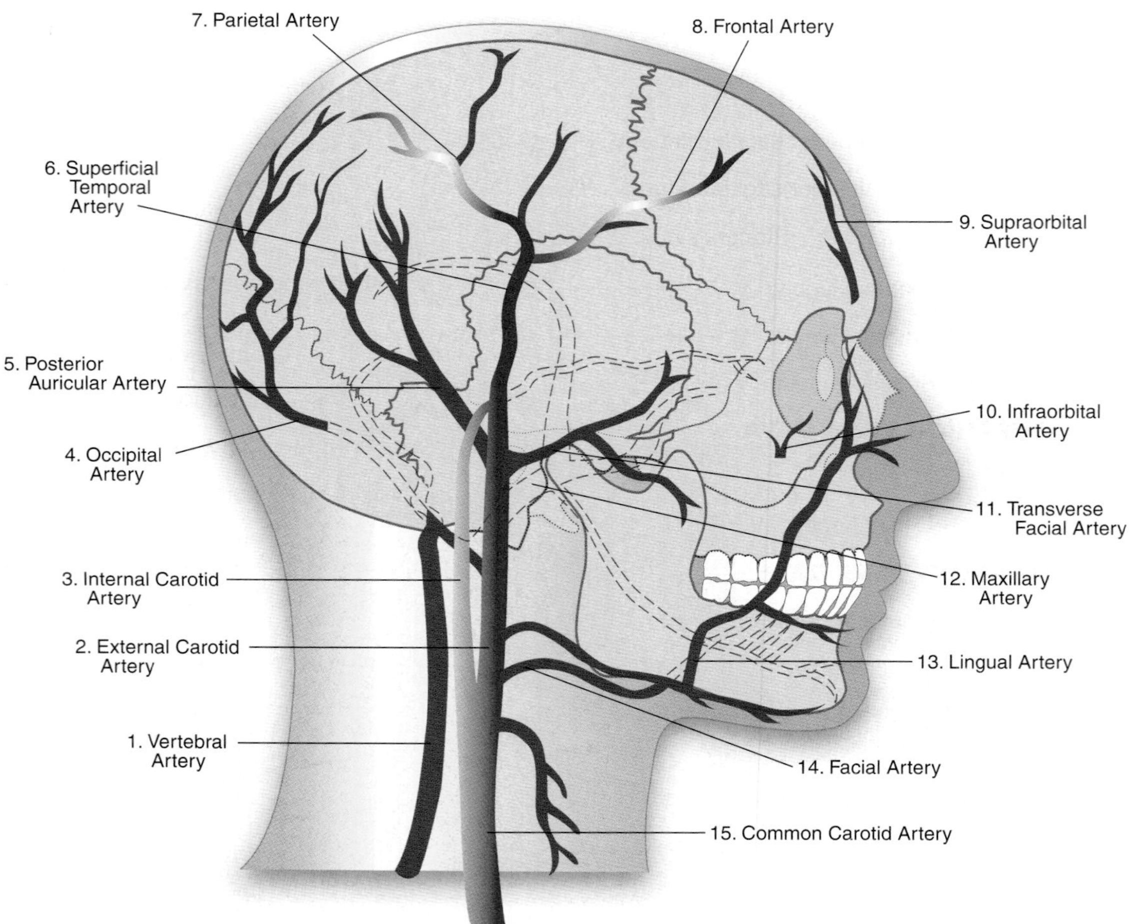

FIGURE 5–50 Arteries of the head, face, and neck.

Arteries of the Head, Face, and Neck

The common carotid arteries are the main sources of blood supply to the head, face, and neck. They are located on either side of the neck, and each artery divides into an internal and external branch. The internal branch of the common carotid artery supplies the cranial cavity, whereas the external branch supplies the superficial parts of the head, face, and neck. The arteries, like the muscles and nerves, are named in accordance with the parts of the body that they serve (Figure 5-50).

Table 5.6 presents the names and functions of the important arteries of the body.

Table 5.7 presents the names and functions of the important veins of the body.

TABLE 5.6

IMPORTANT ARTERIES OF THE BODY	
NAME	FUNCTION
Head and Neck	
Facial Artery	Supplies blood to face and pharynx
Temporal Artery	Supplies blood to forehead, masseter muscle, and ear

Common Carotid Arteries:	
Internal branch	Supplies blood to cranial cavity
External branch	Supplies blood to surface of head, face, and neck
Branches of External Carotid Artery	
Ophthalmic artery	Supplies blood to the eyes
Supraorbital artery	Supplies blood to the eye socket, forehead, and side of the nose
Frontal artery	Supplies blood to forehead
Parietal artery	Supplies blood to the crown and the sides of head
Posterior auricular	Supplies blood to the scalp and back of ear artery
Submental artery	Supplies blood to chin and lower lip
Superior labial	Supplies blood to upper lip and center of nose
Trunk	
Aorta	Forms main trunk of arterial system and subdivides to form large and small branches
Subclavian artery	Supplies blood to neck, chest, and upper part of back
Coronary artery	Supplies blood to heart muscles
Common iliac artery	Supplies blood to abdominal wall
External iliac artery	Supplies blood to lower limb
Internal iliac artery	Supplies blood to pelvic organs and inner thigh
Upper Extremities (The following arteries are for one side of the body.)	
Axillary artery	Supplies blood to shoulder, chest, and arm
Brachial artery	Supplies blood to the arm and forearm
Radial artery	Supplies blood to forearm, wrist, and thumb side of hand
Ulnar artery	Supplies blood to forearm, wrist, and small finger side of hand
Lower Extremities (The following arteries are for one side of the body.)	
Femoral artery	Supplies blood to lower part of abdominal wall, pelvic organs, and upper thigh
Popliteal artery	Supplies blood to knee and leg
Anterior tibial artery	Supplies blood to leg
Posterior tibial artery	Supplies blood to leg, heel, and foot
Dorsalis pedis artery	Supplies blood to foot

TABLE 5.7

IMPORTANT VEINS OF THE BODY

NAME	FUNCTION
Head and Neck	
Facial vein	Receives blood from face and empties into internal jugular vein
Internal jugular vein	Receives blood from cranial cavity and from surface of face and neck
External jugular vein	Receives blood from deep parts of face and from the surface of cranium
Temporal veins	Receive blood from the temporomaxillary region of the head
Maxillary anterior	Receives blood from the anterior portion of the face vein
Ophthalmic vein	Receives blood from the eyes
Supraorbital vein	Receives blood from the forehead and eyebrows

TABLE 5.7 (continued)

Frontal vein	Receives blood from the anterior portion of the scalp
Superior and inferior	Receives blood from the upper and lower lips labial veins
Trunk	
Innominate (brachiocephalic) veins	Receive blood from internal jugular and subclavian veins
Coronary veins	Receive blood from heart muscles
Common iliac vein	Receives blood from external and internal iliac veins and empties into inferior vena cava
Inferior vena cava	Receives blood from abdomen, pelvis, and lower limbs
Superior vena cava	Receives blood from head, neck, thorax, and upper limbs
Upper Extremities (The following veins are for one side of the body.)	
Cephalic vein	Receives blood from radial side (front) of arm
Basilic vein	Receives blood from ulnar side (outside) of arm
Axillary vein	Returns blood from arm to heart
Lower Extremities (The following veins are for one side of the body.)	
Great saphenous	Receives blood from the inner side of front leg veins
Small saphenous	Receives blood from back of leg vein
Popliteal vein	Receives blood from anterior and posterior tibial veins
Femoral vein	Receives blood from feet, legs, and thigh

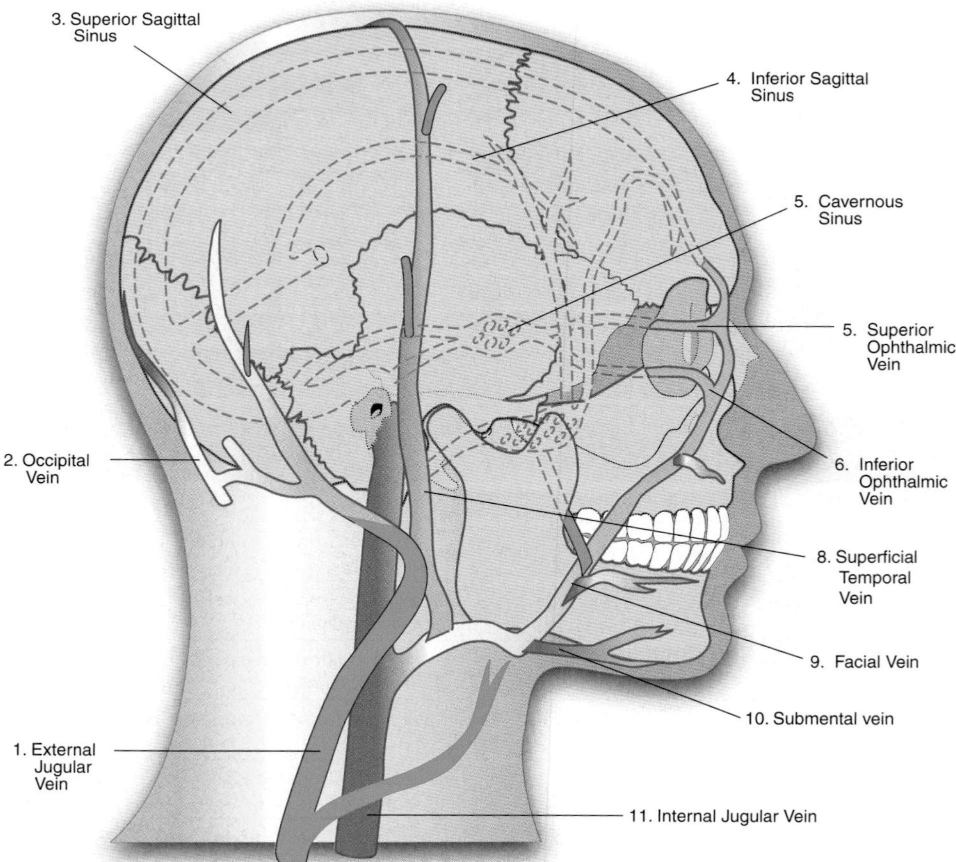

FIGURE 5–51 Veins of the head, face, and neck.

The Circulation of the Blood

The blood is in constant circulation from the moment it leaves until it returns to the heart. There are two systems involved in circulation: pulmonary and systemic.

Pulmonary Circulation

Pulmonary circulation is the blood circulation from the heart to the lungs and back again to the heart. During pulmonary circulation, the deoxygenated blood is pumped from the right ventricle of the heart, through the pulmonary arteries, to the capillaries of the lungs where carbon dioxide is replaced by oxygen. The exchange is continuous: freshly oxygenated blood returns to the left atrium of the heart through the pulmonary veins.

pulmonary circulation

is the blood circulation from the heart to the lungs and back again to the heart.

General or Systemic Circulation

General or **systemic circulation** is the blood circulation from the heart throughout the body and back again to the heart.

general or systemic circulation

is the blood circulation from the left side of the heart throughout the body and back again to the heart.

The course that blood travels is as follows:

1. The right atrium or auricle receives oxygen-poor blood from the large superior and inferior vena cava.
2. From the right atrium, the venous blood passes through the tricuspid valve into the right ventricle.
3. From the right ventricle, the venous blood is pumped through the pulmonary semilunar valve and is carried through the pulmonary arteries to the lungs to be oxygenated.
4. The freshly oxygenated blood is collected from the capillaries into the pulmonary veins and returned to the heart.
5. The left atrium receives the oxygenated blood from the pulmonary veins.
6. From the left atrium or auricle, the oxygenated blood passes through the bicuspid or mitral valve into the left ventricle.
7. From the left ventricle, the blood is pumped through the aortic semilunar valve and into the aorta.
8. From the aorta, the blood is distributed to the major arteries throughout the body, except for the lungs. The blood moves into ever-smaller branches of the arterial system until it flows into the arterioles.
9. From the arterioles, the blood moves into the thin-walled capillaries, where the oxygen, nutrients, and fluids move into the tissue spaces and the metabolic wastes and carbon dioxide are reabsorbed into the bloodstream.
10. The blood is then collected from the capillary beds into the venules and then into larger and larger veins until the blood finally flows into the inferior or superior vena cava.
11. This cycle is repeated as the venous blood is brought back again to the right atrium or auricle of the heart (Figure 5-52).

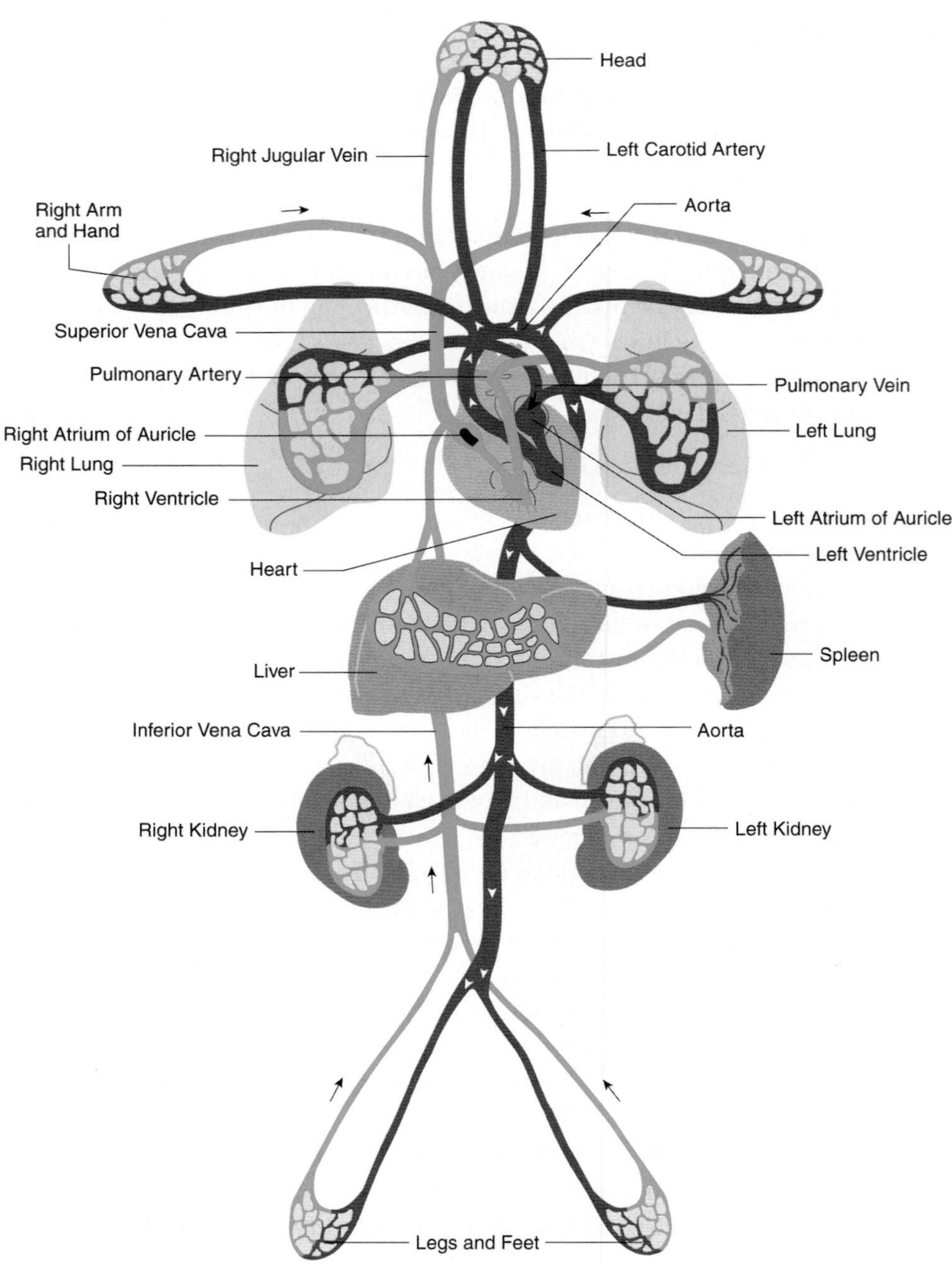

FIGURE 5-52 Circulation of the blood.

Disorders of the Blood Vessels

Atherosclerosis

Atherosclerosis is characterized by an accumulation of fatty deposits on the inner walls of the arteries. The development of the deposits, called *plaque*, seems to relate to the level of cholesterol in the blood. The deposits can interfere with blood flow or create a surface where blood clots may form. The walls of affected arteries tend to thicken, become fibrous, and lose their elasticity in a condition called *arteriosclerosis* (ar-**TEER**-ee-o-skler-**O**-sis).

Having a family history of atherosclerosis, high blood pressure, a high cholesterol level, a sedentary lifestyle, and smoking increase the chances of developing atherosclerosis. There are really no outward symptoms of atherosclerosis until it has progressed to the point that a related condition appears. Occlusion of a coronary artery is common and results in *angina pectoris* or a heart attack (myocardial infarction). If atherosclerosis causes a thrombus (blood clot) to form or if the clot breaks free to become an embolus, the embolus can become lodged in an artery, and the tissues supplied by that artery will stop functioning. If that happens in the brain, a stroke results; in the heart, a heart attack occurs. If it happens in the lungs, a pulmonary embolism can result. Advanced atherosclerosis can also affect the aorta, renal arteries, the carotid arteries, or the peripheral arteries of the legs by restricting blood flow to the structures that they supply.

Circulatory massage is contraindicated for persons with advanced or diagnosed atherosclerosis. If a prospective client is under a doctor's care or is taking any kind of medication for circulatory conditions, be sure to obtain medical clearance from the physician before proceeding with massage.

Phlebitis and Thrombophlebitis

Phlebitis is an inflammation of a vein that can result from injury, surgery, or infection. Symptoms include pain and inflammation along the course of the vein and swelling. *Thrombophlebitis* signifies the presence of a blood clot (thrombus) in an inflamed vein. It is difficult to determine whether the clot is the cause or the result of the inflammation. Thrombophlebitis usually occurs in the lower extremities and can affect the superficial or deep veins.

A major concern with thrombophlebitis is that a portion of the blood clot could break free to become an embolus that travels through the veins back to the heart, and then to the lungs to cause a pulmonary embolism, which could be life threatening.

Symptoms for thrombophlebitis vary. In fact, the first symptoms can be those of a pulmonary *embolism*: shortness of breath, pain in the lungs, and coughing. Thrombophlebitis in a superficial vein can be accompanied by signs of inflammation. The vein is tender to the touch and feel like a hard cord. Deep vein thrombophlebitis is often accompanied by a deep ache in the area of the clot and edema distal to the location of the clot because the venous blood flow is inhibited, causing fluid to remain in the tissues. Thrombophlebitis is a serious condition that requires immediate medical attention. Massage is systemically contraindicated.

Aneurysm

An *aneurysm* is a local distention or ballooning of an artery from a weakening wall. It most commonly occurs in the abdominal or thoracic cavity and occasionally in the cranium. It is generally asymptomatic but can cause a feeling of pressure, pain, or edema, depending on the location. The most serious consideration with an aneurysm is that it could rupture, causing internal bleeding and possibly death. Massage is contraindicated.

Cerebrovascular Accident

A *cerebrovascular accident* (CVA) or stroke is caused by a disturbance in cerebral circulation. This can be due to an embolism, atherosclerosis, hemorrhage, or a ruptured aneurysm. Symptoms vary according to the area of the brain affected and can include unilateral weakness, paralysis, numbness, dizziness, confusion, and blurred or double vision. The aftereffects of a stroke depend on the severity and which portion of the brain was involved. About 25 percent of strokes have no lasting effects. Fifty percent result in some physical impairment, and twenty-five percent of strokes are fatal. Disability from a CVA can include partial to full paralysis to one side of the body, possible memory loss, vision loss, loss of the ability to speak, and/or personality changes that can range from mild to extreme. The onset of a CVA requires immediate medical attention. Massage in the acute stage is contraindicated but can be very beneficial during rehabilitation under a physician's supervision.

Myocardial Infarction

Commonly known as a heart attack, a *myocardial infarction* is the result of a reduced blood flow in the coronary arteries supplying the heart muscle due to atherosclerosis, narrowed vessels, or an embolus. The reduced blood flow causes a lack of oxygen and nutrients that damages or kills the portion of the heart muscle supplied by the occluded artery. The seriousness of the heart attack is determined by the location and the extent of the damaged heart tissue. Symptoms include pressure or aching around the heart, often radiating into the left arm, back, or jaw. If symptoms are experienced, immediate emergency medical care is required to increase the chance of survival. Nearly one half of those who experience myocardial infraction die before getting to the hospital. Massage is contraindicated during the acute stage but can be incorporated during rehabilitation under a doctor's supervision.

Varicose Veins

Varicose veins are characterized by protruding, bulbous, distended superficial veins, particularly in the lower legs. Extensive back pressure in the veins from prolonged standing or blockage causes the veins to enlarge and stretch to the point that the valves become incompetent. The weight of the blood further distends the veins, and more valves become dysfunctional, perpetuating the condition. Increased pressure in the veins also increases pressure in the capillaries and often results in edema. Severe varicose veins are contraindicated for all but the lightest massage. Darkened veins that are not elevated or painful and small, isolated spider veins are safe for moderate or light massage.

Hematoma

hematoma

is a mass of blood trapped in some tissue or cavity of the body and is the result of internal bleeding.

A **hematoma** is the result of bleeding under the epidermis and sometimes deep within the tissues of the body. A superficial hematoma, commonly referred to as a *bruise*, is recognized by its black-and-blue or purplish color and localized pain. The color fades to a greenish yellow as macrophages move into the site to clean up the debris. Deep hematomas or bleeding deep between the muscle sheaths might show discoloration but are painful to the touch. Massage is contraindicated during the acute stages of a hematoma; however, it can be applied gently around the periphery to sooth the area and promote circulation in the subacute stages.

Edema

Edema is a condition of excess fluid in the interstitial spaces. Edema is characterized by swelling of the tissues because of excess fluid. The cause of edema is an imbalance in fluid pressures within the capillaries. The pressure imbalance can be caused by obstructions in the veins or lymph vessels, high capillary pressure or porosity, or kidney malfunction that results in fluid retention. Edema can be associated with a weakened heart, congested liver, chemical imbalance, or a local injury or infection. Edema is a local contraindication for classic massage techniques. Some types of edema respond well to specialized lymph massage techniques. (See Chapter 16, Lymph Massage.)

The Blood

Blood is the nutritive fluid circulating throughout the blood-vascular system. It is salty and sticky, has an alkaline reaction, and maintains a normal temperature of 98.6°F (37°C). The amount of blood varies according to a person's size as well as other factors. An average-sized man (about 160 lbs) will have approximately 11 pints of blood, or about 1/16 to 1/20 of the body's weight. The skin can hold as much as one half of all the blood in the body.

Chief Functions of Blood

1. The blood carries water, oxygen, food, and secretions to all areas of the body.
2. It carries away carbon dioxide and waste products to be eliminated through the excretory channels.
3. It helps to equalize the body temperature, thus protecting the body from extreme heat and cold.
4. It aids in protecting the body from harmful bacteria and infections through the action of the white blood cells.
5. It coagulates (clots), thereby closing injured blood vessels and preventing the loss of blood through hemorrhage.

Composition of Blood

The blood is a liquid connective tissue consisting of a fluid component (blood plasma) and a solid component that consists of red corpuscles, white corpuscles, and blood platelets. Plasma constitutes from 50 to 60 percent of the blood volume.

Blood Cells

Red corpuscles (red blood cells) or *erythrocytes* (e-**RITH**-row-sites) are double concave disk-shaped cells colored with a substance called **hemoglobin** (hee-mow-**GLOW**-bin). The function of the red corpuscles is to carry oxygen from the lungs to the body cells and transport carbon dioxide from the cells to the lungs. The red blood cells are confined to the blood vessels and do not circulate outside the blood-vascular system. The red blood cells are formed in the red bone marrow. They are far more numerous than the white blood cells and account for as much as 98 percent of the blood cells.

The blood itself is bright red in the arteries (except in the pulmonary artery) and dark red in the veins (except in the pulmonary vein). This change in color is due to the color change of hemoglobin as the result of a gain or loss of oxygen as the blood passes through the lungs and other tissues of the body.

red corpuscles

or erythrocytes, carry oxygen from the lungs to the body cells and transport carbon dioxide from the cells to the lungs.

hemoglobin

an iron-protein compound in red blood cells capable of carrying oxygen from the lungs to the cells and carbon dioxide from the cells.

white corpuscles

or leukocytes, protect the body against disease by combating infections and toxins that invade the body.

White corpuscles (white blood cells), also called *leukocytes,* differ from red blood cells in many respects. They are larger in size, colorless, and can change their shape and other properties according to their location and function. White corpuscles are produced in the spleen, lymph nodes, and the red marrow of the bones. Leukocytes can squeeze between the cells that compose the capillary walls and move through the intercellular spaces with an amoeba-like motion. The most important function of these cells is to protect the body against disease by combating different infectious and toxic agents that can invade the body. Most leukocytes actually engulf and digest harmful bacteria and other foreign elements in a process called **phagocytosis** (fag-o-sigh-**TOE**-sis). Our bodies also manufacture specialized leukocytes that produce antibodies that protect us from specific disease organisms and are an important part of our **immune system.**

phagocytosis

is a process in which leukocytes engulf and digest harmful bacteria.

immune system

helps to protect the body and keep it safe from pathogens and diseases.

Blood platelets or *thrombocytes* are colorless, irregular bodies, much smaller than the red corpuscles. They are formed in the red bone marrow. These bodies play an important role in the clotting of the blood over a wound (Figure 5-53).

blood platelets

or thrombocytes, are colorless, irregular bodies, much smaller than red corpuscles.

Blood Coagulation or Clotting

When a blood vessel is damaged, several things happen to prevent severe blood loss. The blood platelets adhere to the ragged edges of the injured vessel, especially to the collagen fibers surrounding the blood vessel. They immediately begin to change shape as protrusions form from their cell membranes and they stick together to create a platelet plug. Platelets also release *serotonin* (seer-o-**TOE**-nin), which is a vasoconstrictor that causes a vascular spasm that temporarily closes the blood vessel.

The tissue damage causes an enzyme to be released that acts on one of the components in the plasma (fibrogen) to activate and form threads of *fibrin.* The fibrin tends to stick to the damaged blood vessels, forming a meshwork that entraps other platelets and blood cells in a *blood clot.*

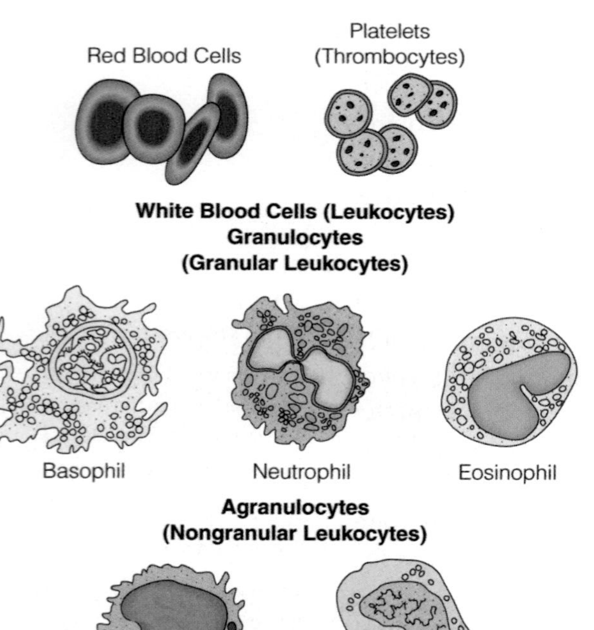

FIGURE 5-53 Blood cells and platelets.

Plasma

Plasma is the fluid component of the blood, straw-like in color, in which the red corpuscles, white corpuscles, and blood platelets are suspended. Approximately 90 percent of plasma is water. The remaining plasma is made up of about 7 percent proteins and 1.5 percent other substances. It functions to regulate fluid balance and pH and to transport nutrients and gases. Plasma is derived from the food and water taken into the body (Figure 5-54).

Diseases of the Blood

Hemophilia

Hemophilia is a disease characterized by extremely slow clotting of blood and excessive bleeding from even very slight cuts. This disease is hereditary, but men are the chief sufferers. Women can transmit this blood condition to their sons, however.

Anemia

Anemia refers to several conditions in which there is a rapid loss or inadequate production of red blood cells. In this condition, the oxygen-carrying capacity is reduced, resulting in a lack of body strength and paleness of the complexion.

Anemia is more a symptom of a condition than an actual disease. Some forms of anemia are related to nutritional deficiencies that inhibit red blood cell production. *Nutritional anemia* can be due to dietary deficiencies of iron, folic acid, or B12, all of which are essential for the production of hemoglobin. Severe lack of protein or copper can also contribute to this symptom. If the deficiency is due to inadequate amounts of the nutrient in the diet, replenishing the missing nutrient can reverse the anemia. In *pernicious anemia,* perhaps the most serious nutritional anemia, the stomach does not produce enough intrinsic factor needed to assimilate B12. B12 supplementation, usually in the form of monthly injections, is required.

Nutritional anemia is not a contraindication for massage; however, no amount of massage can improve the condition until the proper nutrients are restored to promote red blood cell production.

Hemorrhagic anemia is the result of excessive blood loss either from large wounds or internal bleeding such as bleeding ulcers or excessively heavy menstruation.

Aplastic anemia occurs when the bone marrow slows or stops the production of blood cells. Infection, exposure to certain types of radiation or poison, cancer, or autoimmune disease can inhibit the bone marrow's ability to produce red and white blood cells and platelets. In some cases, if the disease is detected early enough, a bone marrow transplant can successfully reverse aplastic anemia.

General massage is systemically contraindicated for hemorrhagic, hemolytic, and aplastic anemia.

Secondary anemia is a complication of or accompanies other serious conditions such as hepatitis, leukemia, kidney disease, bleeding ulcers, or other acute infectious diseases. The anemia usually dissipates as the associated condition heals. Massage is contraindicated as long as the primary condition and the associated anemia persist.

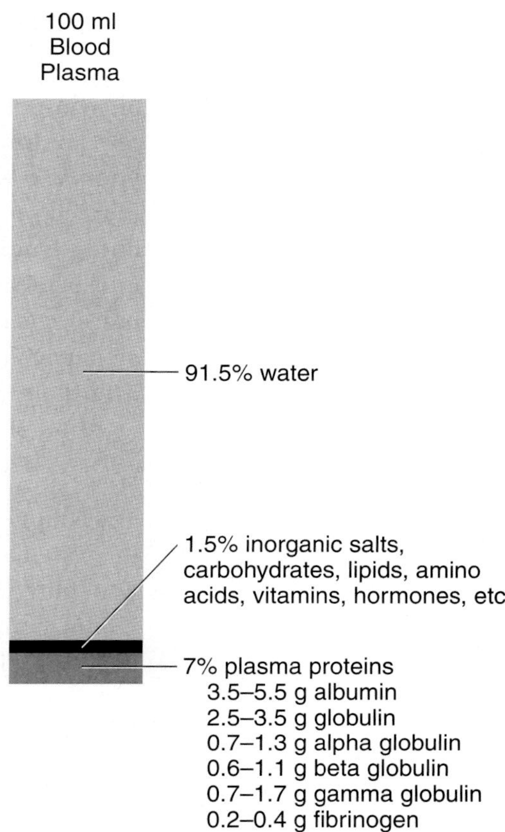

FIGURE 5-54 Composition of plasma. Plasma, which is primarily water, contains about 7 percent protein and 1.5 percent other substances.

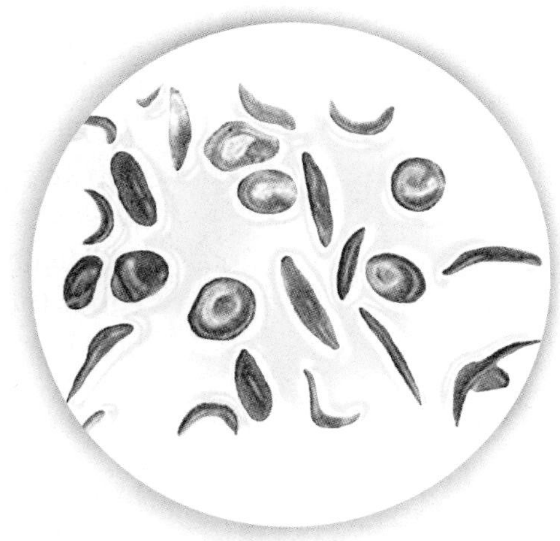

FIGURE 5-55 Sickle cell anemia is an inherited disorder in which abnormal hemoglobin causes red blood cells to assume a sickle shape.

Leukemia

Leukemia is a form of cancer in which there is an uncontrolled production of white blood cells. These cells do not fully mature, and they remain virtually nonfunctional. As a result, the person's resistance to disease is reduced. There are two major types of leukemia: myeloid leukemia begins in the bone marrow, and lymphoid leukemia begins in the white cell–producing portions of the lymphoid tissue. The leukemic cells soon metastasize into other areas of the body, producing leukemic cells and demanding excessive amounts of metabolic elements, resulting in severe tissue degeneration. Common effects are severe anemia, spontaneous bleeding, a tendency toward infections, and eventually death.

The Lymph-Vascular System

The lymphatic system acts as an aid to, and is interlinked with, the blood-vascular system. Lymph is derived from the blood and interstitial fluid and is gradually shifted back into the bloodstream. The lymph-vascular system includes the lymph, lymphatics, lymph ducts, lymph nodes, and lacteals. Also considered a part of the lymph system are the tonsils, spleen, and thymus gland.

Function of the Lymph System

The lymphatics collect excess tissue fluid, invading microorganisms, damaged cells, and protein molecules that are too large or too toxic to return directly to the blood system through the capillary walls. These materials are transported from the interstitial spaces through the lymph vessels, are filtered through the lymph nodes, and eventually rejoin the blood near the junction of the subclavian and jugular veins. The lymphoid tissue contains vast numbers of lymphocytes, white blood cells that are an important element of the body's immune system (Figure 5-56a and b).

Lymph and Tissue Fluid

Lymph is a straw-colored fluid that is derived from and is very similar to the tissue fluid or interstitial fluid of the body part from which it flows. By bathing all cells, tissue fluid acts as a medium of exchange, trading to the cells its nutritive materials and receiving in return the waste products of metabolism. Most of the fluid that filters through the capillary walls to surround the cells is eventually reabsorbed into the capillaries. Approximately 10 percent of the fluid enters the lymph capillaries and returns to the blood through the lymph system, however.

Lymph-collecting Vessels

lacteals

are lymphatic capillaries located in the villi of the small intestine.

Lymph capillaries are located throughout the body, with the exception of the epidermis of the skin, the CNS, the bones, and the endomysium of most muscles. **Lacteals** (**LAK**-tee-als) are lymphatic capillaries located in the villi of the small intestine. The walls of the lymph capillaries are constructed of endothelial cells that overlap at the edges yet are not securely attached. The endothelial cells have fine filaments that anchor the lymph capillaries in the tissue and help the capillaries to open in response to fluid pressure or the gentle stretching and relaxation of the tissues. This arrangement creates flap-like valves that allow fluid from the tissue spaces to enter the lymph capillaries (Figures 5-57 a and b).

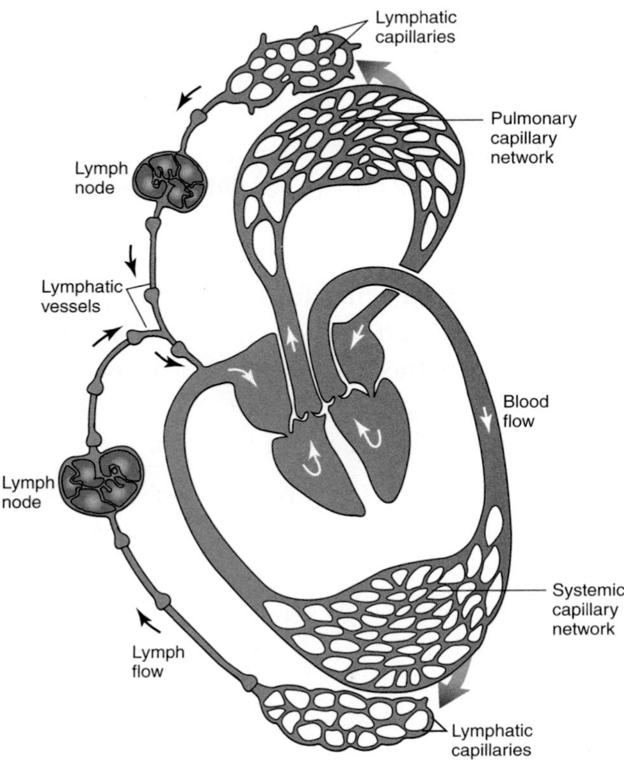

FIGURE 5-56 A Interaction of blood and lymph system.

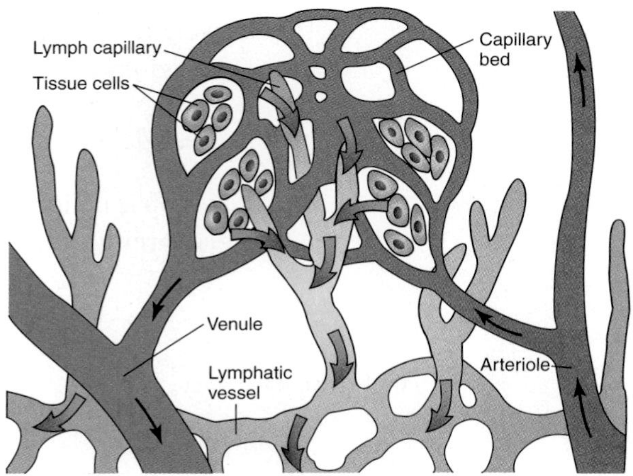

FIGURE 5-56 B Lymph capillaries begin as closed-end tubules in the tissue spaces near blood

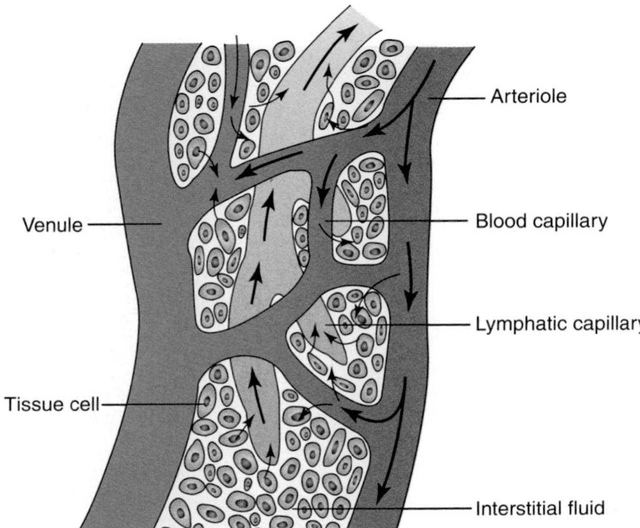

FIGURE 5-57 A Relationship of lymph capillaries, tissue cells, and blood capillaries.

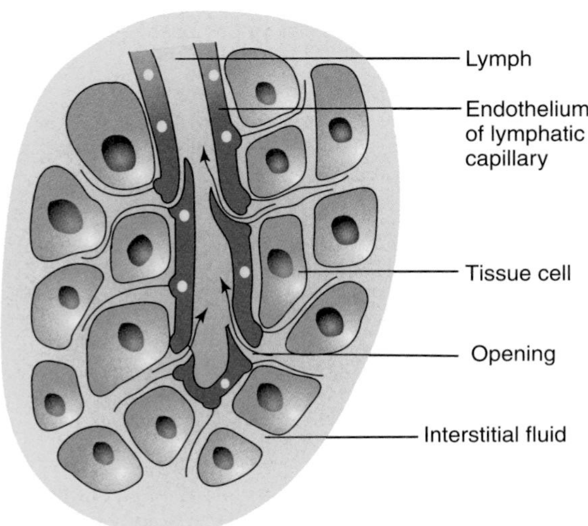

FIGURE 5-57 B Lymph capillary in tissue cells showing valves and filaments.

Lymph Pathways

lymphatics

are small, intermediate lymph vessels.

After being collected in the lymph capillaries, lymph flows into **lymphatics,** which merge into larger and larger lymphatics. The pathways of the lymphatics are closely associated with the veins of the body. The lymphatics continue to merge until the lymph flows into one of two large lymph ducts and finally back into the blood.

thoracic duct

is the largest lymph vessel that collects lymph from both legs and the left side of the rest of the body.

Lymph from the legs, abdomen, left arm, left side of the head, neck, and chest flows into the **thoracic duct** *(left lymphatic duct).* Lymph from the thoracic duct reenters the bloodstream through the left subclavian vein and from there flows into the superior vena cava and into the right atrium of the heart. Lymph from the right side of the head, neck, chest, and the right arm flows into the right lymphatic duct. Lymph from the right lymphatic duct reenters the bloodstream at the right subclavian vein.

Unlike the blood-vascular system, in which the blood flows through a relatively closed circuit of arteries, capillaries, and veins, lymph moves through a closed-end system from the body tissues to the heart (Figure 5-58a and b).

The Movement of Lymph

Lymph is collected from the interstitial spaces into the lymph capillaries. It travels through the lymphatics and lymph nodes, into the right or left lymphatic

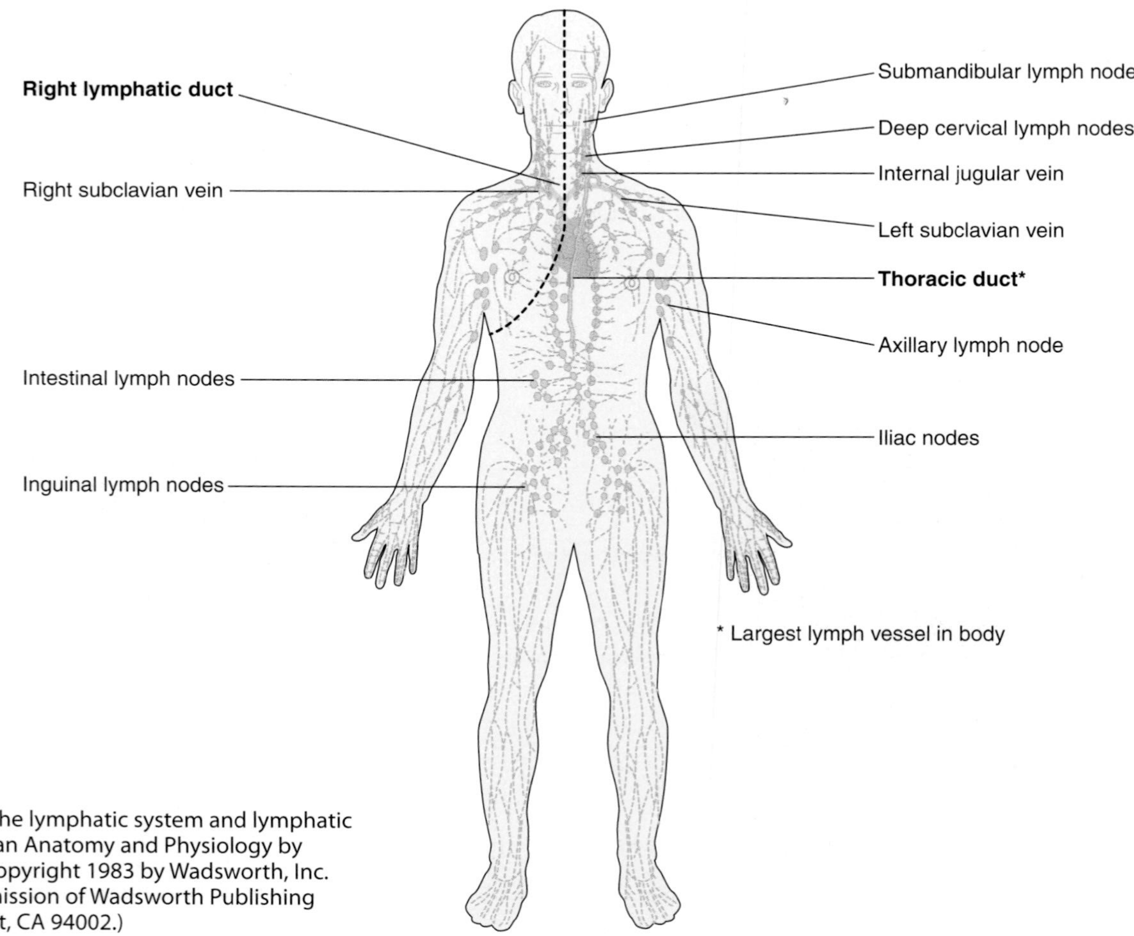

FIGURE 5-58 A The lymphatic system and lymphatic ducts. (From Human Anatomy and Physiology by Joan G. Creager. Copyright 1983 by Wadsworth, Inc. Reprinted by permission of Wadsworth Publishing Company, Belmont, CA 94002.)

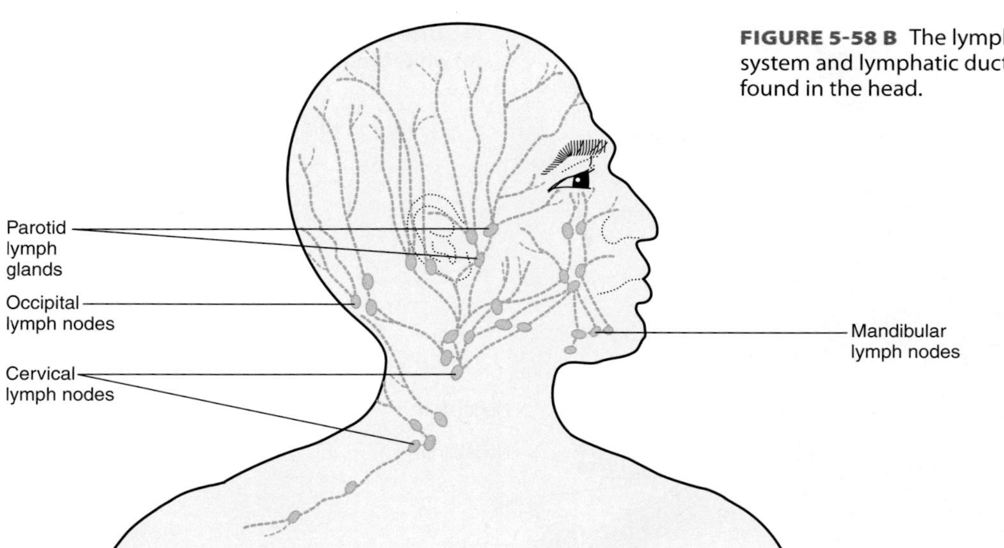

FIGURE 5-58 B The lymphatic system and lymphatic ducts found in the head.

duct, and finally back into the bloodstream. Unlike the blood-vascular system, in which the heart pumps the blood, the lymph system has no internal pump. The structure and arrangement of lymphatics resemble those of the veins except that the lymphatic capillaries are closed, whereas the veins are a continuation from the arteries and capillary beds. Also resembling the veins, the lymph vessels contain a system of valves that allow fluid movement in only one direction. The walls of the larger lymphatics are similar to veins. The inner surface is a thin layer of endothelial cells; the middle layer is made up of smooth muscle tissue surrounded by tough connective tissue. The action of the smooth muscle combined with external forces on this extensive system of valves creates a *lymphatic pump.*

Beginning in the smallest lymph capillaries, the endothelial cells that form the capillary walls overlap in such a way that they form microscopic valves that allow the movement of fluids into the capillary, but the slightest back pressure closes the openings so that once inside, the fluid does not escape. Within the lymphatics, flaplike valves protrude from the inside of the vessel walls to prevent backflow (Figure 5-57b).

When a segment of a lymph vessel is compressed, the pressure on the fluid in that segment forces the previous valve to close and the next one to open as the fluid moves through the valve and progresses toward the heart. The external pressure that activates the lymphatic pump is supplied primarily from the contraction of the skeletal muscles. Other factors that can contribute are the movement of body parts, breathing, contractions of smooth muscles in the larger lymph vessels, arterial pulsation, and compression of tissues from outside the body (e.g., massage).

Lymph Nodes

Lymph nodes are made of *lymphoid tissue* and are located along the course of the lymphatics. They are oval or rounded masses from the size of a pinhead to an inch in length and resemble the shape of a bean. Lymph nodes contain a large concentration of lymphocytes and serve to filter and neutralize harmful bacteria and toxic substances collected in the lymph, thereby preventing the spread of infection to other parts of the body (Figure 5-59).

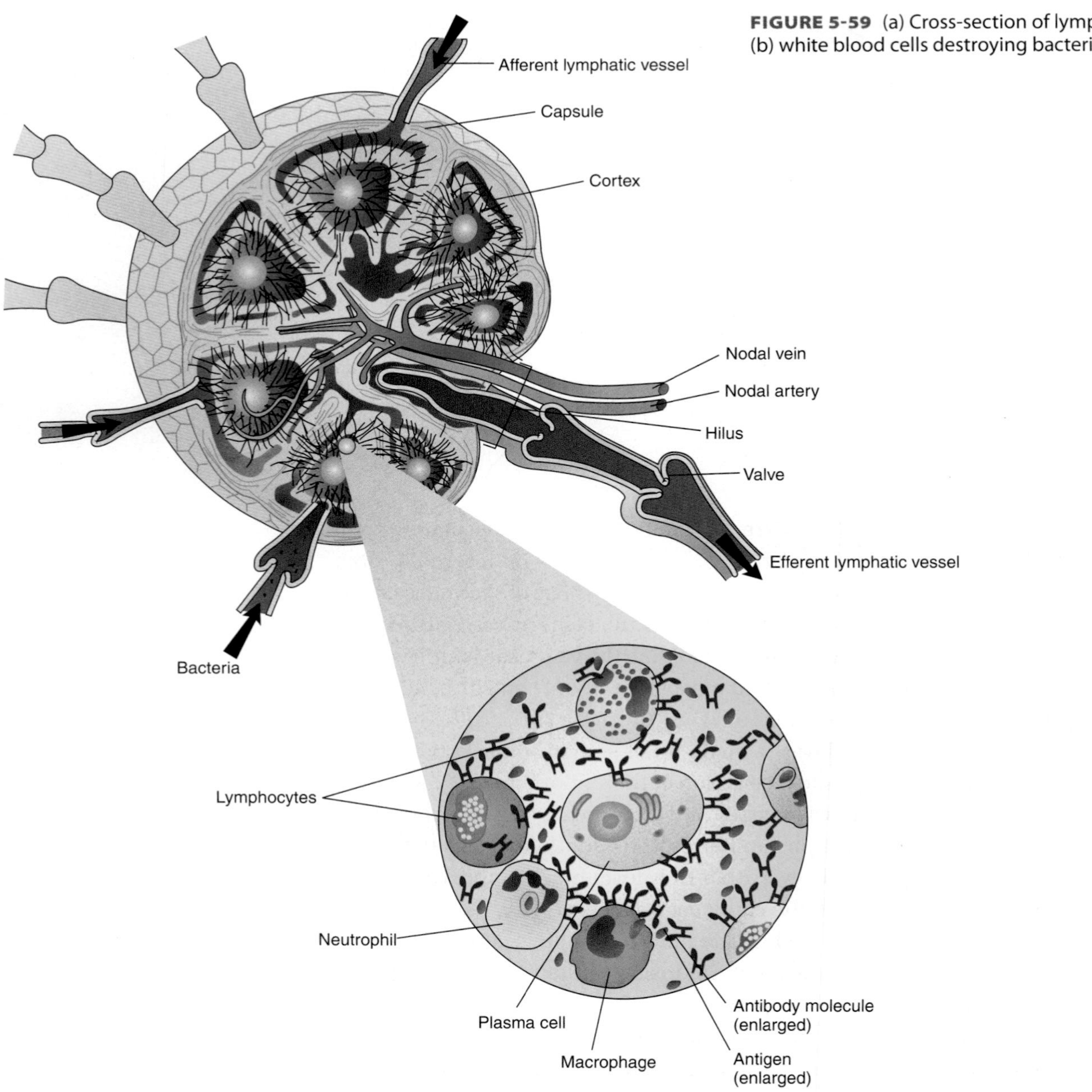

FIGURE 5-59 (a) Cross-section of lymph node; (b) white blood cells destroying bacteria.

Lymph nodes are found in the following regions of the body:

1. Back of the head, draining the scalp
2. Around the neck muscles, draining the back of the tongue, pharynx, nasal cavities, and the roof of the mouth
3. Under the floor of the jaw, draining the floor of the mouth
4. Upper extremities, in the bend of the elbow, under the armpit, and under the pectoral muscle
5. Abdomen and pelvis, along the blood vessels in these regions
6. Lower extremities, in back of the knee, and the groin

Regional lymph nodes are named according to their location in the body:

Node	Location
Submandibular	Beneath the mandible
Occipital	Base of the skull
Axillary	Armpit
Inguinal	Groin
Supratrochlear	Elbow
Popliteal	Behind the knee
Mammary	Breast
Femoral	Thigh
Tibial	Leg
Cervical	Neck

Healthy tissue depends on good lymph circulation. Correct massage can increase lymphatic circulation and clear the lymph spaces as well as drain sluggish lymph nodes. The purpose of lymph drainage is to cleanse and regenerate the tissues and organs of the body. Massage stimulates the movement of lymph and the formation of lymphocytes that produce antibodies, increasing the body's resistance to infection (see Lymph Massage, Chapter 16).

IMMUNE SYSTEM

The immune system is a remarkable system that helps to keep people safe from a variety of "foreign" invaders and diseases. This system consists of a complex array of organs, cells, and molecules distributed throughout the body. Keeping infection-causing organisms such as bacteria and viruses, as well as parasites and fungi, out of the body and destroying any that get in is the mission of the immune system.

Specialized white blood cells (lymphocytes) play a major role in the immune response. White blood cells originate in bone marrow. Some migrate to the thymus, where they develop into specialized types of immune cells (*T-cells*). From the bone marrow and thymus, white blood cells are transported through the blood and lymph and gather in lymph nodes and other immune organs, including the spleen, tonsils, adenoids, appendix, and small intestine, where they can encounter antigens. (An **antigen** is anything that can trigger an immune response.)

antigen
is anything that can trigger an immune response.

Lymphatic vessels and blood vessels transport white blood cells throughout the body to sites of infection. Lymphatic vessels also transport lymph-carrying microorganisms and dead cells from distant infections into lymph nodes, where they can be digested and eliminated.

Lymphocytes, called *B-cells* and *T-cells*, are the main types of immune cells and bear the major responsibility for immune response. They recognize and coordinate an attack against specific microorganisms.

The B-cell is responsible for the production of antibodies (proteins that can bind to specific molecular shapes), and the T-cell (two types) is responsible for helping the B-cell to make antibodies and for killing damaged or "different" cells (all foreign cells except bacteria) within the body. The two main types of T-cells are the "helper" T-cell and the cytotoxic T-cell (CDT cell).

The immune system is amazingly complex. It can recognize millions of different enemies and produce secretions and cells to match up with and wipe out each one of them. Whenever any foreign substance or agent enters the body, the immune system is activated. Both B- and T-cell members respond to the threat, which eventually results in the elimination of the foreign substance or agent from the body.

The marvel of the immune system is its ability to distinguish between what is "you" and belongs from what is "foreign" and does not belong. Every substance—from a dust mite to the flu virus to one of your own cells—carries its own "chemical ID card," marked by a unique molecular pattern on its surface. All of your body's cells have the same molecular pattern. White blood cells learn to recognize and ignore cells identified by the body's own pattern and react strongly against antigens. They become the "soldiers" in the "immune army."

In abnormal situations, the immune system can mistake self for nonself and attack itself. The result is called **autoimmune disease.** Some forms of arthritis and diabetes are autoimmune diseases. In other cases, the immune system responds inappropriately to a seemingly harmless substance such as ragweed pollen or cat hair. The result is allergy, and this kind of antigen is called an **allergen.**

autoimmune disease

occurs when the immune system mistakes self for nonself and attacks itself.

allergen

an antigen that can cause an allergic response in some people.

B-Cell System

B-cells work chiefly by producing antibodies. When a B-cell intercepts an antigen, it produces a specific antibody that fits to and disables the invading body. Each B-cell is designed to make a specific antibody, and each antibody is designed to battle a specific microorganism. B-cells also develop into plasma cells that manufacture millions of identical antibody molecules and pour them into the bloodstream. An antibody matches an antigen much as a key matches a lock. Whenever antibody and antigen interlock, the antibody marks the antigen for destruction by other scavenging cells of the immune system. Other B-cells transform into rapidly multiplying memory cells that circulate throughout the body, preparing it for the next encounter with this antigen.

T-Cell system

T-cells coordinate immune defenses and kill organisms in cells on contact. T-cells are active against bacterial infection, fungi, cancerous cells, transplanted tissue, and wounded cells harboring pathogens. T-cells produce lymphokines, which draw macrophages, neutrophils, and eosinophils toward sensitized T-cells, and activate macrophages, which then inhibit viral reproduction.

T-cells originate in the thymus and also become localized in lymphoid organs. A variety of T-cells have been identified:

- Killer T-cells attack antigens directly.
- Helper T-cells enable the other T-cells and most B-cells to perform their functions. They activate B-cells, causing the appropriate ones to transform into plasma cells and flood the bloodstream with antibodies. T-cells are destroyed by the HIV virus in AIDS, resulting in a depressed immune response that allows infection by a variety of microorganisms and the growth of certain tumors.
- Suppressor T-cells monitor and adjust the level of antibodies and counteract the action of helper T-cells.

Other White Blood Cells

Other important types of white blood cells associated with the immune system, including macrophages and granulocytes, remove neutralized antibody-antigen complexes and organisms by *phagocytosis*, a process of engulfing and digestion. **Phagocytes,** the name for these large white blood cells, comes from the Greek word meaning "eaters." Their main function is to gobble up foreign bodies—a speck of dust or pollen to a virus. The macrophage is one type of phagocyte that migrates out of the bloodstream into the tissue spaces. As scavengers, macrophages rid the body of worn-out cells and other debris. They also play a vital role in initiating the immune response. Other white blood cells—neutrophils, eosinophils, and basophils—are also "cell eaters." In addition, they release powerful chemicals that destroy microorganisms. Mast cells are responsible for the recruitment of other inflammatory cells, mainly through releasing their contents of inflammatory mediators, such as histamine, protein-breaking enzymes, leukotrienes, and heparin. They are most important in allergic disorders.

phagocytes

blood cells that are able to engulf and digest cellular debris and foreign bodies in the tissues.

How the System Works

The immune system responds to external factors such as bacteria, viruses, toxins, and foreign proteins, and internal ones, including potential tumors and damaged normal tissue. In addition, many diseases, such as some forms of diabetes and arthritis, can result from altered immune processes that target healthy normal tissue. The term *antigen* is short for "antibody-generating." An antigen can be any type of molecule that is encoded in such a way that the body does not recognize it as one of its own and therefore provokes an immune response. The immune system responds by producing antibody proteins that selectively bind to and usually inactivate the antigen.

When an antibody binds to an antigen, a complementary set of chemical reactions is initiated. The sequence of events involved in this kind of immune response can be summarized in this series of steps:

- Invading microorganisms initially encounter whichever macrophages, neutrophils, or B- and T-cells might be present in the immediate vicinity.
- Pathogenic destruction by local phagocytes produces chemical messengers.
- Inflammation is initiated.
- Chemical signals are sent to the bone marrow, where the production of white blood cells and phagocytes increases.
- More macrophages, neutrophils, and lymphocytes are drawn to the site of invasion.
- Any antibodies present at the site of infection lock onto their antigen.
- T-cells are brought into action, directly killing some pathogens and making others more susceptible to attack by phagocytes.
- Debris from this interaction produces strong attracting signals for more phagocytes and lymphocytes.
- The killer T-cells attack antigens directly, and T-cells begin to produce lymphokines.

Immunity, Natural and Acquired

Immunity refers to all the physiologic mechanisms used by the body as protection against foreign substances. These foreign substances include such common infectious organisms as bacteria, viruses, and parasites (e.g., fungi, worms, and single-cell protozoa), as well as drugs, foods, chemicals, and various inhalants (e.g., pollens).

innate immunity

is present from before birth.

Innate immunity is present from before birth, consisting of many nonspecific factors and blood-based immunity from the mother.

acquired immunity

results from an encounter with a new substance, which triggers events that induce an immune response specific to that particular substance.

Acquired immunity, a more specialized form of immunity, is the result of an encounter with a new substance, which triggers events that induce an immune response specific against that particular substance. This involves B-lymphocytes, T-lymphocytes, and macrophages. When people are exposed to a new antigen, it usually takes several days to a week for the immune system to develop an immunity, which corresponds to the time needed for the B-lymphocytes to be mobilized and activated for antibody production to counteract the antigen invasion. Whenever T-cells and B-cells are activated, some of the cells become *memory cells.* The next time a person encounters the same antigen, the immune system is set to stop the infection before it starts.

vaccine

contains microorganisms that are either dead, weakened, or altered forms of a live infectious organism that stimulates an immune response without causing an illness.

When you are vaccinated**, vaccines** containing microorganisms that are either dead, weakened, or altered forms of a live infectious organism stimulate an immune response, usually without causing the accompanying illness. The resulting memory cells provide immunity for years or even a lifetime.

Protective Functions of the Immune System

Fever

Fever is an abnormally high body temperature that is an immune system response to a viral or bacterial infection, or sometimes it is a response to major tissue damage. Normal body temperature is 98.6°F (37°C), although it can fluctuate a degree higher or lower. A body temperature above 99.8°F is considered a fever. Fevers of 104°F or more are serious and require medical care. Sustained fevers of 107°F or higher can cause permanent brain damage or death. If a fever is accompanied by any of the following signs, a doctor should be consulted immediately:

- Significant stiff neck and pain when bending the head forward
- A severe headache
- Persistent vomiting
- Difficulty breathing
- Severe swelling of the throat
- Unusual skin rash
- Unusual sensitivity of the eyes to bright light
- Mental confusion
- Extreme listlessness or irritability
- Abdominal pain or pain when urinating

A fever is an indication that the body is working to get rid of a pathogen. Although uncomfortable, unless it is dangerously high or lasts more than 48 hours, it is advantageous to allow the fever to eradicate the invader. For instance, viruses that cause colds and other respiratory infections thrive in cooler temperatures. By creating a fever, the body is helping to eliminate the virus. Common complications of prolonged fever are dehydration and acidosis (bloodstream that is too acidic), so it is important to drink plenty of water and get plenty of rest.

When an infectious virus or bacteria enters the body, it is attacked by certain white blood cells. In response, the white blood cells produce a substance called *interleukin-1* that travels to the brain, where a series of chemical reactions cause—among other things—the hypothalamus to reset the body's thermostat. The muscles and glands of the body respond, metabolism increases, superficial blood vessels constrict, shivering and "chills" begin, and the body's core temperature begins to rise. The increased body temperature helps to fight the invading pathogens by increasing the production of T-cells, which stimulates B-cells to produce antibodies. The heart rate increases to increase the distribution of white blood cells. The antiviral agent interferon becomes more active.

A fever usually resolves itself as the pathogen is controlled. As the fever breaks, the body often responds by sweating to cool the body down. This is a sign that health is being restored.

Massage is contraindicated during a fever.

Inflammation

Inflammation is an immune system response to a local infection or injury that acts to isolate and resolve the damage and protect the body from invasion. Inflammation is a reaction to tissue damage. The damage can be from trauma, a burn, laceration, toxic chemical, or an infectious agent. When a cell is damaged, it releases certain proteins such as histamines and cytokines that set off a chain reaction:

- Immediately, vasoconstriction occurs to prevent excessive bleeding.
- This is soon followed by a period of vasodilation, in which the capillaries dilate and become more permeable, allowing white blood cells, antibodies, clotting factors, and other important substances to flood the area. This accounts for the inflammatory heat and swelling.
- Platelets and fibrin begin to form clots to close off broken blood vessels. This not only stops blood loss but also prevents pathogens and other harmful substances from entering the bloodstream.
- Neutrophils and macrophages neutralize and phagocytize pathogens.
- Fibroblasts migrate to the area and begin producing collagen fibers to start mending the torn and damaged tissues. Collagen produces scar tissue that continues to form after the initial acute inflammation subsides.

The first four steps represent the acute inflammation stage. The classic signs of acute inflammation are pain, heat, redness, swelling, and sometimes loss of function and itching. The acute inflammatory stage for an injury such as a wound or sprain/strain is usually 24 to 72 hours. The subacute stage of scar tissue formation and repair can take days, weeks, months, or even years, depending on the nature and extent of the injury.

Massage during the acute stage of inflammation, when swelling, pain, and heat are present, is contraindicated. Massage during the subacute stages, when scar tissue is forming and the tissues are rebuilding, can be invaluable to ensure that strong, pliable, and flexible tissue develops.

Dysfunctions of the Immune System

When the immune system is weakened or overwhelmed, a variety of conditions can occur:

- Allergy—This response is an overreaction by the immune system to an otherwise harmless substance such as pollen or pet dander. Contact with an allergy-causing substance, or allergen, triggers production of a specific kind of antibody that causes immune cells in the mucous lining of the eyes and airways to release inflammatory substances, including histamine. Release of histamine leads to the familiar symptoms of allergy and asthma—redness and swelling of the eyes, sneezing, coughing, difficult breathing, nasal congestion, and hives. A more severe allergic reaction is anaphylactic shock, which can occur in previously sensitized persons as a result of a bee sting, a food reaction, or an injected or ingested drug. In this case, the bronchioles constrict, breathing becomes difficult, and cardiac failure can result unless emergency treatment is given with an injection of epinephrine to dilate the airways and stimulate the heartbeat.

- Autoimmune diseases—In these conditions, the body makes antibodies and T-cells directed against its own cells. Insulin-dependent diabetes, for example, can be partly caused by an attack on the pancreas by a person's own antibodies. Self-destructive antibodies are also associated with chronic muscle weakness (myasthenia gravis), rheumatoid arthritis, and multiple sclerosis. No one knows what causes the immune system's recognition process to break down this way. Scientists think that multiple factors—heredity, viruses, certain drugs, or even sunlight—might play a role.
- Cancers of the immune system—When immune cells reproduce uncontrollably, the result is a cancer of the immune system such as leukemia, multiple myeloma, or lymphoma.
- Immune-deficiency diseases—These conditions occur when one or more parts of the immune system are deficient or missing. These defects can be inherited or acquired from a viral infection such as AIDS. They also can be caused by the toxic effects of radiation or some drugs.

HIV/AIDS

HIV disease occurs when the human immunodeficiency virus (HIV) enters a person's body. HIV specifically infects CD4+ lymphocytes, the very cells necessary to activate both B-cell and cytotoxic T-cell immune responses. Without helper T-cells, the body cannot make antibodies properly, nor can infected cells containing HIV (an intracellular pathogen) be properly eliminated. Consequently, the virus can multiply, kill the helper T-cell in which it lives, infect adjacent helper T-cells, and repeat the cycle, until eventually there is a substantial loss of helper T-cells, and the body's ability to fight infection weakens.

A person with HIV infection can remain healthy for many years. During this time, enough of the immune system remains intact to provide immune surveillance and prevent most infections. Eventually, when a significant number of CD4+ lymphocytes have been destroyed and when production of new CD4+ cells cannot match the rate of destruction, failure of the immune system leads to the appearance of clinical AIDS. The term *AIDS* applies to the most advanced stages of HIV infection.

According to the Centers for Disease Control (CDC), a diagnosis of AIDS is made when the count of CD4+ T-cells falls below 200 per cubic millimeter of blood. (Healthy adults usually have CD4+ T-cell counts of 1,000 or more.)

In addition, the definition of AIDS includes 26 clinical conditions that can affect people with advanced HIV disease. Most AIDS-defining conditions are opportunistic infections that rarely cause harm in healthy people. In people who have AIDS, however, these infections are often severe and sometimes fatal, because the immune system is so ravaged by HIV that the body cannot fight off certain bacteria, viruses, and other microbes. HIV infection always evolves to clinical AIDS over time, although the speed at which this evolution occurs varies.

The first cases of AIDS were noticed in 1980. HIV was first identified in 1984 by French and American scientists, but the human immunodeficiency virus did not get its name until 1986.

HIV is spread most commonly by sexual contact with an infected partner or through contact with infected blood. Women can transmit HIV to their fetuses during pregnancy or birth. HIV also can be spread to babies through the breast milk of infected mothers. Although researchers have detected HIV in the saliva of infected people, no evidence exists that the virus is spread by contact with saliva, such as by kissing. Scientists also have found no evidence that HIV is spread through sweat, tears, urine, or feces. HIV is not spread through casual contact such as the sharing of food utensils, towels, bedding, swimming pools, telephones, or toilet seats. Biting insects such as mosquitoes or bedbugs cannot spread HIV either.

In the health care setting, workers have been infected with HIV after being stuck with needles containing HIV-infected blood or, less frequently, after infected blood contacts the worker's open cut or splashes into a mucous membrane (e.g., the eyes or inside the nose). This risk can be reduced if health care workers follow Universal Precautions, treating all blood, semen, or vaginal secretions, no matter from whom the fluid comes, as if they contained HIV. Health care workers must wash their hands between patients; wear gloves, masks, gowns, and eyewear when performing certain procedures; and disinfect or sterilize appropriate equipment.

Massage is not contraindicated for people with HIV unless they are severely ill with one of the many opportunistic diseases. Precautions must be taken because the client has a weakened immune system and risks picking up infections from the therapist. The therapist must avoid any open lesions or wounds and be cautious of any bodily fluids. Massage should not be performed if the therapist has cuts or abrasions on her own hands unless wearing gloves for protection. When massaging people in the advanced stages of AIDS, work under the direction of the physician. With strict hygiene precautions, touch and massage are valuable therapies for people afflicted with HIV and AIDS.

SECTION QUESTIONS FOR DISCUSSION AND REVIEW

1. Name the important parts composing the circulatory system.
2. What are the two divisions of the circulatory system?
3. What is the function of the heart?
4. Name the protective covering of the heart and describe its function.
5. Name the chambers of the heart in the order that blood passes through them.

6. Which nerves regulate the heartbeat?
7. What is the function of the arteries?
8. What is an arteriole?
9. Which nerves control the movements of the arterial walls?
10. What is the function of the capillaries?
11. What is the function of the veins?
12. What is a venule?
13. What is the purpose of the venous pump?
14. Name the main artery of the body.
15. Name two circulatory systems of the blood-vascular system.
16. Which vein carries freshly oxygenated blood?
17. Which constituents are found in the blood?
18. What is the primary function of the red blood cells?
19. What is the primary function of the white blood cells?
20. Which substances are carried by the blood to the body cells?
21. Which substances does the blood carry away from the body cells?
22. How does the blood protect the body?
23. What is the normal temperature of the blood?
24. Name the parts of the lymph system.
25. What is the major function of the lymph-vascular system?
26. What is the major function of the lymph glands or nodes?
27. Which regions of the body contain lymph nodes?
28. From what is lymph derived?
29. Into which blood vessels does the lymph return?
30. What is meant by lymph drainage?
31. What are lacteals?
32. How is massage of value to the health of the lymphatic system?
33. What determines the names of lymphatics?
34. What is the lymphatic pump and how does it work?
35. Trace the flow of lymph from just before it enters the lymph system until it leaves.

REVIEW

Important Veins of the Body

Matching Test I

Insert the letter of the proper term in front of each definition.

______	**1.**	receives blood from eyes	a.	femoral vein
______	**2.**	receives blood from heart	b.	ophthalmic vein
______	**3.**	receives blood from face	c.	coronary veins
______	**4.**	receives blood from outer arm	d.	facial vein
______	**5.**	receives blood from legs	e.	basilic vein

True or False Test I

Carefully read each statement and decide whether it is true or false; draw a circle around the letter T or F.

1. T F Both the internal and external jugular veins return blood from the head, face, and neck to the heart.

2. T F The inferior vena cava receives blood from the abdomen and upper limbs.

3. T F The popliteal vein is located in the lower extremities.

4. T F The innominate (brachiocephalic) veins are found in the upper extremities.

5. T F The superior vena cava receives blood from the head, neck, thorax, and upper limbs.

Important Arteries of the Body

Matching Test II

Insert the letter of the proper term in front of each definition.

______	**1.**	supplies blood to heart	a.	ophthalmic artery
______	**2.**	supplies blood to eyes	b.	subclavian artery
______	**3.**	supplies blood to face	c.	frontal artery
______	**4.**	supplies blood to forehead	d.	coronary artery
______	**5.**	supplies blood to chest	e.	facial artery

True or False Test II

Carefully read each statement and decide whether it is true or false; draw a circle around the letter T or F.

1. T F The posterior auricular artery supplies blood to the scalp.

2. T F The aorta does not form large and small branches.

3. T F The axillary artery supplies blood to the shoulder, chest, and arm.

4. T F The external branch of the common carotid artery supplies blood to the cranial cavity.

5. T F The external iliac artery supplies blood to the upper limbs.

SYSTEM 5 THE NERVOUS SYSTEM

The nervous system controls and coordinates the functions of other systems of the body so that they work harmoniously and efficiently. The nervous system is composed of the brain, spinal cord, and peripheral nerves. The primary function of the nervous system is to collect a multitude of sensory information; process, interpret, and integrate that information; and initiate appropriate responses throughout the body.

neuron

is the structural unit of the nervous system.

nerve cell

is the same as a neuron.

nerve fibers

projections from the body of the nerve cell that carry nervous impulses.

dendrites

connect with other neurons to receive information.

axon

conducts impulses away from the cell body.

synapse

the junction where nerve signals jump from one nerve to another.

neurotransmitter

is a chemical that sends a nerve signal across a synapse.

sensory neuron

carries impulses from sense organs to the brain.

motor neuron

carries nerve impulses from the brain to the effectors.

interneuron

carries impulses from one neuron to another.

The functions of the nervous system are:

1. To rule the body by controlling all visible and invisible activities.
2. To control human thought and conduct.
3. To govern all internal and external movements of the body.
4. To give the power to see, hear, move, talk, feel, think, and remember.

Neurons and Nerves

A **neuron** is the structural unit of the nervous system. A neuron is the **nerve cell** (cell body) including its outgrowth of long and short projections of cytoplasm, called **nerve fibers.** There are two types of nerve fibers. A neuron has numerous multibranched **dendrites** that connect with other neurons to receive information, and a single **axon** that conducts impulses away from the cell body. The axons of most nerves are covered by a myelin sheath that is made of fatty Schwann cells. The myelin insulates the nerve and aids in the conduction of the nerve impulse. The nerve cell stores energy and nutrients that are used by the cell processes to convey nerve impulses throughout the body. Neurons have the ability to react to certain stimuli (irritability) and to transmit an impulse generated by that stimulus over a distance or to another neuron (conductability). Impulses are passed from one neuron to another at a junction called a **synapse** (**SIN**-aps). When an impulse reaches the end of an axon, a chemical **neurotransmitter** is released at the synapse that acts on the membrane of the receptive neuron to pass the impulse along (Figure 5-60).

Functionally, there are three types of neurons:

Sensory neurons (afferent neurons) originate in the periphery of the body and carry impulses or messages from sense organs to the brain, where sensations of touch, cold, heat, sight, hearing, taste, or pain are interpreted and experienced.

Motor neurons (efferent neurons) carry nerve impulses from the brain to the effectors (the muscles or glands that they control).

Interneurons (internuncial neurons) are located in the brain and spinal cord and carry impulses from one neuron to another. They function to transmit and direct impulses from one place in the spinal cord or brain to another.

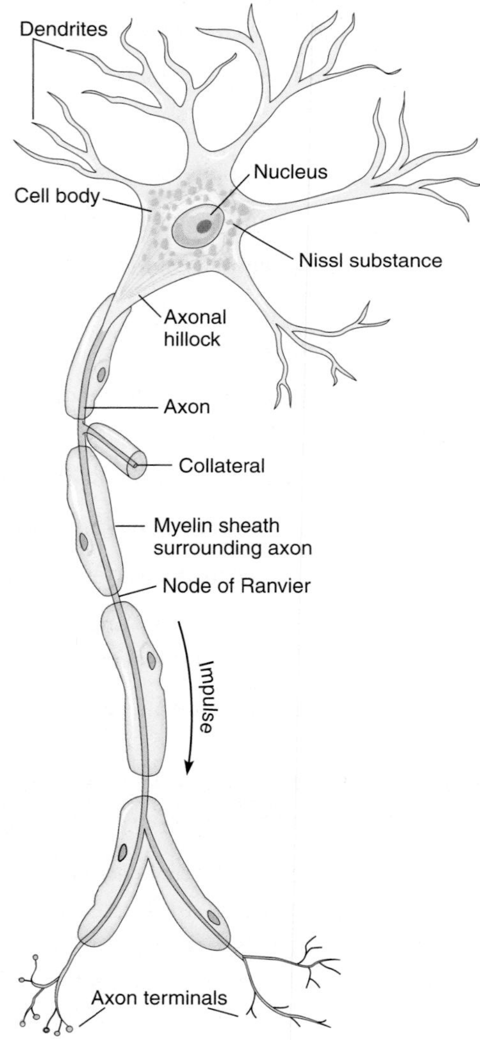

FIGURE 5-60 Common neuron.

A nerve fiber is the extension from a neuron. A **nerve** is a bundle of nerve fibers held together by connective tissue that extends from the CNS to the tissue that the neurons innervate. Nerves have their origin in the brain and spinal cord and distribute branches to all parts of the body.

Sensory nerves, or **afferent nerves,** carry sensory impulses from a variety of sensory receptors toward the brain or spinal cord. *Motor nerves,* termed *efferent nerves,* carry impulses from the brain or spinal cord to the muscles or glands. Most nerves contain both sensory and motor fibers and are called *mixed nerves.*

Anatomically, the nervous system is divided into two main divisions: the CNS and the peripheral nervous system.

nerves

are bundles of fibers held together by connective tissue that originate in the brain and spinal cord and distribute branches all over the body.

afferent nerves

carry impulses toward the spinal cord and brain.

central nervous system

consists of the brain and spinal cord.

meningitis

is an acute inflammation of the pia mater and arachnoid mater around the brain and spinal cord.

dura mater

is the outer layer of the meninges.

pia mater

is the innermost layer of the meninges.

arachnoid mater

is the middle space of the meninges.

Central Nervous System

The CNS is the main control center for the human organism. It is responsible for our thoughts and emotions, for receiving and interpreting incoming sensory information, and for disseminating appropriate motor responses to maintain safety and homeostasis. The CNS consists of the *brain* and *spinal cord.* The CNS is surrounded by bone and is covered by a special connective tissue membrane called the **meninges** (me-**NIN**-jeez). More specifically, the brain is housed in the cranium, and the spinal cord is housed in the vertebral canal of the spine. The meninges have three layers. The outer layer, the **dura mater** (**DOO**-ruh **MAY**-ter), which translates as "tough mother," is a protective fibrous connective tissue sheath covering the brain and spinal cord. The **pia mater,** which means "delicate mother," the innermost layer, is attached to the surface of the brain and spinal cord and is richly supplied with blood vessels to nourish the underlying tissues. Between the dura and pia mater is a thin netlike membrane called the **arachnoid mater,** which means "spider layer" and is sometimes referred to as the *arachnoid space.* The arachnoid mater provides a space for the blood vessels and the circulation of cerebrospinal fluid (Figure 5-61).

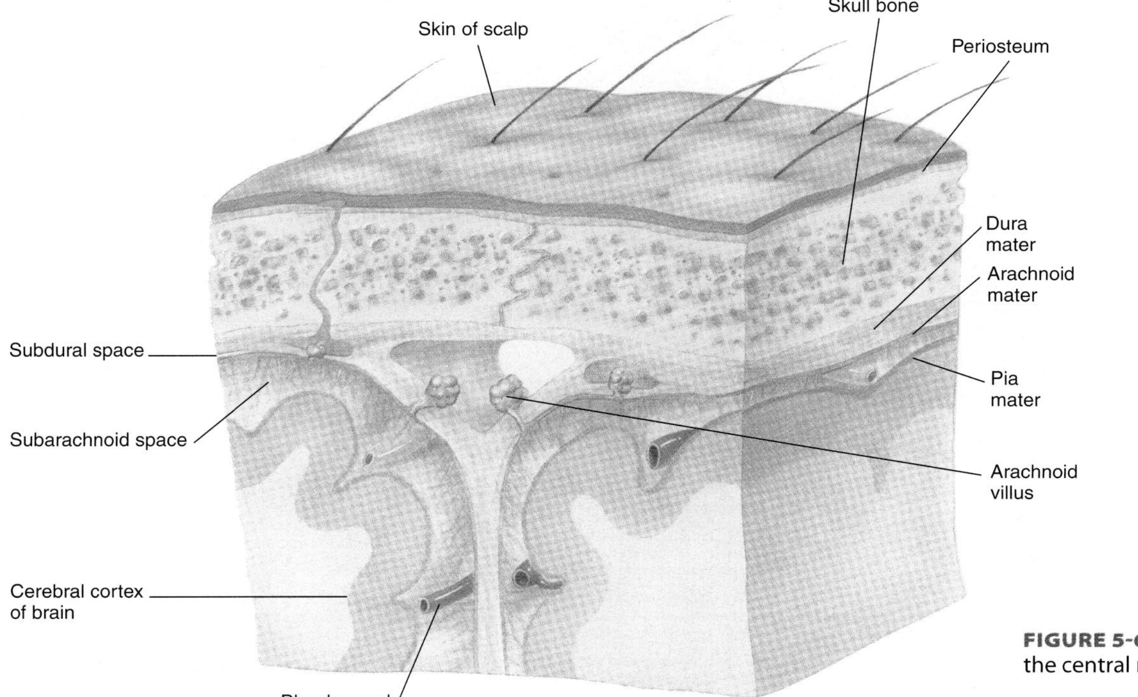

FIGURE 5-61 Meninges of the central nervous system.

cerebrospinal fluid

flows through and around the brain and spinal cord to nourish and protect them.

Cerebrospinal fluid is a clear fluid derived from the blood and secreted into the inner cavities or ventricles of the brain. The fluid circulates through the ventricles and then down through the central canal of the spinal cord and into the arachnoid space. The brain and spinal cord are surrounded by cerebrospinal fluid and indeed seem to be suspended by the fluid. Cerebrospinal fluid carries some nutrients to the nerve tissue and carries wastes away, but its main function is to protect the CNS by acting as a shock absorber for the delicate tissue.

The Brain

The *brain,* the principal nerve center, is the body's largest and most complex nerve tissue, containing in excess of 10 billion neurons and innumerable nerve fibers (Figure 5-62). It is located in and protected by the cranium. It controls sensations, muscles, glandular activity, and the power to think and feel (emotions). The brain includes the following:

1. The *cerebrum,* the largest portion, making up the front and top of the brain, presides over such mental activities as speech, sensation, communication, memory, reasoning, will, and emotions. The cerebrum is divided by a central fissure into right and left cerebral hemispheres, which are connected by bundles of nerve fibers called the *corpus callosum* that provide communication between the right and left hemispheres. It is interesting to note that sensory and motor functions from the right side of the body are processed on the left side of the brain and the sensory and motor activities from the left side of the body are processed and controlled by the right side of the brain.

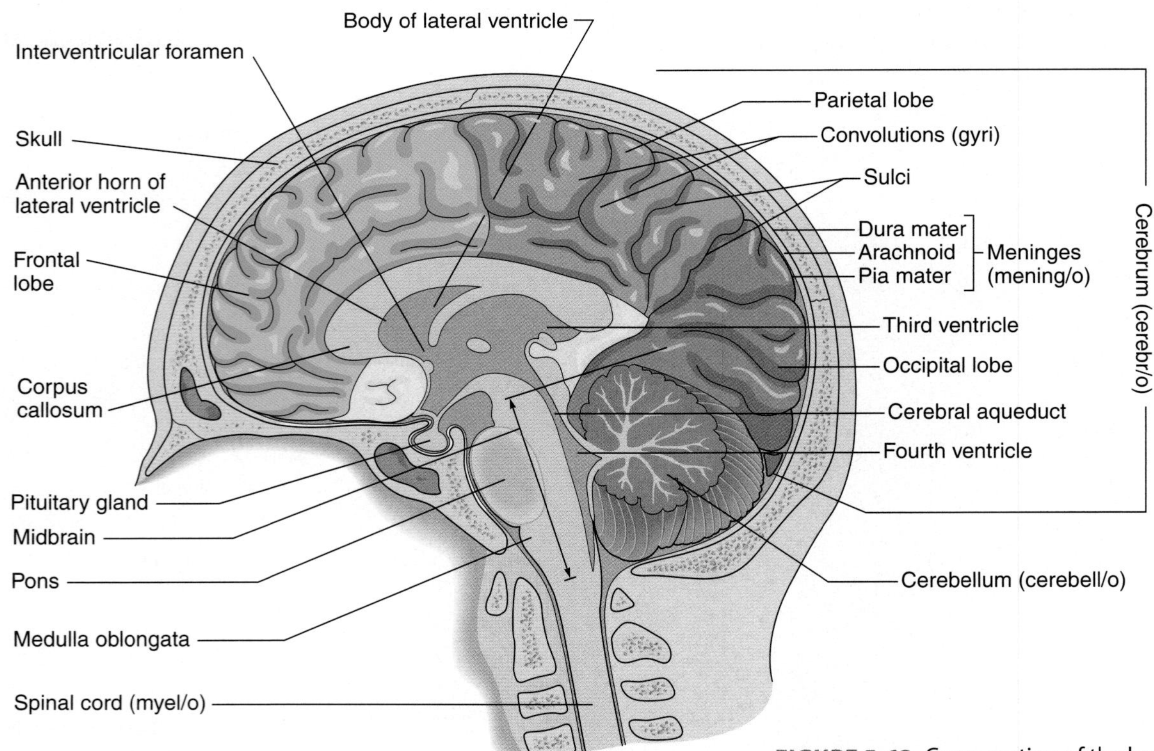

FIGURE 5-62 Cross-section of the brain.

2. The *cerebellum,* the smaller part of the brain, located below the cerebrum and at the back of the cranium, helps to maintain body balance, coordinates voluntary muscles, and makes muscular movement smooth and graceful.
3. The *diencephalon,* which includes the hypothalamus, thalamus, and pineal and pituitary glands, is located in the center of the brain. The thalamus is a relay center for sensory information coming into the brain. The hypothalamus governs the pituitary gland, thereby having a regulatory effect on the autonomic system and the endocrine glands. The pituitary gland, considered to be the master gland because its hormones control other endocrine glands, is located at the base of the brain in the sella turcica of the sphenoid bone.
4. The *brain stem* has three parts: the midbrain, the pons, and the medulla oblongata. These contain intricate masses of nerve fibers that relay and transmit impulses from one portion of the brain to another.

The midbrain contains the main nerve pathways connecting the cerebrum and the lower nervous system as well as certain visual and auditory reflexes that coordinate head and eye movements with things seen and heard.

The pons, located between the midbrain and the medulla oblongata, relays nerve impulses between the cerebrum and the medulla and from the cerebrum to the cerebellum.

The medulla oblongata is an enlarged continuation of the spinal cord that extends from the foramen magnum to the pons and connects the brain with the spinal cord. Control centers within the medulla oblongata regulate movements of the heart and control vasoconstriction of the arteries and the rate and depth of respiration.

Spinal Cord

The spinal cord extends downward from the brain and is housed in and protected by the vertebral column. The spinal cord extends down from the medulla oblongata to the level of the first lumbar vertebrae. The spinal cord consists of 31 segments, each segment being the site of attachment of a pair of spinal nerves. The spinal cord functions as a conduction pathway for nerve impulses traveling to and from the brain, as well as a reflex center between incoming and outgoing peripheral nerve fibers (Figure 5-63).

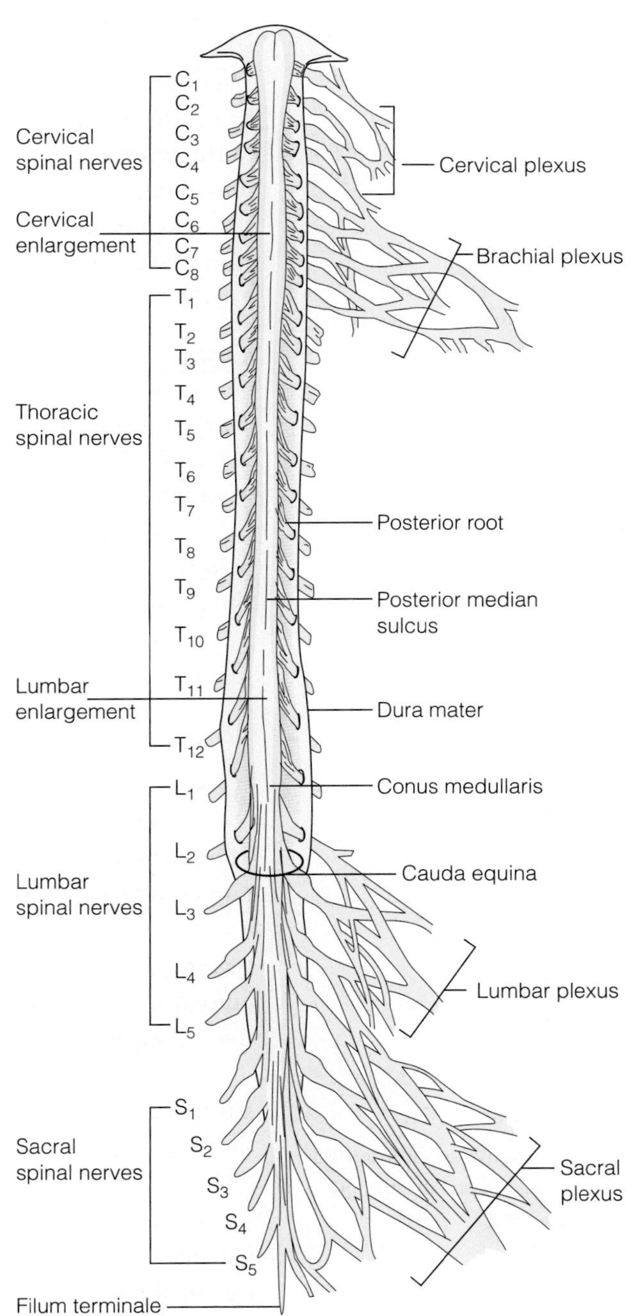

FIGURE 5-63 Spinal cord and spinal nerves.

The Peripheral Nervous System

peripheral nervous system

peripheral nervous system consists of all the nerves that connect the CNS to the rest of the body.

autonomic nervous system

regulates the action of glands, smooth muscles, and the heart.

somatic nervous system

consists of the nerves that connect the central nervous system to the voluntary muscles and skin.

The **peripheral nervous system** consists of all of the nerves that connect the CNS to the rest of the body and includes the spinal nerves, the cranial nerves, and all of their branches. Peripheral nerves send sensory impulses to the brain and spinal cord and transmit motor impulses from the brain to the muscles, glands, and visceral organs. The peripheral nervous system is divided into the **autonomic nervous system** and the **somatic nervous system.** Basically, the somatic system involves those nerves connecting the CNS, the voluntary muscles, and skin; the autonomic nervous system connects the CNS to the visceral organs such as the heart, blood vessels, glands, and intestines.

Cranial Nerves

cranial nerves

twelve pairs of nerves that emerge from the brain through openings in the base of the cranium.

There are 12 pairs of **cranial nerves** that connect directly to some part of the brain surface and pass through openings called *foramina* on the sides and base of the cranium. They are classified as *motor* or *sensory* nerves and *mixed* nerves, which contain both motor and sensory fibers.

The cranial nerves are named numerically according to the order in which they arise from the brain, and by names that describe their type, function, or location (Figure 5-64 and Table 5.8).

Spinal Nerves

Thirty-one pairs of spinal nerves emerge from the spinal cord and are numbered according to the level of the vertebra where they exit the spine. All spinal nerves are mixed nerves that contain both sensory and motor nerve fibers to provide two-way communication between the CNS and the body. Each spinal nerve has an anterior and a posterior root. The anterior root contains motor neurons, and the posterior root contains sensory neurons.

Spinal nerves number

- Eight pairs of cervical nerves
- Twelve pairs of thoracic nerves
- Five pairs of lumbar nerves
- Five pairs of sacral nerves
- One pair of coccygeal nerves

cervical plexus

consists of the four upper cervical nerves that supply the skin and control the movement of the head, neck, and shoulders.

brachial plexus

is composed of four lower cervical nerves and the first pair of thoracic nerves that control arm movements.

lumbar plexus

is formed from the first four lumbar nerves.

sacral plexus

is formed from the fourth and fifth lumbar nerves, and the first four sacral nerves.

sciatic nerve

is the largest and longest nerve in the body.

The four upper cervical nerves form the **cervical plexus,** which supply the skin and control the movement of the head, neck, and shoulders.

The four lower cervical nerves and the first pair of thoracic nerves form the **brachial plexus,** which controls the movement of the arms by way of the musculocutaneous, radial, median, and ulnar nerves. The next 11 pairs of thoracic nerves supply the muscles, skin, and organs in the thorax.

The first four lumbar nerves form the **lumbar plexus,** the nerves of which supply the skin, the abdominal organs, hip, thigh, knee, and leg. The femoral and obturator nerves reach the upper parts of the leg.

Portions of the forth and fifth lumbar nerves, and the first, second, third, and fourth sacral nerves form the **sacral plexus.** The spinal nerves that form the sacral plexus divide and merge to form several collateral nerves and one main branch, the **sciatic** (sigh-**AT**-ic) **nerve.** The sciatic nerve is the largest and longest nerve in the body. The sciatic nerve consists of two nerves within the same nerve sheath: the common peroneal nerve and the tibial nerve. The sciatic nerve serves the hamstrings and the lower leg and foot.

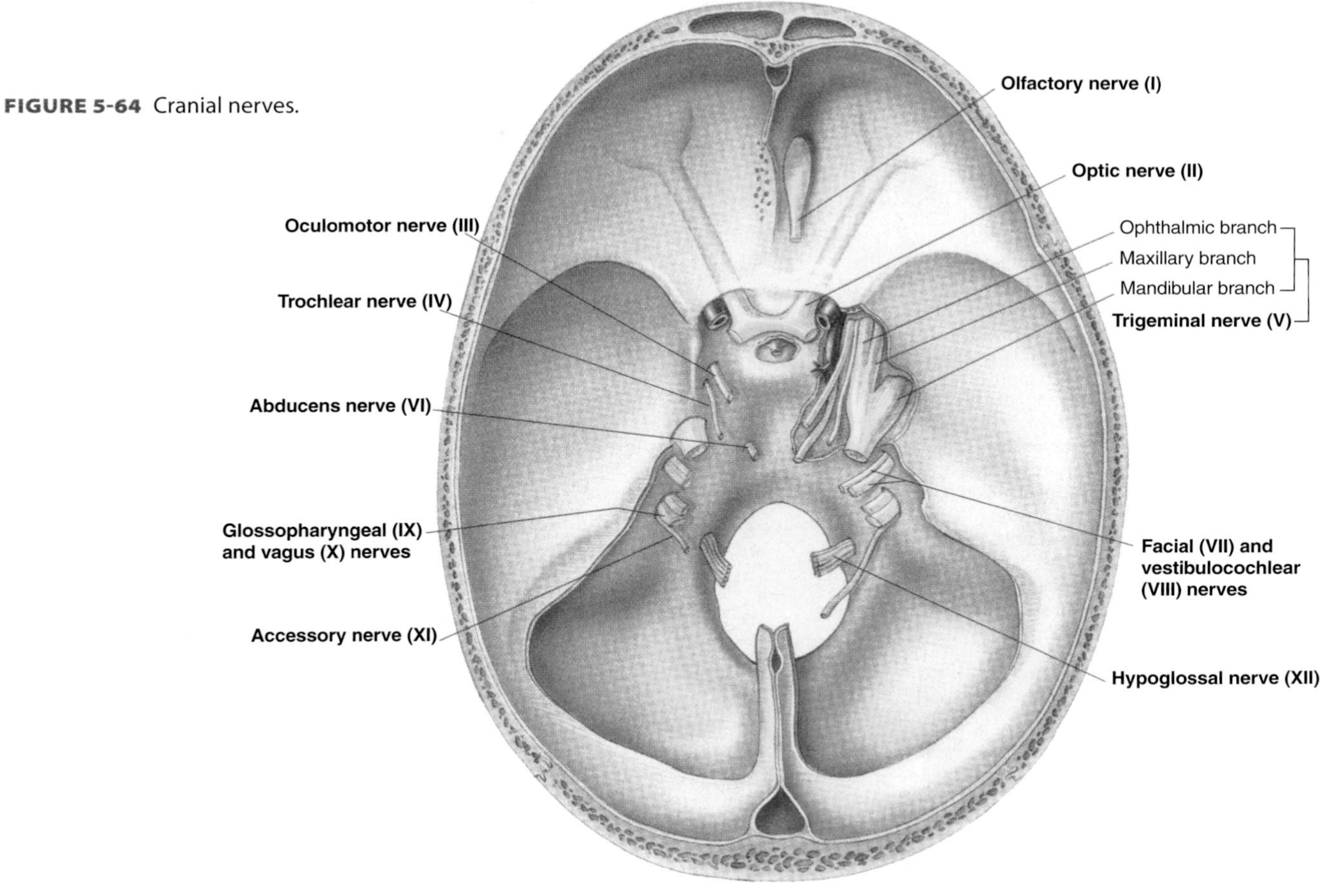

FIGURE 5-64 Cranial nerves.

TABLE 5.8

CLASSIFICATION OF CRANIAL NERVES				
	CRANIAL NERVE	TYPE OF NERVE	LOCATION	FUNCTION
i.	Olfactory nerve	Sensory nerve	Nose	Sense of smell
ii.	Optic nerve	Sensory nerve	Retina of eye	Sense of sight
iii.	Oculomotor nerve	Motor and sensory (proprioceptive) nerve	Muscles of eye	Controls eye movements
iv.	Trochlear nerve	Motor and sensory (proprioceptive) nerve	Superior oblique muscle of eye	Rotates eyeball downward and outward
v.	Trigeminal or trifacial nerve	Motor and sensory nerve	Face, teeth, and tongue	Controls sensations of the face and movements of the jaw and tongue
vi.	Abducent nerve	Motor and sensory (proprioceptive) nerve	Recti muscles of eye	Rotates eyeball outward
vii.	Facial nerve	Motor and sensory nerve	Face and neck	Controls facial muscles of expression and some muscles of the neck and ear
viii.	Acoustic or auditory nerve	Sensory nerve	Ear	Sense of hearing
ix.	Glossopharyngeal nerve	Motor and sensory nerve	Tongue and pharynx	Sense of taste
x.	Vagus or pneumogastric nerve	Motor and sensory nerve	Pharynx, larynx, heart, lungs, and digestive organs	Controls sensations and muscular movements relating to talking, heart action, breathing, and digestion
xi.	Spinal accessory nerve	Motor nerve	Shoulder	Controls movement of neck muscles
xii.	Hypoglossal nerve	Motor nerve	Tongue and neck	Controls movement of the tongue

coccygeal plexus

is formed from a portion of the fourth sacral nerves, the fifth sacral nerve, and the coccygeal nerve.

Another portion of the fourth sacral nerves, the fifth sacral nerve and the coccygeal nerve, forms the **coccygeal plexus** (kok-**SIJ**-ee-al **PLEK**-sus). The coccygeal nerves supply the skin and muscles around the coccyx (Figure 5-65 to Figures 5-66 a and b).

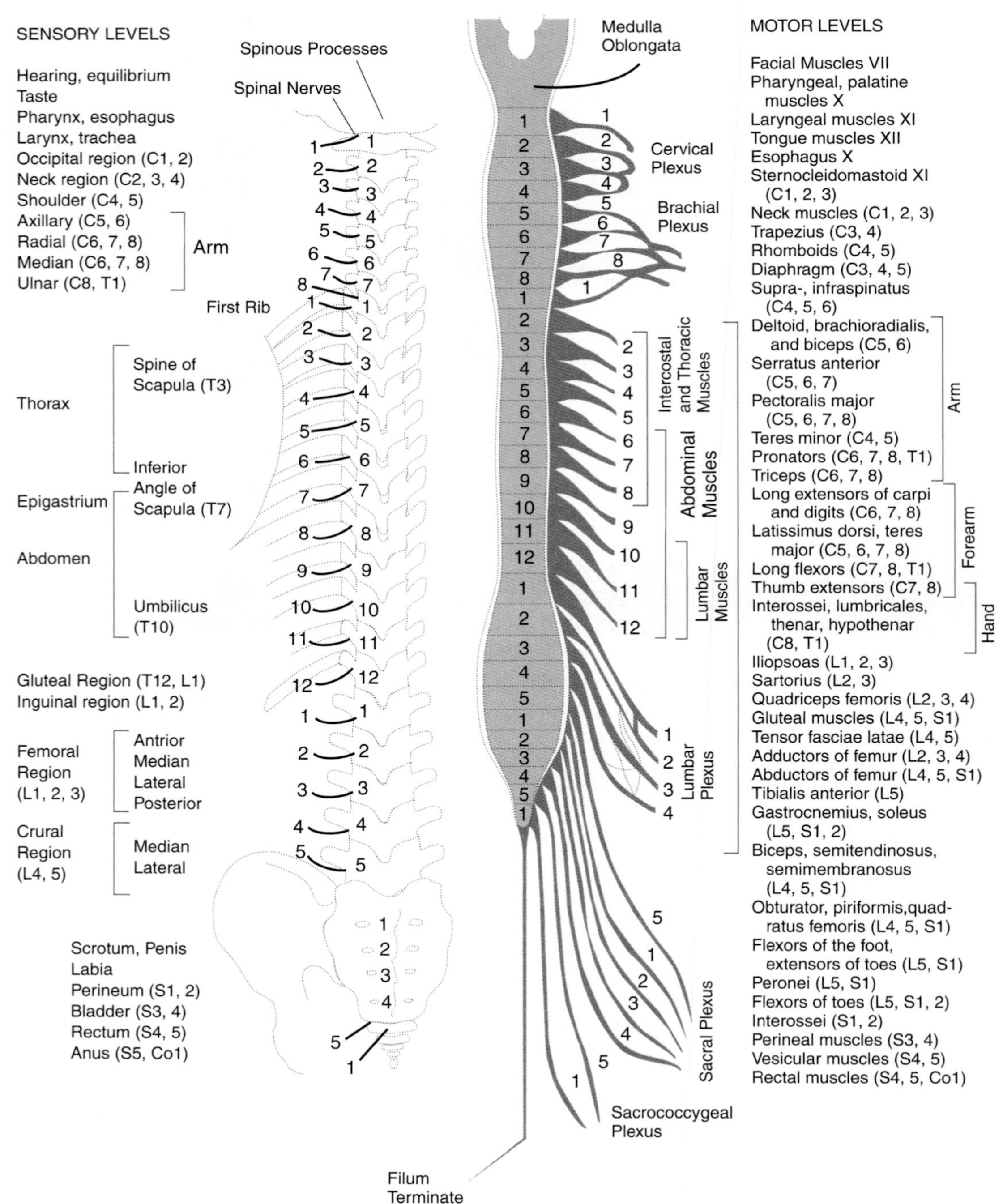

FIGURE 5-65 Spinal nerves showing plexuses, and motor and sensory functions.

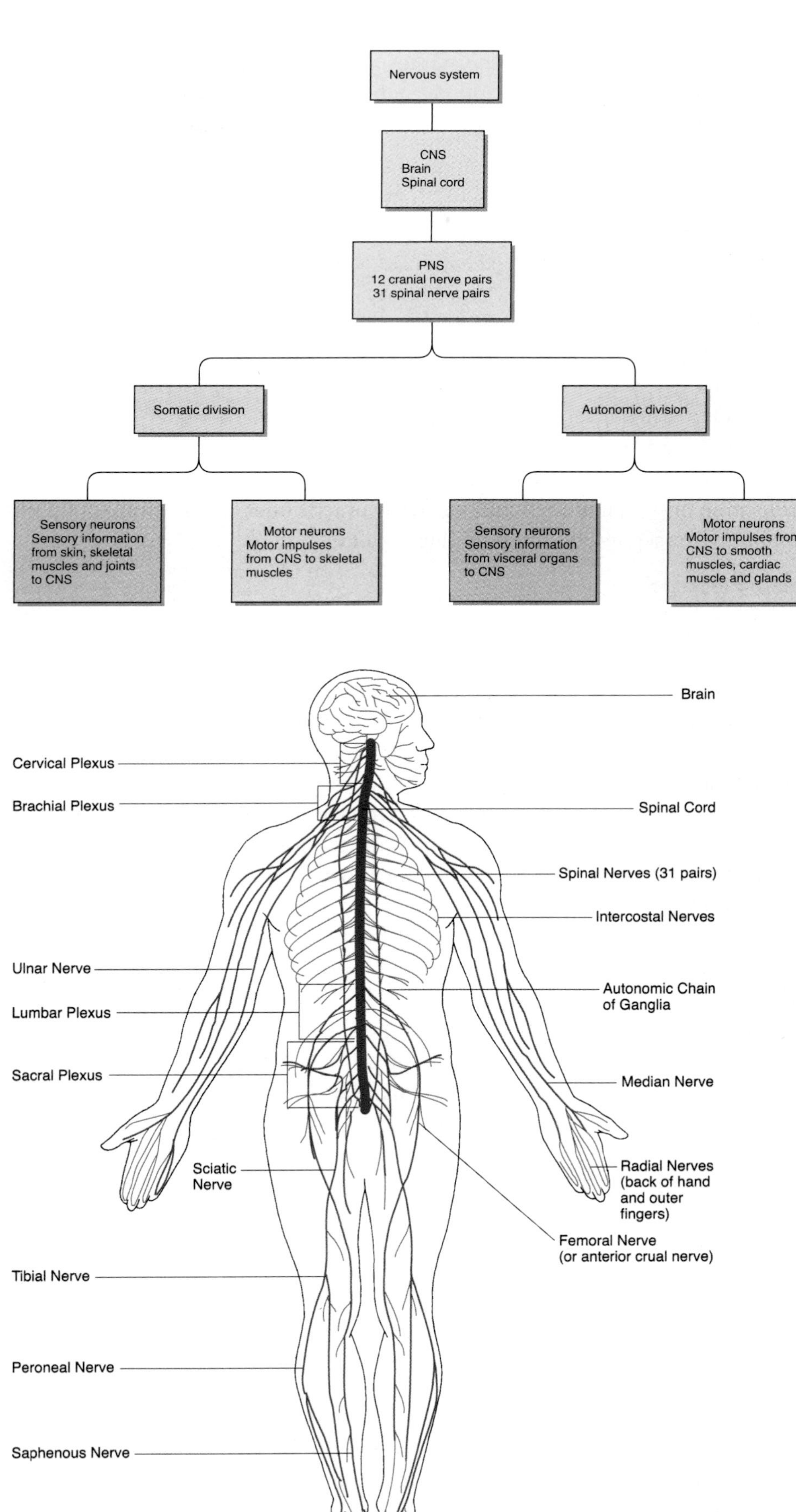

FIGURE 5-66A Divisions of the nervous system.

FIGURE 5-66B The nervous system.

dermatome

is an area of the skin supplied by nerve fibers originating from a single spinal nerve root.

Tables 5.9 to 5.15 present the names, functions, and distribution of the nerves of the neck, chest, head and face, abdomen, back, the arms and hands, and legs and feet, respectively.

Dermatomes

The entire surface of the body is innervated by the spinal nerves in a specific, segmented pattern. With the exception of C-1, every spinal nerve supplies a specific skin segment called a **dermatome.** Most of the face is innervated by the fifth cranial nerve (the trigeminal nerve). On the thorax and abdomen, the dermatomes are stacked to form consecutive bands that can overlap slightly, so that if a single nerve supply is interrupted, there is no loss of sensation. On the arms and legs, the pattern is more longitudinal. Although the dermatome pattern is similar on everyone, there are always some minor individual variations. It is helpful to be familiar with the location of dermatomes so that if there is lack of sensation or pain in a particular area, the practitioner can be aware of which spinal nerve or segment is involved (Figure 5-67).

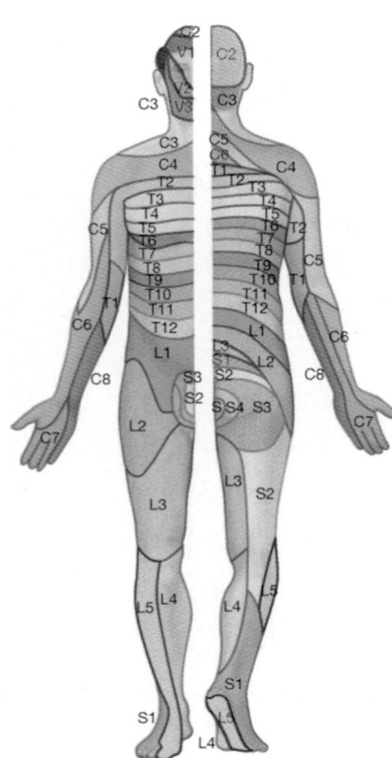

FIGURE 5-67 Dermatomes of the body.

Sensory Receptors

Sensory input from a neuron is initiated from a variety of sensory receptors. They can be categorized as mechanoreceptors, thermoreceptors, photoreceptors, chemoreceptors, and nociceptors.

Mechanoreceptors respond to mechanical stimulation or tissue distortion such as touch, pressure, vibration, and stretch. Examples of mechanoreceptors include the Ruffini end organs, Pacini corpuscles, and Merkel disks in the skin and the proprioceptors located in the muscles, fascia, and joints. The latter include the muscle spindle cells and the Golgi tendon organs.

Thermoreceptors are located in the skin and in the mouth. Two types of thermoreceptors detect heat or cold.

Two types of *photoreceptors* located in the retina of the eyes, rods, and cones are sensitive to light and detect color. They give us the ability to see color and form.

Chemoreceptors, located in the mouth and nose, are sensitive to certain chemical stimuli and give us the sense of taste and smell. Chemoreceptors in certain arteries are sensitive to carbon dioxide and pH changes in the blood and affect respiration and other involuntary functions to maintain homeostasis.

Nociceptors detect pain and are located in nearly every tissue in the body except the brain. They respond to extreme stimuli (i.e., pressure, sound, heat, and cold) and tissue damage. Nociceptors serve as a protective function by informing us that when something is wrong, it hurts. Usually pain is felt where the nociceptors are affected; however, at times pain can be referred—such as with trigger points or with visceral pain.

The Autonomic Nervous System

autonomic nervous system

regulates the action of glands, smooth muscles, and the heart.

Autonomic means self-governing. The **autonomic nervous system** regulates the action of glands, smooth muscles, and the heart. It controls the circulation of blood, the activity of the digestive tract, respiration, and body temperature. These activities are not under conscious control and are considered involuntary.

TABLE 5.9

NERVES OF THE NECK		
NAME	FUNCTION	DISTRIBUTION
Auricular, great	Sensation	Skin of neck
Colli, superficial	Sensation	Skin of neck and throat
Dental, inferior	Sensation-Motion	Mylohyoid muscle
Digastric	Motion	Stylohyoid and posterior portion of digastric muscle
Hypoglossal	Motion	Geniohyoid and omohyoid muscles
Mylohyoid	Motion	Mylohyoid and anterior part of digastric muscle
Spinal accessory	Motion	Neck muscles
Stylohyoid	Motion	Stylohyoid and posterior part of digastric muscle
Suboccipital	Motion	Muscles of back and neck
Cervical	Sensation	Skin of front of neck superficial
Occipital, greater	Sensation-Motion	Muscles of back of neck
Pneumogastric	Sensation-Motion	Larynx or voice box

TABLE 5.10

NERVES OF THE CHEST		
NAME	FUNCTION	DISTRIBUTION
Pneumogastric	Sensation-Motion	Heart and lungs
Phrenic	Motion	Diaphragm
Suprasternal	Sensation	Skin over top of breastbone
Thoracic, external	Motion	Pectoralis major anterior
Thoracic, internal	Motion	Pectoralis major and minor anterior
Thoracic, external	Motion	Serratus anterior posterior
Thoracic, spinal	Sensation-Motion	Muscles and skin of chest
Cervical (8)	Sensation-Motion	Trunk and upper extremities
Dorsal (12)	Sensation-Motion	Muscles and skin of chest and trunk

The autonomic nervous system consists of motor neurons that originate in the CNS. The autonomic nervous system is further subdivided into the *sympathetic* and *parasympathetic* nervous systems. Neurons from both systems supply the same visceral organs (except the adrenals) and are said to be complementary. The sympathetic system excites and the parasympathetic system inhibits in such a way as to maintain internal homeostasis in an ever-changing external environment.

The nerves of the **sympathetic nervous system** originate in the thoracolumbar (thoracic and lumbar portions of the spine) between T-1 and L-2 and enter a double chain of small *ganglia* (**GANG**-glee-uh; masses of neurons) that extend along the spinal column from the base of the brain to the coccyx. Within these ganglia, neurons synapse with other neurons before continuing to their target organs. These ganglia are connected with each other and with the CNS by nerve fibers. The sympathetic nervous system supplies the glands, involuntary muscles of internal organs, and walls of blood vessels with nerves.

sympathetic nervous system

supplies the glands, involuntary muscles of internal organs, and walls of blood vessels with nerves and prepares the body for energy-expending circumstances.

The activity of the sympathetic system is primarily to prepare the organism for energy-expending, stressful, or emergency situations. Stimulation of the sympathetic nerves can bring about rapid responses, such as increased respiration, dilated pupils, and increased heart rate and cardiac output.

TABLE 5.11

NERVES OF THE HEAD AND FACE		
NAME	FUNCTION	DISTRIBUTION
Auriculotemporal	Sensation	Side of scalp
Auditory	Sensory nerve of hearing	Ear
Abducent	Motion	Obliquus externus muscle of eye
Trochlear	Motion	Obliquus superior muscle of eye
Auricular, anterior	Sensation	Skin of external ear
Auricular, great	Sensation	Side of neck and ear
Auricular, posterior	Motion	Epicranius and auricularis posterior muscle
Buccal	Motion	Buccinator and orbicularis oris muscles
Dental, inferior	Sensation-Motion	Teeth of lower jaw and skin of chin
Facial	Sensation-Motion	Muscles of expression
Frontal	Sensation	Skin of forehead
Glossopharyngeal	Sensation-Motion	Muscles and mucous membranes of pharynx and back of tongue
Infraorbital	Sensation	Skin of cheek and lower eyelid
Infratrochlear	Sensation	Skin of lower eyelid and side of nose
Mandibular	Sensation-Motion	Teeth and skin of lower jaw and cheeks
Masseteric	Motion	Masseter muscle
Maxillary	Sensation	Nasal pharynx, teeth of upper jaw and skin of cheek
Mental	Sensation	Skin and mucous membrane of nose
Occipital, greater	Sensation-Motor	Skin over back part of head
Occipital, lesser	Sensation	Skin behind ear and on back of scalp
Oculomotor	Motion	Levator palpebrae superioris, recti muscles and obliquus inferior muscle of eye
Olfactory	Sensory nerve of smell	Nose
Ophthalmic	Sensation	Tear glands, eye membrane, skin of forehead and nose
Optic nerve	Sensory nerve of sight	Retina of eye
Orbital	Sensation	Skin of temple
Supraorbital	Sensation	Skin of forehead
Pterygoid, external	Motion	External pterygoid muscle
Pterygoid, internal	Motion	Internal pterygoid muscle
Trigeminal or	Sensation-Motion	Skin of face, tongue, teeth and muscles of trifacial mastication
Supratrochlear	Sensation	Skin of upper eyelid and root of nose
Pneumogastric	Sensation-Motion	Pharynx
Temporal	Motion	Temporal muscle

TABLE 5.12

NERVES OF THE ABDOMEN		
NAME	FUNCTION	DISTRIBUTION
Hypogastric	Sensation-Motion	Muscles and skin of abdominal wall
Iliohypogastric	Sensation-Motion	Muscles and skin of lower abdomen
Ilioinguinal	Sensation-Motion	Obliquus internus abdominis muscle and skin of groin
Intercostal	Sensation-Motion	Muscles and skin of upper abdomen
Lumbar (5)	Sensation-Motion	Front of lower abdomen, hip, thigh and leg
Pneumogastric	Sensation-Motion	Stomach
Thoracic, spinal	Sensation-Motion	Muscles and skin of chest
Cervical (8)	Sensation-Motion	Trunk and upper extremities
Dorsal (12)	Sensation-Motion	Muscles and skin of chest and trunk

TABLE 5.13

NERVES OF THE BACK		
NAME	FUNCTION	DISTRIBUTION
Coccygeal	Sensation-Motion	Coccygeus muscle and skin over coccyx of spine
Gluteal, inferior	Motion	Gluteus maximus muscle
Gluteal, superior	Motion	Gluteus medius muscle
Intercostal	Sensation-Motion	Muscles and skin of back
Subscapular	Motion	Latissimus dorsi muscle
Suprascapular	Motion	Supraspinatus and infraspinatus muscles
Spinal accessory	Motion	Trapezius muscle
Supra-acromial	Sensation	Skin over shoulder
Iliac	Sensation	Skin of gluteal region
Sacral (5)	Sensation-Motion	Multifidus muscles of spine and gluteal region

TABLE 5.14

NERVES OF THE ARMS AND HANDS		
NAME	FUNCTION	DISTRIBUTION
Cervical (8)	Sensation-Motion	Upper extremities
Circumflex	Sensation-Motion	Deltoid, teres minor, shoulder joint, and overlying skin
Cutaneous,	Sensation	Skin of inner part of forearm internal
Interosseous,	Motion	Deep flexor and pronator muscles of forearm anterior
Interosseous,	Sensation-Motion	Muscles and skin of back of forearm and wrist posterior
Median	Sensation-Motion	Pronator and flexor muscles of forearm, external lumbricales, and skin of fingers
Musculocutaneous	Sensation-Motion	Flexors of upper arm and skin of external part of forearm
Musculospiral	Sensation-Motion	Extensor muscles of entire arm and hand, and skin of back of forearm
Radial	Sensation	Back of hand and outer fingers
Subscapular	Motion	Teres major and subscapularis muscles
Ulnar	Sensation-Motion	Flexor carpi ulnaris and flexor digitorum profundus muscles, elbow and wrist joints, and skin of fingers

TABLE 5.15

NERVES OF THE LEGS AND FEET		
NAME	FUNCTION	DISTRIBUTION
Crural	Sensation	Skin of upper thigh
Musculocutaneous	Sensation-Motion	Peroneal muscles and skin of external part of leg lower leg and foot
Obturator	Sensation-Motion	Adductor muscles of thigh, hip, and knee joints, and skin of inner portion of thigh
Pectineal	Motion	Pectineus muscle
Popliteal, external	Sensation-Motion	Extensor muscles of lower leg and foot and Peroneal, common overlying skin
Popliteal, internal	Sensation-Motion	Flexor muscles of lower leg and foot and overlying skin
Sacral	Sensation-Motion	Muscles and skin of lower extremities
Saphenous, external	Sensation	Skin of foot and toe
Saphenous, internal	Sensation	Skin of inner part of knee, leg, ankle, and dorsum of foot
Sciatic, great	Sensation-Motion	Flexor muscles of thigh, leg, foot, and skin of calf and sole
Sciatic, small	Sensation	Skin of back of thigh
Tibial, anterior	Sensation-Motion	Extensor muscles of foot and toes and skin of dorsum of foot
Tibial, posterior	Sensation-Motion	Flexor muscles of foot and toes, and skin of sole
Cutaneous, dorsal	Sensation	Top of foot
Plantar	Sensation-Motion	Sole of foot, deep muscles of foot and toes

Blood vessels dilate, and the liver increases conversion of glycogen to glucose for more energy. There is increased mental activity and production of the adrenal hormones epinephrine and norepinephrine. All of these activities prepare the body to meet emergencies.

parasympathetic nervous system

functions to conserve energy and reverse the action of the sympathetic division.

The **parasympathetic nervous system** counteracts the action of the sympathetic system. The general function of the parasympathetic division is to conserve energy and reverse the action of the sympathetic division. The effects of parasympathetic activity are reduced heart rate, respiration, and blood pressure, and increased digestion and elimination. The parasympathetic nervous system is most active when the person is calm and in a state of relaxation.

Parasympathetic nerve fibers that serve the organs and glands of the thorax and abdomen are part of the vagus nerve. Pelvic portions of the parasympathetic system arise from the second, third, and fourth sacral spinal nerves. Parasympathetic nerve fibers associated with parts of the head are included in cranial nerves III, VII, IX, and X (Figures 5-68a and b).

Reflexes and Reflex Arcs

neurologic pathway

is the route that a nerve impulse travels through the nervous system.

A **neurologic pathway** is the route that a nerve impulse travels through the nervous system. The usual nerve path consists of a stimulus that initiates an impulse along a sensory nerve fiber to the spinal cord to communicate with an indeterminable number of interneurons (depending on how complicated or intricate the response) and finally a response impulse along motor nerves to the associated effectors, producing the resultant action.

reflex

is the simplest form of nervous activity, which includes a sensory and motor nerve.

reflex arc

is the nerve pathway of a reflex.

The simplest form of nervous activity that includes a sensory and motor nerve and few if any interneurons is called a **reflex.** The nerve pathway of a reflex is called a **reflex arc.** A simple reflex, such as a knee jerk, involves just two neurons (sensory and motor) that pass into and out of the spinal cord without influencing any other nerve centers. Another type of reflex, called the withdrawal *reflex* (*flexor reflex*), occurs when a person touches something sharp or hot and immediately pulls away, thereby preventing excessive injury. Reflexes are automatic, unconscious, involuntary responses to a stimulus and are responsible for many of the body's activities, such as sneezing, coughing, and swallowing, as well as many involuntary activities such as heart rate, breathing rate, and blood pressure. More complex reflexes affect parts of the body distant from the point of stimulation (Figure 5-69).

The areas of the body that are particularly sensitive to reflex influences are:

1. The skin of the back between the shoulders.
2. The side of the chest between the fourth and sixth ribs.
3. The skin at the upper and inner portion of the thigh.
4. The skin overlying the gluteal muscles.
5. The sole of the foot.

Proprioception

exteroceptors

record conscious sensations such as heat, cold, pain, and pressure throughout the body.

Peripheral nerves are classified as either motor nerves or sensory nerves. Sensory nerves can be further classified as exteroceptors and proprioceptors, according to their location and the sensations they record. **Exteroceptors** are located throughout the body and record conscious sensations such as heat, cold, pain,

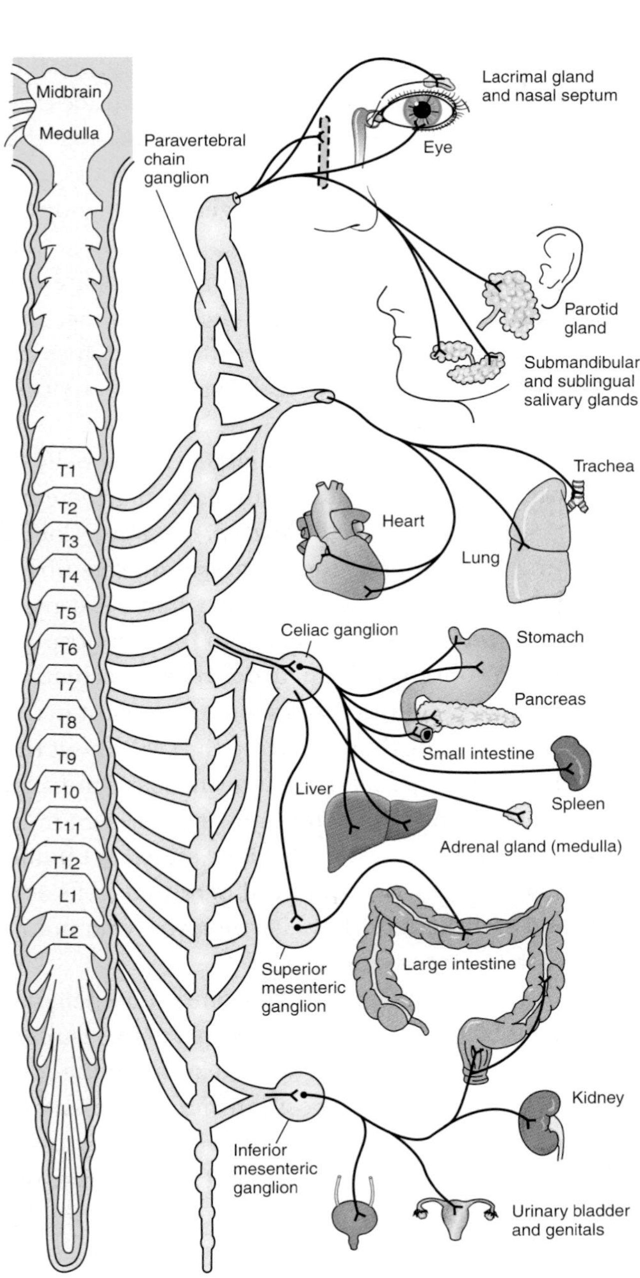

FIGURE 5-68A Nerves of the sympathetic division of the autonomic nervous system communicate through a chain of ganglia located along each side of the spine.

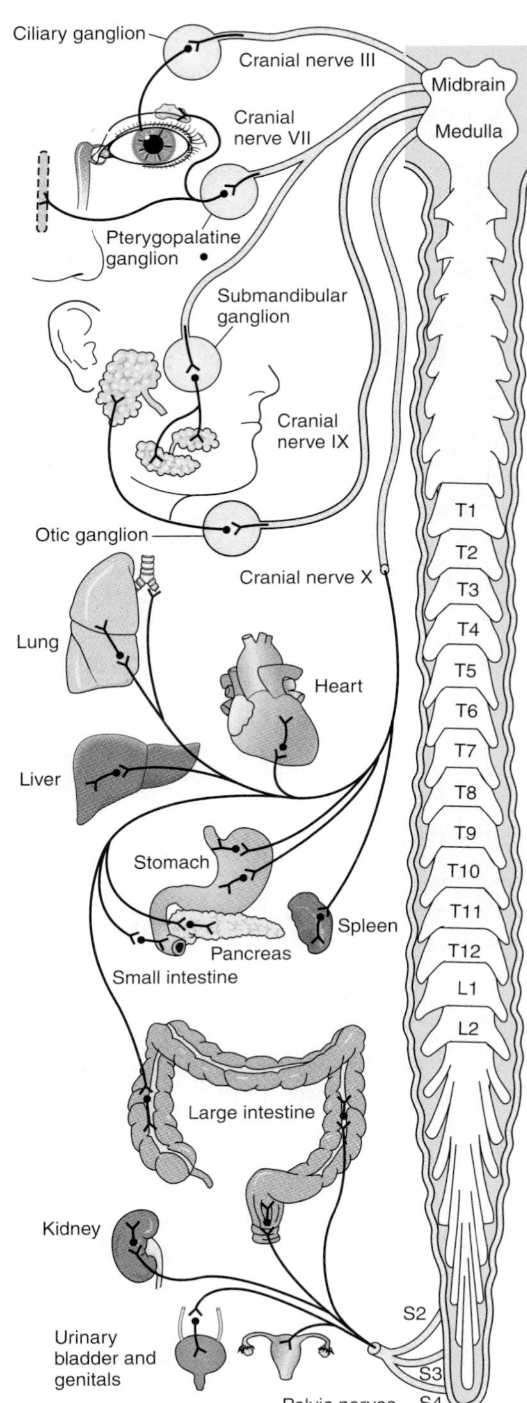

FIGURE 5-68B Nerves of the parasympathetic division of the autonomic nervous system.

and pressure. **Proprioceptors** respond to the unconscious inner sense of position and movement of the body known as *kinesthesia* (kin-es-**THEE**-zee-uh). They sense where the body is and how it moves.

proprioceptors

sense where the body is and how it moves.

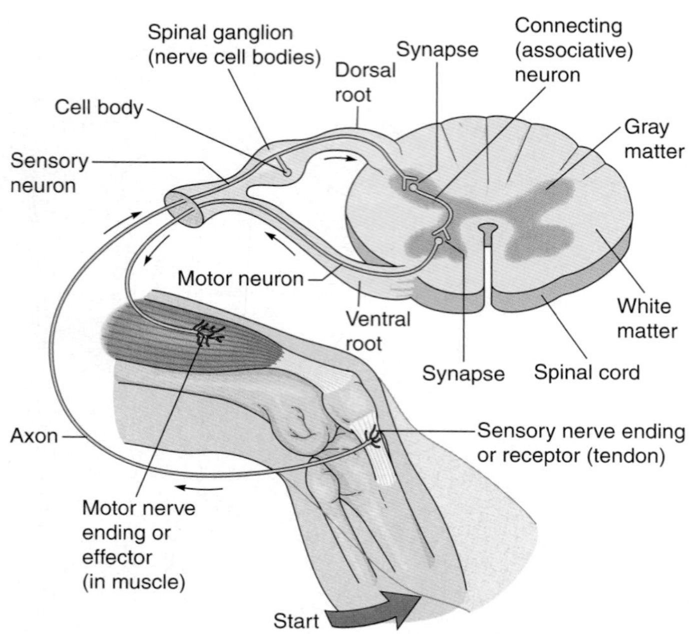

FIGURE 5-69 Simple reflex arc; knee-jerk reflex.

Proprioception is a system of sensory and motor nerve activity that provides information to the CNS about the position and rate of movement of different body parts. Proprioception also provides information about the state of contraction and position of the muscles and in so doing helps to prevent injury to the joints and muscles from excessive stretches or contractions and makes possible the coordination of smooth and accurate motion.

Proprioceptors are specialized nerve endings located in the muscle, tendons, joints, or fascia. Three major categories of proprioceptors are the **muscle spindle cells, Golgi tendon organs,** and joint proprioceptors. Their sensory input goes no farther than the brain stem, so that their activity is all unconscious.

Spindle cells are located largely in the belly of the muscle. They are made up of specialized contractile tissue called *intrafusal muscle fibers.* Coiled around the center of the intrafusal muscle fibers are the *annulospiral* or *primary receptors.* A secondary sensory nerve receptor, often referred to as a *flower-type receptor*, is located adjacent to the annulospiral receptor. These sensory nerve ends of proprioceptive neurons relay information directly to the spinal cord. These receptors continuously sense movement in the spindles and in the muscle fibers surrounding them, alerting the CNS about the length and stretch of the muscle as well as how far and fast the muscle is moving.

muscle spindle cells

sensory organs in muscle that detect the rate of stretch in muscles.

Golgi tendon organs

are multibranched sensory nerve endings located in tendons.

The *Golgi tendon organs* (GTOs) are multibranched sensory nerve endings located in the musculotendinous junction, where muscle fibers attach to tendon tissue. The GTOs measure the amount of tension produced in muscle cells as a result of the muscle's stretching and contracting. They also monitor the amount of force pulling on the bone to which the tendon attaches.

The proprioceptive receptors located in and around the joints sense angulation and pressure. The two main types of joint proprioceptors are *Pacini's corpuscles* and *Ruffini's endings.* These are mechanoreceptors located in the connective tissue or fascia surrounding the joints that sense the position and movements of the joints. When the joint moves, soft tissue on one side of the joint compresses and the soft tissue of the other side stretches. The mechanoreceptors sense the deformation and send impulses to the CNS. Based on the pattern of stimulation, the brain is able to determine the position of the body part. Other pressure-sensitive nerve endings are situated throughout all planes of connective tissue, and together these supply sensory information to the CNS to give a concise body image of soft tissue and of joint position and movement (Figure 5-70).

How Proprioceptors Work

Proprioceptors sense tissue distortion. Each time the tissue is compressed, decompressed, twisted, or distorted in a specific way, or there is a pressure on or movement in the body, these nerves record that change with the CNS. These messages feed the integrative areas of the brain with richer and more detailed

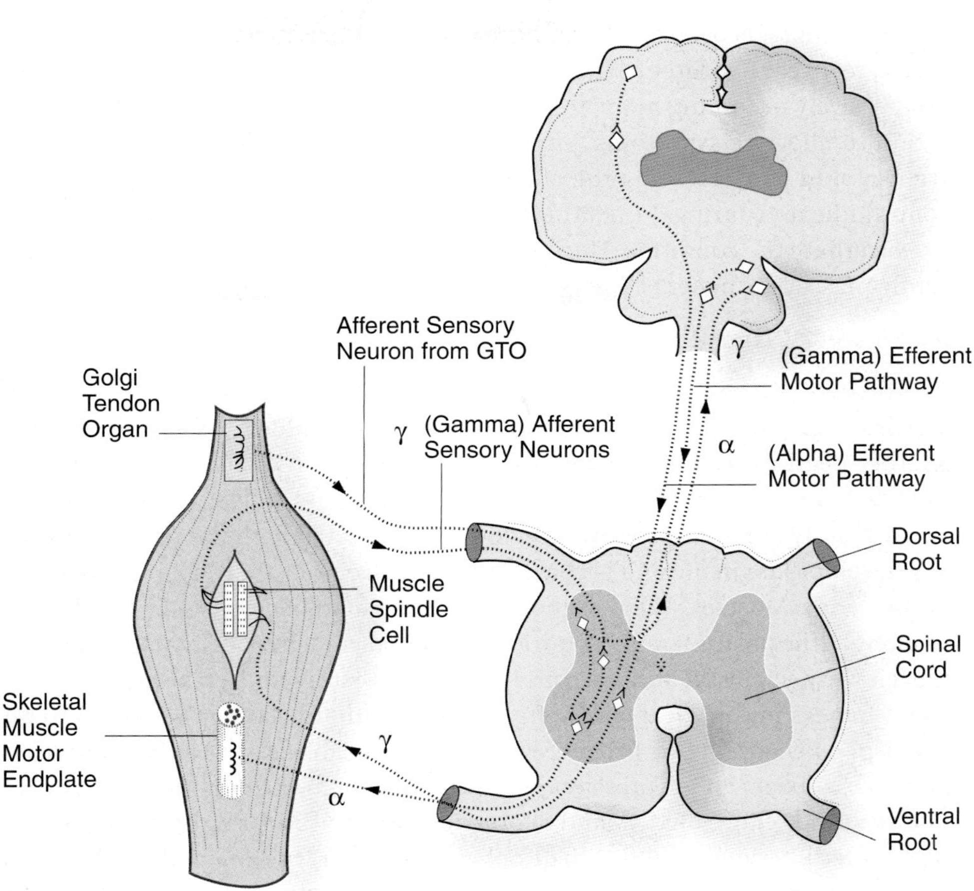

FIGURE 5–70 Proprioceptors' role in coordination of muscle movement.

information about every body part. The information is continually assembled into an overall body image that is the brain's way of knowing what the body is doing.

Neurologic Disorders

Diseases of the nervous system have many causes. They can result from birth defects, trauma, or degenerative disease. They can be caused by infection, blood clots, tumors, or hemorrhage. Some diseases manifest as abnormal muscular activity, whereas others affect functional and mental activities. Only physiologically based diseases are discussed here.

Multiple Sclerosis

Multiple sclerosis (MS) is a degenerative nerve disease that affects the body's ability to control the muscles. MS usually occurs in young adults between the ages of 20 and 50 and is the result of the breakdown of the myelin sheath that surrounds the nerves, which inhibits nerve conduction. Symptoms vary from minor to debilitating, depending on the area of the brain or spinal cord affected and the extent of damage to the myelin sheath or nerves. Symptoms include muscle weakness, spasticity, loss of coordination or balance, and loss of bladder control. Speaking becomes difficult, vision is affected, and patients can experience memory loss and difficulty concentrating. The progress of the disease varies with periods of remission and exacerbation. A person can have an

multiple sclerosis

occurs in young adults and results from the breakdown of the myelin sheath.

episode, totally recover, and never have another attack, or a person may have an attack, recover, then later have another attack, followed by another and another, progressively becoming more and more debilitated. There is no cure, but medication to alleviate symptoms, physical therapy, and psychological counseling are useful in counteracting the effects of the disease. Massage is systemically contraindicated during the acute stages, when the extra stimulation would tend to exacerbate the condition. During the subacute phase and when in remission, gentle massage is beneficial to counter stress, spasticity, and depression.

Parkinson's Disease

Parkinson's disease occurs as a result of the degeneration of certain nerve tissues that regulate body movements.

Parkinson's disease occurs as the result of the degeneration of an area of the cerebrum that produces the neurotransmitter dopamine. Without dopamine, another nearby area of the cerebrum loses the ability to balance the activity of the prime movers and their antagonists, resulting in the lack of coordination and difficulty in moving experienced by those afflicted with the disease. It usually develops late in life and is characterized by tremors and shaking, especially in the hands. Muscles stiffen as movement slows and becomes more deliberate as many of the postural reflexes are lost. A gradual and progressive rigidity of the muscles, especially the flexors, cause a stooped posture and a labored, shuffling gait. Changes in the vocal cords affect speech until it becomes little more than a whisper. Because of the progressive nature of the disease, it is usually accompanied by anxiety and depression. Massage is useful to maintain flexibility, relax muscles, and relieve anxiety and depression. The massage therapist must work under the supervision of the client's physician when working with people with Parkinson's disease.

Amyotrophic Lateral Sclerosis

Amyotrophic lateral sclerosis (ALS), also known as *Lou Gehrig's disease,* is a progressive and eventually fatal neurologic condition that causes the motor neurons of the brain and spinal cord to degenerate and die, causing weakness, spasticity, and atrophy of the voluntary muscles. It usually attacks people between the ages of 40 and 60, although there have been cases reported in people older and younger. It affects nearly twice as many men as women. Early symptoms can be weakness or twitching of a leg, arm, or hand or slurred speech, depending on which nerves are involved. As the disease progresses, more muscles throughout the body become involved, affecting the ability to move, speak, swallow, and even breathe. There is no known cure for ALS. Fifty percent of those diagnosed die within 3 to 5 years, and 90 percent succumb within 10 years, usually from complications of paralysis or the loss of respiratory function. ALS attacks only the motor neurons and does not affect the intelligence, memory, or personality, or the ability to taste, smell, and hear or the sense of touch. In the earlier stages of the disease, massage can be helpful to relieve spasticity and stress. Because ALS is not contagious, does not spread through the blood and lymph, or affect the sensory nerves, massage is not contraindicated and can provide a great amount of comfort and relief. As the disease progresses, massage should be given under the physician's supervision and in coordination with the health care team.

Spinal Cord Injury

A *spinal cord injury* (SCI) is caused by trauma or disease to the vertebral column or to the spinal cord itself. Most injuries are caused by trauma to the vertebral column that results in pinching, bruising, or tearing of the spinal cord. The injury affects the ability of the nerve fibers in the cord to transmit impulses to and from the brain and results in loss of sensation and movement of the parts of the body that are controlled by the spinal nerves that exit the spinal cord below the site of the injury. Each spinal cord injury is different according to the level of the injury and the extent of damage to the spinal cord. Injury of the cervical spine (C-1 through T-1) results in *tetraplegia* or **quadriplegia,** affecting the neck, shoulders, arms, hands, and legs. If the injury is between T-2 and S-5, and only the mid-to-lower chest, stomach, legs, and feet are affected, the condition is called **paraplegia.** The higher the level of injury, the more sensory and motor deprivation occurs. An SCI is a *complete injury* when there is no motor or sensory function below the injury level and *incomplete* when not all the spinal nerve fibers are affected and there is still some sensory and motor function below the injury site.

quadriplegia

is paralysis of the arms and legs caused by a stroke or spinal cord injury.

paraplegia

paralysis of the lower extremities; does not affect the arms or hands.

Massage can be very beneficial for people with an SCI, but it requires some special consideration. Massage applied above the injury level, where there is normal sensation and mobility, is similar to massage on an able-bodied person and is helpful in addressing compensation patterns that accompany living in a wheelchair. Below the injury level, there is no or impaired sensation, and muscle tissue is atrophied, spastic, or brittle. The feet and ankles can be edematous because of lack of movement. Massage directed toward the muscles is generally contraindicated. Light massage or **skin brushing** can help to reduce edema and improve the quality of the skin. If done regularly, gentle range of motion can help to maintain flexibility, prevent contractures, and reduce spasms. Because of mobility impairments, special care must be taken when transferring a client with an SCI to and from the massage table. Clear communication can help to determine how much assistance is needed and how to provide it. (See Chapter 19, *Massage for Special Populations* for more information)

skin brushing

a light, brisk brushing using a dry vegetable bristle bath brush.

Stroke (CVA)

Stroke or **cerebrovascular accident** (CVA) is the result of a blood clot or ruptured blood vessel in or around the brain and the subsequent destruction of nerve tissue. It is the third leading cause of death in the United States after cancer and heart disease and is the leading cause of adult-onset disability. The effect of the stroke depends on the location and extent of damaged tissue. There can be loss of vision in one or both eyes, loss of the ability to speak or understand language, loss of memory, or personality changes. Often, a stroke causes paralysis on one side of the body, opposite the side of the brain in which the damage occurred. The extent of the paralysis is relative to the extent of the neurologic damage. The condition of unilateral paralysis caused by a stroke is called **hemiplegia.** Massage can be a beneficial part of stroke rehabilitation when given under medical supervision and with consideration of related cardiovascular precautions. Because hemiplegia can involve sensory deprivation and muscle paralysis, deep massage directed toward the muscles is contraindicated.

cerebrovascular accident

or stroke, is caused by a blood clot or ruptured blood vessel in or around the brain that subsequently destroys nerve tissue.

hemiplegia

is unilateral paralysis caused by a stroke.

epilepsy

is a neurologic condition in which there is an abnormal electrical activity in the CNS without apparent tissue abnormalities.

Epilepsy

Epilepsy is a neurologic condition in which there is abnormal electrical activity in the CNS without apparent tissue abnormalities. Epilepsy is characterized by seizures, some of which are so mild that they are barely noticeable, whereas others can be so extreme that the person loses consciousness and is thrown into uncontrollable convulsions. People with epilepsy generally can live normal, productive lives with the use of appropriate medication. Massage is inappropriate during a seizure; however, massage is indicated for a person with a history of a seizure disorder.

Viral or Bacterial Infections

Many diseases that affect the nervous system are the result of an invading virus or bacteria. Causes of such infections can vary from contaminated wounds and bites from animals or insects to infections elsewhere in the body. Viral infections include poliomyelitis, encephalitis, and shingles.

Polio

Poliomyelitis (po-lee-o-my-e-**LIE**-tis), or *polio,* is a crippling or even deadly disease that affects the motor neurons of the medulla oblongata and spinal cord, resulting in paralysis of the related muscle tissues. Symptoms of polio include fever, gastrointestinal discomfort, stiff neck, and headache. If detected early, its devastating effects can be minimized. The development of the Salk and Sabin vaccines has nearly eradicated this terrible disease. Post-polio syndrome occurs in polio victims years or even decades after the initial infection and causes degenerative muscle weakness and fatigue. Massage is beneficial in both polio and post-polio syndrome as part of a physician-directed treatment.

Encephalitis

Encephalitis (en-sef-a-**LIE**-tis) refers to several related viral diseases that cause an inflammation of the brain or the meninges. The infection is sometimes spread by a carrier such as an animal or bird, by a mosquito bite, or it can arise as a secondary infection from measles, mumps, or chickenpox. Symptoms include headache, fever, disoriented behavior, and often seizures. Serious cases can result in nerve or brain damage and can result in paralysis, emotional disturbances, or even death.

Meningitis

Meningitis (men-in-**JIGH**-tis) is an acute inflammation of the pia and arachnoid mater around the brain and spinal cord. This is often a secondary infection from bacteria traveling from the middle ear, upper respiratory tract, lungs, or sinuses, or it can be from polio or mumps viruses. Symptoms include severe headache, stiff neck, high fever, chills, delirium, and often convulsions or even coma. Antibiotic treatment is usually effective. If untreated, permanent brain damage usually results, with possible blindness, deafness, retardation, or paralysis.

Diagnosis of encephalitis and meningitis is made with a spinal tap or lumbar puncture, in which a hollow needle is inserted into the spinal canal in the lumbar area to determine the constituents and pressure of the cerebrospinal fluid. Massage is systemically contraindicated during the active stage of encephalitis or meningitis. For a client with a history of either who has no current symptoms, massage is quite appropriate, however.

Shingles

Shingles is an acute inflammation of a nerve trunk and the dendrites at the end of the sensory neurons by the herpes zoster virus. The symptoms include a band of pain around the torso and a rash with water blisters that erupt in a confined area on one side of the body. Seldom does the rash cross the midline of the body. Shingles can develop from an exposure to herpes or chickenpox viruses, a reaction to a medication, or trauma. Massage is contraindicated because of the risk of infection and because it would be very painful. Immediate medical attention is recommended.

Neuritis

Neuritis literally means inflammation of a nerve. Neuritis is not a disease but a symptom of some other condition such as a herniated disk, herpes zoster, or diabetes mellitus. Neuritis affects the nerves of the peripheral nervous system. Because most peripheral nerves are both sensory and motor, neuritis can cause weakness or paralysis and can be painful. The pain associated with neuritis is called *neuralgia*. Generalized neuritis affecting several nerves (polyneuritis) can be due to nutritional deficiency, alcoholism, chemical poisoning, allergies, and viral or bacterial infections. Usually the symptoms of neuritis subside when the cause is resolved. Rest, a diet rich in B vitamins, and therapy such as massage are helpful. The appropriateness of massage depends on the cause of the neuritis and should be decided on a case-by-case basis. Local massage is contraindicated in the area of the inflamed nerve.

Sometimes neuritis affects a specific nerve (mononeuritis). Pain or partial paralysis along the course of the affected nerve could be the result of disease or pressure on or injury to the nerve. A common form of neuritis is the result of injury or pressure on the sciatic nerve called *sciatica*. The sciatic nerve is exposed to many sites of possible irritation as it exits the spine and courses through the pelvis and down the leg. Depending on the severity, sciatica results in burning pain or paresthesia (pins and needles) through one buttock and down the back of the leg and into the foot that can be accompanied by muscle weakness or paralysis. Skilled massage is very effective to relieve sciatica if it is caused by soft tissue conditions of the muscles or ligaments. MHowever, if the sciatica is caused by a herniated disk, spondylosis (bone spurs on the vertebrae), or other conditions within the spine, massage is contraindicated A diagnosis and clearance from a physician before proceeding are essential.

A *pinched nerve* can refer to any of a wide variety of conditions in which pressure on a nerve is responsible for pain, numbness, or a reduction of function in the tissues supplied by the nerve. The pinched nerve could be a result of *nerve compression* or *nerve entrapment.*

Nerve compression or impingement is due to bone or cartilage pressing against the nerve such as a herniated vertebral disk pressing against a spinal nerve. Symptoms include sharp pain at the site of the lesion, radiating pain along the course of the nerve, tingling, numbness, or weakening of the affected muscle.

Nerve entrapment is caused by soft tissue such as muscle, fascia, tendon, or ligament putting pressure against a nerve. The nerve can be trapped within constricted soft tissue as a result of overuse or injury, or constricted soft tissue could be pressing the nerve against bone, as in thoracic outlet syndrome. Symptoms of nerve entrapment vary according to nerve involvement and severity, from mild to intense local or radiating pain, numbness, burning, or weakness in the affected muscles. Massage is indicated to relieve the constricted soft tissues responsible for the entrapment.

Thoracic Outlet Syndrome

Thoracic outlet syndrome (TOS) is caused by a compression or entrapment of the brachial nerve plexus and/or blood vessels going to or from the arm that results in pain, paresthesia, numbness, and/or weakness in the shoulder, neck, and arm. The brachial plexus originates as the spinal nerves C-5 to T-1. The nerves travel through the spinal foramen, between the anterior and medial scalene muscles, between the clavicle and first rib, under the pectoralis muscle near its attachment to the coracoid process, and down the arm. The axillary artery and the subclavian vein lie parallel to the nerve between the clavicle and first rib, under the pectoralis muscle and through the axilla. Compression along the course of the nerve or blood vessels causes symptoms in the arm or along the course of the nerve. Occasionally, the cervical nerve is impinged by a spinal misalignment, bulging disk, or bone spur on the vertebra. Hypertonicity of the scalene muscles can compress the brachial nerves, whereas tension in the pectoralis minor muscle can compress the nerves and blood vessels against the first rib, causing TOS symptoms down the arm. TOS caused by muscular involvement can be effectively relieved with massage. If the TOS is from bone spurs, a herniated disk, or pressure from a cervical rib, massage can offer little or no relief, however.

Carpal Tunnel Syndrome

Carpal tunnel syndrome (CTS) is the result of compression of the median nerve as it passes through the anatomic tunnel of the wrist, causing pain and weakness in the thumb and/or first three fingers. There are different conditions that cause CTS. A common cause is the same activity of the hand and wrist repeated hour after hour, day after day (*repetitive stress injury*) such as meat cutting, typing, or cashiering, activities that result in hypertrophy of the tendons passing through the carpal area or fibrosis of the connective tissues. This causes pressure on or irritation to the median nerve. Fluid retention and edema can also cause pressure on the nerves in the wrist, causing CTS. Other conditions can mimic CTS, such as herniated disks, TOS, or shoulder and wrist injuries. It is important to have a definitive diagnosis before providing massage to a client with CTS symptoms. Edematous CTS responds well to gentle massage to drain the excess fluids from the arm. CTS due to fibrotic buildup or hypertrophy might not respond to massage. Always work conservatively. If massage around the wrist exacerbates the symptoms, stop immediately! If the client experiences relief and improvement, proceed slowly and cautiously.

SECTION QUESTIONS FOR DISCUSSION AND REVIEW

1. What is the primary function of the nervous system?
2. Name the main parts of the nervous system.
3. Name and describe the general structure of a nerve cell.
4. Which abilities do neurons have that enable them to transmit nerve impulses?
5. What is a synapse?
6. Describe three types of neurons.
7. Describe the structure of a nerve.
8. What is an efferent nerve?
9. What is an afferent nerve?
10. What is a mixed nerve?
11. What are the two divisions of the nervous system?
12. What is the CNS and where is it located?
13. Define *meninges* and name its layers.
14. What is cerebrospinal fluid and what is its function?
15. What are the main parts of the brain?
16. Where is the peripheral system located?
17. What are the divisions of the peripheral nervous system?
18. How many pairs of cranial nerves branch out from the brain?
19. Identify the cranial nerves by name and number.
20. How many pairs of spinal nerves branch out from the spinal cord?
21. Describe how the spinal nerves are numbered.
22. What is a nerve plexus?
23. Name the important spinal nerve plexuses and the body areas that they supply.
24. What is the function of the autonomic nervous system?
25. Name and contrast the two divisions of the autonomic nervous system.
26. Which organs are supplied by the sympathetic nervous system?
27. What is a reflex action?
28. What is proprioception?
29. Name two categories of proprioceptors, including where they are located and the information that they record.

REVIEW

Nerves of the Head and Face

Matching Test I

Insert the letter of the proper term in front of each definition.

______	1.	sense of hearing	a.	facial nerve
______	2.	sense of smell	b.	trifacial nerve
______	3.	sense of sight	c.	auditory nerve
______	4.	supplies skin of face	d.	olfactory nerve
______	5.	supplies muscles of expression	e.	optic nerve

True or False Test I

Carefully read each statement and indicate whether it is true or false; draw a circle around the letter T or F.

1. T F The great auricular nerve supplies the epicranius muscle.
2. T F The frontal and supraorbital nerves supply the skin of the forehead.
3. T F The abducent nerve supplies the obliquus superior muscle of the eye.
4. T F The trigeminal nerve supplies the muscles of mastication.
5. T F The auriculotemporal nerve supplies the side of the scalp.

Nerves of the Neck and Chest

Matching Test II

Insert the letter of the proper term in front of each definition.

______	1. supplies neck muscles		a.	greater occipital nerve
______	2. supplies front of neck		b.	phrenic nerve
______	3. supplies back of neck		c.	pneumogastric nerve
______	4. supplies heart and lungs		d.	superficial cervical nerve
______	5. supplies diaphragm		e.	spinal accessory nerve

True or False Test II

Carefully read each statement and decide whether it is true or false; draw a circle around the letter T or F.

1. T F The cervical nerves supply the trunk and the lower extremities.
2. T F The suboccipital nerve supplies the back of the neck.
3. T F The dorsal and spinal thoracic nerves supply the muscles and skin of the chest.
4. T F The pneumogastric nerve supplies the heart and lungs but not the larynx.
5. T F Branches of the thoracic nerve supply the pectoralis major, pectoralis minor, and serratus anterior muscles.

Nerves of the Abdomen and Back

Matching Test III

Insert the letter of the proper term in front of each definition.

______	1. supplies lower abdomen		a.	supra-acromial nerve
______	2. supplies upper abdomen		b.	iliohypogastric nerve
______	3. supplies shoulders		c.	pneumogastric nerve
______	4. supplies stomach		d.	spinal accessory nerve
______	5. supplies trapezius muscle		e.	intercostal nerve

True or False Test III

Carefully read each statement and decide whether it is true or false; draw a circle around the letter T or F.

1. T F The sacral, coccygeal, and suprascapular nerves supply various muscles of the spine.
2. T F The subscapular and suprascapular nerves supply the same muscles of the back.
3. T F The lumbar nerves supply the upper part of the abdomen.
4. T F The superior gluteal nerve supplies the gluteus medius muscle.
5. T F The subscapular nerve supplies the latissimus dorsi muscle of the back.

Nerves of the Arms and Hands

Matching Test IV

Insert the letter of the proper term in front of each definition.

______	1.	supplies elbow joint	a.	median nerve
______	2.	supplies shoulder joint	b.	ulnar nerve
______	3.	supplies skin of back of arm	c.	circumflex nerve
______	4.	supplies deltoid muscle	d.	radial nerve
______	5.	supplies muscles of forearm	e.	subscapular nerve

True or False Test IV

Carefully read each statement and decide whether it is true or false; draw a circle around the letter T or F.

1. T F The subscapular nerve supplies the teres minor muscle.
2. T F The cervical nerves supply the upper extremities.
3. T F The musculospiral nerve supplies the extensor muscles of the entire arm and hand.
4. T F The musculocutaneous nerve supplies the pronator muscles of the upper arm.
5. T F The ulnar nerve supplies the skin of the fingers.

Nerves of the Legs and Feet

Matching Test V

Insert the letter of the proper term in front of each definition.

______	1.	supplies soles of foot	a.	small sciatic nerve
______	2.	supplies upper thigh	b.	obturator nerve
______	3.	supplies inner portion of thigh	c.	crural nerve
______	4.	supplies back of thigh	d.	external saphenous nerve
______	5.	supplies foot and toe	e.	plantar nerve

True or False Test V

Carefully read each statement and decide whether it is true or false; draw a circle around the letter T or F.

1. T F The obturator nerve supplies the hip and knee joints.
2. T F The internal popliteal nerve supplies the extensor muscles of the lower leg and foot.
3. T F The sacral nerve supplies the muscles and skin of the lower extremities.
4. T F The anterior tibial nerve supplies the flexor muscles of the foot and toes.
5. T F The dorsal cutaneous nerve supplies the top of the foot.

SYSTEM 6 THE ENDOCRINE SYSTEM

The endocrine system comprises a group of specialized glands that affect the growth, development, sexual activity, and health of the entire body, depending on the quality and quantity of their secretions.

The major function of the endocrine system is to assist the nervous system in regulating body processes.

Glands of the Body

exocrine

or duct glands possess tubes or ducts leading from the gland to a particular part of the body.

endocrine

or ductless glands depend on the blood and lymph to carry their secretions to various affected tissues.

Glands are specialized organs that vary in size and function. The circulatory and nervous systems closely interact with the glands. The glands act as chemical factories, with the ability to remove certain constituents from the blood to produce specialized secretions. There are two main classifications of glands. **Exocrine** (**EK**-sow-krin) or *duct glands* possess tubes or **ducts** leading from the gland to a particular part of the body, such as the sweat glands. Various skin and intestinal glands belong to this group. The other group, known as *ductless* or **endocrine glands,** depend on the blood and lymph to carry their secretions to various affected tissues.

The chemical substances manufactured by the endocrine glands are known as *hormones*. Hormones, sometimes referred to as the body's chemical messengers, are specialized so that they act on specific tissues (target organs) or influence certain processes in the body. Some hormones stimulate other endocrine or exocrine glands. Some have a profound effect on physical or sexual development. Others regulate metabolism or body chemistry (see Table 5.16 on glands and their associated hormones.) The endocrine glands operate cooperatively with one another and the nervous system to maintain a state of homeostasis within the organism. Some of the endocrine glands exert a regulatory influence over the other glands. The effect of their hormones can either stimulate or restrain the activity of another gland. Under- or overfunctioning of any ductless gland upsets the delicate balance of the entire chain of endocrine glands.

Among the important endocrine glands are the pituitary, thyroid, parathyroid, adrenal, and sex glands (gonads), and the pancreas. Other organs that have hormone-producing tissue include the pineal gland, the hypothalamus, the kidneys, the placenta, and intestinal mucosa.

TABLE 15-16

ENDOCRINE GLANDS AND THEIR HORMONES

GLAND	HORMONE	PRINCIPAL FUNCTIONS
Anterior pituitary	ACTH (adrenocorticotropin)	Stimulates adrenal cortex to produce cortical hormones; aids in protecting body in stress situations (e.g., injury, pain)
	TSH (thyroid-stimulating hormone)	Stimulates the thyroid to produce thyroxin
	FSH (follicle-stimulating hormone)	Stimulates growth and hormone activity of ovarian follicles; stimulates growth of testes; promotes development of sperm
	HGH (human growth hormone)	Promotes growth of all body tissues
	LH (Luteinizing hormone)	Causes development of corpus luteum at site of ruptured ovarian follicle in women; stimulates secretion of testosterone in men
	Lactogenic hormone (prolactin)	Stimulates secretion of milk by mammary glands
Posterior pituitary	ADH (antidiuretic hormone; vasopressin)	Promotes reabsorption of water in kidney tubules; stimulates smooth muscle tissue of blood vessels
	Oxytocin	Causes contraction of muscle of pregnant uterus; causes ejection of milk from mammary glands
Pineal	Melatonin	Melatonin's function in humans is unclear but seems to be related to regulation of the 24-hour circadian rhythm.
Thymus	Thymosin	Important in the development of T-lymphocytes, a major part of the immune system
Adrenal cortex	Cortisol (95% of glucocorticoids)	Aids in metabolism of carbohydrates, proteins, and fats; active during stress
	Aldosterone (95% of mineralocorticoids)	Aids in regulating electrolytes
	Sex hormones	Can influence secondary sexual characteristics in male subjects
Adrenal medulla	Epinephrine and norepinephrine	Increase blood pressure and heart rate; activate cells influenced by the sympathetic nervous system plus many not affected by sympathetics
Pancreatic islets	Insulin	Aids transport of glucose into cells; required for cellular metabolism of foods, especially glucose; decreases blood sugar levels
	Glucagon	Stimulates the liver to release glucose, thereby increasing blood sugar levels
Parathyroids	Parathormone	Regulates exchange of calcium between blood and bones; increases calcium level in blood
Thyroid gland	Thyroid hormones (thyroxine and triiodothyronine [T3])	Increase metabolic rate, influencing both physical and mental activities; required for normal growth
	Calcitonin	Decreases calcium level in blood
Ovarian follicle	Estrogens (e.g., estradiol, estriol, estrone)	Stimulate growth of primary sexual organs (i.e., uterus, tubes) and development of secondary sexual organs such as breasts; also involved in various aspects of the menstrual cycle.
Corpus luteum (in ovaries)	Progesterone	Stimulates development of secretory parts of mammary glands; prepares uterine lining for implantation of fertilized ovum; aids in maintaining pregnancy
Testes	Testosterone	Stimulates growth and development of sexual organs (i.e., testes, penis, others) plus development of secondary sexual characteristics such as hair growth on body and face and deepening of voice; stimulates maturation of sperm cells
Placenta	Chorionic gonadotropn	Stimulates the ovaries to release progesterone during early pregnancy
	Estrogen and progesterone	Helps to keep the uterus receptive to the fetus and placenta during pregnancy

The hypothalamus is part of the brain positioned at the inferior portion of the diencephalon that plays a major role in controlling the secretions of the pituitary gland. The hypothalamus, situated just superior to the pituitary and connected by a series of minute capillaries, produces neural and chemical signals by releasing *hormones* or *inhibitory hormones* that either stimulate or inhibit the release of particular hormones by the pituitary gland. Likewise, the hypothalamus is influenced by the presence of hormones from the endocrine system that are in the bloodstream. Much of the relationship between the nervous and endocrine system is maintained or controlled within the hypothalamus and the pituitary gland.

hyperactive glands

oversecrete hormones owing to lack of regulation or glandular tumors.

pituitary gland

is a small gland, often called the master gland, because the hormones it secretes stimulate or regulate other glands.

Most diseases or dysfunctions of the endocrine system are the result of overactivity or underactivity of one or more glands. Overactive or **hyperactive glands** oversecrete hormones because of lack of regulation or glandular tumors. Underactive or hypoactive glands secrete insufficient amounts of their hormones. Hypoactive glands can be diseased or underdeveloped; injured by trauma, surgery, or radiation; or not receiving proper stimulation and regulation. Individual glands are discussed as to their primary function and some effects of hyper- or hypoactivity (Figure 5-71).

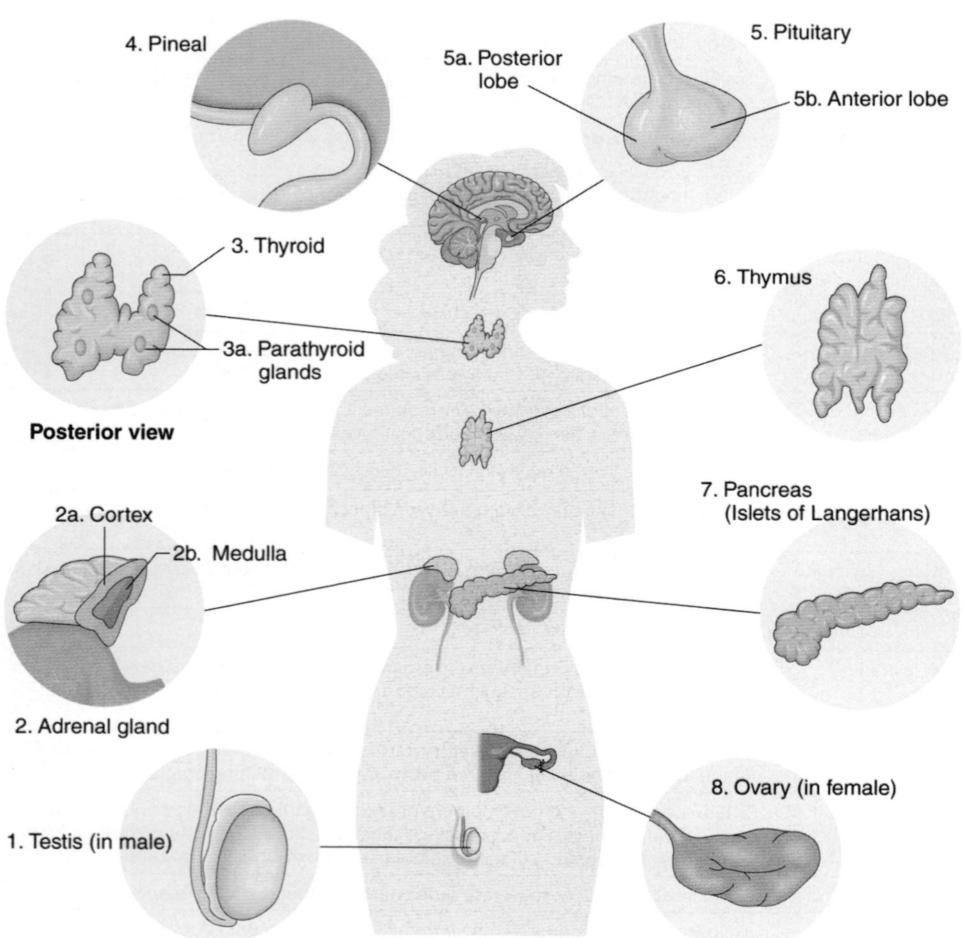

FIGURE 5–71 The endocrine system.

The Pituitary Gland

The pituitary gland is a small gland about the size of a cherry that produces several hormones that regulate many body processes. The pituitary gland is located in a depression on the sphenoid bone called the *stella turcica* just behind the point where the optic nerves cross. The **pituitary gland** is often called the *master gland* because many of the hormones it secretes stimulate or regulate other endocrine glands. The pituitary gland is regulated by impulses and secretions from the hypothalamus. It has an anterior and posterior lobe, each of which secretes different hormones.

The anterior lobe of the pituitary produces and secretes the following:

- *Somatotropic or growth hormone.* This hormone stimulates the growth of bones, muscles, and organs. A deficiency of this hormone inhibits mental and physical growth.
- *Thyroid-stimulating hormone (TSH).* This hormone regulates the thyroid gland.
- *Adrenocorticotropic hormone (ACTH)* stimulates the adrenal cortex.
- *Gonadotropic hormones* regulate the development and function of the reproductive systems in women and men.
- *Prolactin* stimulates the production of milk in a woman's breast.

The posterior lobe of the pituitary stores and secretes the following:

- *Antidiuretic hormone* stimulates the kidneys to reabsorb more water, thereby reducing urine output.
- *Oxytocin* causes the uterus to contract (during and after childbirth) and causes the letdown of breast milk.

Hyperpituitarism (high-per-pi-**TOO**-i-tar-izm) is most notably observed as the production of excessive amounts of growth hormone. If the hypersecretion occurs before puberty, the activity in the growth plates of the bones is accelerated and produces a giant, a condition known as *giantism.* If the hyperpituitarism occurs after puberty, when a person has reached full height, the effects are different. The bones of the hands, feet, face, and spine enlarge in a condition called *acromegaly* (ak-row-**MEG**-a-lee). There is excessive growth in some soft tissues as the lips and nose enlarge and the lower jaw protrudes. Hyperactivity of the pituitary is usually caused by a tumor.

Hypopituitarism can result from inadequate stimulation from the hypothalamus or from destruction of the pituitary gland. Because the secretions of the pituitary gland act to stimulate other endocrine glands, deficient pituitary secretions inhibit the actions of the target glands. This can affect a wide variety of bodily functions such as blood pressure, reproduction, growth, or failure to thrive, depending on which hormones are deficient.

The Thyroid Gland

The thyroid gland, situated on either side of the trachea, produces three hormones. **Thyroxin** and **triiodothyronine** (trigh-ioh-do-**THIGH**-ro-neen) both act to stimulate the metabolic rate of the body. Thyroid hormones regulate the cellular consumption of oxygen and therefore the production of heat and energy in body tissues. The proper manufacture of these hormones requires adequate iodine in the blood. Proper diet ensures adequate iodine, which helps to prevent goiter (enlarged thyroid).

thyroxin
stimulates the metabolic rate of the body.

triiodothyronine
stimulates the metabolic rate of the body.

Secretions from the pituitary gland control the rate of production of thyroxin. When the level of thyroxin in the blood is low, the pituitary releases *thyroid-stimulating hormone (TSH),* which stimulates the thyroid to produce more thyroxin to be secreted directly into the bloodstream. When there is an adequate level of thyroxin in the blood, the pituitary stops releasing TSH into the blood, and thyroxin production is inhibited.

The thyroid also produces **calcitonin** (kal-si-**TOE**-nin), a hormone that is antagonistic to the parathyroid hormone and helps to control the calcium level of the blood.

calcitonin
is a hormone that controls the level of calcium in the blood.

Hyperthyroidism is the excessive functional activity of the thyroid gland. Often the thyroid gland enlarges to create a *goiter*. Symptoms of hyperthyroidism include heart palpitations, rapid pulse, profuse sweating, insomnia, nervousness, and excitability. Graves disease, a form of hyperthyroidism, is characterized by a strained, tense facial expression and bulging eyes.

Hyperthyroidism is generally treated by destroying some or all of the thyroid gland with radioactive iodine therapy or by surgically removing part or all of the thyroid gland.

Hypothyroidism is a condition of deficient thyroid activity. Symptoms are the opposite of hyperthyroidism, with patients having a slow heart rate; sluggish mental and physical activity; bloated, edemic appearance; and muscle weakness. **Cretinism** (**KREE**-tin-izm) is congenital hypothyroidism caused by an error in fetal development in which the thyroid fails to develop or is underactive. Thyroxin is essential to physical and mental health and development. Lack of it in young children results in a dwarfed stature and mental retardation. Hypothyroidism is easily treated with oral thyroxin supplementation.

cretinism

is caused by a lack of thyroxin during fetal development and results in a dwarfed stature and mental retardation.

Parathyroid Glands

Two pairs of parathyroid glands, situated on each lobe and behind the thyroid, produce **parathormone,** which regulates the blood level of calcium. When the blood calcium is low, the parathyroid secretes parathormone, which stimulates the activity of the osteoclasts in the bones. Thus, calcium from the bones is absorbed into the blood. When blood calcium levels are high, calcitonin has an opposite effect, and calcium is deposited in the bones. In this way parathormone and calcitonin have an antagonistic yet cooperative action in maintaining proper calcium levels in the blood.

parathormone

regulates the blood level of calcium.

Hyperparathyroidism causes loss of calcium from the bones and excessive excretion of calcium and phosphorus from the kidneys. The bones become brittle and prone to fracture, and there is a tendency toward kidney stones and disease.

Hypoparathyroidism results in low blood calcium. The low blood calcium makes the nervous activity hypersensitive. The main characteristic of hypoparathyroidism is **tetany,** a sustained muscle contraction that usually affects the hands and feet.

tetany

a sustained muscle contraction that usually affects the hands and feet.

The Thymus

The thymus is located behind the sternum and above the heart. It has endocrine and lymphatic functions and in most people is active until puberty, at which time it begins to diminish. The thymus produces several related hormones that are essential in developing and maintaining our immune system. The main purpose of the thymus is to stimulate lymphoid tissue to produce T-lymphocytes.

The Pancreas

The pancreas is located behind the stomach and has both endocrine and exocrine functions. Producing digestive enzymes that are excreted into the small intestine through the pancreatic duct is the exocrine function. Scattered throughout the pancreas are small groups of specialized cells called *islets* **(islets of Langerhans)** that produce the hormones *insulin* and *glucagon,* which are secreted directly into the bloodstream.

Islets of Langerhans

found in the pancreas, produce insulin and glucagon.

Insulin regulates the movement of glucose across the cell membrane so that when there is an increased level of glucose in the blood (e.g., after meals) secretion of insulin into the blood causes a rapid intake of glucose by most tissues in the body, especially the muscles, liver, and adipose tissue. Insulin also plays an important role in protein and fat transport and metabolism.

Diabetes mellitus is a condition caused by decreased output of insulin by the pancreatic islets. When insulin is deficient, blood glucose is elevated, and glucose is not transported across the cell membrane, so there is not enough glucose in the cells for proper cell metabolism. Because the glucose is not used by the cells, blood glucose remains high, and glucose is discharged by the kidneys into the urine. Glucose in the urine is the major sign of diabetes. Without being able to use glucose for metabolism, the body resorts to the abnormal breakdown of proteins and fats. Long-term fat and protein breakdown lead to serious complications of diabetes. Fat metabolism causes an increase in the lipids in the blood and a decrease in pH. The decrease in pH can cause the person to go into a coma. Increased blood lipids cause artherosclerosis. Circulation is generally poor, and occluded arteries in the heart can cause heart failure. Poor circulation to the retina of the eyes results in blindness. Vascular disorders in the legs result in poor healing and often gangrene, which sometimes leads to amputation.

diabetes mellitus
is caused by decreased output of insulin by the pancreas.

Treatment of diabetes is in the form of controlled diet, exercise, and a controlled program of insulin injections.

Glucagon, also produced by specialized cells in the islets of Langerhans, has an effect that is antagonistic, or the opposite of insulin. When the glucose level in the blood is low, glucagon acts to convert glycogen stored in the liver into glucose, thereby increasing the glucose level in the blood.

The Adrenal Glands

The *adrenal glands* are situated on top of each kidney. The adrenal glands each have two distinct parts, the *medulla* and the *adrenal cortex,* that produce different hormones.

The two principal hormones produced by the medulla are *epinephrine* (ep-i-**NEF**-rin; also called adrenaline) and *norepinephrine.* Stimulation of the adrenal medulla comes from the sympathetic nervous system, and the actions of adrenaline and norepinephrine cause a similar effect throughout the body as direct stimulation to the organs by the sympathetic nervous system. Known as the "fight-or-flight" hormones, they cause the bronchioles to dilate, the heart rate to increase, the blood pressure to elevate, and glycogen to convert to glucose, flooding the bloodstream and preparing the muscles to do an extraordinary amount of work to respond to any emergency situation.

The adrenal cortex produces a group of hormones called *corticosteroids* (kor-ti-ko-**STEER**-oyds). More than 30 steroids have been identified. One group, called *mineralocorticoids,* affects the extracellular electrolytes—especially sodium and potassium. The most important of these is *aldosterone* (al-**DOS**-ter-own), which regulates the sodium/potassium balance in the extracellular fluid and in the blood. In the absence of mineralocorticoid secretions, potassium levels increase, sodium levels fall, and the volume of blood decreases. Without the administration of aldosterone or mineralocorticoid therapy, the patient would go into shock and die in a matter of days.

Another group, the *glucocorticoids*, affects carbohydrate, protein, and fat metabolism. The body produces increased levels of these hormones in response to stress. The most important steroid of this group is *cortisol* (**KOR**-ti-sol), also known as *hydrocortisone*. These hormones have the ability to repress or resolve conditions of inflammation and enhance the rate of healing of damaged tissue.

The production of hormones by the adrenal cortex is stimulated by the adrenocorticotropic hormone (ACTH) from the pituitary gland.

Hyperadrenalism is the excessive release of adrenal hormones into the bloodstream. The effects and symptoms of hyperadrenalism depend on which hormones are secreted in excess. **Cushing's syndrome** results from excess glucocorticoid production and is characterized by obesity (especially in the trunk), muscle weakness, elevated blood sugar, hypertension, and arteriosclerosis.

Cushing's syndrome
results from excess glucocorticoid production and is characterized by obesity, muscle weakness, elevated blood sugar, and hypertension.

Hypoadrenalism, also called *Addison's disease*, is due to the failure of the adrenal cortex to produce aldosterone and cortisol. The disease is characterized by weight loss, muscle fatigue or atrophy, low blood pressure, and darkened skin pigmentation.

The Sex Glands

The sex glands (gonads) are both duct and ductless glands. The male and female sex glands manufacture the reproductive cells and sex hormones that are required for fertility and reproduction. In men, the **testes** produce **testosterone,** a potent androgen that is primarily responsible for the development of the reproductive structures. Another function involves the development of secondary sexual characteristics such as a deeper voice, body hair, and body structure.

testes
are two small, egg-shaped glands that produce the spermatozoa.

testosterone
is a male hormone responsible for development of secondary sexual characteristics.

Estrogen and **progesterone** are the two essential hormones produced in the **ovaries** of the female reproductive system. In women, estrogen nearly parallels the actions of testosterone regarding the development of secondary sexual characteristics. Estrogen also regulates the development of the reproductive organs, the mammary glands, and menstruation.

estrogen
is a female hormone responsible for development of secondary sexual characteristics.

progesterone
a female hormone that prepares the uterine lining for implantation, aids maintaining pregnancy, and stimulates development of mammary glands for nursing.

ovaries
are glandular organs in the pelvis that produce the ovum and female sex hormones.

When a woman becomes pregnant, the placenta assumes a minor endocrine role by producing small amounts of estrogen, progesterone, and chorionic gonadotropin to help keep the uterus receptive to the fetus and placenta during pregnancy.

SECTION QUESTIONS FOR DISCUSSION AND REVIEW

1. What is the composition of the endocrine system?
2. What is the major function of the endocrine system?
3. What is an important difference between a duct and ductless gland?
4. Why do the glands depend on an adequate nerve and blood supply?
5. Are sebaceous (oil) glands classified as duct or ductless glands?
6. What is the function of a ductless or endocrine gland?
7. Which glands function as both duct and ductless glands?
8. Which glands produce hormones?
9. Why are hormones important to the body?
10. Name the endocrine glands.
11. What is the nature of most endocrine dysfunctions?
12. Why is the pituitary gland called *the master gland*?

13. What are the two hormone-producing parts of the adrenal glands?
14. What is the endocrine function of the sex glands?

REVIEW

Matching Test I

Match the hormone in the left list with the gland that produces it by writing the appropriate letter in the space provided.

______	1. gonadotropic hormone	a.	pituitary gland
______	2. adrenaline	b.	thyroid gland
______	3. insulin	c.	parathyroid
______	4. antidiuretic hormone	d.	thymus gland
______	5. thyroxin	e.	adrenal cortex
______	6. testosterone	f.	adrenal medulla
______	7. ACTH	g.	pancreas
______	8. cortisol	h.	ovaries
______	9. progesterone	i.	testes
______	10. aldosterone		
______	11. somatropic hormone		
______	12. glucagon		
______	13. epinephrine		
______	14. parathormone		
______	15. TSH		

Matching Test II

Match the hormone with the best description of its function by writing the appropriate letter in the space provided.

______	1. gonadotropic hormone	a.	stimulates the thyroid
______	2. TSH	b.	affects growth
______	3. glucagon	c.	regulates blood calcium
______	4. thyroxin	d.	stimulates metabolic rate
______	5. epinephrine	e.	promotes carbohydrate metabolism
______	6. ACTH	f.	stimulates adrenal cortex
______	7. somatropic hormone	g.	fight or flight response
______	8. cortisol	h.	converts glycogen to glucose
______	9. insulin	i.	resolves inflammation
______	10. parathormone	j.	affects sex organs

SYSTEM 7 THE RESPIRATORY SYSTEM

To carry on the vital functions of the organism, the cells of the body require a continual supply of oxygen and the removal of carbon dioxide. Without a constant supply of oxygen, a human being dies within a matter of minutes. The vital exchange of oxygen and carbon dioxide is accomplished by the respiratory system.

The respiratory system includes the nose, nasal cavity, pharynx, larynx, trachea, bronchial tubes, and the lungs. The lungs are composed of spongy tissue, blood vessels, connective tissue, and microscopic air sacs called *alveoli* (al-**VEE**-o-ligh). A network of very fine capillaries brings the blood into close contact with the thin walls of alveoli (Figure 5-72).

Respiration

Respiration is the exchange of carbon dioxide and oxygen that takes place at three levels in the body:

1. External respiration is the exchange between the external environment and the blood and takes place in the lungs.
2. Internal respiration is the gaseous exchange between the blood and the cells of the body.
3. Cellular respiration or oxidation occurs within the cell.

Respiration begins as air is inhaled through the nose and passes through the nasal cavity, where it is warmed, moistened, and filtered. Air then passes through the pharynx and larynx and into the trachea. The trachea divides into two bronchi, which subdivide into smaller and smaller branches of the *bronchial tree.* The air moves through the *bronchioles* until it reaches the ends of the air passages that terminate in clusters of air sacs called *alveoli.* The thin porous walls of the alveoli are surrounded by capillaries of the pulmonary circulatory system. The blood entering the lungs through the pulmonary arteries has a high concentration of carbon dioxide, which has been picked up from the cells of the body, and a low concentration of oxygen. The concentration of oxygen in the alveoli is greater than in the blood. Likewise, concentrations of carbon dioxide in the blood are higher than in the alveoli. Through the process of diffusion, therefore, carbon dioxide moves from the blood to the lungs and is exhaled while oxygen moves from the lungs into the bloodstream and is carried by the red blood cells back to the heart and then circulated throughout the body.

Oxygenated blood moves into the capillaries of the systemic circulation. Differences in concentration of the gases between the blood and tissue fluid cause oxygen to diffuse into the tissue fluid while carbon dioxide diffuses out of the fluid and into the blood. A similar diffusion process takes place between the tissue fluid and the cells.

Once in the cells, the oxygen is used in cellular respiration to produce energy. The cell uses some of that energy to function; the rest is in the form of heat. The waste products of cellular respiration include carbon dioxide and water, which migrate back into the bloodstream to be eliminated. The carbon dioxide is carried by the red blood cells and the plasma to the lungs, where it diffuses out of the blood into the alveoli, to be expelled from the lungs with the next exhalation.

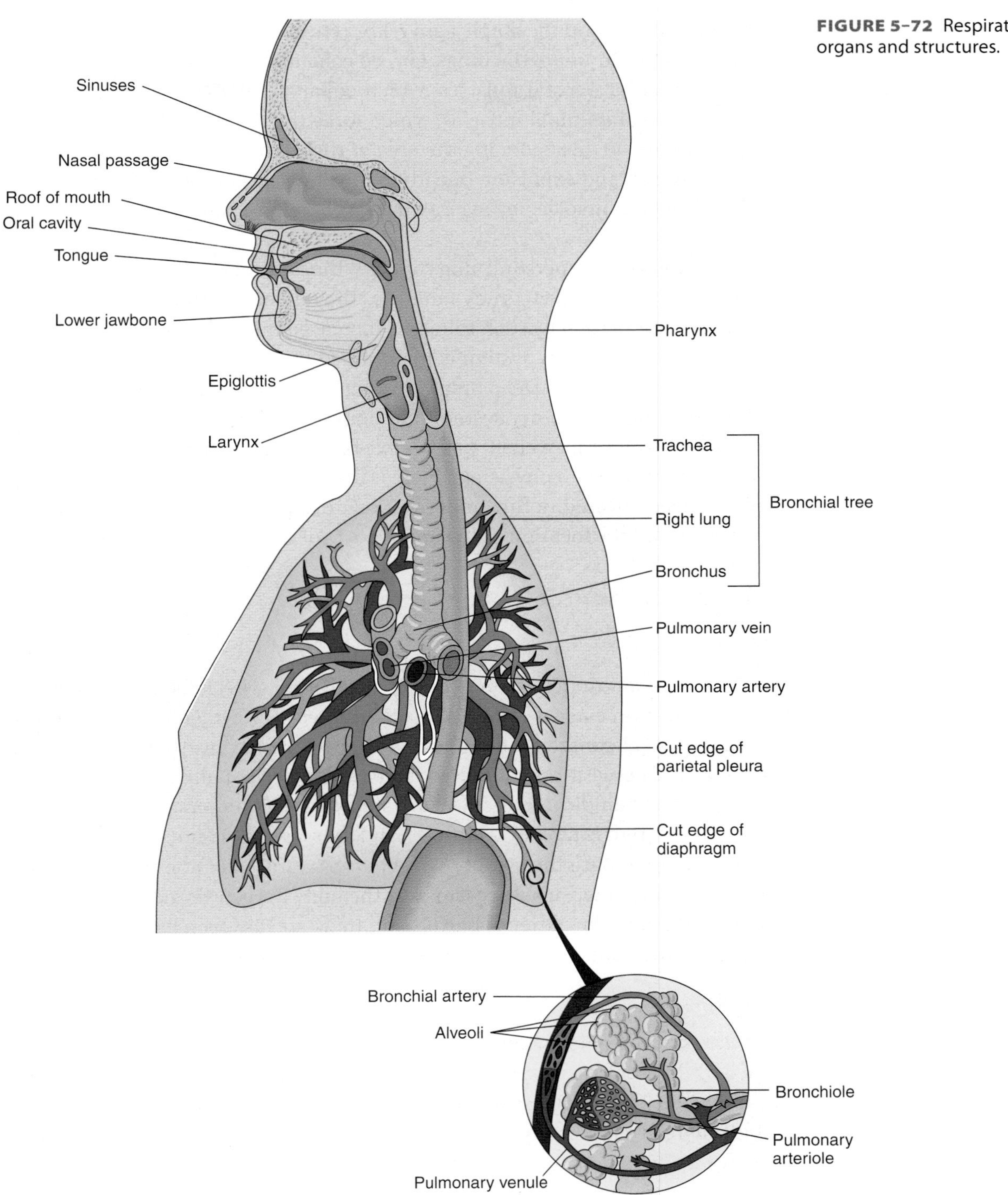

FIGURE 5–72 Respiratory organs and structures.

Breathing

External respiration, also called *ventilation* or *breathing*, involves the act of inhaling and exhaling air, resulting in an exchange of gases between the blood and alveoli. With each inhalation, the intercostal muscles contract, raising the ribs and expanding the thoracic cavity. At the same time, the diaphragm contracts and is pulled down, causing the lungs to draw in air. Exhalation occurs as the intercostals and the diaphragm relax, returning to their neutral positions and pushing the air out of the lungs. Forced exhalation involves the contraction of the internal intercostal muscles, which collapse the rib cage, and the contraction of the abdominal muscles, which force the abdominal viscera against the diaphragm, further reducing the area of the thoracic cavity. The maximum intake of oxygen and expulsion of carbon dioxide is accomplished during deep breathing, which involves exaggerated movements of both the ribs and diaphragm.

Depending on the person's lung capacity, the natural rate of breathing for an adult is between 10 and 20 times a minute. The rate of breathing is increased by the demand for oxygen by such things as increased muscular activity.

A healthy respiratory system is maintained by avoiding air pollution, toxic chemicals, and smoking. Deep breathing, regular exercise, and a healthy diet all help to keep the respiratory system functioning normally. Should the massage practitioner notice that a client has trouble breathing normally, it is wise to suggest that the client see a physician. There is much more to the respiratory system than has been covered in this brief overview. Study Figure 5-71 to be sure that you understand the location of the major parts of the respiratory system.

Disorders of the Respiratory System

The Common Cold

Also known as an upper respiratory tract infection (URTI), the common cold is a viral infection caused by over 200 different viruses, which is usually spread through physical contact. A cold has a variety of symptoms that include nasal discharge and congestion, mild fever, sore throat, dry coughing, and headache. Massage is contraindicated in the acute stage of the common cold, because the respiratory system is already overtaxed and massage only tends to stir up more toxins and exacerbate the symptoms. When the viral infection has progressed to the postacute stage, massage can help the body to recover more quickly. It is important to gain the patient's permission to do so, however, because massage at this stage can cause the patient to feel as if he is experiencing a relapse.

Influenza

Influenza, or the flu, is a viral infection that is similar to the common cold but caused by different viruses. The flu can also be spread through physical contact, but unlike a cold, it can be spread by airborne viruses as well. Flu symptoms include high fever and body aches, both of which should last no more than three days. After the fever subsides, symptoms such as coughing, sneezing, congestion, and general malaise cnacan follow for up to two weeks. A common complication of influenza is that with the body in a weakened condition, the possibility of secondary bacterial infections (e.g., bronchitis or pneumonia) increases. This is a particular concern for those with preexisting lung conditions, or elderly or very young persons. Massage is contraindicated for all stages of the flu except the very end of the subacute stage when it can help to flush out residual toxins and help the body to recover more efficiently. Even at this stage, massage can cause the patient to feel as if a relapse is occurring, and so it is important to inform the client and gain permission before proceeding.

Pneumonia

Pneumonia and *pneumonitis* are terms to describe any type of inflammation of the lungs. There are many different viruses and types of bacteria that cause pneumonia. Symptoms vary widely from coughing, chills, high fever, and body aches to chest pains, cyanosis, and thickened yellow/green or blood-streaked phlegm. There is a different medical treatment for each type of pneumonia, but massage treatment is the same for any type of pneumonitis. Massage should be applied to pneumonia patients only when the infection has reached the subacute stage, and even then only under medical supervision. Percussive massage, especially cupping over the thorax, has proved helpful in loosening phlegm from alveoli into the bronchial tubes. Massage is contraindicated in any other stage of infection.

Sinusitis

Sinusitis refers to the swelling or inflammation of the paranasal sinus cavities. This condition can occur as a reaction to allergies, nasal obstructions, or infection. Symptoms include localized tenderness, pressure headaches, runny nose, congestion, or facial and tooth pain. As long as no viral or bacterial infection is present, massage can be beneficial to a patient suffering from sinusitis; however, in any case in which infectious acute sinusitis is suspected, massage is contraindicated.

Tuberculosis

Tuberculosis is a highly infectious airborne disease that can begin in the lungs and spread to other parts of the body. Tuberculosis (TB as it is commonly called) is caused by an infection of the *Mycobacterium tuberculosis* bacteria. It begins as a bacterial infection that can incubate in the body without detection by sealing itself away in fleshy pockets called *tubercles.* Tubercles are most likely to form in the lungs; however, the bacteria can be transported through the bloodstream, with tubercles forming in other parts of the body such as the bones and kidneys. Once the infected body's immune system weakens, the bacterial infection turns into a disease that is highly contagious. The World Health Organization thought the disease was wiped out by the 1970s, but in the late 1980s, it made a frighteningly successful comeback with a new mutation that is surprisingly drug resistant. AIDS patients, cancer patients undergoing chemotherapy, and anyone who has a severely weakened immune system is at a higher risk of contracting the disease from the bacteria, whereas a person with a strong immune system might have the infection for many years before actually contracting the disease.

The bacterial infection rarely has any symptoms. The disease, however, has a wide variety of symptoms, including night sweats, fatigue, and a cough that will start dry but later begin to be productive of bloody or pus-filled phlegm. Massage is contraindicated for tuberculosis in either form because it can assist in spreading tubercles throughout the body, thereby having a devastating effect on the patient. Therapists also have their own health to consider; they would not be beneficial to any of their clients if they were to contract the disease.

SECTION QUESTIONS FOR DISCUSSIOIN AND REVIEW

1. What are the major organs of the respiratory system?
2. What is the function of the respiratory system?
3. What is the physical appearance of the lungs?
4. What are the three levels of respiration, and where do they take place?
5. What is an alveoli and what is its function?
6. What is breathing?
7. What is the natural rate of breathing for an adult?
8. What is the diaphragm, and which function does it perform?

SYSTEM 8 THE DIGESTIVE SYSTEM

The human body is a living organism made up of millions of cells that perform a multitude of different tasks. Each cell must receive a continuous supply of nutrients to provide fuel for energy and nutritional elements for growth and regeneration. These nutrients come from the food that we eat. Food that enters the mouth must undergo many changes before it can be used by the cells for nourishment. This process is carried on by the digestive system. The main functions of the digestive system are **digestion** and **absorption.** *Digestion* is the process of converting food into substances capable of being used by the cells for nourishment. *Absorption* is the process in which the digested nutrients are transferred from the intestines to the blood or lymph vessels so that they can be transported to the cells.

digestion

is the process of converting food into substances capable of being used by the cells for nourishment.

absorption

is the process in which the digested nutrients are transferred from the intestines to the blood or lymph vessels.

The digestive system is composed of the **alimentary canal** and **accessory digestive organs.** The alimentary canal, also known as the *gastrointestinal* or *digestive tract*, consists of the mouth (oral cavity), pharynx (throat), esophagus, stomach, small intestine, and large intestine. The accessory organs include the teeth, tongue, salivary glands, pancreas, liver, and gallbladder.

alimentary canal

consists of the mouth, pharynx, esophagus, stomach, and small and large intestines.

accessory digestive organs

consist of the teeth, tongue, salivary glands, pancreas, liver, and gallbladder.

The *alimentary canal* is a muscular tube that is about five times as long as a person is tall and extends from the lips to the anus. The tube forms a continuous barrier so that material in the digestive tube can be acted on by the digestive juices, although it is not yet part of the body or its cellular makeup.

The process of digestion changes the food into a nutritious fluid capable of being absorbed by the blood. Digestion is accomplished through physical and chemical means. The physical means involve the teeth, tongue, and involuntary muscles of the pharynx, esophagus, stomach, and small intestine. The teeth tear and grind the food into small pieces while the tongue mixes and moves the food. After the food is swallowed, the involuntary muscles mix the food with digestive juices and propel it through the alimentary canal. Enzymes and a variety of digestive juices act on the food to break it down chemically from complex food substances into simple nutritional molecules that can be absorbed into the bloodstream and through the cell membranes.

The Path of Digestion

oral cavity

or mouth, prepares food for entrance into the stomach.

The mouth, called the **oral cavity,** prepares the food for entrance into the stomach. In the mouth, the food is masticated (chewed) by the teeth and

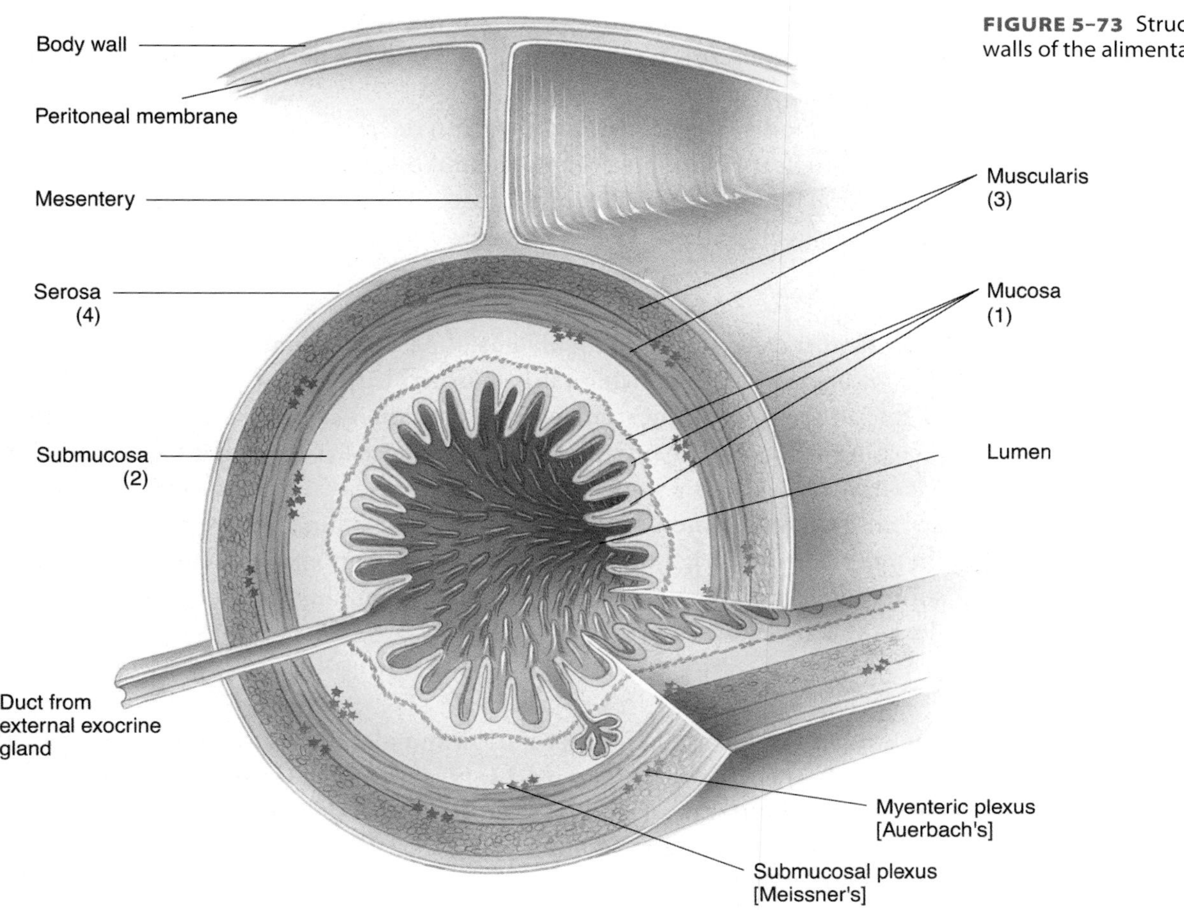

FIGURE 5-73 Structure of the walls of the alimentary tract.

mixed by the tongue with secretions from the *salivary glands.* **Saliva** contains enzymes that begin to digest carbohydrates. The action of the teeth, tongue, and saliva prepares the food into a soft ball called a *bolus* that slides into the throat and is swallowed by voluntary and reflex actions of the muscles of the pharynx.

saliva

produced by the salivry glands in the mouth and contains enzymes that begin to digest carbohydrates.

Structure of the Alimentary Canal

From the throat to the anus, the walls of the alimentary canal are similar in structure except for specialized modifications that perform particular functions. The wall of the alimentary canal consists of four distinct layers (Figure 5-73):

1. The *mucosa* (myoo-**KO**-suh), or mucous membrane, is made up of epithelial cells, connective tissue, and a variety of digestive glands. This layer protects the underlying tissues and functions to carry on secretion and absorption.
2. The *submucosa* consists of connective tissue, nerves, and blood and lymph vessels that serve to nourish the surrounding tissues and carry away the absorbed material.
3. The *muscular layer* has two layers of smooth muscle. The muscle fibers of the inner layer encircle the tube so that when they contract, the diameter of the tube decreases. The outer layer of muscle fibers is arranged longitudinally so that when they contract, the tube shortens.

4. The *serous layer* is the outer covering of the tube. On the stomach and intestines, this layer is continuous with the peritoneum that lines the abdominal cavity.

When food passes from the throat into the esophagus, the smooth muscles of the alimentary canal are stimulated and begin to produce a rhythmic, wave-like motion that propels and churns the food throughout the length of the canal. The wavelike muscular action is called **peristalsis** (per-i-**STAL**-sis).

peristalsis

is the wavelike muscular action of the alimentary canal.

The Stomach

After food travels down the esophagus, it passes through the *cardiac sphincter* and enters the stomach, where it is churned with gastric juices secreted from glands in the wall of the stomach that contain *hydrochloric acid* and protein-digesting enzymes. The mixture of digestive juices, mucus, and food material is called *chyme.* From the stomach, the chyme passes through the *pyloric sphincter* and into the duodenum of the small intestine. Sphincters are muscular valves that allow the passage of food substances in only one direction. The pyloric sphincter also plays an important role in determining how long food is held in the stomach.

The Small Intestine

The *small intestine* is the longest part of the alimentary canal and consists of three parts: the *duodenum* (doo-o-**DEE**-num), *jejunum* (je-**JOO**-num), and *ileum* (**IL**-ee-um). Thousands of glands in the intestinal walls produce *intestinal digestive juices.* In addition to the intestinal juices, secretions of bile from the liver and *pancreatic fluids* from the pancreas are poured into the duodenum. Bile from the liver and gallbladder is carried through the *common bile duct* and is essential for the breakdown of fats. Pancreatic fluid enters the duodenum by way of the *pancreatic duct* and contains enzymes that act to digest proteins, carbohydrates, and fats (Table 5.17).

The small intestine is lined with small, fingerlike projections covering the intestinal walls called *villi* (**VIL**-eye) that greatly increase the surface area available for absorption. Each microscopic villus contains a network of blood capillaries and lymph capillaries (lacteals). The end products of digestion pass through the intestinal wall and are absorbed into the blood vessels and the lacteals. Nutrients absorbed into the bloodstream are carried to the liver. Nutrients absorbed by the lymph flow through the cisterna chyli and the thoracic duct before entering the systemic circulation.

The Large Intestine

After the digestive processes have been completed in the small intestine, the waste (unusable) materials (water and solids) move through the *iliocecal valve* into a small, pouchlike part of the large intestine called the *cecum* (**SEE**-kum). The large intestine (colon) continues upward along the right side of the abdomen to form the *ascending colon.* Then it travels across the abdominal cavity and forms the *transverse colon.* It continues downward on the left side of the abdomen to become the *descending colon.* As the colon reaches the left iliac region, it forms an S-shaped bend known as the *sigmoid colon,* which empties into the rectum. The *rectum* is a temporary storage area for waste. The distal part of the

TABLE 5.17

GLANDS, DIGESTIVE JUICES, AND ENZYMES			
GLANDS AND JUICE	LOCATION	ENZYMES	CHANGES IN FOOD
Saliva (3) Salivary gland	Mouth	Salivary Amylase (ptyalin)	Begins digestion of starch into simple sugars
Gastric juice Stomach	Stomach wall	Pepsin	Begins digestion of protein into amino acids
Pancreatic juice Pancreas	Small intestine	Amylase Trypsin Lipase	Starches, proteins, fats
Juice from small intestine	Small intestine	Lactase Maltase Sucrase	Breaks down complex carbohydrates to simple sugars
Bile from liver	Small intestine	No enzymes	Breaks down fats into fatty acids

large intestine is the *anal canal,* which ends with the anus, from which fecal matter is expelled.

The functions of the colon include storing, forming, and excreting waste products of digestion and regulating the body's water balance. The colon aids in regulating the body's water balance by absorbing large amounts of water from the undigested material back into the body. Through a process of water

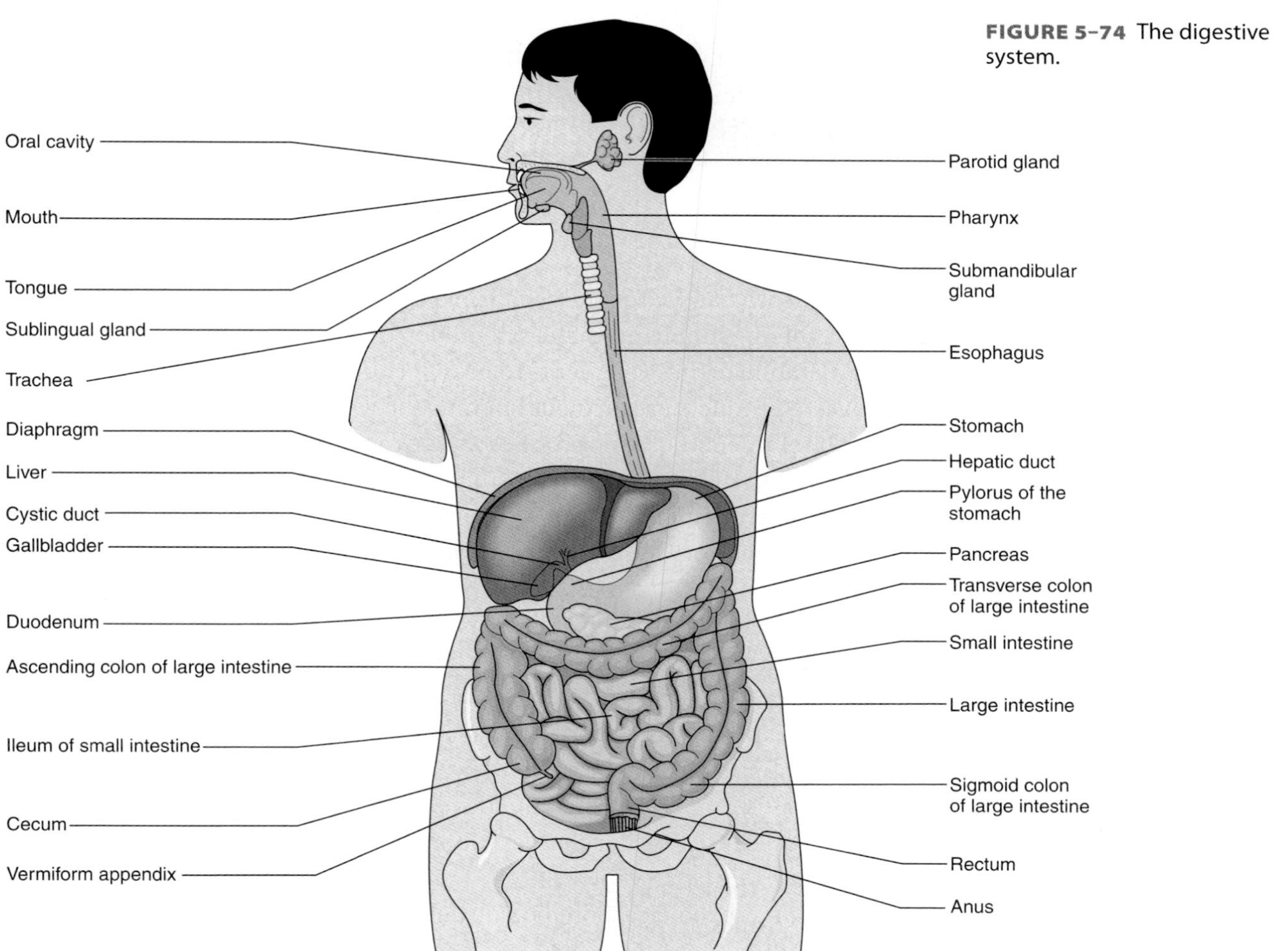

FIGURE 5–74 The digestive system.

absorption and bacterial action, the liquid state of the undigested and indigestible material in the colon is transformed into the semisolid feces, which are eliminated or defecated from the rectum. The bacterial action in the colon also synthesizes some B-complex vitamins and vitamin K, which is reabsorbed into the bloodstream (Figure 5-74).

SECTION QUESTIONS FOR DISCUSSION AND REVIEW

1. Which structures compose the digestive system?
2. What is the function of digestion?
3. What is absorption?
4. What are the physical processes of digestion?
5. Which chemical agents in the digestive juices aid digestion?
6. Which digestive changes occur in the mouth?
7. Describe the general structure of the alimentary canal.
8. What is peristalsis or peristaltic action?
9. Which digestive changes occur in the stomach?
10. Name the three parts of the small intestine.
11. Which glands supply digestive secretions to the small intestine?
12. Which digestive changes occur in the small intestine?
13. Which structures absorb the end products of digestion?
14. From which organ is the undigested food eliminated from the body?

SYSTEM 9 THE EXCRETORY SYSTEM

The Excretory Organs

metabolic wastes

are products formed from cell metabolism.

The food that we eat, water that we drink, and air that we breathe all play an important role in supplying the elements for the body's metabolic activity. As the cells metabolize these elements to produce their specialized substances and energy, waste products are formed that must be carried away and excreted from the body. If retained, these **metabolic wastes** tend to poison the body.

The function of the excretory system (including the urinary system) is to eliminate or excrete metabolic wastes and undigested food from the body. The organs of the excretory system are the kidneys, liver, skin, large intestine, and lungs.

1. The kidneys excrete uric acid, urea, electrolytes, water, and other wastes through the process of urination.
2. The liver produces urea, which is returned to the blood to be excreted by the kidneys. The liver also discharges bile through the gallbladder and into the intestines.
3. The skin eliminates water and heat through the process of perspiration.
4. The large intestine discharges food wastes through the process of defecation.
5. The lungs exhale carbon dioxide and water vapor through external respiration.

Urinary System

The *urinary system* includes two kidneys, two ureters, the bladder, and a urethra. The **kidneys** are bean-shaped organs located at the back of the abdominal cavity, between the tenth thoracic and third lumbar vertebrae, and kept in place by fibrous connective and fatty tissues. The kidneys are an efficient blood filtration system. The **nephron** (**NEF**-ron) is the functional unit of the kidney (Figure 5-75). There are 2 to 3 million nephrons in the kidneys. Each day, the nephrons filter 40 to 50 gallons of plasma from the blood. Ninety-nine percent of this fluid is reabsorbed into the bloodstream. The kidneys excrete the remaining water and waste products through the *ureters.* As the kidneys filter the blood, they remove a certain amount of water and nitrogenous waste products of metabolism (e.g., urea, uric acid, ammonia, and some drugs). The ureters are tubes that carry urine from the kidneys to the **bladder,** where the urine is stored. The *bladder* is a hollow organ constructed of walls of elastic fibers and involuntary muscles that acts as a reservoir for the urine until it is excreted from the body. When the bladder accumulates about a pint of urine, sensors indicate that it is time to urinate. Voiding or emptying the bladder is accomplished by a voluntary relaxation of a sphincter muscle at the mouth of the urethra and the involuntary contraction of the muscles of the bladder. As the bladder contracts, urine is forced through the *urethra* and out of the body (Figure 5-76).

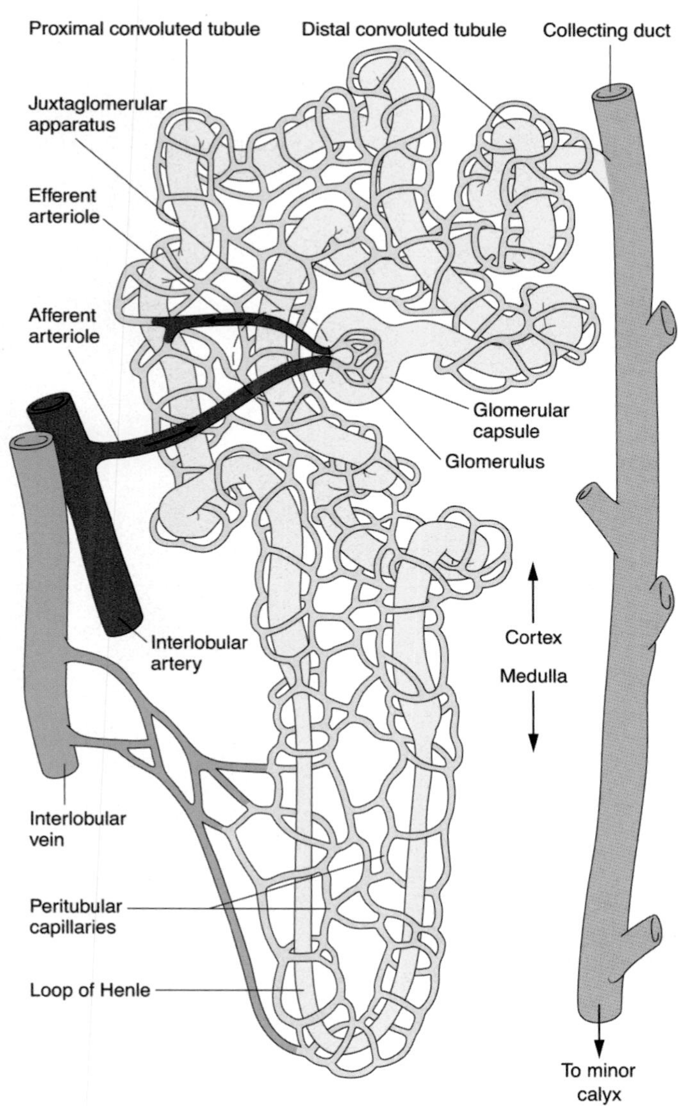

FIGURE 5-75 Anatomy of the nephron, the functional unit of the kidney.

A *urinalysis* is a chemical examination of the urine that is often part of the routine examination given by most physicians. The presence of white blood cells, blood, glucose, or other chemicals in the uriny can be an indication of metabolic imbalance, infection, or numerous other conditions. Normal, healthy urine is a clear yellowish fluid. A change in the color of the urine, such as a reddish or brownish colory can indicate infection or other problems.

The kidneys also function to maintain the body's water balance and acid-base balance. Another function of the kidneys is the production of the hormone *renin,* which acts to regulate blood pressure. When the blood pressure is low, the kidneys are stimulated to release more renin into the bloodstream, which causes blood vessels to contract, thereby raising the blood pressure (Figure 5-77).

kidneys

are bean-shaped glands that filter the blood.

nephron

is the functional unit of the kidney.

bladder

is an organ where the urine is stored.

The Liver

The *liver* is one of the largest organs of the digestive system and is situated on the upper right side of the abdomen, immediately below and in contact with the diaphragm. The liver performs many of the body's chemical functions. The liver

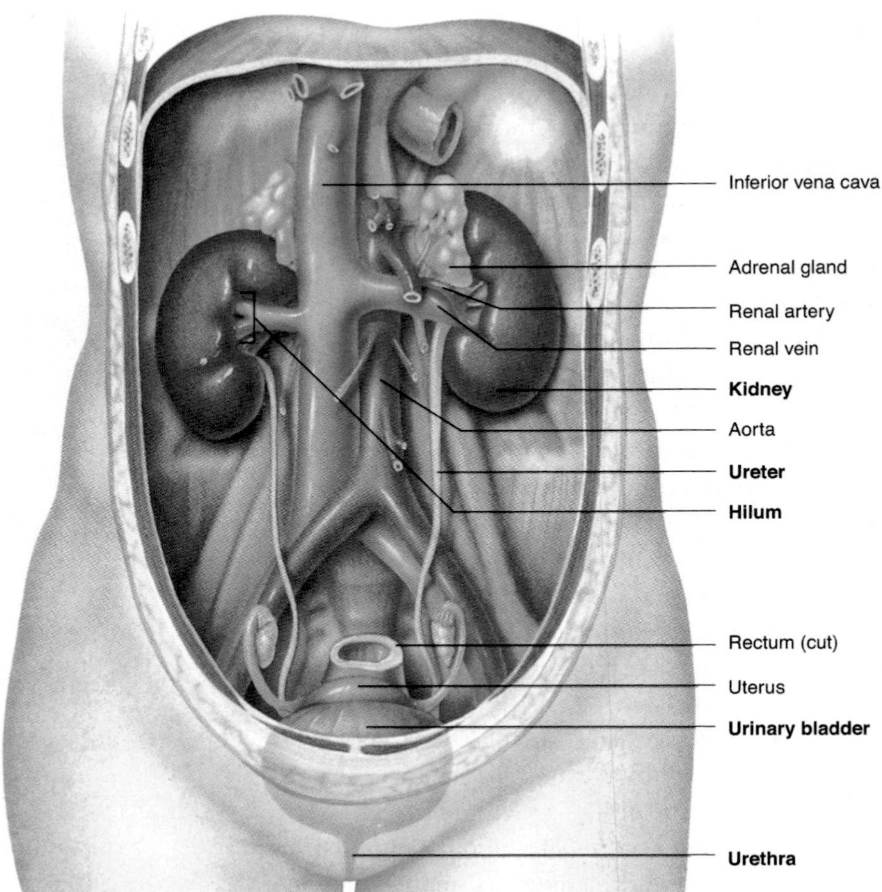

FIGURE 5-76 Organs of the urinary system.

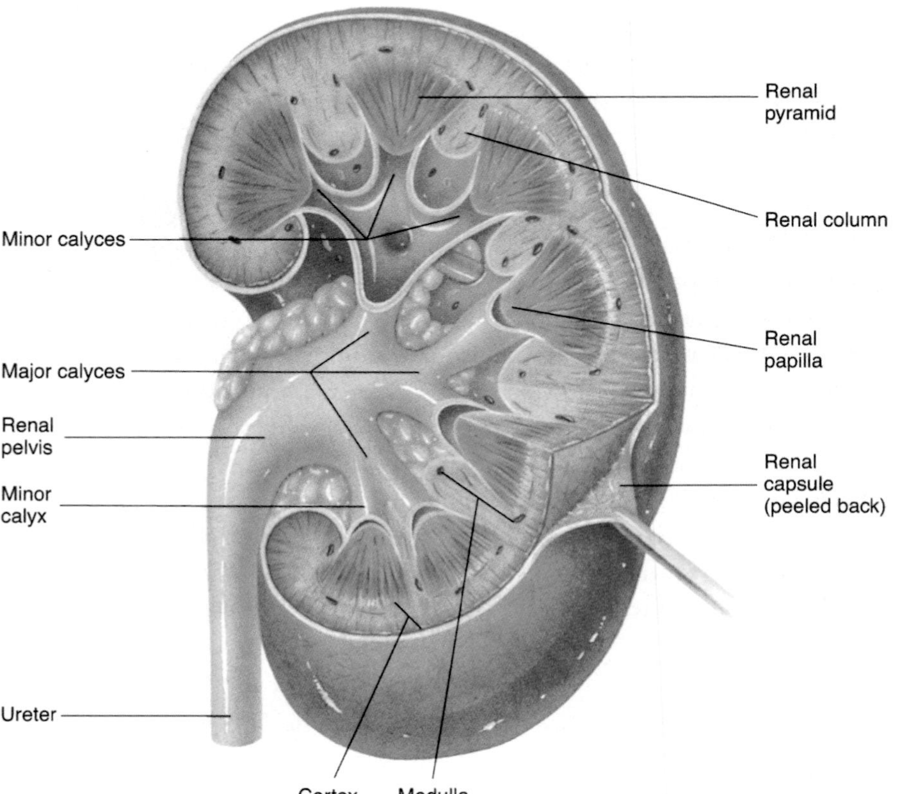

FIGURE 5-77 Internal anatomy of the kidney.

neutralizes or detoxifies toxic substances thae notherwise might be absorbed from the intestines such as alcohol, food additives, and drugs. The liver functions include many other metabolic processes that include converting glucose to glycogen, changing lactic acid to glucose, producing glucose from noncarbohydrates, changing carbohydrates and protein to fats for storage, producing cholesterol lipoproteins, and breaking down and reforming damaged red blood cells. The liver stores vitamins A, B, and B12 and glycogen. The main excretory function of the liver is the formation of urea, which is returned to the bloodstream to be excreted by the kidneys. The liver also produces bile, which is stored in the gall bladder until it is excreted through the bile duct into the duodenum of the small intestines. **Bile** is a bitter, alkaline, yellowish-brown fluid secreted from the liver through the gallbladder and into the duodenum, and contains water, bile salts, mucin, cholesterol, lecithin, and fat pigments. Bile aids in the emulsification, digestion, and absorption of fats and the regulation of alkalinity of the intestines (Figure 5-78).

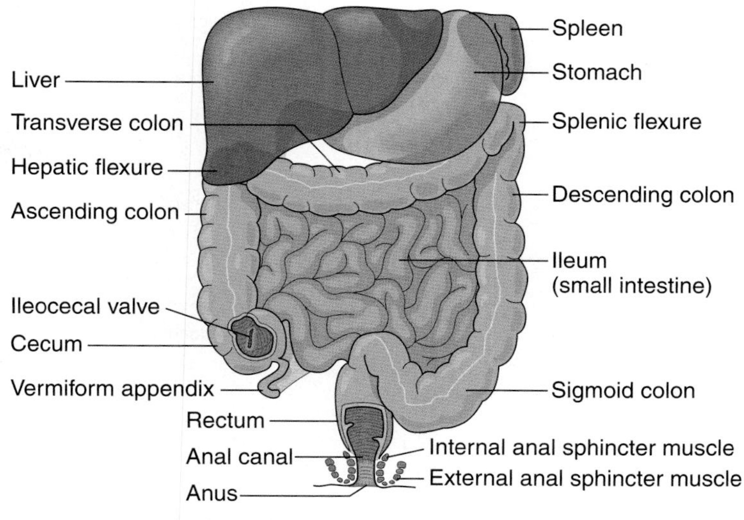

FIGURE 5-78 The liver.

bile
is a bitter, alkaline, yellowish-brown fluid secreted by the liver that aids in fat digestion.

SECTION QUESTIONS FOR DISCUSSION AND REVIEW

1. Name the five important organs of the excretory system.
2. What happens if waste products are retained within the body instead of being eliminated?
3. What is the function of the excretory system?
4. Name the parts of the urinary system.
5. What is the functional unit of the kidney?
6. Why do most physicians include urinalysis aa part of a routine physical checkup?
7. Which colors of urine indicate a problem that needs checking by a physician?
8. Which organ of the body secretes bile?
9. What is the excretory function of the liver?

SYSTEM 10 THE HUMAN REPRODUCTIVE SYSTEM

The reproductive system is the generative apparatus necessary for organisms to reproduce organisms of the same kind and ensure the continuation of their species.

Lower forms of life, such as one-celled organisms, do not need a partner to reproduce. They do so by nonsexual means, which is called *asexual reproduction.*

In humans (and most multicellular organisms), reproduction is sexual and requires a male and female, each having specialized sex cells. *Gamete* is the term

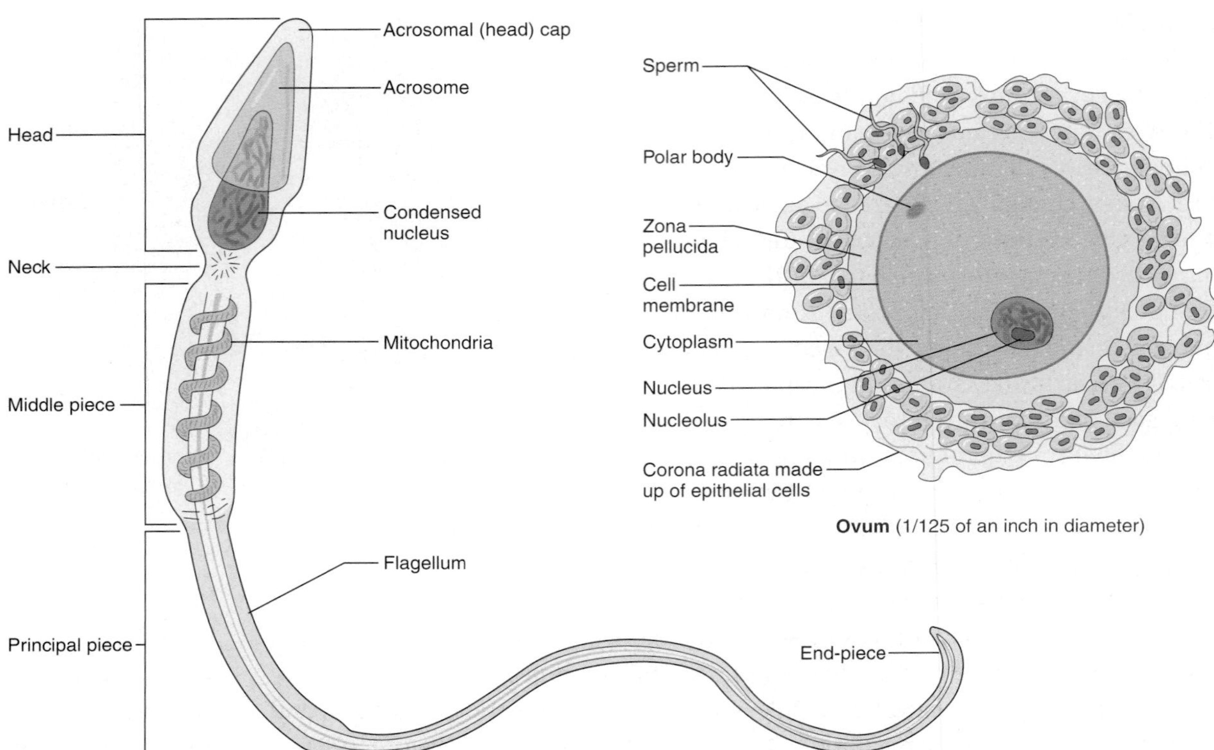

FIGURE 5-79 Human sperm and ovum.

used to describe a reproductive cell that can unite with another gamete to form the cell (zygote) that develops into an embryo. In the male, these cells are *spermatozoa* (sper-ma-to-**ZOE**-uh) and in female, *ovum.* A *zygote* is the fertilized ovum, the cell formed by the union of a spermatozoon with an ovum. A *gonad* is a sex gland that produces the reproductive cell. In the human female, the gonad is the *ovary.* In the human male, it is the *testes* (Figure 5-79).

It is not within the scope of this book to describe in detail the entire process of human reproduction. The following is intended as a brief summary.

The Male Reproductive System

The functions of the male reproductive system are the production of sperm, the production of the male hormones, and the performance of the sex act. The reproductive system is men includes two testes, two vas deferens, two seminal vesicles, a prostate gland, the bulbourethral glands (Cowper's glands), and the penis.

The male gonads are located outside the body in a pouch situated at the base of and beneath the penis called the *scrotum.* The *testes* are two small, egg-shaped glands made up of minute convoluted tubules calles *seminiferous tubules* where the sperm cell is produced in a process called *spermatogenesis.* Spermatogenesis takes place in the tubules as specialized stem cells near the outer membrane divide to produce cells called primary spermatocytes (PRYE-mary spur-MAT-oh-sightz). These cells undergo cellular reduction division or *meiosis* and become secondary spermatocytes, where their stored genetic information has been divided in half. (In humans, the 46 chromosomes have been divided to 23.) These secondary spermatocytes undergo another division so that the original cell becomes four *spermatids* thal soon develop into mature sperm cells or *spermatozoa.* The soft connective tissue between ths seminiferous tubules contains special groups of cells known as the *interstitial cells of Leydig* (LYE-dig) which produce the male sex hormone **testosterone.** Because the testes produce both sperm and testosterone, they are considered both endocrine (without ducts) and exocrine (with ducts) glands.

testosterone

is a male hormone responsible for development of secondary sexual characteristics.

Testosterone is essential to the development of the male sexual characteristics, including body hair, a masculine voice, sex organs, and sperm production. *Spermatozoa* are tiny detached cells, egg-shaped and equipped with a tail that enables them to be motile or to swim. Of the millions of spermatozoa released during ejaculation, only one fertilizes the reproductive cell (egg) produced by the woman. The others die within a short time.

The male reproductive system includes a duct system, tubes that transport the spermatozoa from the testes to the outside of the body.

The *epididymis* (ep-i-**DID**-i-mis), located in the scrotum, receives sperm from the testes and stores the sperm until it becomes fully mature. This tube extends upward to become the left or right *vas deferens (ductus deferens)* and continues through a small canal behind the abdominal wall and behind the urinary bladder. The sperm collects in the vas deferens until it is expelled from the body. The vas deferens join with the ducts of the seminal vesicles to form the *ejaculatory ducts.* These two ducts enter the prostate gland, where they empty into the urethra.

The Accessory Glands

The glands of the male reproductive system produce secretions that combine with the sperm to form *semen,* which is excreted from the body during ejaculation.

Seminal vesicles are two convoluted, glandular tubes located on each side of the prostate that produce a nutritious fluid that is excreted into the ejaculatory ducts at the time of emission. The secretions of the seminal vesicles contain simple sugars, mucus, prostaglandin, and other substances to help nourish, protect, and aid the sperm as it travels into the female reproductive system. The *seminal fluid* forms most of the semen when ejaculated.

The *prostate gland* lies below the urinary bladder and surrounds the first part of the urethra. The prostate secretes an alkaline fluid that enhances the sperm's motility (ability to swim). The fluid also neutralizes the acidic vaginal secretions, thereby protecting the sperm and increasing its chances of reaching and fertilizing the ovum. Ducts from the prostate enter the ejaculatory ducts. The prostate gland is supplied with muscular tissue that reflexively contracts during ejaculation.

The *Cowper's (bulbourethral) glands* are two pea-sized glands located beneath the prostate gland. They are mucus-producing glands that serve to lubricate the urethra.

The *urethra* serves to convey urine from the bladder and to carry reproductive cells and secretions out of the body.

The *penis* is the male organ of copulation, consisting of erectile tissue that can become engorged and erect to deposit the sperm-containing semen deep within the woman's vagina (Figure 5-80).

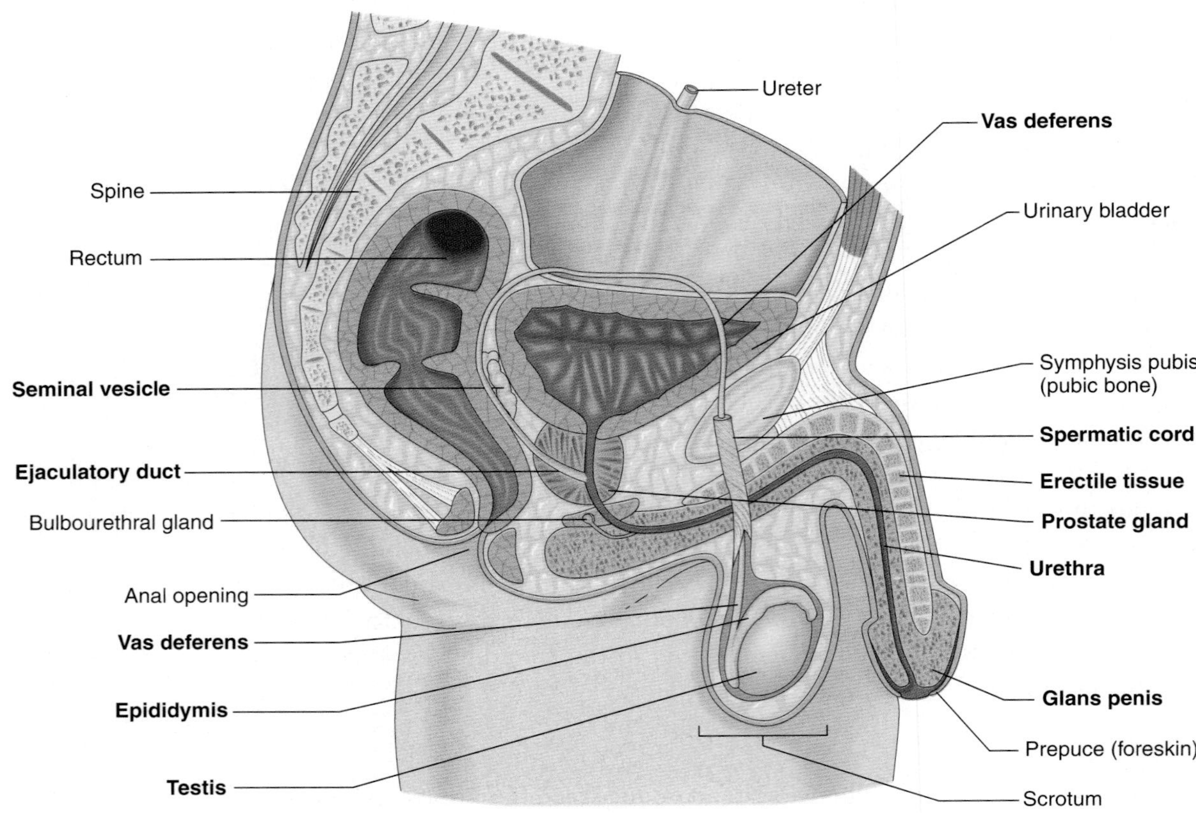

FIGURE 5-80 The male reproductive system.

The Female Reproductive System

The functions of the female reproductive system are to produce the ovum and female hormones, to receive the sperm during the sex act, and to carry the growing fetus during pregnancy.

The reproductive system in females includes two ovaries, two fallopian tubes (oviducts), a uterus, a vagina, and the vulva or external genitalia.

The *vulva* forms the external part of the female reproductive system. It includes the outer lips called the *labia majora* and the inner, smaller lips called the *labia minora.* On a virgin, within the vulva, a fold of connective tissue, the *hymen,* partially covers the external orifice of the vagina. The *clitoris* is a small sensitive body of erectile tissue located at the anterior junction of the labia.

The *mons pubis* is a pad of fatty tissue over the pubic symphysis.

The Female Internal Organs

vagina
is a muscular tube leading from the vulva to the cervix and is the lower part of the birth canal.

The **vagina** is a muscular tube or canal leading from the vulva opening to the cervix and is the lower part of the birth canal. The vagina is the organ that receives the penis and the ejaculated semen during sexual intercourse. Near the vestibule of the vagina are mucus-producing glands called *Bartholin's glands.*

FIGURE 5-81 The female reproductive system.

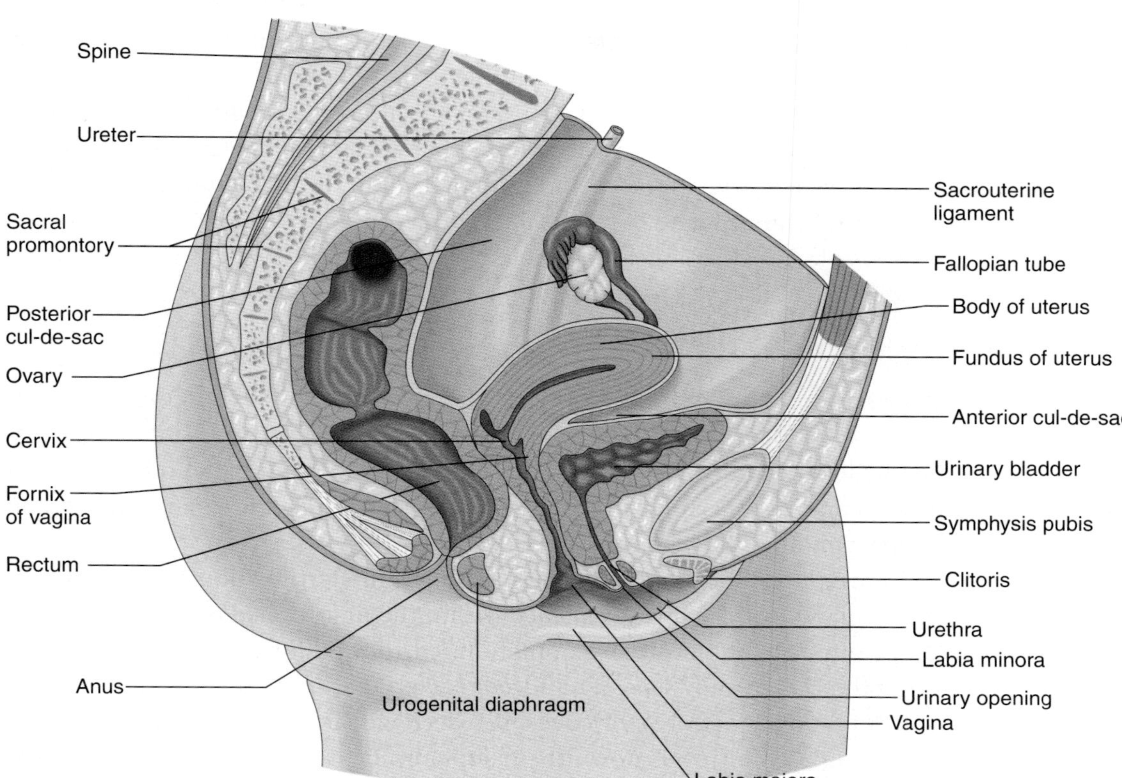

The **uterus** is a pear-shaped, muscular organ consisting of an upper portion, the body, and the cervix or neck. The uterine cavity is small and narrow except during pregnancy, when it expands to accommodate the fetus and a large amount of fluid.

uterus

is a pear-shaped, muscular organ that expands during pregnancy to accommodate the fetus.

The *oviducts,* also called *fallopian tubes,* are the egg-carrying tubes of the female reproductive system. They extend from the uterus to the ovaries. The **ovaries** (female gonads) are a pair of glandular organs located within the pelvic area. The ovaries perform two functions. They produce the ovum and the female sex hormones, *estrogen* and *progesterone.* The *ovum* is the egg cell capable of being fertilized by a spermatozoon and developing into a new life (Figure 5-81).

ovaries

are glandular organs in the pelvis that produce the ovum and female sex hormones.

During each *menstrual cycle* (the regularly recurring series of changes that take place in the ovaries, uterus, and related structures in women), a follicle develops in the ovary and produces estrogen (female hormone) as an ovum (egg) matures. Usually only one follicle matures each cycle (approximately every 28 days). **Ovulation** is the discharge of a mature ovum from the follicle of the ovary. A hormone from the pituitary gland called *luteinizing hormone* transforms the follicle into the *corpus luteum.* This is a yellowish endocrine body formed in the ruptured follicle of the ovary that produces estrogen and progesterone. These hormones promote the lining of the uterus to thicken in preparation to receive the egg if it should be fertilized. Estrogen also controls the development of secondary female sexual characteristics (i.e., breast development, female body contours).

ovulation

is the discharge of a mature ovum from the follicle of the ovary.

The ovum is carried into the fimbriated ends of the oviducts by the action of cilia, which produce a current in the peritoneal fluid. The ovum travels down the oviduct toward the uterus. If the ovum (egg) is fertilized by a sperm cell, pregnancy results. If the ovum is not fertilized, the built-up lining of the uterus sloughs off and is expelled along with the menstrual blood and secretions.

menstruation

is the cyclic, physiologic uterine bleeding that occurs at about four-week intervals during the reproductive period of the female.

Menstruation is the cyclic, physiologic uterine bleeding that normally occurs at about four-week intervals (except during pregnancy) during the reproductive period of the human female. Menstruation begins at puberty and continues until **menopause,** which occurs at about ages 45 to 55. Menopause is the physiologic cessation of the menstrual cycle and therefore the end of the childbearing years.

menopause

is the physiologic cessation of the menstrual cycle.

Pregnancy

pregnancy

or gestation, is the physiologic condition that occurs from the time an ovum is fertilized until childbirth.

gestation

is the same as pregnancy.

Pregnancy, or **gestation** (jes-**TAY**-shun), is the physiologic condition that occurs from the time an ovum is fertilized until childbirth. During pregnancy, the fertilized egg develops in the mother's uterus or womb from a single cell through many stages to a full-term infant. The duration of pregnancy in women is approximately 280 days, or 40 weeks.

Embryonic life begins at conception, with the fertilization of the ovum by the sperm, which usually takes place within the first three days after ovulation and the first few hours after copulation. Of the millions of sperm deposited within the vagina, only several hundred reach the ovum. Of those that reach the ovum, only one penetrates the covering to fertilize the egg. After fertilization, the developing zygote travels down the fallopian tubes and becomes embedded in the uterine wall. The developing form first receives nourishment from the uterine fluids, and then the wall of the uterus until a placenta develops. From about the 12th week, the developing fetus, enclosed in a protective fluid-filled amniotic sac with its own circulatory system, receives nourishment and disposes of its wastes by way of the placenta. The mother's blood and the blood of the fetus never interchange. From the beginning of the third month of pregnancy until birth, the developing child is called a **fetus.** During pregnancy, the mother's metabolism changes because of the demands made on her body systems. Her lungs must provide more oxygen, and her heart must pump more blood. The kidneys must excrete nitrogenous wastes from the fetus and the mother's body.

fetus

is the developing child from the third month of pregnancy until birth.

During pregnancy, the mother needs proper nutrition to provide for the growth of the fetus as well as to maintain the health of all organs as the body prepares for labor and birth.

After childbirth, the mother should maintain her health and that of her child by attention to nutritional needs and by specific exercises to tone and strengthen her muscles.

SECTION QUESTIONS FOR DISCUSSION AND REVIEW

1. What is the reproductive system?
2. What is the difference between asexual and sexual reproduction?
3. What is a gonad?
4. What is a zygote?
5. What are the parts of the male reproductive system?
6. What are the functions of the male reproductive system?
7. What are the parts of the female reproductive system?
8. What are the functions of the female reproductive system?
9. What is the difference between an embryo and a fetus?
10. What is ovulation?
11. What is the approximate duration of pregnancy in women?

PART 3

MASSAGE PRACTICE

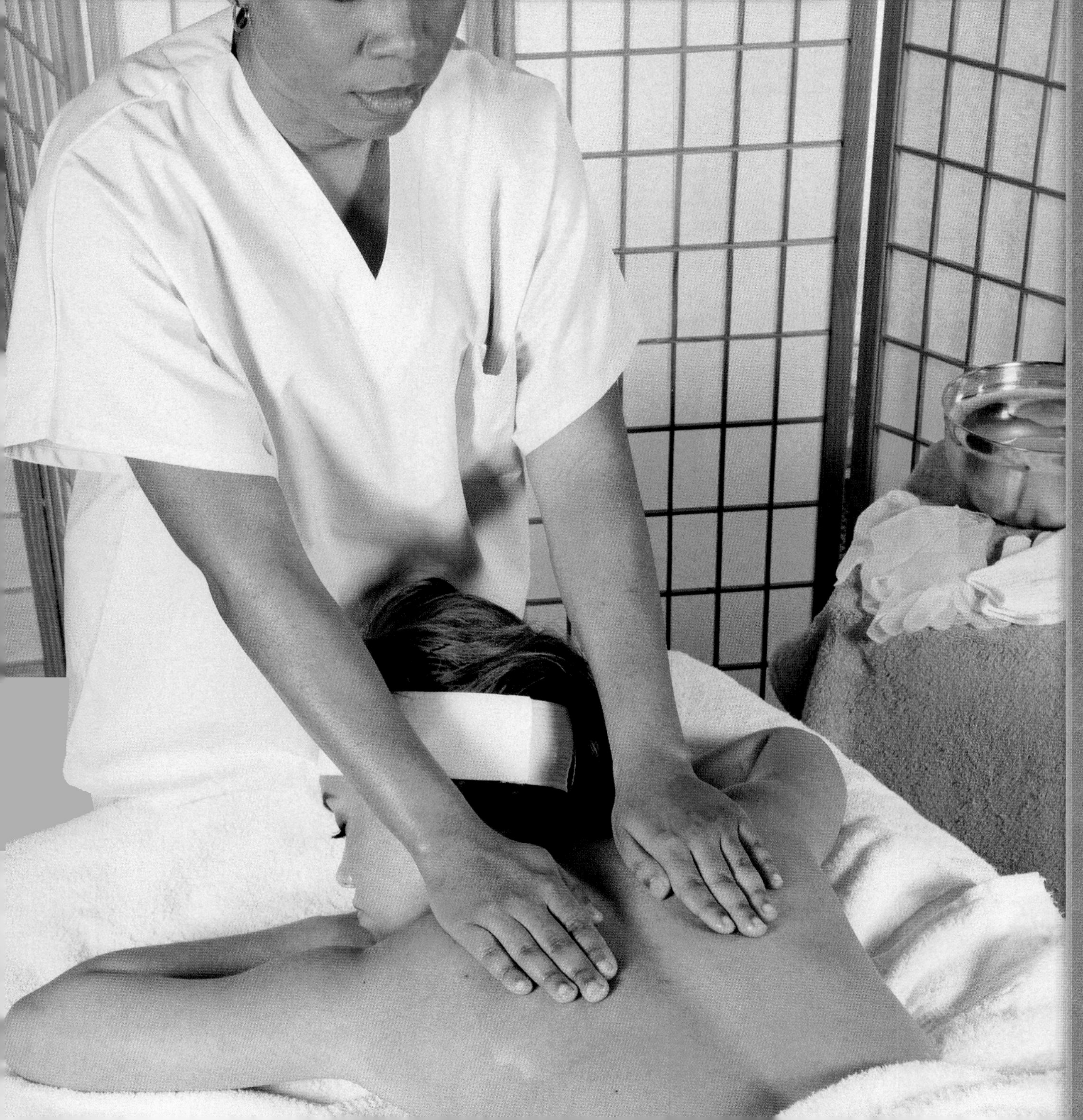

CHAPTER 6

Effects, Benefits, Indications, and Contraindications of Massage

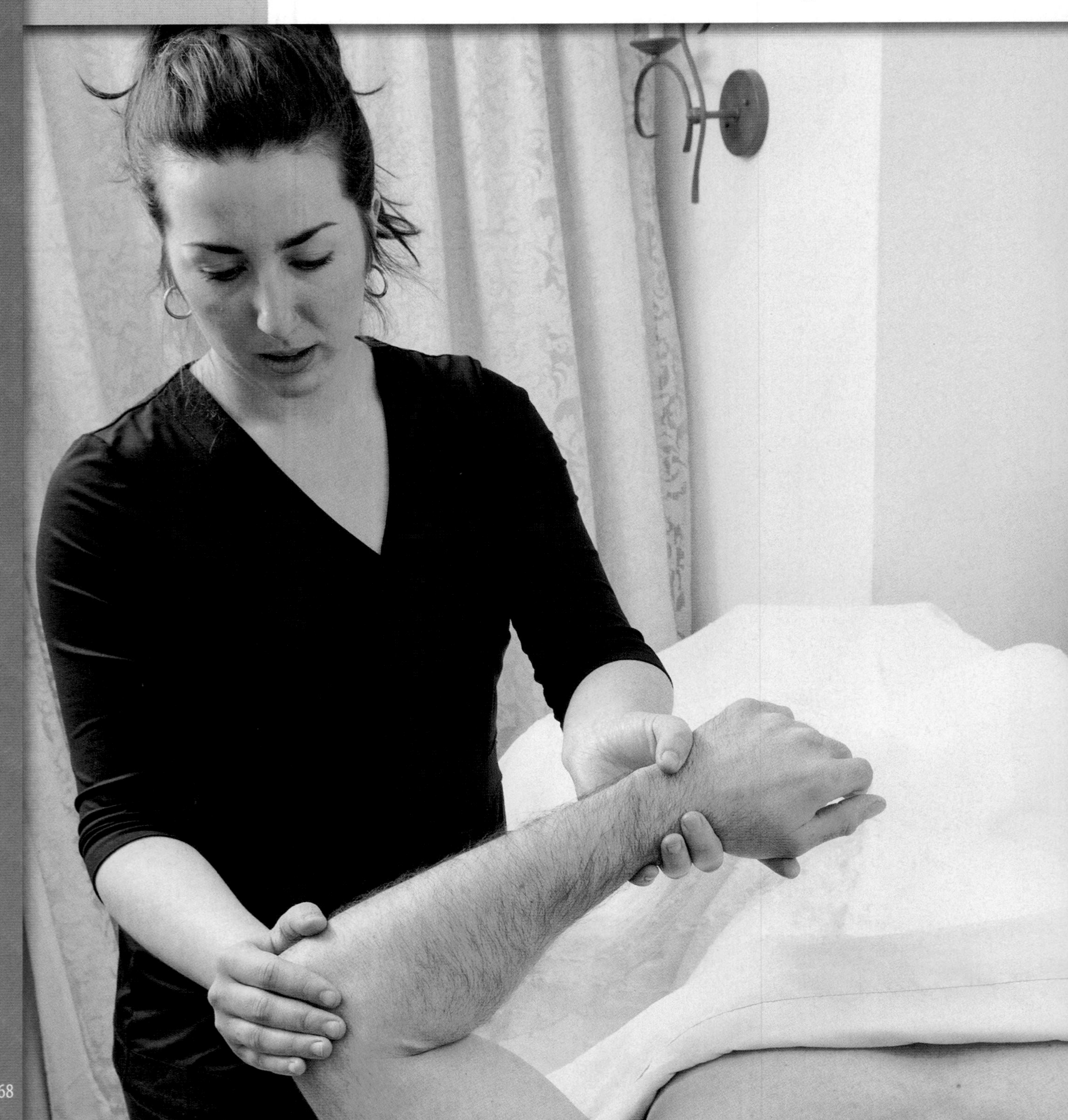

LEARNING OBJECTIVES

After you have mastered this chapter, you will be able to

1. **Explain the physiologic effects and benefits of massage.**
2. **Explain the psychological effects and benefits of massage.**
3. **Describe the effects of massage on the circulatory, muscular, and nervous systems of the body.**
4. **Describe the effects of massage on the skin.**
5. **Explain the main contraindications for massage.**
6. **Differentiate among absolute, regional, and conditional contraindications.**
7. **Identify the major endangerment sites on the body.**

INTRODUCTION

There is much historical evidence to indicate that massage was one of the earliest remedial practices for relief of pain and for the restoration of healthy body functions. Massage is a natural and instinctive method by which minor aches and pains can be soothed away while bringing relief from nervous tension and fatigue.

The term *massage* is applied to different practices. In the following chapters, the techniques of traditional Western, or what is commonly termed Swedish massage and selected soft tissue manipulations of therapeutic massage are considered. The effects of massage differ from one client to another, depending on the needs of the individual client and the goals and intentions with which the massage is administered. This is why massage on two different people can render different results. In addition to physical effects from massage therapy, the client also can experience mental and emotional reactions. Many healthy people believe that frequent massage helps them to remain physically, mentally, and emotionally fit. They enjoy the relaxed, refreshed, and invigorated feeling that they get from a therapeutic massage.

Although massage is not a magic cure-all, it is safe and beneficial for everyone from infants to elderly people, except when there are certain contraindications. A **contraindication** is any physical, emotional, or mental condition that could cause a particular massage treatment to be unsafe or detrimental to the client's well-being. Simply stated, a contraindication is a medical reason not to massage. When there is doubt on the part of the practitioner whether to give massage in the presence of a questionable condition, the client should be referred to her primary health care provider and obtain the physician's recommendations in writing. If the client does not have a primary physician, the practitioner may recommend an appropriate health care professional known to be familiar with and supportive of the practice of massage therapy.

contraindication
is a medical reason not to massage.

EFFECTS AND BENEFITS OF MASSAGE

Massage has direct psychological and physiologic benefits. Physically, massage increases metabolism, hastens healing, relaxes and refreshes the muscles, and improves the functions of the lymphatic system. Massage helps to prevent and relieve muscle cramps and spasms and improves the circulation of blood and lymph, thereby improving the delivery of oxygen and nutrients to the cells as it enhances the removal of metabolic wastes. Because blood carries nutrients to the skin, massage is beneficial in keeping the skin functioning in a normal, healthy manner. Massage therapy is effective in pain management in conditions such as arthritis, neuritis, neuralgia, labor and delivery, whiplash, muscular lesions, sciatica, headache, muscle spasms, and many other conditions.

Psychologically, massage relieves fatigue, reduces tension and anxiety, calms the nervous system, and promotes a sense of relaxation and renewed energy.

There are indications that massage is beneficial in numerous conditions; however, in cases of injury or disease, the client's physician must be consulted before massage treatments are given. Massage has been credited with being of great benefit in helping patients to recover from various illnesses or injuries. In some cases, the client's physician might recommend modalities that use heat, light, cold, and water. A physician can recommend massage for both its physical and psychological benefits.

Physiologic Effects of Massage

Skillfully applied massage is an effective means of influencing the structures and functions of the body. The specific effects of any massage vary according to the intent with which it is given, the selection of techniques used, and the condition of the client. Depending on the type and manner of manipulation, a sense of mild relaxation, stimulation, or refreshment can follow massage. Under no circumstances should massage be applied with such intensity that it causes the client to feel exhausted or results in bruised or injured tissues.

There are two physical effects of massage, mechanical and reflex, which can occur separately or together.

- Mechanical effects are direct physical effects of the massage techniques on the tissues that they contact.
- Reflex effects of massage are indirect responses to touch that affect body functions and tissues through the nervous or energy systems of the body.

Gentle stimulation of the sensory nerve endings in the skin, as in superficial stroking, results in reflex effects, either locally or in distant parts of the body. When pressure is applied to the muscles, blood, and lymph vessels, or to any internal structure, both reflex and direct mechanical effects are experienced. Pressure on reflex points, active trigger points, and other pressure points reflexively affects functions or areas of the body away from the actual point of contact.

The immediate effects of massage are noticeable on the skin. Friction and stroking movements heighten blood circulation to the skin and increase the activity of the sweat (sudoriferous) and oil (sebaceous) glands. Accompanying the increased flow of blood, there is a slight reddening and warming of the skin. Nutrition to the skin is improved. Massage treatments over time impart a healthy radiance to the skin, making it softer, suppler, and of finer texture.

The physiologic effects of massage are not limited to the skin. The body as a whole benefits by the stimulation of muscular, glandular, and vascular activities. Most organs of the body are favorably influenced by clinical massage treatments.

Effects of Massage on the Muscular System

Muscles are the primary targets for many Swedish, neuromuscular, and myofascial techniques. These techniques have both mechanical and reflex effects on the muscular system. Mechanical effects enhance circulation to and from the muscles, deform sensory and proprioceptive nerve endings, and stretch and compress various connective tissues. Reflex effects relax or reset muscle tone, cause **hyperemia** (high-per-**EE**-mee-eh), and warm the tissues. Massage is also an effective means of relaxing tense muscles, releasing muscle spasms and reducing trigger point activity.

hyperemia

hyper = increased or excessive; -emia = blood; increased blood in an area of the body.

The supply of blood to the muscles is proportional to their activity. It is estimated that blood passes more rapidly through muscles being massaged than muscles at rest. Petrissage or kneading and compression movements create a pumping action that stimulates venous blood and lymph circulation away from the tissues and brings a fresh supply of blood to the muscles. Because it has been shown to increase circulation, massage aids in the removal of metabolic waste products and helps to nourish tissues.

Massage prevents and relieves stiffness and soreness of muscles. Muscles fatigued by work or exercise are more quickly restored by massage than by passive rest of the same duration.

Muscle tissue that has suffered injury heals more quickly with less connective tissue buildup and scarring when therapeutic massage is applied appropriately and regularly. Massage is contraindicated during the acute inflammatory stage following a soft tissue injury. When the initial swelling has subsided, however, appropriate massage enhances the healing process. Massage can release fascial restrictions and reduce the thickening of connective tissues (hyperplasia), allowing more flexibility and easier, pain-free movement. Friction massage, when properly applied, prevents and reduces the development of adhesions and excessive scarring after trauma.

Massage can have positive effects on the range of motion (ROM) of limbs that have a limited range because of tissue injury, inflammation, muscle tension, or strain. The client might have experienced discomfort or pain, resulting in limited use of a limb, or he might have stopped using the limb completely. The limb must be taken through the ROM passively and carefully and the range increased gradually.

Passive movement is the method by which joints are moved through their ROM with no resistance or assistance by any muscular activity on the part of the client. Passive massage movements benefit circulation of the blood and lymph, nourish the skin, relax and lengthen the muscles, soothe the nerves, and lubricate the joints.

Active joint movement in massage refers to exercises in which the voluntary muscles are contracted by the client and either resisted or assisted by the therapist. Active joint movements have beneficial effects similar to exercise. They help to firm and strengthen muscles, improve circulation, and aid the function of related internal organs.

Effects of Massage on the Nervous System

nervous system
controls and coordinates all the body systems and includes the nerves, spinal cord, and brain.

central nervous system
consists of the brain and spinal cord.

peripheral nervous system
consists of all the nerves that connect the CNS to the rest of the body.

sympathetic nervous system
is responsible for preparing the body to expend energy in response to emergency situations. .

parasympathetic nervous system
functions to conserve energy and reverse the action of the sympathetic division.

The **nervous system** consists of the **central nervous system** (CNS, brain and spinal cord) and the **peripheral nervous system**. The peripheral nervous system includes the autonomic nervous system, the cranial nerves, and the spinal nerves. The cranial and spinal nerves are made up of somatic (motor) nerves and sensory nerves. The autonomic nervous system is composed of the **sympathetic nervous system** and the **parasympathetic nervous system**.

The sensory nerves and their associated nerve receptors provide input to the central nervous system about what is happening in the body and the surrounding environment. These are the nerves that are influenced by massage. Information from sensory input is processed in the CNS, then appropriate responses are sent out by various neurotransmitters, the somatic nerves, and the autonomic nervous system, to maintain homeostasis.

The effects of massage on the nervous system depend on the direct and reflex reaction of the nerves stimulated. The nervous system can be stimulated or soothed, depending on the type of massage movement applied.

Stimulation of the peripheral nerve receptors can have reflex reactions affecting the autonomic nervous system, neurotransmitters in the brain, pain perception, or the underlying joints and muscles of the areas being massaged.

1. Stimulating massage techniques
    a. Friction (light rubbing, rolling, and wringing movements) stimulates nerves.
    b. Percussion (light tapping and slapping movements) increases nervous irritability. Strong percussion for a short period excites nerve centers directly. Prolonged percussion tends to anesthetize the local nerves.
    c. Vibration (shaking and trembling movements) stimulates peripheral nerves and all nerve centers with which a nerve trunk is connected.
2. Sedative effect of massage techniques
    a. Gentle stroking produces calming and sedative results.
    b. Light friction and petrissage (kneading movements) produce marked sedative effects.
    c. Holding pressure (ischemic compression) on a sensitive trigger point desensitizes the point and helps to release the pathophysiologic reflex cycle that maintains hypertension in the associated muscle.

Effects of Massage on the Autonomic Nervous System

The effects of massage on the autonomic nervous system are mostly reflexive. The autonomic nervous system is divided into the sympathetic nervous system and the parasympathetic nervous system. The sympathetic nervous system is responsible for preparing the body to expend energy in response to emergency situations, commonly referred to as "fight-or-flight" preparation. Activation of the sympathetic nervous system is related to stress, real or perceived. Sympathetic stimulation initiates an accelerated heart rate, blood is diverted to the muscles, elimination and digestion are inhibited, adrenal secretions of **epinephrine/adrenaline** and **norepinephrine** are increased, sweat glands are activated, and the body is more alert and attentive.

The parasympathetic system is responsible for counteracting the effects of the sympathetic system and establishing the normalizing and restorative functions of a non-alarm state. Stimulation of the parasympathetic system causes a reduced heart rate, increased digestion and elimination, and increased circulation to the internal organs in a relaxation/restorative response. The sympathetic and parasympathetic nervous systems work together to maintain **homeostasis**.

epinephrine

"fight" or "flight" hormone that prepares the body to respond to emergencies.

norepinephrine

"fight" or "flight" hormone that prepares the body to respond to emergencies.

homeostasis

is the internal balance of the body.

Initially, massage seems to alert the sympathetic nervous system. Short, invigorating massage, such as pre-event sports massage or 15-minute chair massage, tends to stimulate the body, leaving it more alert and energized. Longer, relaxing massage, however, seems to affect the autonomic nervous system by sedating the sympathetic nervous system and stimulating the parasympathetic nervous system. As a result, blood levels of epinephrine and norepinephrine are reduced, heart rate and blood pressure are reduced, and the relaxation response is increased.

Effects of Massage on Neurotransmitters

Various studies by Tiffany Fields and her associates at the Touch Research Institute (TRI) in Miami, Florida, have provided compelling evidence that massage promotes relaxation and relieves stress. One study at the institute showed that people who received 15-minute massages twice a week exhibited a decreased beta wave and an increased delta wave when given an electroencephalogram (EEG). These same subjects performed better on math tests, completing the tests in significantly less time and with significantly fewer mistakes. Job-related stress, anxiety, and blood levels of cortisol (the stress hormone) were also reduced (Field, Ironson, Scafidi, et al., 1996). Massage therapy reduces anxiety while it enhances EEG patterns of alertness and the ability to do math computations (*International Journal of Neuroscience, 86,* 197–205, 1996).

Research has shown that massage influences the levels of several neurochemicals or elements related to, or that regulate, various physiologic functions. As mentioned previously, massage reduces the blood levels of the stress-related adrenal hormones epinephrine and norepinephrine. Studies also indicate that massage has been found to increase the levels of serotonin, dopamine, endorphins, and enkephalins — neurochemicals related to elevated moods and pain control.

Epinephrine/adrenaline and norepinephrine/noradrenaline are produced in the adrenal medulla and are excreted into the bloodstream in response to stimulation of the sympathetic nervous system. These hormones are also neurotransmitters that stimulate alertness and attentiveness in response to fear or in preparation for the fight-or-flight response. Epinephrine functions in the body; norepinephrine is active in the brain.

Mental and emotional stresses are directly related to increased levels of adrenaline/epinephrine. Low levels of epinephrine and norepinephrine cause drowsiness, low energy, fatigue, and sluggishness.

Short invigorating massage tends to stimulate the production of epinephrine and norepinephrine, whereas a full, relaxing, one-hour rhythmic massage decreases the levels of epinephrine and norepinephrine and encourages relaxation.

dopamine

is a neurotransmitter that controls fine movement, emotional response, and the ability to experience pleasure and pain.

Dopamine is a neurotransmitter that affects brain functions that control fine movement, emotional response, and the ability to experience pleasure and pain. Elevated levels of dopamine lead to feelings of pleasure and excitement, improvement of mood, alertness, and sex drive. A decline of dopamine in the brain is linked to cognitive and movement problems. Parkinson's disease is caused by the body's inability to produce dopamine.

serotonin

is a neurotransmitter that helps to regulate nerve impulses and influences mood, behavior, appetite, blood pressure, temperature regulation, memory, and learning ability.

Serotonin is a neurotransmitter that is synthesized in the brain and found in the brain, bloodstream, and intestinal walls. Serotonin has a broad range of influences, including mood, behavior, appetite, blood pressure, temperature regulation, memory, and learning ability. Serotonin seems to modify behavior in a way that counterbalances the effects of norepinephrine. Whereas norepinephrine is released in response to stimulants, stress, and anxiety, serotonin promotes a sense of calm and well-being. It seems to regulate moods in a quieting, comforting manner. Serotonin also suppresses outbursts and irritability while reducing cravings for food or sex. A low level of serotonin is implicated in depression, eating disorders, personality disorders, sleep disturbances, and schizophrenia.

Massage increases levels of available serotonin and dopamine. Increased levels of serotonin and dopamine indicate decreased stress and depression and an elevated mood.

Massage increases the secretions of endorphins and enkephalins in the CNS. These elements are mood elevators and natural painkillers. Endorphins interact with pain receptors in the brain in a manner very similar to that of morphine and codeine. Besides reducing the sensation of pain, enkephalins and endorphins are related to feelings of euphoria, appetite control, and enhancement of the immune system.

Effect of Massage on Pain

gate control theory

the positive effects of relaxing massage interrupts the transmission of pain sensations of affected nociceptors from entering the central nervous system by stimulating other cutaneous receptors.

Massage is effective in reducing pain owing to several neurologic processes and conditions. The positive effects of relaxing massage interrupt the transmission of pain sensations of affected nociceptors from entering the CNS by stimulating other cutaneous receptors, because of what is known as the **gate control theory**. According to the gate control theory, painful impulses are transmitted along small- and large-diameter nerve fibers from nociceptors to the spinal cord and on to the brain. Stimulation of thermo- or mechanoreceptors by rubbing, massaging, icing, or other means is transmitted along the larger fibers and suppresses the pain sensations at the gate, where the fibers enter the spinal column. Evidence of this theory can be witnessed in the instinctive practice of briskly rubbing a part of the body that has been bumped or struck by an object to relieve the intensity of the pain.

As mentioned before, massage also reduces the sensation of pain by increasing the concentration of endorphins and enkephalins and other pain-reducing neurochemicals in the CNS and bloodstream.

Massage can relieve referred myofascial pain and reduce ischemia-related pain by releasing hypersensitive trigger points and restoring circulation to hypertonic muscle tissue.

Certain massage techniques affect the proprioceptive mechanisms of the muscles' spindle receptors and the Golgi tendon organs. Techniques such as compression, positioning, stretching, and pressure alter the feedback circuits and allow new pain-free possibilities for muscle length and function.

Effects of Massage on the Circulatory System

Clinical massage affects the quality and quantity of blood coursing through the various parts of the circulatory system. With the increased flow of blood to the massaged area, better cellular nutrition and elimination are favored. The work of the heart is lessened because of the improvement in surface circulation. Blood pressure and heart rate are temporarily reduced at the same time the systolic stroke volume is increased and capillary beds dilate and become more permeable. Under the influence of massage, the blood-making process is improved, resulting in an increase in the number of red and white blood cells (Figure 6-1). In 1992, studies at Touch Research Institute showed an increase in the presence and activity of T4 killer cells in the bloodstreams of people with HIV after receiving massage, indicating that massage might strengthen the immune system.

An important principle to remember in Swedish massage is to always massage **centripetally** or toward the heart. Massage movements should be directed upward along the limbs and lower parts of the body and downward from the head, thereby facilitating the flow of venous blood and lymph back toward the heart and other eliminatory organs.

centripetal

referring to a direction, toward the center (heart).

Massage can influence the blood and lymph vessels either by direct mechanical action on the vessel walls or by reflex action through the vasomotor nerves. Pressure against the vessels not only tones their muscular walls but also propels the movement of the blood. The vasomotor nerves, by controlling the relaxing and constricting of the blood vessels, determine the amount of blood that reaches the area being massaged.

Massage movements affect blood and lymph channels in the following ways:

1. Light stroking produces an almost instantaneous, although temporary, dilation of the capillaries, whereas deep stroking brings about a more lasting dilation and flushing of the massaged area.
2. Light percussion causes a contraction of the blood vessels, which tend to relax as the movement is continued.
3. Friction hastens the flow of blood through the superficial veins, increases the permeability of the capillary beds, and produces an increased flow of interstitial fluid. This creates a healthier environment for the cells.
4. Petrissage or kneading stimulates the flow of blood through the deeper arteries and veins.

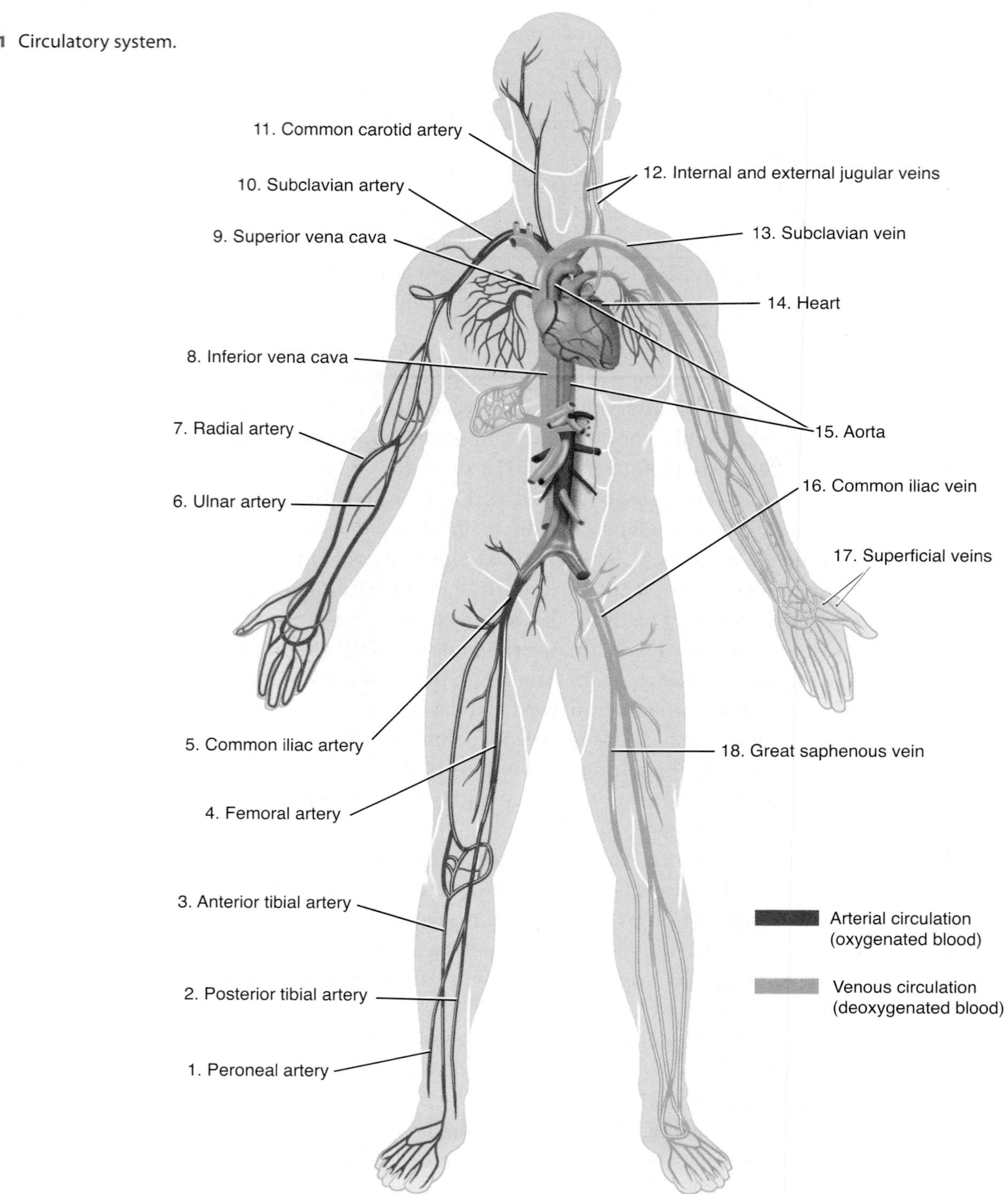

FIGURE 6-1 Circulatory system.

5. Properly applied, light massage enhances lymph flow and reduces certain types of edema.
6. Compression produces a hyperemia or an increase in the amount of blood stored in the muscle tissue.

Psychological Effects of Massage

The psychological effects of massage should not be underestimated. If the client feels healthier, invigorated, and more energetic, the massage has been worth the effort. In treatment centers for addictions, massage has proved to be an effective therapeutic tool to rebuild a more positive self-image and sense of self-worth. Victims of sexual abuse and rape indicate having an improved self-image and a reduction of an aversion to touch after receiving therapeutic massage. Massage has also been shown to reduce depression and anxiety in adolescents who have experienced sexual or verbal abuse (Fields 1993). People have regular massages as much for psychological as for physical benefit.

Many people suffer from stress and find that massage promotes relaxation and mental alertness as it soothes away minor aches and pains. For some clients, regular massage keeps them feeling more youthful and encourages them to pay more attention to proper nutrition, exercise, and good health practices.

Massage helps clients to become more aware of where they are holding tension, and where they have tight muscles or painful areas. The practitioner can discover areas that the client might not have been aware of previously. By getting in touch with or becoming aware of these conditions, the client can begin to focus on relaxing them both during the massage and on a daily basis. Becoming aware of these trouble spots and responding to them is considered a part of preventive maintenance.

CONDITIONS GENERALLY RELIEVED BY MASSAGE

Almost all healthy people occasionally have some physical condition that can be improved by massage. When relief is obtained, there is also a renewed sense of well-being. No matter how well a client is, a good massage can leave that person feeling even better.

The following conditions are most frequently relieved by regular massage treatment:

1. Stress and tensions are relieved. With the relief of tension and stress, the client feels better able to cope with day-to-day situations.
2. Mental and physical fatigue is relieved, leading to renewed energy and ambition.
3. Pain in the shoulders, neck, and back (when caused by strained muscles or irritated nerves) is relieved.
4. Muscles and joints become suppler, and soreness and stiffness are relieved.
5. Muscle soreness from overexertion can be reduced or prevented.
6. Circulation is improved, thus improving delivery of nutrients to and removal of wastes from the tissues.
7. Digestion, assimilation, and elimination are often improved.
8. Facial massage helps to tone the skin, helps prevent blemished skin, and softens fine lines.
9. Headache and eyestrain are often relieved.
10. Deep relaxation is induced, and insomnia is often relieved.

11. Muscular spasms are relieved.
12. Obesity (being overweight) and flabby muscles can be improved when combined with proper exercise, diet programs, and massage.
13. Pain in joints, sprains, and poor circulation are relieved.
14. Increased circulation of nourishing blood to the skin and other parts of the body encourages healing.
15. Mental strain is reduced, resulting in better productivity.
16. Mildly high blood pressure is temporarily reduced.
17. Renewed sense of confidence and control is experienced.
18. Constrictions and adhesions can be reduced or prevented as traumatized muscle tissue heals.
19. Joint mobility can be increased.

CONTRAINDICATIONS FOR MASSAGE

Although there are many benefits from therapeutic body massage, there are also contraindications of which the professional practitioner must be aware.

Contraindication means that the expected treatment or process is inadvisable. In massage, it means that conditions exist in which it would not be beneficial to apply massage to a part or all of the body. Contraindications can be absolute, regional, or conditional.

- A contraindication is absolute when massage is absolutely not appropriate, such as in cases of severe, uncontrolled hypertension; abnormally high fever; shock; acute pneumonia; or toxemia during pregnancy.
- Regional or partial contraindications prohibit administering massage to only a local part of the body, such as local contagious conditions, open wounds, or acute neuritis or arthritis, but massaging other areas is fine.
- Conditional contraindications require the practitioner to adjust the massage when there are health concerns for which certain massage techniques might cause discomfort or have adverse effects, although other therapeutic applications are very beneficial.

The practitioner must know not only when massage is advised but also, more important, when it should be avoided, or when certain strokes or movements should not be used.

When you define massage as a form of touch that is applied in a therapeutic manner, then it is true that massage of some form is beneficial to nearly everyone. There are situations, however, in which particular manipulations might not only be uncomfortable for the client but also could be dangerous. There are numerous styles and modalities of massage and bodywork ranging from deep tissue techniques that test a person's tolerance, to gentle techniques using the lightest pressure against the skin. Some modalities are directed toward body structure and some toward fluid circulation, whereas others focus on the body's energy fields. The reason that a client comes for a massage and the client's current health condition determine the therapist's choice of massage techniques.

Many conditions are both indicated and contraindicated for massage. Many conditions respond favorably to massage, whereas others can be aggravated or worsened by specific massage techniques. Certain movements could do more harm than good, and such techniques are therefore contraindicated. It is the responsibility of the practitioner to understand fully the indications and contraindications for massage.

During the first interview or consultation with a client, it is important to obtain information about the state of the client's health and determine any reasons why massage treatments might be inadvisable. A client intake form that includes a medical history is helpful. Careful questioning about the client's condition is essential in determining whether contraindications exist. When these conditions exist, the client is usually already under the care of a doctor. Most contraindications are conditional. When a client is under the care of a physician, the client should inform the doctor about receiving massages and request a written recommendation that includes both precautions and indications for massage. In this way, the practitioner becomes part of a health care team, and massage becomes an integral part of the client's health program. In many cases, the physician might not be aware of massage procedures and their benefits. With the client's permission, the practitioner can confer with the physician regarding the client's condition, the effects and benefits of massage, and any precautions or recommendations that the doctor might have. It is important for the practitioner to follow any recommendations that the physician might have.

Often during the interview or during the course of a massage, conditions that the client might be unaware of become apparent. When these are contraindicated or a medical concern, they should be referred to the attention of a physician. When in doubt, caution is the best policy. The client can be asked (tactfully) to supply a physician's report or recommendations before beginning or continuing treatments, or the practitioner could, again after receiving the client's consent, ask the client's physician first when there are questionable circumstances.

Because massage requires a great deal of physical energy on the part of the practitioner, mechanical and electrical apparatus have been devised as aids to manual massage. The hand vibrator is an example. The same contraindications for manual massage also apply when any kind of aid apparatus is used.

The major contraindications include the following:

- *Abnormal body temperature:* 98.6° F (Fahrenheit), or 37° C (Celsius), is considered normal body temperature, but this can vary depending on the time of day or other factors. Normal body temperature can vary from 96.4° to 99.1°F (35.8° to 37.3°C). Some doctors and therapists say that massage is not recommended when temperature exceeds 99.4° F. If the client feels abnormally warm or feverish, the temperature should be taken to ascertain the advisability of massage treatment. Massage is contraindicated when the client has a fever. Generally, a fever indicates that the body is trying to isolate and eliminate an invading pathogen. The body is stepping up its own action to confine, narrow down, and eliminate the problem. Massage in this case would tend to work against the body's defense mechanisms.

- *Acute infectious disease:* Typhoid, diphtheria, severe colds, influenza, and similar illness preclude massage. Giving a massage to a person who is coming down with an acute viral infection (cold or flu) tends to intensify the illness and also exposes the therapist to the virus. Massage is systemically contraindicated, and the client should contact her physician.
- *Inflammation:* When there is acute inflammation in a particular area of the body, massage is inadvisable because it could further irritate the area or intensify the inflammation. This is particularly true for spreading or penetrating types of massage manipulations. Inflamed joints do not indicate massage of the joint itself; however, there are some pressure point applications that are useful. Therapeutic touch, which is simply placing your hands on or near the inflamed area, can be helpful.

Although working directly on an area might be contraindicated, working on a reflex or related area or working in an area proximal to the affected area can be useful because it tends to stimulate circulation and the natural healing properties of the body. A reflex point is an area that is distant to the affected area that when stimulated has an effect on that area.

There are numerous types of inflammations. A word having the suffix -itis pertains to inflammation. For example, arthritis is an inflammation of the joints; neuritis is an inflammation of a nerve or nerves; dermatitis is inflammation of the skin. Caution must be used when a client has any kind of inflammation that could be aggravated by massage.

Inflammation from tissue damage: When tissue is damaged, the body's natural response is inflammation. Inflammation is characterized by swelling, redness, heat, and pain.

Signs of Inflammation

- swelling
- redness
- heat
- pain

If the tissue damage is of a traumatic nature and severe enough, blood vessels can be damaged, resulting in a hematoma (hee-muh-**TOE**-muh). The area becomes swollen and discolored. The bluish color is from blood escaping from the damaged blood vessels. Any reddening is a sign of inflammation. Inflammation is the body's natural defense mechanism for protecting and speeding healing to the tissues.

Inflammation from bacterial infestation: If there is pus or a pus pocket formed, massage is definitely contraindicated. *Pus* is a combination of dead white blood cells and bacteria. If it is disturbed, there is a chance of spreading the infection. If the pus gets into the bloodstream, there is a chance of a serious systemic infection.

Osteoporosis: This condition leads to deterioration of bone. In advanced stages, bones become brittle, sometimes to the point that they are easily broken. Osteoporosis is prevalent in elderly people and in certain kinds of diseases. The symptoms of osteoporosis include frailty and stooped shoulders. In women, osteoporosis can be from reduced estrogen levels. It is best to obtain the advice of the client's physician before giving massage when osteoporosis is indicated (Figure 6-2).

Varicose veins: Varicose veins is a condition in which the valves in the veins break down because of back pressure in the circulatory system. The veins bulge and rupture, usually in the legs. The development of varicose veins is often the result of gravity or obstructed venous flow, as the result of certain postures that inhibit circulation to or from the legs. Varicose veins are often hereditary or can be the result of standing for long hours. In women, the pressure on the large veins in the pelvic area during pregnancy often contributes to this condition.

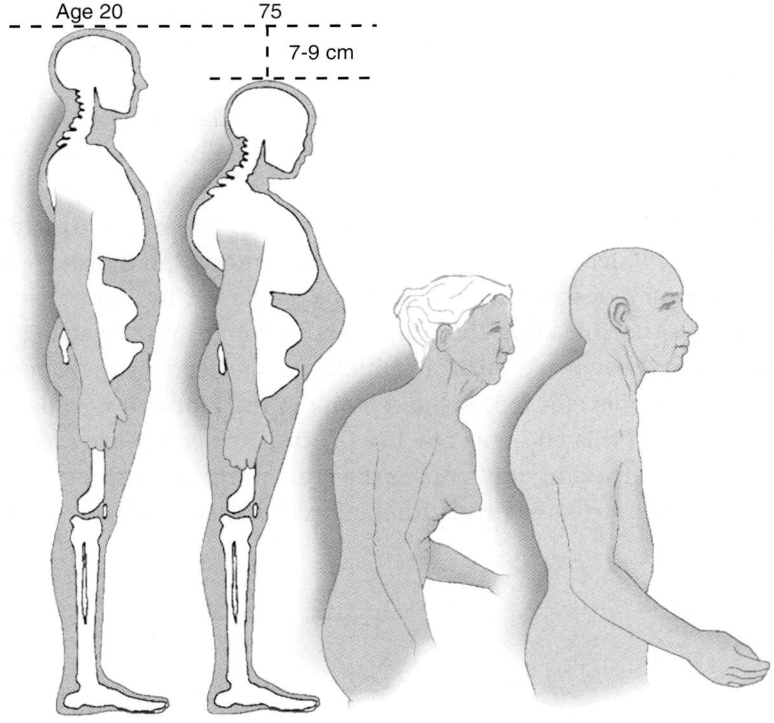

FIGURE 6-2 Symptoms of osteoporosis often include stooped shoulders.

Blood is pumped through the veins by means of pressure originating in the heart and is helped along by contractions of muscle surrounding the veins. Veins are basically tubes consisting of a layer of endothelial lining and smooth muscle and are covered with connective tissue. Many veins, especially those in the arms and legs, have a system of valves that prevent blood from flowing backward in the vein and act as a *venous pump* to move the blood toward the heart. These valves are flaplike structures that protrude from the inside walls of the vein in such a way that blood moving toward the heart pushes past the valve, but if the blood attempts to move in the reverse direction, pressure against the valve forces it closed and blood cannot pass. The venous pump is a phenomenon that results when muscles contract and exert external pressure on the veins, which tends to collapse them. As the vein is repeatedly collapsed, the blood is forced along through the system of valves toward the heart (Figure 6-3).

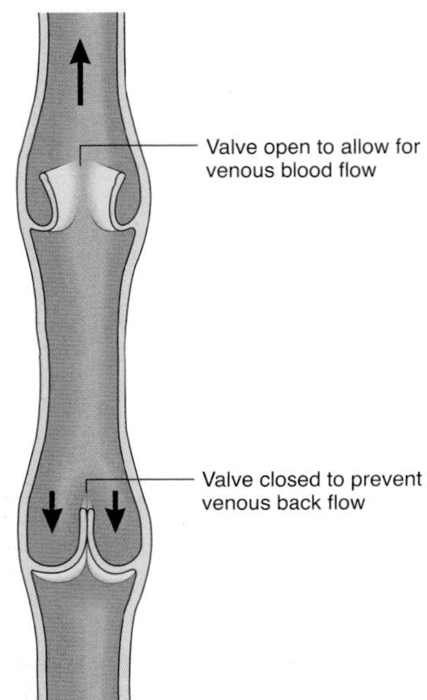

FIGURE 6-3 A vein valve.

Extensive back pressure in the veins from prolonged standing or blockage causes the veins to enlarge and stretch to the point that the valves become incompetent. The weight of the blood further distends the veins and more valves become dysfunctional, perpetuating the condition. When veins become abnormally dilated from excessive back pressure, they rupture and are called *varicose*. Blood then accumulates in enlarged portions of the vein. If the flow of blood becomes obstructed, clotting can occur. When this condition is accompanied by inflammation, it is painful and potentially dangerous. Increased pressure in the veins also increases pressure in the capillaries and often results in edema.

The practitioner can recognize varicose veins as bluish, protruding, thick, bulbous, distended superficial veins usually found in the lower legs. Also to be considered with caution are the small reddish groupings of broken blood vessels that often surround a small, protruding vein. Any deep massage on these areas could set a blood clot loose in the general circulation and cause a serious problem (Figure 6-4).

It is easy to see why massage would be contraindicated in cases of varicosities. Massage proximal to the affected area might be very helpful, however, especially superficial (barely touching) techniques.

phlebitis

is an inflammation of a vein accompanied by pain and swelling.

thrombophlebitis

is the inflammation of veins from blood clots.

embolus

is a piece of a clot that loosens and floats in the blood.

Phlebitis: Inflammation of a vein accompanied by pain and swelling is called **phlebitis** (fle-**BY**-tis). Phlebitis can be the result of surgery, can be secondary to an infection or injury, or can have no apparent precursor. In many cases of phlebitis, a blood clot forms along the wall of the inflamed vein, causing the dangerous condition known as **thrombophlebitis,** or deep vein thrombosis (DVT). If a piece of this clot loosens and floats in the blood, it is called an **embolus** (**EM**-bo-lus). If this embolus reaches the lungs, it can cause death by pulmonary embolism. If the embolus reaches the brain or the nourishing vessels of the heart, it can cause stroke or myocardial infarction (heart attack).

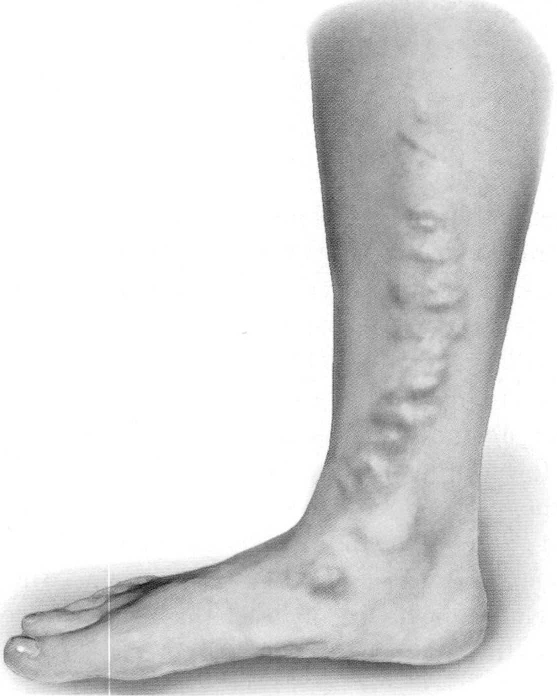

FIGURE 6-4 Varicose veins appear as bluish, protruding, thick, bulbous, distended superficial veins usually found in the lower legs.

Postsurgical: Always obtain the physician's permission before applying massage following surgery. The possibility of thrombosis is increased for a while following surgery. Massage over a fresh incision is contraindicated; however, after the initial healing has taken place, specialized connective tissue massage can help to reduce excessive scar formation and adhesions. If an incision has already healed, creating excessive scar tissue and adhesions to the neighboring fascia, muscles, or skin, specialized scar tissue massage can be applied to break down the adhesions and reduce the associated pain and discomfort.

Aneurosa: An *aneurosa* (an-yoo-**RO**-suh) or **aneurysm** (**AN**-yoo-rizm) is a localized dilation of a blood vessel or, more commonly, an artery. It can be caused by a congenital defect, arteriosclerosis, hypertension, or trauma and is generally located in the aorta, thorax, and abdomen or sometimes in the cranium. Although this condition can appear, it is rarely encountered in massage, and if suspected, should be referred to medical attention.

aneurysm

is a local distention or ballooning of an artery due to a weakening wall.

Hematoma: A **hematoma** is a mass of blood trapped in some tissue or cavity of the body and is the result of internal bleeding. **Contusions** (kun-**TOO**-zhuns) or bruises are common types of hematomas that are generally not too serious. Contusions usually occur as a result of a blow that is severe enough to break a blood vessel. The escaping blood leaves the familiar black-and-blue spot. The blood quickly clots, and over time the body naturally reabsorbs the cellular debris. The bruise changes color to shades of green and yellow and eventually disappears.

hematoma

is a mass of blood trapped in some tissue or cavity of the body and is the result of internal bleeding.

contusion

or bruise is a common type of hematoma that is generally not too serious.

When the hematoma is in the acute phase, massage is contraindicated because of the risk of reinjuring the tissue. After the bruise begins to change colors, light massage enhances circulation to the area and actually assists the healing.

A cranial hematoma is a serious condition that is usually the result of a blow to the head. A broken blood vessel inside the cranium forms a tumor-like mass that puts pressure on the brain. Depending on the location and severity of the hematoma, symptoms range from headache, confusion, and drowsiness, to paralysis, loss of consciousness, and death. The only treatment for cranial hematoma is surgery to remove the pressure.

Edema: **Edema** (e-**DEE**-muh) is a circulatory abnormality that generally appears as puffiness or swelling in the extremities but is sometimes more widespread. Edema is an excess accumulation of fluid in tissue spaces; it has numerous causes. In some instances, massage is indicated, and in others, it is not. If edema is the result of back pressure in the veins from immobility, massage and mild exercise can prove helpful. Conversely, if edema is the result of protein imbalance because of breakdown in the kidneys or liver, or is the result of increased permeability (allowing passage especially of fluids) of the capillaries from inflammation, massage is contraindicated.

edema

is a condition of excess fluid in the interstitial spaces.

When edema is suspected, it can be easily detected by pressing a finger into the area. When the finger is removed and an indentation remains, edema is present. This indentation will take several seconds to return to the level of adjoining skin. This is called *pitting edema.* Local circulatory massage is contraindicated for all cases of pitting edema.

Edema can result from an imbalance of factors that regulate the interchange of fluids between the capillaries and tissue spaces. Other causes can be related to heart or kidney disease, poison in the system (affecting histamine levels that cause increased capillary permeability), or an obstruction of lymph channels. If edema is related to pregnancy and is caused by toxemia (poisons in the blood), massage is definitely contraindicated.

Obviously, such conditions should be brought to the attention of a physician. The reason for the edema must be known before massage is performed on the edematous tissue.

lymphedema

is an accumulation of interstitial fluid, or swelling, in the soft tissues caused by inflammation, blockage, or removal of the lymph channels.

Lymphedema: **Lymphedema** is swelling, usually in an extremity, when fluid accumulates in the interstitial spaces because it is unable to pass into and through the lymph channels. *Primary lymphedema* is a congenital or genetic condition in which a portion of the lymphatic system does not develop completely. *Secondary lymphedema* is the result of trauma, surgery, radiation, infection, or some other event that damages lymph tissue or otherwise interferes with the lymph transport system. Lymphedema is a localized condition. Generalized or deep massage on the limb with lymphedema is contraindicated; however, massage on the rest of the body is fine. Light massage on the affected limb should be performed last and directed distally to proximally. The most appropriate form of massage to be performed on the affected area is *manual lymph drainage massage*, as taught by the Vodder School or other similar methods.

high blood pressure

refers to an elevated pressure of the blood against the artery walls.

High blood pressure: **High blood pressure** refers to an elevated pressure of the blood against the walls of the arteries. In a client with a history of high blood pressure, the physician should be consulted before treatment. The client might be taking medication to bring the condition under control. Unless it is severe, massage can be of assistance in relieving some of the hypertension that accompanies high blood pressure. Any massage that involves high blood pressure should be soothing and sedating.

Low blood pressure is not a contraindication for massage; however, the client might experience dizziness when turning over or sitting up following the massage.

cancer

is the uncontrolled growth and spread of abnormal cells in the body.

Cancer: **Cancer** is a conditional contraindication for massage. Many types of cancer spread or metastasize through the blood or lymph channels. Because massage enhances circulation, the application of massage must be modified when working with people with cancer. Massage has proved to have many benefits for people with cancer, including relaxation, pain relief, easing of side effects from cancer treatments, and support of the immune system. Of course, it is essential to consult with the client's physician and to be a part of the health support team prior to any treatment. (See Chapter 19, Massaging People with Cancer.)

Fatigue: In cases of chronic fatigue, the excretory system is already overburdened, and there is little to nourish those overworked and exhausted tissues. When a client is suffering from chronic fatigue, massage should be extremely light and superficial to induce rest and relaxation. Over time, massage helps to restore the client's energy.

Intoxication: Intoxication is a contraindication because massage can spread toxins and overstress the liver.

Psychosis: Psychosis is another condition in which it is advisable to work directly under the supervision of the patient's doctor.

Medication and drugs: Sometimes a client is taking specific medications or drugs such as blood thinners or pain medication, and massage may or may not be recommended. All medications used by a client should be listed on the intake form. The client usually can inform the practitioner about medications and the conditions that they treat. If there is any question concerning the client's condition and possible harmful side effects that a massage might cause, the client's physician should be consulted. (See Appendix I for more information on the relevance of massage therapy to different medications.)

Pregnancy: During a normal, low-risk pregnancy, massage has many benefits; however, there are concerns about massage in the first trimester, when the fertilized egg becomes a floating embryo before it embeds in the uterine wall and begins developing into a fetus. The first trimester is also when mothers experience most pregnancy-related ailments such as nausea, vomiting, mood swings, and fatigue. This period is also when most miscarriages occur, and so it might be in the best interests of the mother, baby, and practitioner to postpone the first prenatal massage until after the twelfth week of the pregnancy.

A pregnant client should inform her physician of her desire to receive prenatal massage and obtain a signed and dated statement from the doctor that her pregnancy is normal, or if there are any complications, what they are and which, if any, precautions should be observed. High-risk pregnancies contraindicate massage unless performed under the close supervision of the attending physician.

During the second and third trimesters, special considerations are made for positioning the mother on the massage table. The prone position is contraindicated. A semireclining or side-lying position is preferred. Massage should always be soothing and relaxing, and no heavy percussion or deep tissue massage should ever be done. Likewise, abdominal kneading or other deep abdominal massage is contraindicated. (See Massage during Pregnancy in Chapter 19 for more information on prenatal massage)

Skin problems: The following skin conditions are contraindications. Most conditions are local contraindications. For example, a minor laceration on the hand would not prevent massage of other healthy parts of the body. As has already been stated, however, when a condition is contagious, massage should not be given.

Acne	Impetigo	Skin cancer
Boils	Inflammation	Skin tags
Broken vessels	Lacerations	Sores
Bruises	Lumps	Stings and bites
Burns and blisters	Rashes	Tumor
Carbuncles	Scaly spots	Warts
Hypersensitive skin	Scratches	Wounds

Hernia: Hernia is a protrusion of an organ or part of an organ, such as the intestine protruding through an opening in the abdominal wall surrounding it. This is also referred to as a rupture, and massage is not recommended over or near the afflicted area.

Frail elderly people: Frail elderly people can have fragile bones, very sensitive skin, use numerous medications, and be under the care of one or more doctors.

Gentle massage can be beneficial for older people, however. (See Massage for the Elderly in Chapter 19 for more information about massage for older adults.)

Scoliosis: When a client has scoliosis (sko-lee-**O**-sis), or a crooked spine, massage must be recommended by the client's physician, and caution must be exercised (Figure 6-5).

Specific conditions or diseases: It should be obvious to the practitioner that a client who is suffering from *severe asthma* (a chronic respiratory disorder), diabetes (deficient insulin secretion), or any type or heart, lung, or kidney disease should be under the supervision of a physician. Massage should not be given without the physician's knowledge and advice, which is why it is important to take time during the first consultation (interview) to determine the client's state of health.

When making decisions whether to perform massage on a person who has a medical condition, be conservative. When in doubt, don't! Remember the first and foremost rule: "Do no harm!"

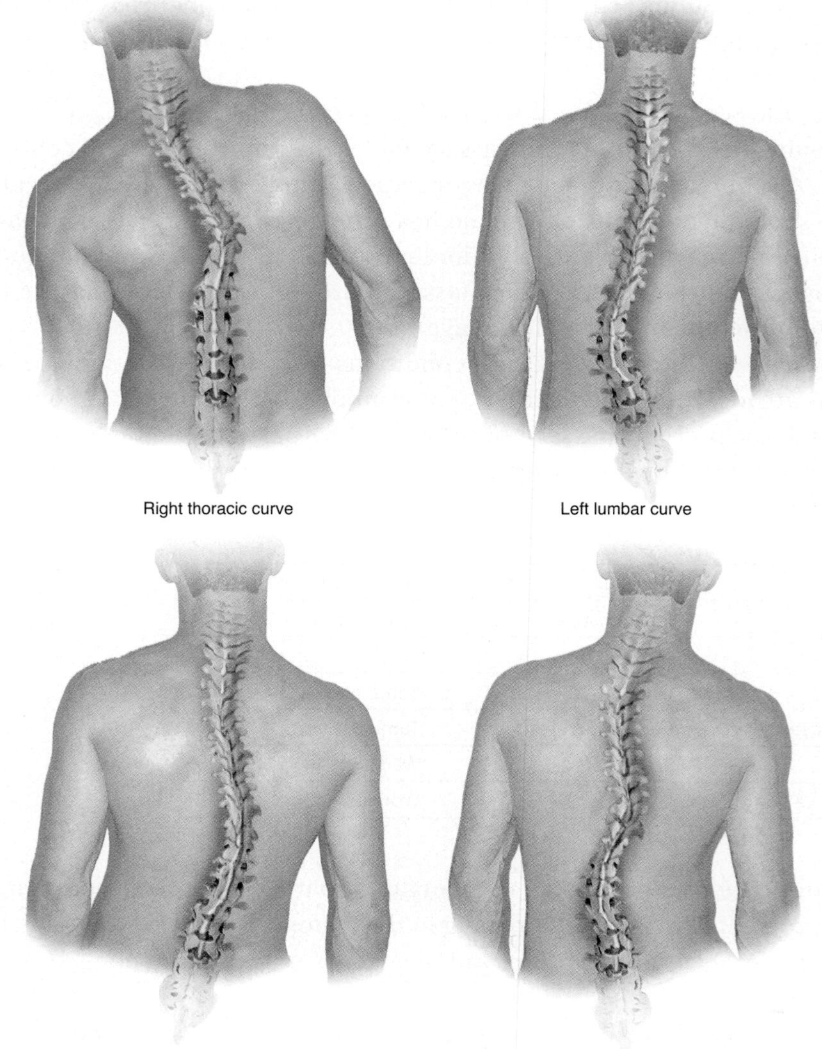

FIGURE 6-5 Scoliosis is an abnormal lateral curve of the spine.

TABLE 6.1

ENDANGERMENT SITES		
ENDANGERMENT SITES	**LOCATION**	**STRUCTURES OF CONCERN**
Inferior to the ear	Notch posterior to the ramus of the mandible	Facial nerve, external carotid artery, styloid process
Anterior triangle of the neck	Bordered by the mandible, sternocleido-mastoid muscle, and the trachea	Carotid artery, internal jugular vein, vagus nerve, lymph nodes
Posterior triangle of the neck	Bordered by the sternocleidomastoid muscle, the trapezius muscle, and the clavicle	Brachial plexus, subclavian artery, brachiocephalic vein, external jugular vein, and lymph nodes
Axilla	Armpit	Axillary, median, musculocutaneous and ulnar nerves; axillary artery; axillary nerve and lymph nodes
Medial brachium	Upper inner arm between the biceps and triceps	Ulnar, musculocutaneous, and median nerves; brachial artery; basilic vein; and lymph nodes
Cubital area of the elbow	Anterior bend of the elbow	Median nerve, radial and ulnar arteries, median cubital vein
Ulnar notch of the elbow	The "funny bone"	Ulnar nerve
Femoral triangle	Bordered by the sartorius muscle, the adductor longus muscle, and the inguinal ligament	Femoral nerve, femoral artery, femoral vein, great saphenous vein, and lymph nodes
Popliteal fossa	Posterior aspect of the knee bordered by the gastrocnemius (inferior) and the hamstrings (superior and to the sides)	Tibial nerve; common peroneal nerve; popliteal artery; popliteal vein
Abdomen	Upper area of the abdomen under the the ribs	Right side, liver and gallbladder; left side, spleen; deep center, aorta
Upper lumbar area	Just inferior to the ribs and lateral to the spine	Kidneys (avoid heavy percussion)

ENDANGERMENT SITES

Certain areas of the body warrant consideration when being massaged because of delicate, relatively unprotected underlying anatomic structures. Because of the possibility of injury to the structures by certain massage manipulations, these areas are sites of potential endangerment. In most of these areas, major nerves, blood vessels, or vital organs are relatively exposed and vulnerable to deep manipulations or direct, sustained pressure. Table 6.1 lists these endangerment sites, their location, and the anatomic structures of concern.

SUMMARY

Massage, in its many forms, has a wide variety of beneficial effects on the body. The effects can differ according to the needs of the client and the intention with the massage is administered. Benefits can be both psychological and physiologic. Psychologically, massage relieves fatigue, reduces tension and anxiety, calms the nervous system, and promotes a sense of relaxation and renewed energy. Physiologically, massage can affect many of the body's systems, relaxing muscles, stimulating circulation and elimination, and managing pain. Massage has direct, mechanical effects on the tissues where it is applied as well as indirect, reflex effects that affect body functions and tissues through the nervous or energy systems of the body. Depending on its application, massage can have either a stimulating or sedating effect. Some of the indirect, reflex effects of massage are due to the response of the autonomic nervous system. Initially, massage stimulates the sympathetic nervous system, resulting in increased energy and alertness. Longer massages stimulate the parasympathetic nervous system, reducing the heart rate and blood pressure and increasing relaxation. Massage has been shown to have an effect on the blood levels of various hormones and neurotransmitters, reducing those associated with stress and increasing those related to pain reduction and relaxation.

Nearly everyone can benefit from receiving a therapeutic massage, and there are innumerable conditions that indicate the application of skillfully applied touch. There are situations and conditions, however, in which massage is contraindicated, meaning that there is a medical reason not to apply massage.

The contraindication can be

- Absolute – meaning that massage should not be given until the condition subsides
- Regional or partial – meaning that massage is prohibited on a portion of the body because of a local condition
- Conditional – meaning there are health concerns for which certain massage techniques are not used because they could have adverse effects whereas other techniques would be beneficial.

Besides contraindications, there are certain areas on the body that require some consideration owing to the delicate structures below the surface that could be adversely affected by some massage techniques. These are called *endangerment sites.* They are areas to avoid or use only superficial techniques when near them. It is the responsibility of the massage therapist to be aware of not only the benefits and indications for applying therapeutic massage techniques but also the contraindications and endangerment areas, to provide a positive and beneficial experience for the client.

QUESTIONS FOR DISCUSSION AND REVIEW

1. What are the main physiologic benefits of massage?
2. What are the main psychological benefits of massage?
3. What are the two physical ways in which massage affects the body?
4. Which body systems are said to benefit from regular therapeutic massage?
5. In which way does the muscular system benefit from massage?
6. Which massage movements promote circulation in muscles?
7. How does massage relieve sore and stiff muscles?
8. Which massage technique prevents the formation of adhesions and fibrosis in muscles?
9. What are the immediate effects of massage on the skin?
10. How does massage affect the nervous system?
11. Which massage movements have a stimulating effect on the nervous system?
12. Which massage techniques have a sedative effect on the nervous system?
13. What is the effect of massage on the circulatory system?
14. Why are most massage movements directed toward the heart?
15. Which massage movements increase the flow of blood and lymph?
16. How does improved circulation of the blood benefit the skin?
17. When should massage be avoided?
18. What is the meaning of *contraindication* as it relates to massage?
19. Why does the practitioner need to take the client's medical history?
20. Why should the therapist keep a fever thermometer on the premises?
21. What should the practitioner do when a client has a condition that appears to be a contraindication to massage?
22. What are the signs of inflammation?
23. How should massage be applied in the case of local inflammation?
24. How can a therapist recognize varicose veins?
25. What is a hematoma, and how is it massaged?
26. Why are certain areas of the body sites of potential endangerment?

CHAPTER

7

Equipment and Products

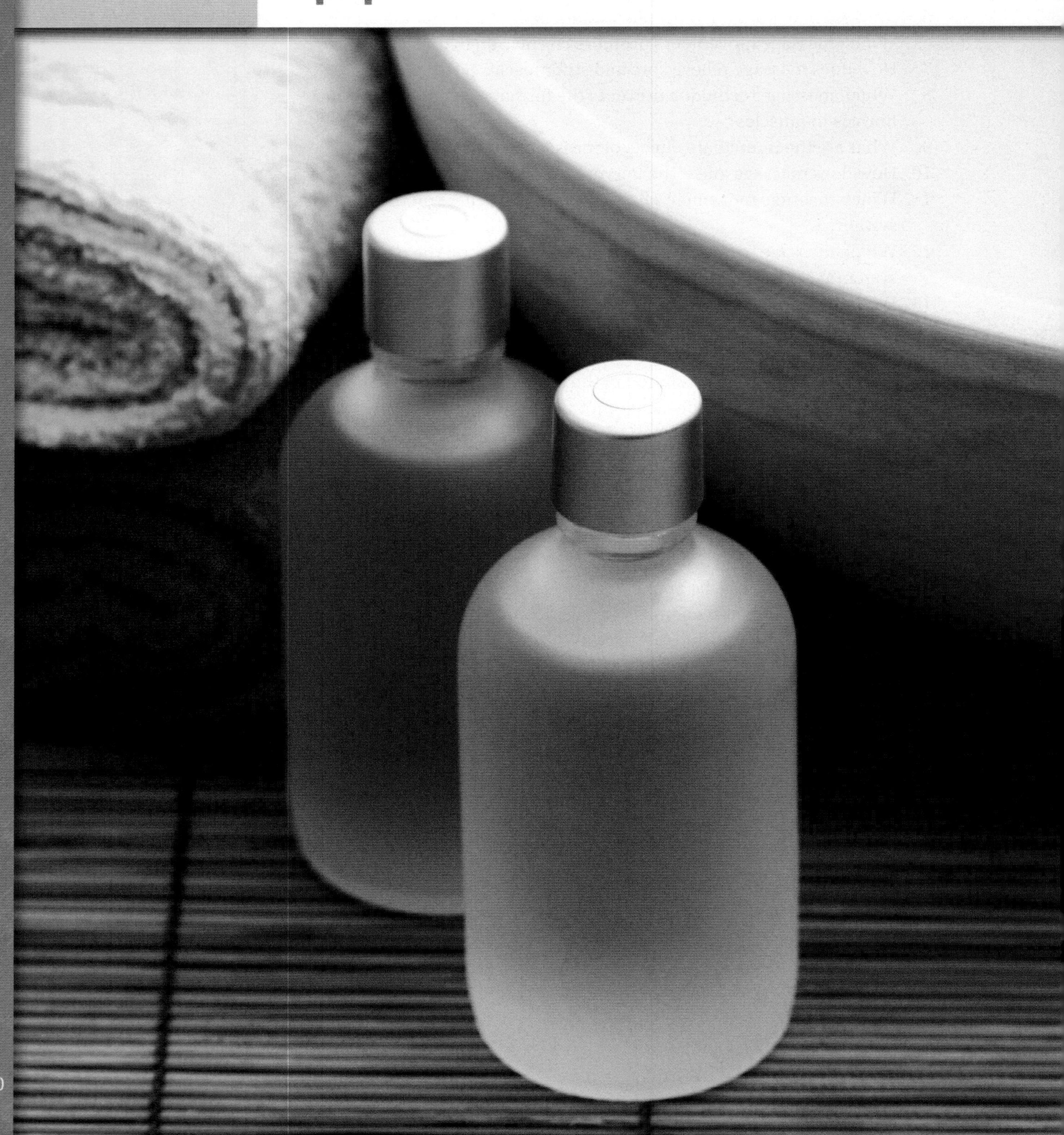

LEARNING OBJECTIVES

After you have mastered this chapter, you will be able to

1. **Prepare a checklist of supplies and equipment needed for therapeutic massage.**
2. **Describe various products and their use.**
3. **Select a massage table.**
4. **Check and adjust lighting for the massage room.**
5. **Check all equipment for safety and readiness.**

INTRODUCTION

The practice of therapeutic massage is a part of the health care profession. For this reason and many others, a practitioner must look and behave in a professional and friendly manner at all times. Professionalism is an attitude that is manifested through therapists and their business. Clients expect a professional image, which is projected by speech, appearance, good manners, the equipment used, and the place of business. Technical competence and a sense of confidence in practice are also professional ingredients.

Generally, a client coming for a massage anticipates a relaxing, rejuvenating experience. To provide such an experience, several conditions are desirable, if not necessary. The professional and friendly manner in which the practitioner presents herself provides the client with a certain confidence. The appearance and atmosphere of the massage facility affect the client's overall response. Cleanliness, a sense of order, and sanitation are essential factors. Comfortable yet professional furnishings add to the client's confidence. Privacy and the absence of distractions or interruptions are important considerations. The facilities in which you work should reflect a professional appearance, yet at the same time they should be comfortable and relaxing.

When considering the comfort of the client, adequate heat, ventilation, and indirect lighting are important. Relaxing music is an option that many practitioners employ. An awareness of the factors that enhance the massage experience enables the practitioner to incorporate these factors when planning the massage facilities.

YOUR PLACE OF BUSINESS

The location of the massage business is an important consideration and is discussed extensively in Chapter 22. The image of a place of business makes an impression on massage clients and therefore must be considered when establishing a business.

A 1990 national survey of massage practitioners conducted by Knapp and Associates indicates that approximately one third of massage therapists operate a private practice out of their home, one third from a private office or clinic, and the remaining third practice in another facility such as a health club, resort, health professional's office or spa. A more recent survey, conducted in 2007 by the Federation of Massage Therapy Boards, shows that nearly 40% of massage therapists work from a private office or clinic, 20% from home, 15% from a spa or fitness facility, and the others from a variety of locations such as chiropractic offices, hospitals, and on site. Regardless of the location of the business, the internal environment of the facility reflects directly on the impression that the client has of the therapist and of the services that the therapist offers.

Clients coming into a place of business are influenced by the environment and the people with whom they come in contact. The decor should be professional yet comfortable, clean yet not sterile, relaxed, and free of distractions and safety hazards. In a massage establishment, space should be allotted for the exclusive practice of massage. Although this is necessary for a client's privacy and comfort, it also gives a more professional image. Some practitioners go to their clients' homes in addition to or rather than maintaining a studio and office space. The equipment used, as well as the appearance and actions of the therapist, when performing in-home massage or outcalls to an office, hotel, or other facility directly reflect on the perception of the client. Whether the massage facility is in the practitioner's home, the client's home, or a separate office, standards of cleanliness, safety, and professionalism must be observed.

Sanitation and Safety in the Workplace

Whether working out of an office in your home, a small salon or studio, or a large, luxurious spa, the space and equipment must be kept clean and neat. The massage facility and the equipment should be checked regularly to eliminate situations that could cause injury to the therapist or client. Passageways must be kept clear. Surfaces and linens must be sanitized and equipment checked against failure. The main concern is the protection of the client's health and comfort. (See Chapter 8, Sanitary and Safety Practices, for more on this important topic.)

Equipment and Supplies

Depending on the extent and dimensions of the massage business, the specific equipment and supplies that are necessary or preferred vary somewhat. There are, however, several items that are essential to a smooth and efficient massage business operation. The actual practice of giving a massage requires the use of certain equipment and supplies. The manner of conducting consultations, record keeping, and other business operations dictate the related equipment and materials. Whether hydrotherapy and bathing are available in the practice influences the selection of equipment and related supplies.

The setting of a massage operation also influences the selection of equipment and supplies. A massage business that is operated out of a home differs from a massage concession on a cruise ship or the athletic massage facility of a professional sports team. Most massage operations have some consistent needs, however. For the purpose of this chapter, consider an independent massage practitioner operating out of the home or a small private office.

There are generally three areas of activity in a massage business: the massage area, the business area, and the bathroom or hydrotherapy area.

The massage area is where the client actually receives the massage treatment. Often in a small operation, the massage area is also where the client disrobes and gets dressed. The massage area must be of an adequate size for the necessary equipment and for the practitioner to move around comfortably while performing the massage.

The business area is where the practitioner keeps records, does consultations, answers the telephone, and carries out other business activities related to the massage practice. All of these activities may take place in the massage room or in an adjacent room, or the activities can be divided so that some things, such as client records and consultations, happen close to the massage area and other activities, such as bookkeeping, take place elsewhere.

Every massage area must have access to a clean restroom. Because massage tends to have a stimulating effect on the urinary and digestive systems, the client might need to use the restroom during or after the massage session. Ideally, there should be a place for the client to shower or bathe before or after the massage. The restroom also provides a facility for the practitioner to wash his hands before and after each massage.

Ancillary services to the actual massage vary widely. The availability of such services as steam baths, showers, exercise facilities, hot packs, or hot baths affect the procedures that the client follows preceding and following the massage. If the ancillary services are part of the massage operation, the required equipment and related supplies will be dictated by the services offered.

Equipment and supplies should be checked frequently to be sure they are in proper condition and that enough are on hand. Each area and massage room should have the appropriate furnishings and equipment for the treatments to be given. All equipment should be checked regularly for fitness and safety. All supplies must be kept in a clean, sanitized condition. Supplies such as oils, linens, and paper products should be selected and ready before the client enters the facility or massage room.

Below are general lists of equipment and supplies for the different areas. The lists might include many optional items, especially in the ancillary areas. Examine the lists, and add items that you think would enhance your massage business.

The Massage Area

- Massage table
- Stool
- Supply storage cabinet
  - Facial tissues
  - Cotton-tipped swabs
  - Alcohol or other sterilizing agents
  - Analgesic oil or gel
- Bolsters or pillows (face cushion)
- Linens (an adequate supply)
  - Sheets and towels for draping
  - Pillow and bolster covers
- Blankets, wraps, and/or robes
- Lubricants, oils, creams, powders, and liniments
- Dressing area (privacy space with chair, hangers, a mirror, and wraps)
- Indirect lighting
- Desk or table and chair
  - Client intake and SOAP forms
- Clock
- Device to play music and a music selection
- Covered wastebasket

The Business Operation Area

Desk and chairs
Business telephone with an answering machine
Appointment book
A secure filing system
Stationery and stamps
Pencils, pens, stapler, tape, and other office supplies

Bathroom/Bathing Area

Antibacterial soap
Paper hand towels
Clean bath towels for each client
Robes or wraps
Shampoo and bath soap
Disposable water cups

Hydrotherapy Area

Hydrotherapy equipment and related supplies
Towels and robes
Sanitation and cleaning supplies

THE MASSAGE ROOM

Studio Space

A massage room needs to be a minimum of 10 feet wide and 12 feet long. This allows enough space for all necessary equipment as well as enough room to move around the massage table. It also allows space for a desk, chair, and supply table or cabinet. A stool is also a handy item to have in the massage room, because there are times when the practitioner can sit down while working on the client's neck, face, feet, or hands. Sitting for a few minutes allows much-needed rest when a therapist is working long hours (Figure 7-1).

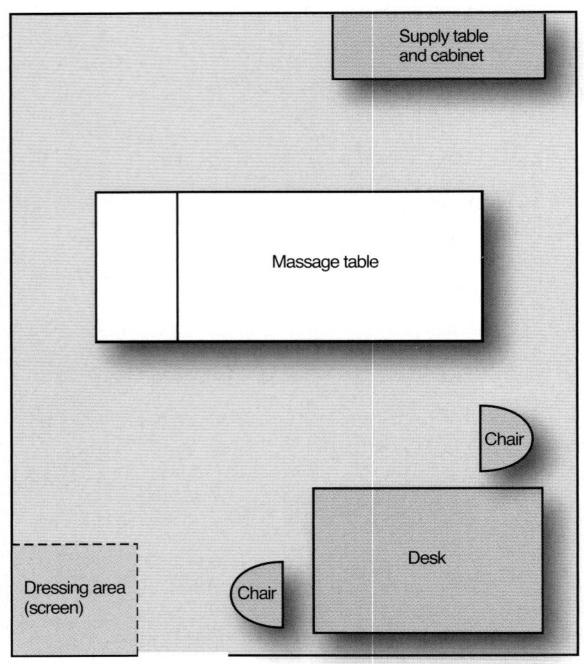

FIGURE 7-1 The minimum size for a massage room is about 10 by 12 feet. This allows room for a table, desk, chairs, supply cabinet, and room to move around the table to perform the massage.

Temperature of the Massage Room

The temperature of the massage room should be comfortable. The room should be warm enough that the client does not chill. If the client becomes chilled, it is very hard for him to relax. About 72° to 75° F is warm enough for most clients and at the same time is cool enough to keep the practitioner from getting uncomfortably warm while working. The room should be warmed in advance, because it is easy for the client to become chilled, especially after oil or lotion has been applied to the skin. In a room that is cooler, auxiliary blankets, electric mattress pads, a small electric heater, or other heating devices can be used to ensure the client's warmth. In hot or humid weather, the room should be equipped with air conditioning or a fan that circulates the air so that it does not become uncomfortably warm.

The massage room must be well ventilated. Performing a massage requires considerable exertion on the part of the practitioner. For proper relaxation, the client needs a good supply of fresh air. With poor ventilation, the room would become stuffy, and the air can acquire an offensive odor. Proper ventilation ensures an abundant supply of fresh air.

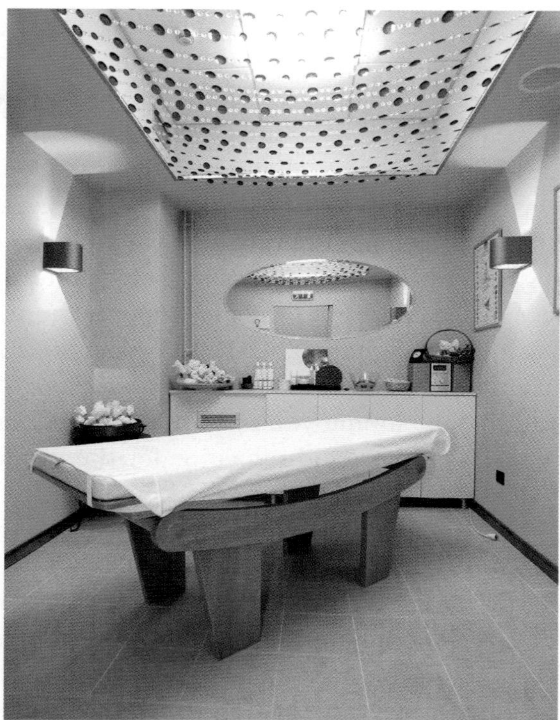

FIGURE 7-2 Avoid direct overhead lighting in the massage room. Soft natural light from a shaded window or indirect light from wall or table lamps is preferred.

Lighting

It is difficult for either the practitioner or the client to be comfortable when the lighting in the room is harsh and glaring. Colored lights such as red or blue can make the client feel uncomfortable, however. Reflective or soft, natural light is preferred. Dimmer switches allow the light to be changed easily. Avoid direct overhead lighting or any light that could shine directly into the client's eyes (Figure 7-2).

Use of Music

A stereo and supply of soothing music can provide another dimension to a relaxing massage. Although the therapist might like music playing while working, some people find it distracting and prefer absolute quiet. Have a selection of soothing music available, and ask the client what he prefers. If there is outside noise that might be distracting, music can mask it. Avoid up-tempo beats, music with lyrics, some classical music, and nature sounds because these might inhibit the client's ability to relax. Obviously, do not attempt to match the rhythm of the massage movements to the tempo of the music.

The Massage Table

As a massage therapist, one of your most important possessions is a massage table that fits your needs. The massage table is the practitioner's main piece of equipment and, next to the hands, is the most important tool for the therapist's comfort and that of his clients. The massage table should be stable, firm, and comfortable. If an office or studio is the site of the business, a stationary table might be the best choice. If your situation is temporary, or if you prefer the freedom of taking your equipment with you, choose a good portable table. The table must be portable and light enough to carry.

Regardless of your choice, check the construction carefully. The table should not shake, rock, or squeak. Seldom does new equipment display these problems, but consider what will happen after the table has been used for several hundred treatments.

A massage table allows you to move about or change positions easily and when necessary, without breaking the rhythm of the massage movements. The optimal height of the massage table depends on several factors, including the kind or style of massage being done, the height of the practitioner, the size of the client, and the personal preferences of the practitioner. The table must be the right height to give proper leverage and to prevent fatigue in the back, neck, arms, and shoulders. The height of the table is determined by your height so that you are not at a disadvantage when reaching and applying pressure. A good indicator for the proper height of a massage table is to stand in an erect yet relaxed manner and measure the distance from the floor to the middle of the palm of the hand. This is approximately the optimal height for the table. Another way to test the height of a table is to stand next to the table and place the palm of the hand flat on the table. While doing this, you should be able to hold your arm straight at your side. If, after a few sessions discomfort is felt in the lower back, the table is probably too low. If the discomfort is in the upper back, shoulders, or arms, the table is probably too high (Figure 7-3).

Several stationary and portable table models have legs that can be adjusted up or down by removing and replacing wing nuts or thumbscrews. These are advantageous if people of different heights use the same table, or if various techniques used require different table heights. Therapists practicing deep tissue techniques or Asian bodywork often prefer a slightly shorter table, allowing them to use their body weight and lean into their technique. Some stationary tables have a height adjustment button and are operated by hydraulic force or electricity. Although costly, this type of table is very useful when dealing with elderly or disabled clients, who might have difficulty getting on a table of normal height, or when several different practitioners use the same table.

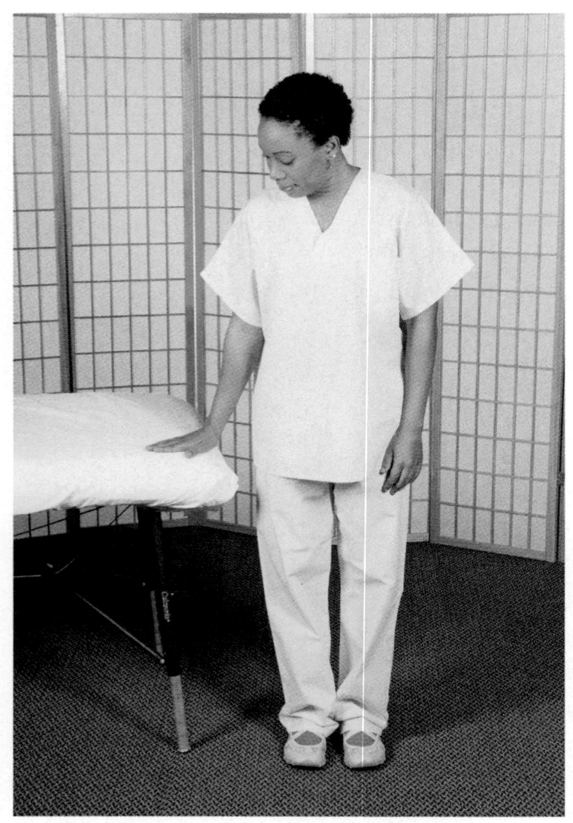

FIGURE 7-3 Measuring proper table height.

The width of a massage table is approximately 28 inches, with an additional inch allowed for padding, or approximately 29 inches wide. Tables narrower than 27 inches do not give enough arm support for larger clients. Tables wider than 30 inches become awkward when the practitioner must reach across to the opposite side of the client. The width of the table depends somewhat on the height of the practitioner. A taller practitioner will find it somewhat easier to reach across a wider table and easier to carry a wider portable table when it is folded. A good length for a massage table is about 76 inches. Most portable tables are about 68 to 72 inches long, which can be too short for taller clients.

The padding on the massage table should be firm so that pressure applied by the practitioner to the client is absorbed by the client's body and not pushed into the table. About 1 to 2 inches of high-density foam is the best material to use. Padding should extend beyond the edge of the framework of the table by approximately one half inch all around to ensure the comfort of the client, who might place a hand or foot over the edge. A good-quality vinyl is the best covering for the massage table because it is durable and easy to keep clean. To care for high-quality vinyl, clean it regularly with water and a mild detergent. Avoid extended contact with massage or body oils, alcohol, or chlorine bleach, because these substances can cause the vinyl to become brittle and crack. Try to avoid exposing the vinyl to extreme temperatures. If the table gets either extremely hot or cold—because it has been stored in a car, for example—allow the vinyl to return to room temperature before using.

Tables come in a variety of designs. Often the surface of a massage treatment table folds up or down in a variety of configurations. This is to accommodate specific therapy situations and can be of no use to the general massage practitioner. An exception is the headpiece that adjusts up or down to alleviate cervical strain. Accommodations for the face can be in the form of a hole in the end of the table or a padded extension to the end of the table called a *face cradle*. These additions allow the client to lie face down with the cervical spine straight, taking the strain off the neck and upper back.

Some massage tables include several accessories, like the face cradle. The face cradle is a valuable addition for the comfort of the client. Many tables have face cradles that adjust to several different positions to ensure comfort (Figure 7-4). Some tables include side extensions to support the arms of larger clients. Another valuable accessory for a portable massage table is a carrying case to protect the table when transporting it from one location to another. Besides protecting the table, the carrying case has extra handles and straps to make lifting and carrying the table easier. Some carrying cases are equipped with wheels to accommodate rolling the table from place to place. Many cases also have a large pocket for carrying linens and supplies.

Because the table is the massage therapist's main piece of equipment, a professionally designed massage table is recommended. Most massage students and new practitioners choose a good-quality portable massage table as their first table. There are several reputable table manufacturers in the United States; tables from these companies tend to be good tables.

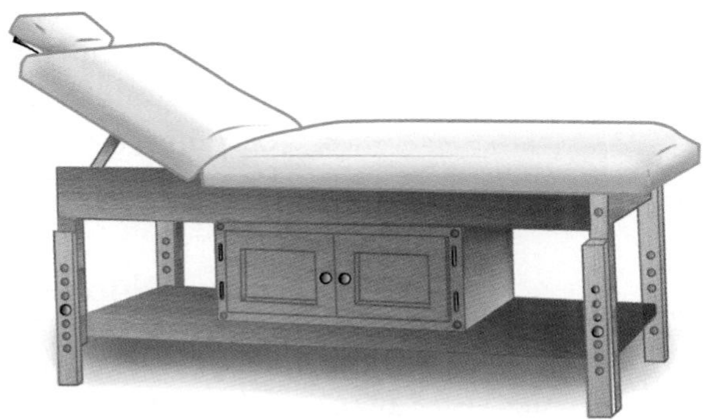

Studio table with adjustable head piece.

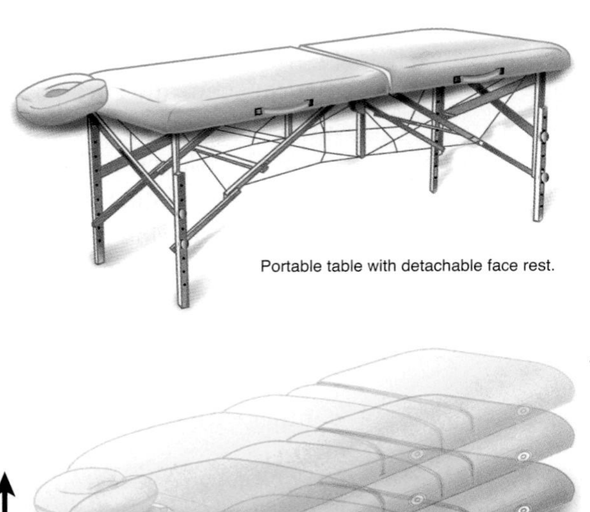

Portable table with detachable face rest.

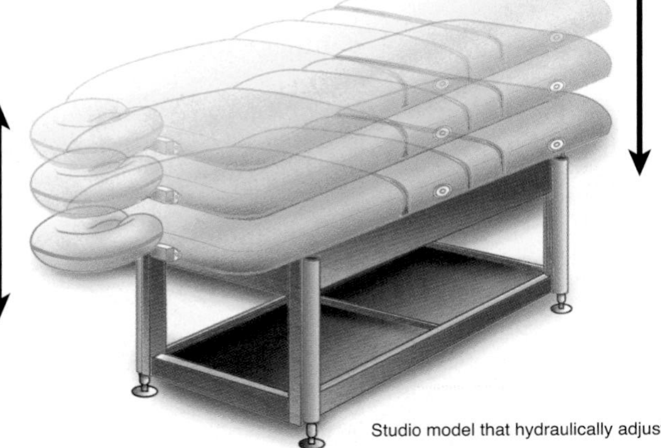

Studio model that hydraulically adjusts the height.

FIGURE 7-4 Massage tables come in a variety of styles.

Most companies have a range of prices depending on accessories, such as adjustable face rest, special covering, or extra foam padding. A few companies have a variety of tables such as portable tables, studio tables, and hydraulic tables. In looking through publications such as the *Massage Magazine* or *Massage Therapy Journal*, the student or practitioner can glean information and phone numbers from numerous table manufacturers. Other sources include catalogues, specialty stores, massage convention exhibits, and online Web sites. One possible source for good used massage tables is online at www.craigslist.org.

Regardless of the company or the price of the table selected, there are several factors to keep in mind when choosing a table. They include but are not limited to

- Adjustable legs
- Appropriate dimensions
- Face rest (some adjustability is a benefit)
- Vinyl covering (for easy cleaning)
- Easy setup and take-down
- Stability and durability
- Carrying case (for easy carrying and for protection)
- Good warranty

Bolsters and Pillows

To position a client comfortably on the massage table, it is helpful to have a variety of supportive devices such as pillows and bolsters (Figure 7-5). Bolsters come in a variety of sizes and shapes. They can be round, half-round, rectangular, or specially shaped to support a particular part of the body. Specially manufactured body support systems are available, as are bolsters that are specially designed to support pregnant clients who receive prenatal massage. Six- or eight-inch round bolsters made of foam and covered with vinyl, which are nearly as long as the table is wide, are very common. These are placed under the client's knees when face up or under the ankles when face down to reduce the strain in the lower back. The vinyl should not come in contact with the client's skin. The bolster can be slipped either under the sheet covering the table or into a pillowcase. Vinyl-covered bolsters can be cleaned with the same mild detergent used to clean the massage table.

It is also a good idea to keep three or four firm bed pillows on hand for special positioning situations such as side-lying positions or for extra support under the abdomen or head. Pillowcases on pillows and bolsters that come in contact with the client's skin must be changed between clients.

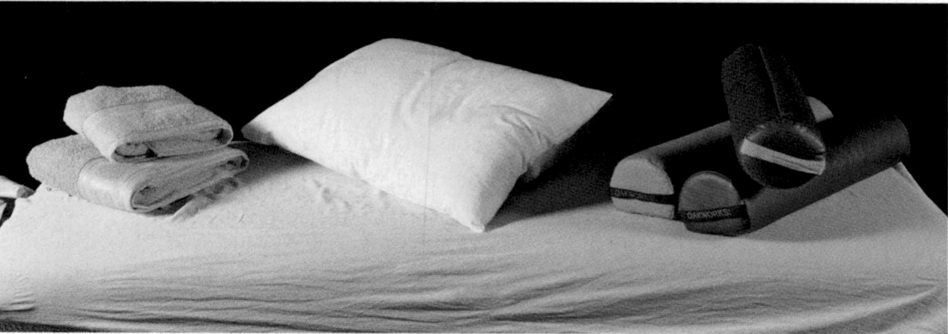

FIGURE 7-5 A variety of bolsters.

Massage Linens

In the practice of massage, linens are used to cover the massage table, the client, the face cradle, bolsters, and pillows. The type of services offered and the style of draping used determine which linens are needed. Single-sized (twin) fitted or flat sheets can be used as table coverings. Single-sized (twin) flat sheets, bath sheets, beach towels, large or regular-sized bath towels can be used as drapes for clients. Pillowcases are used for pillows and possibly for bolsters. Washcloths, hand towels, pillowcases, or specially made covers can be used on face cradles.

Clean linens are used for every client. The amount or number of linens needed depends on the number of clients seen in a day and how often laundry is done. If laundry is done daily, there should be enough linens to last for two days. If laundry is done weekly, there should be enough linens to last one and a half to two weeks.

Popular fabrics for sheets include percale, cotton, cotton blends, and flannel. White, light pastels, and pale floral prints launder and tolerate bleach well. Darker colors tend to fade and show oil stains. When linens become stained or threadbare, they should be replaced. Some oil manufacturers sell products that effectively remove oil stains and odors from linens.

Some practitioners prefer to use towels or a combination of towels and sheets for draping. A variety of towel sizes can be used. A bath sheet or large beach towel can be used as a top cover. A large bath towel can be used in combination with a top sheet to hold it in place or as a partial drape. A small bath towel is used as an upper torso (breast) drape. If the service includes bathing facilities, extra towels must be available for drying.

Besides sheets, towels, and pillowcases, the practitioner should keep a couple of light flannel, cotton, or wool blankets on hand for situations when the client might become chilled. The blanket is used over the top of the usual draping to provide extra warmth, security, and comfort. Even though the blankets do not come into direct contact with the client, they should be of a material that is easy to launder occasionally.

Massage Lubricants

Good-quality lubricants are some of the practitioner's most important products. The primary purpose for using lubricants is to reduce the friction between the practitioner's hands and the client's skin. The choice of lubricant depends on the style of massage, the needs of the client, and the preference of the practitioner. The practitioner may choose a lotion, cream, gel or massage oil. Massage oils and creams are the most commonly used lubricants. There is such a wide variety of massage lubricants available from several manufacturers and distributors that it can be difficult to choose the powders, oils, creams, or lotions you want to stock. Quality is important.

Mineral oils are not recommended for massage because they are a petroleum-based product that tends to dry the skin, deplete nutrients, and clog the pores. A combination of vegetable-based oils such as coconut, sweet almond, apricot, olive, peanut, sesame, grape seed, or sunflower oils are mild and easy to work with and provide natural nutrients to the skin. Some clients or practitioners are allergic to nut products and therefore sensitive to oils such as almond oil. It is important to use fresh oil, because rancid oil has a strong offensive odor and possible health considerations. If oil remains on sheets and sets for a while, it saturates the fibers, and they will develop stains and an offensive odor. Some oil distributors have special laundry products that are effective for removing oil from linens.

Oils, creams, and lotions have different qualities. Lotions provide a more limited glide that decreases as the area is worked. Most lotions absorb into the skin and become sticky, but they provide nutrients to the skin. Lotions are often the choice of deep-tissue practitioners because they allow penetration without irritation. Because it does absorb into the skin so readily, you might need to reapply lotion often.

Massage creams are being offered by more specialty manufacturers as a popular alternative to massage oil. Massage creams often provide special properties that may stimulate, sooth, warm, cool, or provide special nutrients to the area being massaged. Massage creams are often less oily, can be water based instead of oil based, and have gliding properties similar to oils, but creams are usually considerably more expensive.

As a therapist, experiment with different products until you find the ones that you and your clients prefer. Once a preference is established, it is more economical to buy in larger quantities. If you buy oil in bulk, some should be transferred to smaller bottles. These bottles should be kept filled to the top because it is the air space in the bottle that causes the oil to become rancid. When oil does not have a pleasant smell but is not rancid, a few drops of oil of lemon, clove, cinnamon, musk, or some other essential oil can be added. Usually a few drops of concentrate to a cup of oil is enough to give a hint of scent. Use scented oils cautiously. Clients can be sensitive to, allergic to, or simply not like certain fragrances. When an oil or cream is being used as a carrier for an essential oil as an aromatherapy treatment, the oils should be mixed specifically for the client at the time of application. Oils and concentrated fragrances can be purchased from supply houses or specialty stores, or they are usually available at drugstores. Some practitioners like to mix their oils and then place them in unbreakable, easy-to-handle bottles with dispenser tops; this prevents spillage (Figure 7-6). All lubricants must be kept in and dispersed from containers in a manner that prevents contamination.

Some clients have very oily skin or might not tolerate oil. For these clients, a light powder such as cornstarch might be preferred. Talcum powder is another option, but is not recommended because it is a potential lung irritant. You must avoid inhaling talc or other powders when using it for massage by applying it carefully and possibly wearing a mask. Even though powder does not provide the same lubrication as oil, the same massage movements can be done effectively with powder, and some clients prefer powder.

There are excellent creams and lotions on the market. Always read the label to be sure that you know the product's ingredients and that it is safe to use for massage. It is a good idea to have a dictionary of cosmetic ingredients so that you can look up unfamiliar words. When possible, consult a pharmacist or dermatologist. The federal Food and Drug Administration (FDA) endeavors to

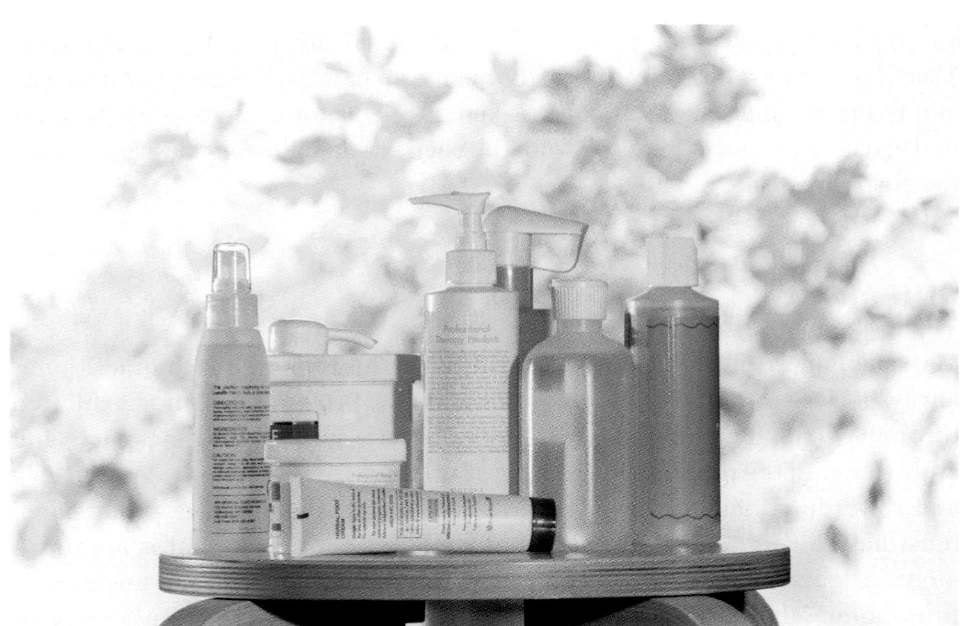

FIGURE 7-6 Oil bottles with a variety of dispenser tops.

control the distribution of products that contain harmful substances; however, what is harmless to most people can cause an allergic reaction in someone with a sensitivity to a particular substance. During the consultation or before applying a substance to the face or body, it is best to determine whether the client is allergic to any substance. When in doubt, do a patch test before proceeding with the application.

To give a patch test, first wash the area of the inner bend of the elbow with mild soap and warm water. Rinse the area, and then apply a small amount of the product to the skin. Allow 15 to 30 minutes to see whether there is a reaction (e.g., signs of itching, inflammation, and sensitivity, or a stinging sensation). If so, do not use the product. If there are no signs of inflammation or the aforementioned sensations, the product is considered safe to use. If the client does begin to have a reaction to a lubricant—for example, the skin where the lubricant was applied becomes inflamed—immediately remove all of the lubricant with soap and water. The client can then decide to discontinue the massage or to continue using a different lubricant. Unfortunately, most reactions happen several hours after the application, after the client has left the facility.

Some people with allergies to fragrances and other cosmetic substances might need to have a patch test 24 hours before a treatment. In such cases, the client is usually aware of any allergies or sensitivities and which products to avoid. They also might be under the care of a physician, who can give guidance on which products to use and which to avoid. Clients who are sensitive to some products sometimes prefer to supply their own lubricants. There are lubricants on the market that are labeled **hypoallergenic**. These products have been tested and found safe for most people even if they do have sensitivities. It is good practice to have some hypoallergenic products on hand to use for clients with known sensitivities to commonly used products.

hypoallergenic

relatively unlikely to cause an allergic reaction.

Most nonprescription products are considered safe for the general public. Most practitioners keep a variety of lubricants on hand to better serve the needs and wishes of their clients. Alcohol is kept available for sanitation purposes. It is also used to remove excess oil from the client's skin following massage, before the client dresses.

SUMMARY

Massage is part of the health care profession, and the massage practitioner always strives to appear and act professionally. Professionalism is exhibited through personal mannerisms and interactions as well as the atmosphere and appearance of the professional business facility. To provide a safe, comfortable and rewarding massage experience for the client, the massage professional must have a variety of equipment and supplies in a facility that is appropriately designed for massage. Massage is offered in a wide range of businesses, from home offices to health clubs to chiropractor's offices to cruise ships to spas. Regardless of where the massage business is located, the equipment and supplies required are essentially the same. Usually the massage takes place in the privacy of a room that is well ventilated and a comfortable temperature, with indirect lighting and few distractions. A massage table of the proper height for the practitioner's comfort and safety and well padded for the client's comfort is draped with appropriate linens. Clean, fresh linens are used for each client to provide warmth and a modest cover while they receive massage. There is enough space in the room for the practitioner to move around all sides of the massage table. There are a variety of bolsters and pillows available to support and position the client for the utmost comfort. There is also a variety of massage oils, creams, or lotions to be used as lubricants when performing the massage. The choice of lubricant is determined by the practitioner's preference as well as the client's safety, preference, and special needs. A clean restroom should be close by and easily accessible to the client. Depending on the type of operation, there might also be a business office with all of the necessary supplies. Regardless of where professional massage services are provided, proper equipment and supplies not only convey a professional image but also give clients confidence that they will have a safe, comforting massage experience.

QUESTIONS FOR DISCUSSION AND REVIEW

1. Which kind of image should a massage practitioner project to clientele?
2. What are some important considerations when preparing a space to do massage?
3. Approximately how much space is optimal for a massage space?
4. Why should equipment and supplies be inspected periodically?
5. Why is it important to prepare a checklist of supplies and equipment?
6. Which kinds of products are usually used for body massage?
7. What is the approximate temperature for the massage room?

8. Why is it important to be able to adjust the height of the massage table?
9. Which type of lighting is preferred in the massage room?
10. Why should the client be asked about background music?

CHAPTER

8 Sanitary and Safety Practices

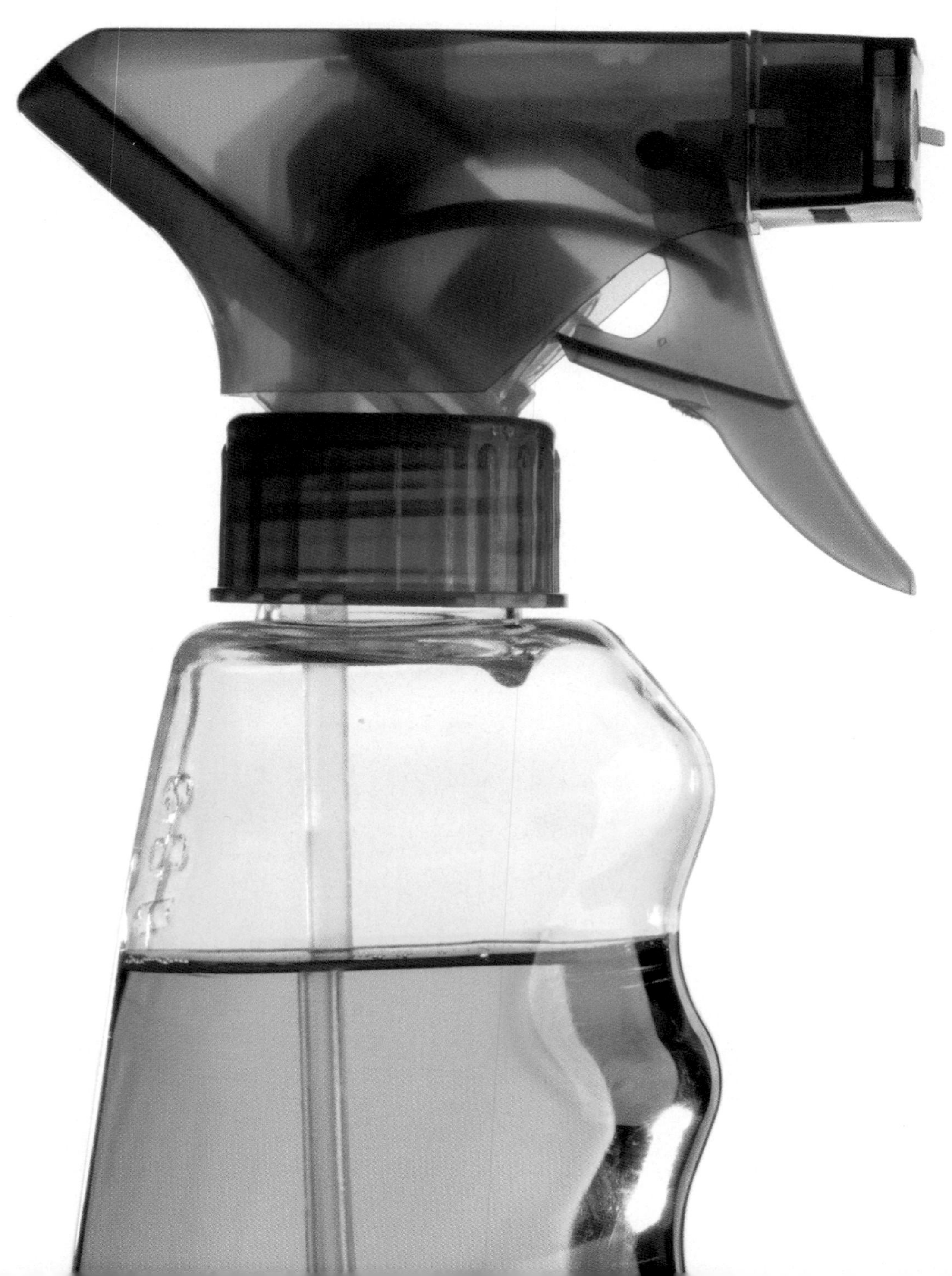

LEARNING OBJECTIVES

After you have mastered this chapter, you will be able to

1. **Explain the need for laws that enforce the strict practice of sanitation.**
2. **Sanitize implements and other items used in massage procedures.**
3. **Explain the difference between pathogenic and nonpathogenic bacteria.**
4. **Explain the importance of cleanliness of person and of surroundings as protection against the spread of disease.**
5. **Describe how various disinfectants, antiseptics, and other products are used most effectively.**
6. **Explain the role of safety in the massage therapy business.**

INTRODUCTION

The everyday practice of sanitation and safety is the activity of protecting the therapist and their clientele against injury or disease. An awareness of hazardous conditions and the elimination of those situations will prevent an injury before it occurs. Likewise the implementation of sanitary practices to curtail the spread of infectious agents reduces or eliminates the possibility of you or a client becoming ill as a result of "picking up a bug" at your place of business.

It is the practitioner's responsibility to provide a safe and sanitary facility. The client depends on and expects this service and will not wish to return to a facility that is unsanitary, cluttered, or unsafe.

In recent years, great progress has been made in the control and prevention of disease. In the medical profession, sanitation and sterilization are required procedures that are taken for granted. Every state has laws that make the practice of sanitation mandatory for the protection of public health. In the personal service professions, every precaution must be taken to protect the health of clients as well as the health of practitioners. The nature of the personal service business determines the extent of the procedures for sanitation and sterilization. For example, in the cosmetology profession, a comb or brush used on one client may not be used on another until it has been thoroughly cleansed and sterilized. The esthetician (skin care specialist) must apply products only with sanitized applicators. The massage practitioner might not use the same kinds of implements or have need for the same sanitation procedures; however, appropriate and recommended procedures must be followed diligently.

The massage practitioner need not be a biologist to have some understanding of transmission of disease and to be aware of the importance of impeccable cleanliness at all times. Contagious diseases, skin infections, and other problems can be caused by the transfer of infectious material by unclean hands and nails and by unsanitary equipment and supplies. Therefore, the primary concern is that any item (e.g., linens, apparatus) that comes in contact with the client is clean and sanitary. The practitioner's hands must be sanitized before touching each client by washing with soap and warm water. The premises also must be clean at all times.

PATHS OF DISEASE AND INFECTION

congenital

a condition or disease that is present from the time of birth.

fomite

an object or material that is likely to carry infection, such as clothing, dirty linens, or used hypodermic needles.

virus

is a class of submicroscopic pathogenic agents that transmit disease.

antigen

a foreign substance or toxin that initiates an immune response such as the creation of antibodies.

The cause or source of disease can be genetic, metabolic, the result of a deficiency, or caused by a cancerous condition. Some conditions may be **congenital** or the result of a traumatic event. Autoimmune disease results when the body's immune system begins attacking its own healthy cells. The discussion in this chapter is concerned with disease that is caused by an infectious agent. Infectious diseases are caused by minute living organisms called *pathogens*. Disease-causing pathogens can be transmitted from an infected host to a new host either directly or indirectly in several ways. Direct transmission occurs when an infected host comes into contact with another subject and the pathogens are transferred to the new host. Indirect transmission can happen when a pathogen from a host is deposited on an object, or **fomite**, such as a doorknob, clothing, or a practitioner's hands and then later picked or transferred to an unwary new host. To infect a new host, a pathogen must make contact with (contaminate) and then find entry into (infect) the organism. Pathogens gain entry to the body in a variety of ways that can be called *paths of infection* or *paths of transmission*. Certain pathogens must enter the body in a specific manner for the body to become infected. Common paths of infection include ingestion, inhalation, direct contact with mucous membranes, skin contact, and invasion through broken skin. Contaminated food or water can contain organisms or parasites that cause illness, including food poisoning, giardia, hepatitis, typhoid, ringworm, and others. Respiratory infections are often the result of inhaling tiny airborne pathogens by simply being close to a contagious person who is coughing, sneezing, or simply talking. The airborne pathogens are inhaled into the respiratory tract and infect the mucous membranes of the upper tract or the more delicate tissues of the lungs. Mucous membranes of the sexual organs are the site of sexually transmitted diseases by either direct contact with infected tissue (i.e., herpes, warts) or with bodily fluids (i.e., syphilis, gonorrhea, HIV).

Healthy skin is a major defense against the invasion of pathogens; however, contact with certain infectious agents can cause an infection or exacerbate conditions like fungal infections and scabies. When the surface of the skin is broken, the possibility of pathogenic invasion increases drastically. Cuts and wounds must be cleaned, covered, and cared for so that they do not become infected.

The massage practitioner is most concerned with infectious diseases that spread by the transmission of pathogens. Pathogens commonly encountered in the massage practice include bacteria, viruses, and fungi.

Bacteria are minute, unicellular microorganisms exhibiting both plant and animal characteristics. They are also called *germs* or *microbes* and are most numerous in dirt, refuse, unclean water, and diseased tissues. Bacteria exist on the skin, in the air, in body secretions, underneath the free edges of the nails, and elsewhere. There are hundreds of different kinds of bacteria that can be seen only under a microscope. Bacteria are classified as either *nonpathogenic* (harmless) or *pathogenic* (harmful). Nonpathogenic bacteria, the beneficial and harmless type, are the most numerous and perform useful functions, such as aiding the digestive process and other bodily functions (Figure 8-1).

Pathogenic bacteria, although not as numerous, are of greater concern because they produce disease. Parasites belong to this group because they require living matter for their growth and reproduction. People involved in health care are primarily concerned with understanding and identifying pathogenic bacteria to handle them more effectively. Figure 8-2 shows the three general forms of bacteria: *cocci* (**KOCK**-sigh), *bacilli* (ba-**SIL**-eye), and *spirilla* (spy-**RIL**-uh). To the right of the name and shape of the bacteria are listed the types of bacteria and the common diseases or conditions with which they are associated (Figure 8-2 to Figure 8-5).

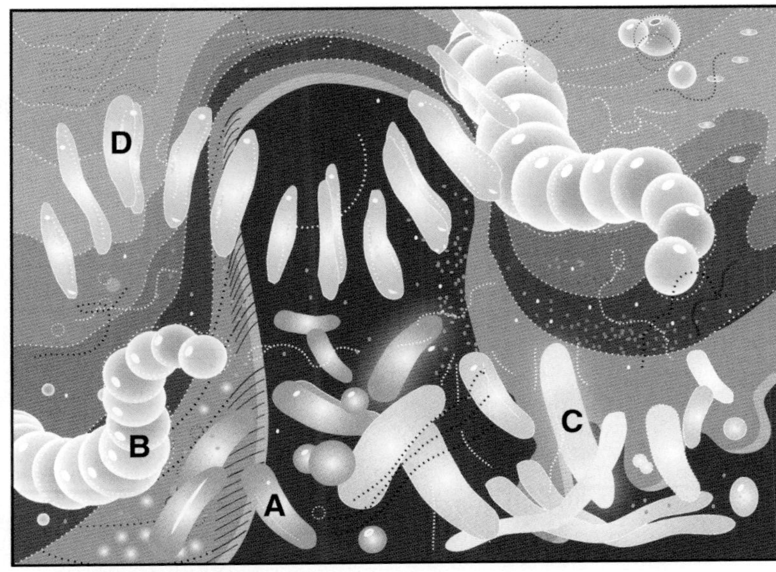

FIGURE 8-1 Nonpathogenic bacteria of many varieties thrive in the large intestine:(A) bacteroides, (B) peptostreptococcus, (C) lactobacillus, (D) eubacterium.

A **virus** is defined as any of a class of submicroscopic pathogenic agents that are capable of transmitting disease. Viruses are parasitic in that they thrive only within the cells of a living host (e.g., plant, animal, or human). They invade living cells and control their activity to produce more viruses, often with toxic substances (Figure 8-6). The cell dies and releases the viruses to invade other cells. A virus can act as an **antigen** and cause the system to produce antibodies. The virus often has the ability to change its characteristics quickly, which makes viral infections hard to treat by chemical means. Viruses are the cause of many diseases such as the common cold, smallpox, some forms of pneumonia, and childhood diseases like mumps and measles. A virus is also the causal agent for AIDS.

Fungi are parasitic organisms that thrive in a warm, moist environment and are found mostly in humans on the skin and mucous membranes. Molds and yeasts are considered fungi. Fungal infections tend to be tenacious and resist treatment. Common fungal infections include athlete's foot, ringworm, candida, and vaginal yeast infections.

fungus (*pl.* fungi) is a diverse group of organisms, potentially capable of causing disease, that thrive or grow in wet or damp areas.

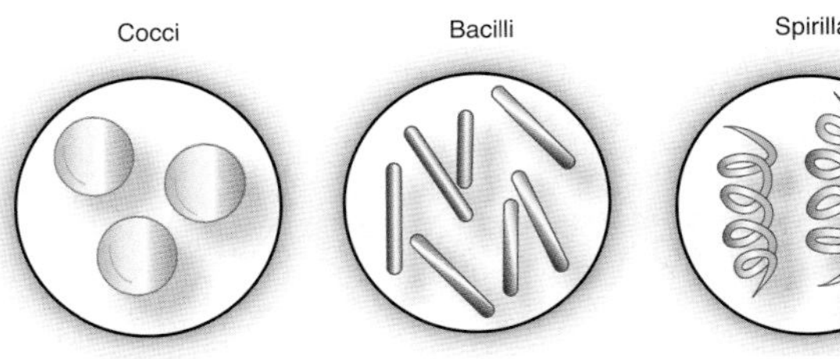

FIGURE 8-2 Three general forms of bacteria.

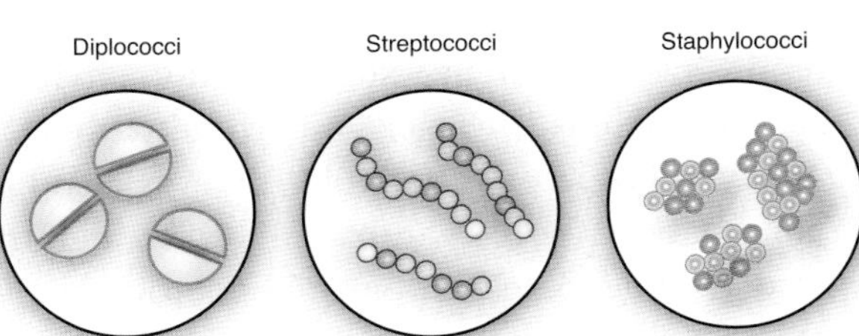

FIGURE 8-3 Groupings of bacteria.

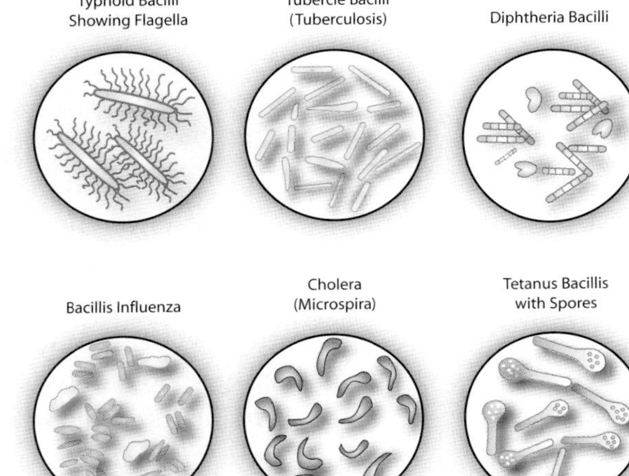

FIGURE 8-4 Six disease-producing bacteria.

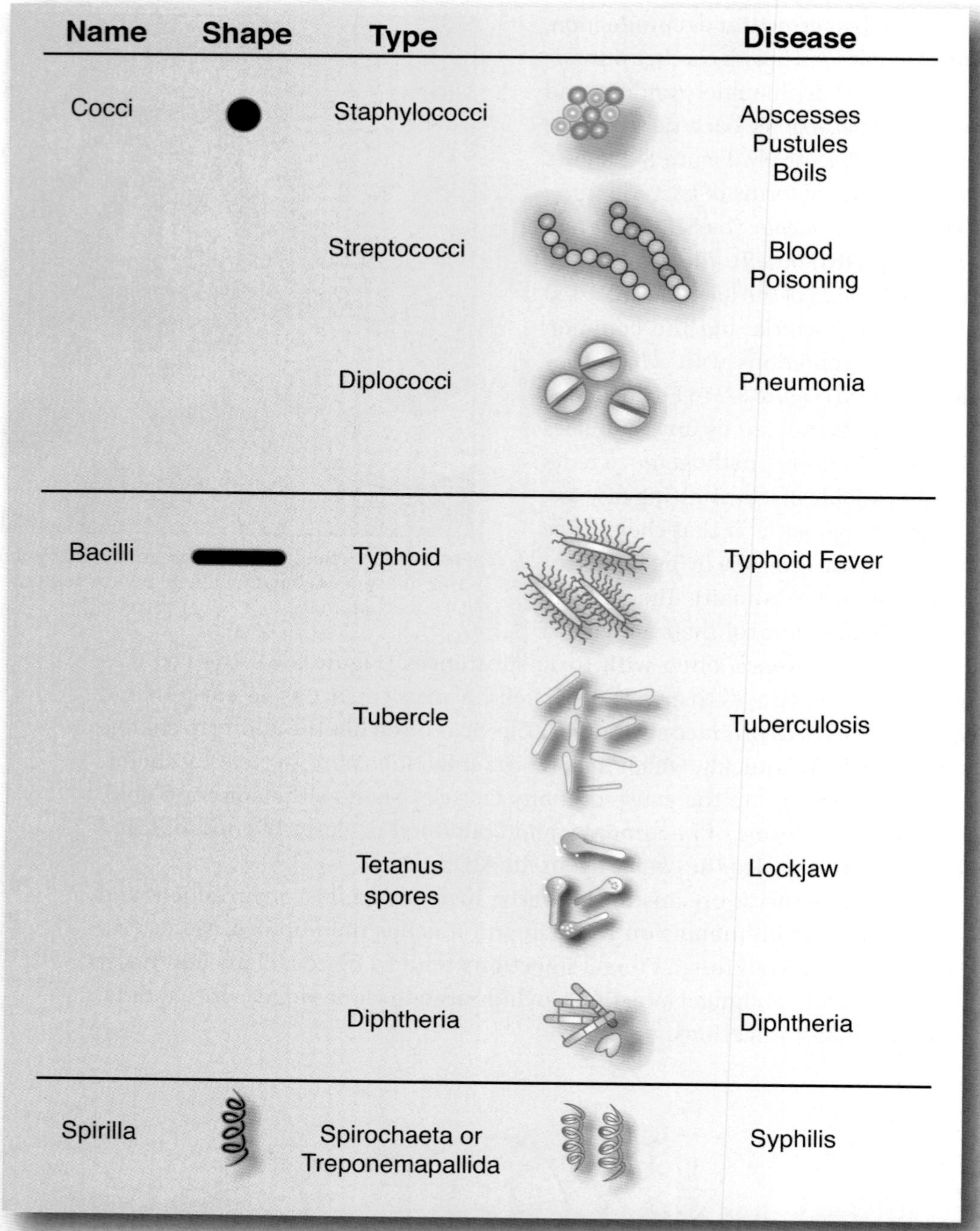

FIGURE 8-5 Pathogenic (harmful) bacteria and the common diseases or conditions with which they are associated.

Name	Shape	Type	Disease
Cocci		Staphylococci	Abscesses Pustules Boils
		Streptococci	Blood Poisoning
		Diplococci	Pneumonia
Bacilli		Typhoid	Typhoid Fever
		Tubercle	Tuberculosis
		Tetanus spores	Lockjaw
		Diphtheria	Diphtheria
Spirilla		Spirochaeta or Treponemapallida	Syphilis

antibodies

are a class of proteins produced in the body in response to contact with antigens that immunize the body.

Pathogens become a menace to health when they are able to invade the body. *Immunity* is the body's natural ability to resist infection by harmful bacteria after they have entered the body. Healthy people are able to resist infection better than those with low resistance or a compromised immune system. Healthy skin is one of the body's most important defenses against invasion of harmful pathogens. Fine hairs in the nostrils, mucous membranes, and tears in the eyes also help to defend against pathogens. Inflammation (redness and swelling) is a sign that white blood cells, or *leukocytes*, are working to destroy harmful microorganisms that have invaded the body. The body also produces antibodies, which inhibit or destroy harmful bacteria. **Antibodies** are a class of proteins produced in the body in response to contact with antigens (e.g., toxins, enzymes) that serve to immunize the body against specific antigens.

The massage practitioner must take special precaution with a client who has a contagious disease or infection and should suggest that the client see a physician. The practitioner also has a duty to protect her own health. For example, the practitioner's hands can pick up bacteria from the client's skin. If hands are not cleaned, bacteria can infect the practitioner or be spread to others with whom the practitioner comes in contact.

The best protection against the spread of infectious disease is to keep yourself and your surroundings clean and sanitary. Maintaining high standards of cleanliness requires constant supervision. Board of health regulations should be observed in maintaining clean massage facilities at all times.

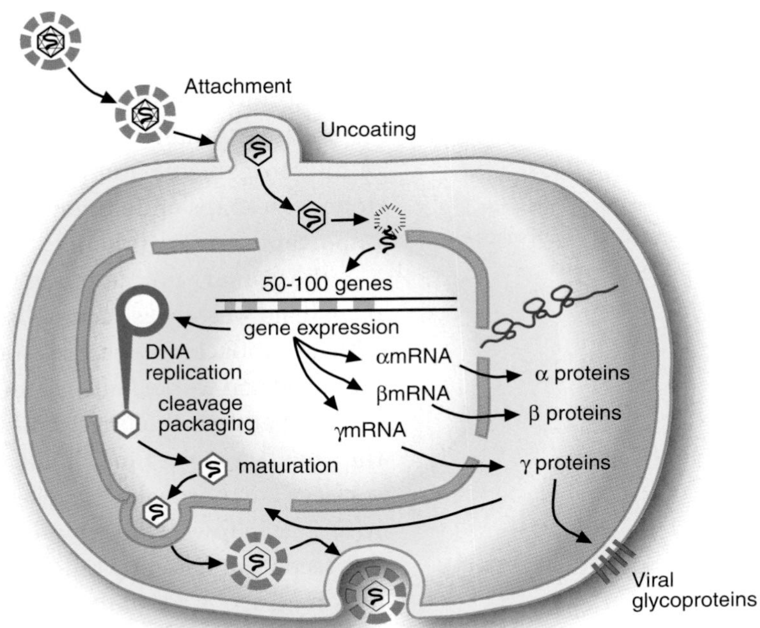

FIGURE 8-6 Schematic of virus replication.

MAINTAINING SANITARY CONDITIONS

The transmission of infectious microorganisms such as bacteria, viruses, and fungi is the cause of many of the diseases that plague humanity. It is not possible or practical to eliminate all of these pathogens from our environment; however, by the practice of sanitary procedures, it is possible to greatly reduce the spread of infectious disease.

There are three main levels of removing pathogens from implements and surfaces: sterilization, disinfection, and sanitization.

sterilization
is the most complete process of removing pathogens; this destroys all living organisms, including bacterial spores.

Sterilization is the most complete process; this destroys all living organisms on an object or surface, including bacterial spores. Sterilization is the process used on surgical instruments in hospitals. This is a difficult and time-consuming process that is generally unnecessary in a massage practice. In fact, it would be impractical if not impossible to sterilize the surfaces in a massage studio.

disinfection
is a medium level of decontamination, nearly as effective as sterilization, but it does not kill bacterial spores.

Disinfection is the next level of decontaminating pathogens, which is nearly as effective as sterilization except that it does not destroy bacterial spores. Disinfectants are powerful substances that disinfect implements and nonliving surfaces. Professional-strength disinfectants must be used with care and according to the manufacturer's instructions. Disinfectants are not used as hand cleaners because they can damage the skin with prolonged or repeated contact.

Federal law requires that manufacturers provide certain information with disinfectants, including instructions for proper use, a list of active ingredients, safety precautions, a list of the organisms against which the product is effective, and a material safety data sheet (MSDS) with information about potentially hazardous materials contained in the disinfectant. Disinfectants, when used properly, are safe and effective. Improperly used, however, they become potentially dangerous. The best way to ensure the proper use of disinfectants is to read and follow the manufacturer's instructions.

Common disinfectants used today are phenols (Lysol), chlorine bleach, and alcohol.

sanitation

is the third level of decontamination practiced in the massage studio and is done with soaps or detergents and water.

The third level of decontamination and the one practiced extensively in the massage studio is **sanitation.** Sanitation significantly reduces the number of microorganisms and pathogens found on a surface. Sanitation is generally done with soaps or detergents and water. Hand washing is a good example of an important sanitary practice.

The primary precaution in infection control is thorough hand washing. Thorough hand washing is accomplished by vigorously scrubbing the hands, preferably with an antibacterial soap and warm water. The hands are first moistened. The soap is applied and worked into a good lather. Special care is given to scrub between the fingers, between the finger and thumb, around the nails, and, if appropriate, up the arms. Hand washing should continue for at least 15 seconds to ensure that all surfaces are thoroughly cleansed. The hands are then rinsed thoroughly and dried with a clean towel. The towel is then used to turn off the water so that the hand is not recontaminated by touching the faucet. If soap and water are not available (e.g., massage at an outdoor athletic event), another option is to use an alcohol based (foam or gel) hand sanitizer. The sanitizer is applied to one hand and then the hands are rubbed together for at least 15 seconds until the hands are dry.

The practitioner's hands should be washed with warm water and soap before and after each session. Washing the hands before the massage protects the client. Thorough hand washing after the massage protects the practitioner and anyone the practitioner might come into contact with later.

There may be situations or conditions in the practice of massage when special hygienic precautions are warranted. As a rule, massage is not performed on clients who have highly contagious or infectious diseases. It is also a rare occasion when the practitioner might be exposed to any body fluids. It is important for the practitioner to recognize these situations and observe Universal Precautions (see discussion later).

The practice of massage might find you working with a client who is in a weak and vulnerable condition or who is in the contagious stage of a disease yet shows no symptoms. Hygienic practices, especially concerning hand washing and protection, are essential to the health and safety of the client, the practitioner, other clients, and personnel associated in any way with the practice.

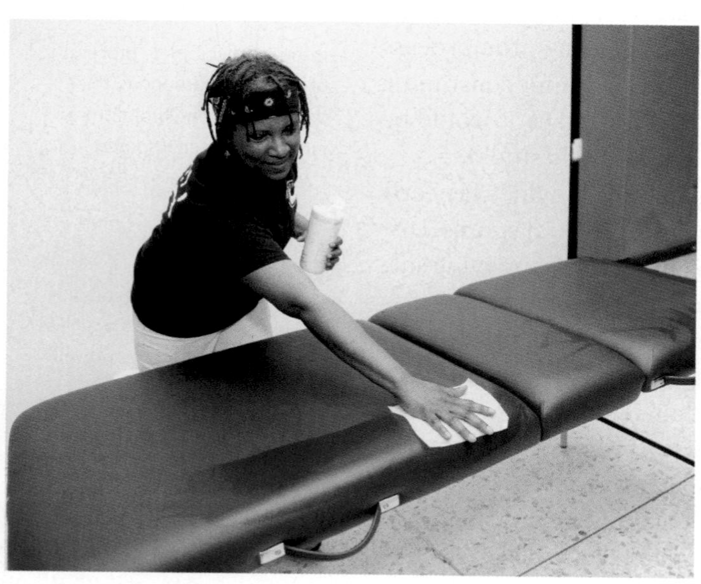

FIGURE 8-7A It is important to keep the massage work area and equipment in a sanitary condition.

It is important to keep the massage studio or work area, dispensary, implements, and equipment in a sanitary condition (Figure 8-7a). Supplies such as towels, blankets, and sheets should be kept in a closed cabinet, away from airbourne pathogens. Clean linens must used for each client. After each use, linens should be stored in a covered container until they can be laundered in hot water and dried in a hot dryer. If there is any concern that the linens have been contaminated, one cup of chlorine bleach can be added to the wash water. Disposable products such as paper towels and sheets are discarded after each use and fresh ones supplied for each client.

Although the massage practitioner might not use a wide range of mechanical aids or electrical equipment, anything that comes into contact with the client's body must be kept sanitized. There are disinfectants, antiseptics, and fumigants that kill or retard the growth of bacteria. Some are commercially prepared, economical to use, and quick acting. General antiseptics are alcohol, hydrogen peroxide, sodium hypochlorite (household bleach), and boric acid. Disinfectants are stronger than antiseptics.

Universal Precautions

Universal Precautions (Box 8.1) is a system of infection control designed to protect persons from exposure to blood and/or bloody body fluids. With Universal Precautions, all blood and body fluids are to be considered potentially infectious for diseases such as HIV, hepatitis A, B, C, and other blood-borne pathogens.

universal precautions

is a system of infection control that protects persons from exposure to blood and bloody body fluids.

Sanitizers

A **wet sanitizer** is any receptacle large enough to hold a disinfectant solution in which the objects to be sanitized can be completely immersed. A cover is provided to prevent contamination of the solution. Wet sanitizers can be obtained in various sizes and shapes (Figure 8-7b).

Before immersing objects such as hand brushes in a wet sanitizer, be sure to wash them thoroughly with hot water and soap, and rinse them thoroughly with

wet sanitizer

is any receptacle large enough to hold a disinfectant solution in which the objects to be sanitized can be completely immersed.

Box 8.1

The Components of Universal Precautions

1. Hand washing with soap and water is mandatory before and after contact with every client. Use disposable paper towels. Hands and other skin surfaces should be washed immediately and thoroughly if contaminated with blood or other body fluids.
2. Gloves must be worn if the skin of the practitioner's hands is not intact. Practitioners who have lesions or weeping dermatitis on their hands should refrain from doing massage until the condition heals.
3. Gloves shall be worn when there is potential for direct contact with body fluids, mucous membranes, nonintact skin of clients, or handling of items or surfaces soiled with blood or body fluids. Gloves shall be immediately discarded after use.
4. Gloves should be put on prior to beginning a task and removed when the task is complete. Hands must be washed after removal of gloves.
5. Linen soiled with blood or body fluids must be gathered without undue agitation and placed in a leak-proof bag for transportation to the laundry or soiled linen container.
6. Laundry: Because the risk of disease transmission from soiled linen is negligible, hygienic and common sense storage and processing of clean and soiled linen is recommended. Soiled linens should be handled as little as possible. Linens should be washed with detergent and one cup of chlorine bleach in hot water and dried in a hot dryer.
7. Housekeeping: Walls, floors, and other surfaces are not directly associated with transmission of infections; therefore, attempts to disinfect or sterilize are not necessary except for the area of a specific spill. Cleaning and removal of soil should be done routinely, however, by using products that, according to the manufacturer's instructions, are effective for the sanitation.

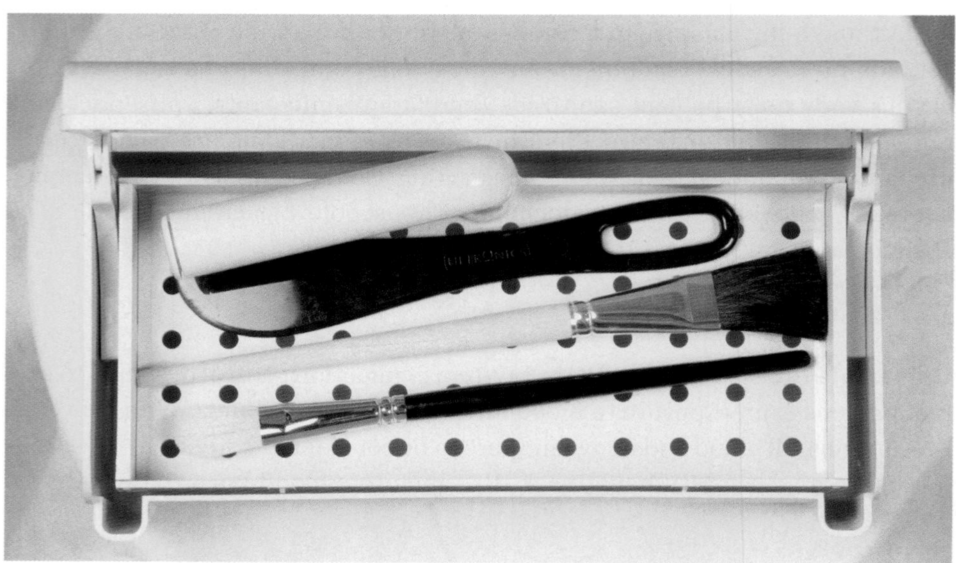

FIGURE 8-7B Wet sanitizer.

clear water. This procedure prevents contamination of the solution. In addition, soap and hot water remove most of the bacteria.

After items are removed from the disinfectant solution, they should be rinsed in clean water, wiped dry with a clean towel, and stored in a dry or cabinet sanitizer until needed.

Some implements can be washed with hot water and soap, immersed in alcohol, wiped dry, and then placed in a sterile container until needed.

Moist heat is the method of boiling objects in water at 212° F (100° C) for about 20 minutes. A vessel known as an *autoclave* is sometimes used in the medical field for sterilization purposes.

Disinfectants

Some disinfectants in general use (Table 8.1) are

- Chlorine bleach
- Ethyl or grain alcohol
- Cresol (Lysol)

Common household chlorine bleach is effective for disinfecting surfaces, implements, and linens. For surfaces and implements, prepare a 1:10 solution by combining one part bleach with nine parts water. Immerse implements for at least 10 minutes. (***Note:*** This bleach solution will discolor dyed material.) For linens, add one cup bleach to hot water during the wash cycle.

Ethyl or *grain alcohol* comes in liquid form. Electrodes and similar implements can be sanitized in 70 percent solution. Alcohol can be used as a rinse to sanitize the hands.

Cresol or Lysol (1 to 5 percent) can be used for cleaning floors, sinks, and restrooms. Commercially prepared solutions are available.

It is important to read directions on all containers when mixing any sanitizing agent.

When in doubt about antiseptics and disinfectants approved for use in your studio or work area, consult your local health department or state board of health.

TABLE 8.1

APPROVED CHEMICALS

NAME	FORM	STRENGTH	HOW TO USE
Sodium hypochlorite (household bleach)	Liquid	10% solution	Immerse implements in solution for 10 or more minutes
Alcohol	Liquid	70% solution	Immerse implements or sanitize electrodes and sharp cutting edges for 10 or more minutes
Cresol or Lysol	Liquid	1% to 5% solution	Use to clean floors, sinks, and restrooms

Proper Practices for Sanitizing Surfaces in a Massage Facility

- Floors
- Massage tables and bolsters
- Restrooms

It is good business practice to keep a massage business facility clean. Clients or patrons expect and appreciate coming into a place that is clean and orderly. For health reasons, it is also important to keep your place of business sanitary. Many different people will pass through your business, and they could be carrying with them a great variety of bacteria and other pathogens. To reduce the possibility of these pathogens being passed on to you or other clients, it is important to exercise good sanitary practices.

Floors

- Carpets: Keep well vacuumed, and shampoo when necessary.
- Solid floors: Sweep daily, sanitize with detergent and water, disinfect with Lysol-type product or a commercial-grade disinfectant.

Other surfaces

- Sanitize all surfaces with cleaning solution (soap and water or commercially prepared solution).

Massage tables and bolsters

- Use spray-type cleaner or soap and water to remove oils.
- Disinfect with disinfectant-type cleaner (10 percent chlorine bleach solution, Lysol, alcohol, or other comparable cleaner/disinfectant).

Restrooms

- Sanitize all surfaces with detergent and water.
- Disinfect with commercial disinfectant or Lysol-type product.
- Use 1:10 solution of chlorine bleach to water.
- Spray or wipe the surface with the recommended disinfectant, then wipe dry. Spray again and allow the surface to air dry. Be sure to wear gloves when using a disinfectant to prevent skin irritation. If using a spray bottle, be sure not to inhale the mists.
- Supply restrooms with paper towels, toilet paper, paper cups (in a dispenser), and a liquid antibacterial hand soap.

All products used in the application of massage services must be stored in closed containers that are clearly labeled. Massage oil should be in unbreakable containers with dispenser tops that allow the practitioner to easily dispense the amount of oil or lotion needed without contaminating the remaining contents of the bottle. Using an unbreakable bottle reduces the risk of spillage or breakage should the bottle slip and fall on the floor.

Salves and creams should be removed from containers with spatulas or other implements rather than with the fingers. Any unused salve or cream must be discarded and not put back into the container. This reduces the chance of the products being contaminated. Lids should be kept on containers, and the outside of the containers should be kept clean.

SUMMARY OF PRECAUTIONS

1. Keep yourself and your clothing clean. If clothing becomes soiled, change clothes between clients. The massage professional may choose to wear medical scrubs when doing massage.
2. Wash and sanitize your hands with soap and warm water before and after every client. A good hand brush should be used for scrubbing, particularly around the nails, and then the hands should be rinsed and wiped dry. If there is cause for suspicion of bacterial contamination, a mild alcohol solution or alcohol-based hand sanitizer can be used to rinse the hands.
3. Keep all products, implements, and areas used during massage in a sanitary condition. This includes the surfaces where items are placed.
4. Keep lubricants (e.g., oils, creams, and lotions) in contamination-proof dispensers and containers. Clean the outside of the lubricant containers after each client.
5. If a jar-type container is used, never remove the product directly with the fingers. Avoid cross-contamination by using a disposable tongue depressor or a spatula that can be sanitized between uses. Discard any unused lubricant rather than returning it to the container. Be sure that all products are correctly labeled to prevent using the wrong product.
6. Use clean linens for every client. Linens and towels should be laundered in hot water and soap and dried in a hot dryer. Chlorine bleach should be added for its germicidal benefits. Clean linens should be stored in closed cabinets. To prevent a rancid odor, sheets and towels should be laundered the same day that they are used. Generally, laundry products and fabric softeners eliminate odor. Once sheets and towels have become rancid, however, they should be discarded.
   Some oils (e.g., peanut, olive, mineral, almond) tend to be hard to remove from fabric. Oil usually washes out if sheets and towels are laundered immediately. When it is not possible to launder as often as needed, practitioners should use disposable sheets. Commercial products are available from most massage oil manufacturers to remove rancid oil and odors from linens.
7. Wear vinyl gloves or another appropriate covering if you have broken skin or infections on your hands.
8. Do not perform massage if you have a contagious illness that could be passed on by contact or being close to others.
9. If a client has a contagious condition, take precautions to protect yourself, your client, and others from spreading the infection. If it is an acute condition, such as a respiratory infection, or accompanied by fever, massage is contraindicated. Rescheduling the appointment might be the best option. If it is a regional condition, avoid the particular area. If it is a general condition

that does not preclude massage and the client is under medical care, consult with the physician or medical team to determine the best way to proceed.

10. Keep all areas of the workplace and furnishings clean and sanitary. This includes restrooms, dressing rooms, and work space.
11. The place of business should be well ventilated and kept at a comfortable temperature. Floors, walls, windows, and furniture should all reflect your concern for cleanliness and pride in your place of business. Practitioners should know and practice all of the rules of sanitation issued by their state board and department of health.

SAFETY PRACTICES AND PROCEDURES FOR MASSAGE THERAPISTS

Massage and massage therapy are personalized health services that usually involve interaction between client and practitioner and do not involve the use of hazardous equipment or practices. There are safety issues that the massage student and practitioner must keep in mind, however. Safety is an attitude put into practice that is concerned with the prevention of situations and elimination of conditions that could lead to injury of the massage practitioner or client. To ensure the health and safety of everyone concerned, safety considerations must focus on (1) the facility and equipment, (2) the massage practitioner, and (3) the client.

The Facilities

The facilities include the building that houses the massage facility, the facility itself, and the equipment and space within the facility. Safety precautions in the facility include housekeeping, sanitation, fire policy, and heating and ventilation.

Housekeeping/Sanitation

- Keep all halls and walkways clear.
- Keep all carpets vacuumed and cleaned.
- Keep all solid floors cleaned and sanitized.
- Sanitize all restroom and bathing facilities.
- Make sure all floors in wet areas are slip proof.
- Sanitize all equipment surfaces that come in contact with clients (i.e., table surfaces, linens, applicators, and vibrators).
- Disinfect hydrotherapy tubs, steam cabinets, shower stalls, and wet tables between each use.
- Maintain hand-washing facilities (e.g., germicidal soap, sanitary or paper towels, clean and sanitary area).
- Linens are commercially laundered or washed in hot water with detergent and dried in a hot dryer. Bleach is available and used when there is any chance of contamination.
- Clean linens are stored in a closed cabinet. Soiled linens are stored in a covered container or stored outside the massage room.

Equipment

- Check all equipment for safety and stability (e.g., tables, stools, chairs,).
- Each time a table is set up, check all hinges and locks for stability.
- Maintain all equipment (e.g., electrical cords, lubrication).
- Store equipment and linens properly.

Fire Safety

- Maintain functioning smoke and carbon monoxide detectors.
- Be familiar with the location and use of fire extinguishers.
- Clearly indicate fire exits.
- Be aware of and practice evacuation procedures.
- Establish a policy regarding the use of open flames, candles, incense, and the like.
- Contact your local fire department for a fire safety inspection.

First Aid

- Keep a maintained first-aid kit on the premises.
- Make sure that all personnel know the location of the first-aid kit.
- As many staff members as possible should learn first aid and cardiopulmonary resuscitation (CPR) techniques.
- Keep emergency information posted in plain view near all telephones, including telephone numbers for the fire and police departments, ambulance, hospital, emergency department, doctors, and taxis.

Heat and Ventilation

The practice of massage requires that the massage room be somewhat warmer than normal. This necessitates either turning up the thermostat or using auxiliary heating devices.

- Maintain and service heating and ventilation systems regularly.
- Use only UL-approved auxiliary heating devices.
- Regularly inspect auxiliary heating devices.
- Turn off auxiliary heating devices when not in use.

Practitioner Personal Safety

- When lifting equipment or clients, use proper body mechanics and lifting techniques to prevent muscle strain and injury.
- Use proper body mechanics and techniques when practicing massage to prevent muscle strain and overuse syndromes resulting in back, shoulder, or arm injury.
- Use equipment and adjunctive modalities properly and according to manufacturers' instructions and recommendations.
- All practitioners should maintain a current first aid and CPR certification.
- Know the location of the first-aid kit.
- Wash hands before and after every treatment.

- Know contraindications for massage and perform only procedures that cause no injury and are within your scope of practice.
- Have a plan in place to deal with or escape from a client who is acting inappropriately or dangerously.
- When doing an in-house massage, inform an associate of the location, name of the client, the time of the appointment, and the time you plan to complete the appointment. When you have completed the appointment, contact your associate to indicate that you have finished.

Client Safety

- Understand the paths of infection and ensure clients' protection with sanitary practices.
  a. Use clean linens with each client.
  b. Wash hands before and after each client.
  c. Provide sanitary bathing facilities and restrooms.
  d. Avoid open wounds and sores.
  e. Do not practice massage if you are ill or contagious.
- Provide safe, clear entryways and passages.
  a. Keep walkways clear and well lighted.
  b. Provide nonskid walkways and floors.
- Assist clients on and off of the massage table.
- Check to make sure that clients are not sensitive or allergic to products used.
- Use proper procedures in dealing with illness and injury. Refer to proper medical authorities when conditions indicate.
- Do no harm!

QUESTIONS FOR DISCUSSION AND REVIEW

1. Why do all states have laws pertaining to sanitation?
2. Why is it particularly important for a massage practitioner to practice rules of sanitation?
3. Why should the practitioner have some knowledge of bacteria?
4. What is the difference between pathogenic and nonpathogenic bacteria?
5. What is the main purpose of the body's production of antibodies?
6. Name three forms of pathogenic (harmful) bacteria.
7. What is the best prevention against the spread of harmful bacteria?
8. What are Universal Precautions and when should they be observed?
9. What should you do before using any disinfectant or antiseptic product?
10. Why are disinfectants used in the practice of massage?
11. What is the best method for keeping the hands and nails clean?
12. Which strengths of cresol or Lysol are most suitable for cleaning floors, sinks, or restrooms?
13. What is sterilization?
14. What is safety?
15. What are the four areas of concern for safety in a massage practice?

CHAPTER

9 Consultation and Documentation

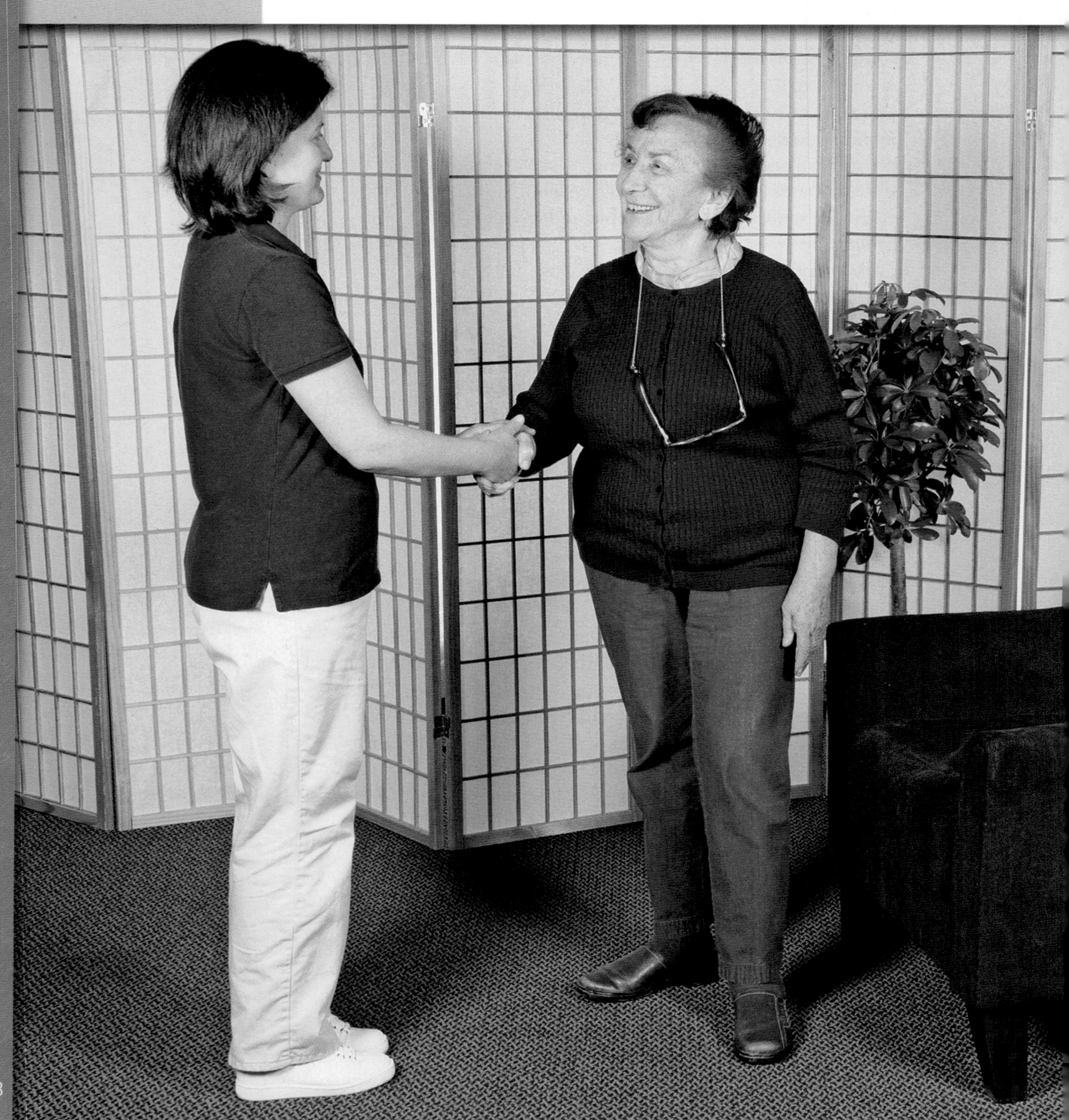

LEARNING OBJECTIVES

After you have mastered this chapter, you will be able to

1. **Explain the importance of the consultation before a massage.**
2. **Demonstrate how to screen clients while making appointments.**
3. **Demonstrate how to determine the needs and expectations of the client.**
4. **Explain why it is important to set policies during the first consultation.**
5. **Define a treatment plan.**
6. **Explain which records should be kept and why they should be updated.**

INTRODUCTION

A consultation is a meeting in which views are discussed and valuable information is exchanged. During preliminary consultations between massage practitioners and prospective clients, the clients give pertinent information about who they are and why they are seeking the services of the therapist. Practitioners inform clients about the services that they provide.

The extent of the consultation depends on the type of massage services offered and the client's reason for coming for the session. A relatively healthy client coming for a general, relaxing, wellness massage will require only a brief consultation to determine the client's preferences, needs, and concerns; review pertinent information from the client intake form; explain policies and procedures; and determine that there are no contraindications. A client coming with a prescription from a doctor, seeking relief from pain acquired from an auto accident, or seeking reimbursement from insurance, however, will require a more extensive consultation, assessment, and record keeping. Consultation practices discussed in this chapter are for practitioners in the wellness, personal service sector. Assessment procedures for therapeutic applications are discussed in Chapter 17, Therapeutic Procedure.

MAKING THE FIRST APPOINTMENT

The first contact between a practitioner and a prospective client is often the first time that the client makes an appointment for a massage. During this first contact, important information can be exchanged to determine whether making the appointment for the massage is appropriate. The prospective client might be looking for services that the therapist does not provide, or it might be determined that massage is contraindicated for the conditions of the would-be client. Screening prospective clients with a few questions can save valuable time for both the would-be client and the practitioner as well as eliminate difficult or inappropriate situations.

Three questions help to screen prospective clients:

- What is your previous experience with massage?
- How did you find out about my services?
- What is your main reason for making this appointment?

Without going into detail, responses to these questions will clarify whether an appointment is desired and appropriate.

THE CONSULTATION

The consultation is a time to gather and exchange information. During the consultation, the therapist has the opportunity to

- Establish open and effective communication with the client
- Explain procedures and state policies
- Determine the client's needs and expectations
- Complete and review intake and medical history forms
- Perform a preliminary assessment
- Formulate a treatment plan
- Obtain informed consent from the client

The consultation is an interview process that helps to determine the course of treatment and sets the tone of the therapeutic relationship between therapist and client. Often, the first consultation is also the first time that the therapist and client meet. First impressions are lasting impressions; the image that the therapist exhibits will influence the client's respect and confidence (Figure 9-1). Be prepared by having everything needed for the interview and massage session organized and ready. Greet the client in a professional and friendly manner. Be courteous and sensitive. Keep the consultation relaxed yet directed toward pertinent information.

An effective consultation depends on clear communication. The practitioner must not only be able to explain policies and procedures so that the client can understand them but also must listen to and understand clearly the needs and wants of the client. To communicate clearly, it is helpful for the practitioner to be aware of the client's level of intelligence and communicating style, as well as the client's emotional and mental condition. Communicate on a level with the client and in a manner that the client comprehends. Some people communicate better

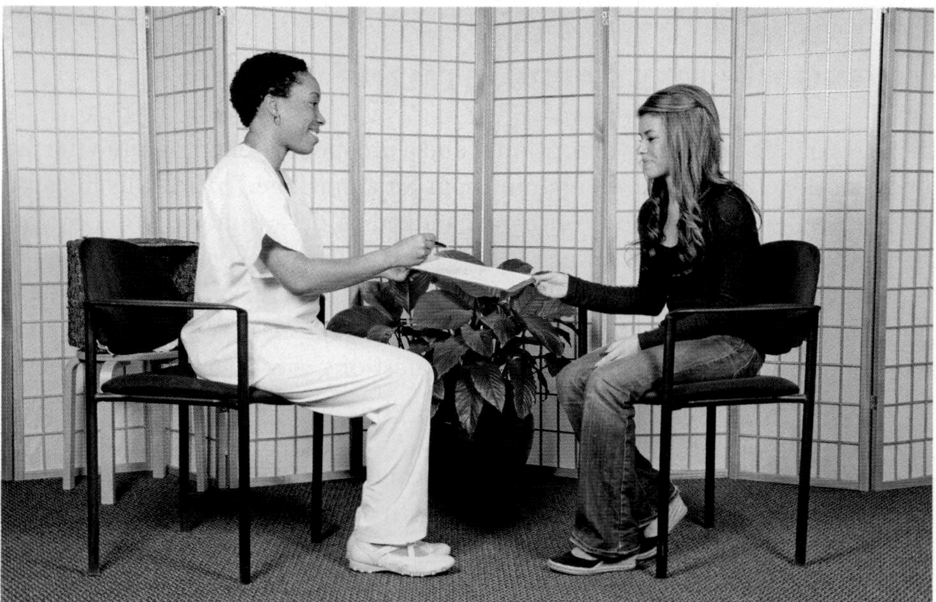

FIGURE 9-1 The consultation allows the therapist to gather information and helps to set the tone of the therapeutic relationship.

by seeing things or by reading or writing information. Others do better talking and listening or by being able to touch and feel things. Be aware of how the client best expresses him- or herself and respond in the same manner. Create an atmosphere of receptivity and develop a rapport with the client by listening carefully and being genuinely interested in any concerns. Personalize the connection by maintaining visual contact, using the client's name and listening attentively during the consultation. Observing and mirroring the client's body language, voice tone, and language can also enhance rapport. Good rapport provides the basis for trust, mutual respect, openness, and harmony, all of which enhance the therapeutic relationship.

Not all communication is by spoken word. **Nonverbal communication** in the way of posturing, gestures, and facial expressions can accompany verbal communication or can be expressed on its own. Nonverbal communication, sometimes known as *body language*, often "speaks louder than words" and provides clues to a person's emotional, subconscious, or even physical condition. Be observant of the way a client holds his body, sits, or moves for clues to where he holds tension or pain, or how confident or uncomfortable he might be. Does the client seem to be open and engaged in the consultation or reserved and reluctant to participate? Sometimes verbal and nonverbal communications are not congruent. The words say one thing, and the body or expression says another. For instance, if a client is telling you how good he feels and how well things are going for him at the same time his head and shoulders are down and his voice is weak and shaky, consider inquiring further into the reasons for seeking massage and provide feedback (tactfully) that his body language is sending a different message.

nonverbal communication also known as body language, is how a person's posturing, gestures, and facial expressions provide information about his mental, emotional, or physical condition.

Nonverbal communication is also an important consideration during the massage. Facial expressions such as serene smiles or grimaces and subtle sounds such as moans and groans provide feedback to the practitioner that the selected massage procedures are appreciated or perhaps too aggressive. Fidgeting, muscle contractions, and flinches indicate discomfort and the need to alter the massage in some way. When a nonverbal message is given and received, the practitioner might want to verbalize feedback to the client to clarify the message and ensure that the interpretation is correct.

As a practitioner, be aware of your own nonverbal expression and body language and how they might affect the client. A practitioner who is attentive and responsive, and who maintains eye contact from the same elevation makes a much better impression than a practitioner who sits across a desk, shuffling papers, or who stands above the client or turns his back while attending to other tasks during the consultation. The practitioner's body language should send the message that the practitioner is open, friendly, confident, and professionally interested in the client during the consultation and throughout the therapeutic relationship.

During the consultation, the practitioner should ask questions to determine client concerns and conditions. Ask pertinent questions and listen closely to the responses. Use open-ended questions that require an explanatory response rather than those that can simply be answered with a yes or no. Questions like, "Describe your areas of discomfort and show me where you feel it" provide more information than "Do you have discomfort?" When you do ask a question, listen attentively to the response and allow as much time as necessary for the client to answer the question completely. To make sure that you understood the client's response, summarize what was said and state it back to the client. This gives the client a chance to agree or clarify what was said. This practice, known as *active listening*, vastly reduces the possibility of misinterpreting any information.

The preliminary consultation is the first opportunity for the client and therapist to meet one another, to clarify their intentions and expectations for the massage, and to agree on some goals. The first consultation is the time for the client to learn about the therapist and the kind of therapies offered and get some idea about the expected outcome. The practitioner is ethically bound to provide information about credentials, training, the massage procedures to be used, and the expected results so that the client can make a choice to participate in those services based on a clear understanding of the information provided. During this first consultation, the therapist learns about the client's conditions, needs, and expectations and determines whether there are any partial or general contraindications for massage, or whether there is any reason to refer the client to another health practitioner. The therapist uses the information gained during the consultation to adapt the massage services to best serve the client's needs. The purpose of the consultation is to exchange information regarding the client's conditions and expectations and the services offered by the therapist and to determine whether they are compatible. During this consultation, enough information is exchanged so that the client can give **informed consent** for the services to be received.

informed consent

is a client's written authorization for professional services based on adequate information from the massage therapist about the massage, including expectations, potential benefits, possible undesirable effects, and professional and ethical responsibility.

The preliminary consultation is the most extensive; forms are filled out, policies set, an assessment done, and a treatment plan created. Each session, however, should begin with a short question-and-answer period to determine any changes in conditions or course of treatment.

EXPLAIN PROCEDURES AND STATE POLICIES

During the first consultation, practitioners clearly explain their operational and client interaction policies. Clearly stating policies concerning such things as missed or late appointments, payment of fees, and sexual boundaries avoids misconceptions and awkward situations. Some practitioners include a disclaimer that their services are not a medical treatment. There is no specific manner to present these policies. They can be posted, printed on the intake forms, or stated verbally. Regardless of how they are expressed, set only those policies that you are willing to uphold.

When the reasons for the client visit are clear and client expectations are stated, practitioners can explain the services that they offer and how those services are of benefit to the client. Practitioners can also explain any procedures that they use during the treatment sessions or procedures that clients need to follow during their visits. It is important to keep clients informed about what is being done and why. This is especially important if it is the client's first visit to the place of business or the first massage. (See Box 9.1.)

During the consultation, the client usually wants to know how the massage treatments will be beneficial. Being able to answer the client's questions adds to the practitioner's credibility as a professional and helps to build client confidence.

Box 9.1

Policies and Procedures

Procedures and policies should be explained during the initial consultation. It is advisable to have policies and procedures printed in a document that the client reads. The therapist can choose to review important policies and procedures to make sure that the client understands them.

Policies and procedures include

- *Type of services offered.* List the modalities or types of therapy offered. Provide an explanation of the benefits, risks, and limitations of the therapy. List any specialty areas, groups, or conditions in which you specialize.
- *Qualifications of therapists.* Provide information regarding schooling, special training, licenses, years of experience, and professional affiliations.
- *Business policies.* Define your appointment policy, including your work schedule, the days and hours available for appointments, and how long in advance an appointment can be made or canceled. State the policy for late or missed appointments and the length of sessions. State that information shared during the session and all client files are confidential except when subpoenaed by a court of law. Before client information is shared for medical or insurance purposes, the client is asked to sign a Release of Medical Information form. State clearly the policies regarding sexual boundaries.
- *Fees.* List the fees for different lengths of sessions or different services. Define the kinds of payment accepted: cash, check, credit card, billing later, insurance accepted (under which circumstances). Do you offer discounts for multiple sessions or referrals? Is there a sliding scale?
- *Session procedures.* Describe a common massage session and what the client can expect. Include the intake and assessment time, undressing and draping procedures, the sequence of the massage, use of oils or lubricants, policy on talking during massage, the use of music or not, and any special or restricted activity following massage.

DETERMINING THE CLIENT'S NEEDS AND EXPECTATIONS

To perform services that directly benefit clients, it is necessary to understand their reasons for seeking your services. What are the client's main and secondary concerns? Has the client received massage previously? Which type of massage does the client prefer? What are the client's expectations for the session? What does the client expect to get out of the treatment; what are the goals? Are those goals reasonable, and what will it take for the client to be satisfied? Which physical conditions might benefit from massage? Are there any conditions that contraindicate massage? Is it necessary to refer the client to another health care provider before providing any massage services?

To obtain an understanding, it is necessary to ask questions and pay close attention to the responses. Two ways of asking questions are written and verbal. Written questions are in the form of intake and medical history questionnaires that the client fills out. When the forms are completed and reviewed, several verbal questions might be appropriate to clarify the written answers or to gain more specific information about clients and their reason for coming. Important responses should be recorded in the client's file (Figure 9-2).

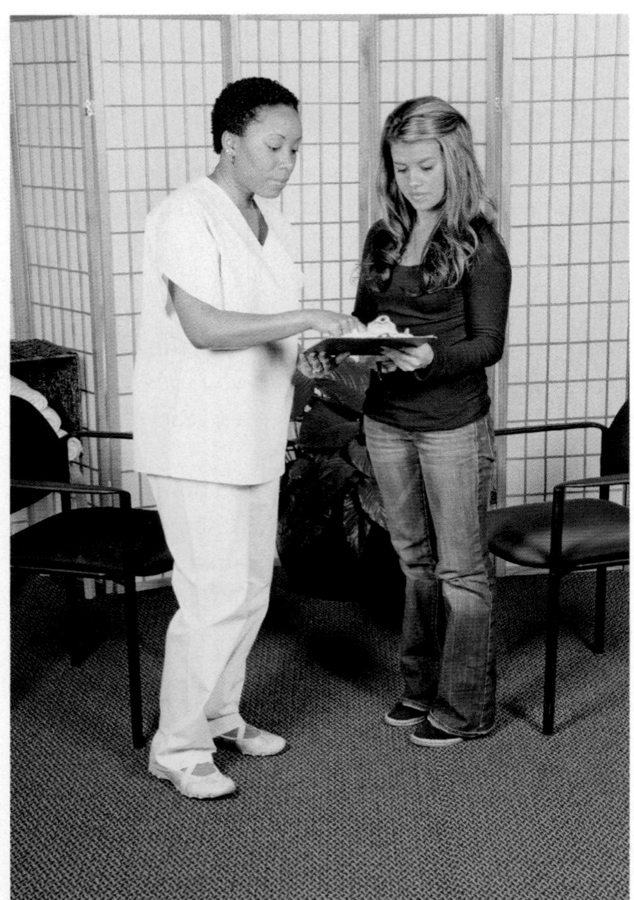

FIGURE 9-2 Review the client's responses on the intake and medical history questionnaires to determine whether further information about the client is needed.

INTAKE AND MEDICAL HISTORY FORMS

Client intake and medical history forms are documents or questionnaires that the client fills out before or during the preliminary consultation. The client intake and medical history forms provide vital information that the therapist uses to formulate a treatment strategy. The information requested on intake and medical history forms varies according to the kind of massage services offered or the needs of the therapist. Examples of intake and medical history forms for relaxation/wellness massage have been included in this chapter to provide ideas or models (Figure 9-3).

By reviewing the forms, the therapist can reduce the time required to interview the client. After the prospective client has filled out the forms and the therapist has reviewed the information, the client is interviewed to elaborate on questions that might need more in-depth consideration. Information gained during the interview is recorded and becomes part of the client's permanent record.

When reviewing consultation forms with the client, be tactful. If a client questions why you are asking certain questions, explain the reasons. For example, if the form is asked, "What do you do with the majority of your time (hobbies, outside work)?" The client's answers can give clues about which area of the client's body that could be carrying stress. The client's answer to the question, "Have you had any surgery?" gives you clues to health problems and contraindications. The question "Have you received massages before?" allows you to determine what the client's expectations and preferences might be. The question "How did you find out about our massage services?" gives you information about which kind of advertising is most effective.

BODY DIAGRAMS

Body diagrams of the male or female figure are helpful when the client has some painful, sore, or stiff areas that require attention. Give the client a few minutes to indicate these areas on the diagram, and then discuss the condition and allow the client to explain any symptoms. After clients have indicated the location of their discomforts on the diagram, ask them to touch or point to the area(s) on their own body. Add notes to the diagram to clarify and record clients' comments about their conditions (Figures 9-4 and 9-5).

The practitioner can direct more questions to assess the situation. Questions specifically relating to the client's condition help to determine the course

Massage Clinic
Client Information Form

Name________________________________ Birth Date ____________________________

Address ______________________________ Telephone ____________________________

______________________________________ Business Phone _________________________

City/State/Zip __________________________ E-mail Address _________________________

Occupation ____________________________ Other Activities_________________________

General Health Condition______________________ Blood Pressure _______________

List any serious or chronic illness, operations, chronic virus infections, or traumatic accidents you have had. ____

Are you in recovery for addictions or abuse?_____________________________________

Are you under a doctor's, chiropractor's, or other health practitioner's care? ________

If so, for what condition(s)? ____

Are you on any medication?_______ If so, what? ______________________________

Do I have permission to contact your doctor/therapist?_____________________________

Names of doctors, chiropractors, or health practitioners:

Name________________________________ Name _________________________________

Address ______________________________ Address _______________________________

Telephone _____________________________ Telephone _____________________________

Why did you come for our services? (relaxation, pain, therapy, etc.)________________

____

What results would you like to achieve with our work? ___________________________

Have you had any massage therapy before?______If so, when and why? ____________

____

How did you find out about our services? _______________________________________

Were you referred to this office? ________ By whom? ____________________________

In case of emergency notify: Name_________________Phone _______________________

I have completed this information form to the best of my knowledge. I understand the massage services are designed to be a health aid and are in no way to take the place of a doctor's care when it is indicated. Information exchanged during any massage session is educational in nature and is intended to help me become more familiar and conscious of my own health status and is to be used at my own discretion.

Our time together is precious, and I agree to cancel 24 hours in advance. Unless there is an emergency, if I miss an appointment, I agree to pay the full appointment fee.

Date__________________ Signature ____

FIGURE 9-3 Sample client intake information form.

that the massage sessions will take. Questions also reveal other conditions that might (or might not) be related to the primary condition. Thorough assessment also exposes any contraindications for massage.

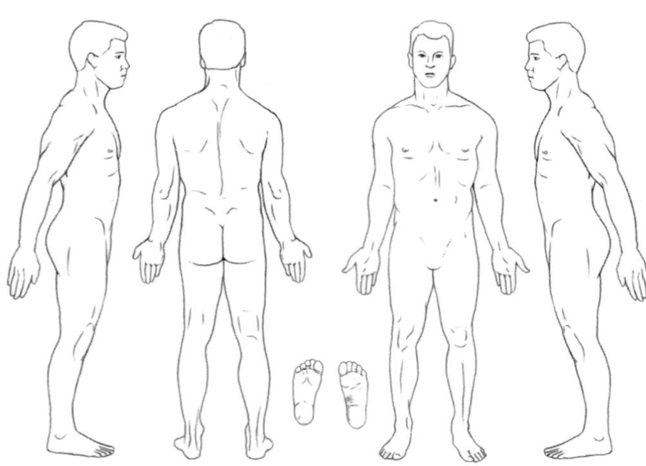

FIGURE 9-4 Male body diagram. On the diagram, mark as follows: Put an X on any painful area. Rate the pain on a scale of 1 to 10. Shade in any stiff or sore areas. Circle areas of other concern and describe the condition.

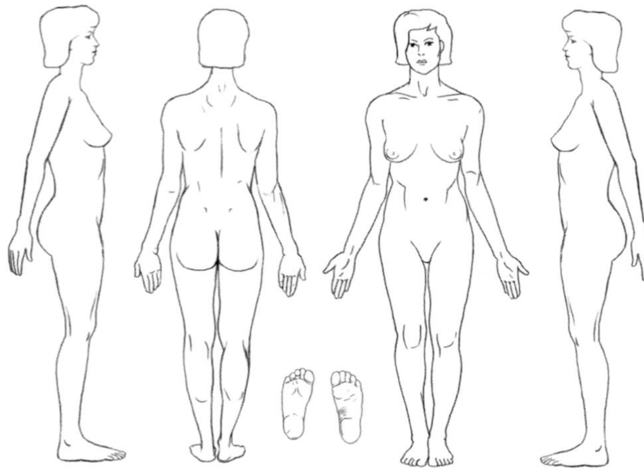

FIGURE 9-5 Female body diagram. On the diagram, mark as follows: Put an X on any painful area. Rate the pain on a scale of 1 to 10. Shade in any stiff or sore areas. Circle areas of other concern and describe the condition.

PRELIMINARY ASSESSMENT

To determine which massage procedures to perform on a prospective client or whether it is advisable to refer the client to another health professional, the therapist must understand as much about the client and his condition as possible. An assessment that includes a client history, observation, and examination can help to disclose problems and the physiologic basis for the client's complaints.

The extent of the assessment depends on the type of massage service being offered. A nonspecific, relaxing body massage, for example, requires a brief assessment to determine any special areas of concern and whether there are any contraindications. A therapeutic massage session to address some specific concerns or musculoskeletal dysfunction would require a more in-depth assessment, however.

The history includes information gained from the medical history form, answers to questions, and descriptions that clients offer. Observation includes noticing how clients hold their bodies and how they move. It includes noticing how they react to questions or manipulative tests. Examination uses various manipulative and verbal tests to help to determine more precisely the tissues or conditions involved. (Assessment for therapeutic application is discussed in Chapter 17.)

The assessment process does not end with the consultation but continues throughout the massage. As the massage proceeds, the practitioner monitors the client and the condition of the tissues and modifies or adapts the massage to best serve the client's needs.

DEVELOP A TREATMENT PLAN

The treatment plan is an outline that the practitioner can follow when giving massage treatments. The plan takes into consideration information from the intake and medical history forms, the interview, and preliminary assessment to formulate session goals and choose massage techniques. A general treatment strategy can cover several sessions, but every session should have a treatment plan.

The intake and medical history forms provide past information about the client. If this is not the first session, records from previous sessions also provide valuable information. The interview provides additional information concerning the client's reasons for coming and preferences. A further assessment will indicate more about the client's current condition.

By combining and reviewing the information, a therapist can develop a strategy or plan of action. The client's needs, wants, and preferences become more apparent. Indications and contraindications are determined, and referral to other professional or health practitioners might be suggested. A discussion between the client and practitioner can prioritize what the client wants to work on,and they can discuss options.

Goals for the session(s) are proposed, and modalities and techniques are chosen accordingly. When the client is informed of, comfortable with, and understands the proposed plan, the client gives informed consent and the plan is put into action.

INFORMED CONSENT

Informed consent is an educational process that ensures that the client has received enough information to understand the nature and extent of the massage services. It is a way for clients to be more in control of their health practice. When the client has received adequate information regarding the practitioner's credentials, the services offered, and policies and procedures used during the sessions, the client is able to give *informed consent.* The practitioner will describe the massage techniques to be employed, with their projected effects and outcomes, including benefits and possible side effects. As the client receives disclosure of the nature of the services being offered, the client can knowledgeably agree to proceed. The client can agree to proceed with the procedure, suggest modifications, or even refuse the treatment. In most situations, the client will consent to proceed with the practitioner's recommended protocol. The client has full right of refusal; that is, the client has the right to modify or withdraw consent to continue treatment at any time during any session. If this happens, the practitioner must comply regardless of any prior consent the client may have given.

The initial informed consent can take place during the initial consultation and again when the initial treatment or care plan is completed. It is preferred, and actually required in some jurisdictions, that an informed consent form be signed and kept in the client's file (see Figure 9-6 for an example of an informed consent form). Consent to proceed can be given many times throughout the therapeutic relationship. After the initial informed consent is completed, the practitioner should continually inform the client at any appropriate time that a new or unexpected procedure is being employed so that the client is aware and can give consent to proceed.

Informed consent is an ongoing process. After the initial informed consent form is signed and filed, future sessions can continue with assessments and the creation of updated treatment plans. The treatment plan includes anticipated outcomes, possible side effects, the number and length of sessions, and the modalities the therapist will use. When the plan is ready, it is discussed with the client for input, and when satisfied, the client can sign it, indicating continued informed consent.

DOCUMENTATION AND CLIENT FILES

The client file is the vehicle that practitioners use to document the work that they have done with the client. The information that a practitioner keeps in the

FIGURE 9-6
Informed consent form. (Copyright ©2006 by Cengage Learning. All Rights Reserved. Permission to reproduce for clinical use granted.)

Informed Consent

I (name of client) ____________________ have received, read and understand the policies and procedures of (name of establishment) ____________________. (Name of therapist) ____________________ has informed me of her/his qualifications, the kind of massage services to be provided, the benefits, risks and the goals of the session(s) that we have agreed upon. I understand that I retain the right to withdraw my consent at any time during any session.

I (name) ____________________ understand that the massage services provided by (name of therapist) ____________________ are intended to promote relaxation and circulation, and relieve stress, muscle tension, spasms and related pain. I understand that the massage therapy is not a substitute for medications or medical treatment and that the massage therapist does not diagnose illness nor prescribe medical treatment or perform spinal manipulations.

I have informed the therapist of my medical and physical condition and of medications I use, and I agree to update the therapist of any changes in my health profile. I release the therapist of any liability if I fail to do so.

If I experience any discomfort or pain during any session, I will immediately inform the therapist so adjustments can be made to the treatment.

Client signature ____________________________________ Date ____________________

Consent to treat a minor

I, the parent or legal guardian of (dependent's name) ____________________ authorize (therapist's name) ____________________ to provide massage treatments to my dependent or child.

Parent or Guardian signature __________________________ Date ____________________

client files varies as much as the massage routines of different practitioners. Information that is often found in a client file includes intake form (e.g., name, address, phone, e-mail address), medical history form, treatment plan, informed consent, Medical Information Release forms, recorded session or SOAP notes, financial records, and billing information. There are numerous reasons for creating and maintaining a system of documentation. Up-to-date records provide quick access to information for contacting clients to confirm or change appointments or informing them of current promotions. Client files are the vehicle to record client's concerns and conditions, what was done during previous sessions, what worked and did not work, and client preferences. They are the basis for creating treatment plans. Concise documentation is the preferred means of exchanging client information with other health professionals and can serve as legal evidence that verifies what took place during a session, thereby reducing a therapist's liability. Keeping accurate records is a tedious but essential part of a professional operation.

SOAP CHARTING

The most popular method of recording client and session information in many health care professions is SOAP notes. The acronym *SOAP* stands for Subjective,

Objective, Assessment or Application, and Planning. SOAP charts are used to document information from the initial interview and then to update information from each session (see Figures 9-7 and 9-8).

Information recorded under each heading of the SOAP notes includes the following:

- *Subjective:* Initial interview; anything that the client tells the therapist—health history, present symptoms, aggravating conditions, what makes it better, what makes it worse, and how it started. Information is derived from intake and client history forms and from the client interview. Update subjective information at the beginning of each session—present condition, changes noticed since the last session. Any information provided by the client or his physician and the client's expectations or goals for the session are recorded.
- *Objective:* Any information that the therapist gathers from history taking, observation, interview, or assessment procedures and tests. The therapist's treatment goals are noted. Information from the subjective and objective assessments is used to design the massage session.
- *Assessment or application:* Records what was done in the session and changes in symptoms or responses by the client to the procedures used in the session. Session goals are reviewed, and subjective and objective changes as a result of the session are recorded. Any progress, either negative or positive, relative to the massage session is documented.
- *Planning:* Records suggestions for future sessions or any recommendations suggested to the client. By taking into account what was done and found during the session, the next session is planned, as well as a more extended treatment plan (frequency and number of sessions) with more long-range goals. (For more detailed information on SOAP charting, refer to *Hands Heal: Documentation for Massage Therapy, 3rd Ed.* by Diane L. Thompson, Lippincott, Williams and Wilkins. 2005.)

UPDATING RECORDS

It is necessary to keep records of all services. Records should be accurate and complete and should provide information about treatments given, products used, the state of the client's health, and accurate financial information. All documentation should be concise and brief. Any unique information regarding the client, reactions to treatment, or changes in the client's condition should be noted. All data should be recorded with each treatment, including any special information that might be needed as a reference.

Keeping accurate records of the client's condition, tolerance, and reactions permits the therapist to render more effective treatments and to achieve better results.

Concern for the client's well-being helps to establish mutual confidence. Reviewing updated records before a client comes in for a return visit refreshes your memory about the client's condition, treatments given, and the client's likes and dislikes. This not only allows you to plan the session but also re-familiarizes

FIGURE 9-7 SOAP chart used during initial consultation.

INITIAL INFORMATION

Name________________________ Date________________________

S **Subjective**

(Symptoms, frequency, duration, intensity, how it started, aggravating/relieving activities, etc.)

Client's experience, expectations, and goals:

O **Objective**

Observations, tests, and results:

Treatment goals:

A **Assessment & Applications**

Massage treatment given:

Changes due to massage:

P **Planning**

Homework:

Plan for next session:

Long-range plans and goals:

you with the client, which impresses the client and increases client confidence. On the other hand, a practitioner who relies on memory and forgets important factors about a client from one session to the next might lose the trust that is so necessary in a therapeutic relationship.

SESSION NOTES

Name ____________ Date ____________

S

O

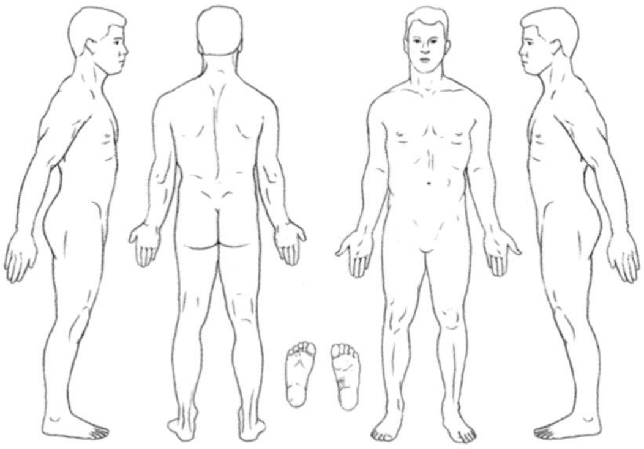

A

P

FIGURE 9-8 SOAP chart used for updating session notes.

The practitioner never discusses or gives out personal information about clients. All records should be kept in a secure place. A practitioner should not divulge information about a client's personal matters without the written consent of the client, and then only when the exchange of such information is for the client's benefit. The practitioner often works closely with a client's physician when working on certain physical conditions; therefore, the confidence of both client and physician must be respected.

When the practitioner thinks that a client's physician should be consulted before beginning massage treatments, the practitioner should talk this over with the client and obtain his written permission.

Confidentiality

As it was discussed in Chapter 3, confidentiality is one of the foundations of a therapeutic relationship. Essentially, confidentially guarantees the nondisclosure of privileged and private information that is shared during a therapeutic session. This means that the identity of a client or any information about them or their condition is kept private and not divulged to any third party. Confidentiality is necessary to build trust within the relationship.

In 2001, the Health Insurance Portability and Accountability Act of 1996 (HIPAA) became effective. This legislation is designed to enhance health care in the United States by restoring trust among consumers, healthcare providers, and organizations delivering the care. Compliance to HIPAA is required by any agency or individual person who stores or transmits personal health information electronically. A major portion of HIPAA concerns maintaining the privacy of individual medical information. Even though a massage therapist might not need to be HIPAA compliant, they can strive to follow the guidelines to maintain a client's trust and privacy.

- Always obtain a signed informed consent before proceeding with treatment.
- Do not divulge client information to any third party without first obtaining a release of information form signed by the client.
- Store client files in a secured (lockable), fireproof cabinet.
- Protect electronic files with appropriate passwords. If the computer is connected to the Internet, use appropriate firewalls.
- Keep client files and appointment books out of view of others.
- Create a *Privacy Policies* notice that outlines how information obtained from clients will be used, stored, and under which conditions it can be shared. Give a copy to each client.

Client files, as well as any information about the client, are kept confidential between the client and practitioner except when pertinent information is shared for the client's benefit, such as with other health professionals whom the client is seeing or with the client's insurance company. In these situations, information is shared only after the client has given their written permission and signed a release of information form. A release of information form contains the client's name, the therapist's name, the name of the person(s) to whom the information is being given, and the time frame in which the information may be released (Figure 9-9). The completed form is signed, dated, and kept in the client files. A copy of the release form is included in the shared information. The only other times information from a client is given out is if it is ordered by a court of law or if there is an imminent threat of physical harm or abuse.

FIGURE 9-9 Release of Information. (Copyright © 2006 by Cengage Learning. All Rights Reserved. Permission to reproduce for clinical use granted.)

Release of Information

I (client's name) ________________ authorize (practitioner's name) ______________ to release and/or exchange information and records concerning my health or health treatments during the time period of ____________ to ____________ with (other professional's name) ______________________. I retain the right to revoke this permission at any time either verbally or in writing.

This authorization is valid until (date) ________________________

Client signature ___________________________________ Date ___________________

SUMMARY

The consultation, which takes place prior to the actual massage, is an opportunity for the practitioner and the client to exchange important information that sets the tone of the therapeutic relationship and determines how the actual massage will proceed. During the initial consultation, the practitioner hears why the client has come for a massage and the client learns about the services that the practitioner offers. The practitioner provides information about their training, as well as the procedures used, fees, and other policies. The client discusses his reason for seeking massage and their expectations. Intake and medical history forms that the client complete provides vital information that helps to formulate the treatment and determine if there might be contraindications for the massage. Further assessment helps to determine which massage procedures could be of most benefit or if referral to another health professional might be more appropriate. Information from the intake, medical history forms, assessment, and the client interview are combined to formulate a plan of action. Goals for the session are proposed and modalities chosen that best address those goals. A treatment plan is developed that can be for a single session or several sessions. When the client is comfortable with the proposed plan, the client gives informed consent, and the plan is put into action.

Updated client files are the means by which the professional massage practitioner documents the work done with a client. Up-to-date files give quick access to client contact information, health history, and what was done during previous sessions. A common method for recording session information is SOAP charts. The acronym *SOAP* stands for Subjective, Objective, Assessment or Application, and Planning. To be useful, client files must be accurate and up to date. Accurate records permit the practitioner to be more effective and achieve better results. Client records as well as all information shared by the client is confidential and is not to be shared with anyone without the client's written permission. Client records, whether on paper or in a computer, must be protected and kept secure.

QUESTIONS FOR DISCUSSION AND REVIEW

1. Why is the consultation important to the success of the massage treatment?
2. What is included in a preliminary client assessment?
3. Why is a preliminary assessment advisable when doing therapeutic massage?
4. What is a treatment plan?
5. How is a treatment plan developed?
6. What is informed consent?
7. Which information is disclosed by whom to obtain informed consent?
8. Why is it important to keep accurate records?
9. Which information is included in a client's file?
10. Why is it important to inform the client of pre-massage procedures?
11. Why should the massage practitioner anticipate any questions that the client might ask and be able to answer them?

CHAPTER

10 Classical Massage Movements

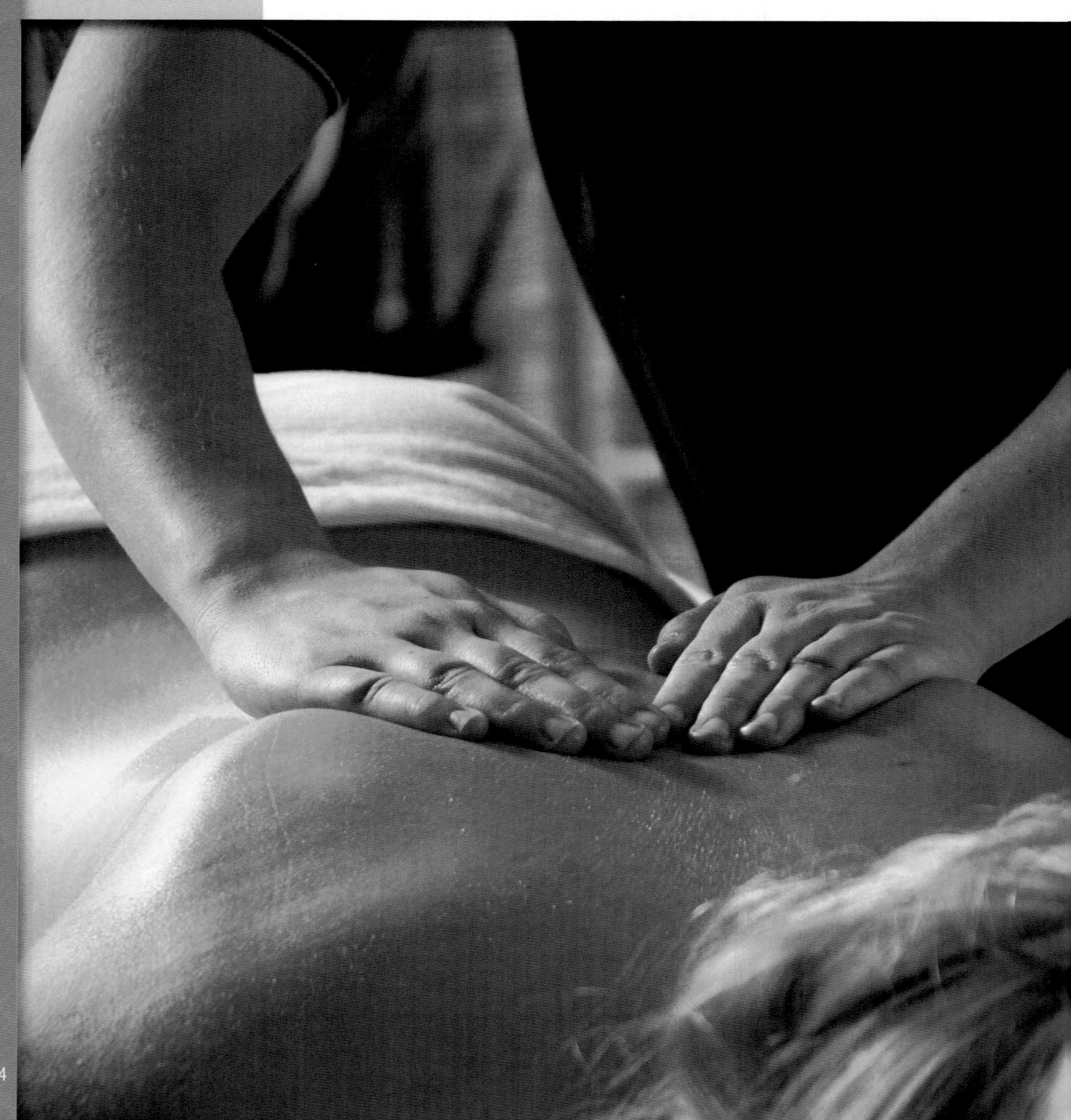

LEARNING OBJECTIVES

After you have mastered this chapter, you will be able to

1. **Describe the six major categories of massage movements.**
2. **Explain Swedish (classic) massage techniques.**
3. **Demonstrate mastery of basic massage movements.**
4. **Demonstrate passive and active joint movements.**
5. **Explain and demonstrate rhythm and pressure as applied to therapeutic body massage.**

INTRODUCTION

Massage movements are to therapeutic massage what words are to language or notes to music. To practice massage, an understanding of the movements is imperative. As a massage therapist, the more mastery you have of the movements, the better you can create a work of art each time that you choose and combine movements according to each client's needs. There are any number of massage manipulations and possible combinations of strokes, so that a massage can be tailored to the specific needs of each client. Regardless of whether a massage routine is standard or specialized for the specific needs of the client, there is much more to applying strokes than the movement of the hands. The continuous interaction of the client and therapist, the purpose for the session, and the intent with which each manipulation is delivered affect the delivery and outcome of the massage.

CLASSIFICATION OF MASSAGE MOVEMENTS

The following movements are the fundamental manipulations used in Swedish massage and are the foundation of most massage styles practiced today. The massage practitioner must understand the indications for and effects of the manipulations. Most massage treatments combine one or more of these movements, as divided into the six major categories:

1. Touch
    a. Superficial
    b. Deep
2. Gliding or effleurage movements
    a. Aura stroking
    b. Superficial
    c. Deep
3. Kneading movements
    a. Kneading or petrissage
    b. Fulling
    c. Skin rolling
4. Friction
    a. Superficial friction

b. Circular friction
c. Transverse or cross-fiber friction
d. Compression
e. Rolling
f. Wringing
g. Chucking
h. Shaking
i. Jostling
j. Rocking
k. Vibration
- Manual
- Mechanical

5. Percussion movements
a. Tapping
b. Cupping
c. Slapping
d. Hacking
e. Beating

6. Joint movements
a. Passive joint movements
b. Active joint movements
- Active assistive movements
- Active resistive movements

The intention with which a massage is given or a technique is applied greatly influences its effect. Each manipulation is applied in a specific way for a particular purpose. The practice of massage becomes scientific only when the practitioner recognizes the purpose and effects of each movement and adapts the treatment to the client's condition for the desired results.

Control over the results of a massage treatment is possible only when the practitioner regulates the intensity of the pressure; the speed, length, and direction of the movement; and duration of each type of manipulation.

UNDERSTANDING MASSAGE MOVEMENTS

The practitioner must understand the movement to be applied to a particular part of the body. For example,

- Light movements are applied over thin tissues or bony parts.
- Heavy movements are indicated for thick tissues or muscular parts.
- Gentle movements are applied with a slow rhythm and are soothing and relaxing.
- Vigorous movements are applied in a quick rhythm and are stimulating.

While applying the movements, the practitioner must pay close attention to the overall response of the client as well as to the response of the tissue or body part to which the movement is being applied and adjust the application accordingly.

An important rule of Swedish massage is that most movements or strokes are directed toward the heart (**centripetal**). Many massage techniques are intended to enhance venous blood and lymph flow and therefore are directed toward the heart and the eliminative organs. Only very light strokes that have little mechanical effect on fluid flow should be directed away from the heart. When a massage movement is directed away from the heart, it is said to be **centrifugal**.

The duration of a massage treatment should be regulated. Usually a therapeutic full-body massage takes about one hour, but some practitioners take more or less time. A prolonged massage can be fatiguing for some clients. When a student is learning massage, a full-body massage can take an hour and a half to two hours. This is not unusual because it takes practice for movements to become smooth and efficient. After a while, an hour will be plenty of time to accomplish the desired results. Because sometimes the practitioner requires more time, the duration of massages varies. Knowledge and experience are prerequisites for judging the client's special need and adjusting the massage session accordingly.

DESCRIPTION OF THE BASIC MASSAGE MOVEMENTS

All hands-on therapies use physical contact as their primary modality. Indeed, it is this caring human contact that makes massage therapy unique.

Touch, in the context of the classification of massage techniques, refers to the stationary contact of the practitioner's hand and the client's body. Touch is the placing of the practitioner's hand, finger, or body part (e.g., forearm) on the client without movement in any direction. The pressure exerted may vary from very light to very deep depending on the intention. Skillfully and purposefully applied, touch achieves physiologic and psychological (soothing) effects.

Gliding is the practice of sliding the hand or forearm over some portion of the client's body, with varying amounts of pressure or contact according to the desired results.

Kneading lifts, squeezes, and presses the tissues.

Friction refers to several massage strokes designed to manipulate soft tissue in such a way that one layer of tissue is moved over or against another.

Vibration is a continuous trembling or shaking movement delivered by either the practitioner's hand or an electrical apparatus. Vibration can be classified as a type of friction.

Percussion is a rapid striking motion of the practitioner's hands against the surface of the client's body, using varying amounts of force and hand positions.

Joint movement is the passive or active movement of the joints or articulations of the client.

APPLICATION OF MASSAGE STROKES

Touch

Touch is the first technique in developing a therapeutic relationship. Touch can be in the form of a handshake or a pat on the shoulder (Figure 10-1). In the course of a massage, touch constitutes the first and last contact of the practitioner with the client. The practitioner begins the massage with a gentle, noninvasive superficial touch to make first contact and enter the client's personal space. This provides the client the opportunity to become more receptive to the practitioner's touch and presence. The practitioner can use this moment of stationary contact to tune in and connect with the client before proceeding with the session. At the conclusion of the session, when the practitioner has finished the final relaxing strokes, a completing gesture of a brief stationary contact provides closure for the practitioner and signals the client that the session is finished.

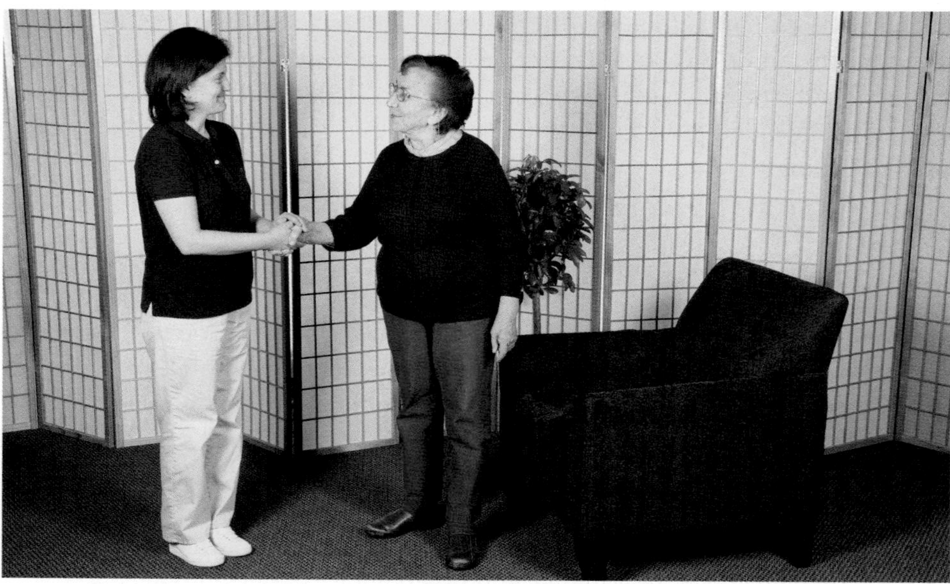

FIGURE 10-1 A friendly greeting conveys a message of confidence and concern.

All massage techniques use physical contact, but the quality and sense of touch convey the intent and the power of the movements. Touch is the primary communication tool used by the massage therapist. The sense of touch tells clients what is happening to their bodies and gives practitioners information about the condition and response of the tissues being working on. The quality of touch continually transmits information from the therapist's hands to the client in direct response to the information communicated by the client (both verbally and with body language).

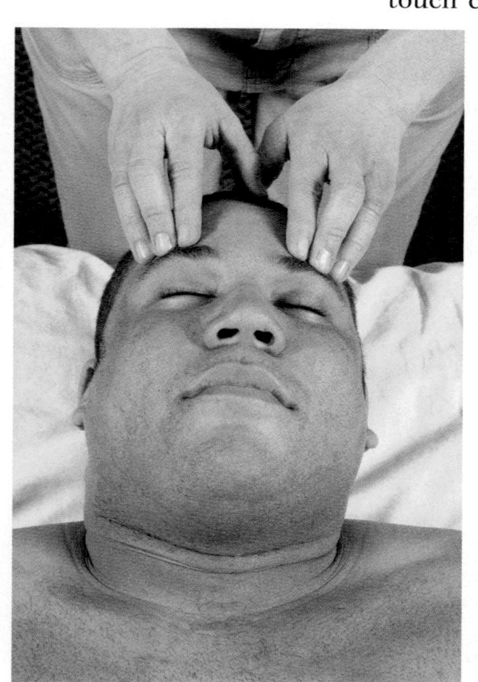

FIGURE 10-2A Gentle contact allows the client to unwind.

Light or superficial touch is purposeful contact in which the natural and evenly distributed weight of the practitioner's thumb, finger(s), or hand is applied to a given area of the client's body. The size of that area can be regulated as necessary by using one or more fingers, the entire hand, or both hands. Some therapeutic techniques employ touch almost exclusively (e.g., *Jin Shin Do*, acupressure, polarity, therapeutic touch, *reiki*). Touch can be remarkably effective in the reduction of pain, lowering of blood pressure, control of nervous irritability, or reassurance for a nervous, tense client. If a person demonstrates contraindications for a basic massage or is in a fragile condition, a complete treatment using light touch exclusively is acceptable. The main objective of light touch is to soothe and to provide a comforting connection that is calming and allows the powerful healing mechanisms of the body to function (Figures 10-2a and b).

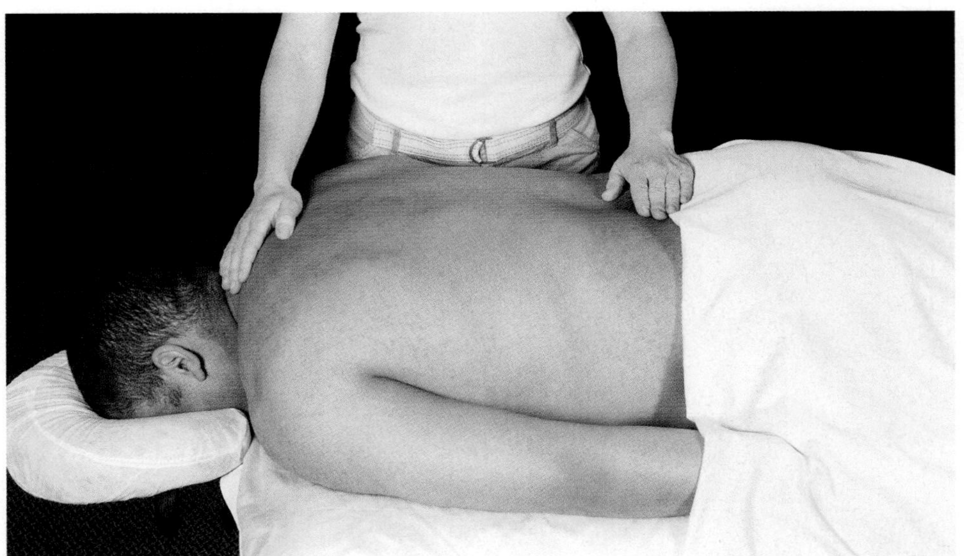

FIGURE 10-2B A light touch at the base of the spine, the base of the neck, or the top of the head is a pleasant way to say hello or good-bye to the client's body.

Touch Using Deep Pressure

Deep pressure is performed with one finger, thumb, several fingers, or the entire hand. The heel of the hand, knuckles, or elbow can be used, according to desired results. The application of deep pressure is used when calming, anesthetizing, or stimulating effects are desired. Deep pressure can be used with other techniques such as cross-fiber friction, compression, or vibration. Deep pressure is useful in soothing muscle spasms and relieving pain at reflex areas, stress points in tendons, and trigger points in muscles. In addition to extensive use in trigger-point therapy, deep pressure is a technique often applied in reflexology, sport massage, acupressure, and *shiatsu* (methods discussed in Chapters 16 and 18). When using deep pressure, the practitioner must use caution to stay within the patient's pain tolerance. Using good body mechanics is essential when applying deep pressure, to prevent injury to the practitioner. Practitioner body mechanics dictate that undue strain should not be exerted to hyperextend any joint. Body mechanics are used in such a way that pressure is delivered through body movement rather than simply by hand and upper-body strength (Figures 10-3a-f).

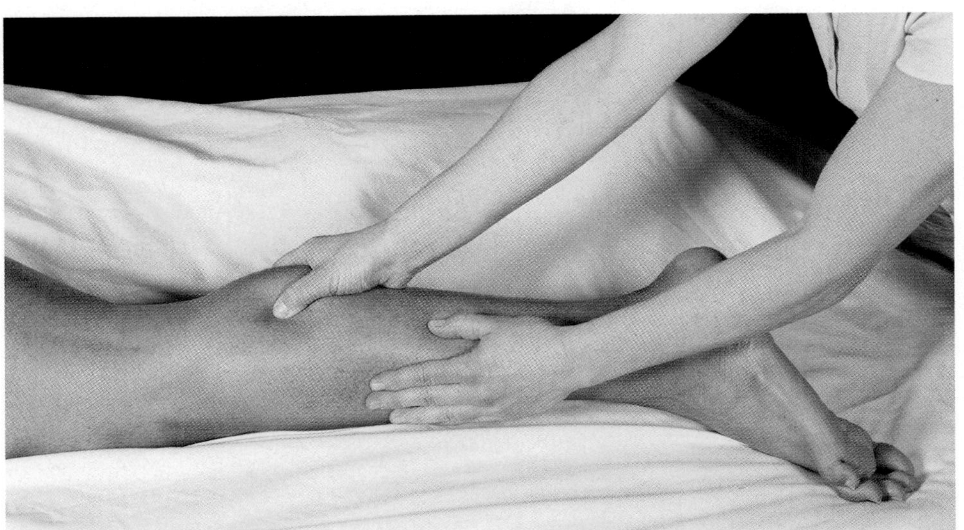

FIGURE 10-3A Deep pressure using thumb. Notice the alignment of therapist's thumb and arm to ensure that pressure is directed into client with minimal stress to therapist's joints.

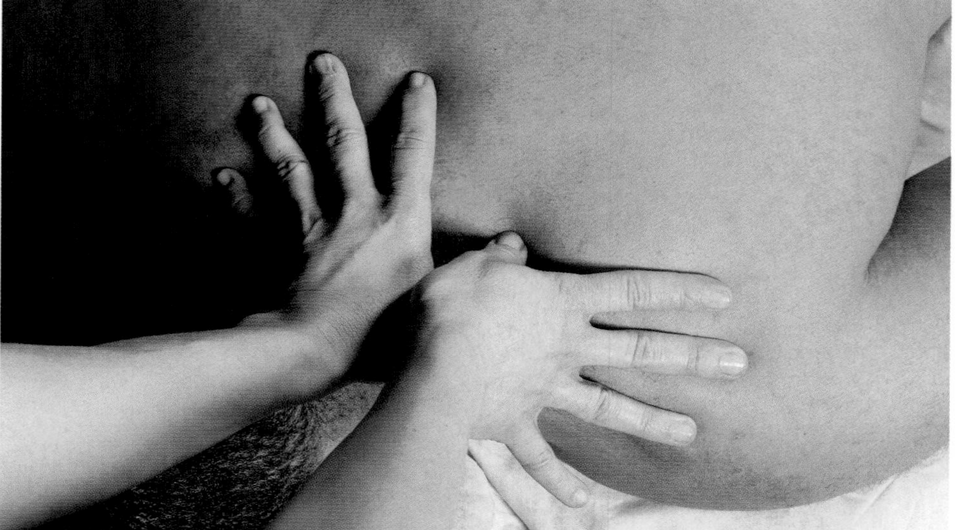

FIGURE 10-3B A braced thumb applies deep pressure.

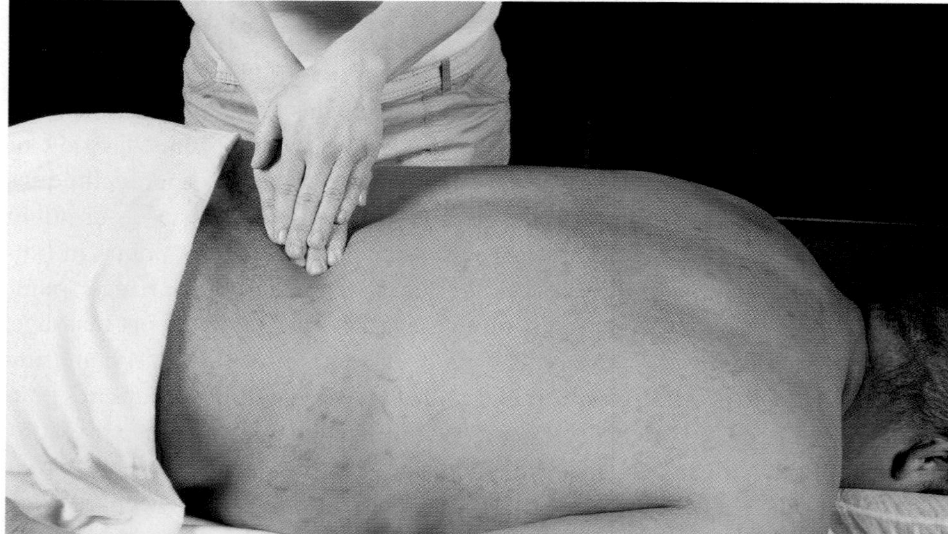

FIGURE 10-3C Deep pressure applied with braced fingers.

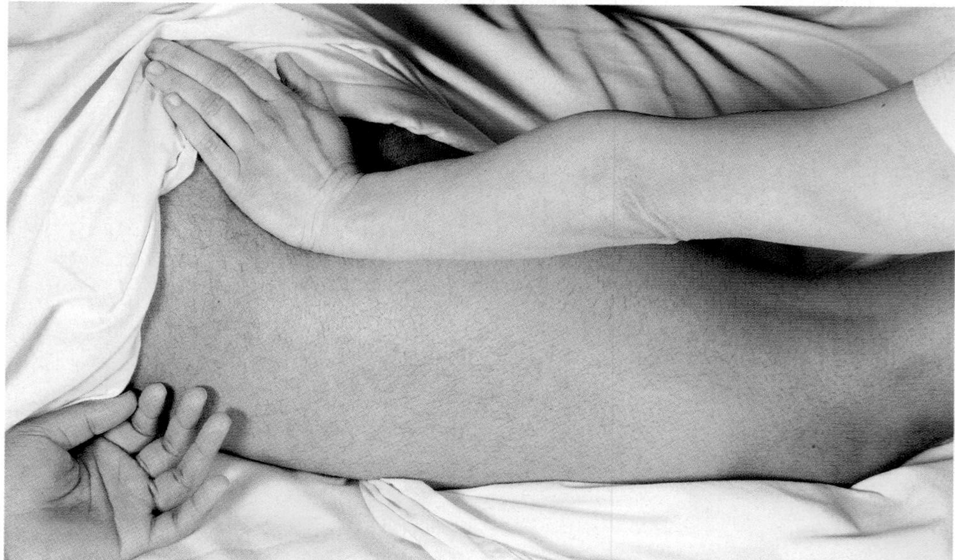

FIGURE 10-3D Deep pressure applied with heel of hand.

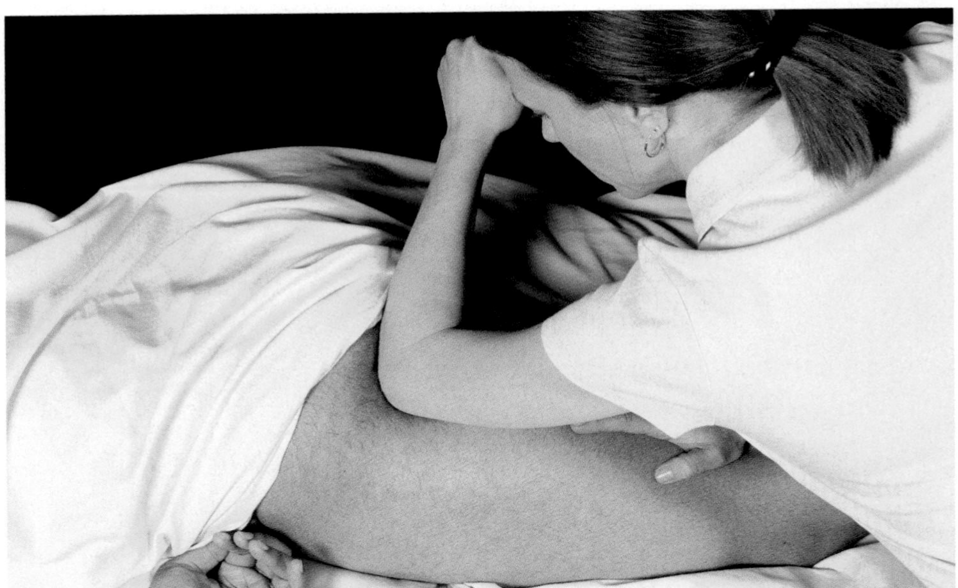

FIGURE 10-3E Deep pressure applied with elbow.

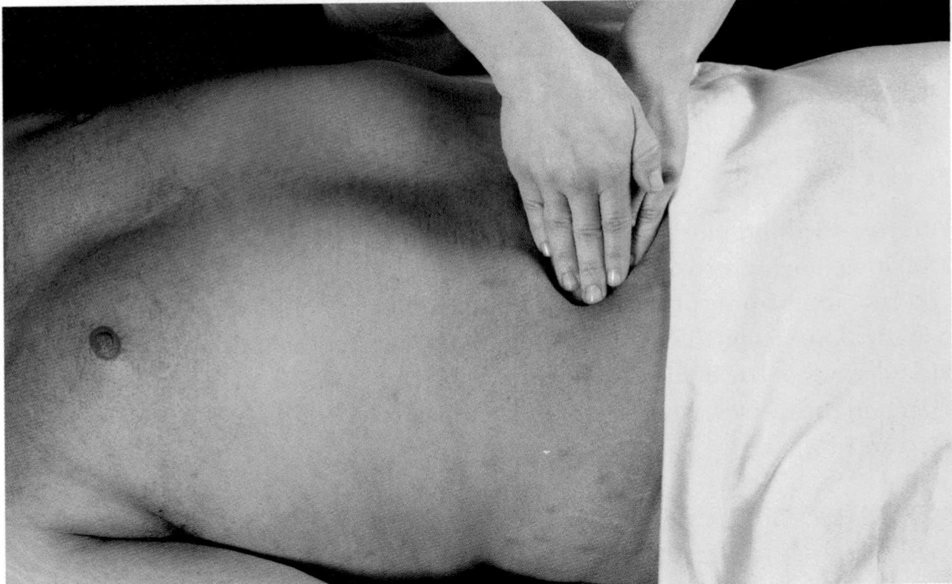

FIGURE 10-3F Deep pressure to the abdominal area.

Gliding Movements

Gliding can be done using a varying amount of pressure and length of strokes. Gliding strokes slide smoothly over the client's body, body part (arm or leg), or a specific area (muscle or reflex).

gliding
is the practice of sliding the hand smoothly over some portion of the client's body with varying amounts of pressure.

Ethereal Body or Aura Stroking

This type of stroking is done with long, smooth strokes wherein the practitioner's hands glide the length of the client's body or body part, coming very close to but not actually touching the body surface. The movement is usually in one direction only, with the return stroke being farther from the body. The intention is to affect the energy fields that, according to some philosophies, surround or permeate the body. The direction of the stroking can be along the surface of the body to enhance or impede the natural flow.

The application of this soothing stroke is done only when the surrounding circumstances are very quiet and relaxed and the patient is receptive. Aura stroking is sometimes used as the final stroke of a massage (Figure 10-4).

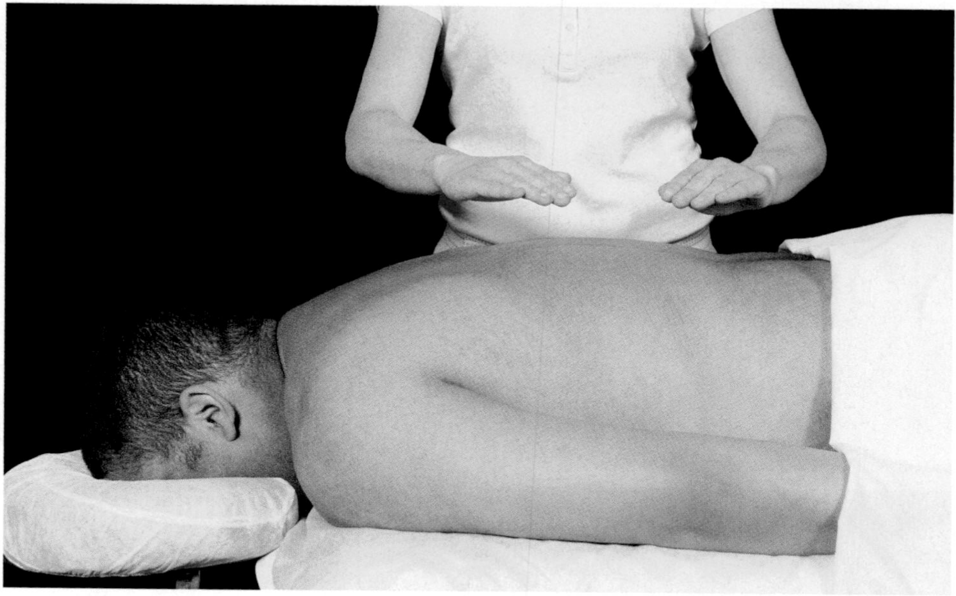

FIGURE 10-4 Ethereal or aura strokes do not touch the surface of the client's body.

Feather stroking

feather stroking requires very light pressure of the fingertips or hands with long flowing strokes.

Feather-stroking movements use very light pressure of the fingertips or hands, with long flowing strokes.

The application of feather stroking, sometimes called nerve stroking, is usually done from the center outward and is used as a final stroke to individual areas of the body. Two or three such strokes have a slightly stimulating effect on the nerves, whereas many repetitions have a more sedating response (Figure 10-5).

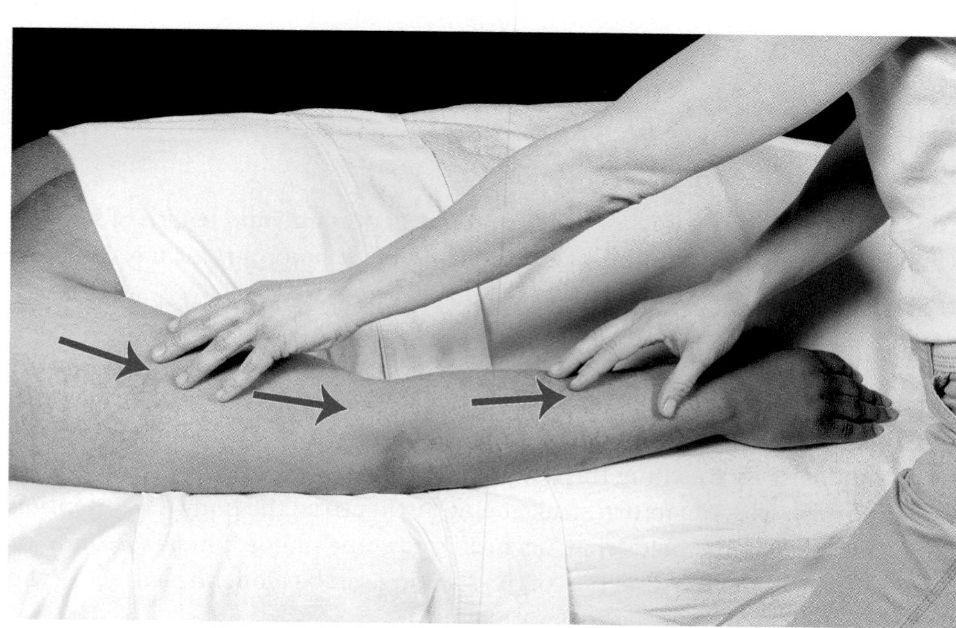

FIGURE 10-5 Feather strokes (nerve strokes) use the lightest touch of the fingertips.

Gliding or Effleurage

Effleurage is a succession of strokes applied by gliding the hand over a somewhat extended portion of the body. Effleurage is perhaps the most frequently used movement in Swedish or Western massage. The term *effleurage* stems from the French verb *effleurer*, meaning to skim or flow. There are two varieties of effleurage: superficial and deep. Superficial effleurage strokes employ a very light touch. In gliding strokes, the pressure becomes firmer as the hand slides smoothly over the surface of the body. The technique of effleurage is accomplished either with the fingers, thumbs, palm of the hand, knuckles, or forearm.

1. Over large surfaces, such as the limbs, back, chest, and abdomen, the gliding movement is performed with the palmar surface of one or both hands.
2. Over small areas, such as the face or hands, the movement is performed with the fingers or thumbs.
3. For very deep gliding strokes, the palms of the hands, thumbs, knuckles, or forearms are used.

effleurage

requires very light pressure of the fingertips or hands with long flowing strokes.

Superficial Gliding

Superficial gliding strokes are generally applied prior to any other movement. The practitioner's hand is flexible yet firm and controlled so that as it slides smoothly over the body, it conforms to the body contours so that there is equal pressure applied to the body from every part of the hand. Superficial gliding strokes accustom the client to the practitioner's contact and allow the practitioner to assess the body area being massaged. Light strokes are used to distribute any lubricant that is used and to prepare the area for other techniques. As the practitioner's hands glide over the tissues, they sense variations that indicate where specific techniques should be applied. Effleurage is interspersed with other techniques to clear the area and soothe the intensity of some deeper movements. In Swedish or Western massage, effleurage is generally the first and the last technique used on an area of the body. Slow, gentle, and rhythmic movements produce soothing effects. Rhythmic strokes should be applied in the direction of the venous and lymphatic flow.

superficial gliding

is when the practitioner's hand conforms to the client's body contours so that light pressure is applied to the body from every part of the hand.

Although superficial stroking appears to be simple, practitioners master this technique only with extensive practice. The practitioner's hand should be relaxed, to mold the surface of the body part being massaged. The pressure and speed of movement should remain constant. On completion of the stroke, the practitioner's hand may be elevated and directed to the starting point. In some cases, the hands stay in contact by exerting more pressure centripetally (toward the heart) and then reduce the pressure and lightly stroke (feather stroke) the body to return to the starting point of the stroke. In this way, the practitioner always maintains contact with the client.

Superficial gliding strokes are a valuable application to help a client to overcome general fatigue or restlessness. This movement is particularly soothing to nervous or irritated people. Clients with nervous headaches and insomnia (sleeplessness) often find relief with gentle gliding strokes of the forehead.

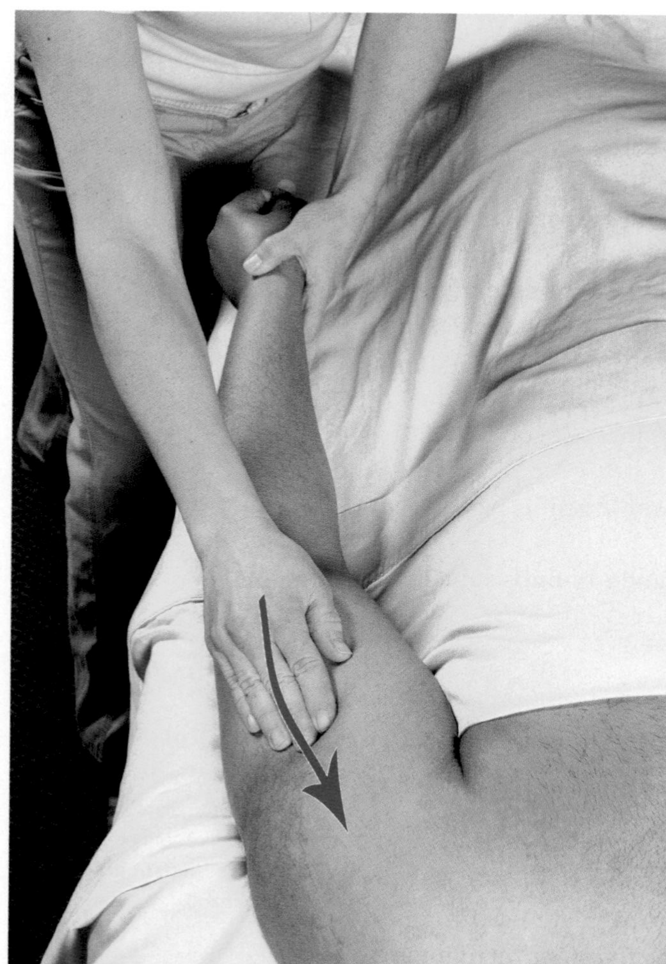

FIGURE 10-6A Effleurage or gliding strokes are applied in the direction of venous blood and lymph flow.

Deep Gliding

The term **deep gliding** indicates that the movement uses enough pressure to have a mechanical effect. The depth of the gliding movement depends on three factors: the pressure exerted, the part of the hand or arm used, and the intention with which the movement is applied. Deep gliding can be applied with the thumb, braced fingers, knuckles, or forearm, depending on the area of the body or tissues involved. Deep gliding strokes do not involve the use of excessive force, however. The pressure should never be forceful enough to cause bruising or injury to the tissues. Deep gliding strokes are especially valuable when applied to the muscles and are most effective when the part undergoing treatment is in a relaxed state. The slightest pressure of the surface is then transmitted to the deeper structures. Deep gliding strokes have a stretching and broadening effect on muscle tissue and fascia and also enhance the venous blood and lymph flow. If the practitioner uses too much force, the client's body responds with a protective reflex that causes muscles to contract, thereby negating the desired effects of the treatment. Deep gliding strokes generally follow the direction of the muscle fibers. On the extremities, the movements are always directed from the end of a limb toward the center of the body (centripetally). The movement is usually toward the heart or in the direction of venous and lymph flow, with the return stroke being much lighter and away from the center of the body. The exception to this rule is deep, short strokes applied to the muscle attachments and tendons. When directed from the tendon toward the muscle belly, these strokes tend to stretch the tendon and cause a reflexive relaxation of the muscle. Indications for the use of deep gliding strokes include increasing fluid movement, stretching underlying tissues, separating and broadening tissues, increasing relaxation, and palpating deeper tissues (Figures 10-6a-g and Figures 10-7a-h).

deep gliding

indicates that the movement uses enough pressure to have a mechanical effect.

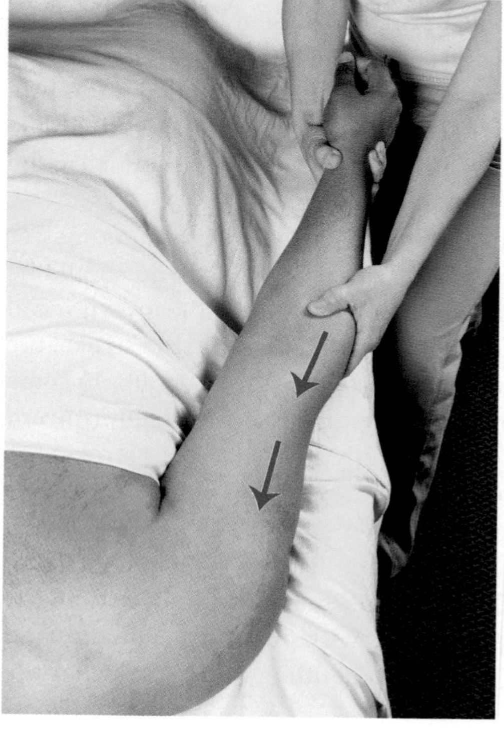

FIGURE 10-6B A V-stroke can be used for superficial or deep gliding strokes.

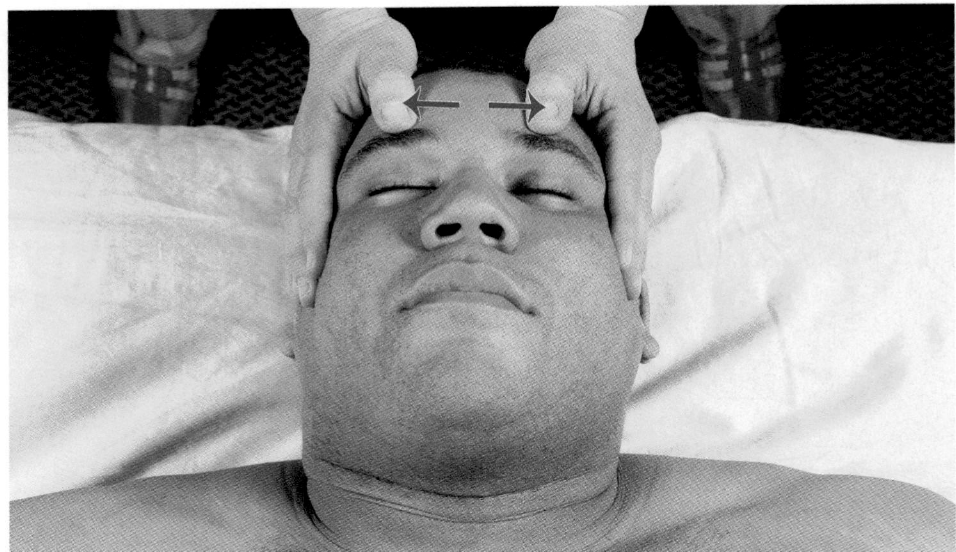

FIGURE 10-6C Digital effleurage to the forehead.

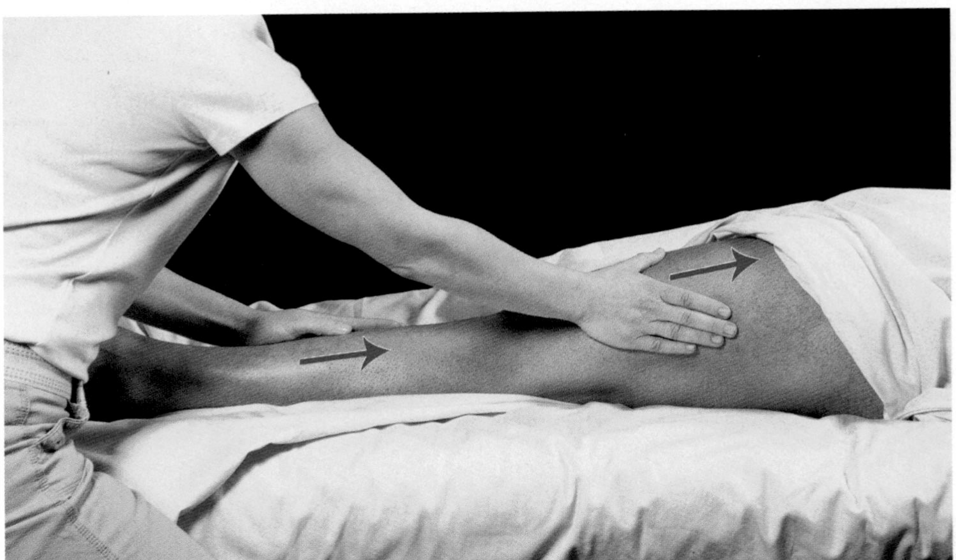

FIGURE 10-6D Direction of effleurage on the lower leg. The stroke can continue all the way up the leg to the hip.

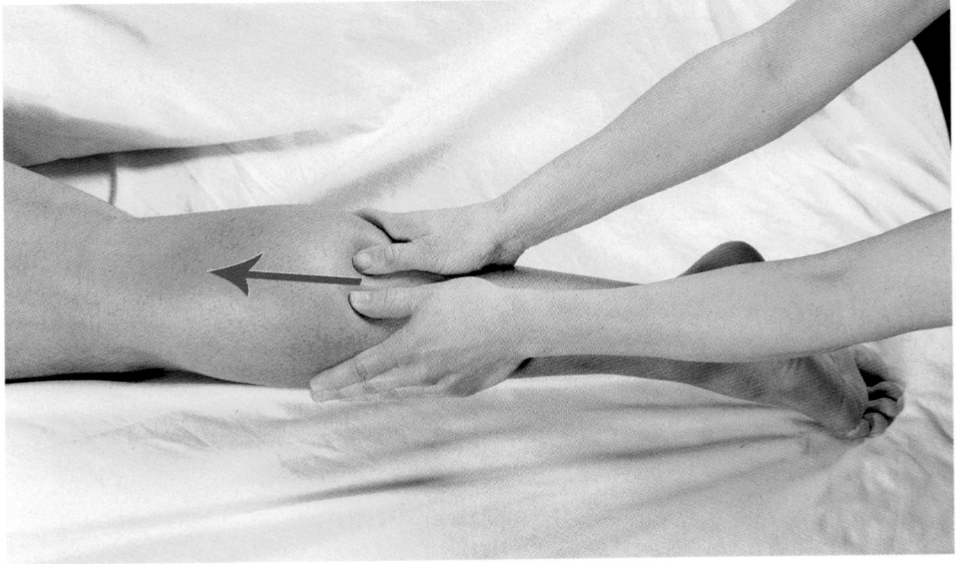

FIGURE 10-6E Gliding strokes applied to the entire length of the leg with two hands.

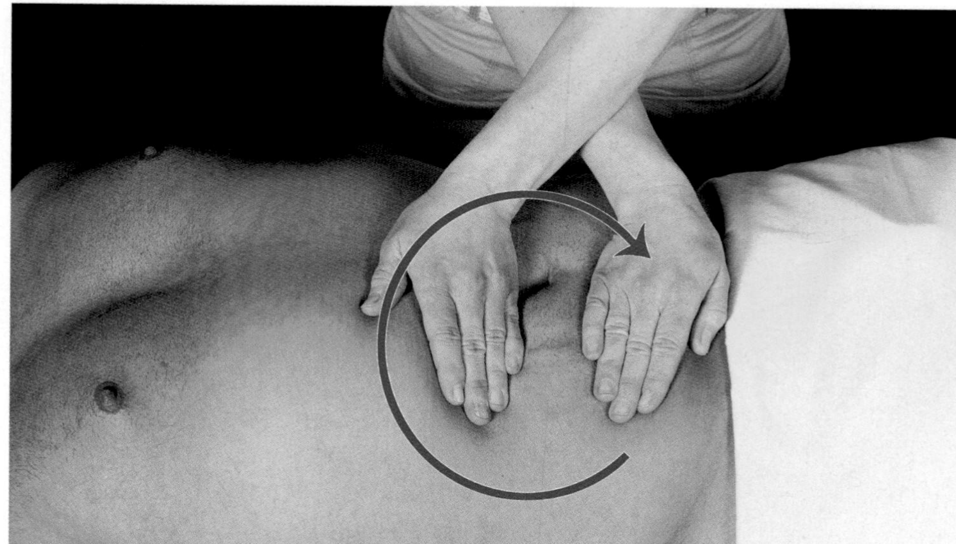

FIGURE 10-6F Effleurage to the abdomen in a circular movement.

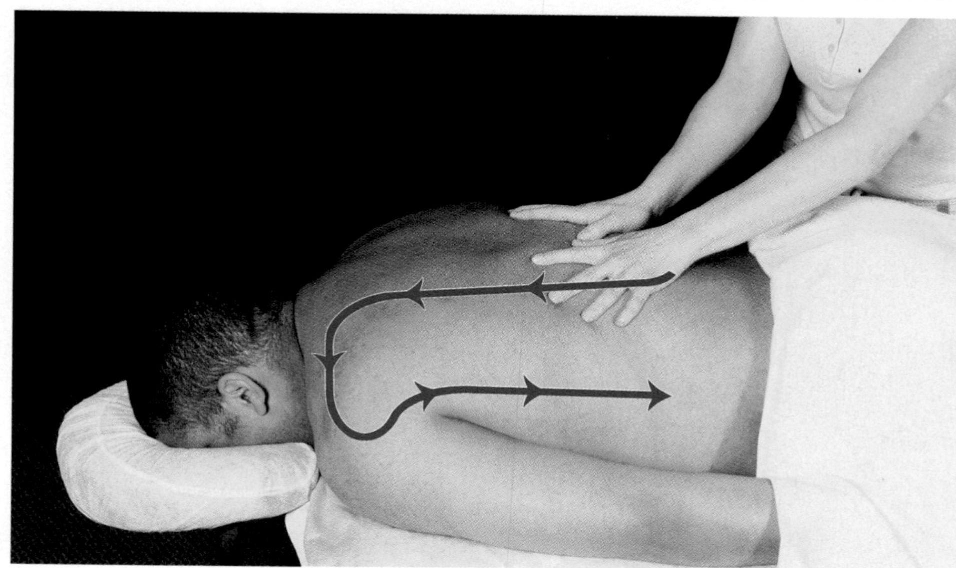

FIGURE 10-6G Gliding strokes applied to the entire back.

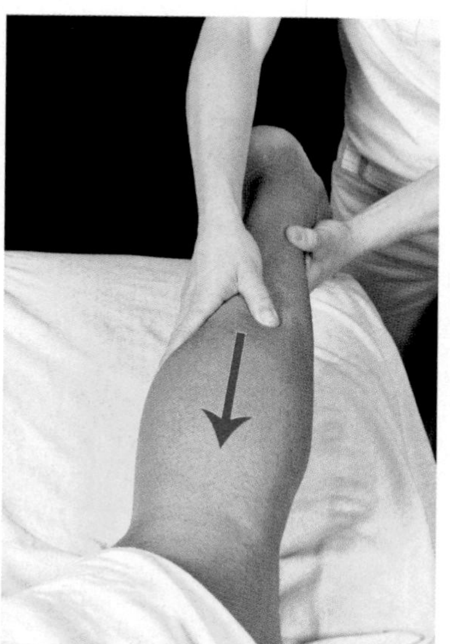

FIGURE 10-7A V-stroke applied to the posterior leg is used for superficial or deep gliding.

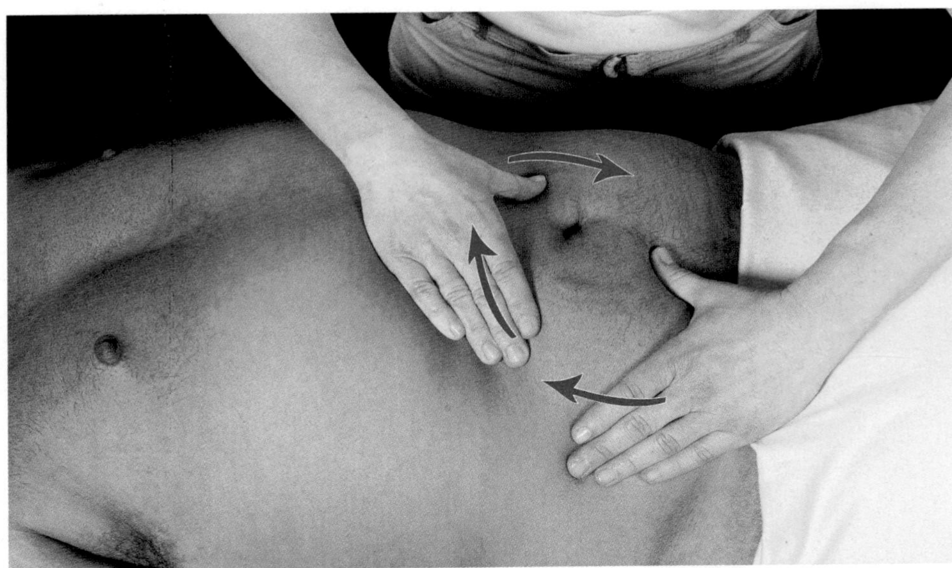

FIGURE 10-7B Circular effleurage should be applied following the path of the colon.

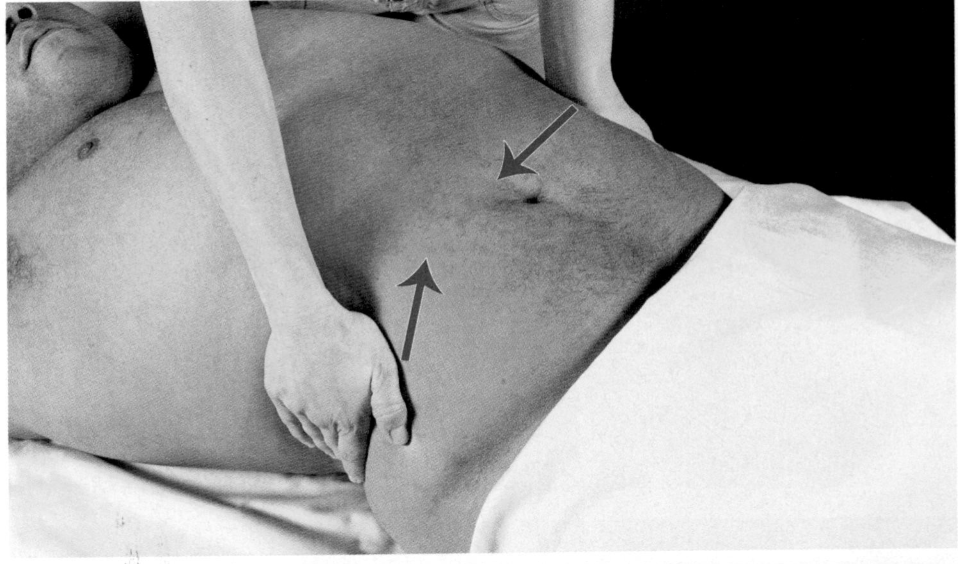

FIGURE 10-7C Inward deep gliding strokes of muscles over the stomach area and the abdominal region.

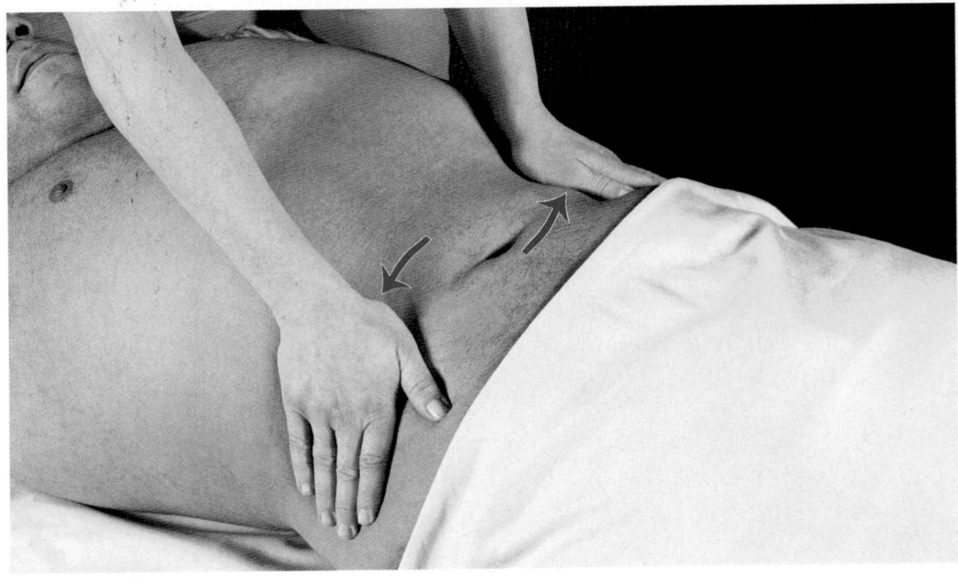

FIGURE 10-7D Outward deep gliding strokes to the muscles of the stomach area and the abdominal region.

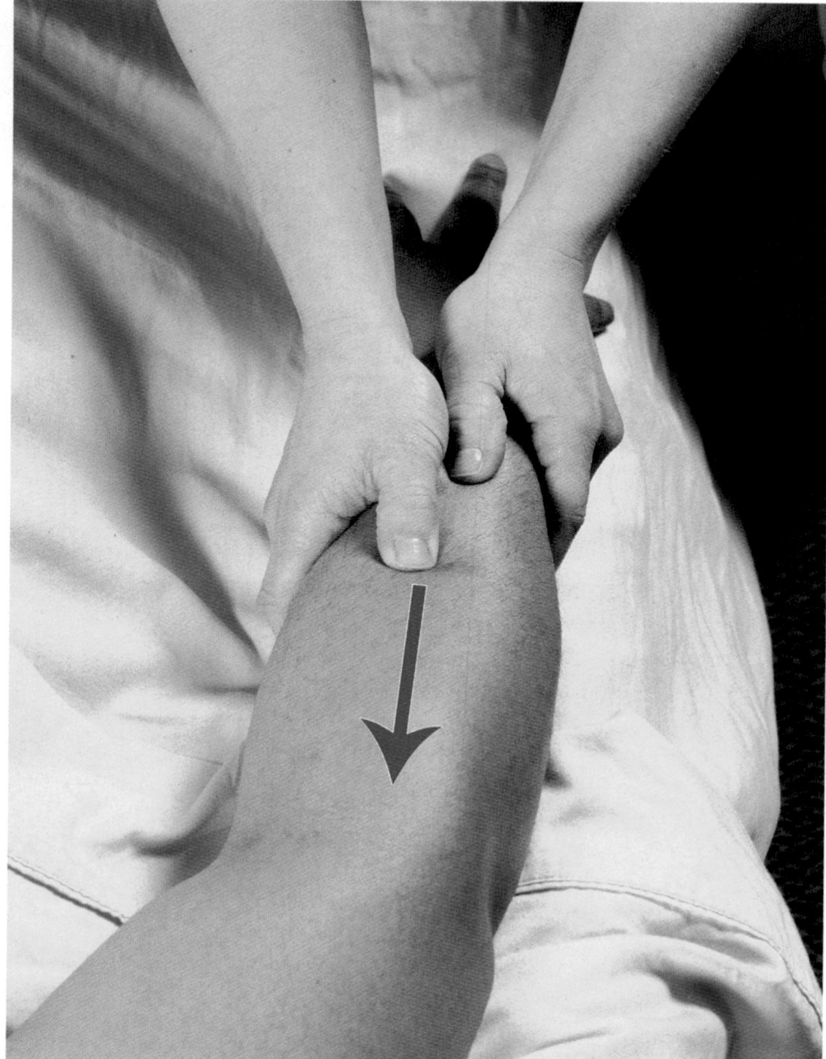

FIGURE 10-7E Deep gliding or "stripping" using the thumb on the forearm.

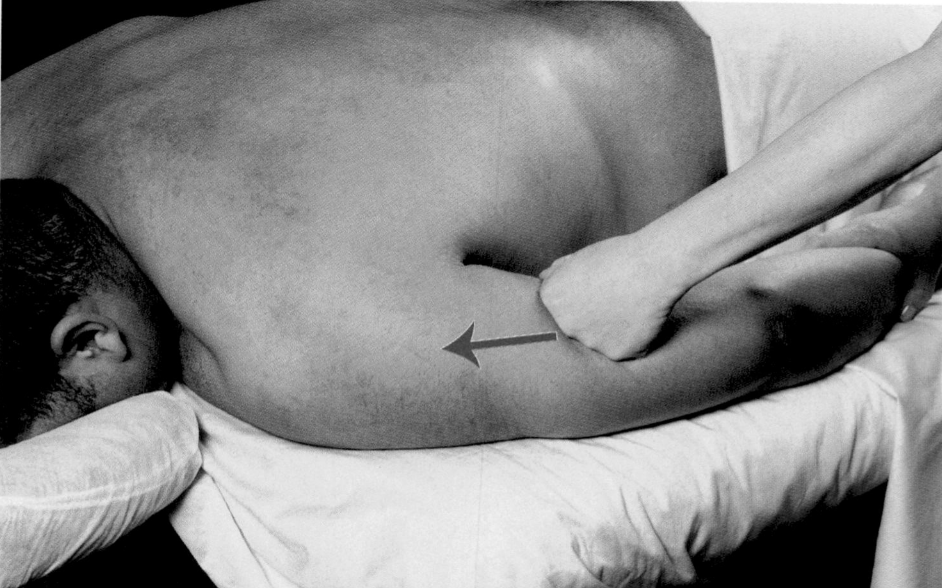

FIGURE 10-7F Deep gliding using a loose fist or knuckles on the triceps.

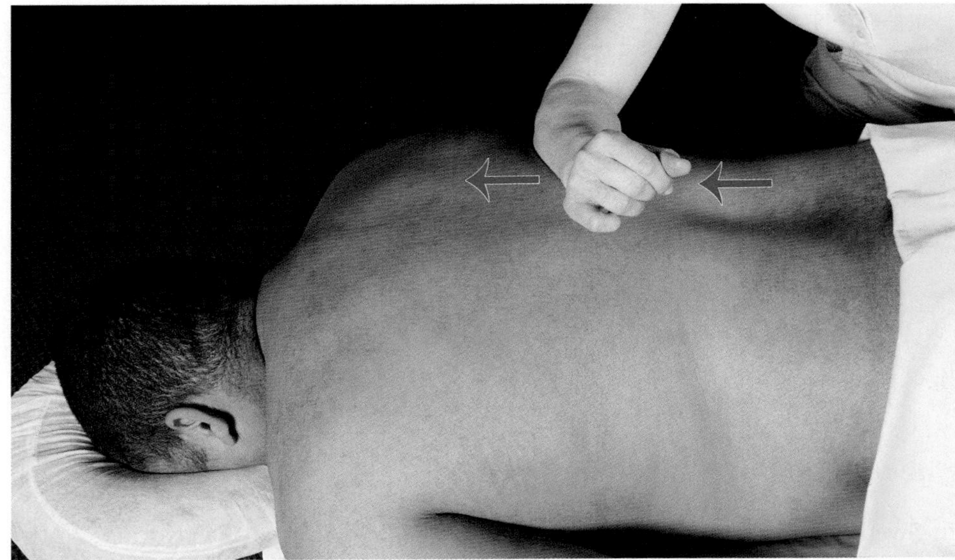

FIGURE 10-7G Deep gliding using the forearm and elbow on the back.

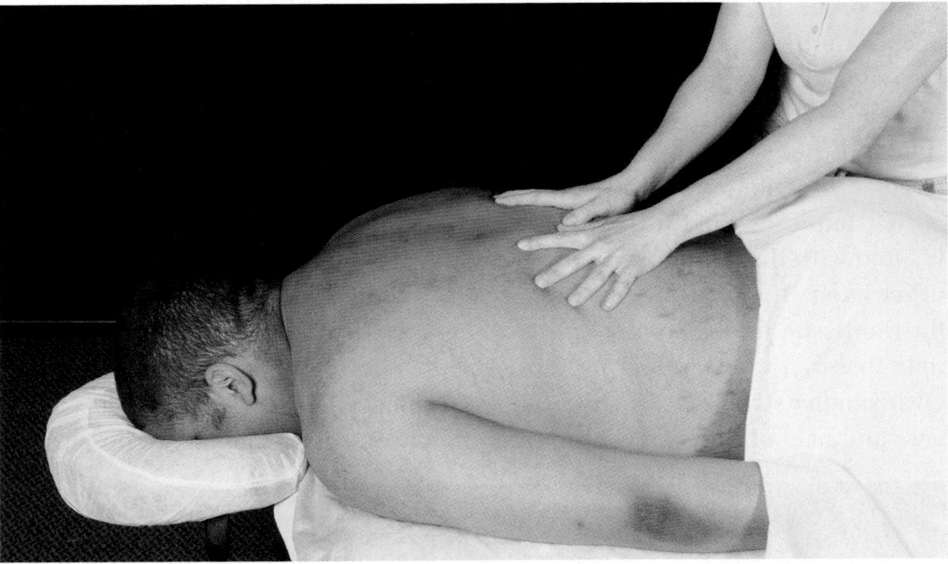

FIGURE 10-7H Deep gliding "stripping" using braced thumbs on the back.

Effect and Benefits of Gliding Strokes

Effleurage or gliding strokes have the following uses or effects:

- Used to spread lubricant evenly
- Used to assess superficial and deeper tissues
- Enhances lymph and venous blood circulation
- Warms the tissue
- Prepares the tissue for deeper work
- Soothes the tissue after deeper work
- Increases circulation to ischemic tissues and aids in removing wastes from congested tissues
- Has a calming effect when done slowly and a stimulating effect when done briskly
- Superficial gliding has more reflexive effects, and deep gliding has more mechanical effects

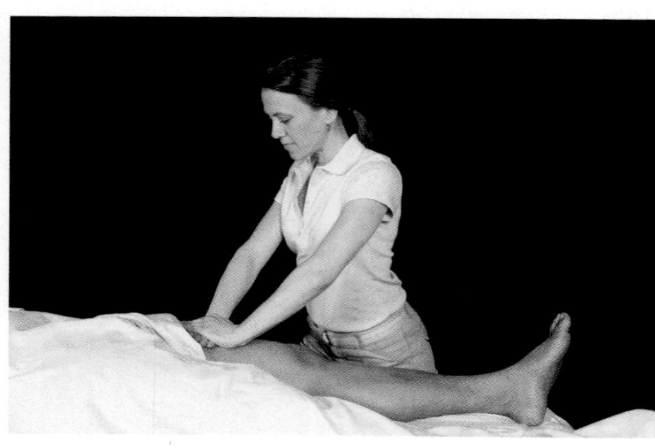

FIGURE 10-8 When using deep techniques, the practitioner must use good body mechanics to direct the manipulation into the client and at the same time protect against injury.

When using deep gliding strokes, the practitioner must use good body mechanics to prevent strain and overuse syndrome injuries. Hand and arm positions should direct the force of the movement into the client. The practitioner's movement should come from the body core. The practitioner's shoulders remain down and relaxed, with the wrists, fingers, or thumbs in proper alignment. Hyperextension of any joint must be avoided (Figure 10-8). When applying long, gliding strokes, the practitioner should shift weight from the back foot to the front foot or take small steps to distribute body weight and maintain consistent pressure throughout the length of the stroke.

Kneading Movements or Petrissage

In Swedish massage, kneading or *petrissage* is used on all fleshy areas of the body. The term *petrissage* comes from the French verb *petrir*, which means to knead or mash. Like deep gliding, kneading enhances the fluid movement in the deeper tissues and can help break up superficial adhesions. Skillfully applied, kneading helps to reduce adhesions and stretch muscle tissue and fascia. In this movement, the skin and muscular tissues are raised from their ordinary position and then squeezed, rolled, or kneaded with a firm pressure, usually in a circular direction.

On large areas of the body, both hands work alternately as a unit. The tissue is lifted with the palmar surface of the fingers of one hand into the palm of the other hand. Then the process is reversed so that the fingers of the other hand lift the tissue into the palm and base of the opposite hand. The hands alternate in a rhythmic circular pattern over the entire body part being massaged. Over smaller structures, such as the arms, the flesh is grasped between the fingers and heel of the hand or the thumb. In both cases, the maximum amount

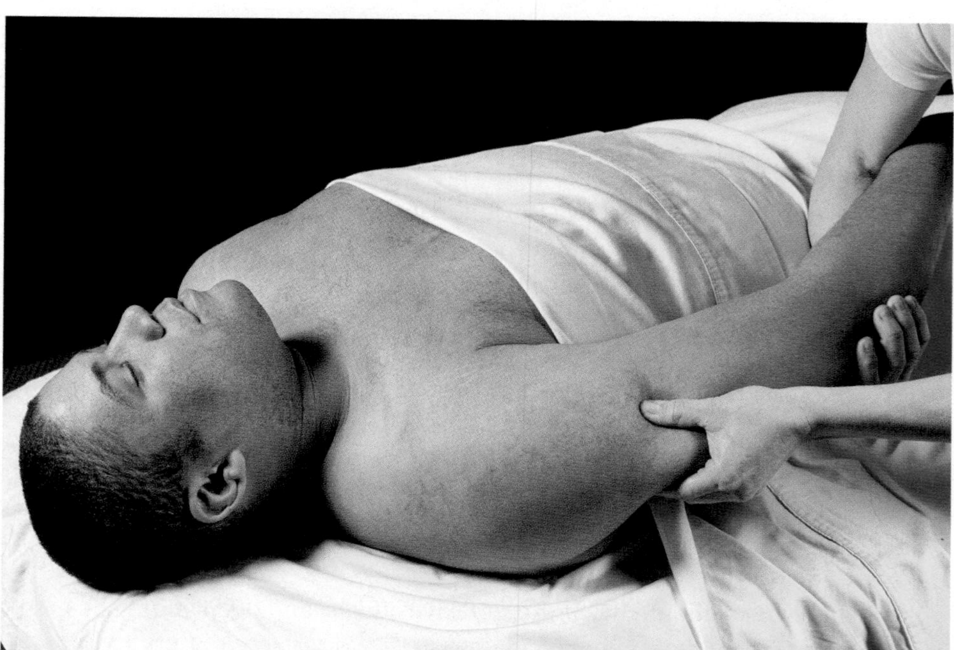

FIGURE 10-9A Kneading the triceps and biceps.

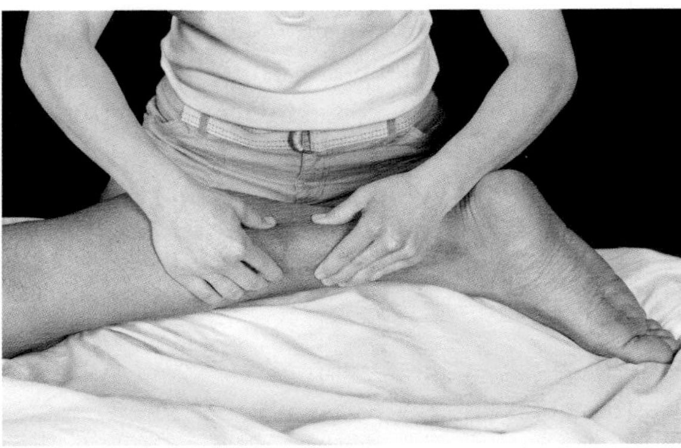

FIGURE 10-9B Kneading the calf muscles.

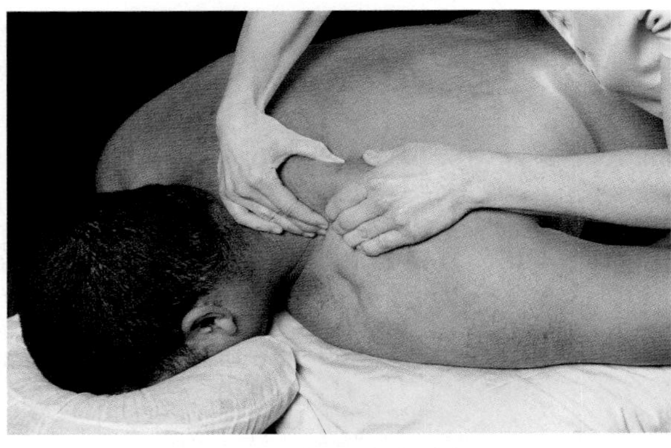

FIGURE 10-9C Petrissage of the trapezius muscles.

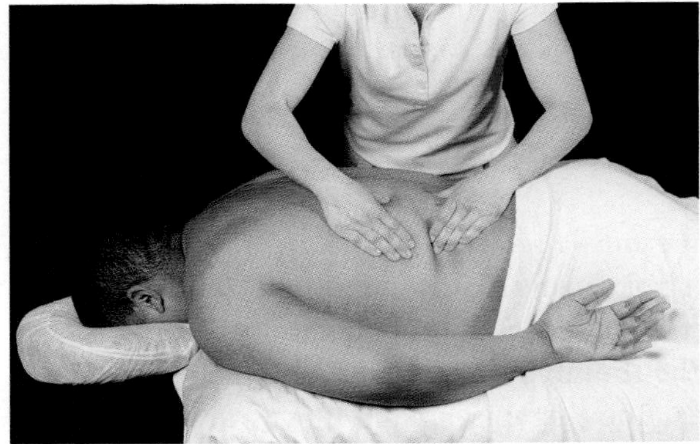

FIGURE 10-9D Petrissage is applied to the entire side that is opposite the practitioner. This takes several passes.

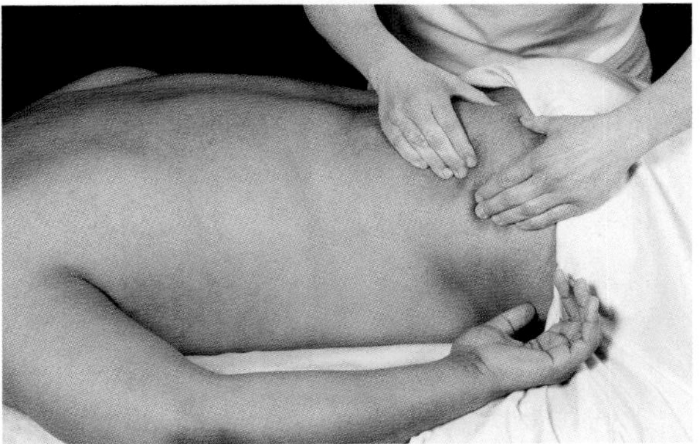

FIGURE 10-9E Kneading over the gluteals.

of flesh is drawn up into the palm and gently and firmly pressed and squeezed, as if milking the tissues. On an area such as the arm, one hand can be used to apply the movement while the other hand stabilizes the arm, or both hands can alternate, grasping the tissue on each side of the arm. On even smaller structures (e.g., the hands or fingers), the flesh is held between the thumb and fingers Figures 10-9a-e).

Fulling is a kneading technique in which the practitioner attempts to grasp the tissue and gently lift and spread it out, as if to make more space between the layers of tissue or muscle fibers. Fulling is applied to the muscular areas of the arm or leg. Often done with both hands simultaneously, the fleshy body part is gathered up between two hands, then raised and separated by the thenar eminence and thumbs as the part is gently stretched across the fibers of the tissue(Figure 10-10).

Skin rolling is a variation of kneading in which only the skin and subcutaneous tissue are picked up between the thumbs and fingers and rolled. As the fingers alternately and continuously pick up and pull the skin away from the deeper tissues, the thumb glides along in the direction of the movement, stretching the underlying fascia. Skin rolling warms, stretches, and begins to separate adhesions between fascial sheaths. When beginning

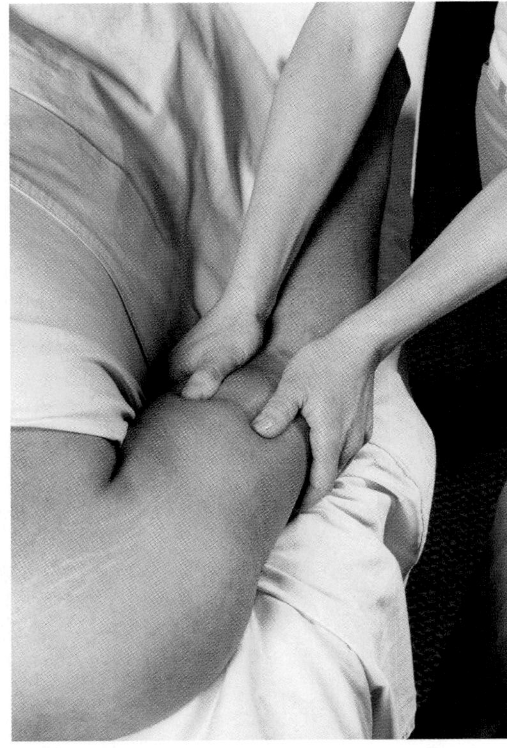

FIGURE 10-10 For fulling movement, grasp the flesh between the fingers and palms of the hand.

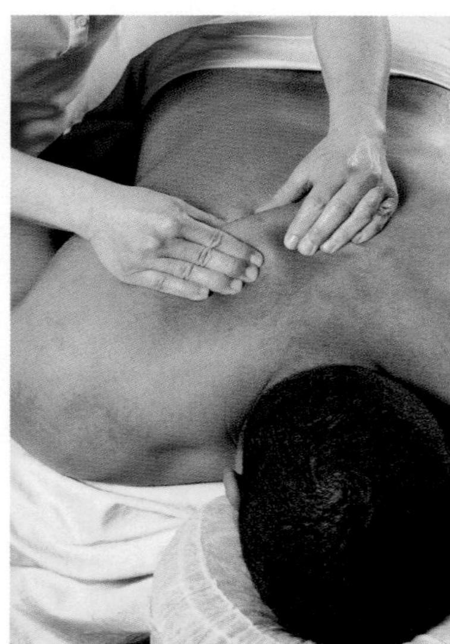

FIGURE 10-11 Skin rolling lifts the superficial tissues away from the muscles and other deeper tissues.

to learn this technique, practitioners should use both hands. Use no lubricant for the technique. Gather up a roll of skin between the thumb and fingers. Continue to gather in more skin with the fingers as you slowly progress along the surface of the body. The thumb supports the roll of skin and slowly slides along as the fingers gather up more skin. Skin rolling is discussed further in Chapter 15 as a myofascial technique (Figure 10-11).

Effect and Benefits of Kneading/Petrissage

Kneading or petrissage has the following effects or benefits:

- Mechanically softens the superficial and deep fascia
- Encourages circulation and flushes out metabolic wastes
- Improves cellular nutrition
- Improves muscle tone, elasticity, and pliability and relaxes muscles
- Improves sensitivity to nerve impulses so that muscle reactions are faster and more coordinated

Friction

Friction strokes can be either superficial or deep. *Superficial friction* is the application of a brisk effleurage-like stroke using a quick back-and-forth movement intended to warm the area and stimulate superficial circulation. Superficial friction is usually preformed with the thumb over a small area or the palm of one or both hands over a larger area. The therapist's hand moves over the client's skin in a quick, rubbing action. When two hands are used, they move back and forth in opposite directions. Lubrication is usually not used. The slight resistance between the surface of the body and the therapist's hand creates heat and warms the superficial tissues (Figures 10-12a,and b)

Deep friction movements involve moving more superficial layers of flesh against the deeper tissues. Whereas kneading is done by lifting and pulling the flesh away from the skeletal structures and squeezing it to milk out the body fluids, friction presses one layer of tissue against another layer to flatten, broaden, or stretch the tissue. Friction is performed in such a way that it also increases heat. As heat increases, the metabolic rate increases. Friction also increases the rate at which exchanges take place between the cells and the interstitial fluids (i.e., fluids situated between the cells and vessels in the tissues of an organ or body part). The added heat and energy also affect the connective

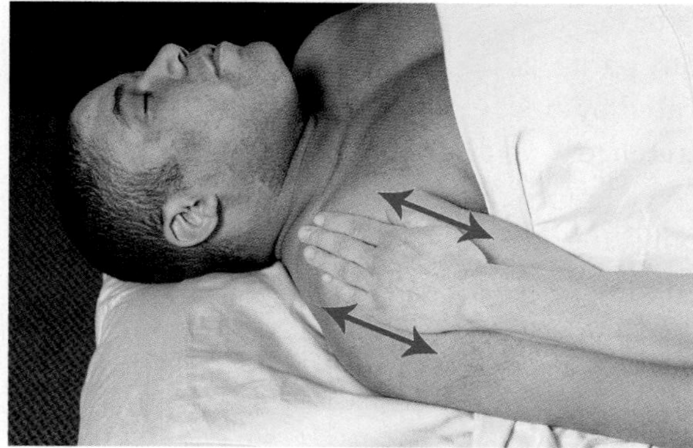

FIGURE 10-12A Superficial friction applied to the upper arm.

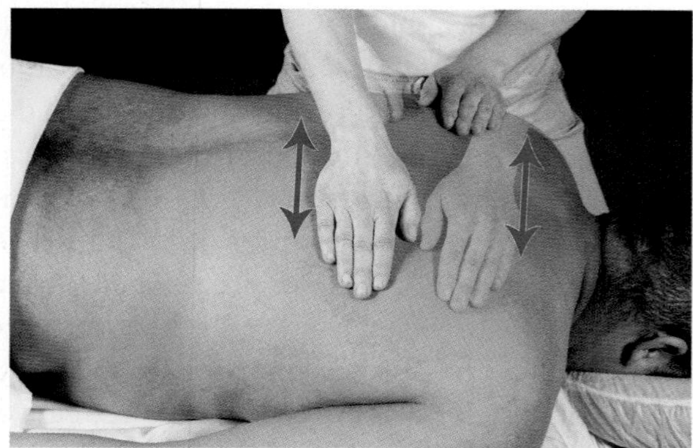

FIGURE 10-12B Two-handed superficial friction on the upper back.

tissue surrounding the muscles, making them more pliable so that they function more efficiently.

Friction helps to separate the tissues and to break down adhesions and fibrosis, especially in muscle tissue and fascia. It softens the amorphous (massed) ground substance between layers of fascia. Friction also aids in absorption of fluid around the joints. Friction has a marked influence on the circulation and glandular activity of the skin. With friction strokes, the area usually becomes red, indicating an increased flow of blood to the area and more blood rushing to the surface of the skin.

Friction strokes involve moving a more superficial layer of tissue against deeper layers of tissue. This requires pressure on the skin while it is being moved over its underlying structures. The skin and the hand move as a unit against the deeper tissues. Over muscular parts or fleshy layers, the palms of the hands, the flat of the fingers, or the thumbs apply friction. Over small surfaces, the fleshy pads of the fingertips or thumbs apply friction.

Friction movements can be circular or directional. In **circular friction**, the fingers or the palm of the hand contact the skin to move it in a circular pattern over the deeper tissues. Circular friction, which is intended to produce heat and stretch and soften the fascia, is a general stroke used to warm the area in preparation for more specific or deeper work. The palm or pads of the fingers make contact with the skin and move the skin and more superficial tissues over the deeper layers in a small circular pattern. When performing circular friction, the fingers or hand do not slide over the skin in a circular manner. The intent is to move the superficial layer of tissue over a deeper layer, resulting in a gentle stretching and warming of the area, although the hand can move along to cover an extended area with circular friction.

circular friction

is movement in which the fingers or palm of the hand move the superficial tissues in a circular pattern over the deeper tissues.

Circular friction is also valuable for palpating an area when assessing the condition of the underlying tissues. When working deeply on an area, circular friction and superficial gliding strokes are useful to soothe and calm the client before, after, and interspersed with deep techniques (Figures 10-13a-d).

Directional friction can be either cross-fiber or longitudinal friction. **Cross-fiber** friction, as the name implies, is applied in a transverse direction across the muscle, tendon, or ligament fibers. Cross-fiber friction is usually applied with the tips of the fingers or the thumb directly to the specific site of a lesion. The intention of cross-fiber friction is to broaden, separate, and align the fibrous tissue, break up adhesions, and soften scar tissue. The stroke is broad enough to cover and deep enough to reach the targeted tissue. When massaging a fibrous band, the cross-fiber friction stroke is not so broad that it snaps across the fiber. The fingers do not move over the skin but move the skin and superficial tissues across the target tissue(see Figure 10-13e). Another method of applying cross-fiber friction in some situations is to apply compression to an affected area and move the limb so that the underlying bone provides the frictioning movement. This technique is especially applicable to points near the elbow by compressing the points and rotating the forearm (see Figure 10-13f).

cross-fiber friction

is applied in a transverse direction across the muscle, tendon, or ligament.

Cross-fiber or transverse friction is a preferred technique for rehabilitation of fibrous tissue injuries. While the injury is healing, transverse friction, when properly applied, promotes the formation of elastic fibrous tissue. At the same time, it reduces the formation of fibrosis and scar tissue, so that the healed injury

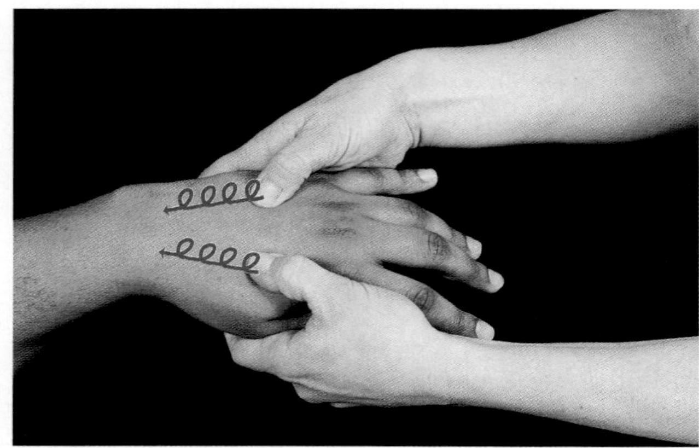

FIGURE 10-13A Circular friction of the muscles of the hand.

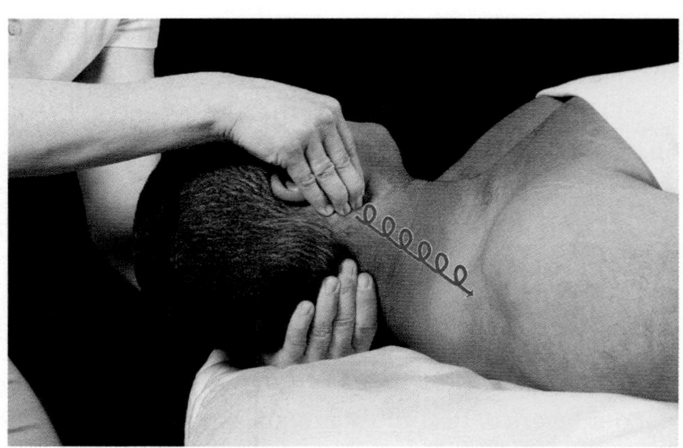

FIGURE 10-13B Circular friction of the back of the neck.

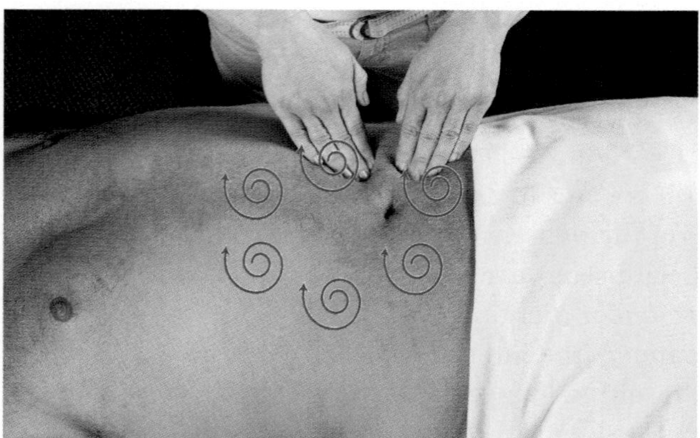

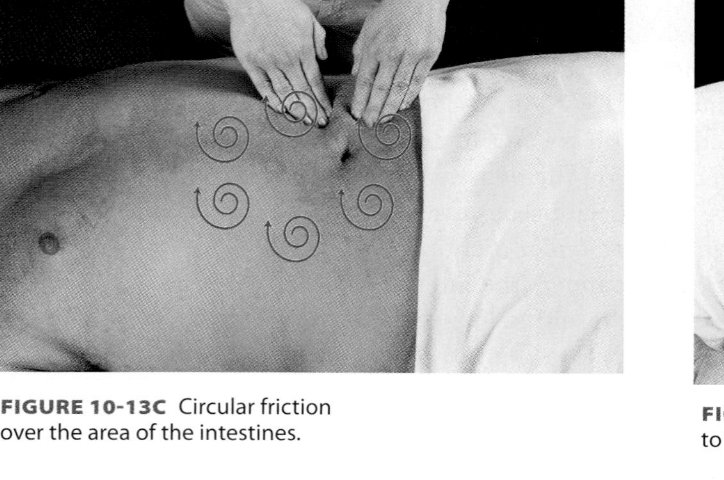

FIGURE 10-13C Circular friction over the area of the intestines.

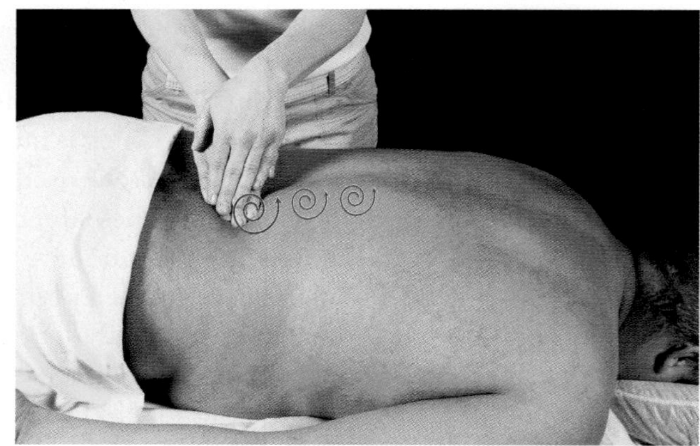

FIGURE 10-13D Friction applied to the muscles along the spine.

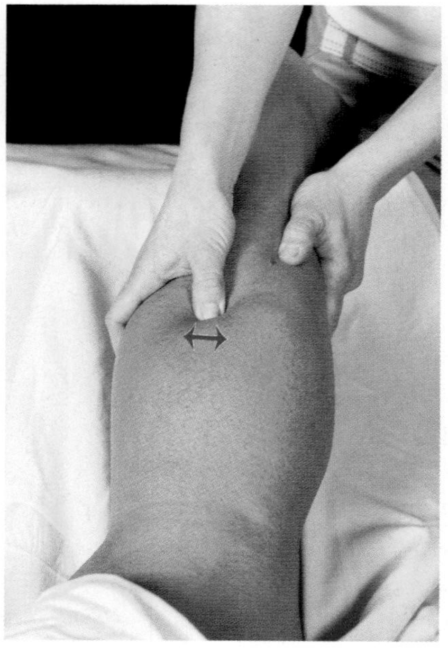

FIGURE 10-13E Cross-fiber friction can be applied to the musculotendinous junction of the posterior leg.

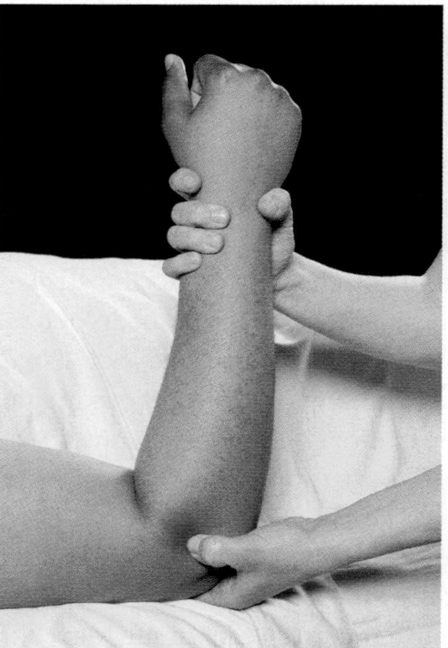

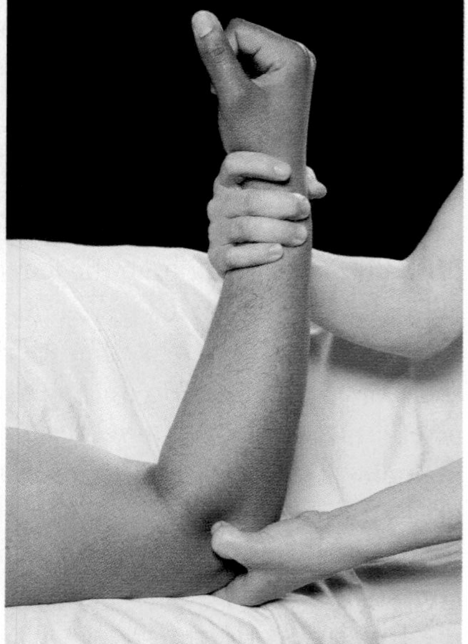

FIGURE 10-13F Cross-fiber friction can be applied by compressing a point and moving the underlying bone.

retains its original strength and pliability. Applied to old injury sites, cross-fiber friction breaks down some of the adhesions and fibrosis, increasing pliability and mobility while reducing the chance of reinjury to the area.

In longitudinal friction, the practitioner's hand moves in the same direction as the tissue fibers. This technique tends to stretch the tissue and align the collagen fibrils within the fascia.

Effect and Benefits of Friction

Friction techniques produce the following benefits and effects:

- Superficial friction causes vasodilation of the superficial blood vessels in the skin
- Moving one layer of tissue against another produces heat in the skin and superficial fascia
- Increases blood and lymph circulation
- Breaks down fascial adhesions and softens scar tissue
- Causes a mild therapeutic inflammation
- Promotes a more pliable scar formation
- Increases circulation in deeper tissues

Another form of friction sometimes classified on its own is **compression**. As the name implies, compression is using rhythmic pressing movements directed into muscle tissue by either the hand or fingers. Palmar compression is done with the whole hand (palm side), the heel of the hand, or a closed fist over the large muscular areas of the body. *Palmar compression* is a rhythmic pumping action directed into the muscle perpendicular to the underlying bone. Compression can be done over clothing and without the use of lubricant. Compression movements cause increased circulation and a lasting hyperemia in the tissue. Compression is a popular movement used in pre-event sports massage. The intention is to bring more blood and fluid into the tissues, preparing them to exert maximum energy sooner and for a longer period (Figure 10-14).

compression is rhythmic pressing movements directed into muscle tissue by either the hand or fingers.

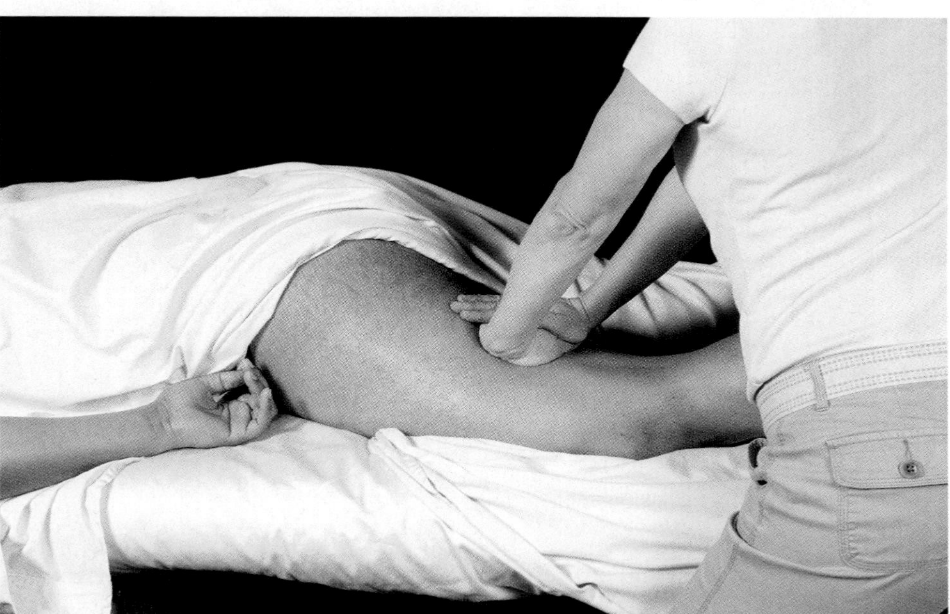

FIGURE 10-14 Two-handed compression applied to the hamstrings.

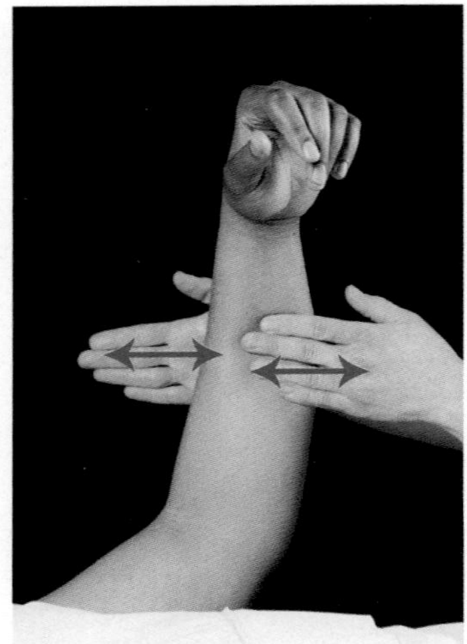

FIGURE 10-15A Rolling the arm.

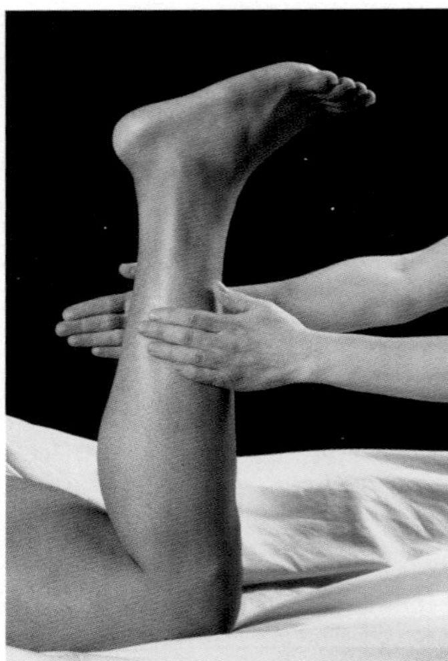

FIGURE 10-15B Rolling the muscles of the leg.

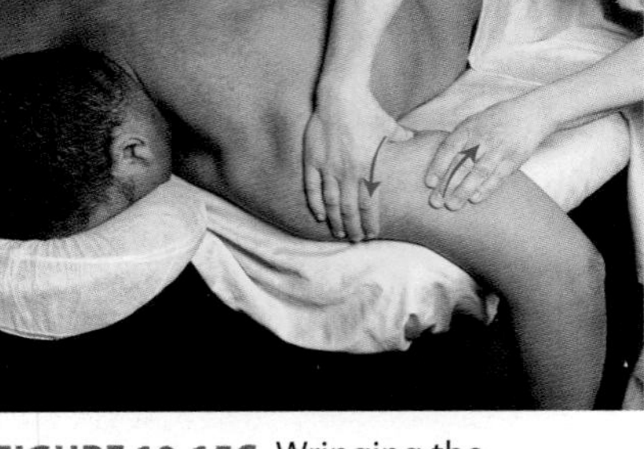

FIGURE 10-15C Wringing the muscles of the arm.

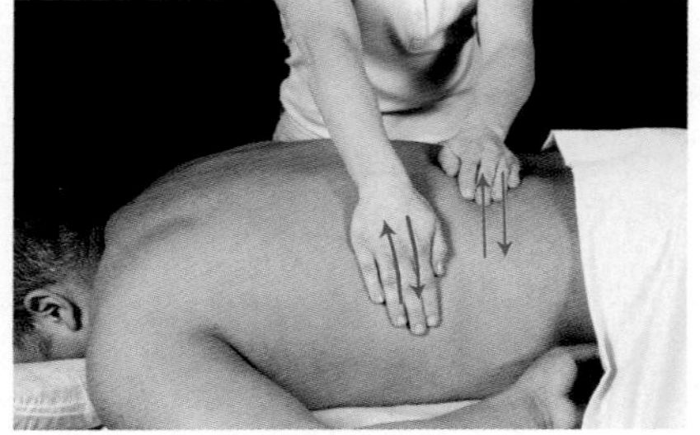

FIGURE 10-15D Wringing the muscles of the lower back in a backward and forward movement.

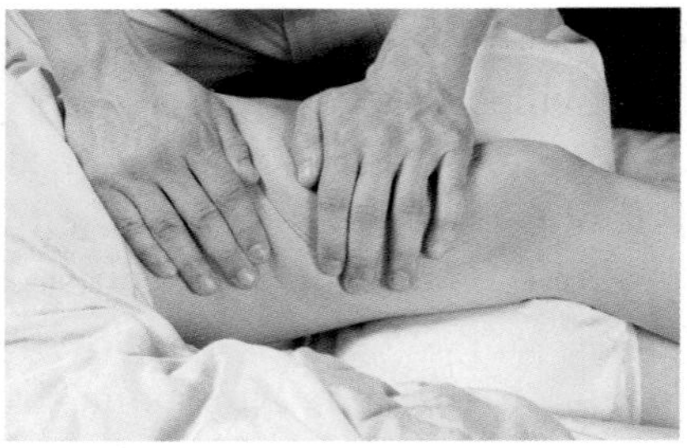

FIGURE 10-15E Wringing the muscles of the leg.

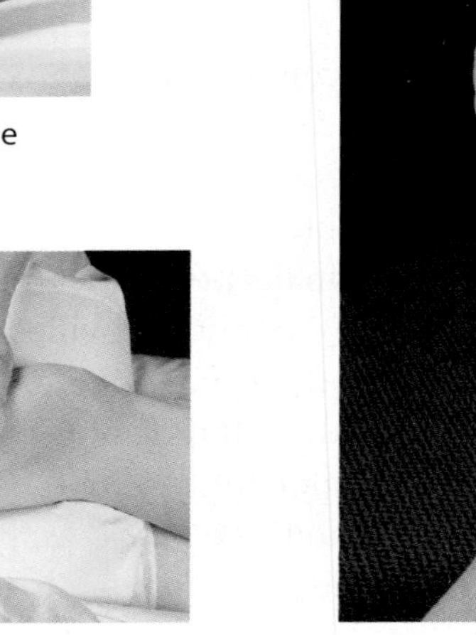

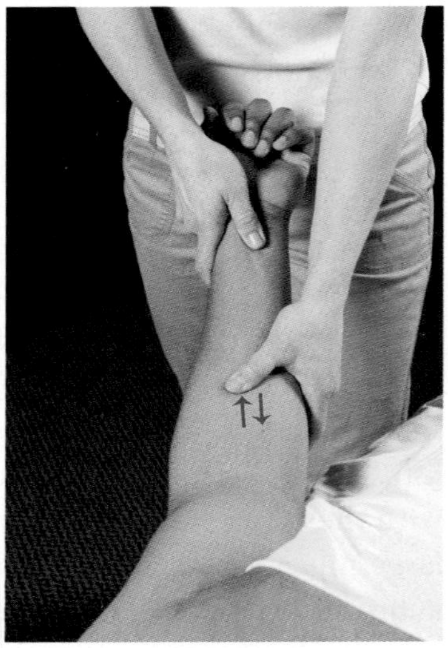

FIGURE 10-15F Chucking the arm.

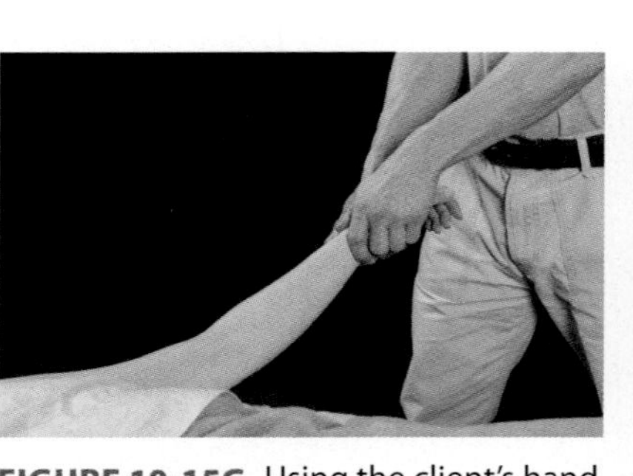

FIGURE 10-15G Using the client's hand as a handle for shaking the hand or during petrissage and applying friction to the hand.

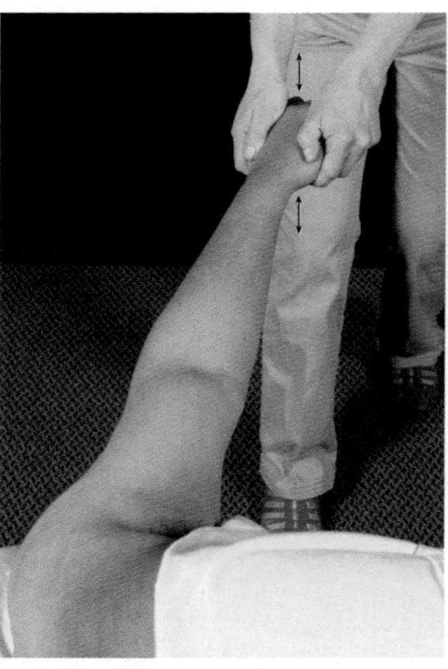

FIGURE 10-15H Shaking applied to the arm.

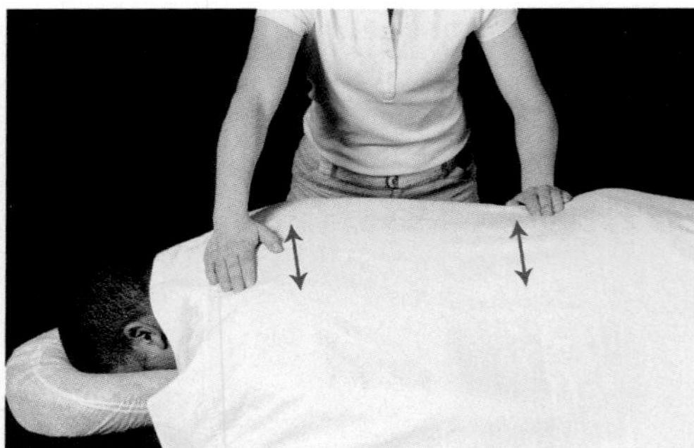

FIGURE 10-15I Rocking applied to the torso.

Other movements that are considered friction include rolling, wringing, chucking, shaking, and vibration. Chucking, rolling, wringing, and shaking are variations of friction employed principally to massage the arms and legs (Figures 10-15a-i).

Rolling

Rolling is a rapid back-and-forth movement with the hands, in which the flesh is shaken and rolled around the *axis*, or the imaginary centerline, of the body part. The intention of rolling is to warm and relax the tissue. Rolling encourages deep muscle relaxation (Figures 10-15a and b).

rolling
is a rapid back-and-forth movement with the hands, in which the flesh is shaken and rolled around the axis of the body part.

Wringing

Wringing is a back-and-forth movement in which both of the practitioner's hands are placed a short distance apart on either side of the limb. The movement resembles that of wringing out a washcloth. The hands work in opposing directions, stretching and twisting the flesh against the bones in opposite directions. The practitioner's whole body is engaged in the movement, and the hands make firm contact in both directions. Pressure is not excessive enough to cause pinching or burning (irritation) of the skin, however. Wringing gently stretches and warms the connective fascia (Figures 10-15c, d, and e).

wringing
is a back-and-forth movement in which both hands are placed a short distance apart on either side of the limb and work in opposing directions.

Chucking

The **chucking** movement is accomplished by grasping the flesh firmly in one or both hands and moving it up and down along the bone. It is a series of quick movements along the axis of the limb (Figure 10-15f).

chucking
involves the flesh being grasped firmly in one or both hands and moved up and down along the bone.

Shaking

Shaking is a movement that allows the client to release tension and at the same time indicates to the practitioner where the client could be storing tension in a part of the body. The relaxed body part is gently yet forcefully shaken laterally or horizontally so that the relaxed flesh flops around the bone. The practitioner observes where the body moves freely and where it seems to be stiff. Rigidness indicates tense areas of the body that require more attention. A type of bodywork known as *Trager* uses extensive shaking and rocking to locate and release tension (Figures 10-15g, and h).

shaking
allows the release of tension by gently shaking a relaxed body part so that the flesh flops around the bone.

Jostling

Jostling releases muscle tension, increases circulation, and relaxes muscles. Jostling is most effective after muscles have exerted themselves, such as after a workout or competition. Jostling is done when the muscle is in a shortened and relaxed position. Grasp across the entire muscle, lift it slightly away from its position, and, while the muscle remains relaxed, shake the muscle quickly across its axis.

jostling
involves grasping the entire muscle, lifting it slightly away from its position, and shaking it quickly across its axis.

Rocking

Rocking uses a push-and-release movement applied to the client's body in either a side-to-side or an up-and-down direction. The body is pushed away slightly and allowed to roll back completely and then pushed away again at a rhythmic rate that is unique to each person. The practitioner can sense the client's rhythm within a few repetitions and then maintains that rhythm and applies it to other movements during the massage. Rocking is perhaps the most soothing and relaxing of all the massage movements (Figure 10-15i).

rocking
is a push-and-release movement applied to the client's body in either a side-to-side or an up-and-down direction.

vibration

is a continuous trembling or shaking movement delivered either by the practitioner or an electrical apparatus.

Vibration

Vibration is a continuous shaking or trembling movement transmitted from the practitioner's hand and arm (or from an electrical appliance) to a fixed point or along a selected area of the body. Vibration is often used to desensitize a point or area. Nerve trunks and centers are sometimes chosen as sites for the application of vibratory movements. Vibration is typically used on larger muscles, avoiding bony areas.

Manual contact vibration is usually done with the pads at the ends of the fingers or the soft touch of the palm of the hand. The therapist makes light contact and shakes the hand back and forth as quickly as possible without moving over the skin where contact is being made.

The rate of vibration should be under the control of the massage practitioner. Manual vibrations usually range from

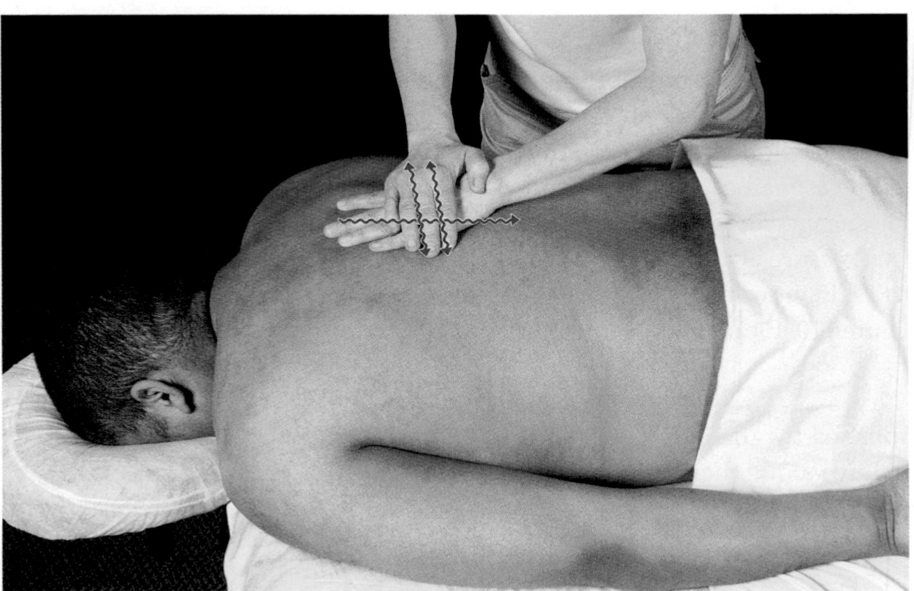

FIGURE 10-16 Vibrating over each vertebra.

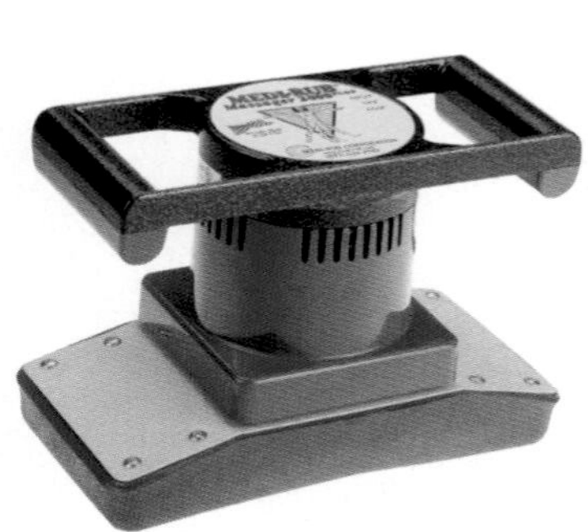

FIGURE 10-17A Popular style of vibrator that uses an orbital movement. (Courtesy of Medi-Rub Corporation.)

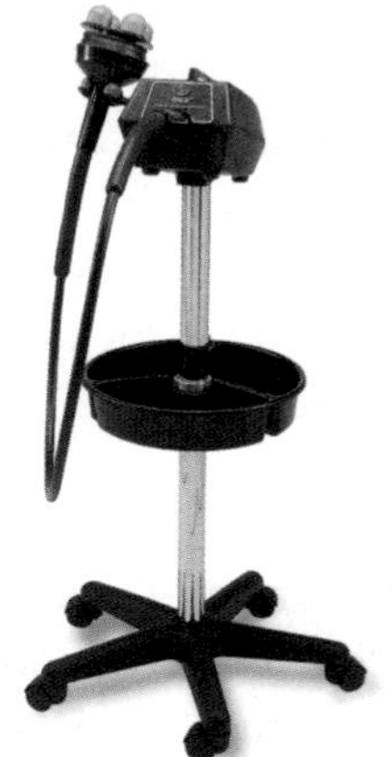

FIGURE 10-17B The floor-standing model has a flexible shaft and a variety of applicator heads. (Courtesy of General Physiotherapy, Inc.)

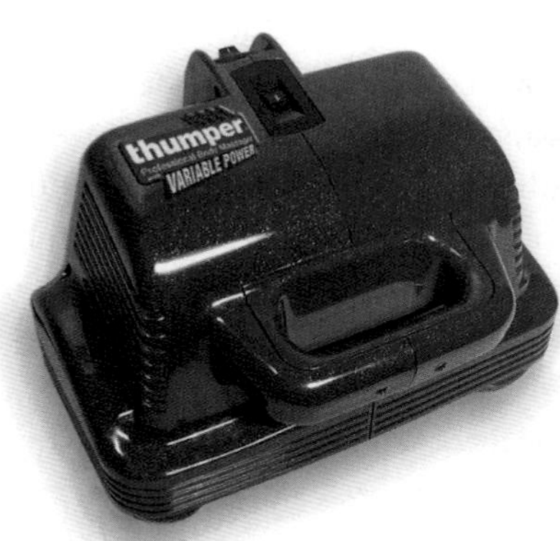

FIGURE 10-17C A type of vibrator that uses a thumping action. (Courtesy of Thumper Massager Inc.)

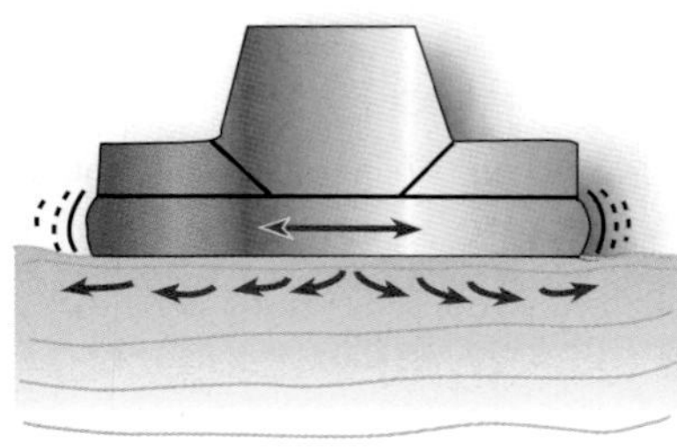

FIGURE 10-18A Oscillating vibrators have a linear back-and-forth action.

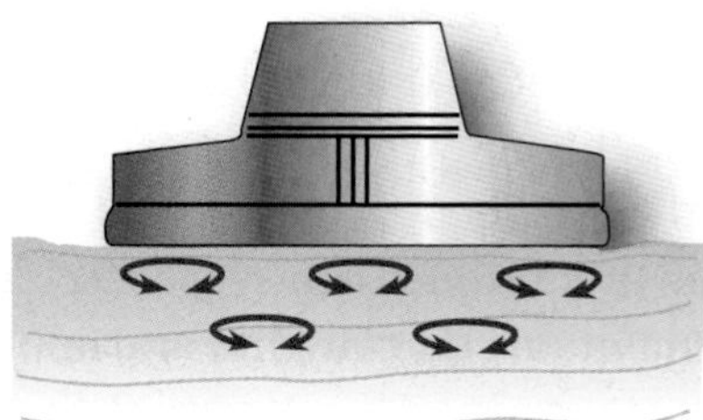

FIGURE 10-18B Orbital vibrators have a circular action.

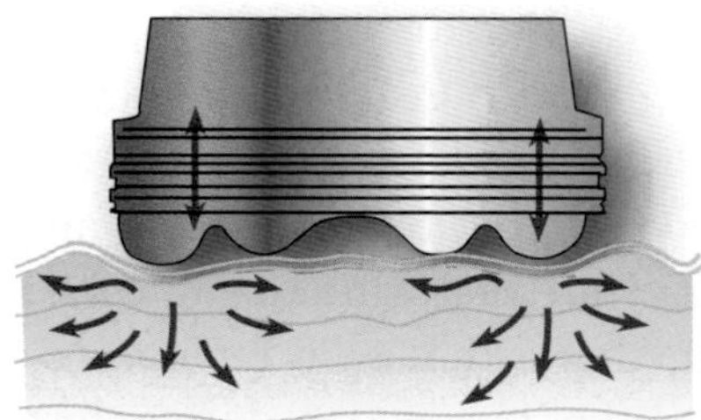

FIGURE 10-18C]"The Thumper" uses a percussion/compression action. (Courtesy of Thumper, Inc.)

5 to 10 times per second; mechanical vibrations can be adjusted to give from 10 to 100 vibrations per second (Figure 10-16).

The variety of mechanical vibrators on the market can be classified by size. A popular small model straps on the back of the practitioner's hand. Another popular size is held (usually with two hands) by the practitioner and moved over the client's body. A larger floor-standing unit uses a flexible applicator arm to deliver its therapeutic effects (Figures 10-17a-c).

Mechanical vibrators can also be classified by the vibrating action that they use. An oscillating vibrator has a back-and-forth movement. An orbital vibrator uses a circular motion. These vibrators produce a shaking movement when applied to the body. Another type of vibrator produces a "thumping" action. This rapid percussion/compression is directed into the tissues rather than laterally along their surface. Using vibrators can enhance the effects of the massage and at the same time reduce the amount of physical exertion required of the practitioner (Figures 10-18a-c).

The effect of vibratory movements depends on the rate of vibration, the intensity of pressure, and the duration of the treatment. This form of massage is soothing and brings about relaxation and release of tension when applied lightly. It is stimulating when applied with pressure. An anesthetizing effect is experienced when vibrations are applied for a prolonged period.

PERCUSSION MOVEMENTS

Percussion movements, traditionally called **tappotement**, include quick, striking manipulations such as tapping, beating, and slapping, which are highly stimulating to the body. Percussion movements are executed with both hands either simultaneously or alternately. They do not use much force. Each time the practitioner's hands touch the body is a glancing contact wherein the practitioner's wrists remain very relaxed.

tappotement

movements include tapping, slapping, hacking, cupping, and beating.

The general effects of percussion movements are to tone the muscles, impart a healthy glow, and stimulate the part being massaged. With each striking movement, the muscles first contract and then relax as the fingers are removed from

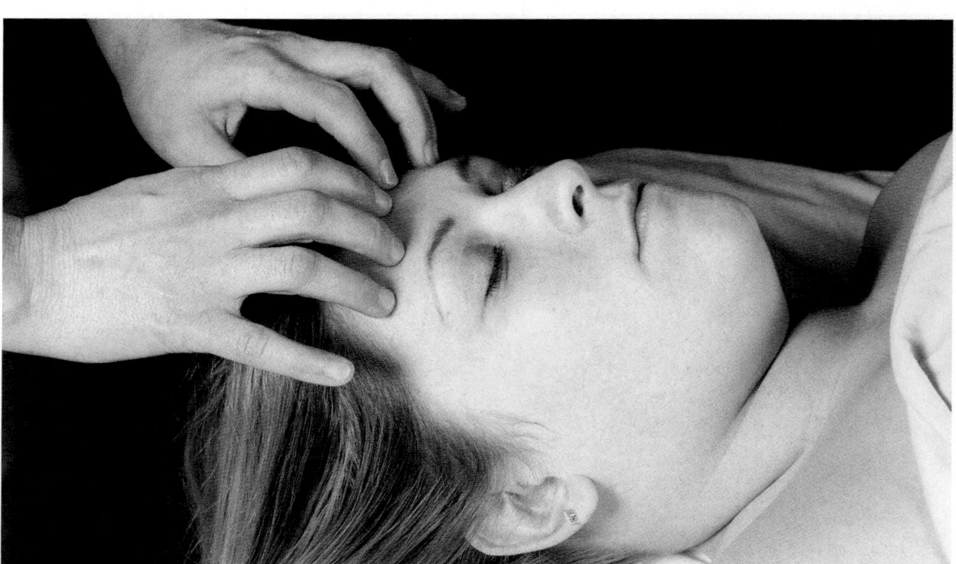

FIGURE 10-19A. Tapping with fingertips on the face.

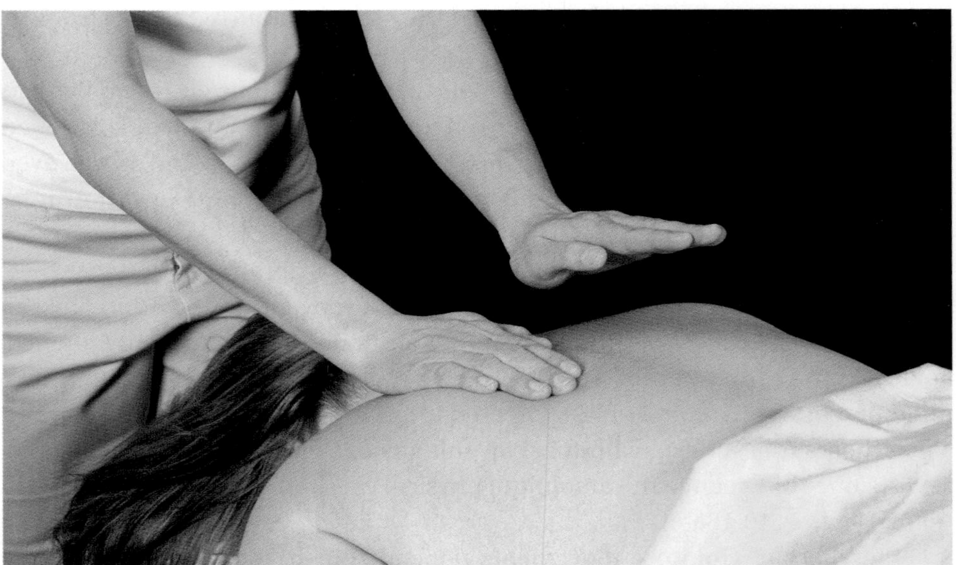

FIGURE 10-19B. Slapping movements on the back.

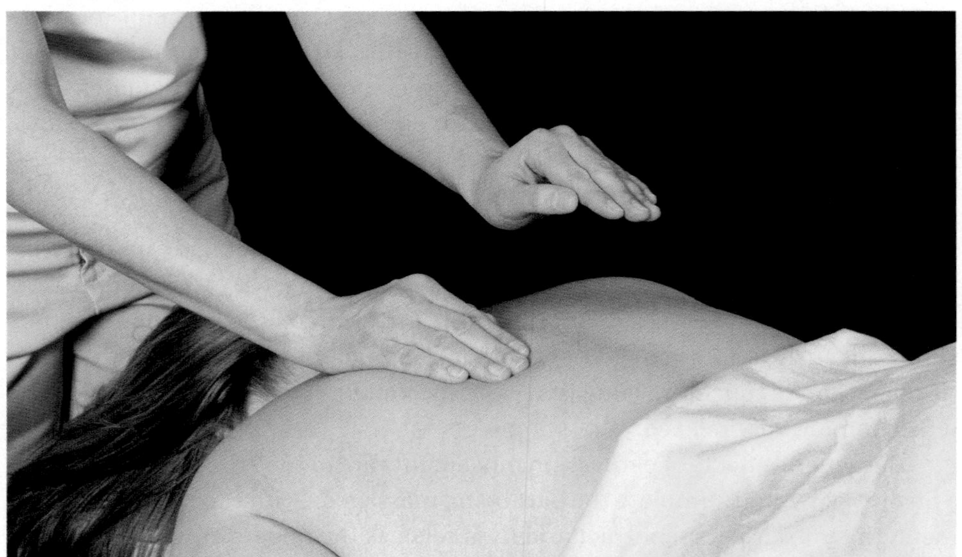

FIGURE 10-19C. Cupping movements on the back.

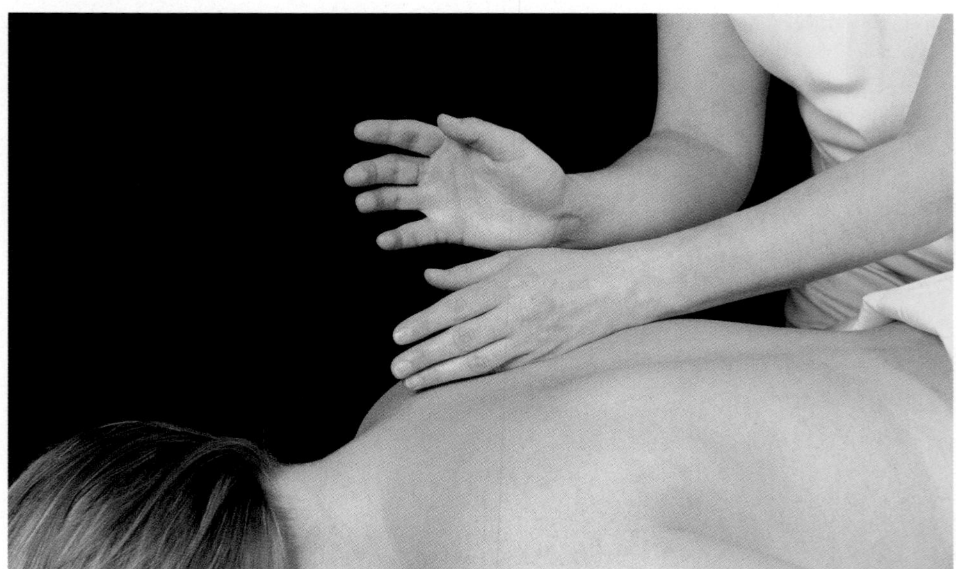

FIGURE 10-19D. Hacking movements on the back.

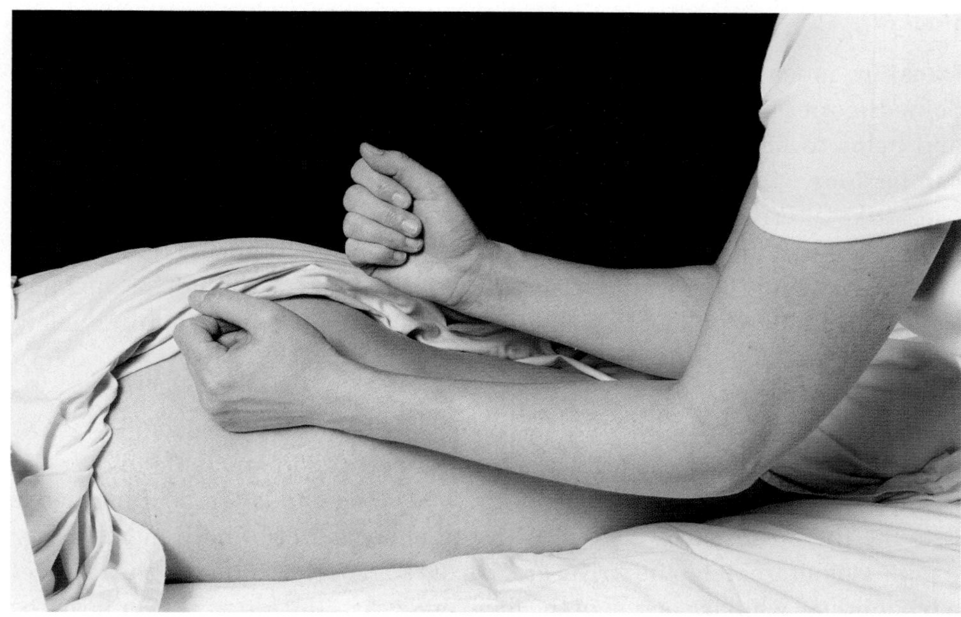

FIGURE 10-19E. Beating the thicker gluteal muscles.

the body. In this way, muscles are toned. Percussion movements should never be applied directly over the spine or muscles that are abnormally contracted, or over any sensitive area such as the kidneys or other endangerment sites (Figures 10-19a-e). The movements can be done in the following ways:

1. Tapping with tips of the fingers
2. Slapping with flattened palm and fingers of the hand
3. Cupping with the cupped palm of the hand
4. Hacking with the ulnar border of the hand
5. Beating with a softly clenched hand

Tapping

Tapping, the lightest, most superficial of the percussion techniques, is used over delicate, sensitive areas such as the face. Only the fingertips are used for tapping. The fingers can be slightly flexed so that only the tips make contact, or, with the fingers held relatively straight, the pads perform a very superficial slapping technique(Figure 10-19a).

tapping

is the lightest, most superficial of the percussion techniques.

Slapping

Slapping is very stimulating and must be used sparingly. Slapping encourages peripheral circulation and gives a "glow" to the area. It is applied with the palmar surface of the fingers and the hand. Slapping produces a crisp smacking sound when done correctly. As with all percussion strokes, the hands and wrists always remain loose and relaxed. Heavy pressure is avoided. Slapping uses a rhythmic, glancing contact with the body (Figure 10-19b).

slapping

uses a rhythmic, glancing contact with the body.

Cupping

Cupping is a technique often employed by respiratory therapists to help break up lung congestion. Cupping is most often employed over the rib cage. To perform cupping, form a cup by keeping the fingers together and slightly flexed and the thumb held close to the side of the palm. On each percussion, the perimeter of the hand contacts the body. The result is a hollow popping sound (Figure 10-19c).

cupping

is a technique used by respiratory therapists to help break up lung congestion.

Hacking

hacking

is a rapid striking movement that can be done with one or both hands.

Hacking, much like vibration, encourages relaxation and local circulation. Some theories claim that hacking stimulates the nerve responses in muscles and helps to firm the muscles. Hacking is a rapid striking movement that can be done with one or both hands. When both hands are used, the hands can strike alternately or together. A quick glancing strike is made with the little finger and the ulnar side of the hand. The wrist and fingers remain loose and relaxed, and the fingers are slightly spread apart. As the side of the hand strikes the body, the fingers come together, causing a slight vibrating effect (Figure 10-19d).

Beating

beating

is the heaviest and deepest form of percussion and is done over the denser muscular areas of the body.

Beating is the heaviest and deepest form of percussion and is done over the thicker, denser, and fleshier areas of the body. The hands are held in a loose fist. The therapist makes contact with the ulnar aspect of both hands either together or alternately. The wrists are relaxed so that the contact is the result of a rebounding, whiplike action of the hand and wrist. The force is never heavy or hard (Figure 10-19e).

Effects and Benefits of Percussion

The effects and benefits of percussion techniques vary according to the variation of the technique used, the area of the body, the intensity and the duration of the application, and include the following:

- Initially has a stimulating effect
- Prolonged application encourages relaxation.
- Prolonged applications have an anesthetic effect on some nerve endings.
- Deeper applications cause vasodilation and increased circulation.
- Cupping aids in breaking up lung congestion.

JOINT MOVEMENTS

There are a great variety of joint movements that can be used to move any joint in the body, including joints of the toes, knees, hips, arms, and vertebrae, or even the less movable joints of the pelvis and cranium.

passive joint movements

stretch the fibrous tissue and move the joint through its range of motion.

The basic classifications of joint movements are passive and active. **Passive joint movements (PJM)** are done while the client remains quietly relaxed and allow the practitioner to stretch and move the part of the body to be exercised. Passive joint movements can be used as an assessment tool to determine normal movement (full range of motion without restriction or pain). Passive joint movements gently stretch the fibrous connective tissue and move the joint through its range of motion. PJMs are used therapeutically to improve joint mobility and range of motion, always working within the client's comfort level.

When performing PJMs, hold and support the limb so that the movement is directed toward the target joint. Move the limb in a normal movement pattern for that joint. Move the limb to the full extent of possible movement within the client's comfort level. If the movement is for assessment purposes, move only to the point of resistance and note the extent and quality of the movement. If the movement is therapeutic, challenge the range of movement by slightly extending or pushing into the end of the movement.

In **active joint movements,** the client actively participates in the exercise by contracting the muscles involved in the movement. In **active range-of-motion** movements, the client moves the limb or the joint without any intervention from the practitioner. This is a common assessment tool to determine which, if any, limitations might exist. The assessment can be done before and after treatment to note any changes. Active joint movements that involve the practitioner can be subdivided into two categories: active assistive and active resistive joint movements.

active joint movements are movements in which the client actively participates by contracting the muscles involved in the movement.

active range of motion the client moves the limb or the joint without any intervention from the practitioner to assess any limitation in the joint movement.

Active assistive joint movements are a therapeutic technique to restore mobility in a limb that has been injured. They are used when a client is unable to move a limb or cannot move it through a full range of motion. When performing active assistive joint movements, the practitioner instructs the client to make a specific movement. This is best done by moving the limb passively through the desired movement. As the client attempts the movement, the therapist assists the limb through that movement as necessary. The movement is repeated several times.

Active resistive joint movements refer to several therapeutic techniques that improve mobility, flexibility, or strength, depending on how the technique is performed. As the name indicates, active resistive joint movements involve a movement made by the client that is in some way resisted by the practitioner. The type and degree of the movement, the extent and direction of the resistance, the duration of the resistance, and the sequence of the actions all have an effect on the outcome of the procedure.

To perform active resistive joint movements to shoulder flexion, instruct the client on the movement by passively moving the arm from a neutral position next to the side to a position high over the head. Instruct the client to repeat the movement on your command. Place one hand on the wrist and the other just above the elbow. Instruct the client to move the arm. Resist the client's movement but allow the movement to take place. Repeat the movement several times, resisting a little more each time but always allowing the full movement to take place. This type of movement builds strength in the specific muscle groups being challenged. Active resistive joint movements can target any specific muscle group in the body.

Joint movements are used to help restore a client's mobility or increase flexibility in a joint. Often, passive and active joint movements are combined. For example, to restore some mobility to a shoulder joint, the client is instructed to raise the arm to the point of discomfort (active unassisted movement). The therapist holds the arm in that position while the client is instructed to push against the therapist and attempt to continue the movement (active resistive joint movement). The client then is instructed to relax as the therapist continues to move the client's arm without help or effort from the client (passive joint movement).

Effects and Benefits of Joint Movements

Passive and active joint movements have beneficial effects on the joint and the soft tissues associated with the joint. Most joint movements are applied to synovial joints. Depending on how they are applied, joint movements:

- Promote relaxation of the related muscles.
- Warm and lubricate the articulating surfaces within the joint capsule and stimulate the production of synovial fluid.
- Affect the proprioceptors and mechanoreceptors in the tissues surrounding the joint and in the associated muscles by manipulating the articulation through its full range of motion and introducing the limb to the possibility of new movement.
- Provide stretch to the fascia of the associated muscles.
- Flex, stretch, and warm tendons and ligaments to become more pliable.
- Help to maintain or increase flexibility and range of motion.
- Stimulate lymph and venous blood circulation because of the movement of the muscles.

Joint movements are most beneficial when performed through the full physiologic range of motion. All joints have normal restrictions or barriers that limit the range of motion. These natural barriers can be classified as anatomic, physiologic, or pathologic. Barriers can be altered by illness, injury, or surgery.

Anatomic barriers limit movement because of the physical structure of the joint. Moving beyond an anatomic barrier can result in damage to the tissues involved.

The physiologic barrier to a joint movement is encountered at the anatomic barrier but usually before it is reached. The physiologic barrier can be due to bone-to-bone contact, such as the extension of the elbow where the movement is stopped when the olecranon of the ulna contacts the humerus. In healthy tissue, the physiologic barrier is usually due to soft tissue, either muscle or ligaments, limiting the movement at the end of a normal range of motion. The barrier can be due to soft tissue approximation, such as flexion of the elbow where the biceps presses against the forearm, restricting further movement. Sometimes the restriction is due to pull on the ligaments, as in the hyperextension of the hip. Most often, however, it is due to the pull of muscles that have reached the extent of their possible stretch.

A pathologic barrier is similar to the physiologic barrier, but it occurs either before the normal end of the range of motion is achieved or is accompanied by pain or discomfort that restricts the movement of that joint. Tense muscles, injured or scarred tissues, inflammation, or other pathologic conditions can restrict the range of motion.

When a therapist is performing joint movements on a client, the limb or joint should move easily and painlessly within its physiologic range of motion. It is beneficial for the practitioner to be familiar with the normal range of motion for the major synovial joints in the body. Keep in mind that normal range of motion varies from person to person. As the practitioner moves a joint so that it approaches its physiologic barrier, the quality of the movement changes.

Text is continued on page 368.

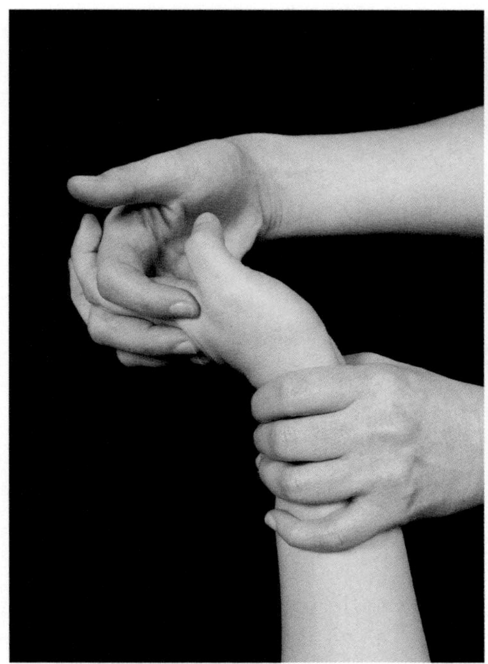

FIGURE 10-20A. Apply joint movements and rotation. Note the interlacing of the fingers.

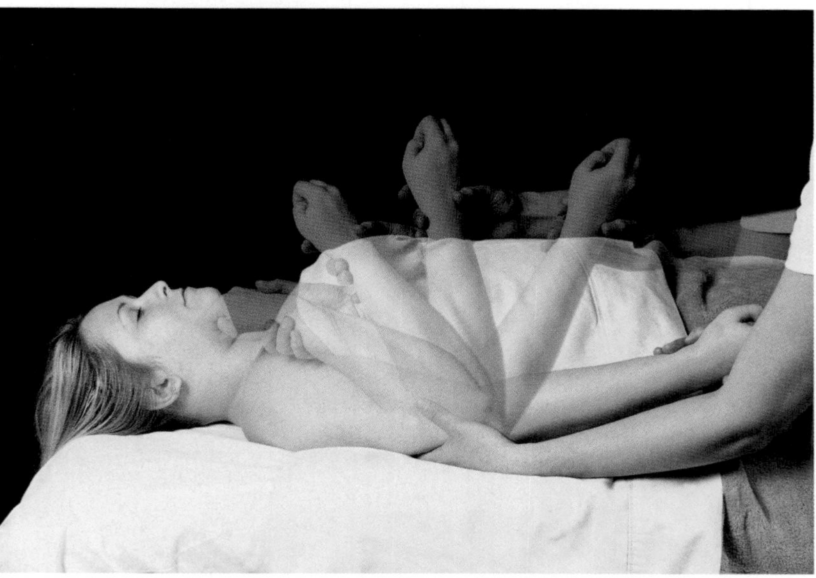

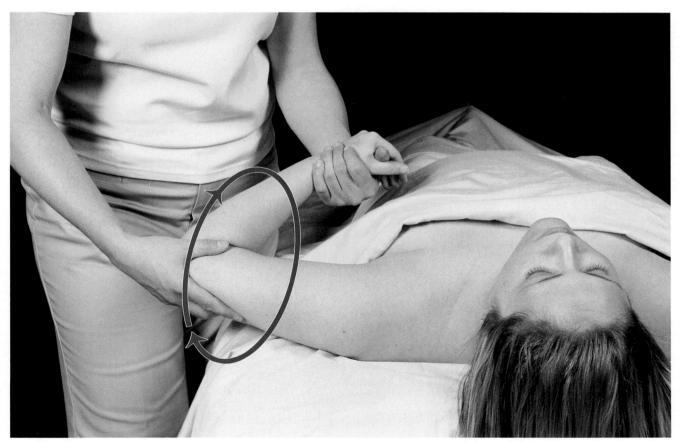

FIGURE 10-20B. Flexion and extension of the forearm.

FIGURE 10-20C. Rotate the shoulder.

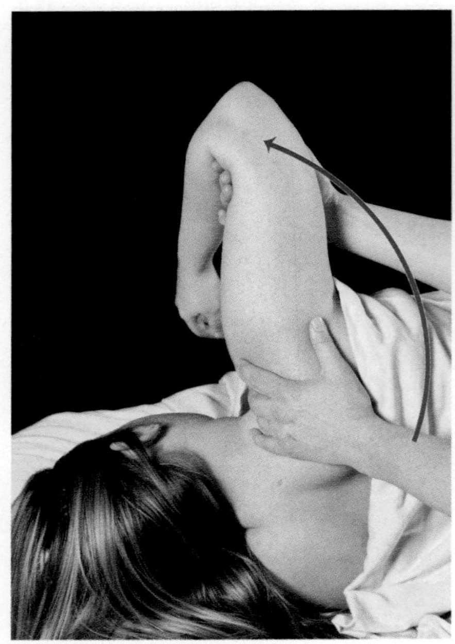

FIGURE 10-20D. Abduction of the arm. This is movement of a part away from the median line of the body.

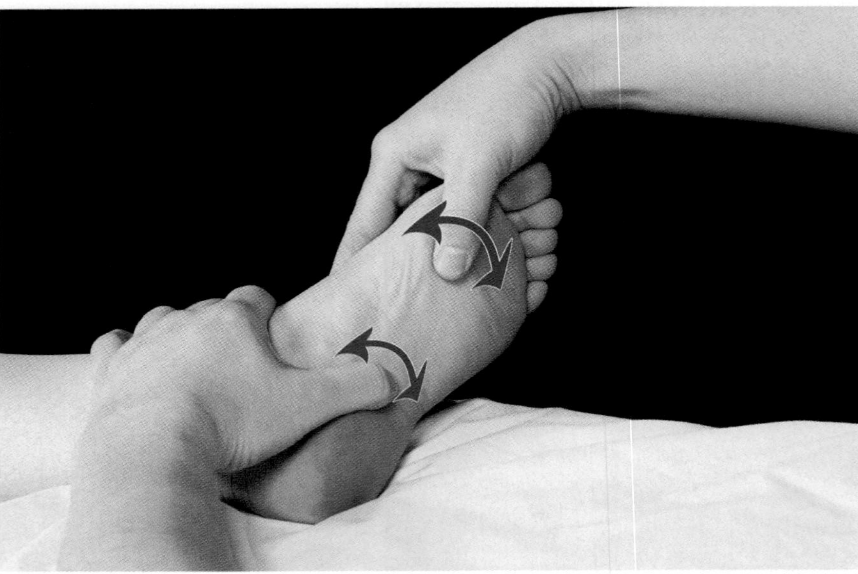

FIGURE 10-20E. Rotate and stretch the tarsals and metatarsals.

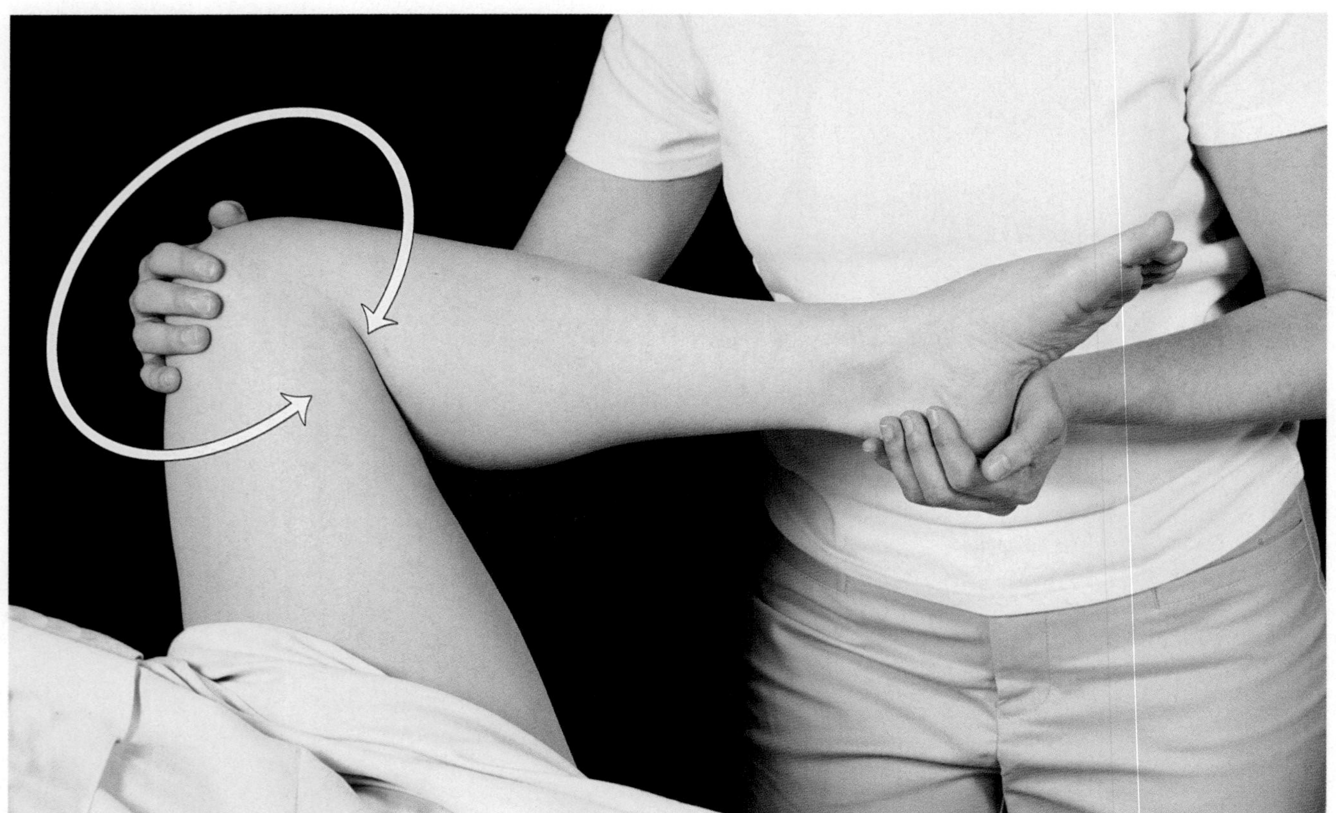

FIGURE 10-20F. Circumduction of the thigh.

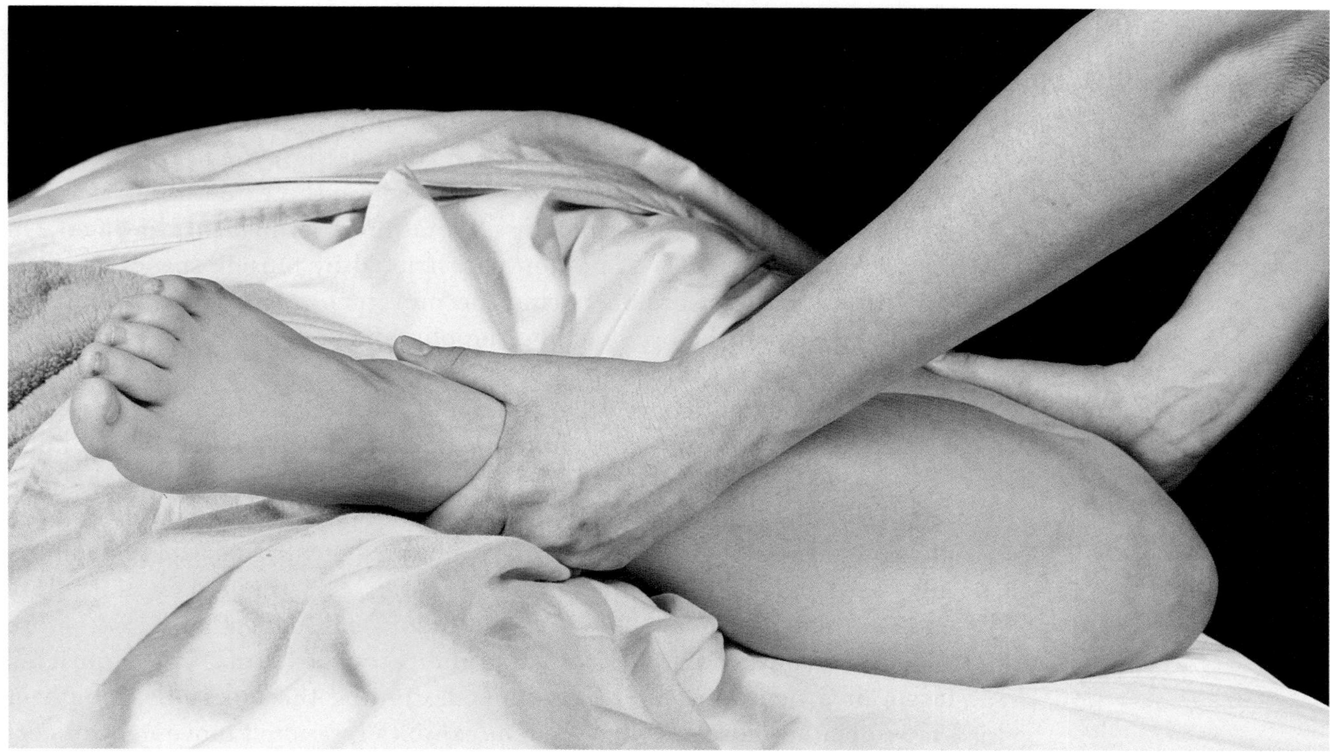

FIGURE 10-20G. Applying joint movements to the knee and hip.

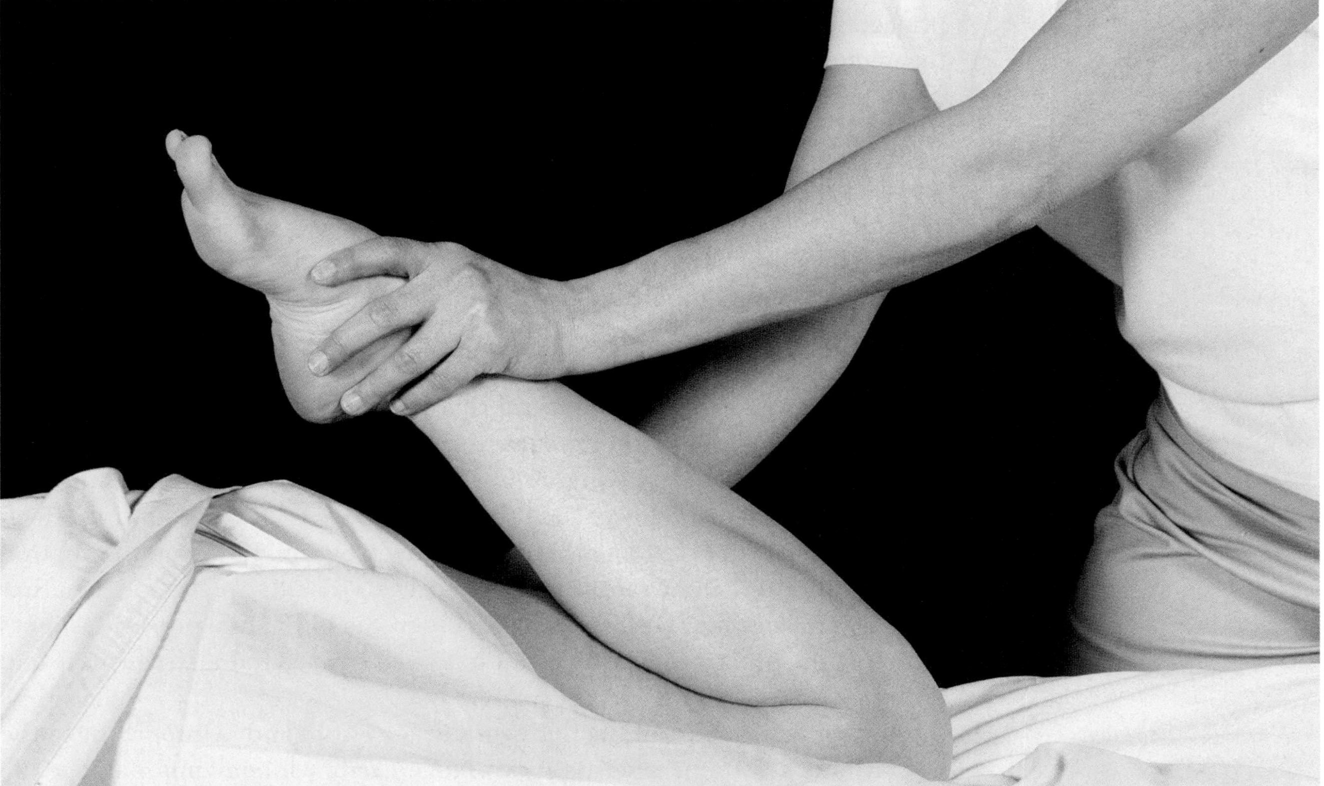

FIGURE 10-20H. Flexing the client's knee, pressing the heel against the gluteals.

end feel

is the change in the quality of the feeling as the end of a movement is achieved.

hard end feel

is a bone-against-bone feeling.

soft end feel

is a cushioned limitation in which soft tissue prevents further movement, such as knee flexion.

empty end feel

is an abrupt restriction to a joint movement caused by pain.

The change in the quality of movement from the first sense of resistance to the extent of the physiologic or anatomic barrier is called **end feel**.

End feel that results in bone-on-bone contact, such as the extension of the elbow, is termed **hard end feel**. Usually, however, the practitioner feels a gradual tightening and springiness in the last few inches of the range of motion owing to the soft tissue's approaching the extent of its possible stretch. This springy, rather painless limitation is termed **soft end feel**. On occasion, normal range of motion is restricted by muscle spasm or other conditions that cause pain during the movement. Abrupt restrictions to a joint movement before reaching the physiologic barrier (due to pain) is known as an **empty end feel**.

Joint movements have great therapeutic benefit as an assessment tool and as a treatment to enhance function and mobility. The practitioner must be aware of the end feel of the joints and the client's reactions when doing joint movements. Hard or soft end feel, without pain and encountered at the physiologic barrier indicates normal function of healthy tissue. Encountering a hard end feel before the normal physiologic barrier or a painful empty end feel indicates abnormal function. A soft end feel encountered before the normal physiologic barrier could indicate restrictions in the muscle's fascia or a neuromuscular guarding, shortening the functional length of an associated muscle. When a client exhibits restricted movement in certain joints, the practitioner can apply specific techniques or movement to increase joint mobility (Figures 10-20a-j).

Joint movements are used extensively in soft tissue modalities such as proprioceptive neuromuscular facilitation (PNF), PNF stretching, muscle energy technique (MET), and position release. These modalities are discussed in more detail in Chapter 13, Therapeutic Techniques.

RHYTHM AND PRESSURE IN MASSAGE

People have individual vibrations and an innate sense of rhythm. The practitioner must remember that some people are high-strung (tense), whereas others are very low-key (relaxed). The goal is to work with people according to their particular needs and not to follow a personal agenda, possibly working against the client's natural rhythm. Consider each individual situation when providing a therapeutic service. Usually someone coming for a massage is seeking a relaxing, rejuvenating experience. The rhythm must be steady and slightly slower than the client's pace to have a sedating effect. If the massage is part of an athletic training program, however, the rhythm can be more upbeat. Practitioners can develop skills to tune in to other people and work more effectively with clients as individual persons. Clients return to the practitioner who is not only well trained but also sensitive and aware.

Breathing is a part of the body's natural rhythm and is important to the practitioner's stamina and ability to move easily while giving massage. Be aware of the client's breathing. As the massage begins, encourage the client to take several full, relaxing breaths. During the massage pay attention to both the client's and your own breathing to be sure both patterns are full and relaxed.

The practitioner must develop an awareness of the right amount of pressure used for various therapeutic situations and techniques. Begin to massage in an area of the body cautiously, gently, and lightly, and then apply more pressure as you become aware of underlying structures and tissue condition This also helps you to note tension and stress buildup and determine how to proceed according to the client's body condition and sensitivity. The pressure varies with the technique used and according to the intended outcome. At no time should the pressure be so forceful as to cause tissue injury. The rule is to begin with a light and sensitive touch and increase the pressure as you work into an area. Encourage verbal feedback from the client about the amount of pressure, and be aware of the client's body language. As tension in the area begins to dissipate and the muscles relax, the client will let you in even deeper. When it is time to leave the area, back out gradually, smoothing the way as you go.

One of the primary indications of tension or dysfunction in the muscles and soft tissue is pain. Massage therapy is one of the best methods of locating and treating these conditions. Many massage techniques directly manipulate the painful areas and therefore can be uncomfortable or even painful. People have different tolerances for pain. You should not work to a point that produces so much pain that the client's pain threshold is crossed. Some deep tissue techniques advise that the most constructive therapy takes place at a depth and intensity that the client can barely tolerate. When the pain threshold is violated, however, the client tenses up and the work becomes less effective. Some bodywork does produce discomfort that is constructive; however, the pressure should never be so deep that it hurts the client. Pain that hurts only can damage the body, it can destroy the client's trust, ruining the therapeutic relationship. When working deeply or in a painful area, encourage verbal feedback from a client in regard to the pressure being used and the client's comfort level. The first rule of massage and bodywork is: **Do no harm**!

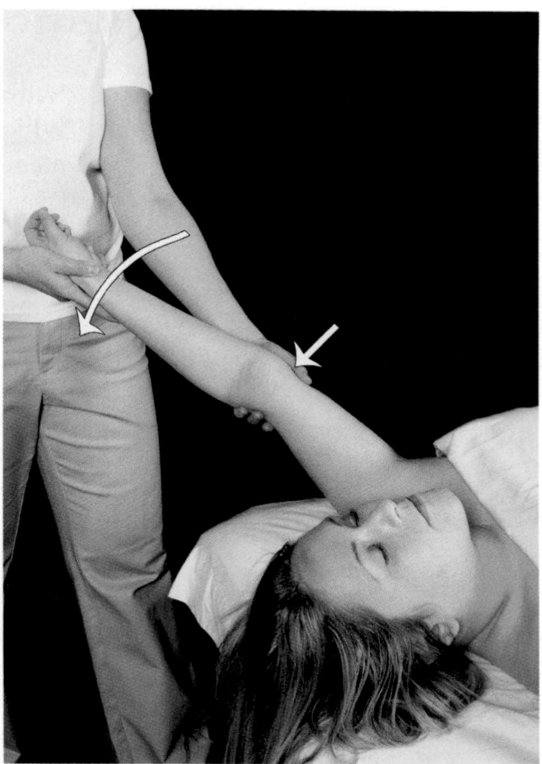

FIGURE 10-20I. Active assistive joint movement: The client tries to move an arm above the head as the therapist assists.

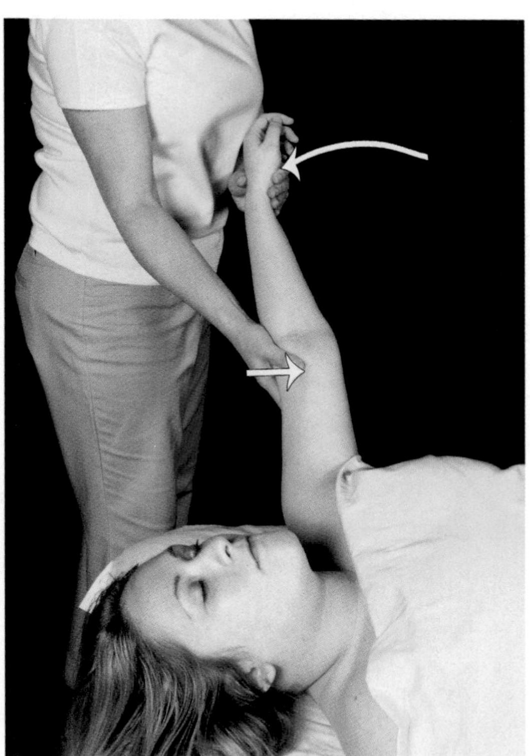

FIGURE 10-20J. Active resistive joint movement: The client attempts to raise an arm as the therapist resists the movement.

QUESTIONS FOR DISCUSSION AND REVIEW

1. Name six basic classifications of movements used in massage.
2. Which control should the practitioner have over the massage treatment?
3. Over which parts of the body are light movements applied?
4. Over which parts of the body are heavy movements applied?
5. In which direction is massage generally applied?
6. When are massage movements directed away from the heart?
7. What is the approximate duration of a full-body massage?
8. In terms of a massage technique, what is touch?
9. How is light touch administered, and what are its effects?
10. How is deep touch given, and when is it used?
11. How is aura stroking performed?
12. What is another name for feather stroking, and how is it used?
13. What is effleurage?
14. Which kind of effleurage requires the lightest possible touch?
15. Which kind of effleurage requires firm pressure?
16. What are the benefits of superficial gliding strokes?
17. What are the benefits of deep gliding strokes?
18. How is the kneading movement applied in massage?
19. What are the benefits of kneading?
20. What is the classical term that means the same as kneading?
21. For what part of the body is the fulling movement recommended?
22. What is the proper way to apply friction movements to the body?
23. What are the effects of friction on the connective tissue?
24. How is cross-fiber friction applied?
25. In what manner are compression movements applied to the body?
26. What are the benefits of compression movements?
27. What is the proper way to apply vibratory movements to the body?
28. What is a safe rate of vibration?
29. How can the practitioner control the effects produced by vibratory movements?
30. Why is excessive vibration harmful?
31. What is the proper way to apply percussion movements to the body?
32. Name the various forms of percussion movements.
33. What are the benefits of percussion movements?
34. To which parts of the body can joint movements be applied?
35. Name two types of joint movements.
36. Describe the difference between active assistive joint movements and active resistive joint movements.
37. What is range of motion?
38. Define end feel.
39. How is pressure regulated during a massage?
40. What is the significance of a pain threshold in the practice of massage?

CHAPTER

11

Application of Massage Technique

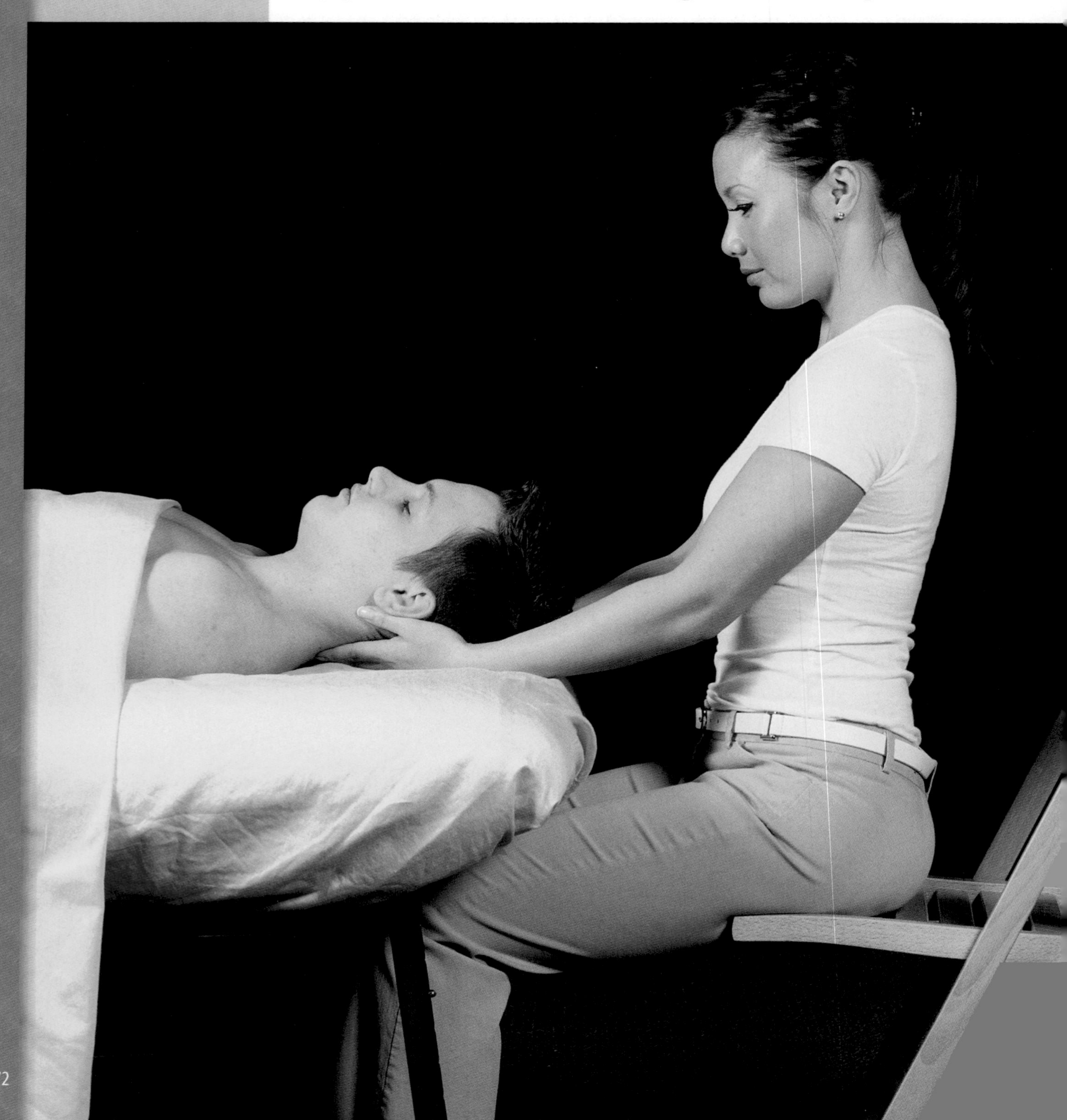

LEARNING OBJECTIVES

After you have mastered this chapter, you will be able to

1. **Demonstrate mastery of various hand exercises specifically for the benefit of massage practitioners.**
2. **Demonstrate correct standing posture and movements specifically for the benefit of massage practitioners.**
3. **Explain why it is necessary and desirable for the massage practitioner to develop coordination, balance, control, and stamina.**
4. **Explain why it is necessary and desirable for the massage practitioner to develop strong, flexible hands.**
5. **Describe the concepts of grounding and centering and how these practices benefit the massage practitioner.**

INTRODUCTION

Recently, the various movements used in body massage have been studied scientifically. Some movements are devised to induce relaxation, whereas others are meant to invigorate and stimulate the body. The massage practitioner is concerned primarily with manual movements that have beneficial effects on the client's body and how to apply these movements correctly and effectively. The correct application of the massage movements described in Chapter 10 requires more than the use of the practitioner's hands against the client's skin. When done correctly, these movements engage the therapist's whole body. The feet are the foundation, the legs are the strength, the pelvis and torso supply the power, the heart supplies the caring and compassion, and the arms and hands supply the intricate dexterity and communication with the client.

Massage is a physically demanding profession. The application of massage technique creates considerable stress on the practitioner's body. Improper posture, poor body alignment, and sloppy technique increase that stress and eventually result in injury, degenerative breakdown, and burnout. Learning good body mechanics while you are learning massage techniques not only reduces fatigue and the chance of injury but also improves the delivery and outcome of those techniques.

The practice of massage requires the therapist to expend a tremendous amount of energy, not only physically but mentally and emotionally as well. If mental and emotional energy are not sustained, replenished, or increased, burnout eventually results. It is important for the practitioner to be grounded, centered, and fully present during each massage session. For therapists to maintain the rigorous schedule necessary to make a living, or even to supplement an income, therapists must be able to conserve, direct, and sustain energy while performing multiple daily massages.

This chapter focuses on techniques and exercises that the practitioner can use to increase the strength and endurance specific to the practice of massage. Exercises to improve mobility and posture are demonstrated and practiced. Finally, body mechanics to increase power, conserve energy, and reduce the chance of injury are studied and incorporated.

BUILDING STRENGTH AND FLEXIBILITY OF THE HANDS

The practitioner's hands are the most important tools used in massage. Hand mobility is important to maintain a regular rhythm and control when performing slow or fast movements. Flexible hands aid in working on the contours of the client's body and in controlling both speed and pressure. In addition to well-trained hands, the practitioner must have a good sense of balance and body control to move efficiently while applying various massage movements. Although the hands are the main implements delivering the manipulations to the client, the positioning and the strength of the entire body are essential to deliver effective massages over an extended period. The exercises shown here help to develop strength, control, and flexibility of the hands (Figure 11-1a to h and Figure 11-2a to d).

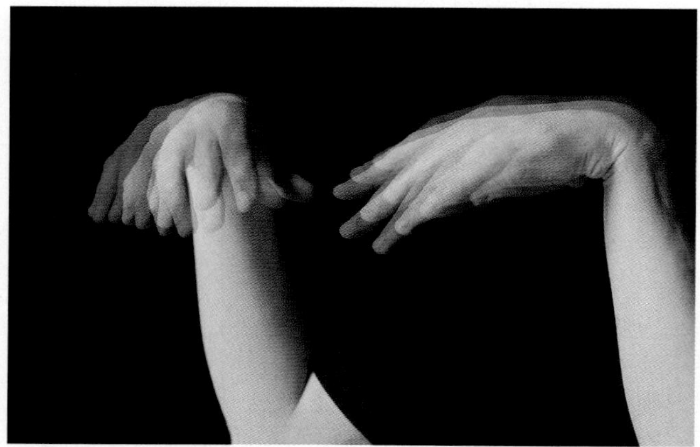

FIGURE 11-1A Hold your hands at chest level and shake them vigorously for about ten counts. This exercise warms and limbers the hands.

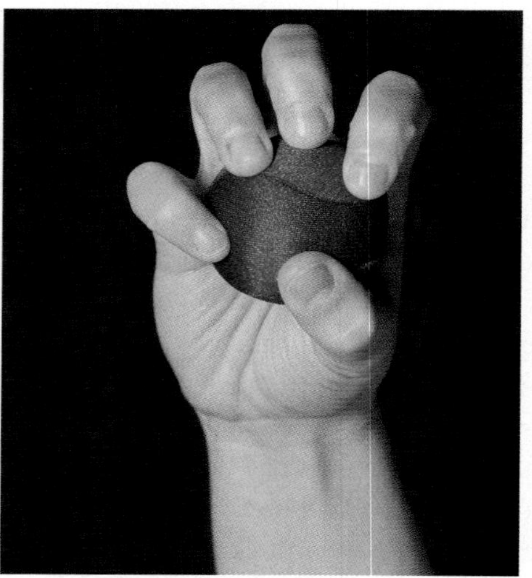

FIGURE 11-1B Hold your hands at chest level. Use a small ball, Thera-Putty, or simply clinch your hands into tight fists. Squeeze the ball or fists as hard as you can and then release ten times. Repeat this exercise several times. This exercise strengthens your hands and wrists.

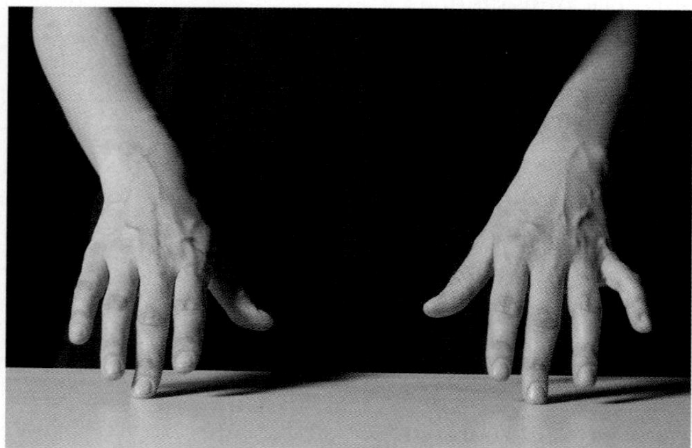

FIGURE 11-1C Place both hands palm down on a flat surface. Begin with the thumbs and count each finger to the little finger and back to the thumbs by raising the digit off the surface as far as possible. This exercise is similar to playing a piano or typing. It is excellent for improving coordination and hand control.

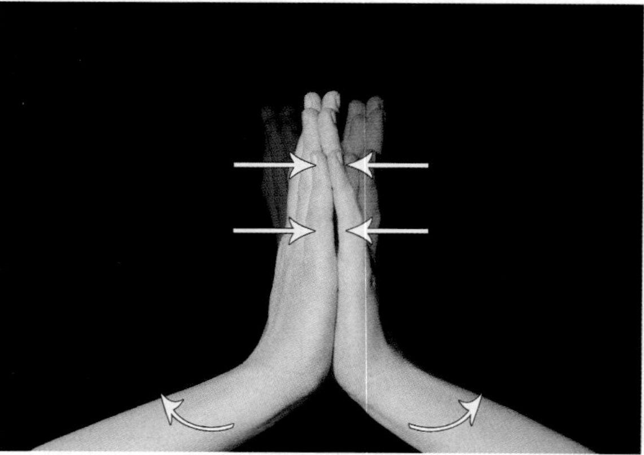

FIGURE 11-1D Place your palms together at chest level. Press one hand against the other back and forth. This makes your wrists supple and strong. Repeat the presses about ten times.

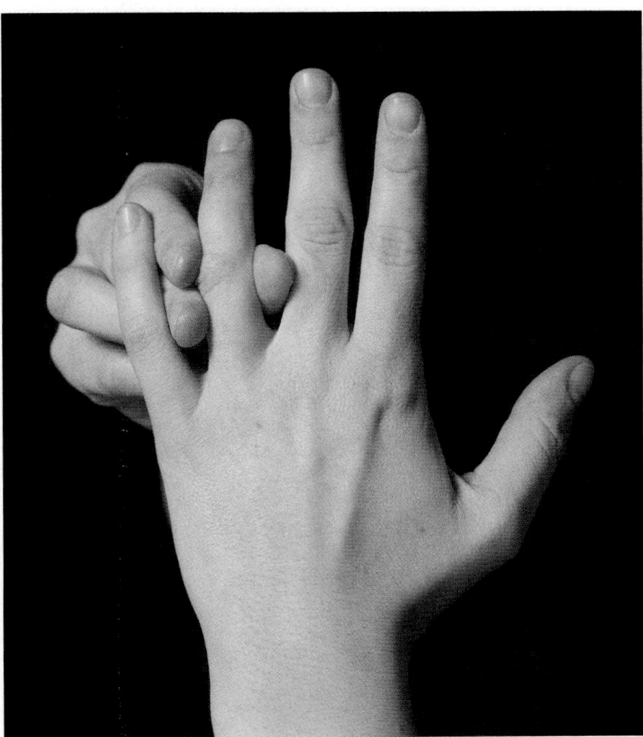

FIGURE 11-1E Beginning with the thumb of the left hand, massage all the fingers of that hand by rubbing each finger from the knuckles of the hand to the tip of the finger. Repeat on the right hand. This exercise stimulates circulation and helps to keep the hands supple.

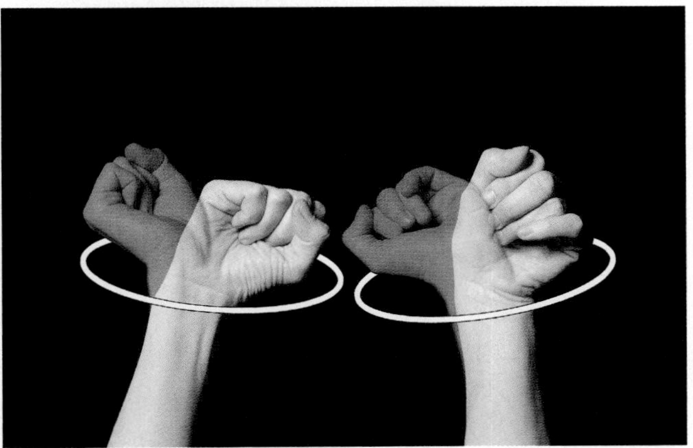

FIGURE 11-1F Hold your hands in fists at chest level. Rotate both hands in circles forward ten times, then reverse ten times. This exercise strengthens and limbers the wrists.

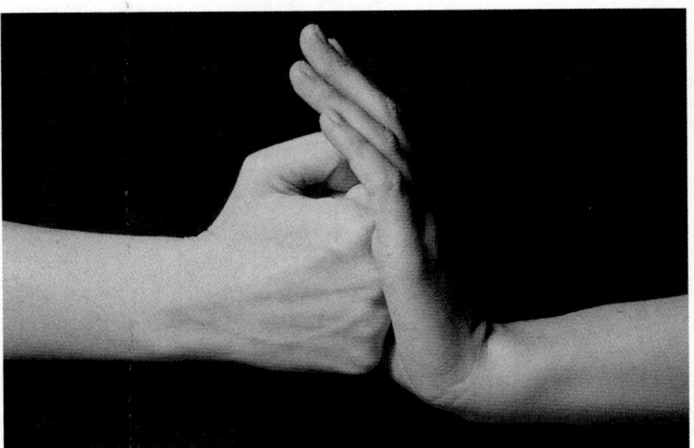

FIGURE 11-1G Press the fist of one hand into the palm of the other, with each hand resisting the other. Do this ten times on each hand. This exercise strengthens the entire arm and the hand.

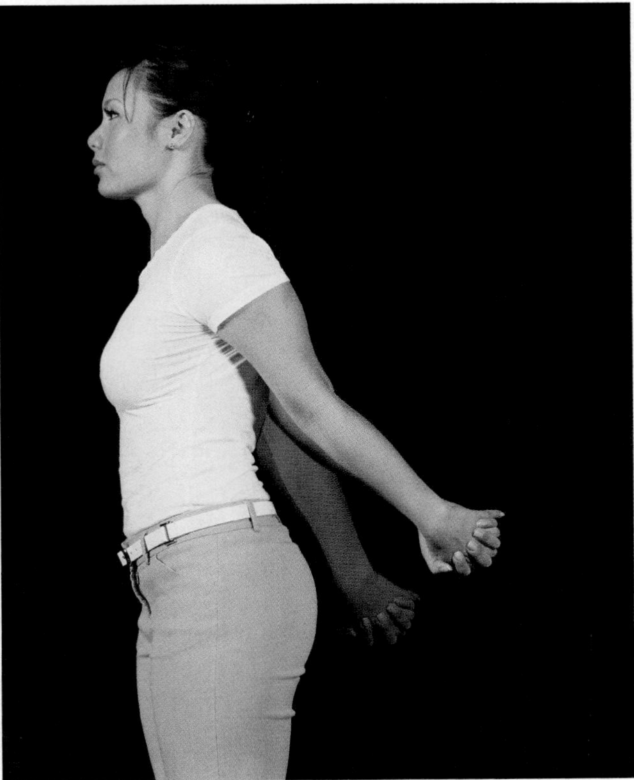

FIGURE 11-1H Clasp your hands just below your waistline at the back of your body. Pull your arms upward while holding the tension for ten counts; then pull your arms downward for ten counts. This exercise strengthens the muscles of your arms, shoulders, and hands.

BODY MECHANICS

The term *body mechanics* means the observation of body postures in relation to safe and efficient movement in daily living activities. Using good body mechanics increases the strength and power available in a movement while reducing the risk of potential injury. In the practice of massage, the hands are the

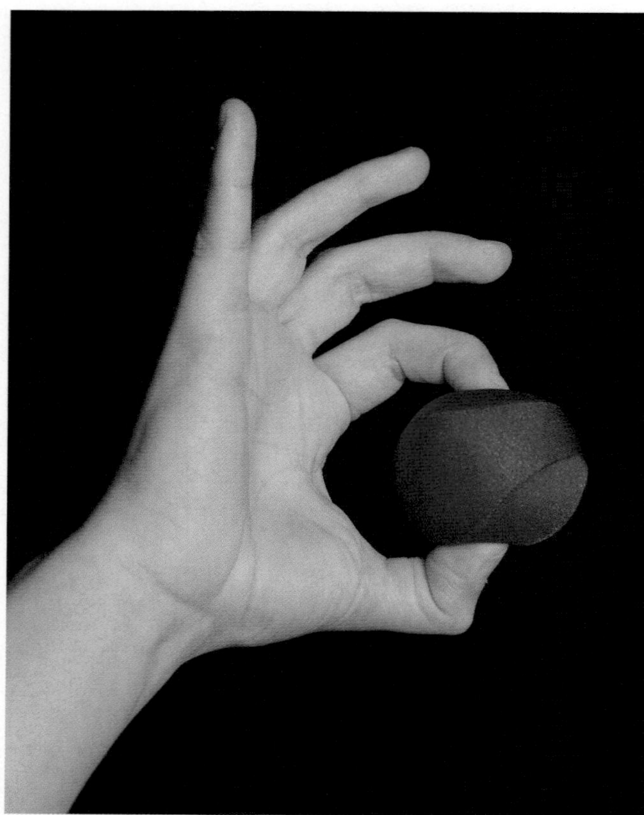

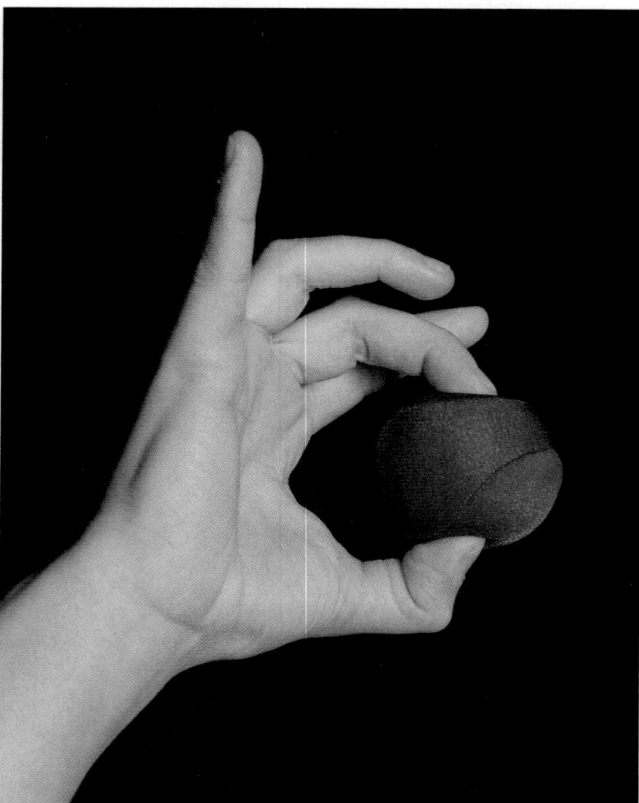

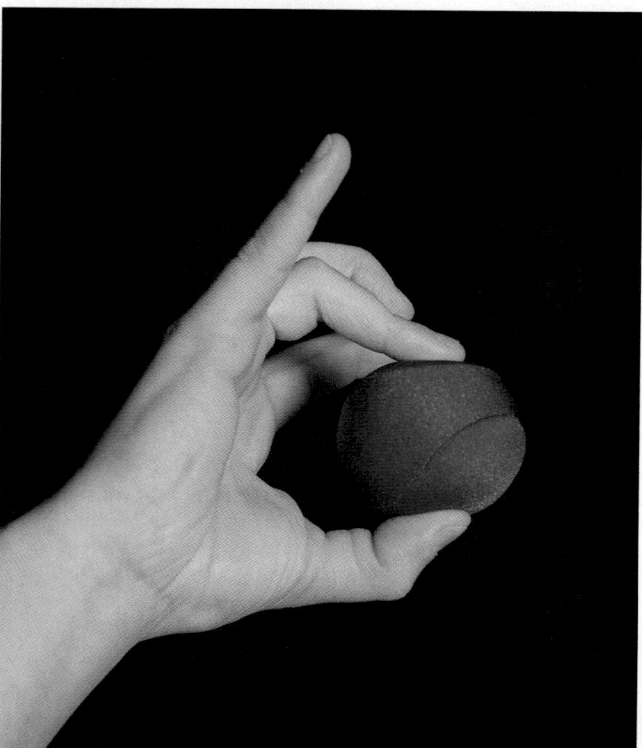

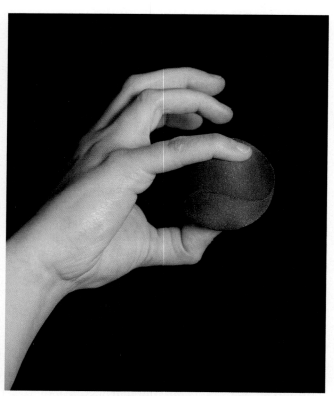

FIGURE 11-2A–11-2D. Hold a semisoft foam rubber ball between the thumb and first finger. Squeeze the ball as hard as possible, ten times. Repeat, squeezing the ball with the second, third, and fourth fingers. Shake and massage that hand and repeat the exercise with the other hand.

primary implements used to touch the client; however, the practitioner's entire body is used to deliver massage movements. Proper positioning of the feet; the strength of the legs; the position of the hips, back, shoulders, and head; and breathing all play important roles in the effective delivery of the massage, the level of fatigue, and the long-term health of the practitioner.

Even though the hands are the point of contact during a massage, if the practitioner depends solely on the hands and arms to do the massage, these parts will fatigue quickly. Tension in the hands and arms reflects into the shoulders and neck. Tension in the shoulders, arms, and hands or a consistent forward posture of the head often results in neck and shoulder pain. Overextending the arms to perform long strokes or reach a distant body part compromises control, force, and pressure. Overreaching usually requires bending or twisting at the waist, which places the back in a strained position.

After years of practice, many massage therapists frequently experience fatigue, pain, and dysfunction in the hands and wrists, neck and shoulders, or lower back. Much of this discomfort can be avoided through the use of good body mechanics and movement. Because the hands are the massage practitioner's most valuable tools, it is important to protect them. Be mindful of the alignment of the wrists, thumbs, and fingers. Maintain proper alignment in the wrists by staying behind the massage movements rather than on top of them. Avoid hyperextending the wrist and using the heel of the hand when applying compressive forces. Use the forearm and elbows when possible to apply deep pressure. When applying pressure with the fingers or thumb, use the cushioned palmar side of the thumb and fingers rather than the tips. Keeping the head up, shoulders down and relaxed, and the arms and hands relaxed as well reduces the strain on the neck. By keeping the hands relatively close to the center of the body and the knees slightly flexed and feet apart, the practitioner can use the muscles in the legs and the movement of the whole body to deliver the strokes. When performing a movement that requires deep pressure or more force, the practitioner keeps the hand and arm in alignment and in a stable position and leans the body into the movement. The practice of keeping the hands in good alignment and using body weight and leverage rather than muscle exertion of the upper body conserves energy and increases the power and strength when performing massage (Figure 11-3a and b).

The risk of injury is directly proportional to the amount of stress and the amount of biomechanical deviation. This is easy to observe in acute injuries such as a sprained ankle or a strained back. If a force is applied when the body is not in proper alignment, the result could be strain or pain in the wrist or fingers; a torn ligament, tendon, or muscle; or even a broken bone. Poor body mechanics practiced over a long time

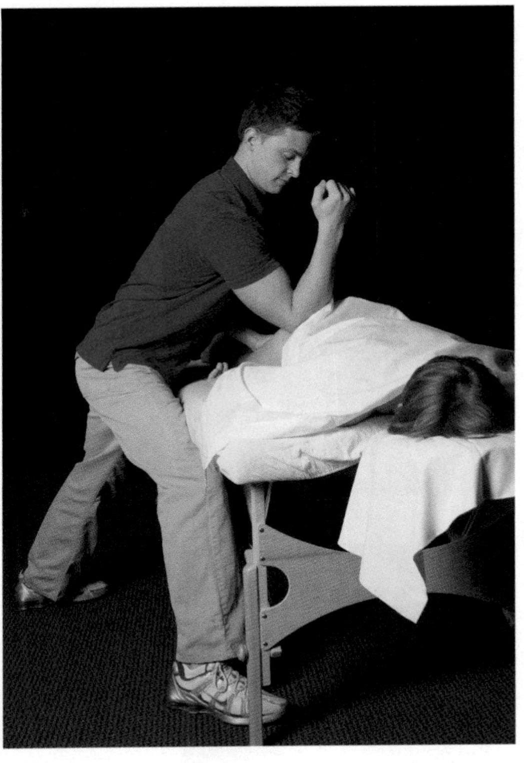

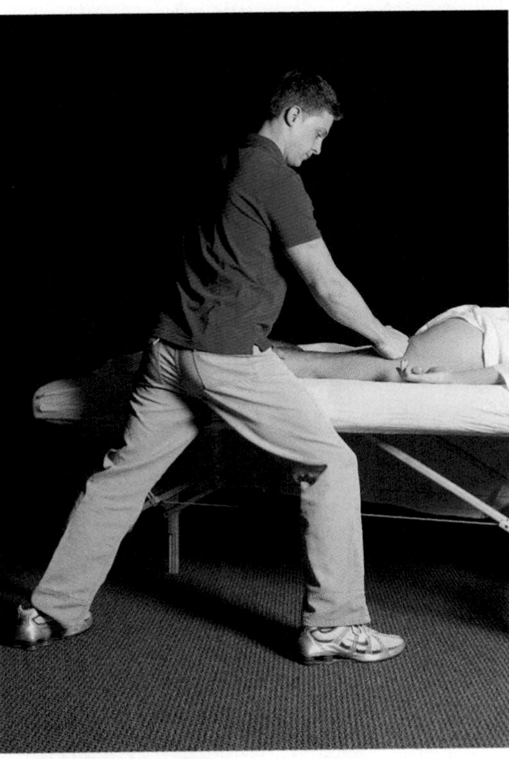

FIGURE 11-3A AND B. Use good body mechanics and lean into the movements to improve efficiency, power, and strength while reducing stress.

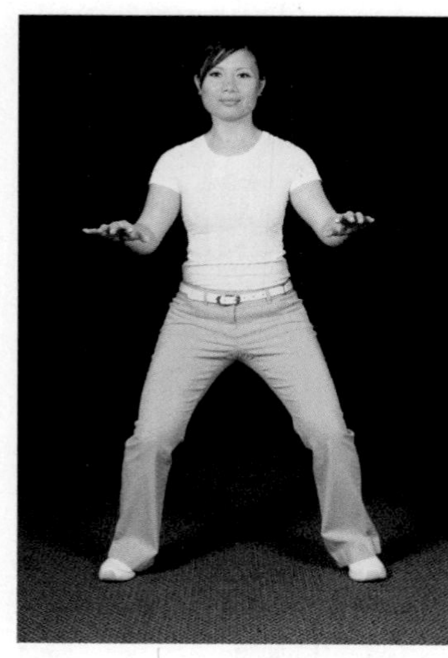

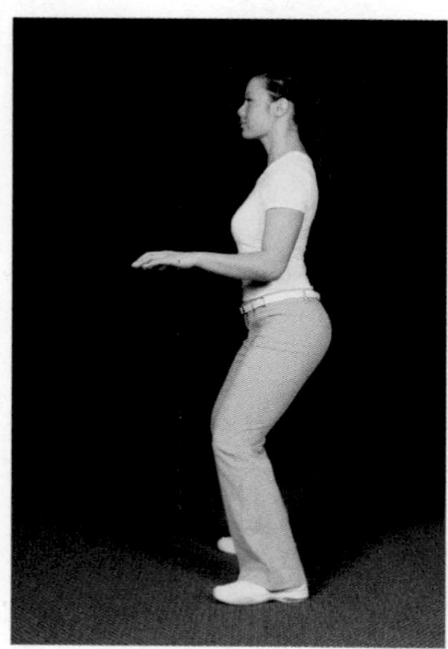

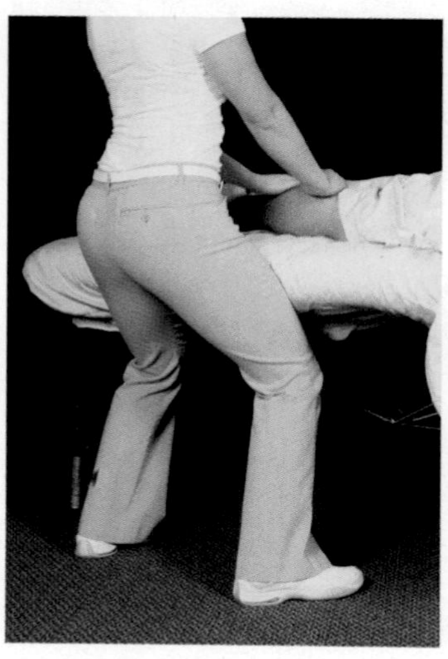

FIGURE 11-4A–C. Horse stance.

become bad postural habits that cause structural (biomechanical) deviations. When the stress of muscular activity or even gravity is added to the biomechanically weak structure, dysfunction, pain, and injury eventually result. This is precisely why many of your clients are seeking relief. The practitioner should avoid positions and practices that put undue stress on the back, neck, shoulders, arms, and hands.

As a massage therapist, you must develop good body mechanics. Using proper body positioning and posture will enable you to deliver powerful strokes and movements with minimal effort. Proper foot position and alignment of the back, shoulders, arms, wrists, and hands, especially when delivering forceful movements, reduces the chance of repetitive stress injuries.

Incorporating proper body mechanics and movement enhances the quality, effectiveness, and efficiency of all massage strokes. Engaging the body when applying stroking, kneading, and friction produces deeper, smoother, and more penetrating results with less effort and fatigue.

POSTURE AND STANCES

Correct posture and stances (foot positions) are important to the practitioner because they aid in balance and allow the delivery of firmer, more powerful, and more direct massage strokes. Proper stances allow the practitioner to lean into and out of the movements to deliver massage strokes that penetrate with minimal effort and maximum effect. Correct posture is essential to conserve strength and prevent repetitive stress injuries caused by improper body mechanics that put too much stress on the practitioner's hands, arms, and shoulders during the massage procedure. Good posture and body mechanics help to sustain energy when it is necessary to perform multiple massages, because they enable the practitioner to move around the table more freely and easily while maintaining the flow of movement and energy.

The most common stances are called **the horse** and **the archer**.

Horse Stance

In the horse stance, both feet are placed in line with the edge of the massage table. This is the most comfortable stance when doing petrissage on the legs or back. The knees are kept slightly flexed so that the therapist can apply firmer pressure to the massage movements by shifting the weight from side to side and leaning into the client, thereby preserving the strength in the arms. The back remains erect and relaxed, with the shoulders comfortably dropped and back. The breathing is deep and full (Figure 11-4a to c).

Archer Stance

The archer stance is the most commonly used position, especially when the practitioner's shoulders are at an angle (rather than parallel) with the edge of the table or when the practitioner is stepping into a movement. For the archer stance, position the feet so that an imaginary line drawn through the center of the back foot at the arch passes through the front foot at mid-heel and the third toe (Figure 11-5). The feet may be close together or a full stride apart. This foot position provides a solid, stable foundation for the therapist to lean into or pull back on a massage movement. By shifting weight from one foot to the other, the therapist can perform long rhythmic strokes without sacrificing good posture. This foot position also provides excellent mobility, so that the therapist can step into or away from a movement smoothly and at the same time maintain contact and pressure. This eliminates the need to bend at the waist. The mobility allows the therapist's hands to remain close to the body, where they retain more control and strength. Mobility uses the muscles of the legs to provide much of the movement and strength for many of the massage strokes. This, with the practice of leaning and stepping into or away from the movement, provides a large portion of the power and energy needed to deliver massage treatments.

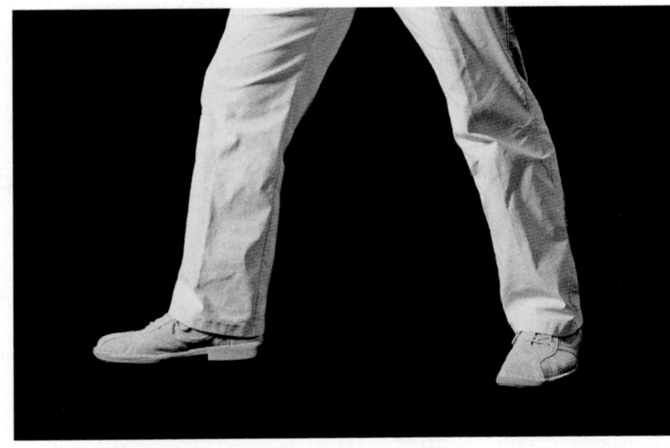

FIGURE 11-5. In the archer stance, the forward foot is pointing in the direction of the movement.

In either stance, the knees and ankles should be kept slightly flexed. Stiff, rigid knees contribute to fatigue, and locking the knees forces a posture that puts the back in danger of injury. The back remains relatively erect and stable.

The tendency when performing massage is often to tighten and raise the shoulders. The shoulders should remain relaxed and dropped to ensure optimal nerve and blood supply to the hands and arms. The breathing should also be deep and full to supply plenty of oxygen and eliminate carbon dioxide.

Correct stances make it easier to shift weight from foot to foot so that movement is smooth, as in dancing. Correct stances give the practitioner more body power when leaning into the movements.

TABLE MECHANICS

Most massages are performed with a client lying on a massage table; however, regardless of whether the massage is done on a mat on the floor, in a chair, in a hospital bed, or in another setting, the practitioner should be aware of any areas of tension or discomfort. The practitioner should practice good body mechanics regardless of the setting. When you are using a massage table, the first consideration is the table height, or more precisely, the height of the client lying on the table. The difference in height of the table with a large client having a wide girth compared with a small, slim client might be several inches and must be considered when preparing for a massage. If the table is too high, the practitioner might have difficulty applying pressure or techniques, causing undue stress and strain in the shoulders. If the table is too low, the practitioner might bend over awkwardly, causing lower back strain and discomfort. Even when a practitioner is the only person using a particular table, the practitioner should be aware of how the body feels and adjust the height of the table to best suit the given situation.

The asymmetric archer's stance is employed for most of the treatment. This stance allows the practitioner to remain mobile and keep the hands close to the

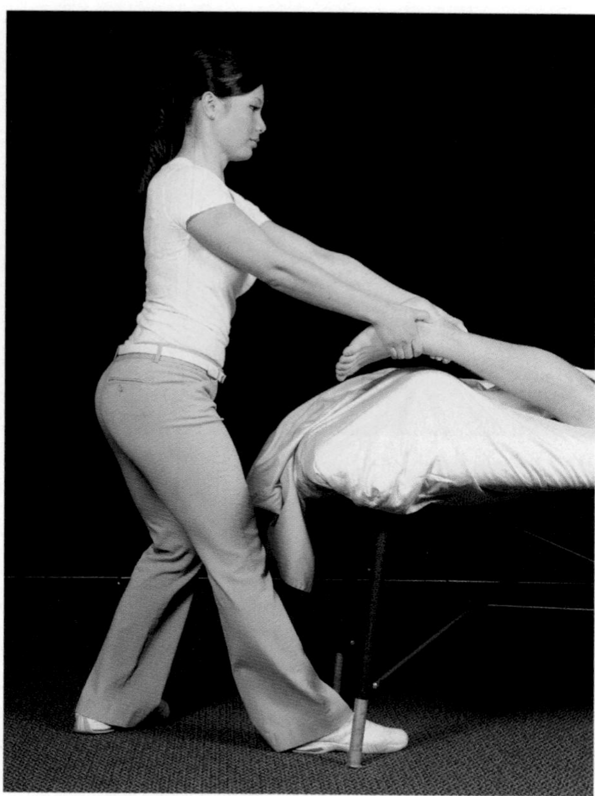

FIGURE 11-6. To apply traction, lean away from the client, using the archer's stance with the weight on the front foot.

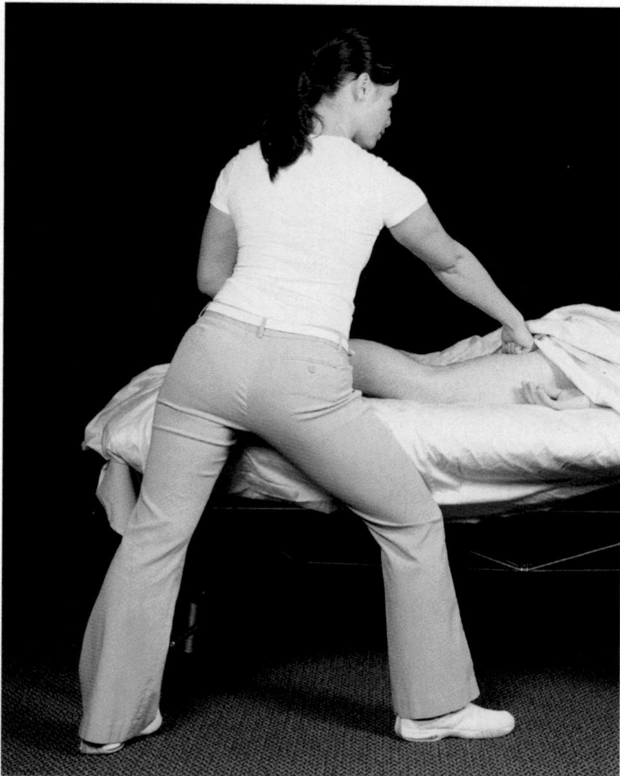

FIGURE 11-7. Proper body mechanics when leaning into a client to apply pressure.

body, being careful not to overreach, especially when applying pressure. When practicing massage, keep your work directly in front of you and avoid twisting or bending. Face where you are working, and keep your shoulders, hips, and feet directed toward where your hands are working. By using the archer's stance, the practitioner can easily use body weight to apply leverage with massage techniques that use traction or deeper pressure. When applying techniques requiring traction, the practitioner grasps the client and leans back, with most of the weight on the front foot. Shoulders remain relaxed, and the back foot is used only for balance (Figure 11-6).

When a massage calls for more or deeper pressure, rather than using muscle strength from the hands or arms, you can apply leverage by leaning into the technique. Again, using the archer's stance, the practitioner's weight is transferred to the back foot. The heel of that foot, the knee, hip, shoulders, and head are all aligned. Use the hand or arm that is contralateral to the back foot to contact the client and apply pressure. The front foot is used for balance (Figure 11-7). For more pressure, raise the front foot, applying more weight to the back foot and to the client. If the hand is the point of contact on the client, avoid hyperextending the wrist or using the heel of the hand to apply pressure. The wrist should remain relaxed, with the angle at the wrist between the hand and the forearm always at more than 110° to protect the nerves and other structures that pass through the carpal tunnel. The practitioner can choose to use the forearm or elbow to apply deep pressure. As a general rule, it is better to stay behind your work rather than on top of it. Maintain an angle of approximately 90° at the shoulder, between the body and the arm. By using proper body alignment and leverage, you can apply controlled pressure with minimal effort.

Be sure to have adequate space around the massage table to allow easy movement and access to every part of the client's body. A general guideline is to have a minimum of three feet of clear space on all sides of the table. This provides enough room to lean, get behind manipulations, and not be too close to perform the massage comfortably.

Practicing massage while standing and moving around a client on a massage table consumes considerable energy, even when practicing good body mechanics. There are portions of a massage, such as working on the head, shoulders, and feet, that the practitioner can easily perform while seated (Figure 11-8). By using a stool at the proper height, the practitioner can maintain good body mechanics and posture while conserving energy.

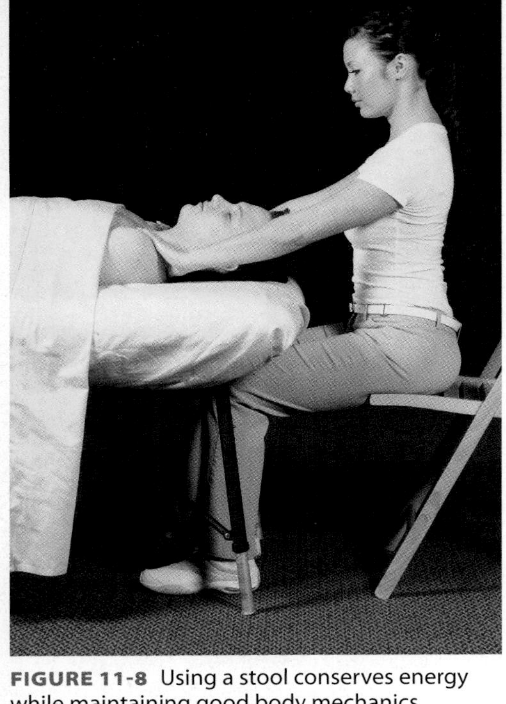

FIGURE 11-8 Using a stool conserves energy while maintaining good body mechanics.

EXERCISES FOR STRENGTH, BALANCE, AND BODY CONTROL

Two techniques called **centering** and **grounding** are important to the practitioner because they provide a psychologic, energetic, and physical base from which to work.

Centering: Centering is based on the concept that you have a geographical center in your body located about two inches below the navel in the pelvic area. The Chinese refer to this as the *tan tein* (don te-in) or the *hara.* Many of the ancient writings about martial arts mention this concept. Having a sense of that center and moving from that center provide a quality of power, balance, and control.

Centering has both a physical and psychoemotional context. Emotionally, being centered refers to a certain confident sense of balance and self-assurance. Being centered means that you feel self-assured and emotionally stable. Being uncentered means you feel insecure and unstable. Feeling centered (in control) is valuable because it is important to be able to handle problems that arise without becoming frustrated or emotionally overwhelmed. Centering is accomplished by focusing awareness on your geographical center (*tan tein*), breathing fully, and being self-assured (Figure 11-9).

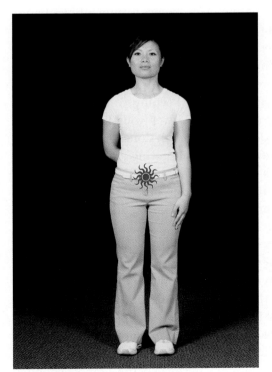

FIGURE 11-9 The *tan tein* is the geographical and energetic center of the body.

Grounding: Grounding is based on the concept that you have a connection with the earth and with the client and that you function as something of a grounding apparatus, helping the client to release unwanted tension and feelings of stress. Grounding is achieved by mentally visualizing yourself as having the ability to draw from a greater power or energy. By being grounded, you become a sort of conduit or conductor that allows the energies to pass through you. The negative energies can pass out of the client, and the positive energies can be directed into the client through you. Grounding allows

centering
is based on the concept that you have a geographical center in your body about two inches below the navel.

grounding
is based on the concept that you have a connection with the earth and with the client and that you function as a grounding apparatus in helping the client to release tension.

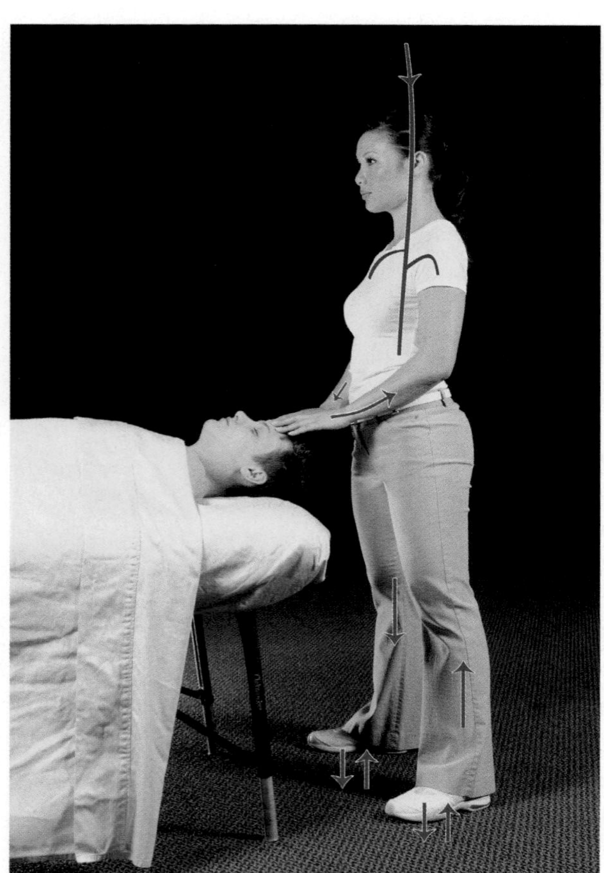

FIGURE 11-10 The practitioner's body serves as a conduit for positive energy to be transmitted into the client and negative energy to be grounded out of the client.

these energy transfers to take place without you, the practitioner, being drained of your own energy or picking up any unwanted tension or stress from the client. Try thinking of yourself as a tree rooted to the ground. Controlled deep breathing is also helpful. The concepts of grounding and centering will become clearer as you master the following exercises (Figure 11-10).

Exercise 1—Grinding Corn

This exercise helps you to reach the full length of the part of the client's body that is being worked on by being able to shift your weight easily from one foot to the other while maintaining good posture and balance. The exercise is called *grinding corn* because the movement is similar to using an old-fashioned hand-operated corn grinder. You can also think of it as a movement similar to polishing a car. Use your imagination to pick the image that works for you.

Procedure: Place your feet apart (about the width of your shoulders) and tilt your pelvis forward and upward. Bend your knees, and sink down until you are in a semi-knee bend, but do not go all the way down to a squatting position. Keep your back straight, and do not allow your head to jut forward. While maintaining this posture, hold your hands in front of your body (palms down) about the level of your waistline. Now begin to move both hands toward the right, forming a wide oval. This position will look as if you are ready for a karate move.

After you get the feel of the standing position and hand movements, begin to move your right hand clockwise and your left hand counterclockwise. Shift your weight from foot to foot. Keep making the ovals (keeping your back straight) until you are comfortable with the movement. Lower your hands about six inches by bending your knees into a deeper knee bend. Continue practicing. As you continue the exercise, become aware of the centering concept previously described and allow your movements to be initiated from the pelvic area (about two inches below the navel), with the rest of your body following through. Remember, your geographical area or center allows your entire body to move with balance and strength (Figure 11-11a to c).

This exercise can be performed while standing next to a massage table. As you practice the movement, glide your hands lightly over the surface of the table. Gradually increase the area that your hands cover until you are able to reach from one end of the table to the other and from one side to the other. To do this, shift your weight from one foot to the other. Be conscious of your balance, and do not compromise your back by extending or leaning too far.

As you master these techniques and continue to practice them, your arms, hands, and shoulders will become less fatigued because of the support supplied by the rest of your body.

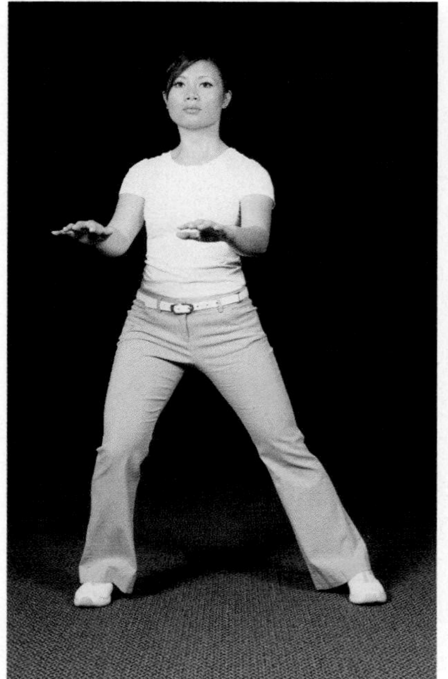

FIGURE 11-11A Grinding corn: Move to the right, making large ovals with your hands and transferring your weight to the right foot.

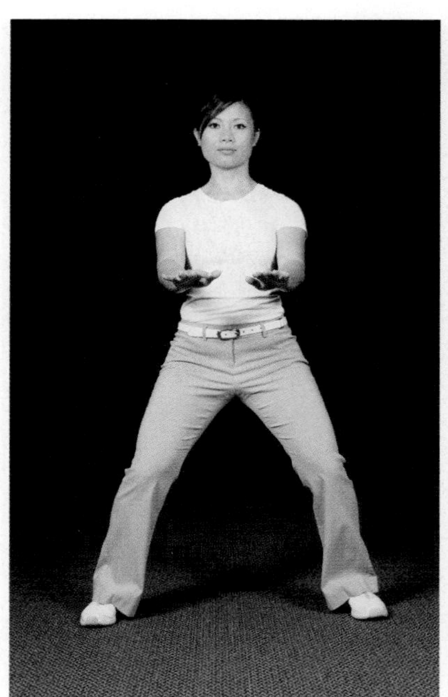

FIGURE 11-11B Grinding corn: Shift weight to the center and then to the left foot, continuing making large ovals with the hands.

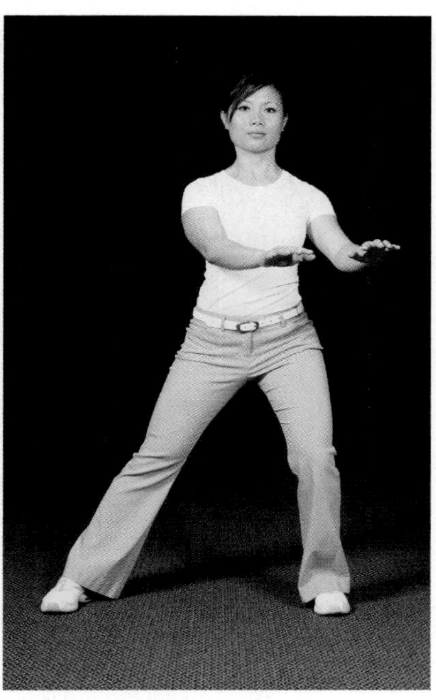

FIGURE 11-11C Grinding corn builds strength in the legs while teaching balance and coordination.

Exercise 2—The Wheel

Procedure: First, take a deep breath and exhale slowly. Repeat this several times; this exercise helps you to relax. Take a comfortable stance with your feet about six inches apart. Turn the left foot out at a 45° angle. Shift most of your weight to the left foot while bending your left knee slightly. With your left heel remaining on the floor, step forward with your right foot. Remember to keep your hips and shoulders facing forward and your knees bent. Your right foot should be forward about 15 to 20 inches. Shift your weight forward to the right foot and then back again to the left smoothly, so that 90 percent of your weight shifts from one foot to the other. Once you have the feel of the stance, take a deep breath and exhale slowly while placing your hands about six inches apart with palms facing one another. Begin making circles with your hands while imagining that you are rotating a large wheel that is suspended in front of you. The top of the wheel is about shoulder level, and the bottom is at the level of your pubic bone. As you shift your weight forward, reach out and rotate the wheel up. Shift your weight back as you rotate the wheel back and down. Continue the movement and breathe deeply and slowly so that with each full revolution of the wheel, you take one full breath (inhale and exhale). Without breaking your rhythm, turn your right foot to a 45° angle and take one step forward. Repeat the exercise several times (Figure 11-12a to c).

To complete the exercise, bring your feet together so that your weight is distributed evenly. Turn your palms facing downward and allow your hands to float down to your sides. Stay in this position for a few seconds to experience the feeling. As you master this movement, you will find that it is best accomplished

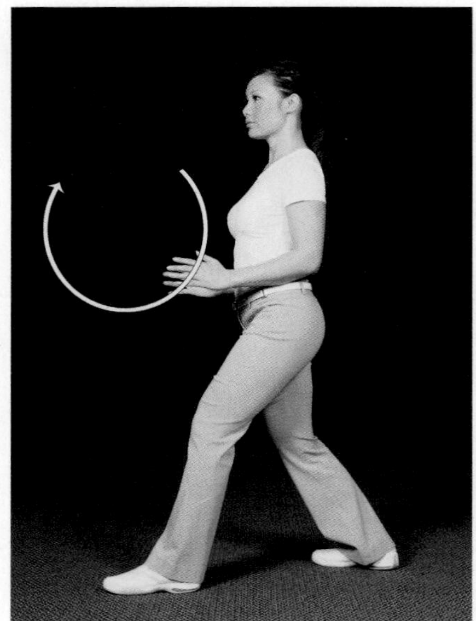

FIGURE 11-12A The wheel is a good centering exercise that teaches deep breathing, balance, and moving from the center (*tan tein*).

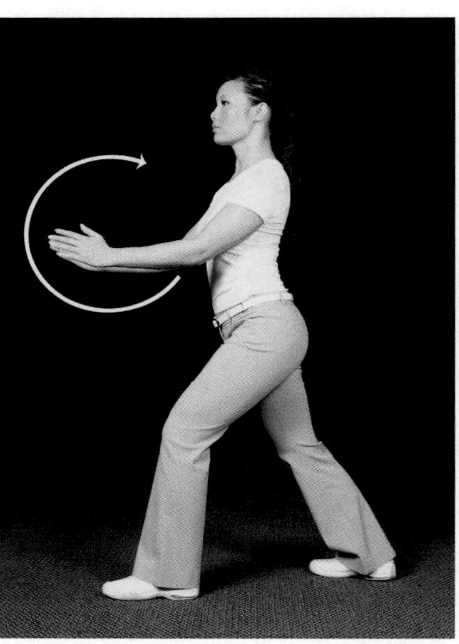

FIGURE 11-12B The wheel: The body weight shifts forward and back from one foot to the other.

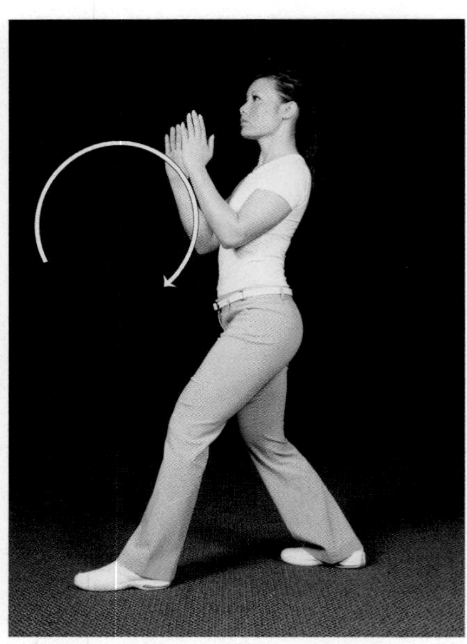

FIGURE 11-12C The wheel: The hands describe a large wheel. Each revolution of the wheel requires one full breath.

by concentrating on originating the movement from the pelvic area (the center or *tan tein*) and moving forward and backward in a straight line while allowing the rest of your body to follow.

Exercise 3—Advance and Retreat

A variation of the wheel is a move that you will find valuable in the practice of massage. As the name implies, *advance and retreat* involves a powerful forward movement followed by a controlled withdrawal.

Procedure: The position of the feet is essentially the same as for the wheel or the archer stance. The back foot is turned approximately 45° while the front foot is pointing in the direction of the movement. The distance that the feet are apart determines the length and the power of the movement. Optimally, the feet should be between 16 and 32 inches apart. The knees remain flexed while 80 percent of the body weight moves from one foot to the other. The hands are positioned at about belt level and close to the side of the body. The primary movement is in the hips and pelvis as they move straight forward and back. The hips do not move up or down but straight forward and back. The torso remains perpendicular, and the hands accentuate the move only slightly. Change the position of the feet, and the hands move to the other side of the body (Figure 11-13a and b).

Advance and retreat can be performed at the side of a massage table to illustrate the usefulness of the maneuver. Stand at the side of a massage table near one end, facing the other end. Turn the foot nearest the table out 45°. Step forward with the outside foot, and bend both knees slightly. Rest both hands on the table beside and slightly in front of you. (Your hands should be close to your body and about the level of the *tan tein.*) Shift your weight from one foot to the

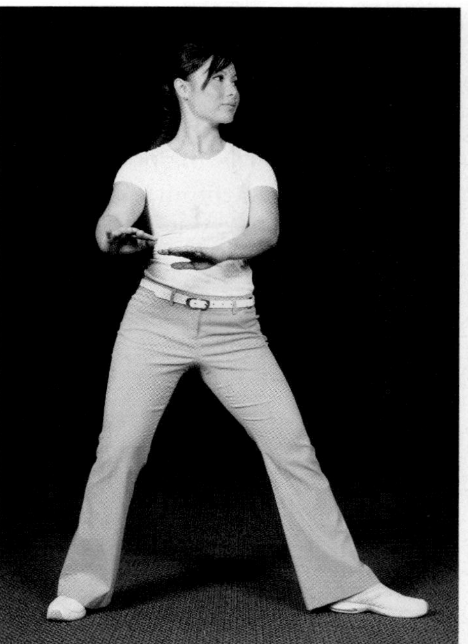

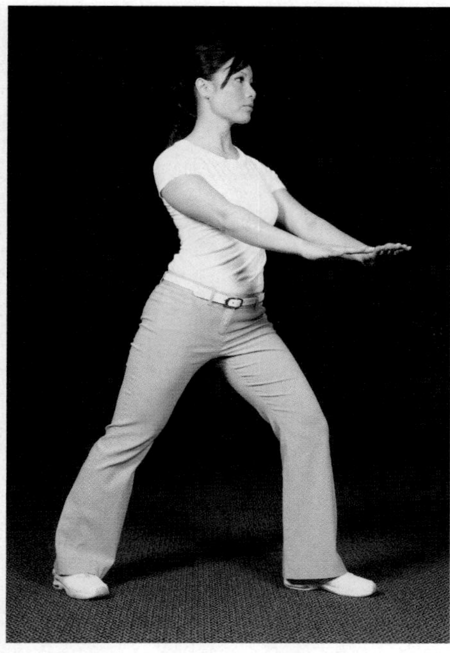

FIGURE 11-13A AND B Advance and retreat: The hands are held at the same height as the *tan tein*. The feet are in a wide archer stance. (a) Retreat: Ninety percent of the weight is on the back foot. Hands are down to one side, and upper body posture is erect. The body weight is shifted smoothly and powerfully forward. (b) Advance: Eighty percent of weight is shifted to the front leg. The arms are extended forward, and the upper body maintains an erect posture.

other. Notice how much of the length of the table you can cover while moving your arms very little (Figure 11-14a and b).

Exercise 4—The Tree

This exercise emphasizes the importance of posture and concentration and can be combined with centering, grounding, and correct breathing.

Procedure: Stand with your feet together, with your shoulders relaxed down and back. Pull your buttocks downward slightly; this will cause your pelvis to tilt upward. Take a deep breath and exhale slowly. Begin the exercise by turning your left foot out (bending the left knee) and shifting all your weight to your

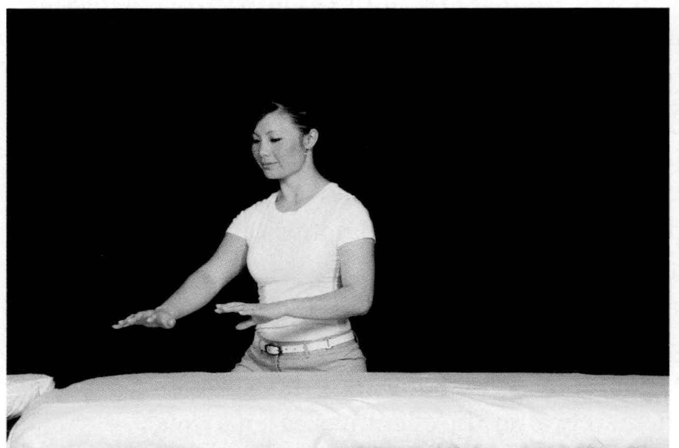

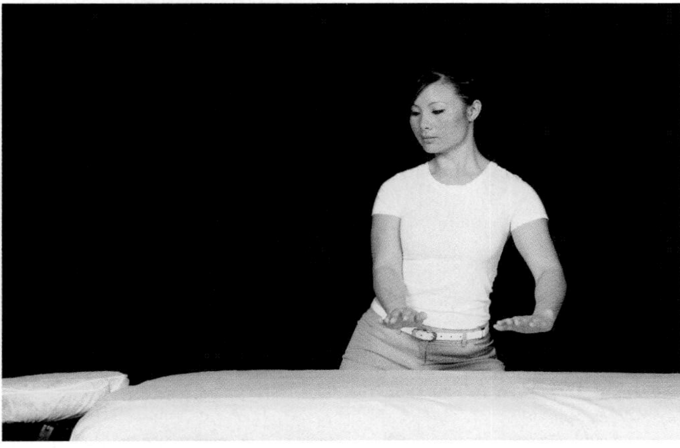

FIGURE 11-14. Using advance and retreat at the massage table allows the practitioner to move the length of the table in one stroke while maintaining good body mechanics.

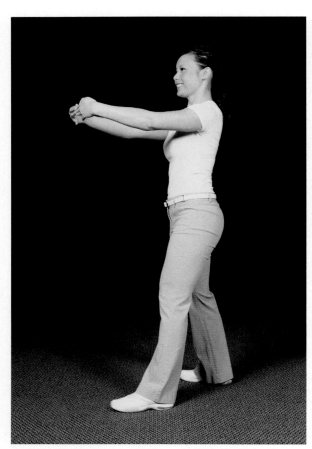

FIGURE 11-15. The tree exercise builds strength and endurance in your legs and shoulders while it encourages concentration and breathing.

left foot. Keep your upper body erect. Move your right foot straight forward so that when your right leg is extended, the ball of your right foot rests lightly on the floor. Bring both arms up to approximately shoulder level to form a circle. This position should look as if you are trying to reach around a large tree. Your fingers will be pointing toward each other, about two inches apart. Keep your head up, chin level, and gaze ahead. As you hold this pose, the leg bearing your weight might begin to feel weak and start to tremble. By maintaining the pose for about three minutes at a time and practicing your breathing exercises, however, you will soon experience a sense of renewed strength and power.

Change the pose to the left foot position (i.e., with the left foot forward) with your weight on your right foot, and continue to breathe deeply, exhaling slowly. Alternate the right and left feet, continuing to practice until you feel completely in control. To finish the exercise, bring your feet to a side-by-side position with your weight distributed evenly and your back straight. Allow your arms to float down to your sides. Take a moment to experience what is happening to your body (Figure 11-15).

Although you may find these exercises tiring and sometimes boring, remember that there is no easy way to accomplish erect posture, body strength, coordination, and proper breathing. Keep foremost in your mind that your goal is to be able to perform efficiently as a master of massage techniques. As you begin to do professional massage, you will see how these exercises increase your feeling of self-esteem.

PROFESSIONAL RULES TO REMEMBER

Knowledge of the restrictions and limitations of massage is as important as knowledge of its proper use. A well-trained practitioner knows when a massage treatment is indicated, how it can be modified for the greatest benefit to the client, and under which circumstances it should not be applied.

Before beginning the massage routines discussed in the next chapter, review the basic rules for safe and effective massage procedures.

1. Everything used in massage treatments should be clean and sanitary.
2. Wash your hands thoroughly with soap and hot water, and rinse and dry them before and after each treatment.
3. Keep your nails short and smooth to avoid scratching the client's skin.
4. Avoid chilling the client by touching with cold hands or by having the temperature of the room too low for comfort.
5. Avoid massage immediately after the client has eaten a meal.
6. Avoid heavy, rapid, or jarring movements that might convey fear of injury to the client.

7. Never use any form of heavy stroking against the venous blood supply.
8. Never apply massage so vigorously that it causes fatigue in the client.
9. Allow the client to have a short rest period before and after the massage.

QUESTIONS FOR DISCUSSION AND REVIEW

1. Why is it necessary for the massage practitioner to develop strong, flexible hands?
2. Define body mechanics.
3. Why is it important for the massage practitioner to practice good body mechanics?
4. How can the practitioner increase the power and strength in a movement and at the same time conserve energy?
5. Why are good posture and the use of proper stances important to the massage practitioner?

CHAPTER

12 Procedures for Complete Body Massages

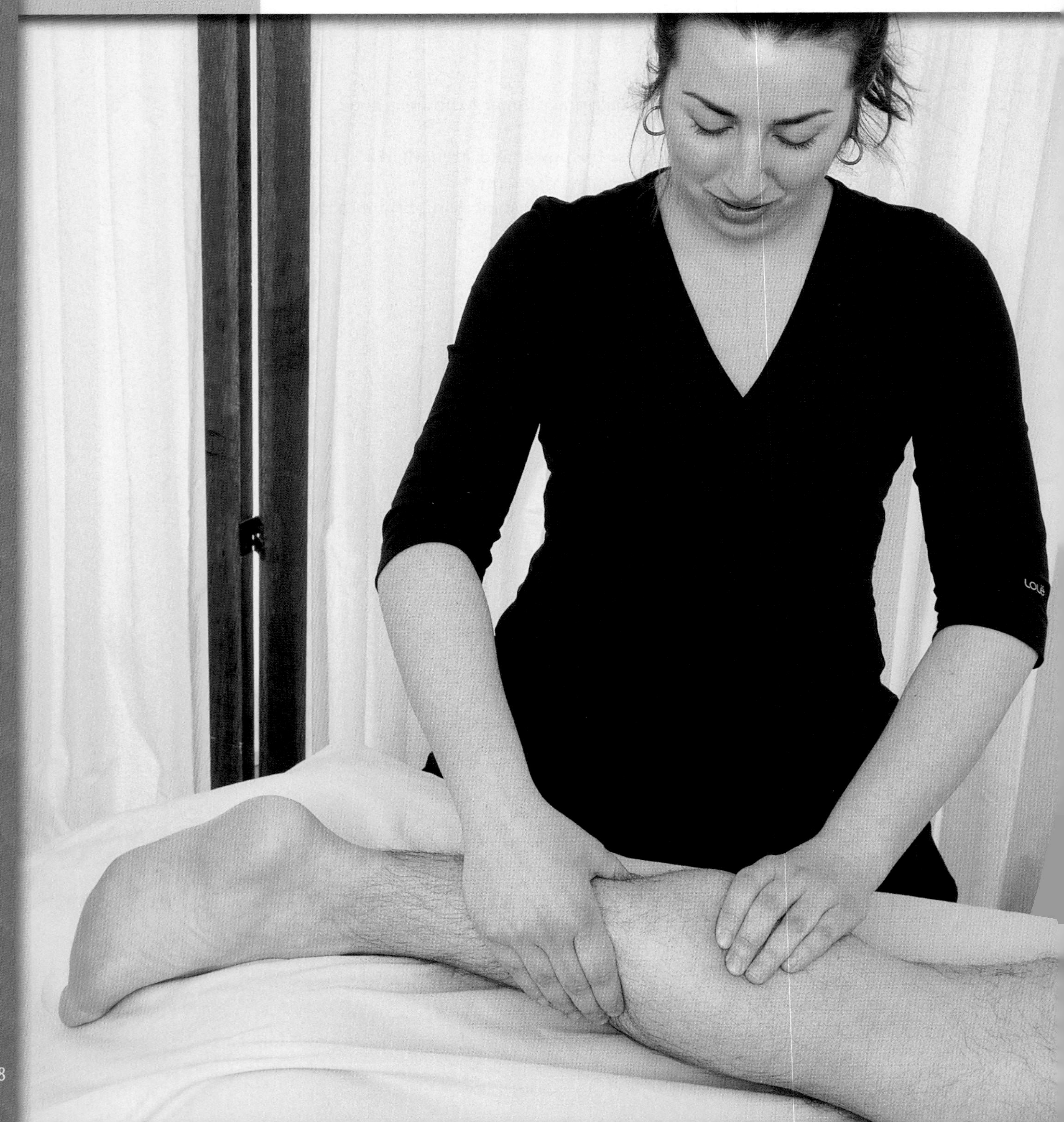

LEARNING OBJECTIVES

After you have mastered this chapter, you will be able to:

1. **Demonstrate the steps in preparing a client for a massage session.**
2. **Demonstrate correct procedures for draping the client.**
3. **Explain the importance of assisting a client onto and off of a massage table.**
4. **Demonstrate a basic body massage (Massage 1).**
5. **Demonstrate massage variations (Massage 2).**
6. **Use correct anatomic terms when describing the part of the body being massaged.**
7. **Demonstrate professional courtesies toward clients before, during, and after massage.**
8. **Understand when and where certain massage movements should and should not be applied.**
9. **Answer client questions concerning any aftereffects of massage.**

INTRODUCTION

Massage procedure is the actual process of performing a massage therapy session. There are as many variations of doing a massage as there are therapists giving and clients receiving massages. Practitioners can adopt a general routine and practice it on every client with minor variations because of specific contraindications or client requests, or the therapist can provide therapeutic services tailored to the specific needs of a client on the day of the appointment. Regardless of the style and content of the massage treatment, guidelines should be followed to ensure that the services received by the client meet high professional standards and the client's expectations. Clients who receive courteous professional services will regard the treatment with respect and will want to repeat the experience and refer others to your service.

PREPARING THE CLIENT FOR THE MASSAGE

When the preliminary interview is finished and the client has completed any necessary forms, it is time to begin the actual massage. If this is the first time you have seen this client or if it is the client's first massage, an explanation of your services and clear instructions about what the client should do will create an atmosphere for relaxation and dispel much of the anxiety that the client might have. At this time the practitioner might obtain a signed informed consent document from the client. This document clearly states the services and qualifications of the therapist, that the client understands the scope of the services, and that the client understands or has received a copy of the therapist's policies. At the end of the preliminary consultation, when the practitioner has ascertained that the client is free of any general contraindications and a strategy for the session has been formulated, briefly explain to the client what you will do and why. Show the client the facilities and explain the use of any equipment, such as steam baths or exercisers, and point out the location of the restrooms. Proceed to the dressing area, which might also be the massage room, and explain the dressing procedures and draping. Clearly explain the draping procedure for the massage, utilizing the method best suited for the client and the facility. This might include the use of a top sheet, a towel or a wrap, to get from the dressing area to the massage table.

Two commonly asked questions are "Do I have to take off my clothes?" and "How many of my clothes do I have to take off?" The most effective way to receive a Swedish relaxation/wellness massage is with all clothing removed. With proper draping, a client's modesty should never be compromised. Many people (especially first timers) are not comfortable removing all clothing, however. The client's comfort is of primary importance. Instruct the client that the best way to receive a thorough and complete massage is with all clothes removed. Stress to the client that draping will be used at all times to ensure modesty and that only that part of the body being massaged is uncovered at any time. Explain that the genitals and breasts (private areas) will be carefully (modestly) covered at all times. Finally, give clients the option to leave on whichever clothing feels most comfortable. Many people choose to wear underwear, but even if the choice is made to remain fully clothed, it is possible to perform a massage through clothing. As time goes on and the client receives more massages, the process and the draping procedure should become more comfortable.

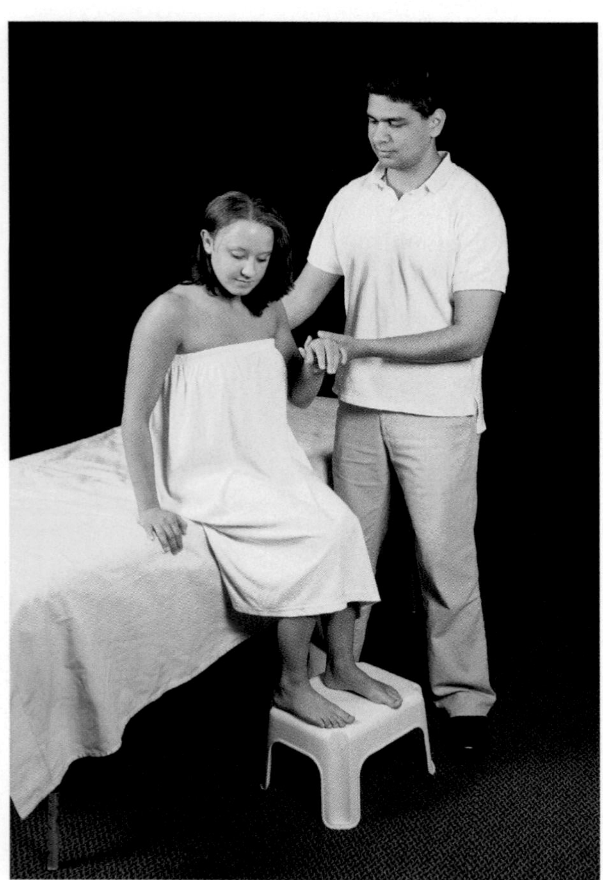

FIGURE 12–1 A stepstool can be used to help the client get onto the table. It is helpful for the therapist to lend a hand as the client gets onto and off of the table.

ASSISTING THE CLIENT ON AND OFF THE TABLE

For reasons of safety and liability, it is advisable that the practitioner be available to assist the client onto the table at the beginning of a massage and into a sitting position and off the table at the end of the massage.

The table might be too high for some clients, or various disabilities might prevent easy access to the table. A footstool is a useful item. It can be used as a step to assist some clients onto the table and by the therapist to stand on for better leverage when performing some techniques (Figure 12-1).

The procedure that you use might require the client to assume a specific position on the table. Careful instruction and physical guidance will ensure that the client is in the proper place. By keeping a hand on clients and guiding as clients sit down on the table and then lie down, you greatly reduce the possibility of injury, and people are more likely to assume the position necessary to perform the massage. Maintaining contact as clients get onto and off of the table also provides a feeling of comfort and security.

Draping procedures must include techniques that allow these movements to be accomplished while keeping the client modestly covered.

POSITIONING THE CLIENT ON THE MASSAGE TABLE

The client should assume a position on the massage table that is comfortable and allows access to the body so that the therapist can perform the massage. Once the client is sitting on the table, instruct and assist the client to lie down either supine, prone, or in a side-lying position, depending on the treatment to be given. The client must be able to relax when lying down.

Some clients cannot comfortably lie on the back or face down without support. For these clients, it is helpful to have foam cushions and bolsters in various shapes and sizes. These are made of fairly high-density foam and are covered with vinyl for easy cleaning.

Bolsters as wide as the table and 4 to 8 inches in diameter can be used under the client's knees when the client is lying on the back to place the lower spine in a more relaxed position. A bolster can be placed under the ankles when the client is lying face down. Bolsters should be covered with a pillow case or placed under the sheets or draping material so that they do not come in direct contact with the client's skin. Positioning with bolsters provides more comfort for the client who has reduced flexibility in the ankles, knees, or lower back. Firm bed pillows can also be used (Figure 12-2).

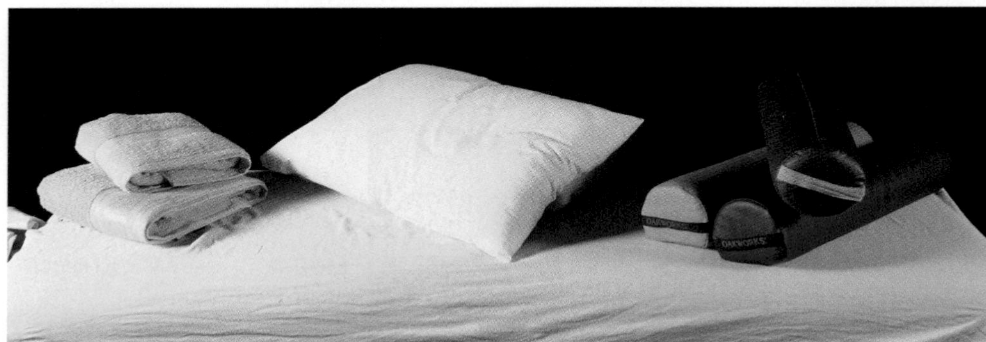

FIGURE 12-2 A variety of bolsters and pillows can be used to position the client for comfort.

Another consideration when positioning the client face down is to have a support to place under the client's chest to take the pressure off the cervical spine while in the prone position. This support should hold the chest 3 to 4 inches off the table while allowing the head to rest forward comfortably. Most modern massage tables have adjustable face cradles that provide comfortable head and neck support for the client in a face-down or prone position. Commercially manufactured Body Support Systems consist of several specifically designed cushions that provide comfortable, full-body support when the client is in the prone position (Figure 12-3a).

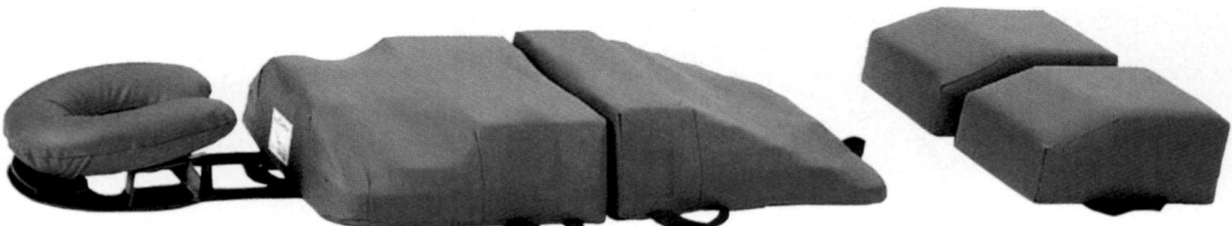

FIGURE 12-3A Body Support Systems provide comfortable whole-body support. (Courtesy of Body Support Systems, Inc.)

Some people need support under the lower abdomen and pelvic region in the face-down position if there is severe low back discomfort. Elevating the mid-section and abdomen 3 to 6 inches in this manner helps you to work on the back more effectively. A person who is unable to lie back with the head resting on the table needs support for head and neck as well as the small of the back and behind the legs (Figure 12-3b-d).

A side-lying position has many advantages when a client is not comfortable in a supine or prone position. When a client is in the side-lying position, one pillow or cushion is placed under the head to keep the cervical and thoracic spine aligned. Another pillow or bolster is placed under the top leg, which is bent at the hip and the knee so that the pelvis is not torqued or twisted. Another pillow can be positioned under the top arm for the client to hug to maintain the arm and shoulder in a comfortable position.

The side-lying position works well for pregnant women in the second and third trimesters and for people with physical conditions who cannot lie flat. The pregnant client is placed in a side-lying or reclining position to prevent the fetus from putting pressure on the abdominal aorta and cutting off circulation to the placenta. This position also provides excellent access when you are working on the inside or outside of the thigh and on the side of the neck (Figure 12-3e).

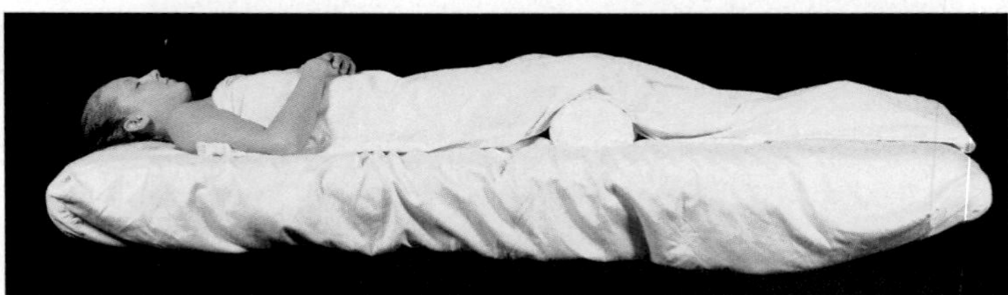

FIGURE 12-3B In the supine position, a bolster behind the knees reduces tension in the back of the legs and the low back.

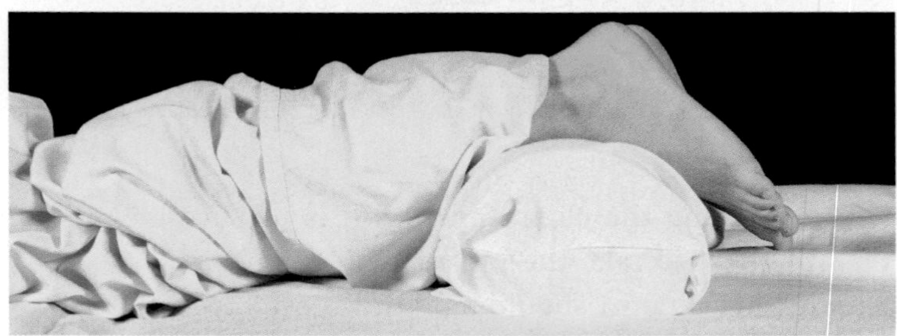

FIGURE 12-3C When a client is in the prone position, a bolster under the ankles prevents hyperextension of the knee and ankle and relieves tension in the lower back.

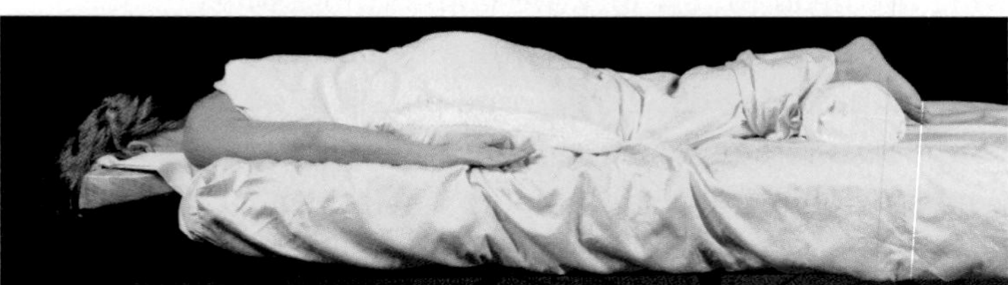

FIGURE 12-3D Support under the abdomen relieves tension in the lower back.

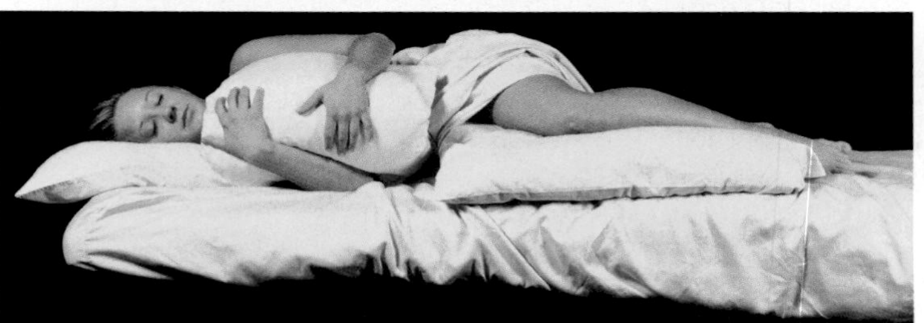

FIGURE 12-3E With the client in a side-lying position, pillows or bolsters are placed under the head and the upper leg. Another pillow is provided for the client to hug.

Clients coming to you for massage will have different problems or concerns. Some clients are unable to lie prone, and others cannot lie flat on their back without some kind of extra support. For this reason, extra supports should be a part of your professional equipment. For example, if a client cannot get up on the massage table or lie down, you can use a chair and pillows to seat the person comfortably. You can then give a massage to the back quite easily (Fig. 12-4a).

A massage chair provides another alternative for a client to receive many of the benefits of an upper body massage in a seated position without removing clothing (Figure 12-4b). (See Chapter 21 for more instruction on Chair Massage.)

Having a variety of supporting pillows or bolsters as part of your equipment enables you to position and support your client when necessary. All bolsters and pillows that come in direct contact with the client must have removable cloth slipcovers. Fresh clean covers are used for each client. You can also place bolsters and pillows under the bottom sheet next to the table to avoid contact with the client's skin.

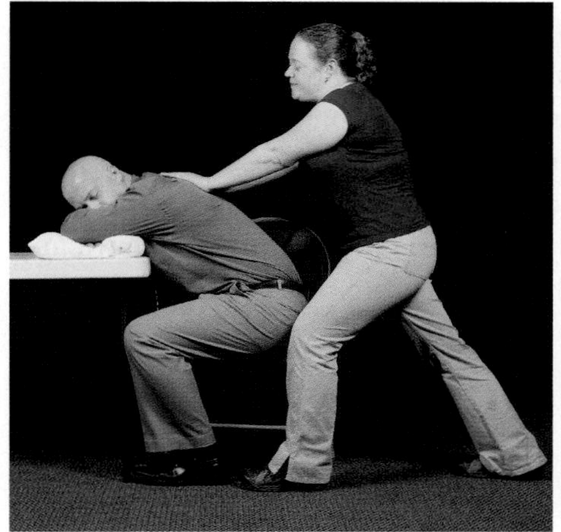

FIGURE 12-4A If using a table is not practical, a supported seated massage is an alternative.

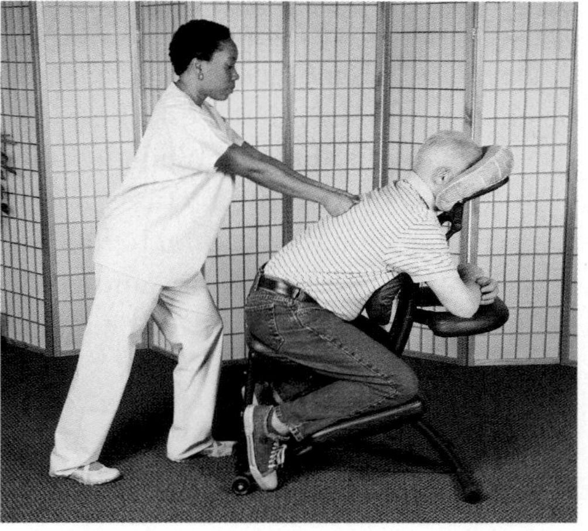

FIGURE 12-4B Seated massage using a massage chair is usually done with the client fully clothed.

DRAPING PROCEDURES

The process of using linens to keep a client covered while performing a massage is called **draping**. This procedure allows the client to be totally undressed and at the same time be covered to retain comfort, warmth, and modesty. It gives the practitioner the freedom to massage all parts of the body unencumbered by the client's clothing.

draping

is the process of using linens to keep a client covered while receiving a massage.

Proper draping ensures that the client stays warm and feels safe and comfortable. Perspiration, massage lubricant, and being in a reclining position all increase the rate at which the body loses heat. Massage stimulates the parasympathetic nervous system, affecting the basal body temperature, which results in the client's becoming chilled more easily. The proper temperature for a massage room is between 72° F and 75° F. If the area is cooler than this, extra precautions should be taken to make sure that the client remains warm. It is much easier for a person to become chilled than to warm up. If a person is chilled, it is nearly impossible to relax.

Two items to keep on hand to prevent a client from becoming chilled are a twin-size electric mattress pad (or a massage table heating pad) to put on the table under the sheet and a flannel blanket or sheet to use once the client is on the massage table and properly draped.

By using proper draping (uncovering only the portion of the body that is being massaged) and by always concealing the client's private parts, the practitioner maintains a professional and ethical practice while preventing embarrassment to either the practitioner or the client.

There are several methods of draping. All methods consist of techniques of maintaining personal privacy while getting the client from the dressing area to the hydrotherapy area or the massage table, using adequate draping while the client receives the massage, and keeping the client well covered while getting up from the massage table and returning to the dressing area.

METHODS OF DRAPING

There are several methods of draping that are easy and effective. This chapter presents two methods. Practice each of these until you are proficient. You may choose one style that works best for you, or you may combine portions of one method with another. While learning these various draping procedures, refer to the step-by-step directions and illustrations included in this chapter. The beginner should be careful to follow directions carefully and practice until able to drape a client smoothly and efficiently. It is also important to know how to instruct the client in how to change positions during the draping procedures.

Method 1—Top Cover Method

The top cover method uses a table covering along with a top covering that is large enough to cover the entire body. A large bath sheet towel or one half of a full or double sheet serves this purpose well. The minimum size for the top cover is 72 inches long and 36 inches wide. It is possible to use two bath-sized towels as a top cover. When the client is lying on the table, the two towels are in a

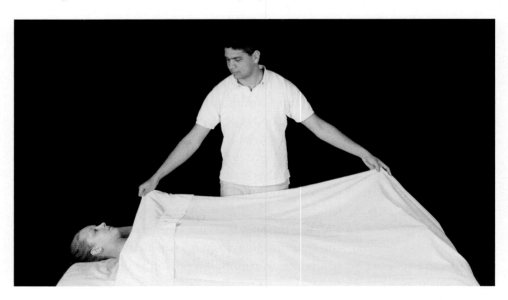

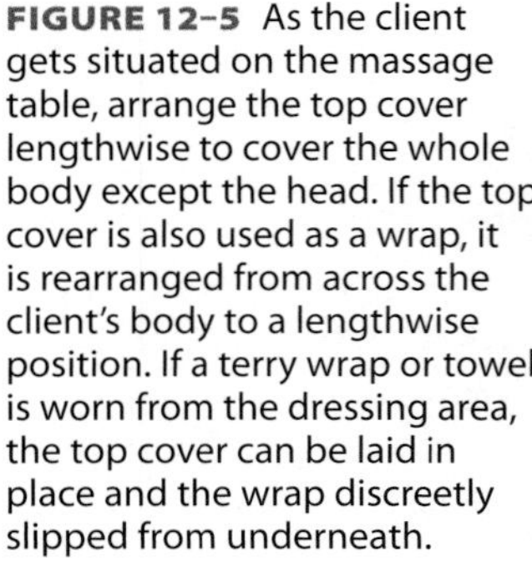

FIGURE 12–5 As the client gets situated on the massage table, arrange the top cover lengthwise to cover the whole body except the head. If the top cover is also used as a wrap, it is rearranged from across the client's body to a lengthwise position. If a terry wrap or towel is worn from the dressing area, the top cover can be laid in place and the wrap discreetly slipped from underneath.

T configuration, with the upper towel lying across the torso and the lower towel covering the lower extremities up to the hips. The lower towel is turned crossways over the central area of the body when it is time for the client to turn over.

The cover sheet also can serve as the wrap that the client uses to get from the dressing area to the table.

The use of this type of draping ensures warmth and modesty while allowing the therapist easy access to each body part (Figure 12-5).

Method 2—Full Sheet Draping

Full sheet draping employs the use of a full-size double flat sheet (minimum width 80 inches) to cover the table and wrap the client. When working with a large client (200 pounds plus), it is necessary to use a queen-size sheet. When using this method, supply an additional wrap for the client to get from the dressing area to the table. After the client is on the table, the wrap is used to secure the sheet and to cover the client when turning over and getting up after the massage (Figure 12-6).

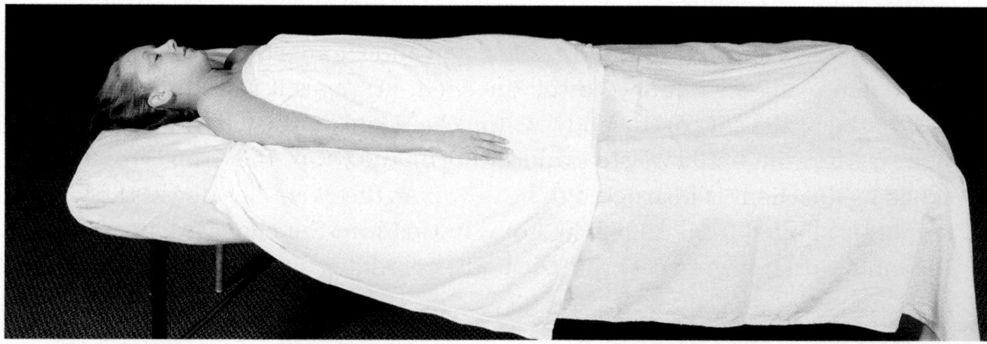

FIGURE 12-6 Full-sheet draping covers the client securely in a cocoon-like wrap, making the client feel safe and warm.

The following items can be used in the draping process:

Sheets

- Full double flat sheets (minimum width 80 inches)
- Cot-sized or twin-sized fitted sheets
- One half of full double sheets, cut and hemmed to use as a table covering or a cover sheet
- Disposable sheets to use as table coverings when laundry is a problem

Towels

- Bath-size towels for draping and for personal use after hydrotherapy
- Bath sheets for body covers
- Terry cloth wraps to wear to and from the dressing area

Miscellaneous

- Pillow cases for covering pillows, bolsters, head rests, or for breast draping
- Washcloths, pillow covers, or specifically manufactured protectors to cover face cradles

- Flannel sheets to use when extra warmth is needed
- Twin-sized electric mattress pad for use on the table when warmth is a problem, such as working in a home where it is too cool

Remember that any materials coming in contact with the client's skin must be freshly laundered and sanitary. Clean linens must be used for each client.

Draping from the Dressing Area to the Massage Table

The first step in the draping process requires some form of wrap to be worn from the dressing area to either the hydrotherapy area or the massage table. The method of draping during the massage, as well as the size and gender of the client, determines the type of wrap to be used. In the top cover sheet method, the cover sheet can be used as the wrap. Terry cloth wraps can be provided instead of a towel for the client to wear in any method of draping. These wraps can be purchased in a department store or uniform store. The women's wrap fastens above the breasts; the men's wrap is a shorter version that wraps around and fastens at the waist. The length is usually just below the knees. These wraps are convenient because they secure and unfasten easily when the client is on the table, and they are easy to put back on after the massage. Wraps are available in small, large, and extra-large sizes for men and women (Figures 12-7a and b).

When using a wrap or a towel, the client arranges it so that the open side is situated at the side of the body. As the client sits on the edge of the table, the wrap is lifted out of the way to avoid sitting on the wrap. The wrap is then unfastened as the client is instructed to lie down. As the client lies down, the wrap is smoothly slipped from under the body. In this way, the client is lying down on the table with the wrap covering the body, not underneath it.

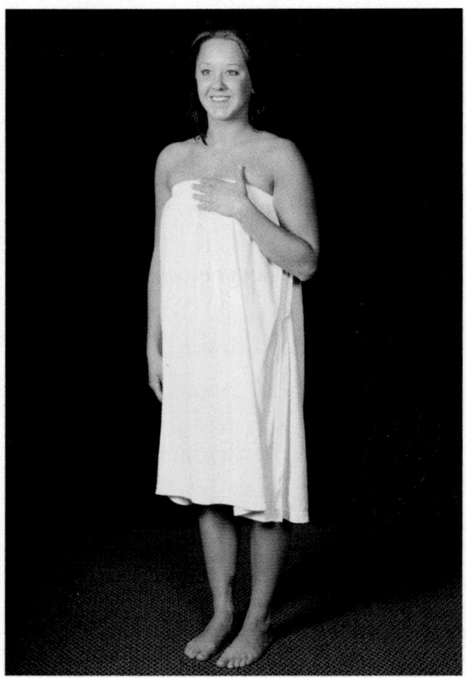

FIGURE 12-7A The female wrap is long enough to cover the body and can be used as a top cover.

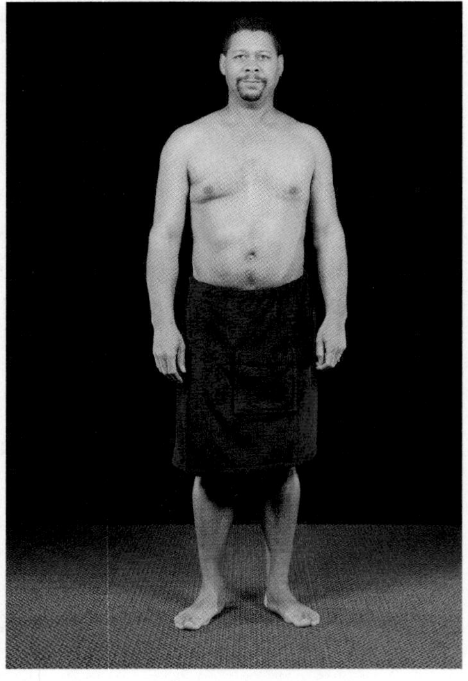

FIGURE 12-7B The male wrap can be smaller but also must act as a modest covering.

An alternative to this procedure is to have the client lie on the table and then unfasten the wrap. Have the client lift the body slightly as you carefully slip the wrap from underneath.

Having gotten the client on the table, lying down, and covered by the wrap, you are ready to proceed with the draping of your choice and the massage.

When the massage has been completed and it is time for the client to get up and get dressed, a procedure must be followed that maintains the client's privacy in a relaxed and efficient manner, while at the same time ensuring the client's safety. The procedure shown in Figures 12-8a-c can be helpful.

It is important to be courteous and attentive toward your clients from the time people enter your place of business until leaving. You should show concern for clients' safety and comfort at all times. Some clients want and expect help when getting on or off the massage table; others might prefer no assistance at all. When in doubt, ask. For example you might say, "May I assist you?" or "Let me help you."

Optional Method

An optional and popular method to get the client undressed and onto the table is for the practitioner to instruct the client on the procedure and then leave the room, allowing the client privacy. The table is prepared with a table covering and a top sheet or large towel. The client is instructed to remove clothing, lie on the

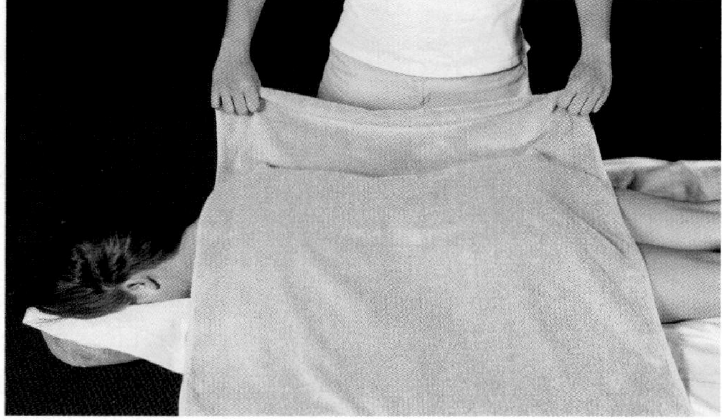

FIGURE 12-8A When the massage is completed, the same wrap that the client wore from the dressing area to the massage table is used. The wrap is placed across the client's body, and other draping is removed. Instruct the client to lie on one side and arrange the wrap in such a way that it covers the back of the body, with most of the wrap in front.

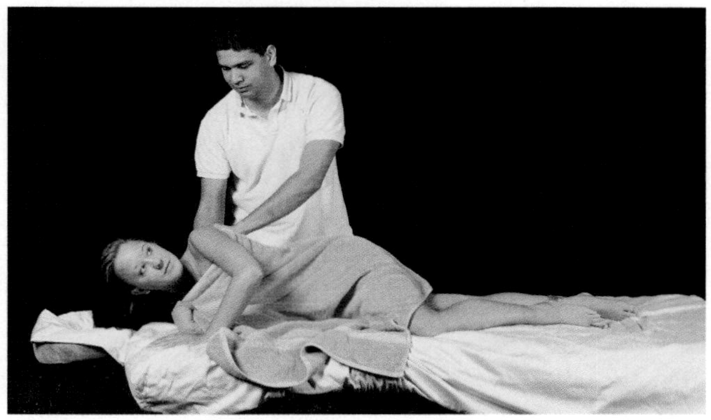

FIGURE 12-8B From the side-lying position, the client draws both knees up so that the feet are just off the side of the table (women hold the wrap over the breasts) and the client uses the top hand and arm to push up while the practitioner assists the client to a sitting position.

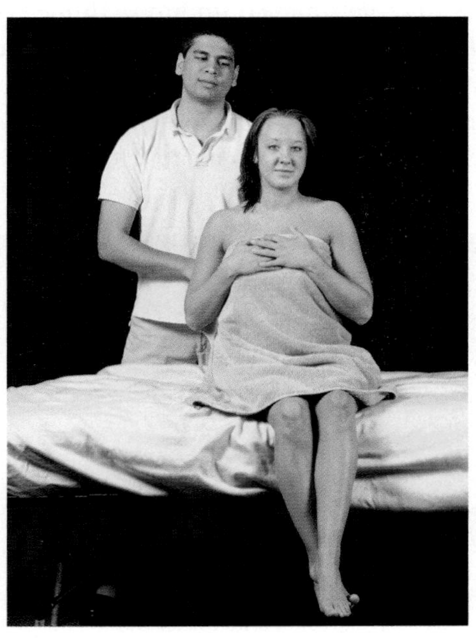

FIGURE 12-8C At this point, the wrap is refastened while the client is given a chance to regain composure. After a moment or two, the client is instructed to stand and return to the dressing area. As the client stands, the practitioner should keep one hand on the client's arm for balance and the other hand on the table to prevent it from tipping.

table in the chosen position, and cover the body with the appropriate drape. The practitioner then leaves the room. The client disrobes, climbs on the table, and covers the body. It is important to give concise but simple instructions so that the client is in the correct position and properly covered when the practitioner reenters the massage room.

When the massage is complete, the practitioner may instruct the client to take a few minutes to relish the experience and then carefully get up and get dressed. The practitioner then exits the room and leaves the client alone to get off the massage table and to get dressed. The author considers this method to be somewhat less professional because it increases the possibility that the client could be injured while getting onto or off of the massage table.

If there is any concern that the client might need some assistance getting up at the end of the session, the practitioner should remain in the massage room to assist the client to a sitting position and then off of the table before leaving the room and allowing the client some privacy to dress. Use proper draping techniques to ensure that the client remains modestly covered while sitting up and getting off the table.

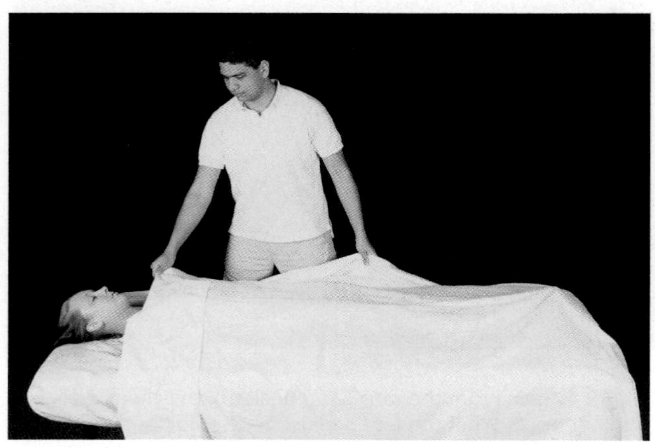

FIGURE 12-9A As the client gets situated on the massage table, arrange the top cover lengthwise to cover all except the head. If the top cover is also used as a wrap, it is rearranged from across the client's body to a lengthwise position. If a terry wrap or towel is worn from the dressing area, the top cover can be laid in place and the wrap discreetly slipped from underneath.

Method 1—The Top Cover Method

Follow the illustrations for the top cover method until you are able to remember how to do the entire procedure smoothly and efficiently (Figure 12-9a-h). Linens required for the top sheet method include a covering for the table, which could be a cot or twin fitted or flat sheet and a top cover. The top cover can be a large bath sheet (beach towel), a twin flat sheet, or one half of a double flat sheet. Two bath towels could also be used as a top cover.

When it is time for the client to turn over, a process is used so that the client stays discreetly covered and does not get tangled up in the drapes (Figure 12-9i-k). The top cover is arranged to cover the client from the shoulders down with the edge of the cover nearest the practitioner draped slightly over the edge of the table. If the top drape is too narrow to overlap the edge of the

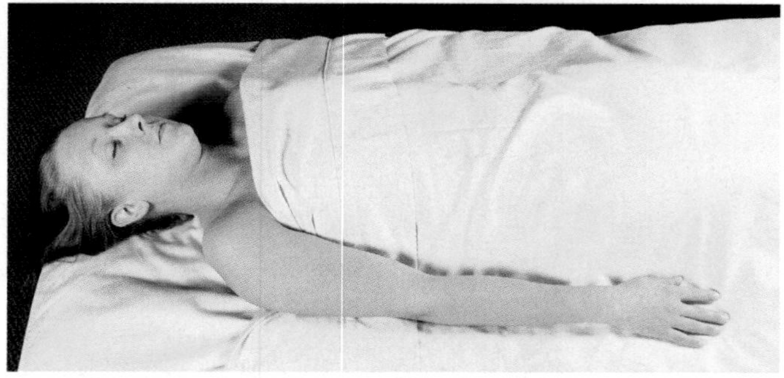

FIGURE 12-9B As each arm is massaged, fold the top cover out of the way, exposing only the limb to be massaged.

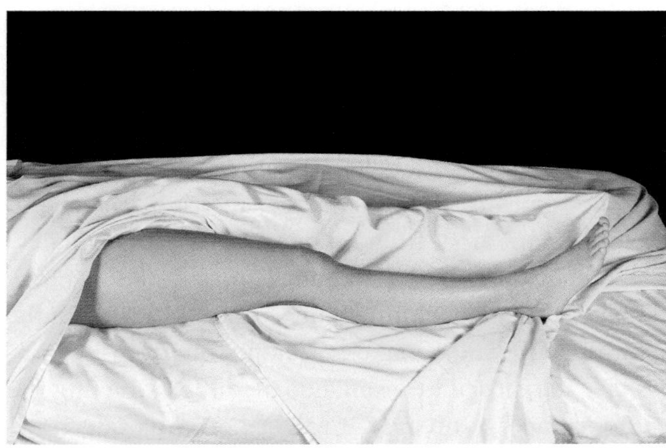

FIGURE 12-9C To massage a leg, uncover that leg only. Lift the knee enough to reach under and pull the drape under the thigh and toward the buttock with one hand while positioning the cover snugly along the inguinal crease with your other hand.

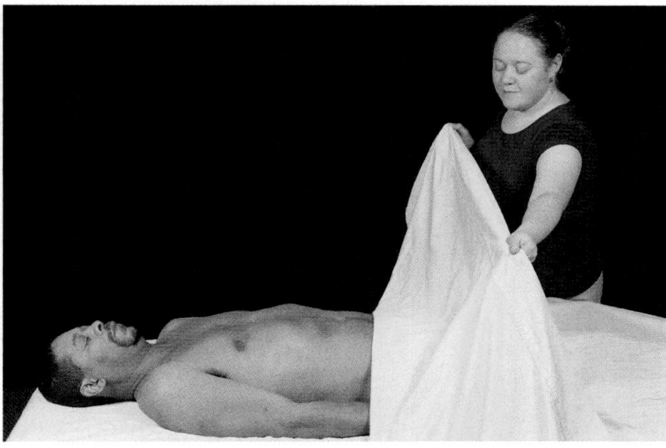

FIGURE 12-9D To massage the chest and abdomen of a man, neatly fold the top cover to the level of the hips.

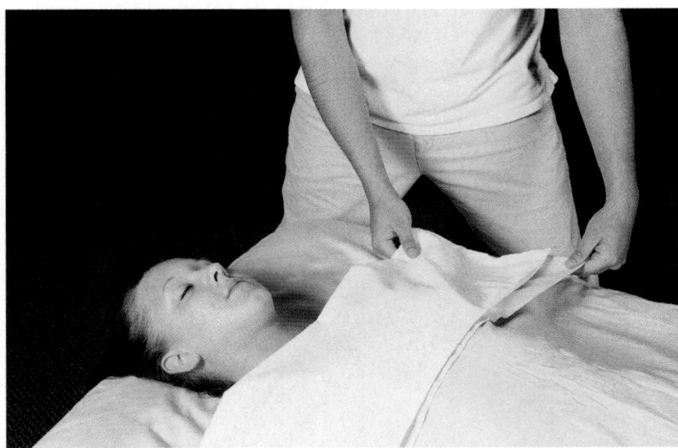

FIGURE 12-9E To work on the abdomen of a woman, breast draping is needed. Fold another towel or pillow case to make a covering for the breasts and place it over the top cover.

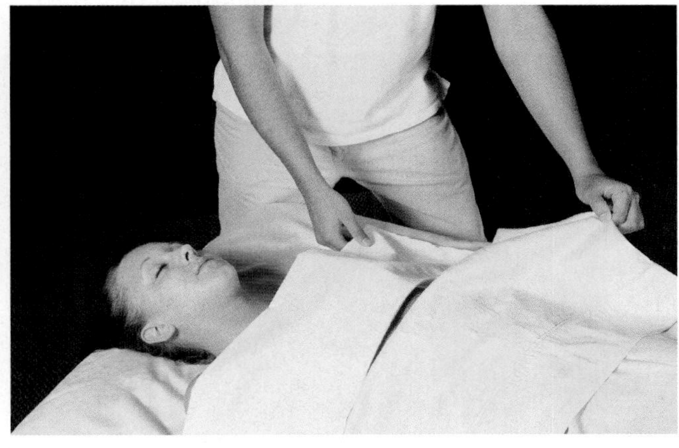

FIGURE 12-9F Peel the top cover down while holding the folded towel or pillowcase in place over the breasts.

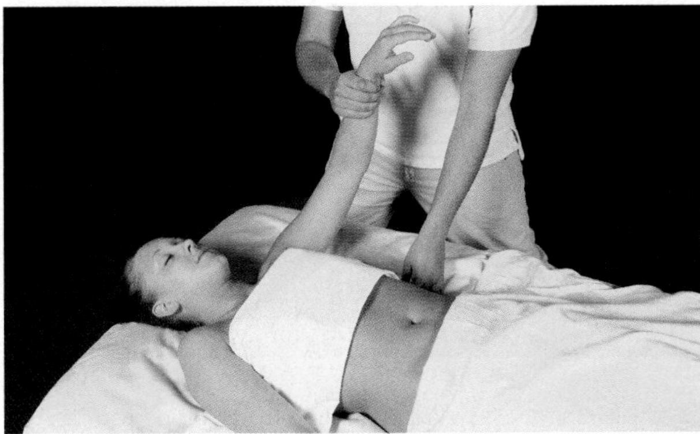

FIGURE 12-9G Raise the client's arm and tuck the towel or pillowcase used for the breast cover neatly under the scapula to hold the ends of the towel securely in place.

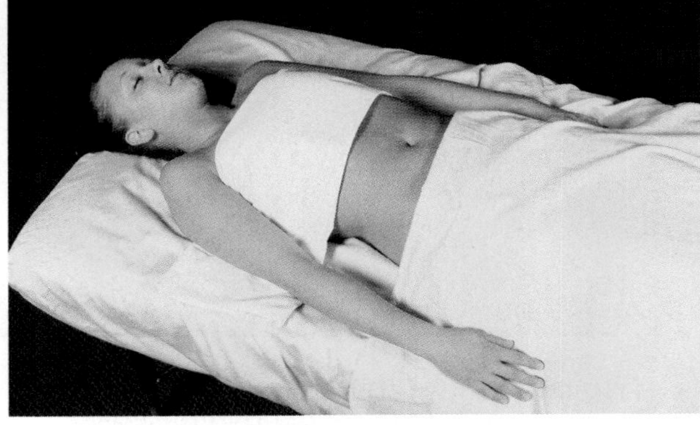

FIGURE 12-9H Place the client's arm down. Tuck the other side of the towel or pillowcase covering the breasts under the other scapula in the same manner. This draping method allows you to work on the abdomen, chest, and sides of the body without exposing the breasts.

table and still cover the client, the drape could be turned sidewise, as long as it still covers the female client from the shoulders to midthigh. The practitioner leans against the side of the massage table to secure the table cover and the top drape with the thighs and reaches across the table to hold the top cover at the level of the shoulder with one hand and below the hips with the other. If the client is turning from supine to prone, the practitioner instructs the client, "Please roll over by turning toward me first, then on over onto your stomach." If a face cradle is used, once on the stomach, the client is instructed to move (slide) up the table until the client's face is comfortably situated in the cradle. Ask whether the client is comfortable, and make any adjustments necessary before beginning back massage. This procedure can also be done by having the client turn away from the practitioner to roll over. It might not be as safe; however, it can be more efficient at securing the client's privacy.

If the client is turning from prone to supine, the practitioner positions and secures the drapes in the same manner and instructs the client to first turn away from the practitioner and then onto the back. As the client turns, the practitioner holds the top and bottom sheet in place by leaning against the table while reaching across the table and supporting the top drape at the level of the client's

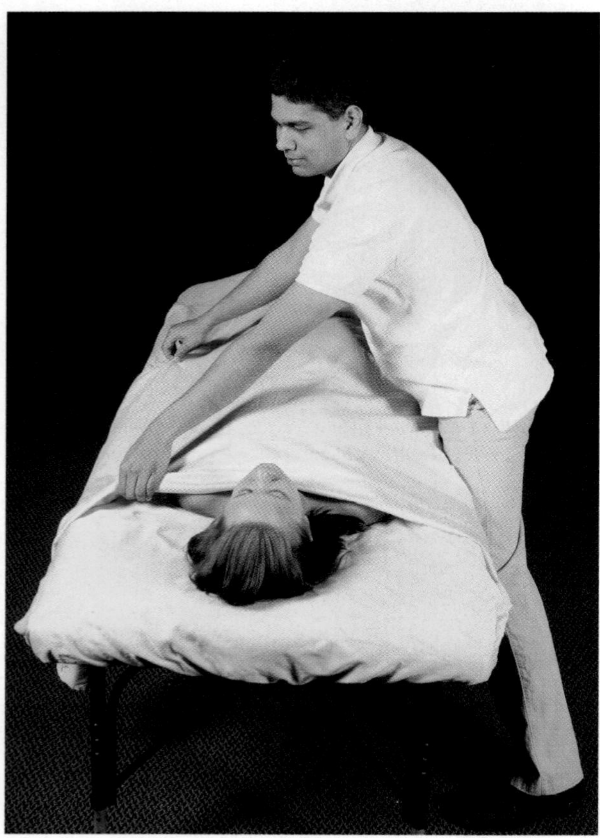

FIGURE 12-9I When it is time to roll over, the drape is repositioned and held in place by the therapist, who leans on the table and grasps the top cover at the level of the client's shoulders and hips.

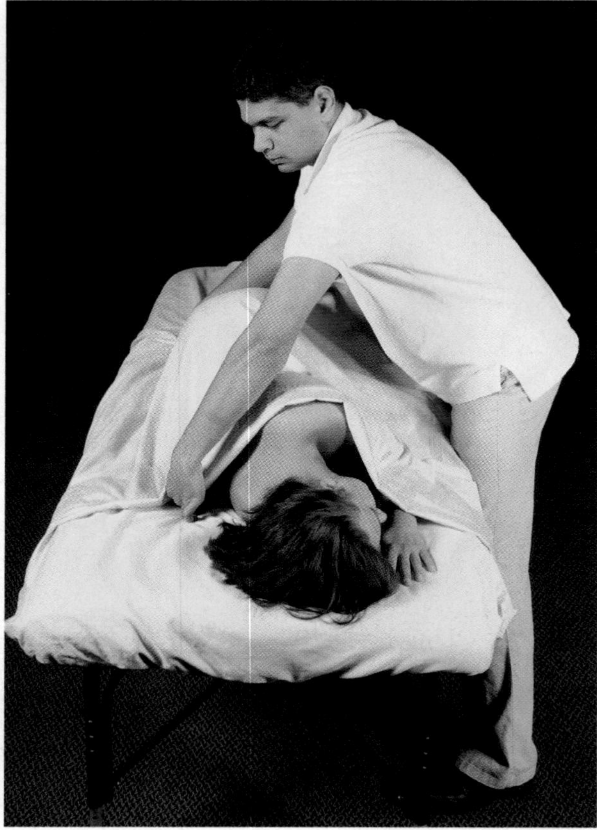

FIGURE 12-9J When rolling from supine to prone, the client is instructed to roll first to face the therapist and then onto the stomach.

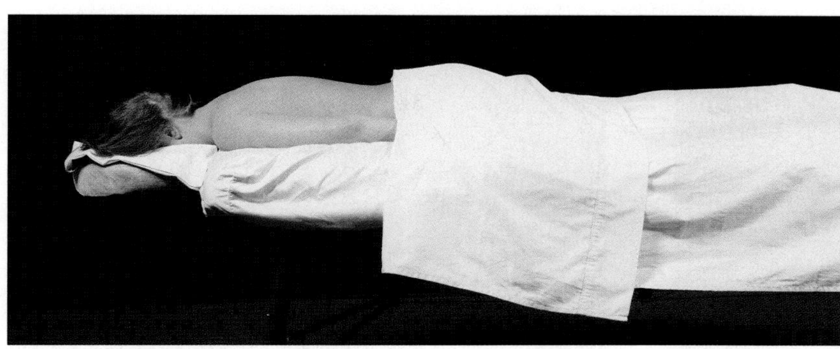

FIGURE 12-9K To massage the back, neatly fold the top cover down to a level two inches below the beginning of the gluteal cleft.

shoulders and upper thigh with both hands as the client turns over. Throughout the process of turning, the practitioner's body should not touch the client's body in any way.

When the massage is complete and it is time for the client to return to the dressing area, use the top cover for a wrap by turning the cover sideways before having the client come to a sitting position. If you choose to use a separate wrap, put the wrap in place and, while holding it with one hand, peel the top cover from underneath the wrap.

Method 2—Full Sheet Draping

The following is a step-by-step description of the full sheet draping method (Figure. 12-10a-o). This method incorporates the use of a double-size flat sheet and a separate wrap or towel. First, prepare the massage table by unfolding the double-size sheet and placing it on the massage table.

Client Assistive Draping

There are several areas in draping where the client can assist in the draping procedure by holding the drape in place while a massage movement is performed. Breast draping, draping of the upper thigh for joint movements,

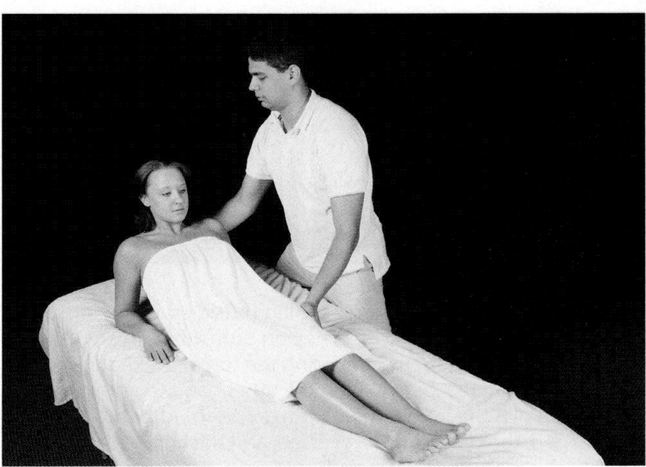

FIGURE 12-10A Assist the client onto the table and into a supine (lying on the back) position. The wrap that the client wore to the table is used as a cover.

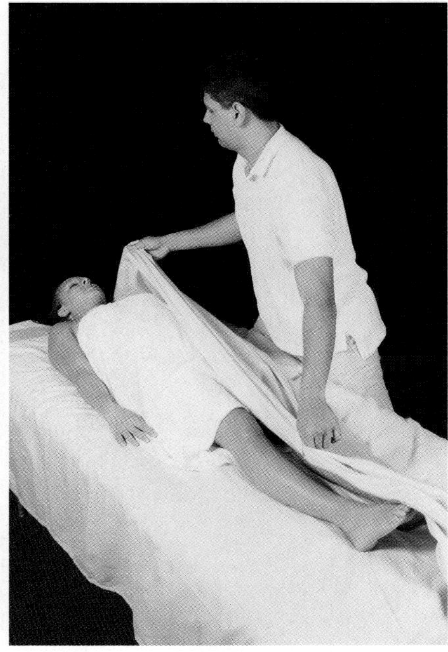

FIGURE 12-10B Drape one side of the flat sheet over the client to cover the entire torso and one leg. The client can choose whether or not to cover the arms.

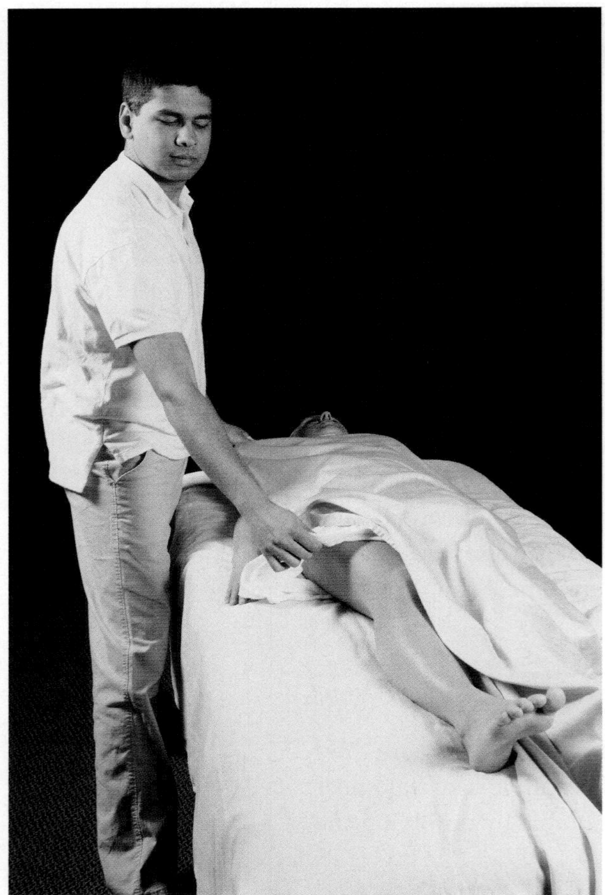

FIGURE 12-10C Discreetly remove the wrap from underneath the draping.

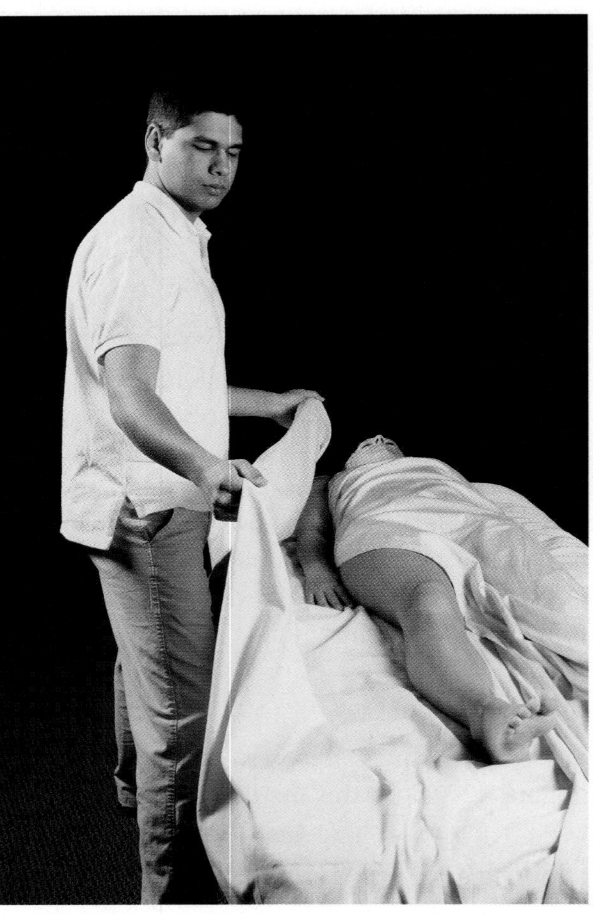

FIGURE 12-10D Drape the other side of the flat sheet over the entire torso and the other leg.

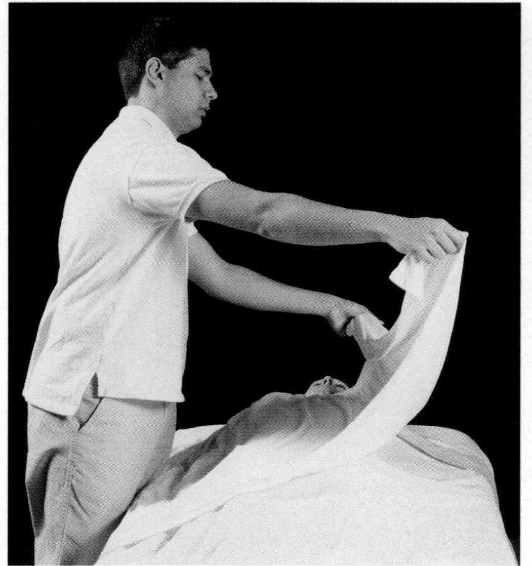

FIGURE 12-10E Place the towel or wrap over the chest area to hold the drape in place. If it is not needed for this purpose, it can be placed aside for later use.

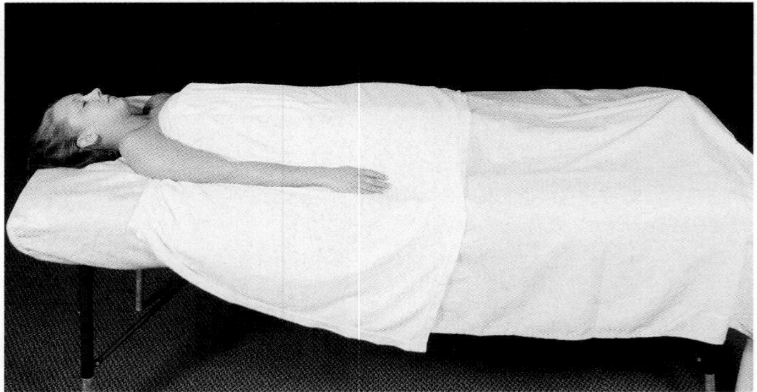

FIGURE 12-10F If the client's arms are left outside the draping, there is no problem. (a) If the client prefers having both arms covered, then proceed with undraping them by holding the top of the draping, lifting it slightly, then reaching in with the other hand to grasp the client's wrist and lift the from beneath the drape. (b) After the arm has been massaged, the procedure is reversed, and the arm is placed back underneath the draping at the client's side.

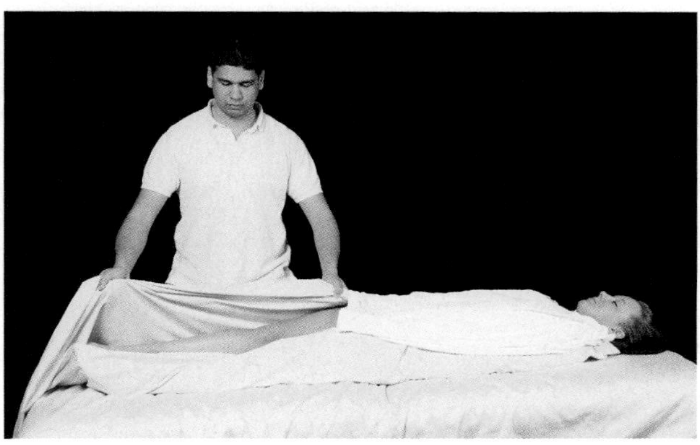

FIGURE 12-10G Undrape the leg, beginning at the foot. Peel the sheet upward all the way to the iliac crest (hip bone). Remember that when initially draping the client, each leg was draped independently and was covered by only one layer of the draping sheet.

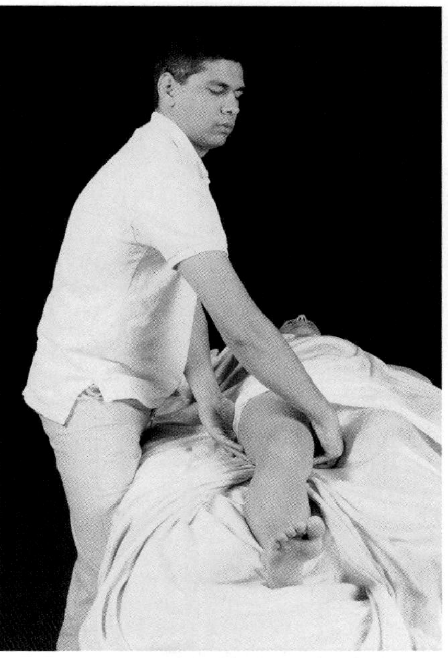

FIGURE 12-10H Carefully tuck the drape covering the opposite leg under that thigh with one hand, while arranging the rest of the draping with the other hand across the torso and the genital area. This method ensures that the client is well covered when massaging upward to the hip bone and when performing leg stretches.

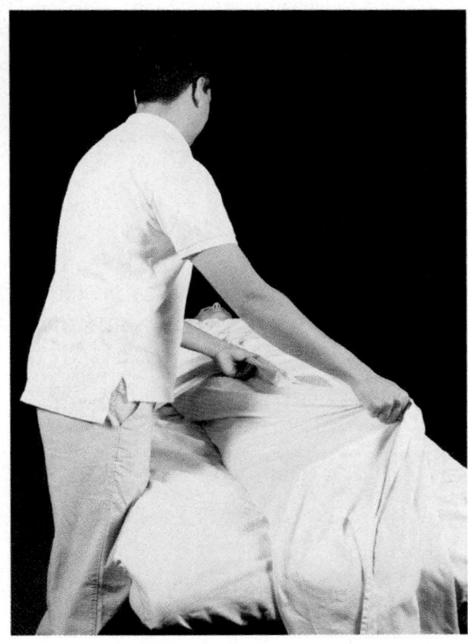

FIGURE 12-10I Re-drape the leg and the entire torso with the sheet on that side of the table, then proceed to the other leg in the same manner.

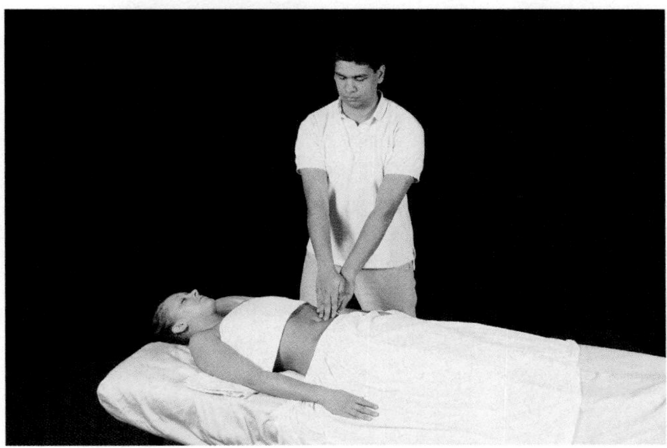

FIGURE 12-10J Prepare to massage the upper part of the body by opening the draping to just above the pubic bone. When massaging a female client, fold the wrap or a pillowcase (or towel) and use it as a breast covering. Use another towel to secure the draping at the level just above the pubic bone.

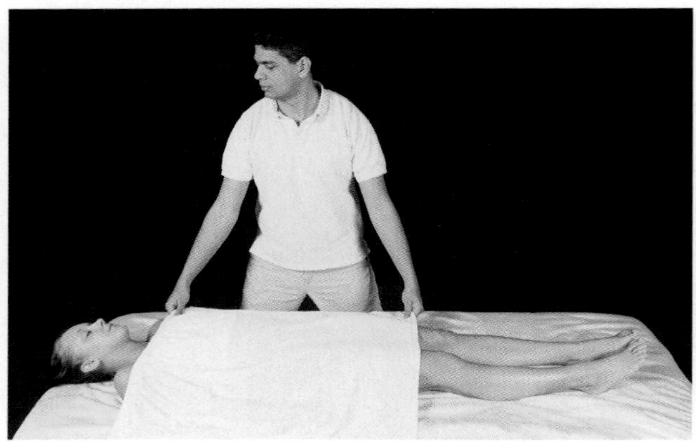

FIGURE 12-10K When it is time for the client to turn over, use the wrap to cover the client from the shoulders to the knees.

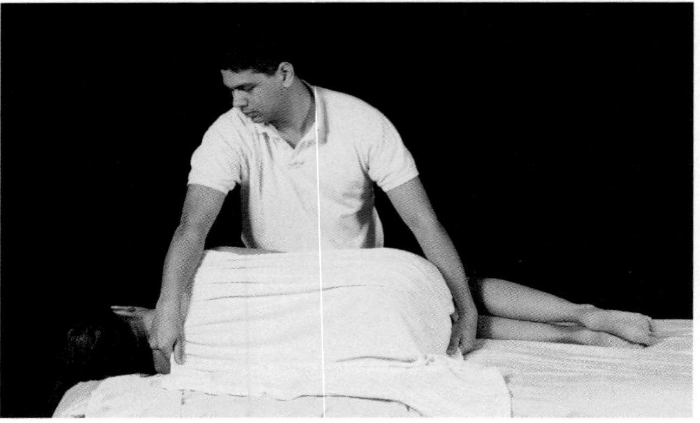

FIGURE 12-10L Instruct the client to turn toward you by lifting the opposite shoulder first; then have the client roll onto the abdomen. Hold the wrap in place with your hands and the flat sheet in place by leaning against the table.

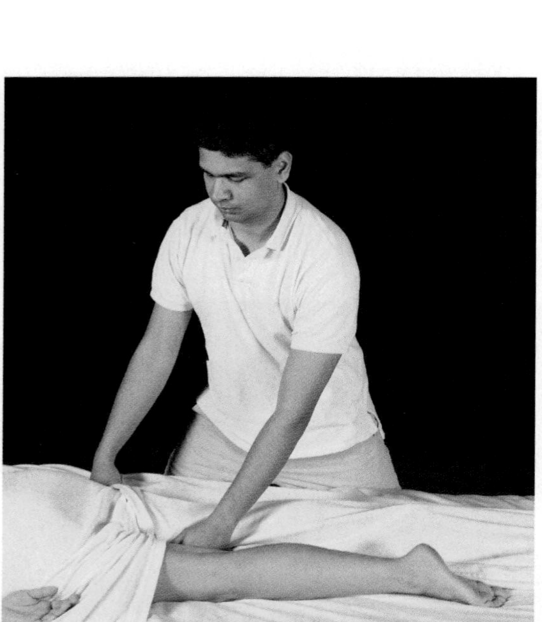

FIGURE 12-10M With the client lying face down, place the wrap so that it covers the back down to the middle of the thighs. Drape the sheet over one leg and the back, and then tuck it around under the same leg. Massage the other leg.

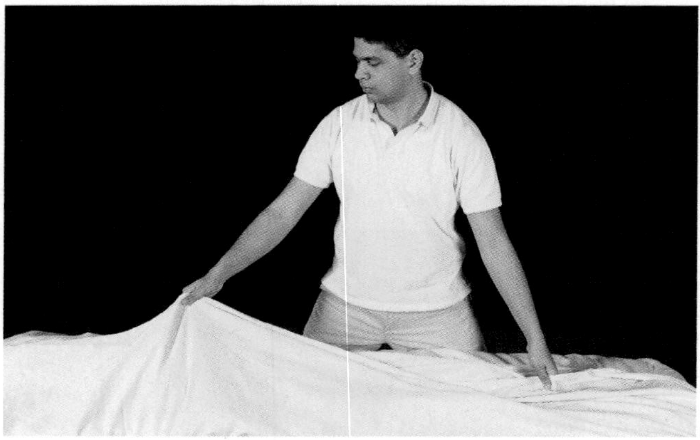

FIGURE 12-10N Drape the leg after massaging it, and then undrape and massage the other leg in the same manner. Re-drape the leg.

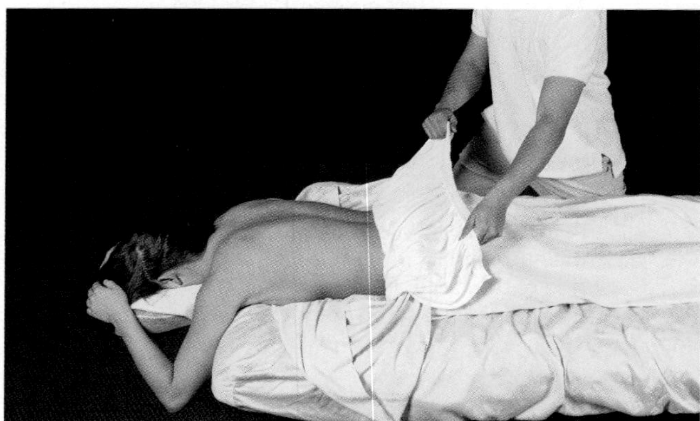

FIGURE 12-10O Prepare to massage the back by peeling the wrap downward to expose the entire back. This method holds the leg draping in place and does not overly expose the gluteal area.

and rearranging draping to secure privacy are examples. When a pillowcase or smaller towel is used to drape the bustline of a woman, the client can place a hand over the drape to keep it secure. When the sheet is tucked under the thigh for joint movement of the hip, the client can hold onto the drape to secure privacy of the pelvic region. Allowing the client to be involved ensures that privacy is of the utmost importance.

CONTACT WITH THE CLIENT AND QUALITY OF TOUCH

In administering a massage, a therapist must be aware of much more than merely the application of strokes to various parts of the client's body. The practitioner must consider contact with the client, the quality of touch, and the constitution or composition of the massage itself.

From the time that a client enters a massage establishment, the practitioner communicates confidence and ability. The confidence shown at the initial contact instills a certain trust in the recipient that encourages relaxation. The success of that communication largely depends on the therapist's quality of touch. Different people exhibit varying qualities in touch, just as there are vast differences in people's voices and the ways in whichpeople communicate. The quality of touch is a key to the way that the client will respond to the therapist and the massage treatment.

Our intentions and attitudes are often communicated through our actions and physical contact with people as much as they are through the spoken word. The massage professional endeavors to promote a sense of relaxation and well-being. Massage is the touch profession. People who come for a massage usually want to "let go" of something and literally be put into the hands of the practitioner. From the time that clients enter the massage office until leaving, clients must feel comfortable and in good hands. The way in which touch is administered to the client determines the success of the massage and is often the reason for a client to return.

MAINTAINING CONTACT WITH THE CLIENT

Before beginning a professional body massage, it is important to "tune in" to the client.

The massage begins when the client is positioned on the massage table and the practitioner comes in contact with the client's body. After undraping and applying massage lubricant to the part of the body to be massaged, remember to keep in contact with the client's body throughout the procedure. Between strokes or during transitions from one body area to another, allow at least one hand to be in continuous contact, maintaining a constant flow without surges or breaks through the entire massage. If the client is in a state of wakeful conversation with eyes open during the massage, then there is verbal and visual contact. If the client is in a state of relaxation with the eyes closed, however, the sense of touch is the only communication. If contact is broken, a vocal reassurance can prevent an immediate reaction of concern on the part of the client, maintaining relaxation and preventing any anxiety. In most cases, the goal is to maintain continuous contact until the massage is finished and the final strokes lightly feathered off.

By maintaining continuous contact, the client is constantly aware of the practitioner's presence and activity, and at the same time has a point of reference and an awareness of the parts of the body that are being massaged. As the various strokes are performed on the body parts, the attention and awareness of the client follow. At some level of consciousness, clients can release the stress and tension in each part of the body and at the same time, tuning out mental stress and tension. With both eyes closed, people float into a state of relaxation anchored by only the touch of the practitioner's hands. If contact is broken, clients immediately lose that point of reference and wonder where the practitioner has gone, what is going on, and which part of the body is going to touched next. When contact is reestablished, it is as though attention has jolted to the new point of contact. If it is necessary to leave a client, this should be explained to the client. Resume contact with the client softly and inconspicuously.

Although continuous contact is important, it must be done in an efficient and unencumbered manner. There should be no element of surprise as the massage moves from one part of the body to another. The therapist accomplishes this through practice and the implementation of a logical massage sequence.

Sequence

sequence

refers to the pattern or design of a massage.

Sequence refers to the pattern or design of a massage. Developing a good sequence is especially important because it coordinates and organizes the massage so that there is smooth progression from one stroke to the next and from one body part to the next. Sequence provides a framework for a well-thought-out, logical progression and at the same time allows for flexibility and creativity. When doing a full-body massage, following a sequence ensures that each and every area of the body is massaged in some logical order.

There are numerous possibilities when formulating a full-body massage sequence, depending on the style of the practitioner, the preferences and needs of the client, and the intentions of the session, among many other considerations. The sequence can begin with the client lying face up, face down, or on either side. The massage can begin at the head, at the feet, or somewhere in between. Generally, a Western or Swedish-style massage is designed so that the client only has to change positions once or maybe twice. A relaxing, wellness massage sequence is designed so that each body area is thoroughly massaged in a logical order so that the entire body is included and the client feels balanced, complete, and relaxed. Some therapeutic applications require the therapist to focus on specific areas of the client's body or to return to an area several times during a session but not even approach other areas of the body. In so doing, the therapist is following a sequence to address the specific needs of the client efficiently. Even in a relaxing full-body massage, the sequence is a guideline that is always flexible enough for the individual needs of the client to be addressed.

Following a massage sequence on a particular body area provides a structure that you, the practitioner, can use to ensure a balanced and complete therapeutic application to that area. In the application of a massage, sequences are built within sequences, and each body part is provided an equal experience. Even during the massage of a body part, there are conditions in which adapting certain sequences proves to be both valuable and therapeutic.

There is a general massage rule to keep in mind: when doing massage, performing a stroke, or working on an area, work from general to specific, then back to general, and from superficial to deep and back to superficial.

Box 12.1

General Massage Rule

When working on an area or performing a stroke,

work from general to specific then back to general,

AND

work from superficial to deep then back to superficial

In working from general to specific, the entire area is relaxed and circulation is stimulated so that more specific massage can relieve congestion and spasm. Ischemic conditions also have a better chance of being relieved. Following specific massage techniques with more generalized massage tends to normalize the area.

Likewise, starting with more superficial effleurage or gliding strokes relaxes the area and encourages the client's confidence to let you work more deeply into the tissues. Following deeper massage techniques, soothing superficial gliding strokes dissipate the tension released from the target tissues and enhance a sense of relaxation.

This can be illustrated by doing a single stroke or a series of strokes—for instance, when doing gliding strokes over an area such as the calf of the leg. Begin with a very light stroke, repeat with a deeper stroke, and get increasingly deeper with each successive stroke until the maximum depth you want is achieved. Then the next few strokes are lighter until the final stroke is nearly as light as the first.

Another example involves a variety of massage strokes that begin with general gliding strokes over an area. An area of tension is palpated. Kneading or petrissage is followed by deeper kneading and deeper gliding. Next are a variety of friction techniques that address the tense tissue more directly and deeply. Deep pressure and transverse friction are applied directly to the tissue. This is followed by jostling, deep gliding, joint movements, more superficial gliding, and finally feather strokes.

Following a sequence when massaging particular conditions and areas provides a structure that allows for creativity and flexibility.

The sequence of the overall massage is designed in a logical progression that leaves the client with a feeling of completeness. Although a sequence might vary according to the situation, a pattern should be used that ensures that every part of the body is massaged properly and thoroughly.

Massage movements for adjacent areas as well as bilateral body parts should follow in sequence. For example, when beginning with the hand, the massage should progress to the arm and then to the shoulder. Then massage the other hand, arm, and shoulder, both shoulders, the neck, and the head. Finally, massage the chest, abdomen, one leg and foot, and then the other leg and foot. This completes the massage for the front of the body.

Developing a sequence also ensures a thorough massage that is balanced between one body part and another. The following is an example of an effective sequence to be used on each body area when giving a relaxing wellness massage.

1. Make contact with and undrape the body part to be massaged.
2. Apply massage lubricant with light effleurage.
3. Apply effleurage to accustom the body to your touch. Effleurage also flushes out the lymph and venous blood.
4. Apply petrissage, kneading the tissues to warm them. This also enables you to become aware of any areas of tension or congestion in the muscles.
5. Apply effleurage to flush the area.
6. Apply friction with any of the recommended friction techniques.
7. Apply deep gliding strokes to areas that seem especially tight or congested.
8. Apply effleurage to the entire area again, flushing the area while linking and integrating the segmented parts back into the whole.
9. Do joint movements to restore mobility by reinforcing the possibility of movement. At the same time, joint movements stretch the muscles and connective tissues and lubricate the joints.
10. Apply effleurage to flush out the loosened debris and to give a feeling of length to the body part.
11. Apply feather strokes. This stimulates the peripheral nervous system, smoothes the energy field, and says good-bye to that part of the body.
12. Re-drape the part of the body that has been massaged, undrape the next part, and continue until the client has been given a thorough massage.

Contact While Applying Lubricant

When you are ready to apply the massage lubricant to the client's skin, lay the back of your hand lightly against the part of the body to be massaged. Put enough lubricant in the palm of your hand to apply a thin film over the body part on which you are to work. Do not apply lubricant directly from the container to the body surface because it will feel cold to the client and cause discomfort. Lightly and briefly rub your hands together to spread the lubricant over both palms and warm the lubricant to body temperature. Warming the lubricant also makes it easier to spread it over the client's skin. Some practitioners prefer to use a massage lubricant holster that straps around the practitioner's waist and holds a lubricant bottle with a dispenser top. When more massage lubricant is needed, one hand maintains contact with the client while the other reaches for a couple of squirts of lubricant. Once the lubricant is obtained, the practitioner briefly rubs both hands together while maintaining contact to warm the lubricant before applying it to the client's body (Figure 12-11).

To apply lubricant efficiently, use long superficial strokes (effleurage) that cover the entire area to be massaged. As the lubricant is smoothed, strokes can become firmer. Effleurage is used to apply the lubricant and at the same time encourage the flow of body fluids toward the center of the body. Strokes should be continuous, pushing in the direction of the heart and then gliding back to the starting point. A good general rule is to keep the hand relaxed yet firm, so that even when passing over an obstacle such as the knee or shoulder, the hand is in complete contact with the client's skin.

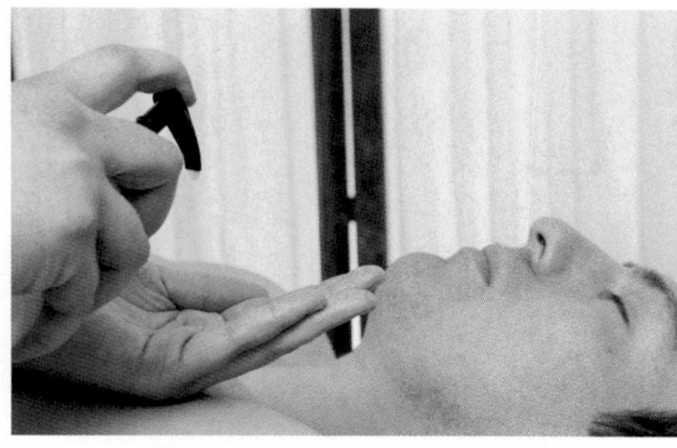

FIGURE 12-11 Before beginning massage movements, undrape the body part and apply the massage lubricant. With the back of your hands, maintain contact with the client's skin as you prepare to apply the massage lubricant.

PROCEDURE FOR A GENERAL BODY MASSAGE

When a student is performing a relaxing, full-body massage, it is helpful to follow a routine to ensure that each area of the body is massaged cohesively. As the student gains experience, the routine is modified to meet the individual needs and goals of the client and the session. Ideally, each massage that the student gives will be unique because every client is different, with individual concerns, needs, and preferences.

The following two massage routines are generalized, full-body routines in which the client begins in a supine position so that the front of the body is massaged and ends with the client in the prone position, concluding the full-body massage with a back massage.

The Massage 1 routine is flexible in that some steps can be omitted and others included. The first massage routine is a basic routine and designed as an introductory massage for both the student and the client. It begins with the hand and arm, the least vulnerable and most safely accessible area of the body. Massage 1 also does not include the face and head so that mussing the hair and makeup are not an issue. The student should follow the instructor's directions. The main objective is to give a beneficial and relaxing massage that is suited to the client's desires and needs.

1. **Preliminary steps:**
    a. Prepare the massage space by collecting all necessary supplies and arranging them as needed.
    b. Perform the consultation to determine the client's needs, determine any contraindications, and obtain informed consent.
    c. See that the client has all the items needed to prepare for the massage.
    d. Direct the client to the dressing room and explain the preparation procedures.
2. **Hydrotherapy (optional):**
    a. Select the bath most suitable for the client.
    b. Adjust the bath equipment and accessories.
    c. Take the temperature of the bath.
    d. Assist the client as necessary during the bath. Give the client water to drink, and take the client's pulse if necessary.

e. Assist the client as needed following the bath.
f. Allow the client to rest for a short period following the bath.

3. **Preparation for body massage:**
   a. Wash and sanitize your hands.
   b. Assist the client onto the massage table and into a supine (face-up) position.
   c. Drape the client's body with sheet or towel, with the exception of the part to be massaged.
4. **Order of treatment (overview):**

   The following procedure is suggested for a basic relaxing massage. It can be varied to suit the convenience of the practitioner and the needs of the client, however. Before beginning the massage, take a few deep, relaxing breaths to be more centered and grounded.
   a. Begin with the hands and arms, right then left.
   b. Proceed to front of the legs and feet, left then right.
   c. Continue movements over abdomen, chest, and neck.
   d. The client will turn over to assume a prone (face-down) position.
   e. Begin with the back of the legs, right then left.
   f. Finish the massage with the back of the body.

Following the massage, the client should be allowed to rest for a short period and then be assisted from the table.

Step-by-Step Procedures for Massage 1

The following step-by-step procedure helps you to learn basic massage techniques quickly. Draping is performed, and all preliminary steps are observed.

General Arm Massage

1. Undrape an arm and apply the lubricant with a light, smooth effleurage stroke from the shoulder to the hand.
2. Apply effleurage to the arm three times.
3. Knead the arm from the shoulder to the elbow.
4. Apply effleurage to the arm from the elbow to the shoulder.
5. Bend the elbow and rest it on the table.
6. Knead the forearm from the elbow to the wrist.
7. Apply effleurage to the forearm from the wrist to the elbow.
8. Apply petrissage and friction movements to the carpals and metacarpals on the back of the hand.
9. Knead the palm of the hand.
10. Knead and circumduct each finger.
11. Apply effleurage to the arm.
12. Roll the arm three times.
13. Apply joint movements to the arm.
14. Apply effleurage to the arm lightly three times.
15. Apply feather (nerve) strokes and re-drape the arm.
16. Move to the other arm and repeat the sequence.

Arm Movements for Body Massage

Depending on the client's requirements, the following movements can be included or omitted (Figure 12-12a-o):

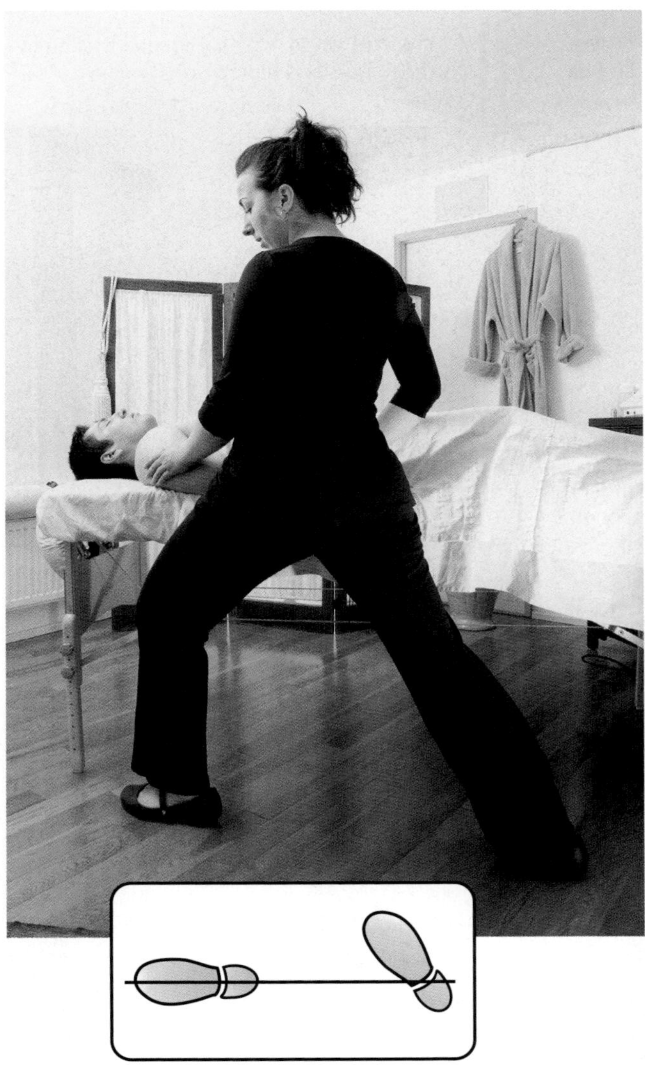

FIGURE 12-12A Proper stance and posture are important. Proper posture reduces fatigue, and proper stance allows mobility and power.

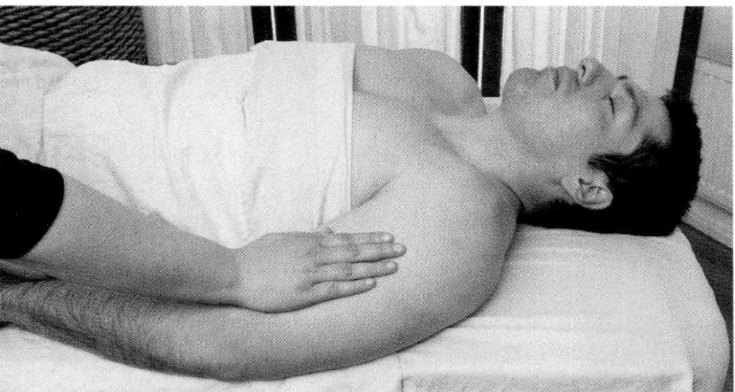

FIGURE 12-12B Apply effleurage to the arm from the hand to the shoulder using firmer pressure. Maintain contact with the arm for the return stroke from the shoulder to the hand, using lighter pressure.

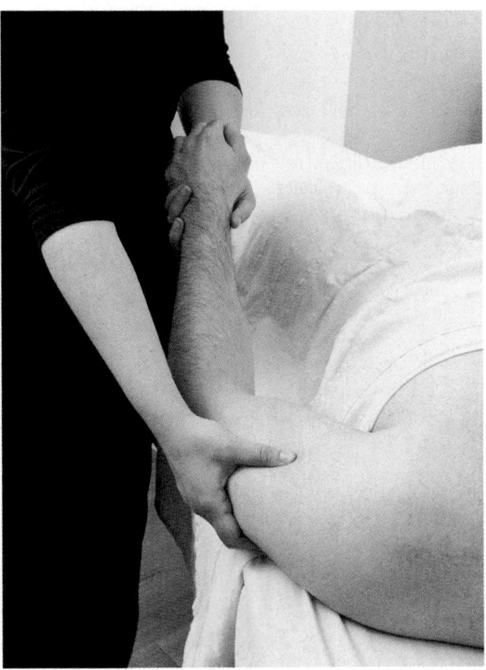

FIGURE 12-12C Apply effleurage to the back of the arm from the wrist to the shoulder with firmer pressure on the upward stroke and lighter pressure on the return.

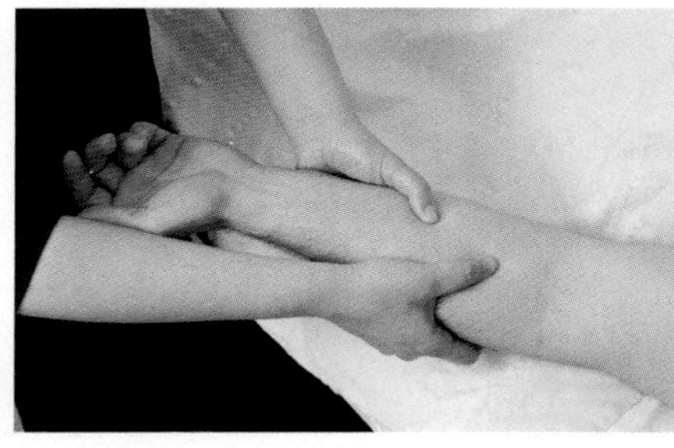

FIGURE 12-12D Knead the entire arm from the shoulder to the wrist.

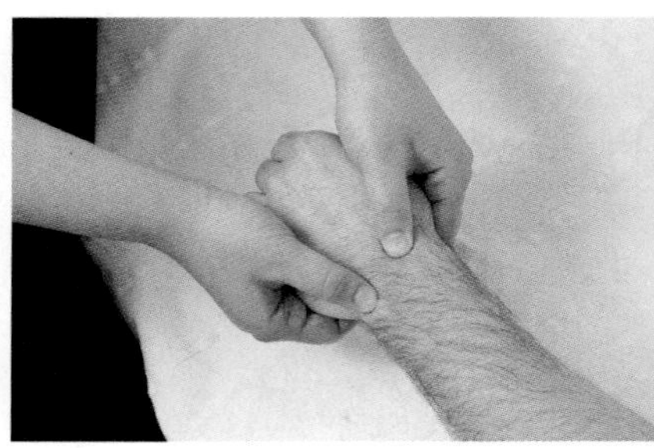

FIGURE 12-12E Knead the carpals and metacarpals of the wrist and hand.

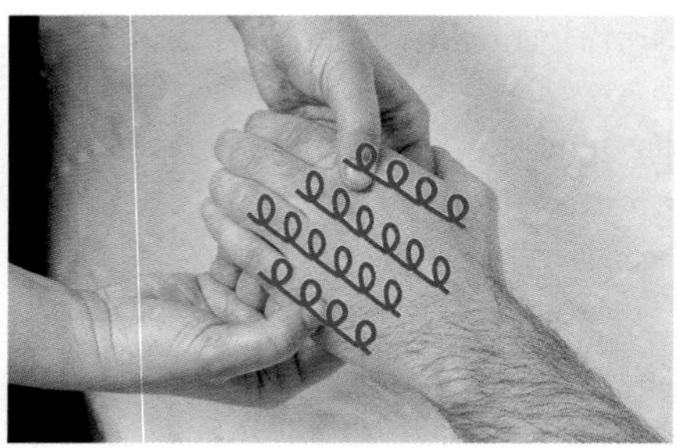

FIGURE 12-12F Apply circular friction to the fingers and hand.

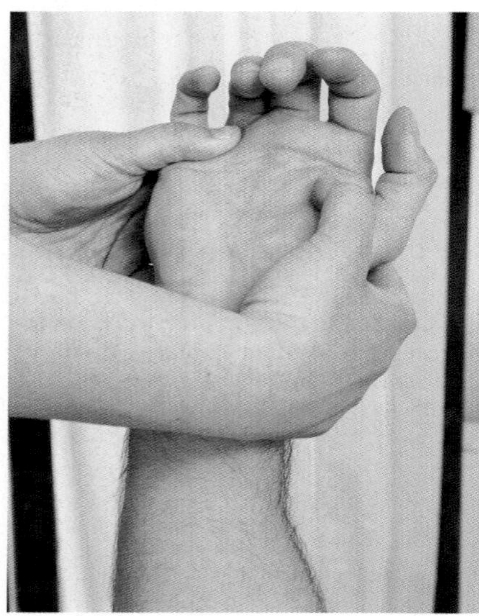

FIGURE 12-12G While holding the client's hand, massage the palm, back of the hand, metacarpals, fingers, and upward over the wrist.

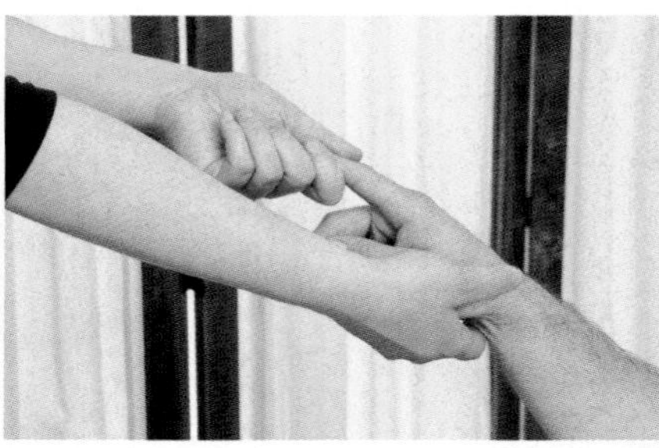

FIGURE 12-12H Hold the forearm firmly. Rotate and circumduct the wrist. Knead and rotate each finger as you circumduct and apply traction.

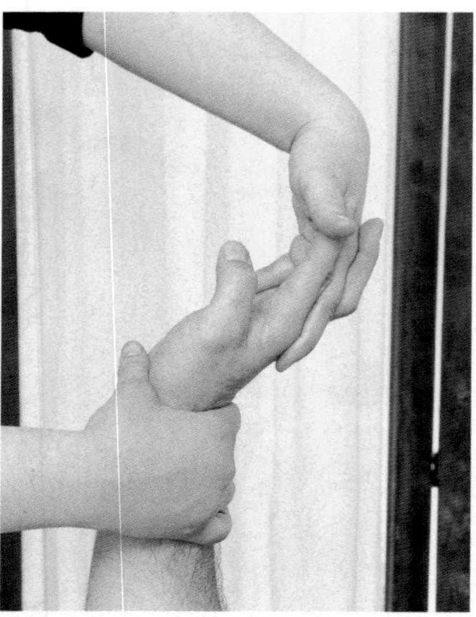

FIGURE 12-12I Apply joint movements and rotation. Note the interlacing of the fingers.

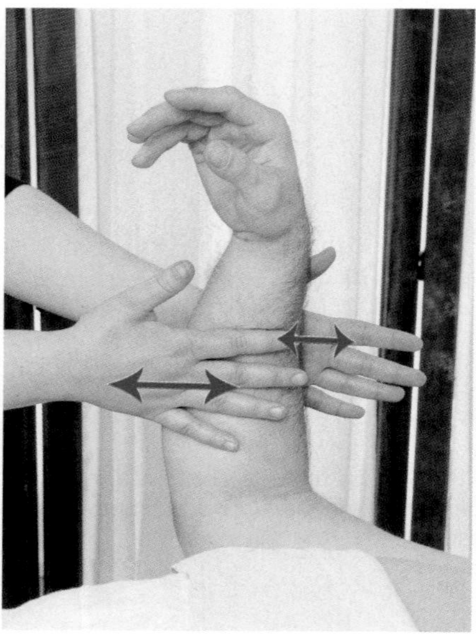

FIGURE 12-12J Roll the arm.

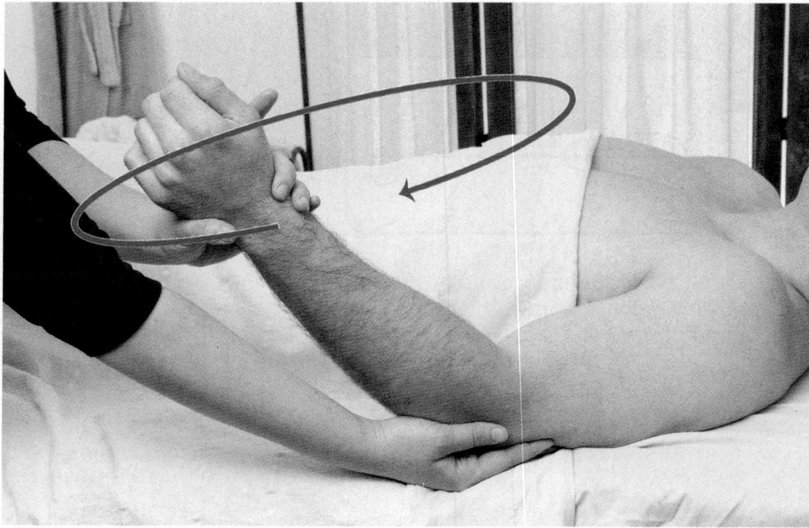

FIGURE 12-12K Rotate the forearm. Note how the fingers are used to steady the client's elbow.

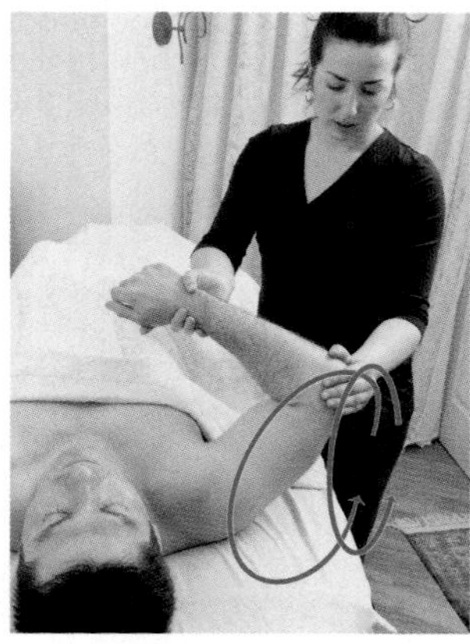

FIGURE 12-12L Rotate the shoulder by moving the elbow. Note how the other hand supports the client's hand.

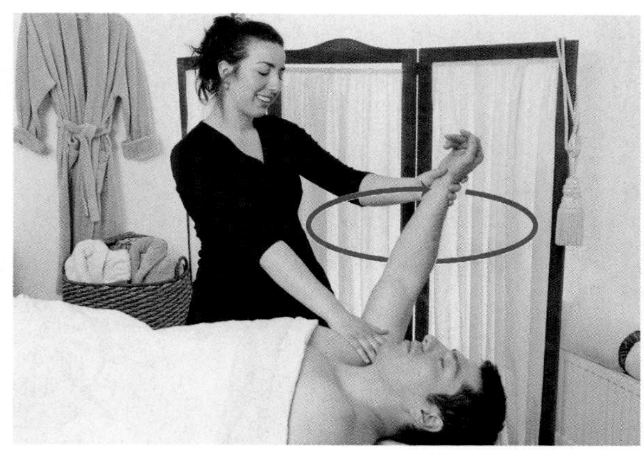

FIGURE 12-12M Circumduct the shoulder.

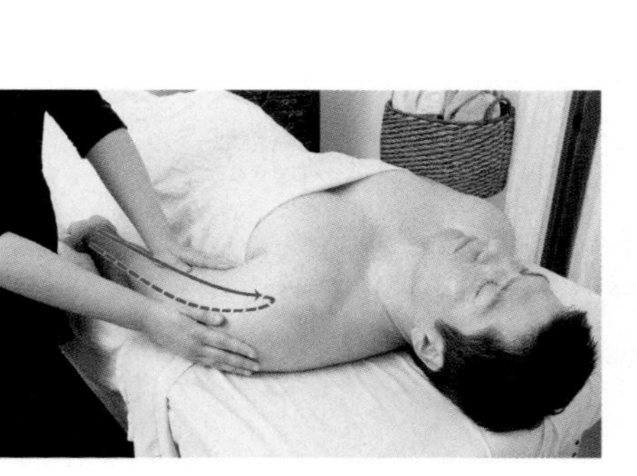

FIGURE 12-12N Repeat gliding strokes to the lateral and medial aspects of the arm.

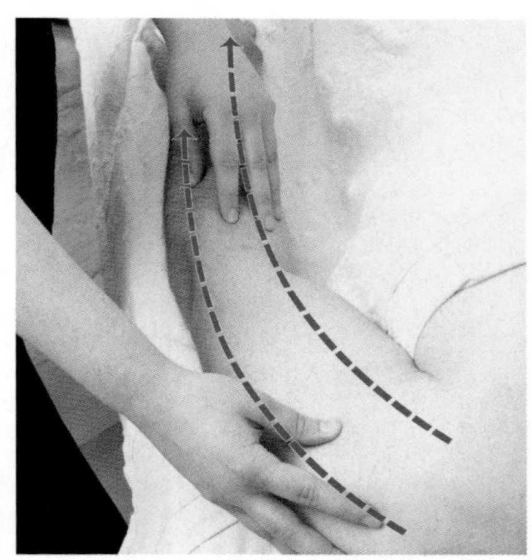

FIGURE 12-12O Apply feather strokes (*nerve strokes*) with your fingertips to complete the massage of the arm. Perform the massage for the other arm using the same sequence of movements.

General Massage for the Foot and Leg

1. Undrape one leg (on the same side of the body as the arm that was just completed) and apply lubricant with a light, smooth effleurage stroke from the foot to the hip and back to the foot.
2. Apply effleurage to the leg three times.
3. Apply kneading or petrissage to the entire foot
4. Apply circular friction between the tendons and other surfaces of the foot.
5. Rotate each toe three times.
6. Apply petrissage to the leg three times.
7. Wring and roll the leg.
8. Apply effleurage to the leg three times.
9. Apply joint movements to the foot, ankle and leg.
10. Apply effleurage to the leg lightly three times.
11. Apply nerve strokes and re-drape the leg.
12. Move to the other leg and complete the sequence.

Massage for the Foot and Leg

Depending on the client's requirements, the following movements may be included or omitted (Figure 12-13a and b and Figure 12-14a-q).

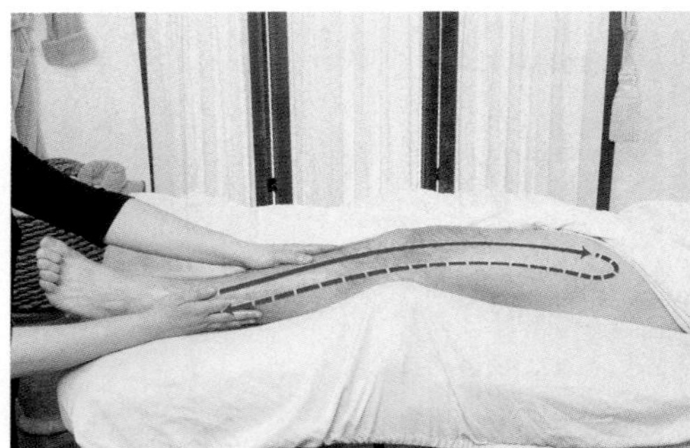

FIGURE 12-13A Apply effleurage to the leg in long movements from the ankle to the hip. Apply more pressure on the stroke up the leg, and maintain light contact as your hands glide back to the starting point.

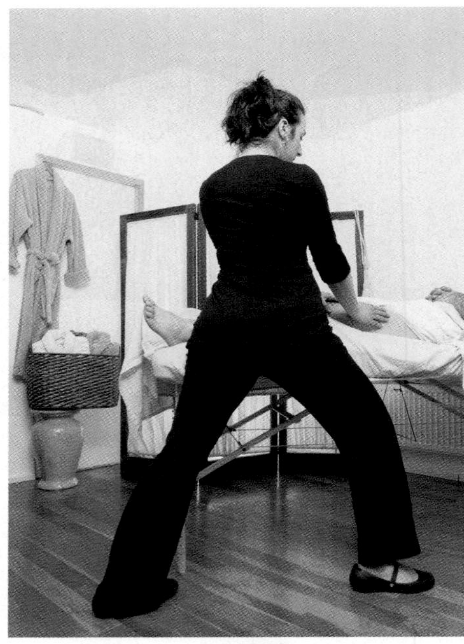

FIGURE 12-13B Use good body mechanics. A wide archer stance allows the therapist to stroke the entire leg.

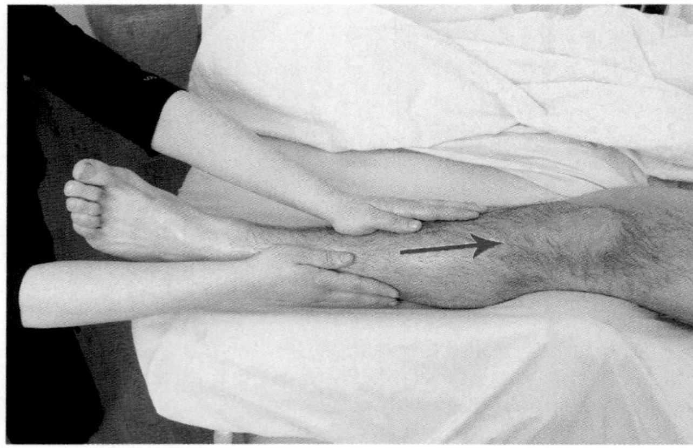

FIGURE 12-14A Apply more pressure on the stroke in the direction of venous blood and lymph flow.

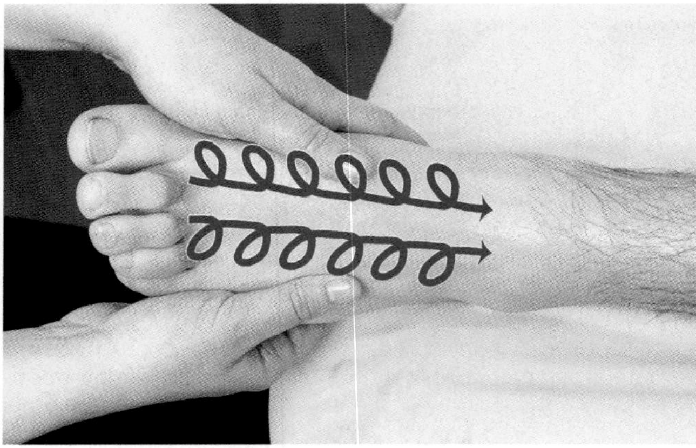

FIGURE 12-14B Knead the top and bottom of the foot.

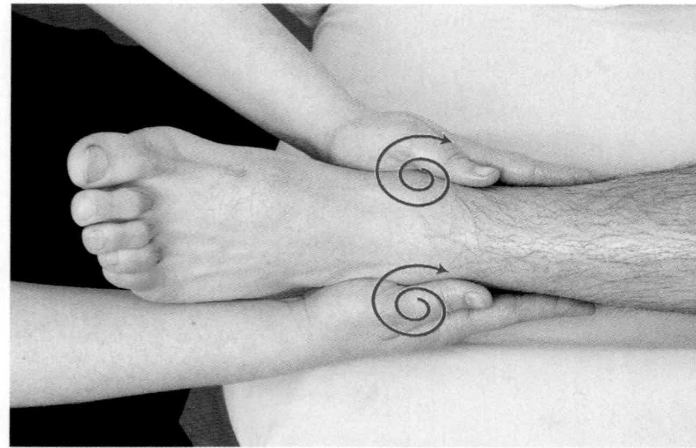

FIGURE 12-14C Warm the foot and ankles with circular rubbing movements.

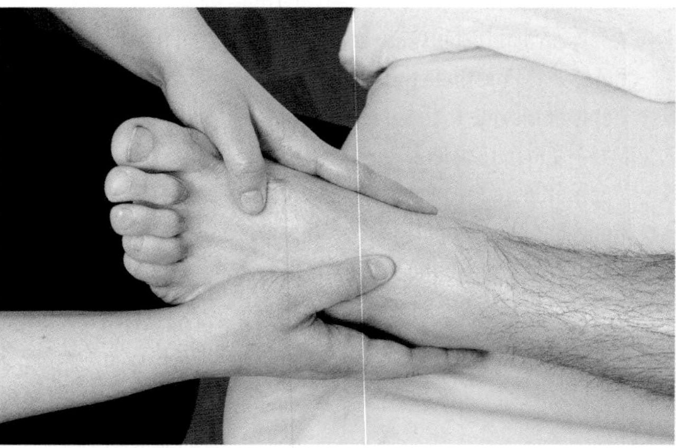

FIGURE 12-14D Apply digital friction between the tendons and bones on all surfaces of the foot.

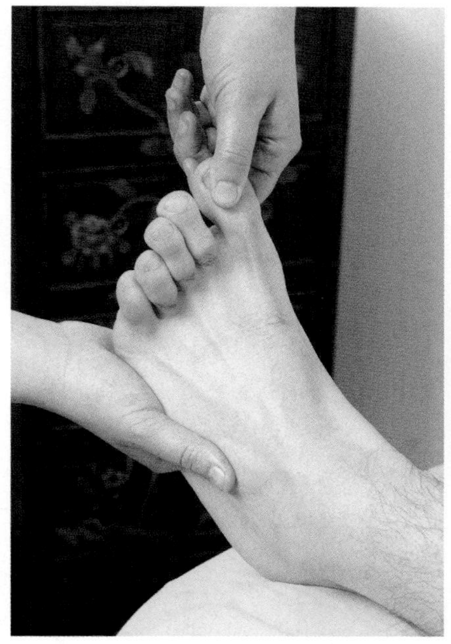

FIGURE 12-14E Massage and rotate each digit.

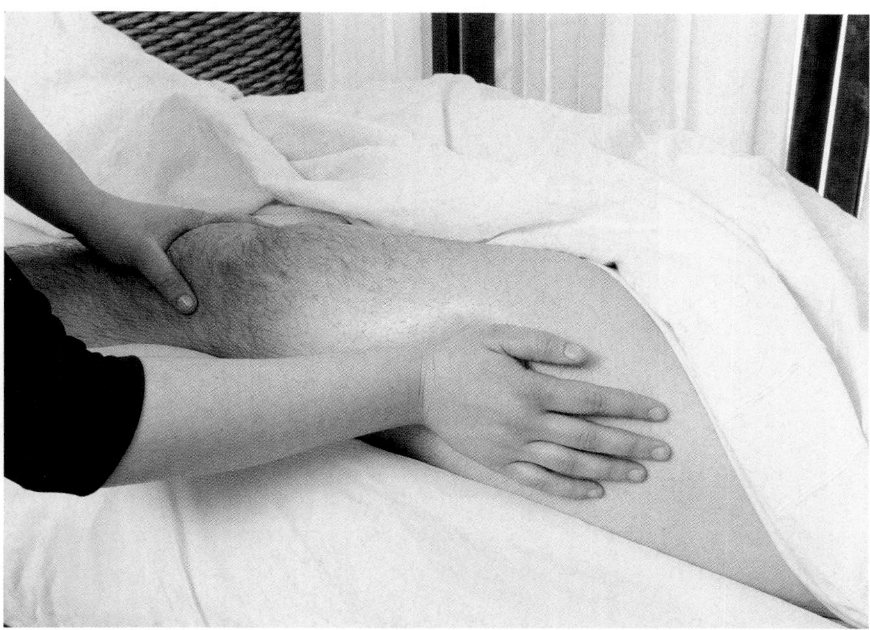

FIGURE 12-14F Knead the leg and thigh in a circular motion.

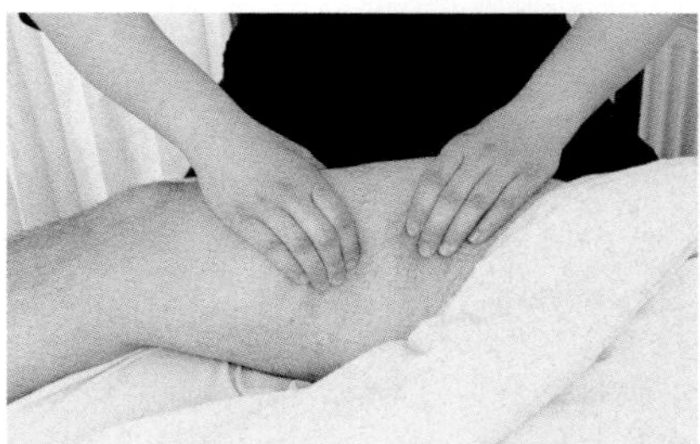

FIGURE 12-14G Apply petrissage to the anterior thigh.

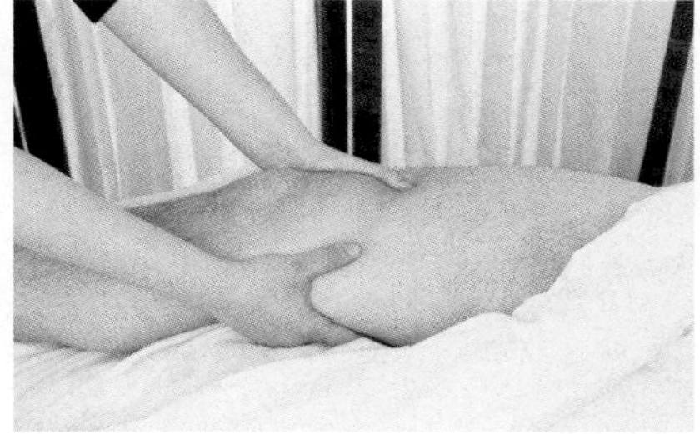

FIGURE 12-14H Apply fulling (compression) movements.

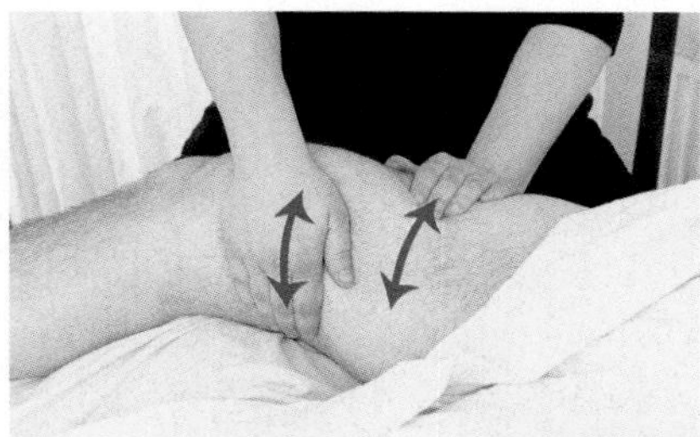

FIGURE 12-14I Wring the muscles of the thigh.

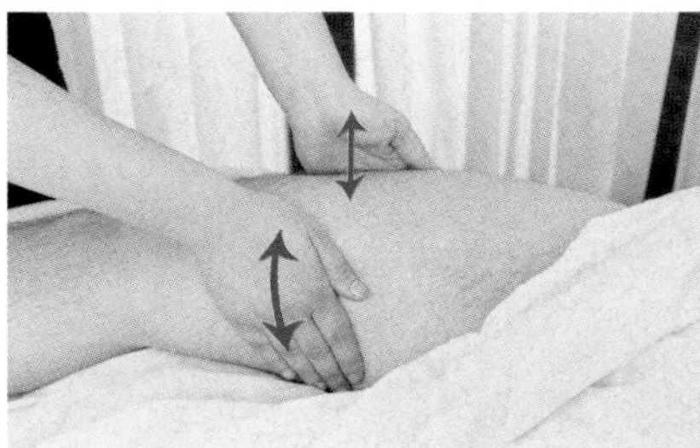

FIGURE 12-14J Roll the muscles of the thigh.

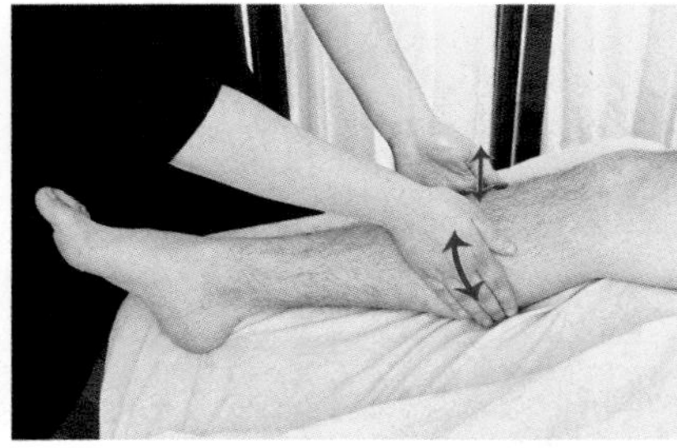

FIGURE 12-14K Roll the muscles of the leg.

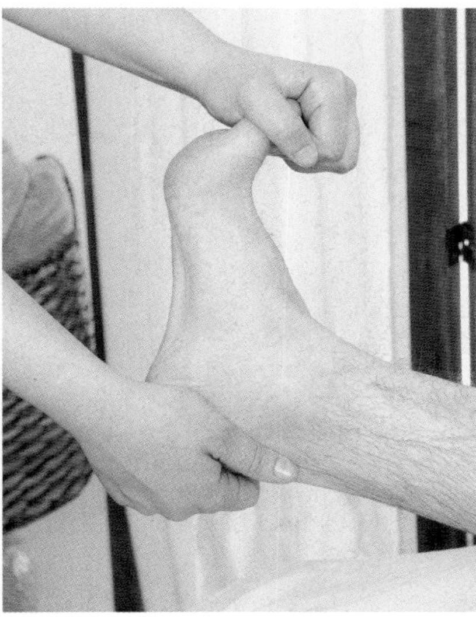

FIGURE 12-14L Stretch the plantar surface of the foot and toes.

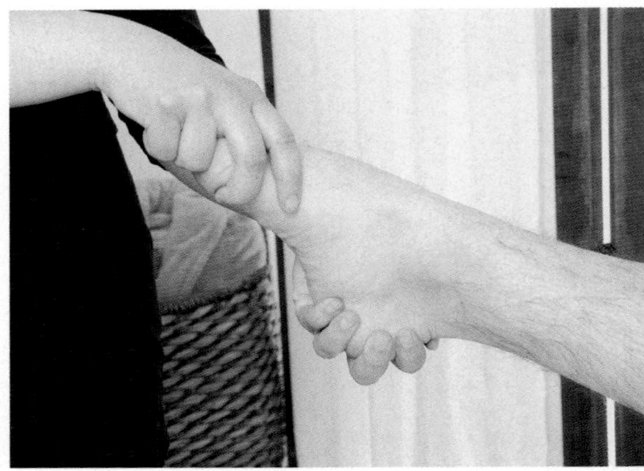

FIGURE 12-14M Stretch the dorsal aspect of the foot and toes.

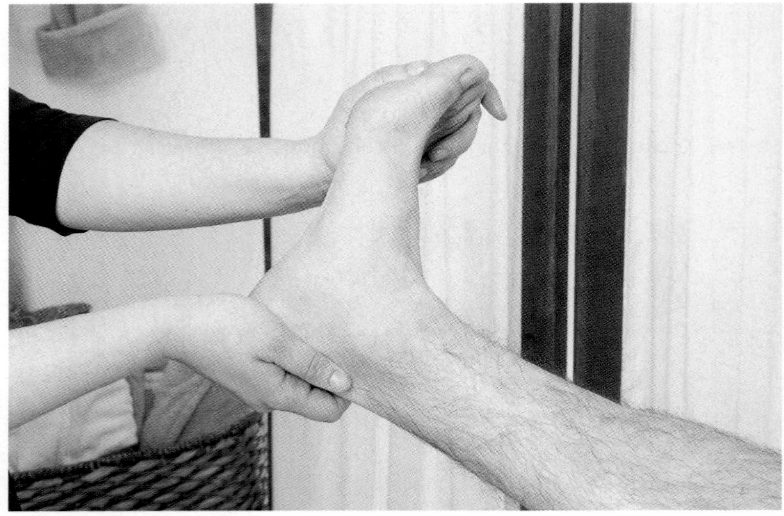

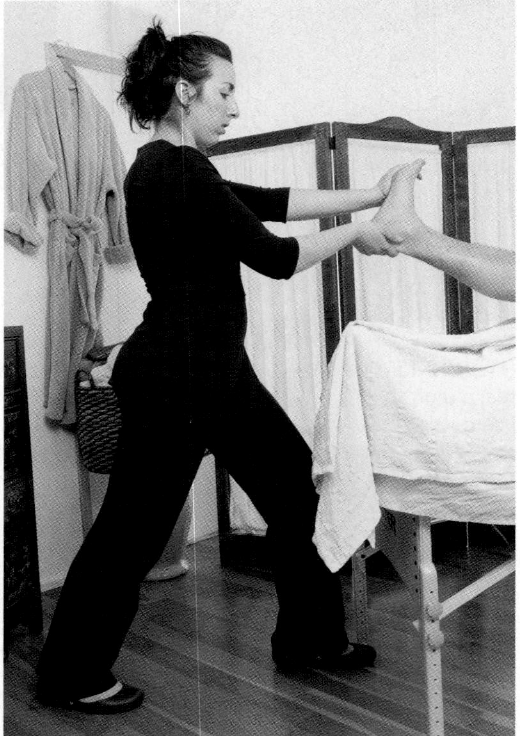

FIGURE 12-14N(1-2) Stretch the Achilles tendon. Note the position of the hands.

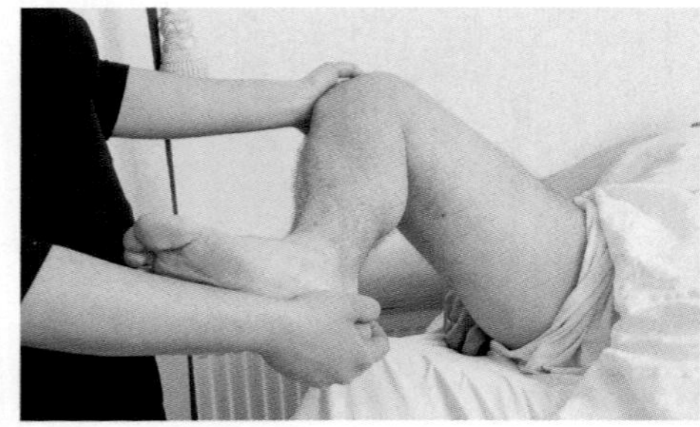

FIGURE 12-14O Apply joint movements. Move the client's knee all the way to the chest. This position also can be used for joint rotations of the hip and knee in the range of motion. Note the position of the hands at the heel and knee.

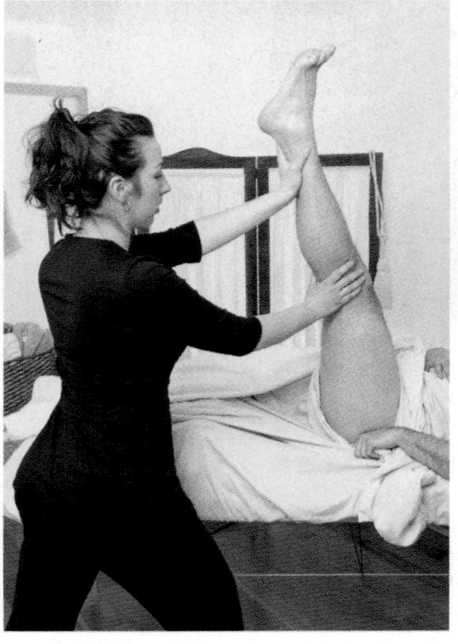

FIGURE 12-14P Apply hamstring stretching movements.

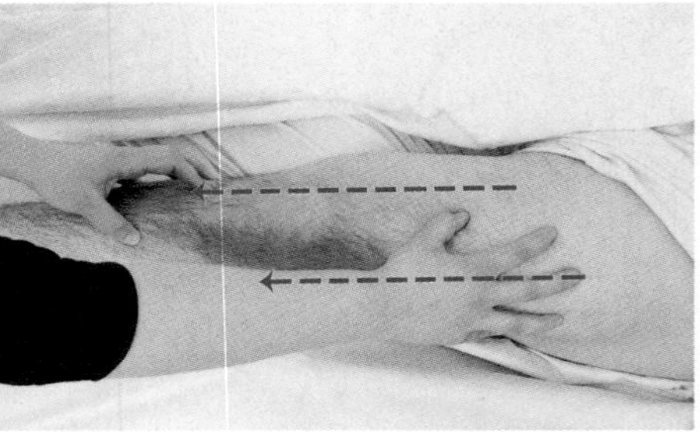

FIGURE 12-14Q Complete the massage of the front of the leg with a nerve stroke, then re-drape and continue to the next part.

General Massage for the Anterior Torso and Neck

1. On a male client, undrape the torso to a level midway between the navel and the pubic bone to expose the abdomen. On a female, use breast draping. Some of the following strokes can be modified to accommodate the breast drape.
2. Standing on the right side of the client, apply circular effleurage on the abdomen in a clockwise direction, following the direction of the colon.
3. Apply deep gliding strokes to the opposite side of the body from near the table to the midline of the body (these repeated gliding strokes are commonly referred to as **shingles**). Begin the first stroke just inferior to the crest of the ilium. When the first stroke is near the midline, begin the next stroke with the other hand. Continue alternating hands moving slowly up the body toward the axilla. In the area of the ribs, flex the fingertips for a raking effect between the ribs. (When using breast draping, proceed up the side of the torso as far as the draping will allow and then back down to the hip.
4. Continue the alternate-hand effleurage (shingles) to the axillary area, over the shoulder and up the neck.
5. Switch sides of the table and continue the shingles stroke down the other side of the torso from the neck to the ilium then back to the axillary area, once again raking over the ribs.
6. Apply petrissage to the pectoral area, first one side, then the other. (Avoid breast tissue on women.)
7. Move to the head of the table. Stroke the chest three times. Stroke down the chest, around to the sides, coming up under each arm, and up and over the shoulders to the neck. (This stroke is not done with breast draping.)
8. Re-drape the torso.
9. From the head of the table, apply effleurage with both hands, beginning at the sternal notch, out over and around the shoulders, up the trapezius to the occipital ridge three to five times.
10. Turn the client's head to one side and apply petrissage and circular friction to the back and sides of the neck and shoulders.
11. Apply deep gliding strokes from the occiput down the shoulders.
12. Turn the client's head to the other side and repeat steps #10 and #11.
13. Repeat step No. 9.

shingles

a short, repeated gliding stroke using alternating hands

Anterior Torso and Neck Movements

Depending on the client's requirements, the practitioner may include or omit any of the following movements (Figure 12-15a-k).

Changing Position

The client turns over to a prone, face-down position. Maintain proper draping to prevent exposure while turning the client.

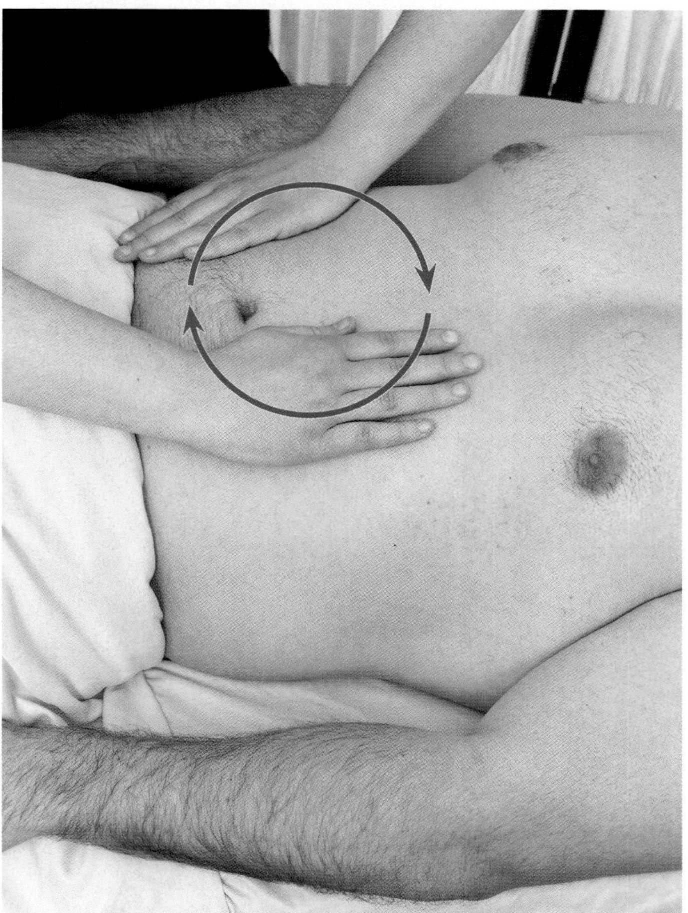

FIGURE 12-15A Apply circular effleurage on the abdomen in a clock-wise direction

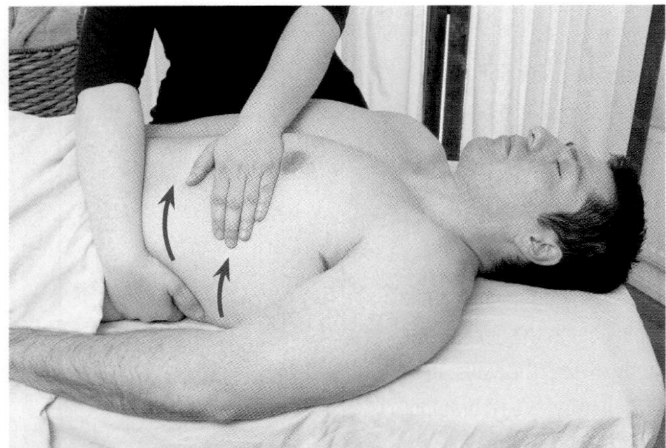

FIGURE 12-15B Apply alternate hand stroking (shingles) from the ilium to the axillary area.

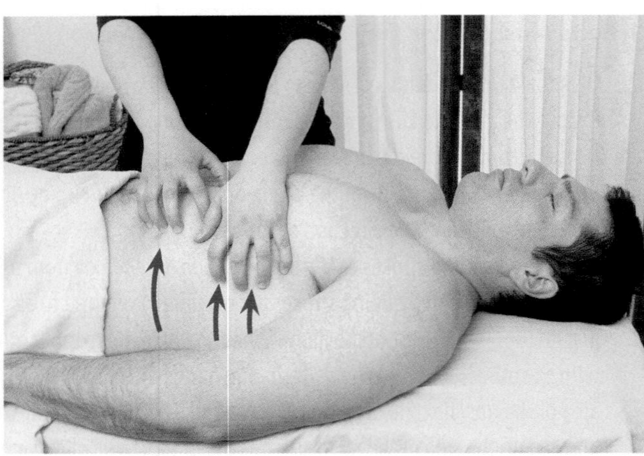

FIGURE 12-15C Raking is done by flexing the tips of the fingers and stroking along the ribs from the table to the midline of the body.

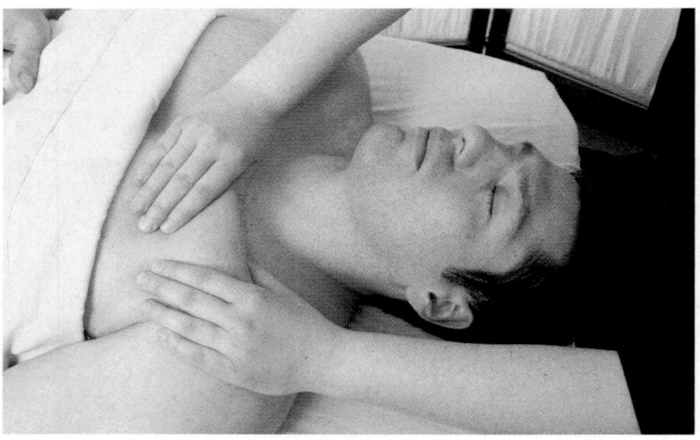

FIGURE 12-15D Apply petrissage and friction to the pectoral muscles.

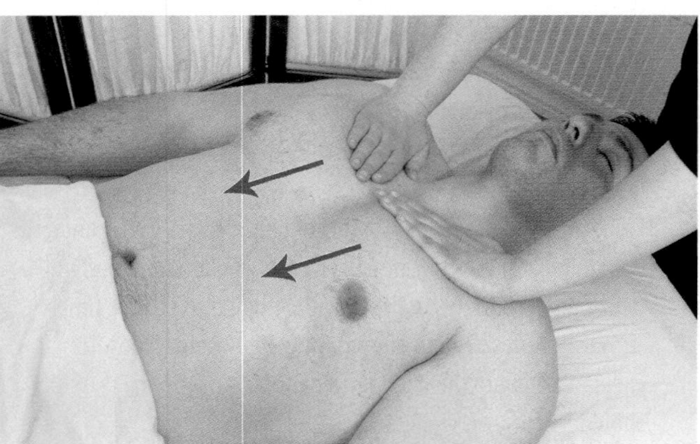

FIGURE 12-15E Using the caring stroke, cover the entire front of the body and the neck. It is not possible to do the full caring stroke on women when using breast draping.

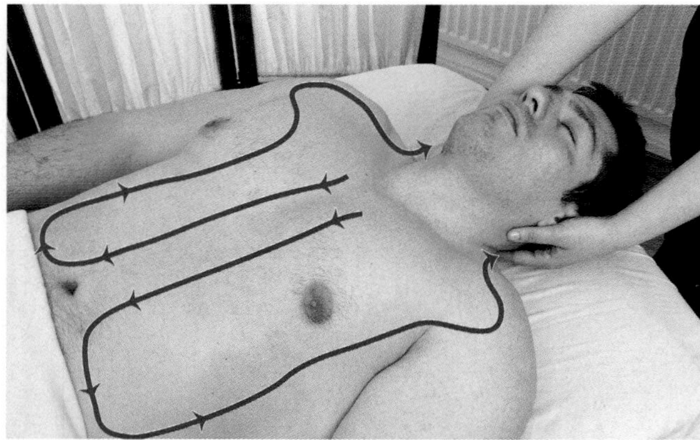

FIGURE 12-15F The stroke begins at the clavicle with a stroke down the front of the body to the pubic bone. Without losing contact with the client, rotate your hands to the sides of the client's body and stroke up to the axillary area. Stroke up, over, and around the shoulders and up the neck.

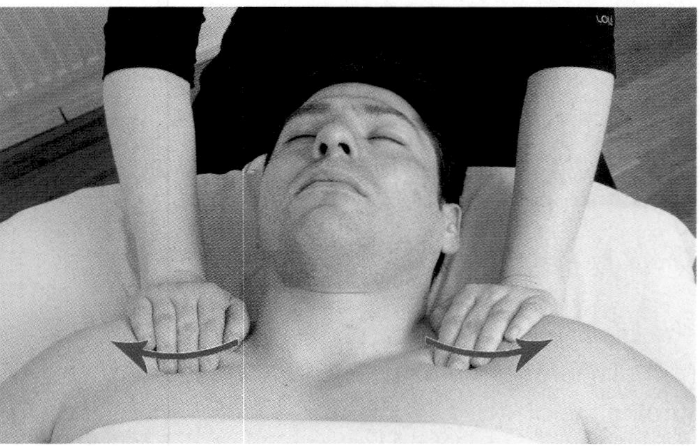

FIGURE 12-15G Apply effleurage from the sternal notch and over the shoulders.

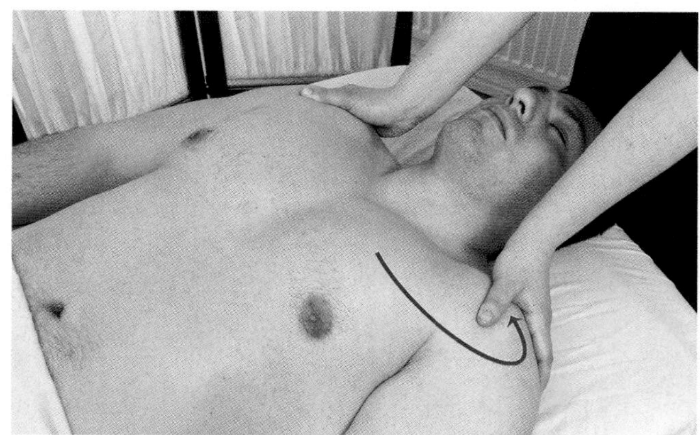

FIGURE 12-15H Continue the movement across the shoulder and around the deltoid.

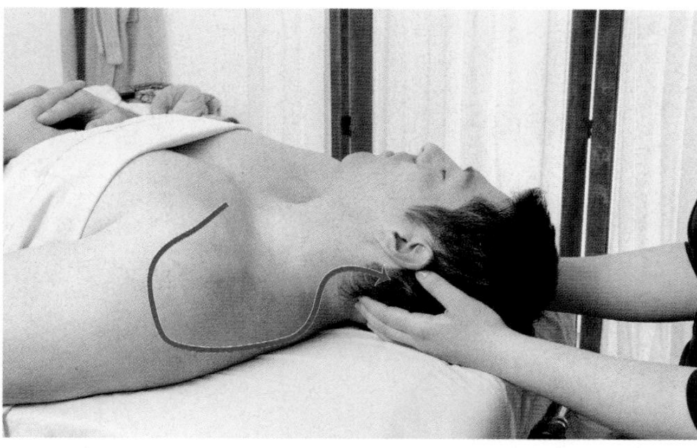

FIGURE 12-15I Continue the movement up the trapezius to the occipital ridge.

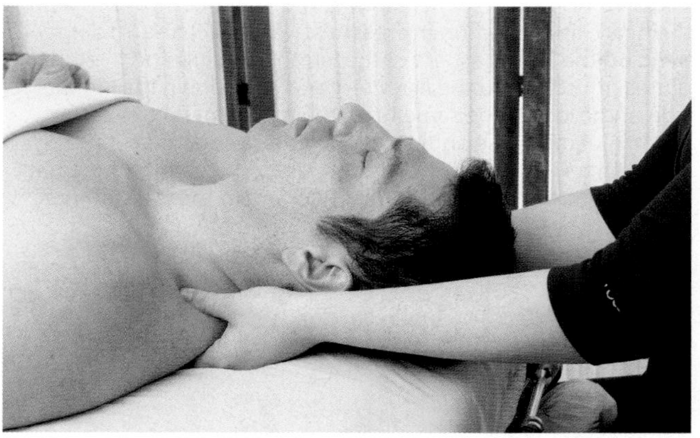

FIGURE 12-15J Apply petrissage to the neck and shoulders.

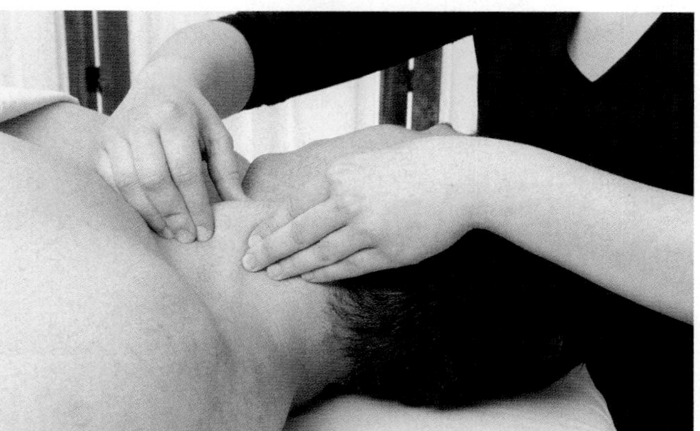

FIGURE 12-15K Apply petrissage to the back of the neck and shoulder region.

General Massage for the Back of the Legs

1. Undrape one leg and apply lubricant.
2. Move the leg closer to the edge of the table and apply effleurage from the heel to the hip three times.
3. Apply petrissage to the leg from the hips to the heels.
4. Knead the bottom of the foot from the heel to the toes.
5. Apply fulling, wringing, and rolling to the lower leg and thigh.
6. Apply effleurage to leg three times.
7. Apply nerve strokes and re-drape.
8. Undrape the other leg and repeat steps 2 - 7.

Back of Leg Movements for Body Massage

Depending on the client's requirements, the following movements can be included or omitted (Figure 12-16a-g).

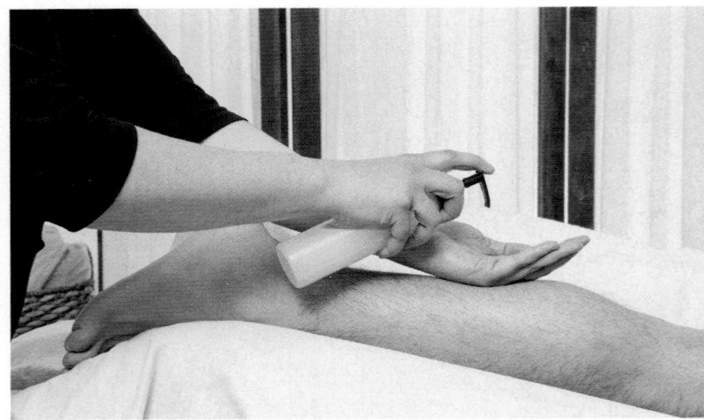

FIGURE 12-16A Before beginning massage movements, prepare the posterior leg by draping and applying lubricant.

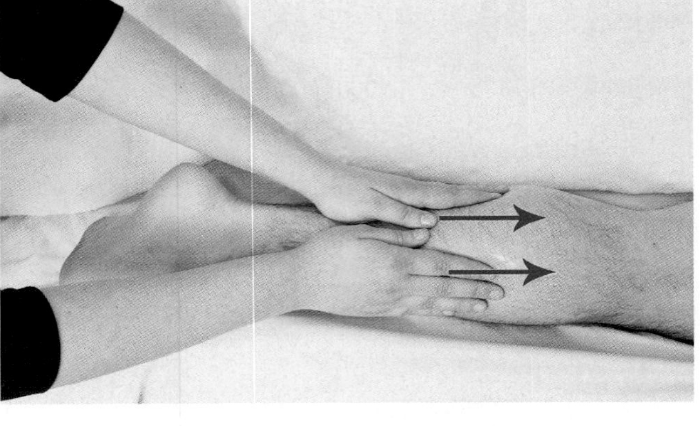

FIGURE 12-16B Apply effleurage to the leg upward with both hands.

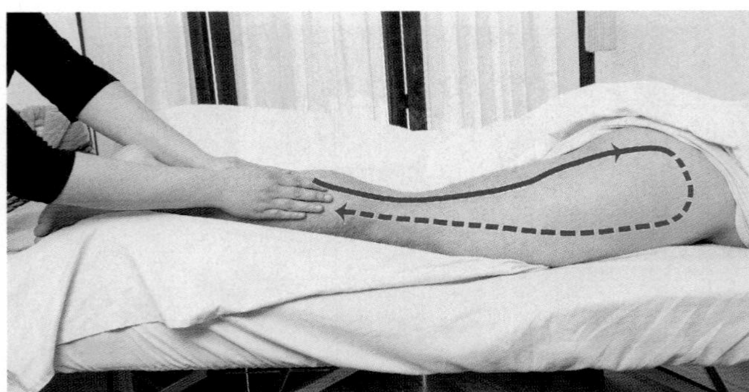

FIGURE 12-16C Apply effleurage movements. Stroke toward the heart, applying firmer **pressure.** *Note:* Place the leading hand on the lateral aspect of the leg to travel up and over the gluteal muscles and the iliac crest and back down the lateral side of the leg. At the same time, the medial hand travels up to the gluteal crease and back down the medial side of the leg. Both hands maintain contact, using much lighter pressure as they return to the starting point to repeat the stroke three or more times.

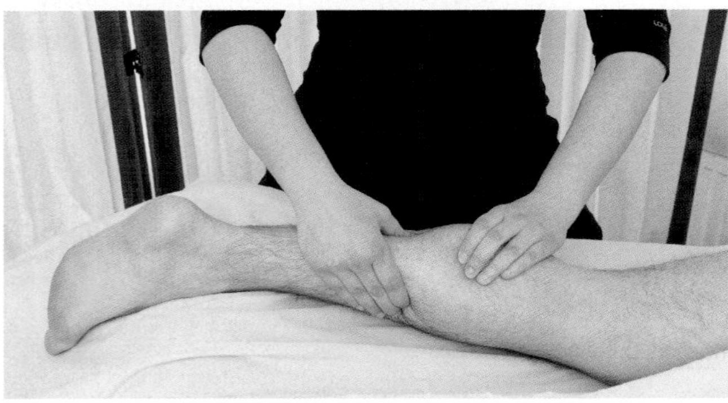

FIGURE 12-16D Knead the calf muscles.

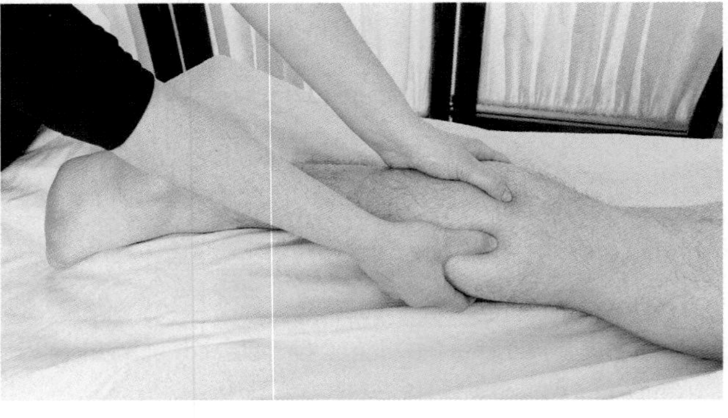

FIGURE 12-16E Apply fulling or compression strokes to the entire leg.

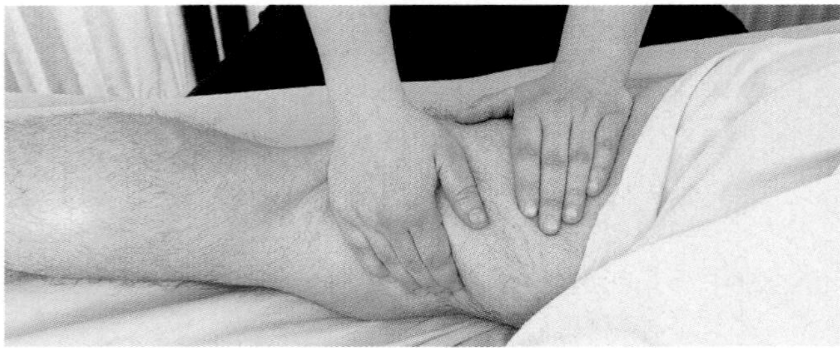

FIGURE 12-16F Apply wringing to the back of the leg.

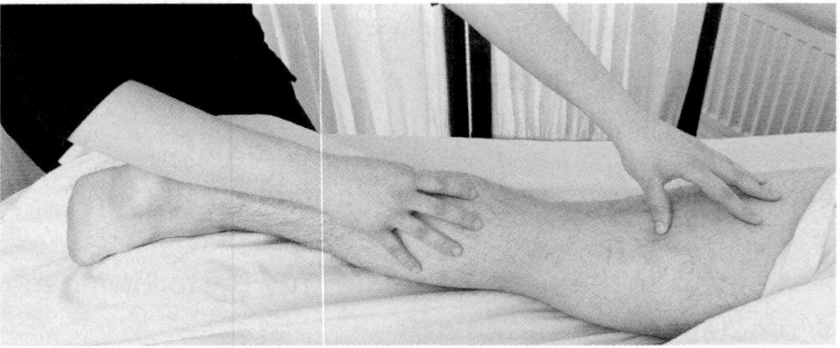

FIGURE 12-16G Complete the massage of the posterior leg with several feather strokes (nerve stroke) from the hip to the foot.

General Massage for the Back of the Body

1. Undrape and apply lubricant to the back.
2. Standing at the side of the client, apply effleurage to the back five times going up along the muscles on each side of the spine and then down on the side of the back.
3. Place the hands flat on each side of the spine at the level of the scapulas and stretch them outward toward the shoulders.
4. Continue step #3 down along each side of the spine to cover the entire back (fan stroke).
5. Vibrate along each side of the vertebral column from the neck to the sacrum.
6. Apply petrissage on the entire back and on each side of the torso.
7. Apply deep gliding strokes on the side of the torso from the table to the center of the back (shingles) from the hips to the shoulders.
8. Move to the other side of the table and repeat step #7.
9. From the head of the table, apply effleurage to the back three times. From the back of the neck, stroke down along the length of the muscles on the side of the spine, around to the side of the body, up the sides, around and over the shoulders up to the neck, and repeat.
10. Move to the side of the table and apply light hacking movements along the muscles along the side of the spine, between the shoulders, over the gluteal muscles, and the back of the legs. Avoid percussion over the kidney area.
11. From the side of the table, apply effleurage to the back lightly several times.
12. Apply nerve strokes to the entire back, from the head all the way to the feet.
13. Re-drape the back and complete the massage.

Back Movements for Body Massage

Depending on the client's requirements, the following movements can be included or omitted (Figure 12-17a-l).

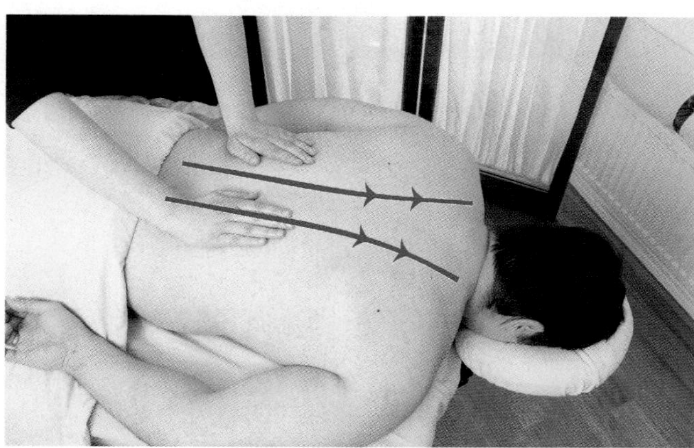

FIGURE 12-17A Begin at the gluteal cleft and apply long strokes up along the muscles on each side of the spine.

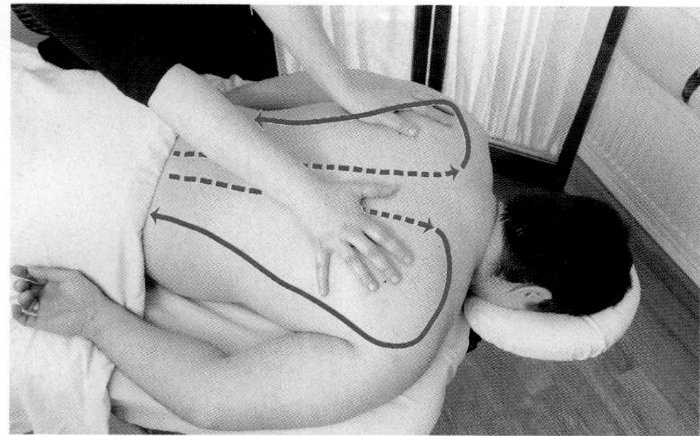

FIGURE 12-17B Continue with effleurage strokes up the back and over the shoulders and down the sides of the back to the hips.

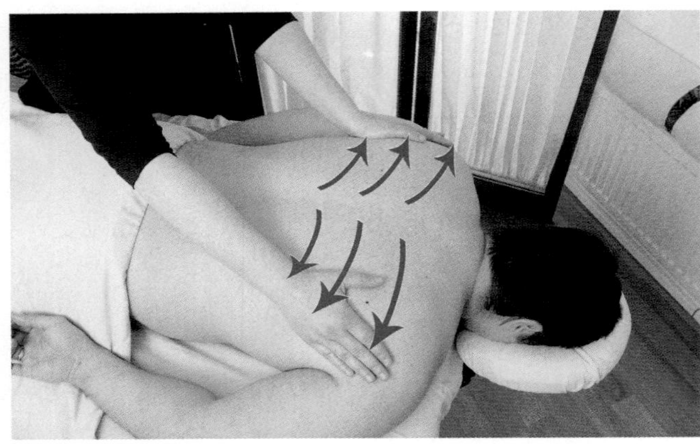

FIGURE 12-17C Stroke the muscles of the back outward.

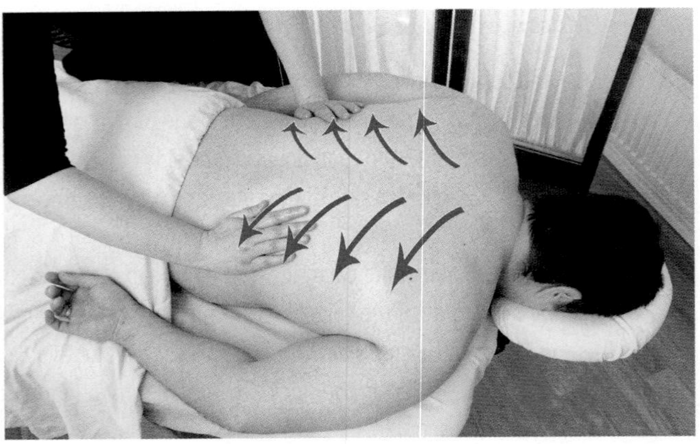

FIGURE 12-17D Use fan stroking on the back.

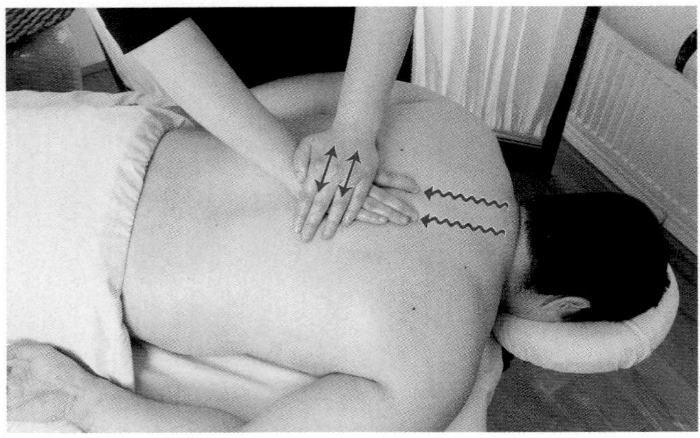

FIGURE 12-17E Apply vibration movements along each vertebra by placing the fingers of one hand on each side of the spinous process and the other hand on top. Vibrate back and forth as you move down along the spine.

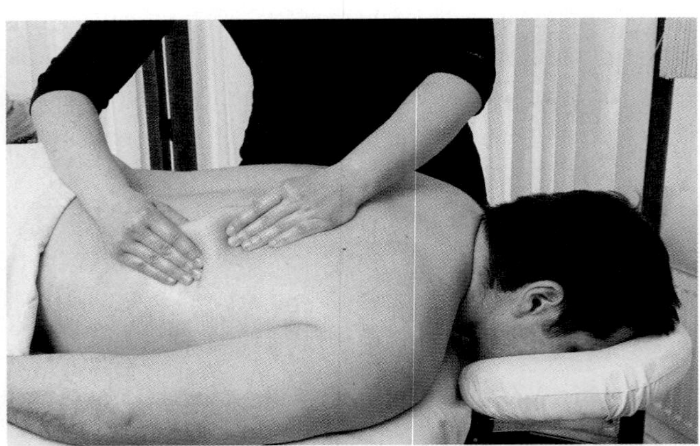

FIGURE 12-17F Apply petrissage to the entire side that is opposite from you. This takes several passes.

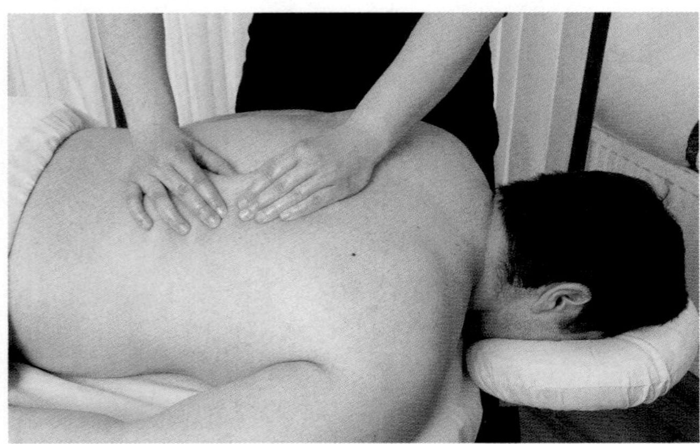

FIGURE 12-17G Knead around the spine.

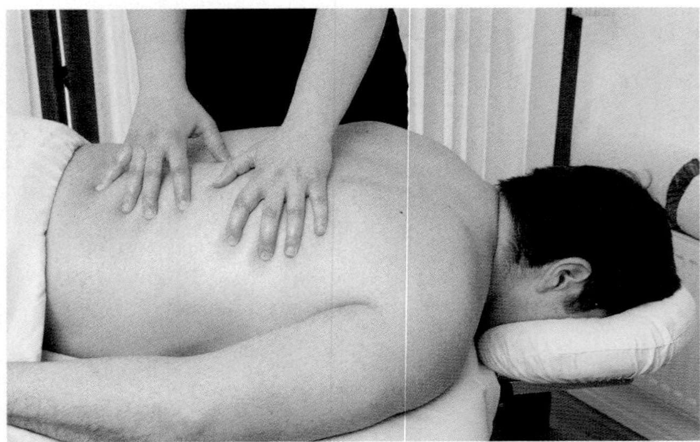

FIGURE 12-17H Apply raking in alternate strokes so that the tips of the fingers glide between the ribs.

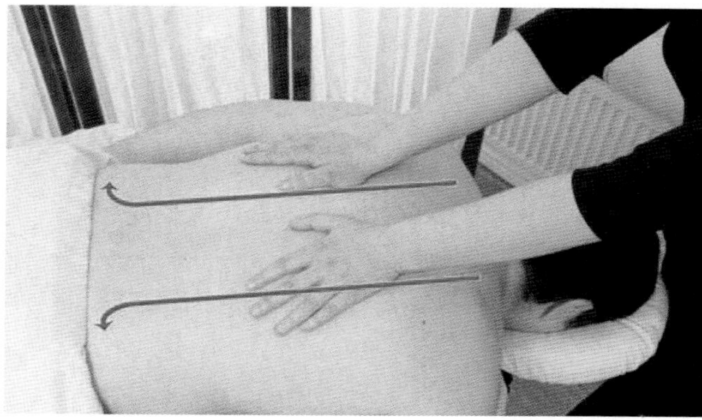

FIGURE 12-17I Apply effleurage movements down the back, over and around the gluteal muscles, back up the sides, then over and around the shoulders to the nape of the neck.

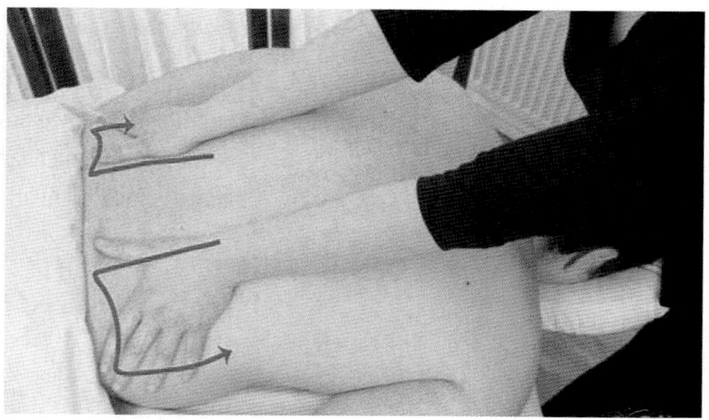

FIGURE 12-17J Continue the caring stroke down the back and over the gluteal muscles.

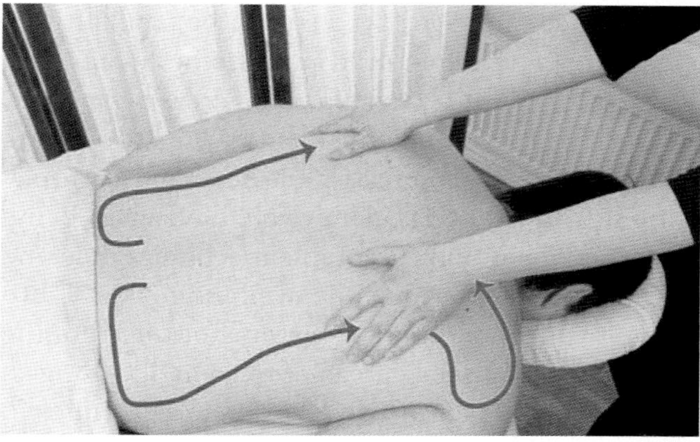

FIGURE 12-17K The caring stroke is a continuous movement that proceeds up the side and around the shoulder to return to the starting point.

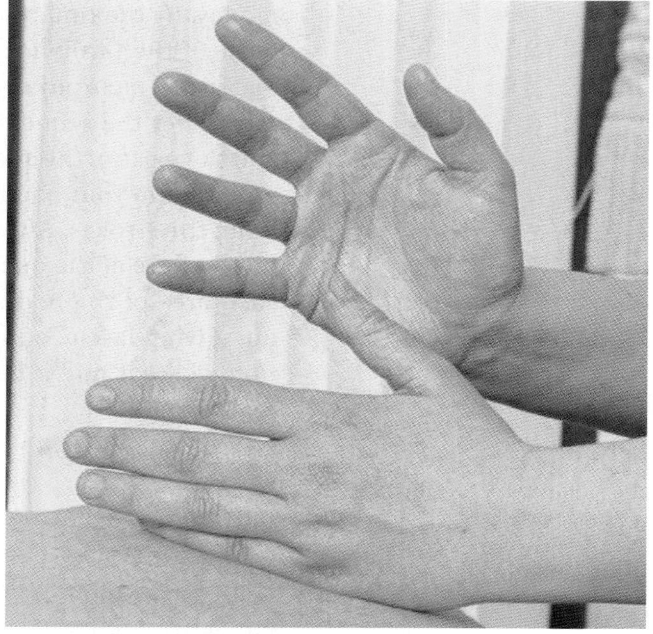

FIGURE 12-17L Apply hacking movements to the back.

Completing the Treatment

1. After completing the final strokes, maintain light contact. Allow the client a few moments to savor the deep relaxation while returning to a more conscious state. Adjust the draping, and suggest that the client turn onto either side. Place a small pillow under the head, bend the knees, and allow the client to rest a few minutes.
2. When it is time to get up, instruct the client to put both legs over the edge of the table and push into a sitting position with the upper arm. Upon sitting up, the client can secure the wrap. You may assist the client by placing a hand under the shoulder and lifting into a sitting position.
3. Suggest supplementary services and answer any questions that the client might have.
4. When the client is totally awake and reoriented, assist the client off the table and indicate where the dressing area is located.
5. After the client is dressed, collect your fees and set up the next appointment.

Final Considerations

1. Complete the client's record or SOAP notes.
2. Place supplies in their proper place; discard used items.
3. See that all equipment and items, including the massage table and bath, are properly prepared before the next client arrives.

PROCEDURE FOR PROFESSIONAL BODY MASSAGE

Massage 2

Massage, like any other skill, requires practice and patience to learn the basics, build speed, and develop new techniques. Each time you give a massage, you will find yourself becoming more innovative and more confident of your techniques. By the time you have learned Massage 1, you should be familiar with most of the terms for the various movements used in basic body massage. Massage 2 incorporates additional techniques to help you increase efficiency, remember the sequence of movements, and readily identify the movements and the parts of the anatomy by their proper names. While doing massage, pay attention to your hand positions, your stance, and how you move when delivering the strokes. Always maintain good body and table mechanics. Become more aware of the qualities of the tissues as you glide over and massage into each area of the body. Be sensitive to the different textures of the skin, the underlying fascia, and muscles. Begin to sense areas of tension and congestion where it might be appropriate to linger or use additional techniques in that area.

Massage 2 enables you to review what you have learned and allows even more creativity in varying massage routines. Before beginning the massage, concentrate on projecting the manner, attitude, and appearance of the professional massage practitioner. Read directions carefully for each step. After you have learned how to give a complete massage correctly and efficiently, you will no longer need to refer to your notes, illustrations, or written guides. Your aim is to be able to give the complete massage knowledgeably and professionally.

Preliminary Steps

1. Prepare the facility and all products.
2. Before the client arrives, take a few quiet moments to prepare yourself with deep breathing, stretching, centering, and grounding.
3. If this is the client's first visit, be ready to greet the client on time and introduce yourself with a handshake. In many places of business, the practitioner is addressed by the first name. For example, when introducing yourself to a new client, you might say, "Good morning, Mrs. Mason, I'm Carolyn. I'll be working with you today." You do not address the client by first name unless it is customary to do so or if the client requests that you do so.

4. The first step with any client is the consultation or interview (see Chapter 9). Have the client fill out the information sheet first, and review it with the client to obtain more direct information. Discuss the client's needs and expectations and the kind of massage that the client prefers. Determine if there are any specific areas of concern . This is the time to observe the client's physical condition and determine which benefits might be derived from the massage or whether the client should be referred to another health care professional.
5. Put first-time clients at ease by showing the facility and explaining the services.
6. Explain to the client how to prepare for the massage. Show the client to the shower or hydrotherapy area, depending on which services that client has decided on. Provide proper draping for the client from the dressing area to the massage table.
7. Assist the client (as necessary) to the massage table and explain the position, either supine or prone, that the client should assume. Drape the client appropriately and provide extra support (towels or bolsters) under the knees or head, if necessary.
8. Attend to the client's comfort:
    a. Ask whether the client is warm enough. Adjust the room temperature or provide an extra blanket if necessary.
    b. Adjust pillows or bolsters so that the client is comfortable on the table.
    c. Encourage the client to speak up at any time the client feels discomfort of any kind so that adjustments can be made.
    d. Observe the client throughout the treatment for any signs of discomfort and ask for feedback if any such signs are noted.

There are many possibilities for varying massage techniques for different clients. Every massage is unique depending on the needs of the client and the practitioner's choices of the combination of massage techniques used during the session. The following massage procedure will help you to become more proficient and creative.

Breathing for Relaxation

When the client is on the table, relaxed and comfortable, encourage the client to breathe fully and deeply. Many people have never done this and might need some basic coaching. Help the client by using some of the following suggestions:

Tell the client to breathe through the nose deeply so that the abdominal area expands first, followed by the chest. Hold for a few counts and then allow the breath to flow outward. Maintain the exhalation for a short time and repeat the exercise a few times. Observe the client's breathing and synchronize your own breathing together. Have the client continue breathing freely for a few minutes to encourage relaxation and stress reduction.

Step-by-Step Procedure for Massage 2

The following procedure is a generalized massage routine designed as a relaxing full-body massage. It is only a guideline, and you can vary or alter it to fit the needs of each individual client and situation.

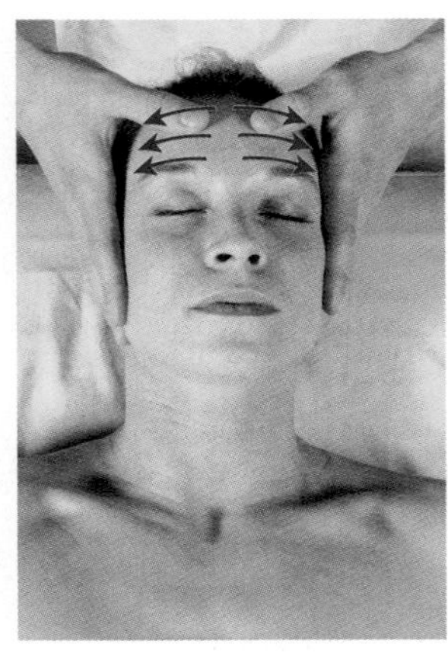

FIGURE 12-18A Apply digital effleurage to the forehead from midline to hairline.

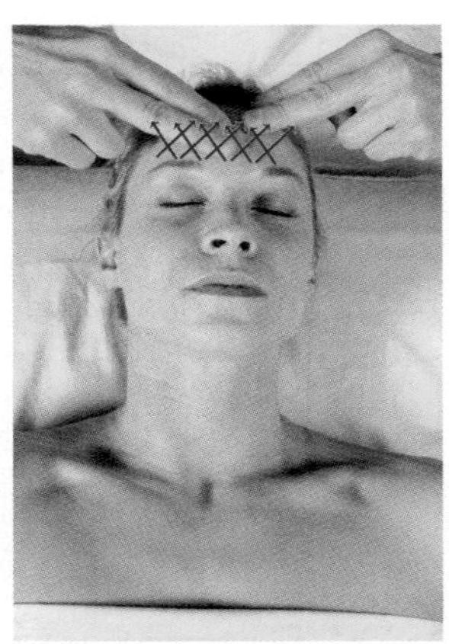

FIGURE 12-18B Use a crisscross movement. Begin at one side of the forehead, making cross movements and then working back.

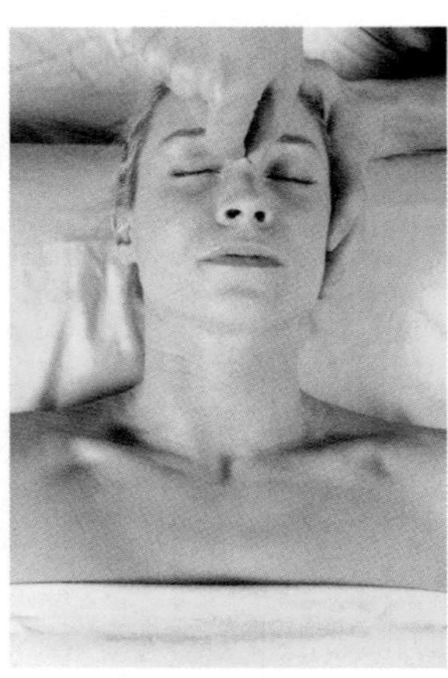

FIGURE 12-18C Grasp the bridge of the nose and apply gentle traction.

The client is positioned face up (supine) on the massage table with a bolster under both knees to relieve any tension in the lower back. The head is resting on the table in a neutral position unless the client exhibits a severe head-forward position, in which case a folded towel or a small pillow can be placed under the head. The practitioner should be standing or seated above the client's head, facing the client.

Face massage can be done as the opening procedure of the massage, or for various reasons, massaging the face may be left out of the massage routine. If the client is wearing makeup, the client might choose to not have a face massage, or to remove the makeup before the session, or to proceed with the massage over the makeup. For sanitary reasons, when a face massage is included, it is usually at the beginning of the massage when the practitioner's hands have been freshly washed. Inform the client that very little lubricant is used, if any at all, for the face massage.

Note: Massaging a client's face, head, neck, and shoulders while positioned above the head can take several minutes. This is a good opportunity for you to get off your feet by sitting on a stool of a proper height that allows you to perform all of the manipulations while maintaining proper body mechanics.

Massage the Face

1. If the massage begins with the face, once both client and therapist are in place, the therapist can take a moment to quiet any thoughts, center and ground the body, and create intention before making initial contact with the client.
2. You can make the initial contact by lightly placing the finger pads of both hands on the frontal eminence of the forehead and resting them there for several seconds. This is a good time to focus on the connection with the client. After a short time, a light pulse can be noted under the fingertips, indicating relaxation of the frontalis muscle and circulation in the area. The practitioner might prefer to make first contact by placing the hands on the client's shoulders if the face is not being massaged.
3. After a moment or when the pulse is noted, gently draw the fingers toward the hairline, gently stretching the frontalis muscle.
4. Place thumbs from both hands in the center of the forehead at the hairline. With slight pressure, glide the thumbs along the hairline to the temples and conclude with gentle circular friction at the temples. Return the thumb to the midline, about a finger's width inferior to the first gliding stroke and repeat. Continue repeating the stroke at finger-width increments down the forehead to the eyebrows (Figure 12-18a).
5. Beginning at one side of the forehead, do alternating diagonal gliding strokes from the eyebrows into the hairline. Begin with the pads of the fingers of one hand placed at the level of the eyebrow, and glide those fingers in the direction of your corresponding shoulder. As soon as the stroke has progressed enough for the fingers of the other hand to be placed in the same place, do so and glide those fingers in the direction of the corresponding shoulder. Continue alternating diagonal strokes across the forehead and back again (Figure 12-18b).
6. Grasp across the bridge of the nose with the thumb and finger and gently traction superiorly and away from the face (Figure 12-18c).

7. Apply light gliding strokes from the nose to the side of the eye socket; first just superior to the supraorbital ridge, then just inferior to the supraorbital ridge, then just inferior to the infraorbital ridge, and finally over the infraorbital ridge. The muscle tissue around the eyes is perhaps the most delicate on the body, so massage movements likewise must be gentle (see Figure 12-18d). (Caution: Avoid strokes around the eyes if the client is wearing contact lenses.)
8. Continue to massage with gentle circular friction, using the pads of the fingers, beside the nose from the eyes to the mouth and laterally beneath the zygomatic arch. Gently press upward under the zygomatic arch with the fingertips. The medial portion of the zygomatic arch is the site of the origin of several mimetic muscles (muscles of expression). Although the friction massage is circular, the intention is to massage these muscles of expression in an upward direction (Figure 12-18e).
9. Massage the masseter muscle with circular friction and gliding strokes with the thumb or fingers from the lateral aspect of the zygomatic arch to the ramus of the mandible. The parotid salivary gland is located over the posterior aspect of the masseter muscle and the temperomandibular joint (TMJ). Avoid pressure over the parotid gland and the TMJ.
10. Tender points or trigger points are common in the masseter muscle on the mandible. These can be addressed with gentle point compression for six to ten seconds, repeated two or three times (Figure 12-18f).
11. Continue to massage along the mandible from the tip of the chin to the ramus of the jaw. The fingers apply gentle circular friction inferior to the mandible while the thumbs gently massage above the ridge. Gently massage under the chin with the pads of the fingers while massaging the area from the lower lip to the chin with the thumbs. Finish with gliding strokes from the chin to the ear (Figure 12-18g).
12. Repeat gliding strokes from the centerline of the face to the side of the head with an upward orientation in increments, starting at the chin, under the lips, above the lips, next to the nose, under the eyes, and over the eyes.
13. Complete the face massage by placing both hands lightly over the entire face, the thenar eminence on the forehead, and fingertips at the outer edge of the lips. Hold still for a moment, allowing the client to sink further into a relaxed state (Figure 12-18h).

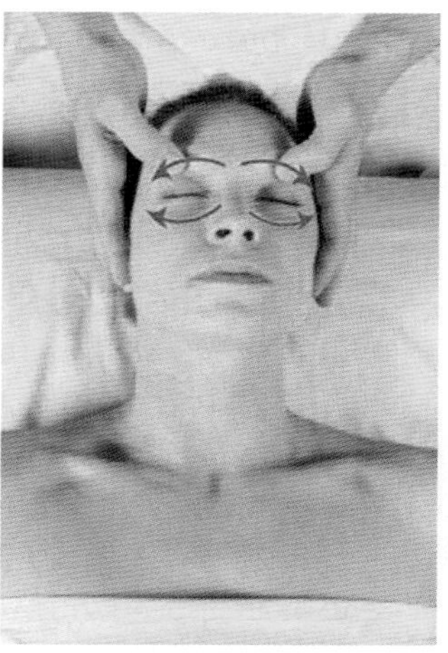

FIGURE 12-18D Apply digital effleurage to the forehead and orbits. Do not put pressure on the eyeballs.

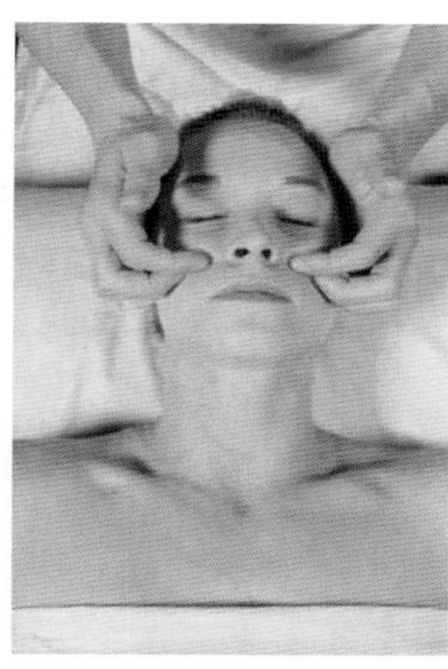

FIGURE 12-18E Apply gentle friction from the nose to under the zygomatic arch bilaterally.

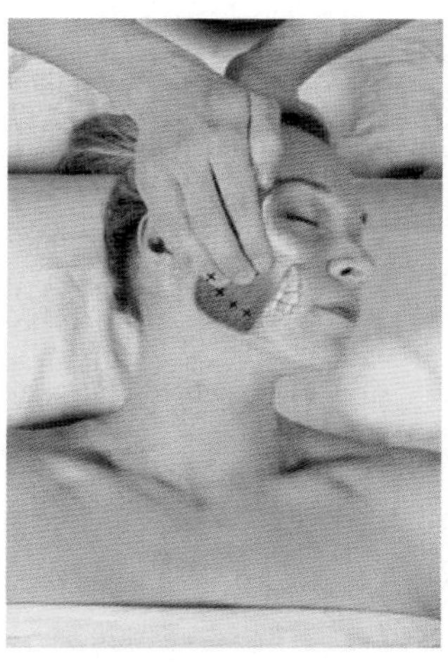

FIGURE 12-18F Treat tender points or trigger points, which are common in the masseter muscle along the ramus of the jaw, with light digital compression.

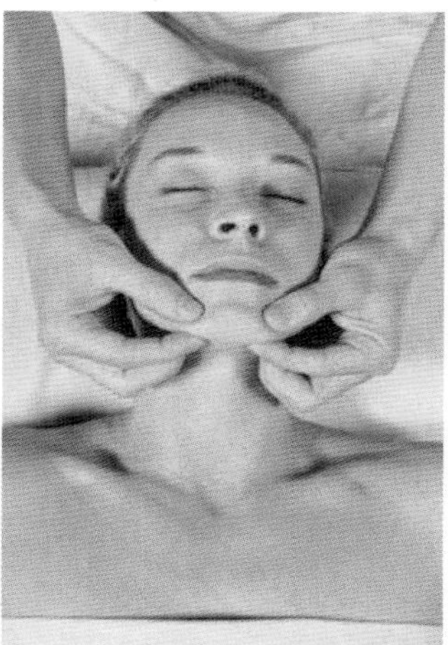

FIGURE 12-18G Apply gentle circular friction inferior to the mandible with your fingers while your thumbs gently massage above the ridge.

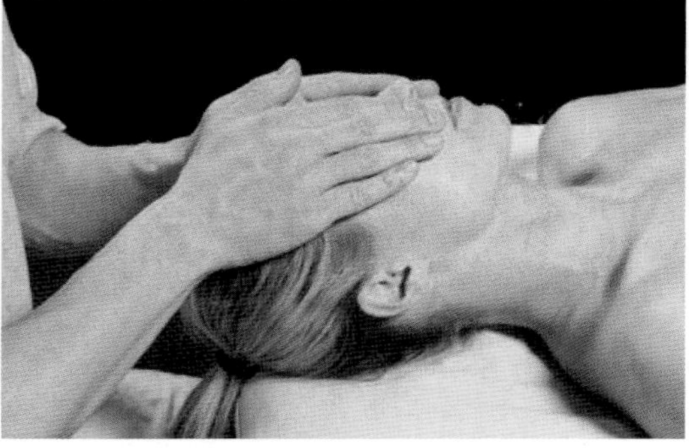

FIGURE 12-18H Complete the face massage by placing both hands lightly over the entire face.

Massage the Scalp

To massage the scalp thoroughly, the therapist turns the client's head first one way, then the other, gently and securely supporting the client's head with one hand while massaging with the other (Figure 12-19).

To support the client's head comfortably, the therapist places one hand on either side of the client's head so that the thumbs are positioned just in front of the ears and the fingers extend behind the ears just beyond the occipital ridge. The palms rest comfortably on the cranium so that the hand encircles the ear but does not cover it. Lift the head slightly and turn it on its axis so that it rests comfortably in the cradle of your hand. By using this cranial handle, the therapist should be able to rotate, extend, flex, and even apply gentle traction to the head and neck easily and securely.

1. Without lubricant and using the fingertips of the top hand, begin just inferior to the occipital ridge on the side of the head that is exposed and massage the scalp with small circular movements. Use moderate pressure, moving the scalp over the underlying tissues, being careful not to pull the hair. Massage thoroughly across the occipital region and continue the movements across and up the back of the head as you proceed toward the top of the head and above the ear. You may want to turn your hand around to continue the circular friction movements around the ear to cover the entire half of the scalp on the side of the head turned upward (Figure 12-20).
2. Change the motion of the hand to a quick vibration with the fingers spread apart, starting at the front hairline and progressing toward the occiput, covering the exposed half of the head.
3. Smooth the hair and scalp by combing through the hair with the fingertips from the front hairline to the back.
4. Lay the upper hand on the cranial "handle" and turn the head the other way, and do the same procedure on the other side of the scalp. When the second side is completed, return the head to a neutral, forward-facing position.

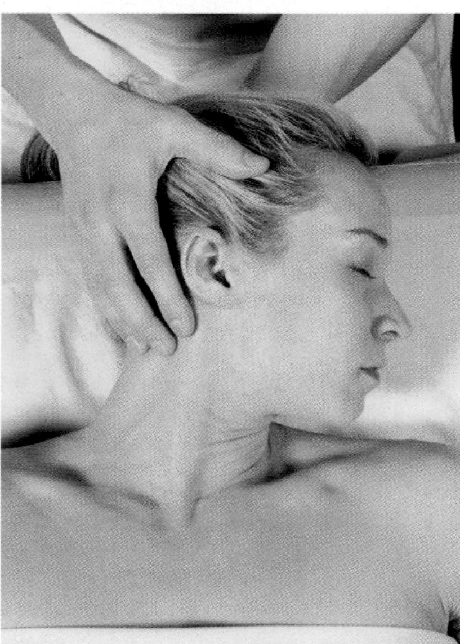

FIGURE 12-19 Note placement of the hands in the "handle" position, supporting the head.

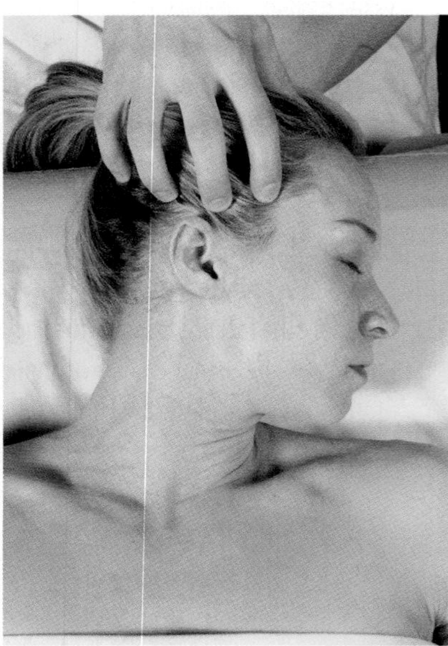

FIGURE 12-20 Massage the scalp by making rotating movements with the fingertips.

MASSAGE THE EAR

The outer ears extend outward from the ear canal, which penetrates the auricular meatus to the delicate tissues of the inner ear. Because the outer ear is made up of cartilage and an abundance of nerves, it is surprisingly sensitive. For this reason, some clients enjoy having the ears massaged, whereas others are uncomfortable with the practice. French and Chinese therapists have developed auricular therapies with the theory that points or areas of the outer ear are reflexively related to every area and organ in the body. Massaging the points in the ear can have stimulating, relaxing, or rejuvenating effects on areas of the body far removed from the ear (Figure 12-21). Both ears can be massaged simultaneously.

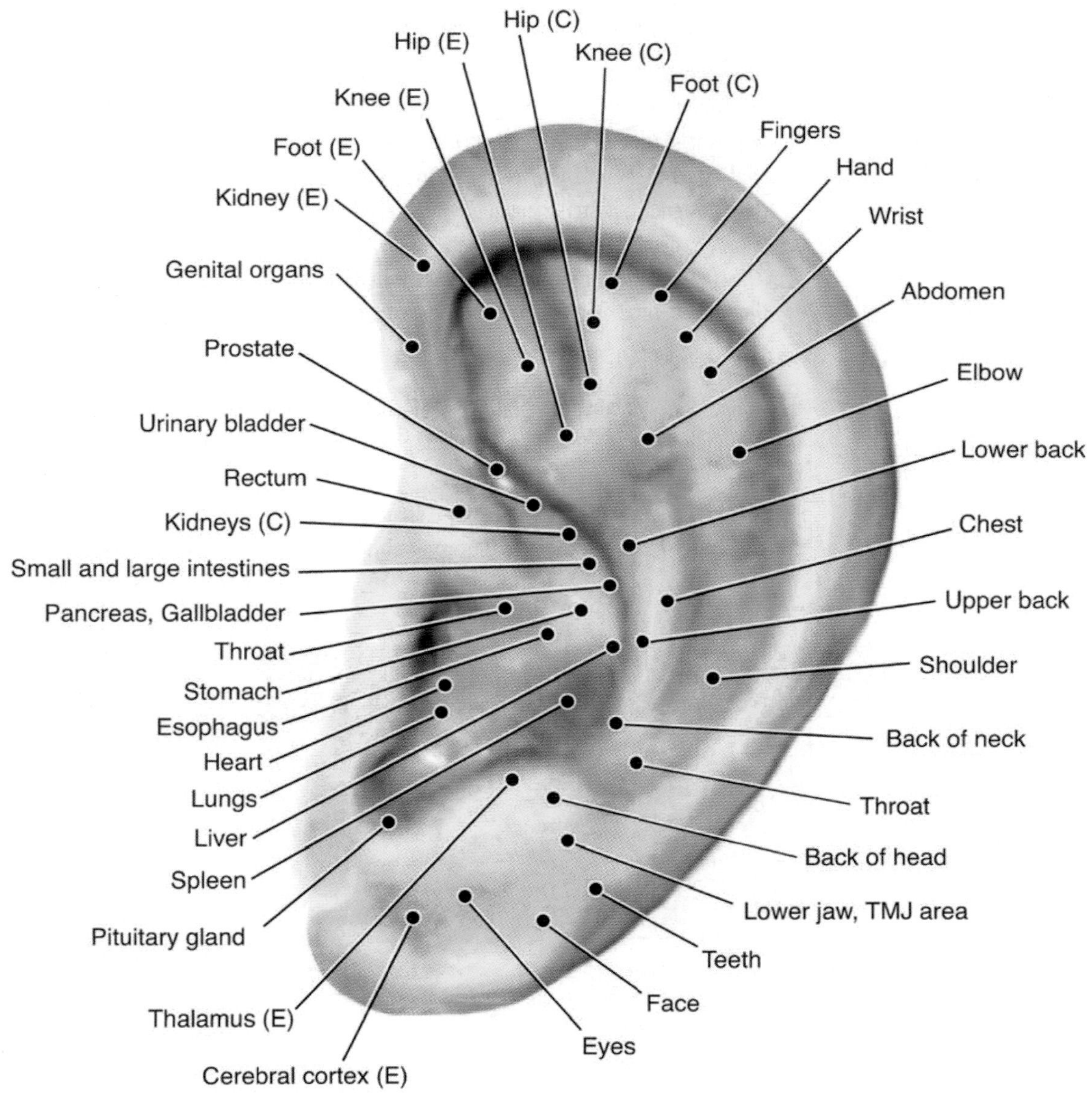

FIGURE 12-21 The Auricular Therapy Ear Chart shows areas in the ear as they relate to other areas of the body. (C) indicates Chinese sources ; (E) European sources.

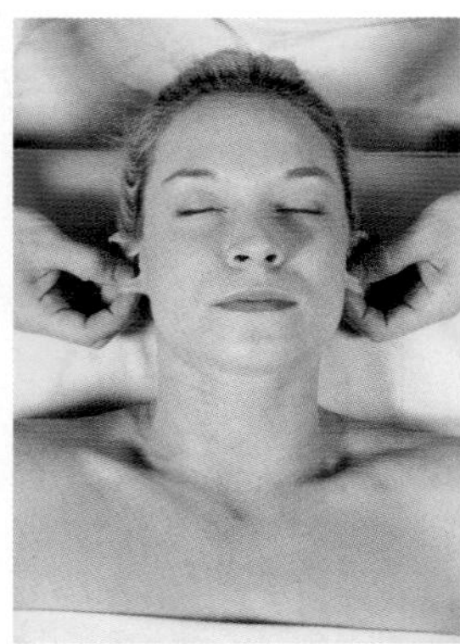

FIGURE 12-22A Unroll the outer edge of the ear.

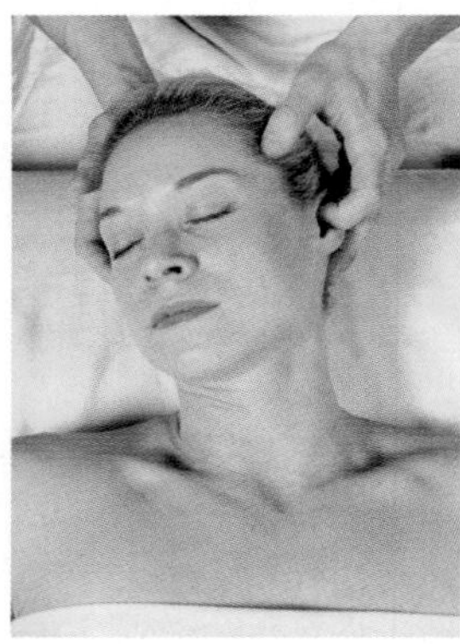

FIGURE 12-22B Massage in and around the ears with light friction movement.

1. Begin by massaging the head all around the ear with circular friction.
2. Glide around the top and back of the ear where it joins to the head with the edge of your finger (two or three repetitions).
3. Beginning at the lower edge of the ear, using moderate pressure, unroll the outer edge of the ear between your thumb and fingers, applying a slight traction and working all the way around to the upper, anterior aspect of the ear (Figure 12-22a).
4. Starting at the top front of the ear, use a fingertip (well-trimmed fingernails always) to trace all the valleys and ridges of the ear carefully and with moderate pressure. The thumb can be positioned behind the ear to provide a backing for the manipulation (Figure 12-22b). If any nodules, granular tissue, or other tissue abnormalities are encountered, or if the client says there are tender points, spend a little extra time stimulating these points. These could be an indication of some condition in a related area of the body. You might want to make a note of the tender point for reference to the body area later in the massage or noted in clients' charts for future treatments.
5. Beginning with the thumbs seated deeply in the center of the ear and the first finger at the base of the ear near the head, grip the ear firmly and slowly pull the ear at an angle away from the head. With digital petrissage, massage the ear between the finger and thumb as you continue tractioning until you reach the outer periphery of the ear. Return the thumb to the center of the ear and repeat the sequence several times, each time in a slightly different direction—inferiorly, inferior-posteriorly, posteriorly, posterior-superiorly, and superiorly.
6. Finish by gently tugging inferiorly on the ear lobes, gently grasping and unrolling the outer edges of the ears, and then, using a gliding stroke with the finger, massage the attachment of the ear to the head. From this point, the massage can continue to the jaw and face or to the neck.

Massage the Neck

1. Apply lubricant with a bilateral-lateral effleurage stroke beginning at the sternal notch and continuing over the shoulders, up the trapezius and the back of the neck, to the occipital ridge (Figure 12-23a-c).

Note: While massaging the neck, avoid the area of the carotid artery and jugular vein because this can impede circulation to and from the brain and cause the client to become faint.

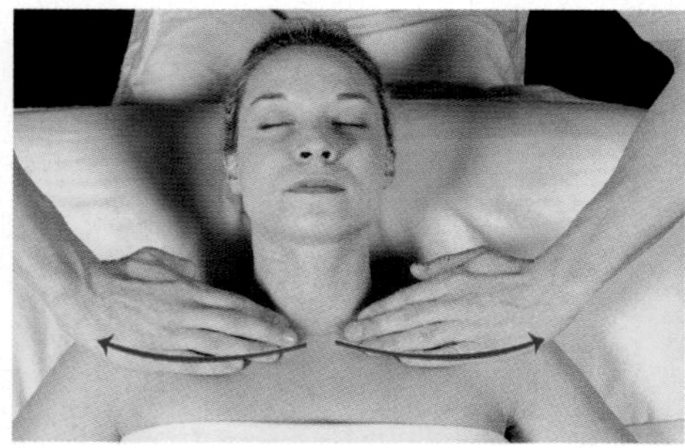

FIGURE 12-23A Apply bilateral effleurage (beginning at the sternal notch). Use the hands simultaneously, leading with the little fingers.

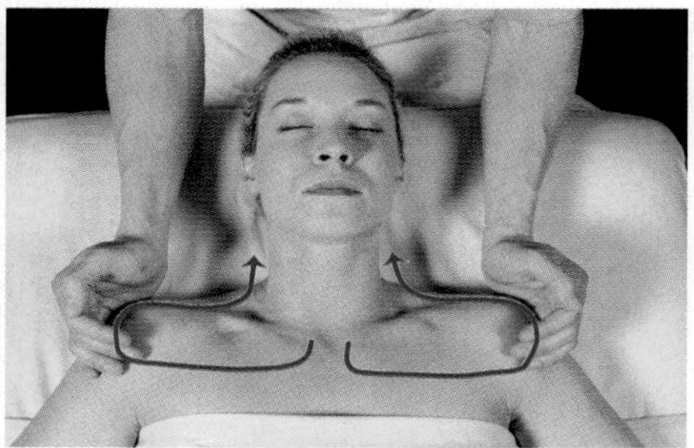

FIGURE 12-23B Continue effleurage from the sternal notch, over the shoulders, and along the trapezius.

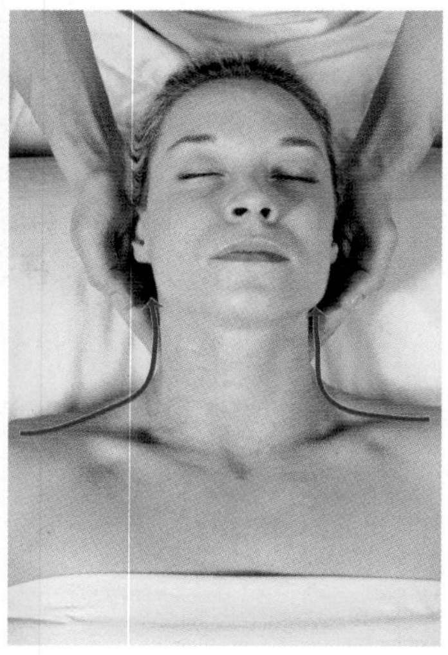

FIGURE 12-23C Continue the movement up to the occipital ridge.

2. Turn the client's head to one side, supporting it with one hand. Leading with the little finger of the other hand, continue light effleurage strokes, beginning just inferior to (below) the mastoid process (the bony bump below and behind the ear). Continue down the lateral aspect of the neck, over the shoulder, and back up the trapezius to the occipital ridge. Repeat three to five times (Figure 12-24a-d).
3. Thoroughly knead the same side of the neck, paying attention to any tight areas.
4. Repeat effleurage strokes to that side of the neck and shoulder.
5. Apply circular friction to any congested or tight areas.

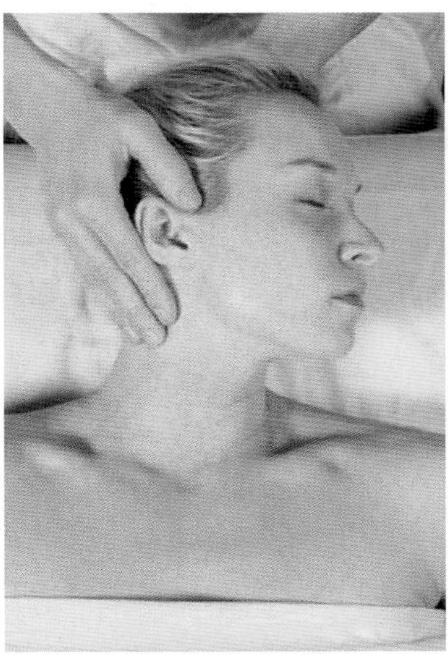

FIGURE 12-24A Note placement of the hands in the "handle" position, supporting the head.

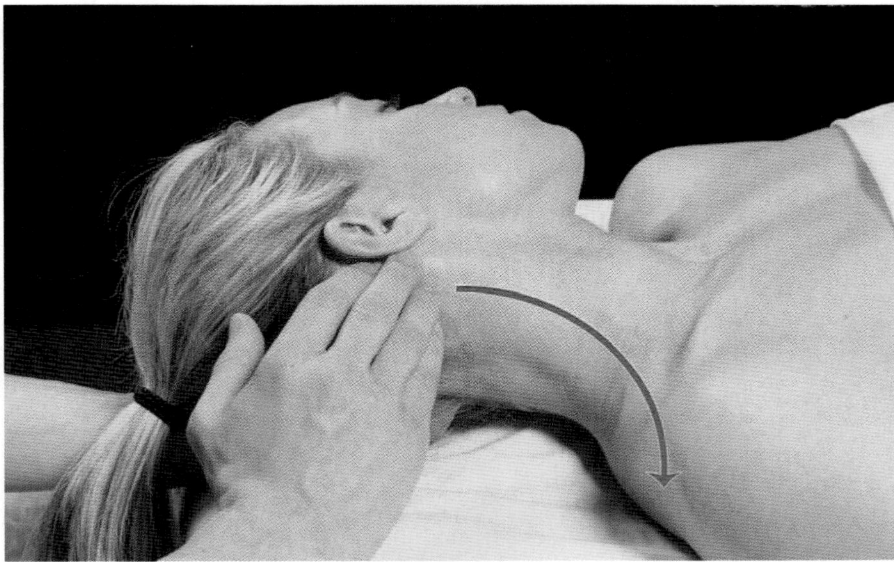

FIGURE 12-24B Apply effleurage, leading with the little finger, just below the mastoid and continue down the neck.

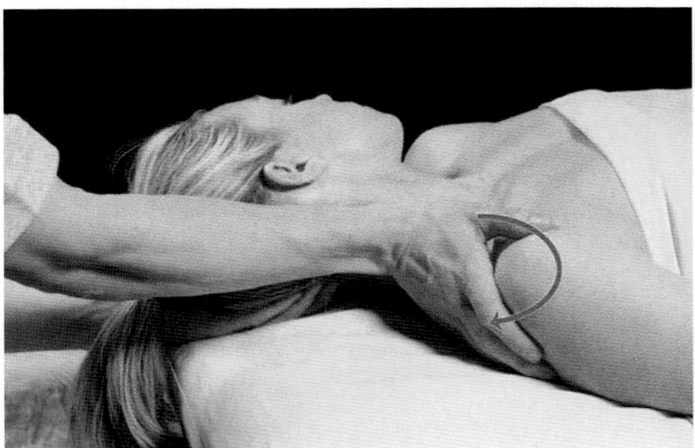

FIGURE 12-24C Continue the movement across the shoulder and around the deltoid.

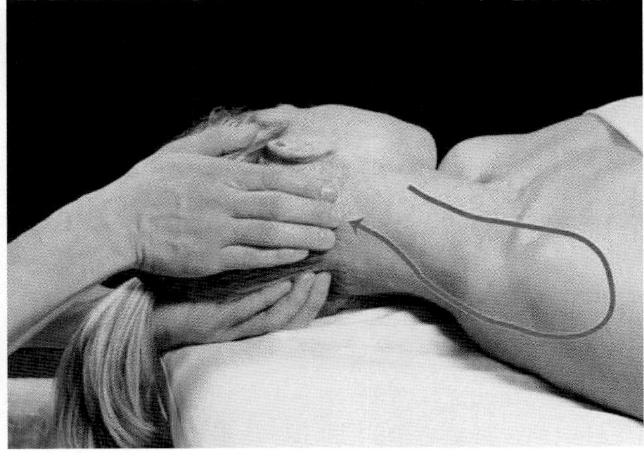

FIGURE 12-24D Hand position at the completion of effleurage stroke.

6. Apply V-stroke effleurage to that side and back of neck (Figure 12-25a-c).
7. Repeat effleurage.
8. Turn the client's head to the opposite side and repeat the movements as you did in steps #2 through #7.
9. Return the client's head to the central position and apply bilateral-lateral petrissage and friction to the neck and shoulders.
10. Do the following joint movements: Tilt the head back with the chin up, then lower the chin to the chest. Laterally flex the neck, moving the ear first toward the right shoulder, then toward the left. Apply a slight traction as the head is returned to a neutral position. Rotate the head to its full range of motion (lateral rotation). The spine remains in a straight line (Figure 12-26a-c).

Note: Joint movements of the neck are contraindicated in cases of osteoporosis.

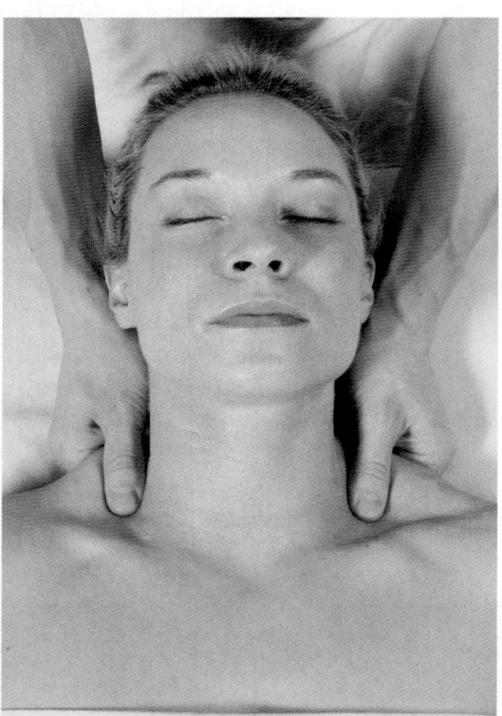

FIGURE 12-25A Apply pertrissage to the neck and shoulders.

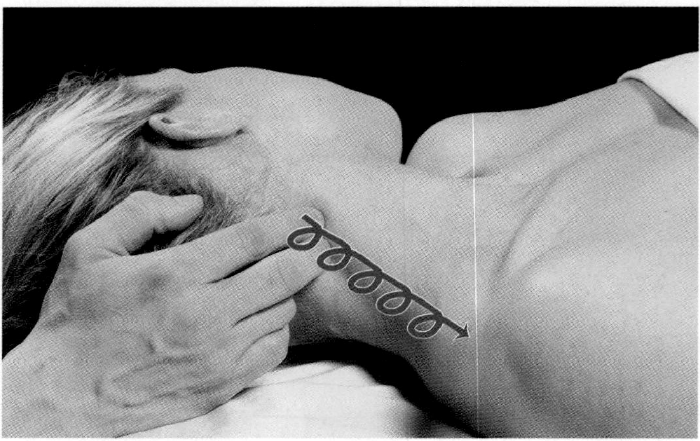

FIGURE 12-25B Apply friction to the neck and shoulders

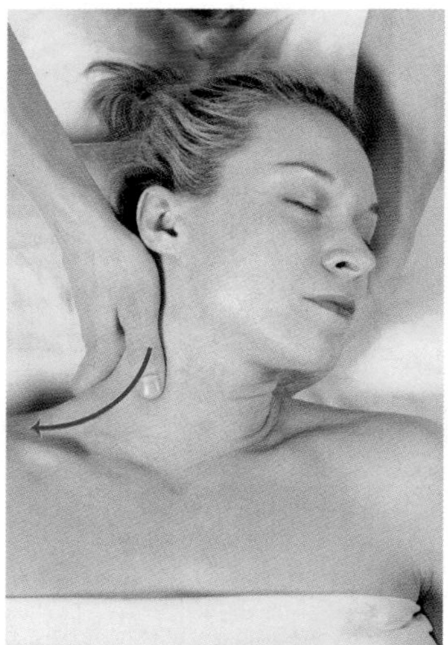

FIGURE 12-25C Apply V-strokes to the neck and shoulders.

11. Hold the occiput in the palm of your hand or hook your fingers under the occiput and apply a slight traction to the neck.
12. Place one hand on each shoulder and alternately push them (gently) toward the feet, providing a gentle rocking motion (Figure 12-27a and b).
13. Repeat the stroking movement in step #1.

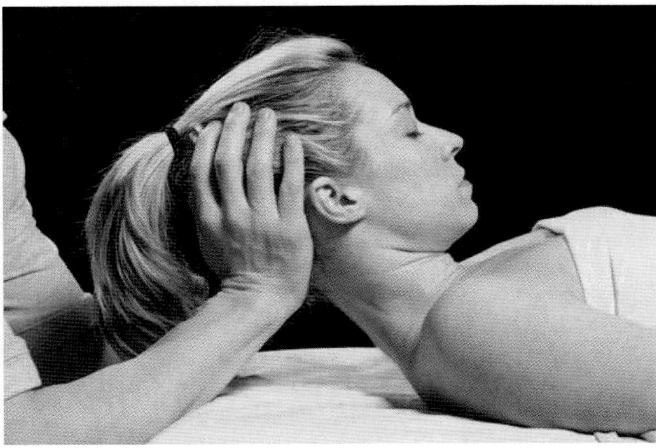

FIGURE 12-26A Apply passive joint movements by rolling the head forward. Note placement of the hands on the client's head.

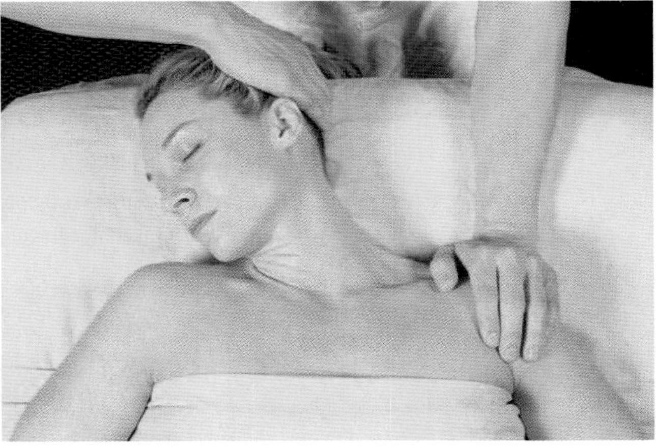

FIGURE 12-26B Apply a passive stretch by supporting the head to the side with one hand and pushing the opposite shoulder toward the feet with the other.

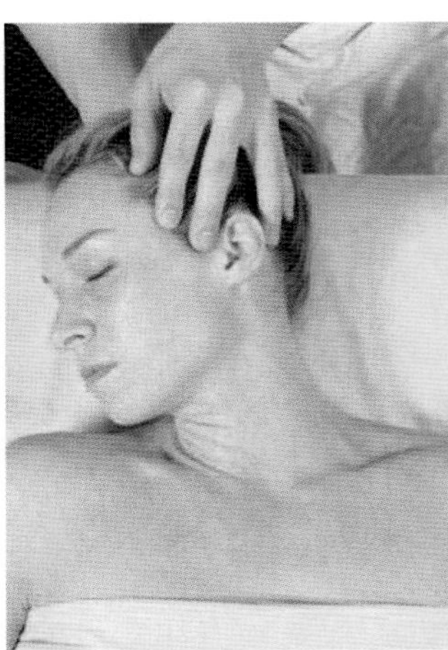

FIGURE 12-26C Apply passive rotation to the neck, being careful to keep the cervical spine straight.

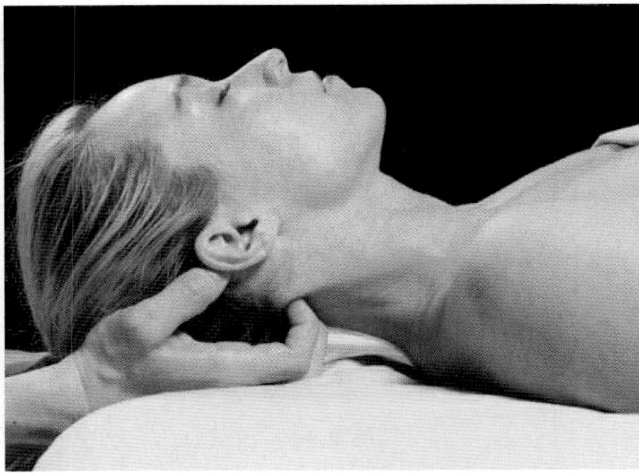

FIGURE 12-27A Apply slight traction to the cervical spine by hooking the fingers under the occiput and pulling.

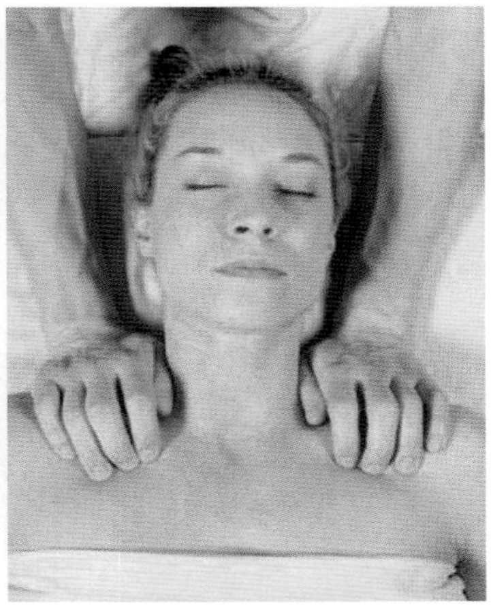

FIGURE 12-27B Apply alternating pressure toward the feet to rock gently and stretch the shoulders.

Massage the Arms

1. Undrape one arm to make contact, and apply lubricant to the client's arm from shoulder to wrist, using light effleurage.
2. Grasp the client's arm at the level of the wrist, and put the client's arm in slight traction by holding it with the wrist handle. (Holding on to the client's wrist provides a good "handle" for the practitioner to apply traction or move the body without slipping.) Hold the thumb side handle (the client's wrist) with the arm that is closest to the client. Apply effleurage to the lateral aspect of the arm. More pressure is applied with the effleurage movement distal to proximal (from wrist to neck); light pressure is applied proximal to distal with the return stroke. Begin from the wrist with a gliding stroke up the arm and over the shoulder. Rotate your hand as it travels over the client's shoulder; at the same time, apply slight traction to the handle. Proceed up the back of the neck and then down under the shoulder (trapezius area); then glide back to the starting point at the wrist. Repeat three to five times (Figure 12-28a-c).
3. Change the handle to the ulnar side of the wrist. Apply effleurage with firmer pressure up the medial aspect of the arm over the shoulder, around and down into the axillary portion of the arm. Then return to the wrist with lighter pressure. Perform effleurage again three to five times (Figure 12-29a-c).

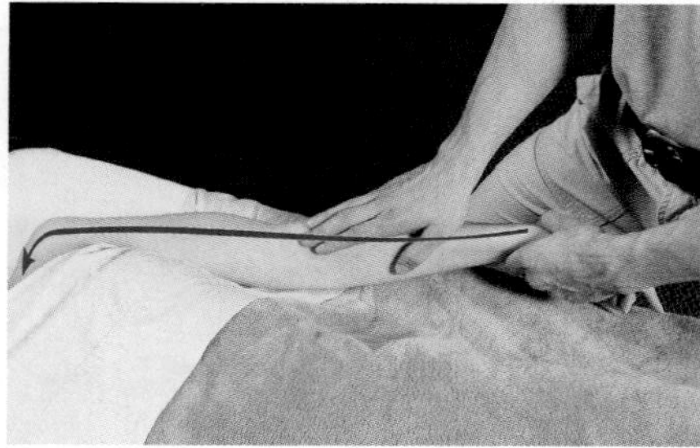
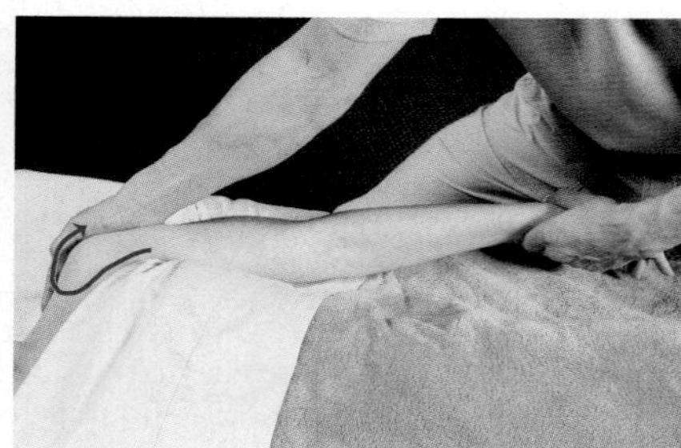
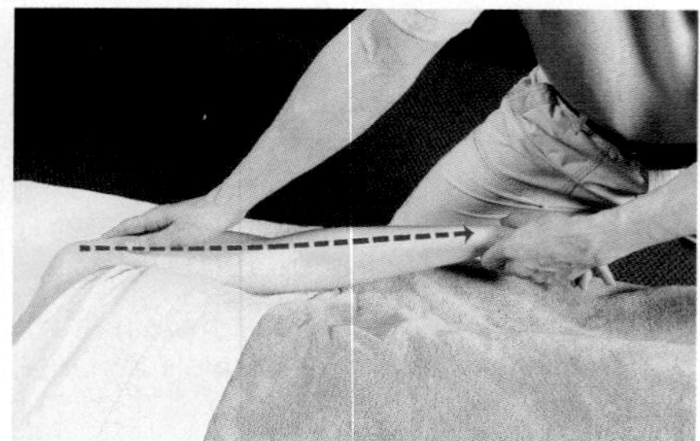

FIGURE 12-28A-C Apply gliding strokes to the lateral aspect of the arm. Note the "handle" and hand position. The stroke is continuous from the wrist, up the arm, over the shoulder, and back to the wrist. Use more pressure on the stroke up to the shoulder and less pressure on the return stroke.

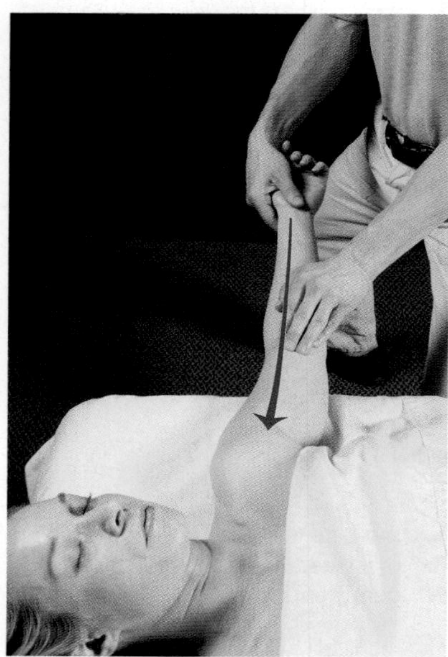

FIGURE 12-29A Continue with effleurage movements on the medial aspect of the arm. Note the "handle" and hand position.

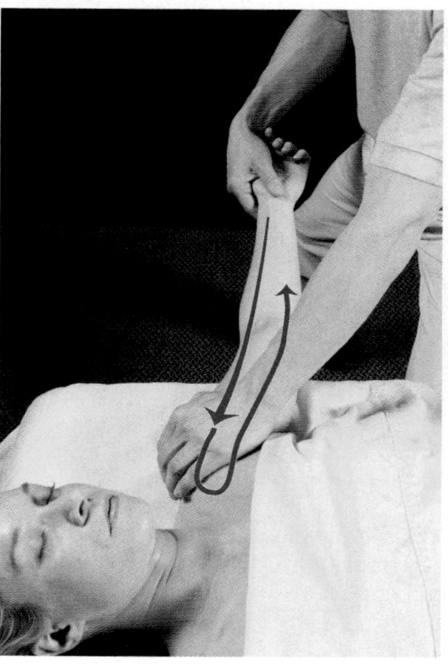

FIGURE 12-29B Continue the effleurage movements up and over the shoulder, and then back down the arm.

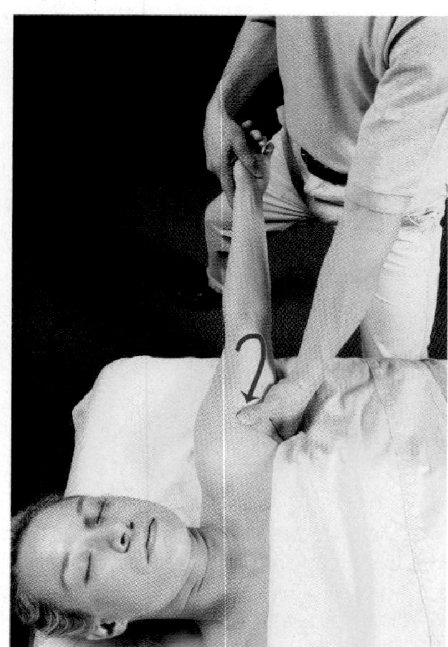

FIGURE 12-29C Continue the effleurage movements up into the axillary area for a slight joint movement and stretch.

4. Using both hands, grasp the arm at shoulder level and apply petrissage, directing individual movements toward the shoulder while moving proximal to distal down the arm to the client's hand. On the upper arm, use both hands to alternately knead the biceps and triceps. On the forearm, alternately knead the wrist flexors and extensors (Figure 12-30a and b).
5. Wring and roll (using both hands) from the shoulder, moving down the arm and giving special attention to the muscles of the forearm (Figure 12-30a-e).
6. Apply V-stroke effleurage from wrist to elbow on the medial and lateral sides of the forearm (Figure 12-31a).
7. Apply fulling to the forearm (Figure 12-31b).
8. Repeat effleurage to the medial and lateral side of the arm.
9. Massage the hand according to the suggestions in the following section, and then do joint movements on the arm and hand.

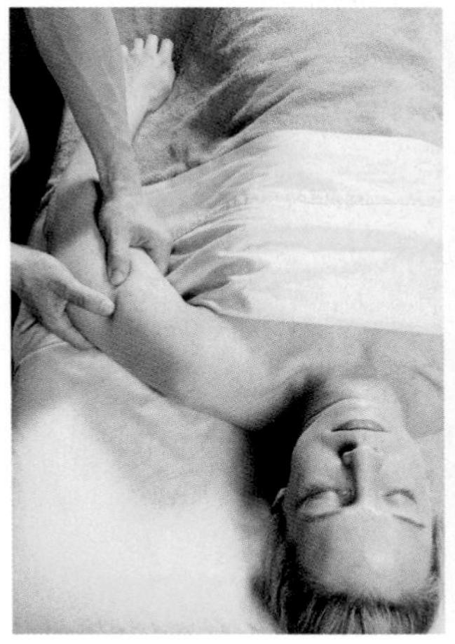

FIGURE 12-30A Apply petrissage from the shoulder and continue down the arm.

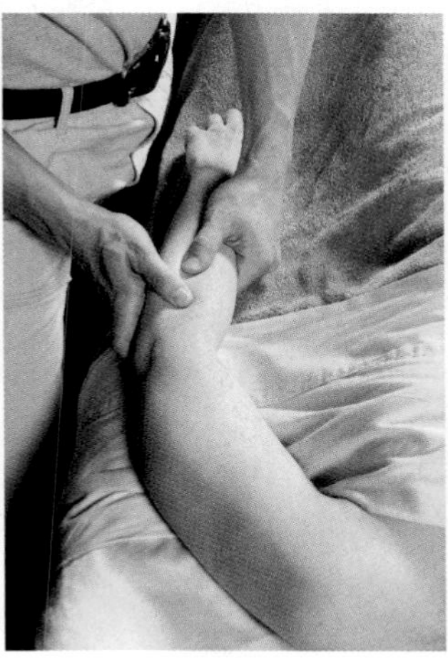

FIGURE 12-30B Continue petrissage down the arm to the wrist.

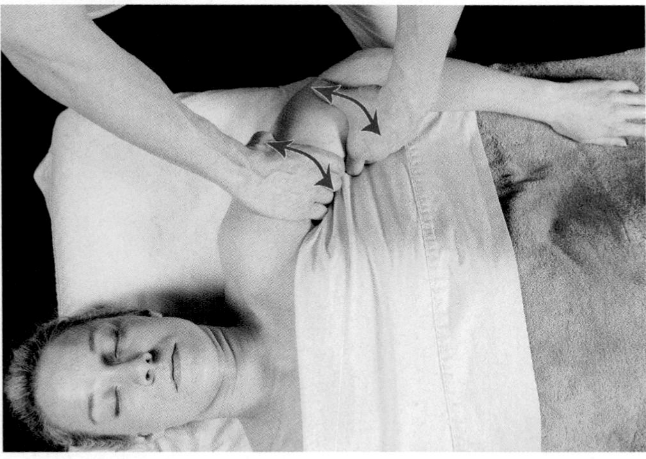

FIGURE 12-30C Apply wringing movements from the shoulder to the wrist.

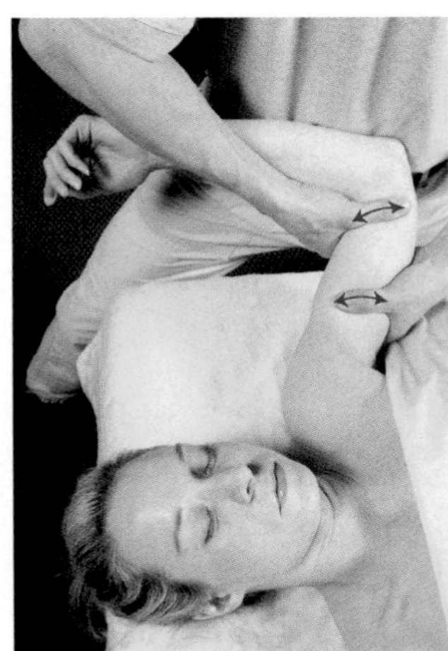

FIGURE 12-30D An alternative position can be used for the wringing movements and kneading.

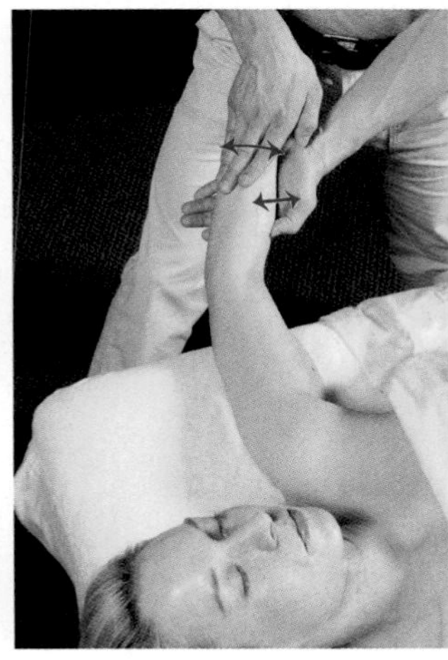

FIGURE 12-30E Do rolling movements from the shoulder to the wrist.

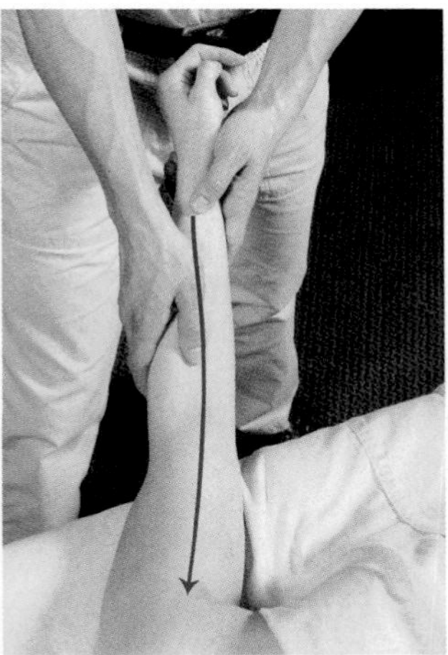

FIGURE 12-31A Note the direction of the V-stroke and position of the arm. Apply the same upward movement when massaging the back of the arm.

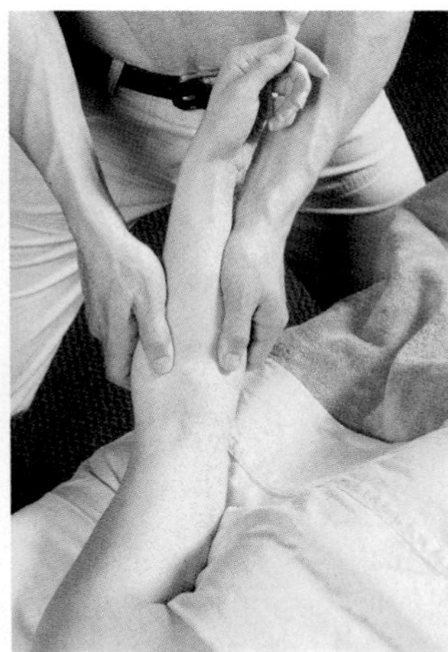

FIGURE 12-31B Apply fulling to the arm.

Massage the Hand

1. Apply petrissage to the palm of the client's hand.
2. Apply friction to the palm.
3. Apply petrissage to the back of the hand.
4. Apply friction to the back of the hand.
5. Do petrissage on each digit, including a joint movement (Figure 12-32a-f).
6. Apply joint movement. Support the client's hand and rotate all fingers both clockwise and counter-clockwise.
7. Extend, flex, and rotate the fingers, wrist, and elbow.
8. Rotate the shoulder joint clockwise and counterclockwise.
9. Extend the arm straight above the client's head to stretch the entire arm.
10. Apply effleurage from elbow past the axillary area (Figure 12-33a-e).

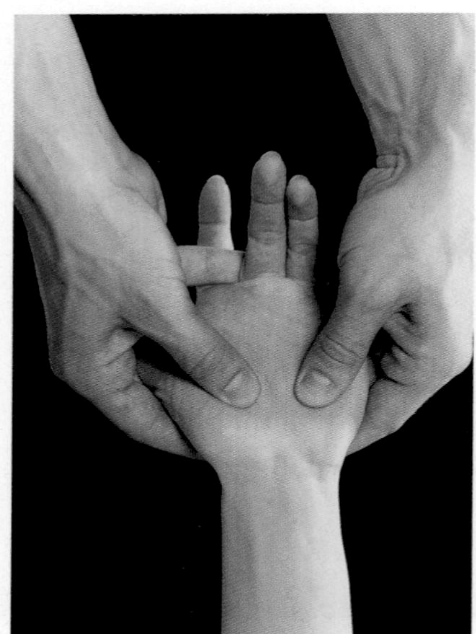

FIGURE 12-32A Apply friction and petrissage to the palm of the hand, spreading the metacarpals.

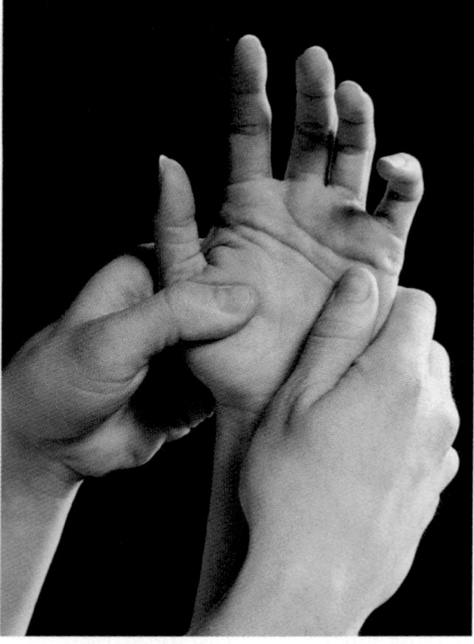

FIGURE 12-32B With the client's elbow resting on the table, hold the hand upright and massage the palm of the hand with your thumbs, using circular movements in alternate directions. This relaxes the hand.

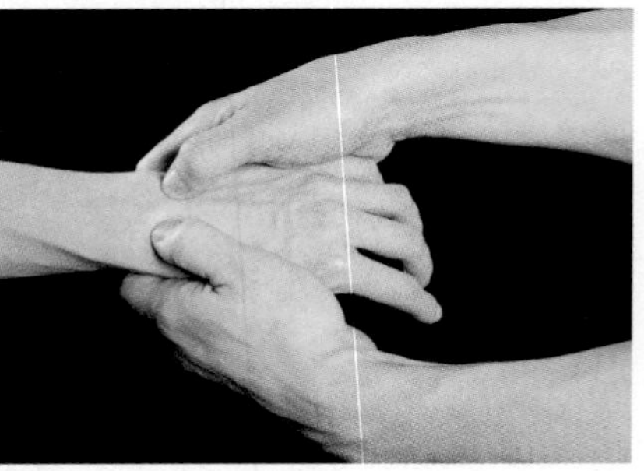

FIGURE 12-32C Apply friction and petrissage to the wrist and muscles of the hand.

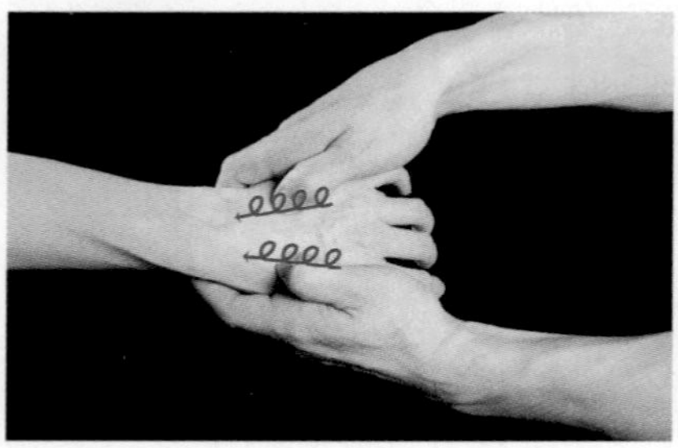

FIGURE 12-32D Apply circular friction to the back of the hand.

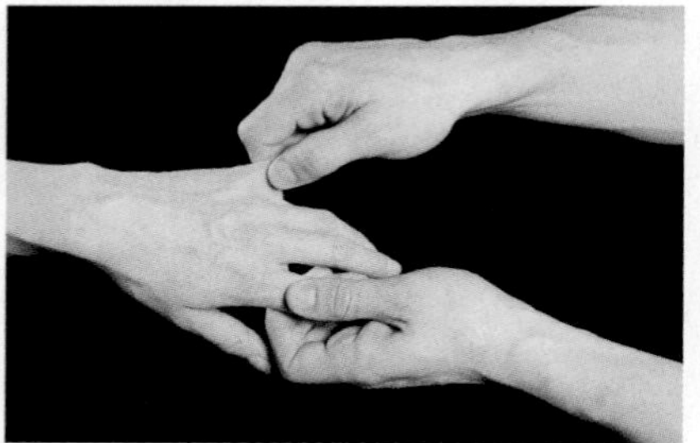

FIGURE 12-32E Beginning at the base of each finger, apply friction and petrissage. Work downward to the tip of each finger.

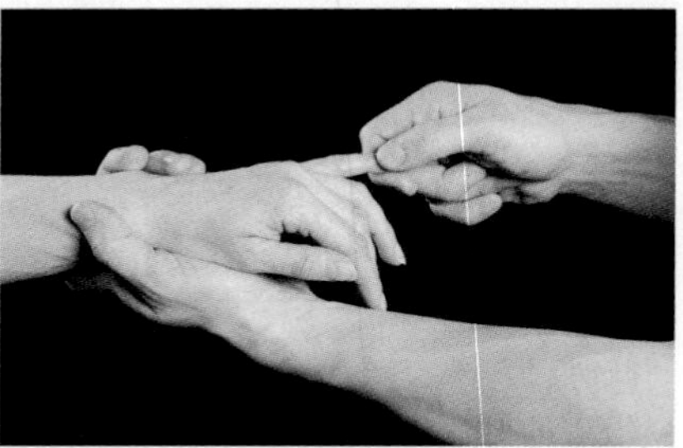

FIGURE 12-32F Squeeze and gently twist each finger, beginning at the base and working toward the tip. Rotate each finger in large circles. Finish each finger with a gentle squeeze of the fingertip.

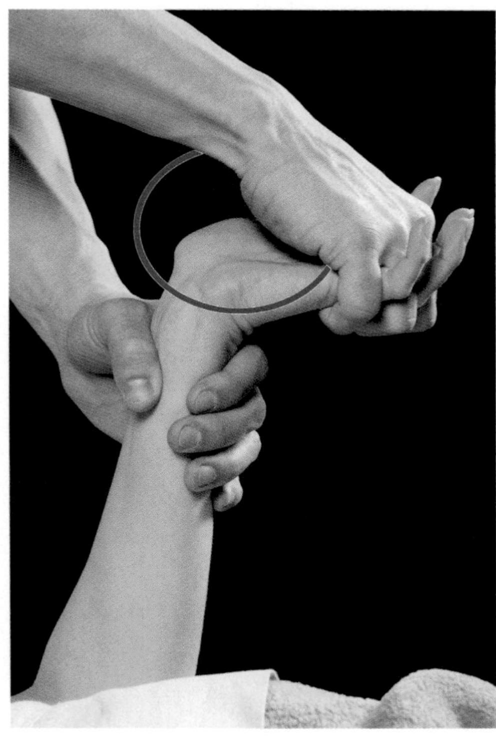

FIGURE 12-33A Apply joint movements and rotation. Note the interlacing of the fingers.

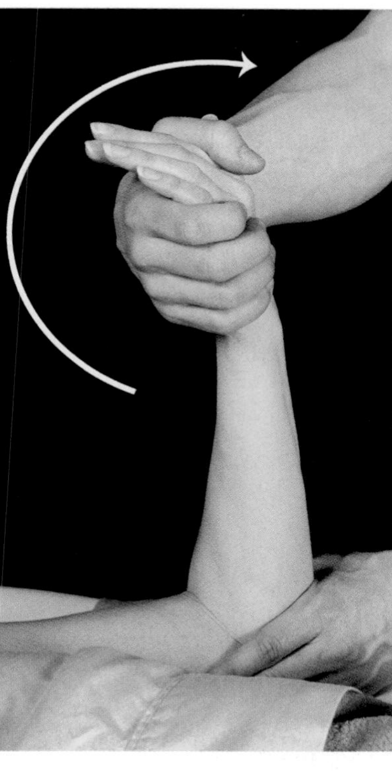

FIGURE 12-33B Rotate the forearm. Note how the fingers are used to steady the client's elbow.

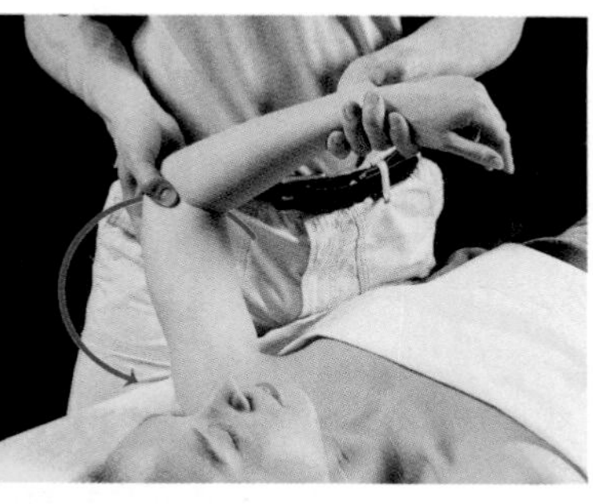

FIGURE 12-33C Apply joint movements to the shoulder by moving the elbow in large circles. Note how the wrist is supported to prevent the client's hand from hitting the face.

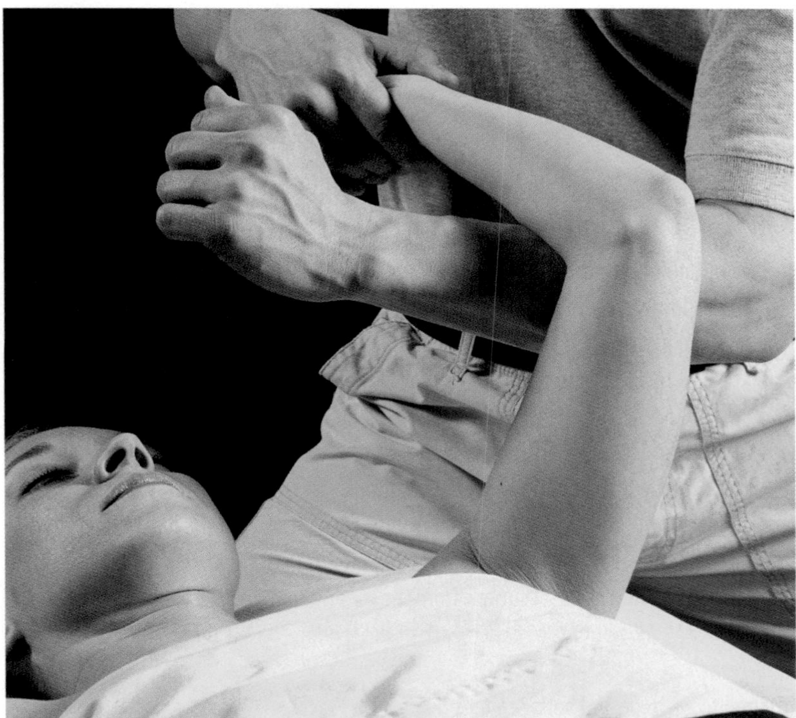

FIGURE 12-33D Stretch the client's arm over your arm. A slight turn or stretch can be done with your hand holding the client's wrist.

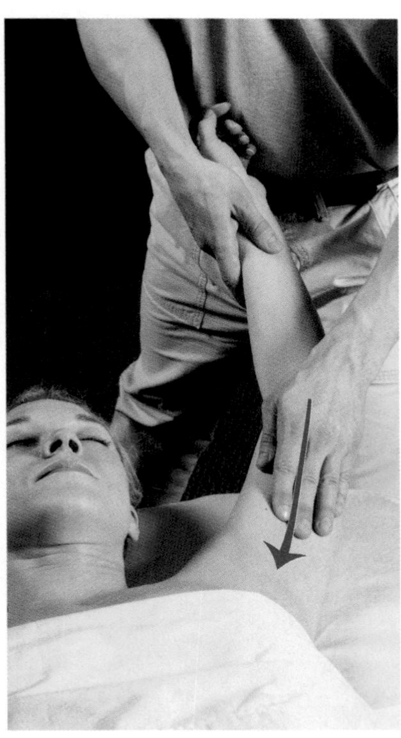

FIGURE 12-33E Apply effleurage or compression to the axillary area.

11. Apply traction at the wrist while moving the arm from a position above the client's head and back down to the side.
12. Shake and vibrate the arm and hand (Figure 12-34a).
13. Apply a final effleurage of the arm and hand and rotate the shoulder.
14. Apply superficial feather (nerve) strokes from the neck, down the arm to the fingertips (Figure 12-34b).
15. Re-drape the client as necessary, and repeat the arm and hand massage for the other arm and hand.

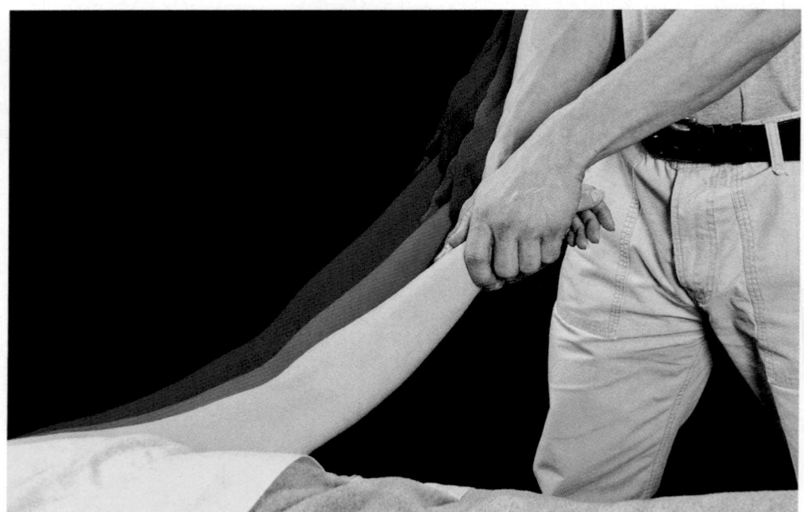

FIGURE 12-34A Grasp the wrist securely, and vigorously shake the arm up and down.

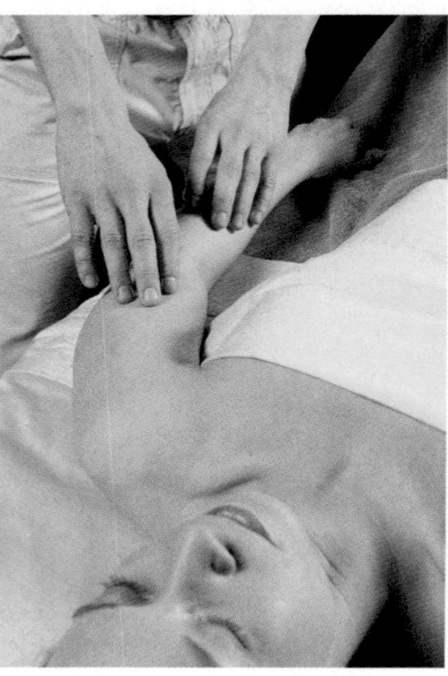

FIGURE 12-34B Apply feather strokes (light effleurage) with your fingertips to complete the massage of the arm. Do the massage of the other arm using the same sequence of movements.

Massage the Feet

1. Move to the feet, maintaining contact by using a light brushing stroke down the side of the body. Pause momentarily to allow the client to sense where you are before you begin massaging the feet. Undrape one foot and leg to the hip.
2. Use just enough lubricant to allow your hands to work smoothly. (Sometimes no lubricant is needed on the feet.)
3. Apply effleurage to each aspect of the foot. Apply gliding strokes distal to proximal ending just past the ankle on the dorsal, medial, and lateral sides, and plantar surface (bottom) of the foot.
4. Apply petrissage and friction to the plantar surface (bottom) of the foot from the ball of the foot to the heel. Use a closed fist or heel of the hand to do deep gliding.
5. Apply kneading movements on the dorsal surface from the toes up to the ankles.
6. Apply small circular friction movements between each of the tendons on the dorsal, medial, and lateral sides of the foot.
7. Apply digital friction to each toe and between toes (Figure 12-35a-f).
8. Beginning with the toes, incorporate joint movements, first individually, then together. Apply plantar and dorsal flexion of the toes, then to the entire foot. Rotate the foot and ankle, then separate the toes (phalanges) and wring and roll the foot (Figure 12-36a-e).

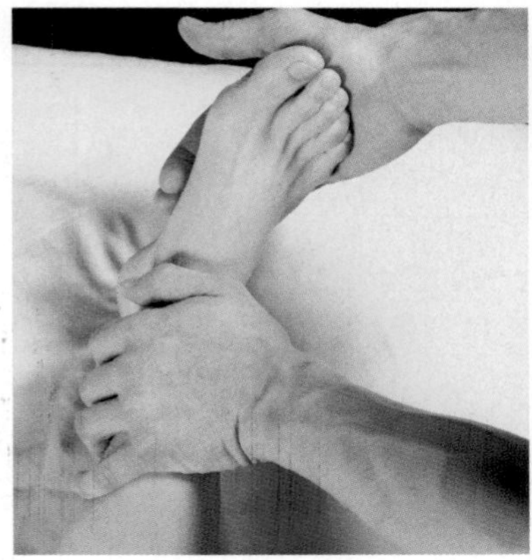

FIGURE 12-35A Apply effleurage to both the top and bottom of the foot, working from the toes upward toward the heart.

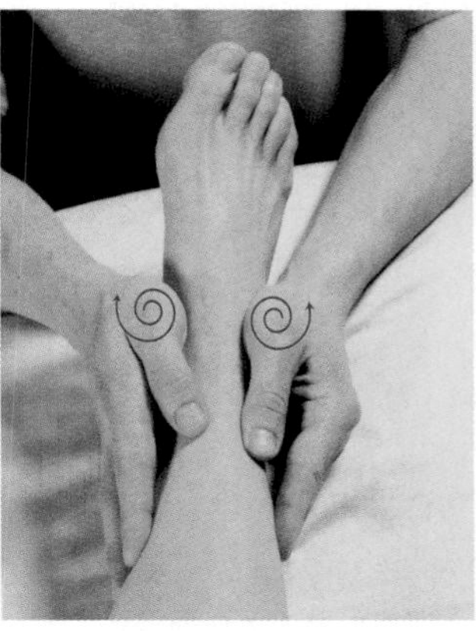

FIGURE 12-35B Warm the foot and ankles with circular rubbing movements.

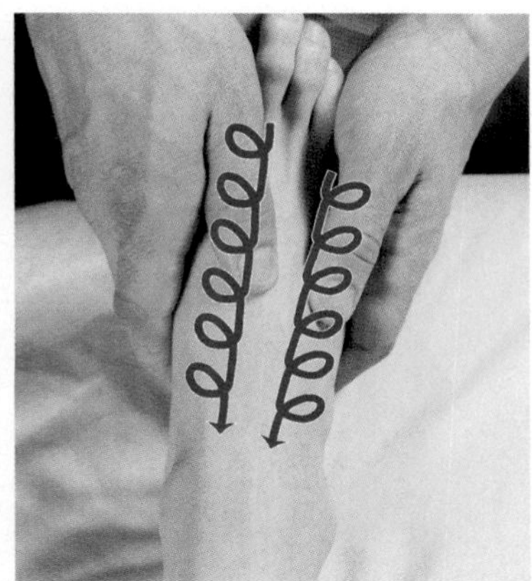

FIGURE 12-35C Knead the foot using circular motions.

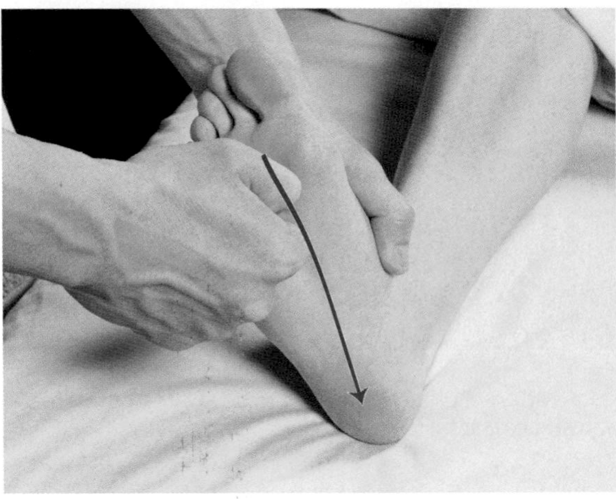

FIGURE 12-35D Apply your knuckles to stroke down the plantar surface of the foot.

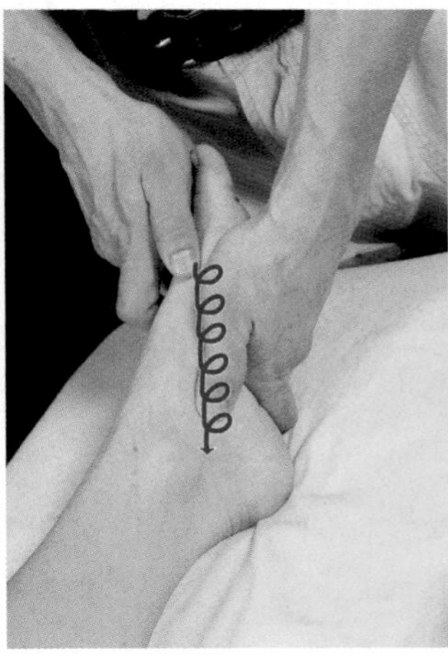

FIGURE 12-35E Apply digital friction between the tendons and bones on all surfaces of the foot.

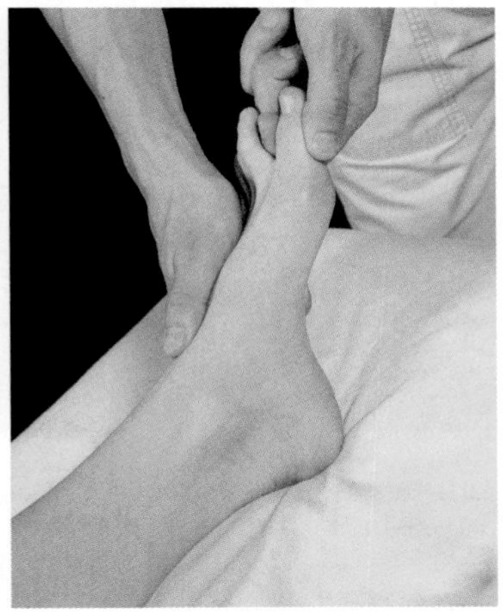

FIGURE 12-35F Massage and rotate each digit.

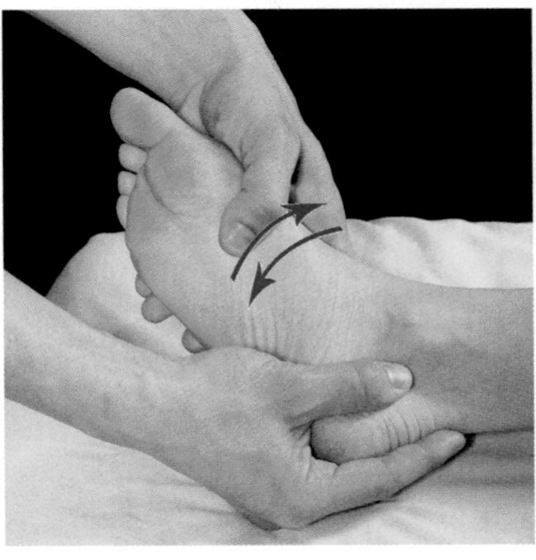

FIGURE 12-36A Rotate and stretch the tarsus and metatarsus.

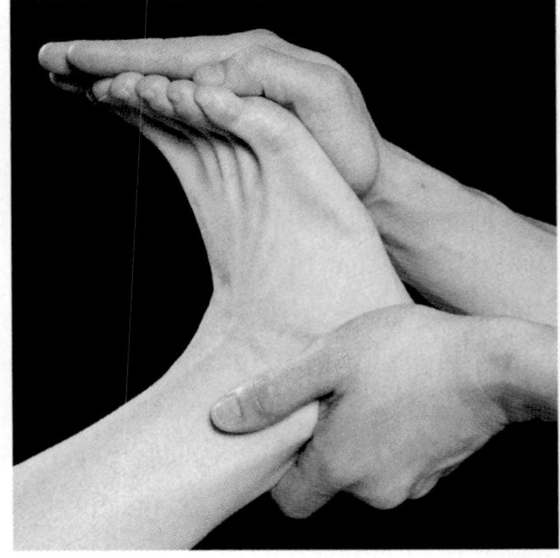

FIGURE 12-36B Stretch the plantar surface of the foot and toes.

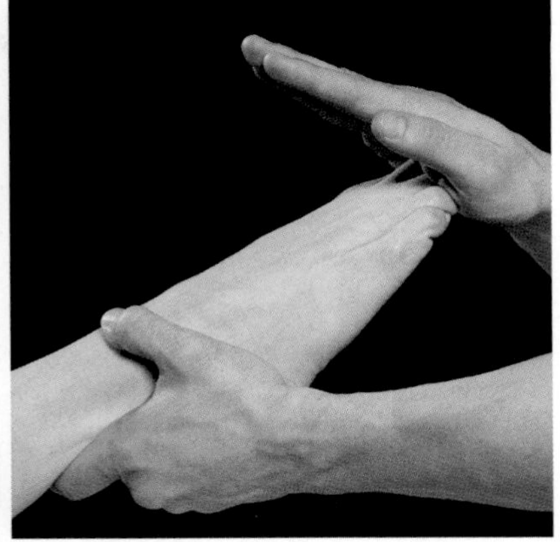

FIGURE 12-36C Stretch the dorsal aspect of the foot and toes.

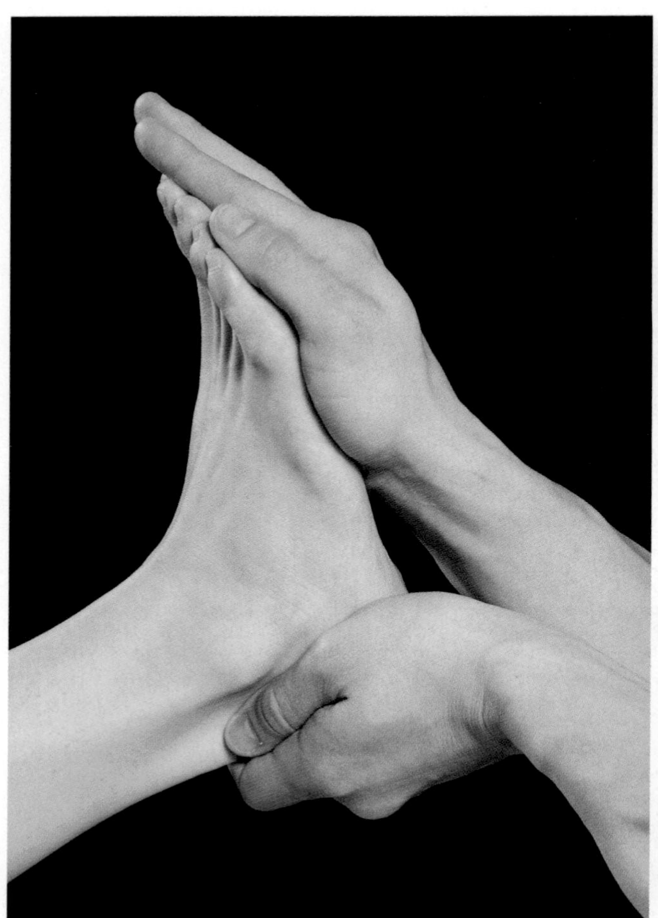
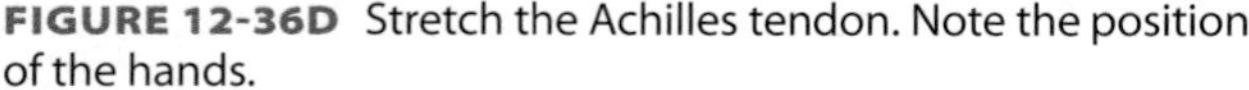

FIGURE 12-36D Stretch the Achilles tendon. Note the position of the hands.

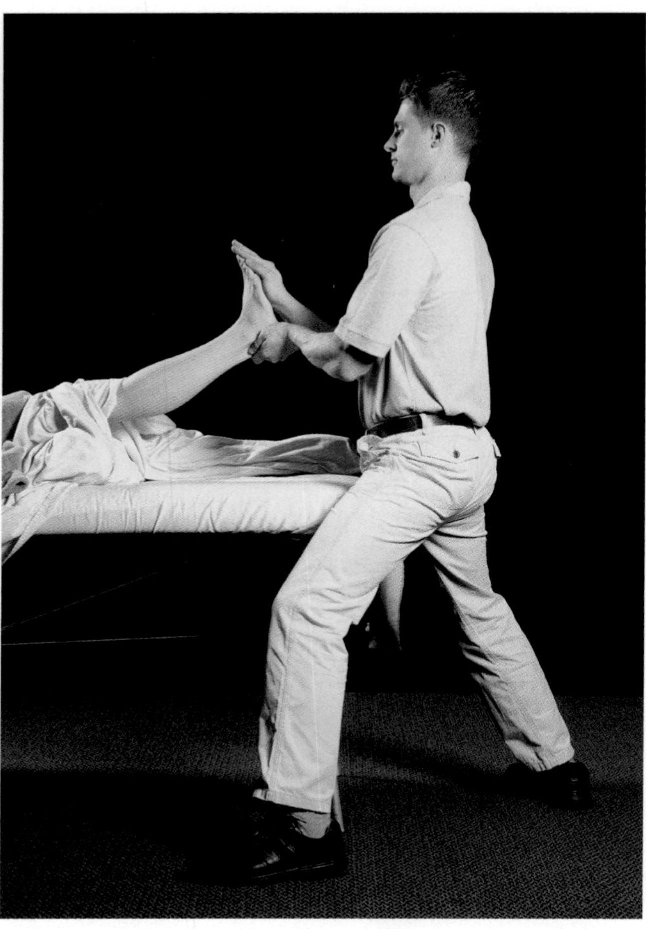

FIGURE 12-36E As a practitioner, always be aware of using proper body mechanics.

9. Repeat this entire procedure on the other foot.

Note: You can choose to work on adjacent parts of the body in sequence (from one part to the adjoining part) rather than interrupting the flow of movement. After working on the foot, proceed directly to the front of the leg. Then continue to the other foot and leg.

Massage the Front of the Legs

1. Apply lubricant with light and continuous effleurage.
2. Apply effleurage with both hands, beginning at the ankle. Apply effleurage to the entire leg by leading with one hand on the lateral side of the leg and the other hand on the medial aspect of the leg. Your hands should span the entire front of the leg. Hand pressure can be increased with each effleurage stroke, returning with light pressure to the starting point. The upward medial hand progresses to the groin and turns as it returns lightly along the medial aspect of the leg to the beginning point at the ankle. The lateral hand starts at the ankle, continues up the lateral aspect of the anterior leg, all the way to the anterior superior iliac spine (ASIS), along the iliac crest, and glides back to the starting point. Repeat these movements three to five times.

Note: The leg is the longest part of the body. Be sure to use proper body mechanics and movement when applying long strokes to the leg (Figure 12.37a-d).

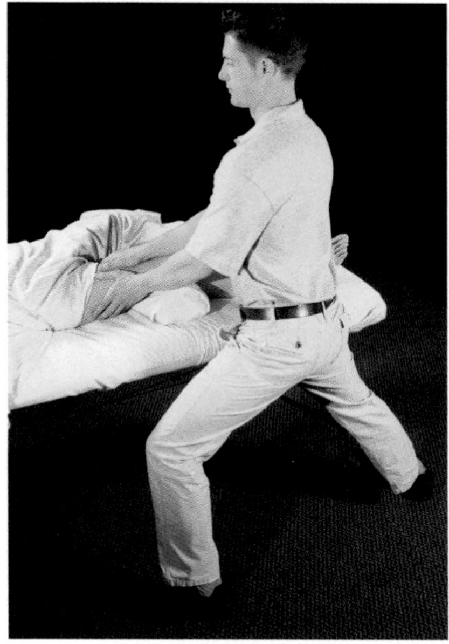

FIGURE 12-37A Apply effleurage to the leg. Maintain good posture and stance, keep the back straight, and flex the knees slightly.

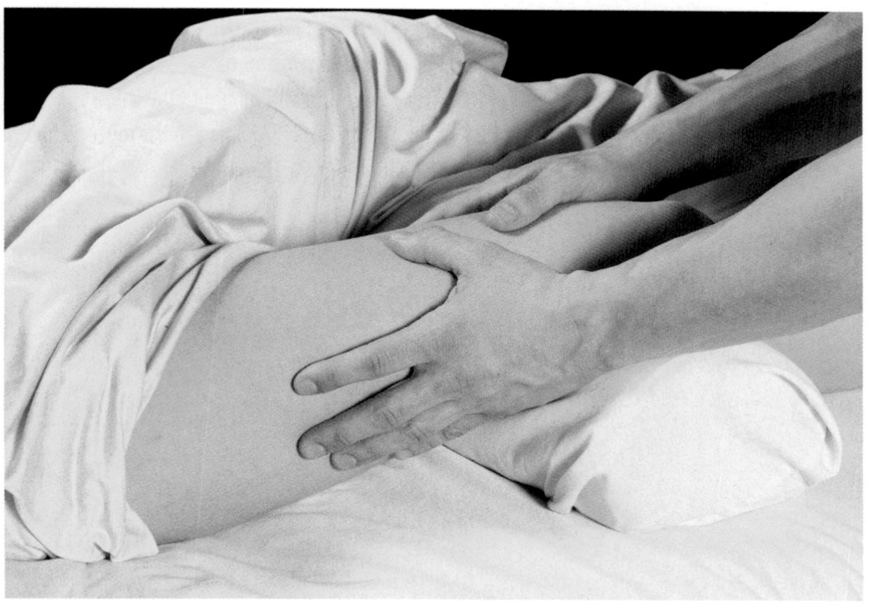

FIGURE 12-37B The leading hand should be on the lateral side of the leg to travel up and over the ilium and return to the starting point.

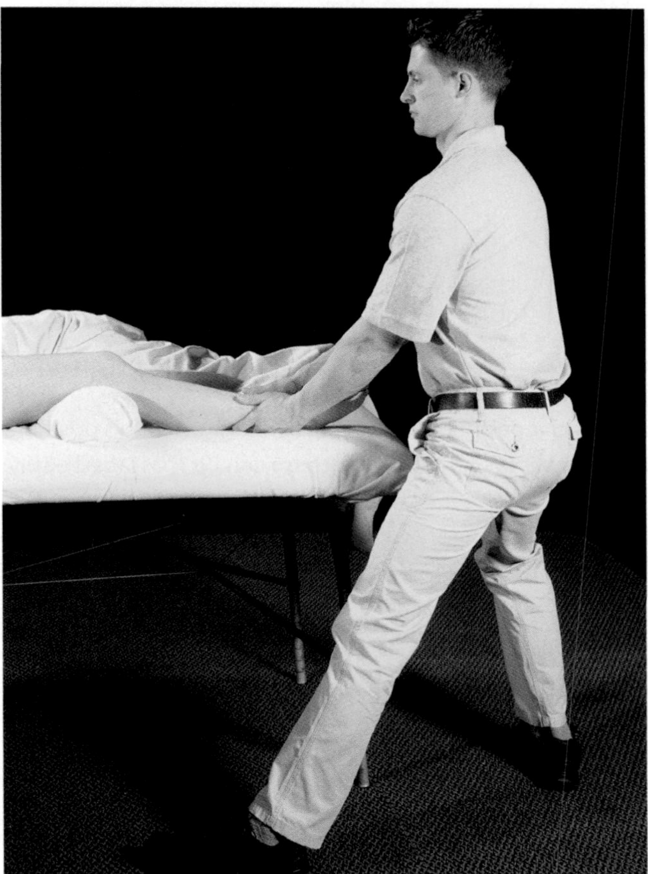

FIGURE 12-37C Note the body position at the beginning of the gliding stroke on the anterior leg.

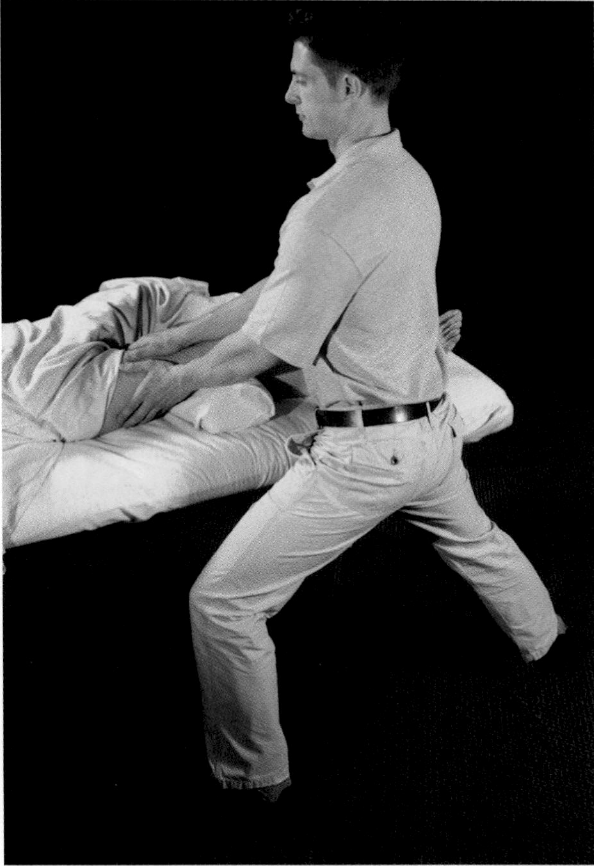

FIGURE 12-37D Note the body position at the end of the gliding stroke on the anterior leg.

3. Apply petrissage to the thigh. The thigh might require several passes up and down with this stroke because it is a large area.
4. Apply wringing and fulling to the thigh.
5. Digital petrissage is applied to the more tendinous areas around the patella and ankle.
6. Repeat effleurage (Figure 12-38a-d).

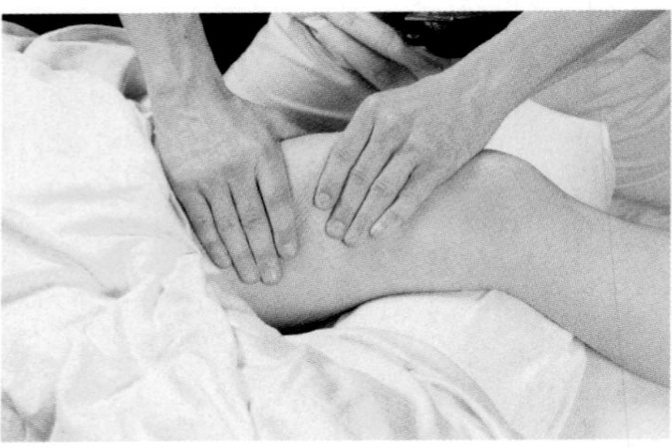

FIGURE 12-38A Apply petrissage to the anterior thigh.

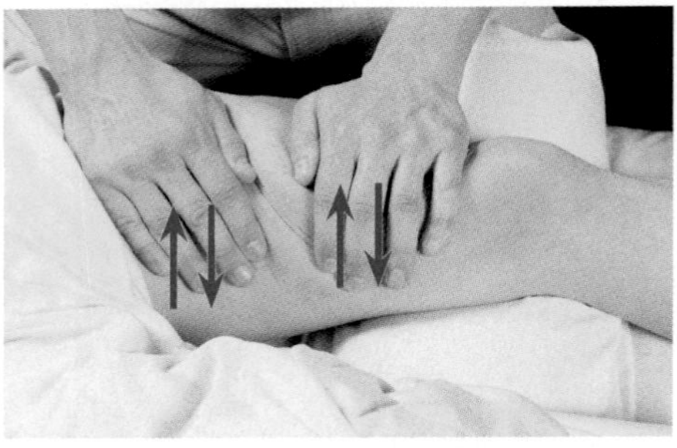

FIGURE 12-38B Continue wringing movements to the thigh.

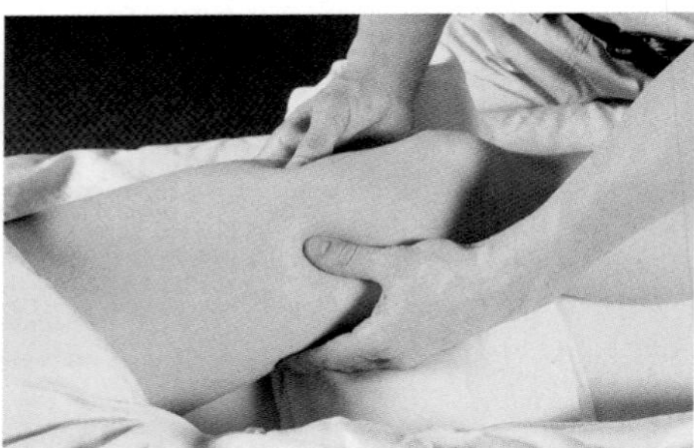

FIGURE 12-38C Apply fulling (compression) movements.

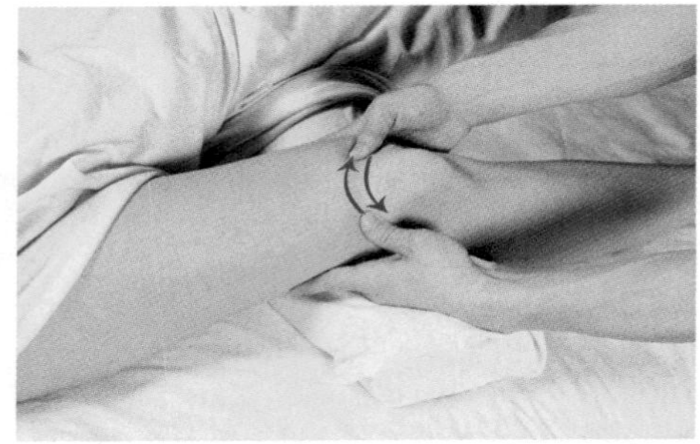

FIGURE 12-38D Manipulate the patella by tracing circles with your thumb in opposite directions.

Optional Position

Bending the Knee: The following is an optional position for leg massage. In this position, the anterior, lateral, and posterior aspects of the calf and thigh can be massaged easily. Position the client's foot flat on the table with the knee bent and the foot 16 to 18 inches from the buttocks. Wrap the foot with the drape, and brace the leg either with your knee or by sitting on the table near the client's toes to keep the leg from sliding. Be sure the draping is secure to ensure modesty of the pelvic area.

1. With the leg in the bent-knee position, apply effleurage from ankle to knee.
2. Apply petrissage from ankle to knee.
3. Repeat effleurage from ankle to knee.
4. While keeping the knee bent, apply a variety of friction techniques from ankle to knee. Pay special attention to areas that seem to be more congested or tight. Apply rolling, wringing, or cross-fiber friction in areas of tension.

5. Repeat effleurage from ankle to knee.
6. Keeping the leg in the bent-knee position apply effleurage from knee to hip.
7. Apply petrissage to the entire thigh. Make several passes to cover the entire circumference of the leg.
8. Apply wringing, rolling, and chucking.
9. Unbend the knee and with the leg resting on the table apply effleurage to the entire leg (Figure 12-39a-e).
10. Apply joint movements. Grasp the ankle with one hand, and place the other hand just below the knee. Move the knee toward the chest while flexing the knee and hips to the maximum. Pay attention to the degree of flexibility, and move the limbs firmly but not forcefully to their maximum range of movement. It is beneficial to have the client breathe deeply and then exhale as you apply downward pressure on the knee toward the chest.

Note: During joint movements of the leg it is essential to practice proper draping to ensure the client's modesty and comfort. Secure the draping across the hip and groin area. This is a good time to have the client assist by holding the draping securely while the practitioner performs the joint movements.

11. Perform hip flexion by moving your hand around to grasp the ankle at the level of the Achilles' tendon; then elevate the foot toward the ceiling to extend the leg and flex the hip. Flex the hip to its maximum range of movement by moving the foot toward the client's head.
12. Hip rotation is performed by flexing the client's knee, bringing it toward the chest; then rotate the bent leg laterally, retaining slight pressure on the knee to maintain full range of motion as the leg rotates outward. Return the leg to the table by continuing the hip rotation and slowly straightening the leg. Your hand should support the back of the leg to prevent hyperextension as the leg is returned to the table. Repeat this procedure twice (Figure 12-40a-e).

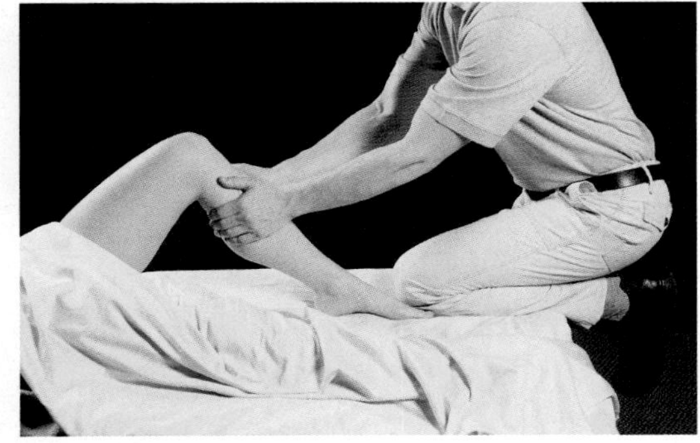

FIGURE 12-39A Support the client's leg in a bent position using your knee.

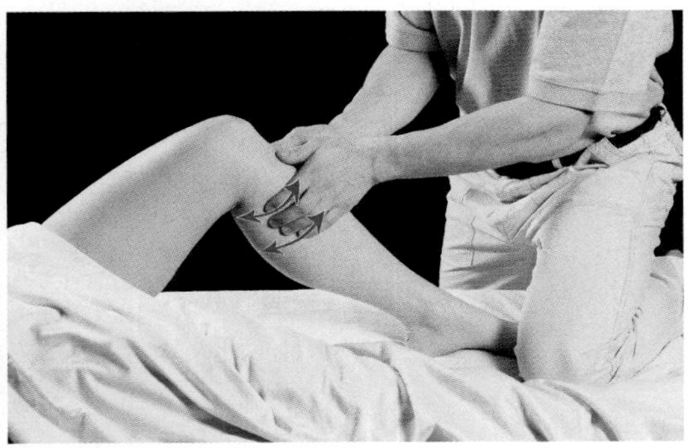

FIGURE 12-39B With the client in the bent-knee position, apply wringing and rolling movements to the calf.

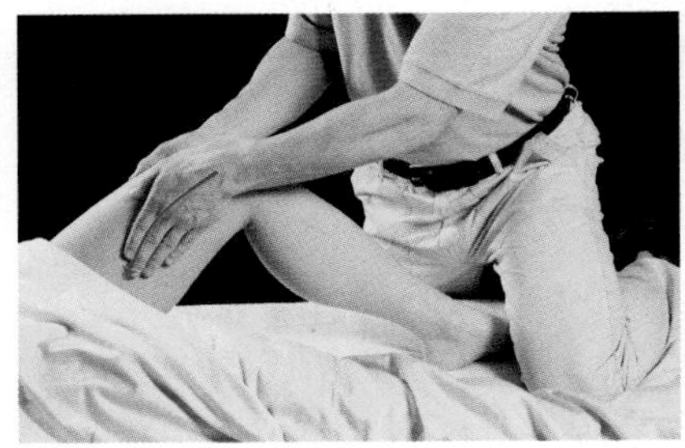

FIGURE 12-39C With the client in the bent-knee position, apply effleurage to the thigh.

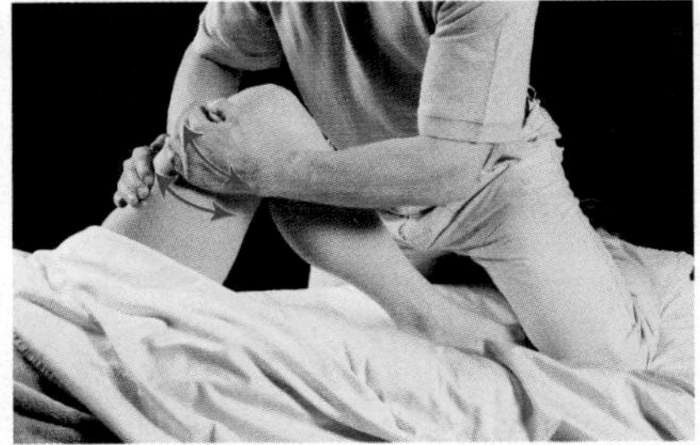

FIGURE 12-39D Knead and wring the thigh while the client is in the bent-knee position.

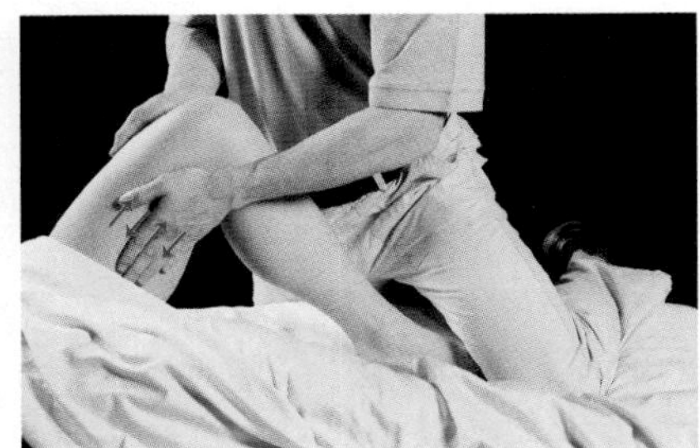

FIGURE 12-39E Apply chucking to the thigh. With the client in the bent-knee position, manipulate soft tissue of the posterior aspect of the thigh and apply effluerage, petrissage, or rolling movements.

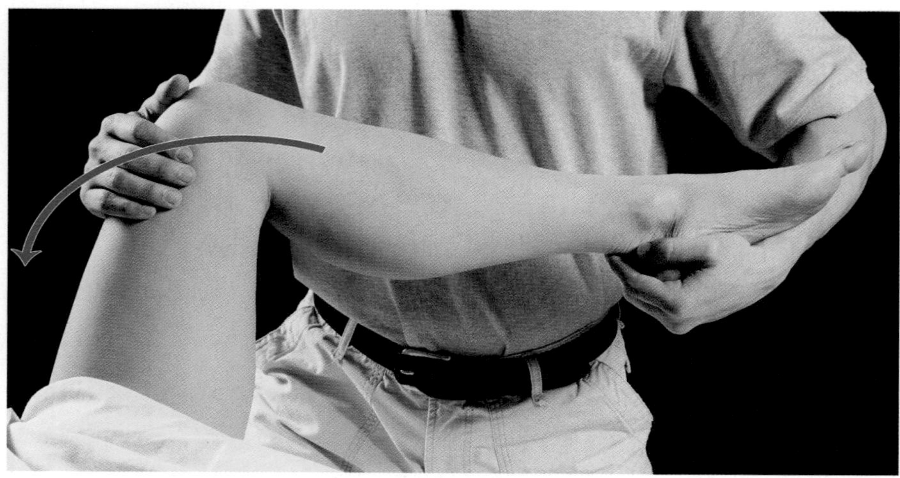

FIGURE 12-40A Apply joint movements. The client's knee can be moved toward the chest, or this position can be used for joint rotations of the hip and knee within its normal range of motion. Note the position of the hands at the heel and the knee.

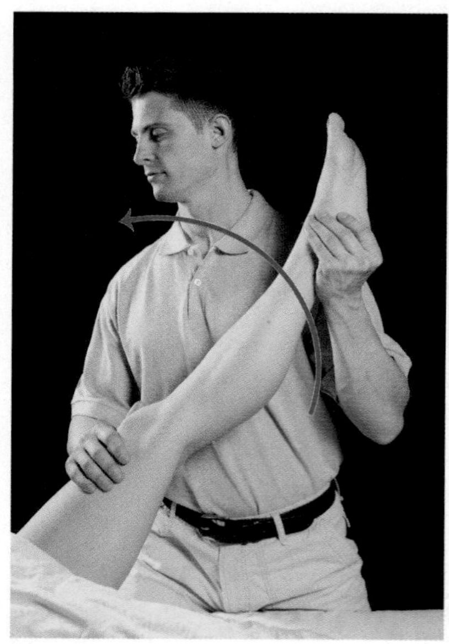

FIGURE 12-40B Stretch the hamstrings by lifting the foot toward the ceiling and straightening the knee.

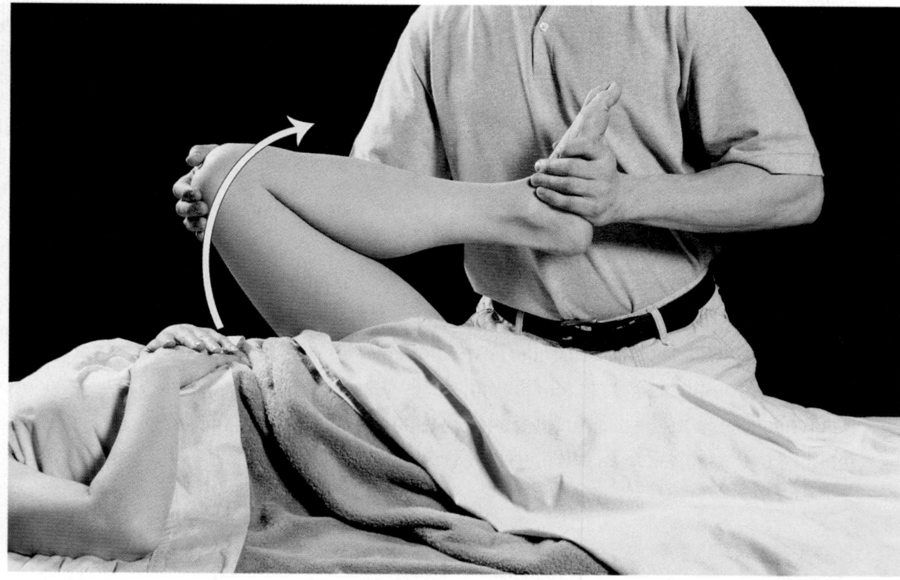

FIGURE 12-40C Move the knee to the chest to stretch the hip and lower back.

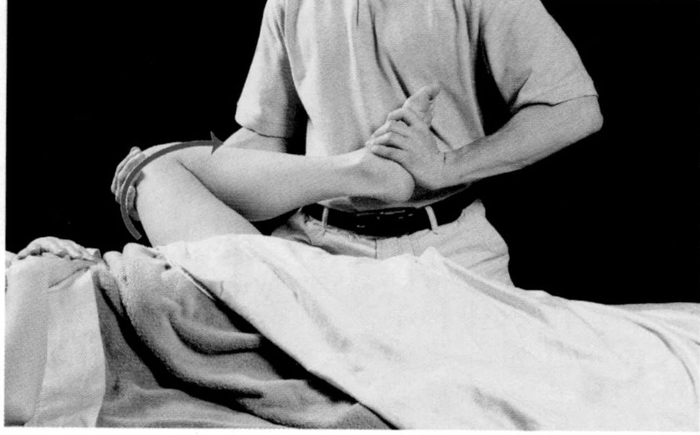

FIGURE 12-40D Abduct, rotate, and circumduct the hip. Note the draping.

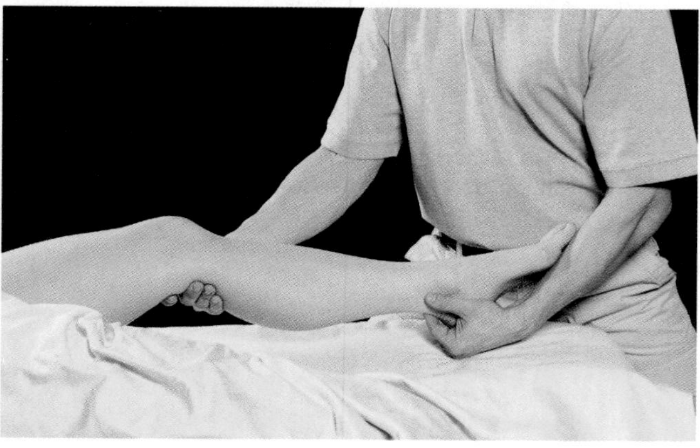

FIGURE 12-40E Support the knee as you return the leg to the table.

13. Move to the foot of the table and grasp the heel (handle) with the lateral hand (the one toward the outside of the leg you were working on). Rotate the foot and leg in the hip socket. This movement is back and forth, and the foot movement resembles that of a windshield wiper.
14. Dorsal flex and plantar flex the foot.
15. Apply traction to the leg by grasping the heel with one hand and placing the other hand over the client's instep to apply slight traction. Maintaining the same hand positions, shake the leg up and down, bouncing the heel on the table to avoid hyperextension of the knee (Figure 12-41a-d).
16. Apply effleurage to the entire leg three to five times.
17. Apply feather (nerve) strokes from hip to toes, three to five times.
18. Re-drape the leg and proceed to the other foot. Repeat the entire procedure on the other leg.

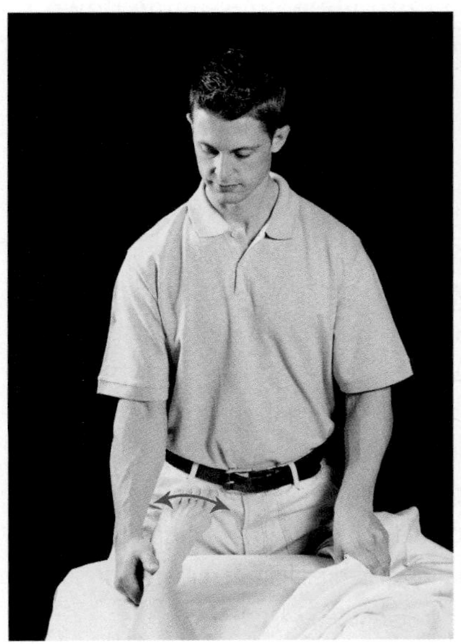

FIGURE 12-41A Rotate the leg medially and laterally with a windshield wiper motion.

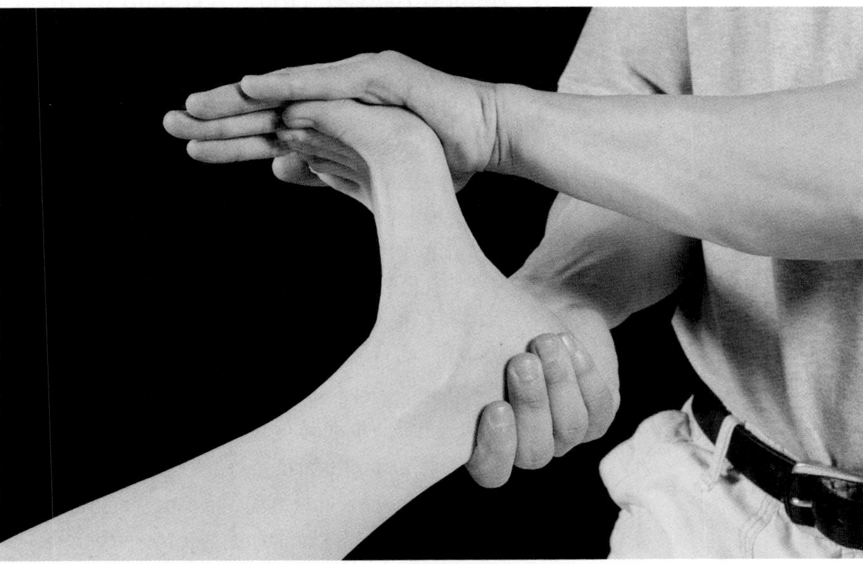

FIGURE 12-41B Stretch the Achilles tendon and calf muscles.

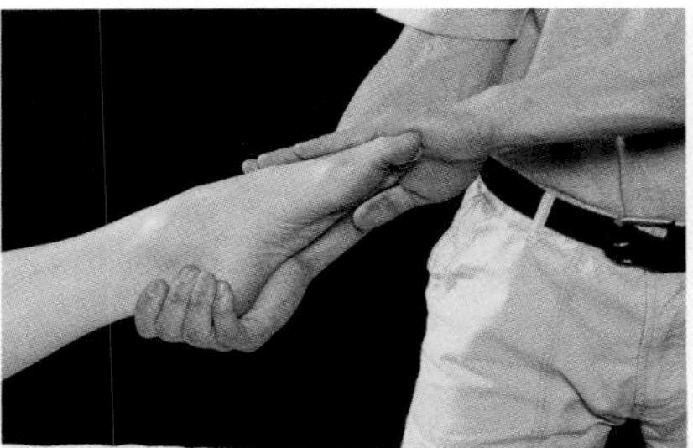

FIGURE 12-41C Plantar flex the foot.

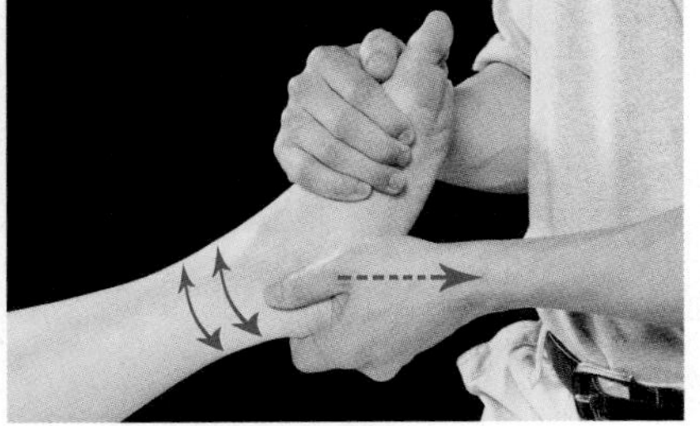

FIGURE 12-41D Apply traction and shaking movements. This completes the sequence of movements for the anterior leg. Re-drape the leg and proceed to massage the other foot and leg.

Massaging the Abdomen and Chest

This part of the massage requires some special considerations. Some clients prefer not to have the abdomen and chest massaged. Always ask before proceeding. The need for draping varies when working with male and female clients. Breast draping is always used on female clients unless informed consent is given prior to the massage for specific procedures in which the breasts will be exposed. In some states, breast draping is a legal requirement. Professional standards recommend that draping procedures (as directed earlier in this chapter) be followed. When asked, some clients opt not to have the abdomen or chest massaged.

The following massage description refers to techniques used on the fully exposed torso, with added comments when using breast draping.

In preparation for massage of the abdominal region, use a bolster or pillow to elevate the client's knees and support them so that the abdominal muscles remain relaxed. Draping should be open enough to allow massaging down to one and one-half inch below the navel, and secure enough to avoid exposure of the genital area (Figure 12-42).

1. To begin, stand to the client's right to apply massage lubricant to the abdomen, chest, and sides of the body.
2. Do effleurage strokes on the abdomen and chest, over the shoulders, around and down the axillary areas, then down the sides of the crest of the ilium. Massage back to the center with a turn of your wrist and repeat the movements. When using breast draping, this stroke glides up as far as the drape allows and then laterally over the ribs and down to the iliac crest. Massage should not be done directly over the sensitive area of the nipples on men or women.
3. Do circular effleurage on the abdomen in a clockwise direction, following the path of the colon. On this stroke, one hand remains in constant contact doing circular massage. The other describes a semicircle beginning at the lower right of the client's abdomen, moving up the right side to the rib cage, across the abdomen just below the rib cage, then down the left side to an area just medial to the hip bone. Abdominal massage should always encourage the natural flow of the large intestines. Repeat the abdominal massage movements several times (see Figure 12-43a).

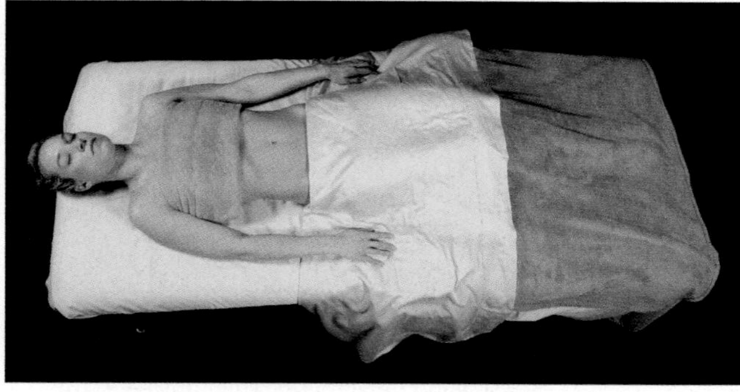

FIGURE 12-42 Note the correct position and draping for massage of the abdomen. Use a folded towel or pillowcase to cover the female client's breasts. Use a bolster to support the knees.

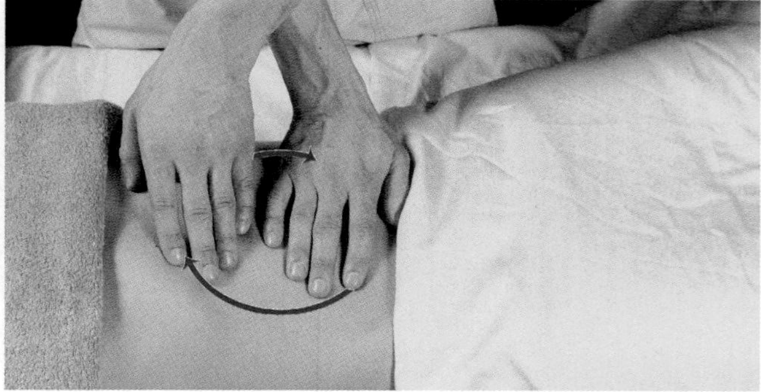

FIGURE 12-43A Stroke the abdomen with deep circular movement in a clockwise direction.

4. Knead the entire abdomen, massaging not only the abdominal muscles but also stimulating the action of the abdominal organs (Figure 12-43b).
5. To massage the large intestine more thoroughly, apply circular friction to its entire length. Begin in the area of the lower left quadrant of the abdomen. The circles should be on an oblique (deviation to the vertical or horizontal line) plane of the surface of the abdomen so that pressure is increased and decreased repeatedly over an area about 2 inches square, and at the rate of about 100 circles per minute. This movement encourages the contents of the colon toward the rectum. Proceed slowly back along the course of the colon all the way to the cecum, the first portion of the colon (Figure 12-43c).
6. Grasp as much of the abdominal tissue as possible and gently lift and shake it (Figure 12-43d).

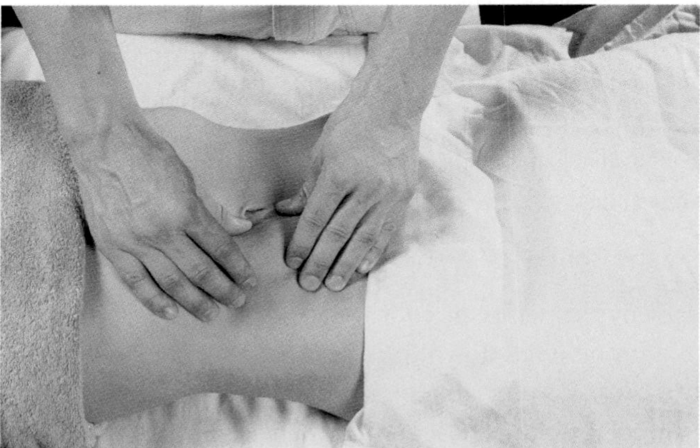

FIGURE 12-43B Apply petrissage to the abdomen.

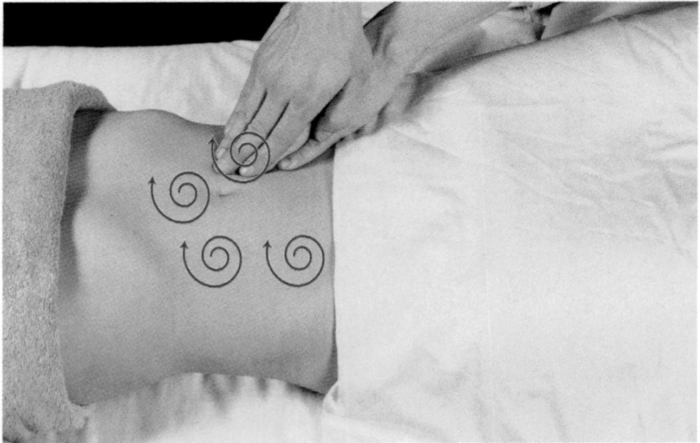

FIGURE 12-43C Apply friction in small circles, following the colon in reverse.

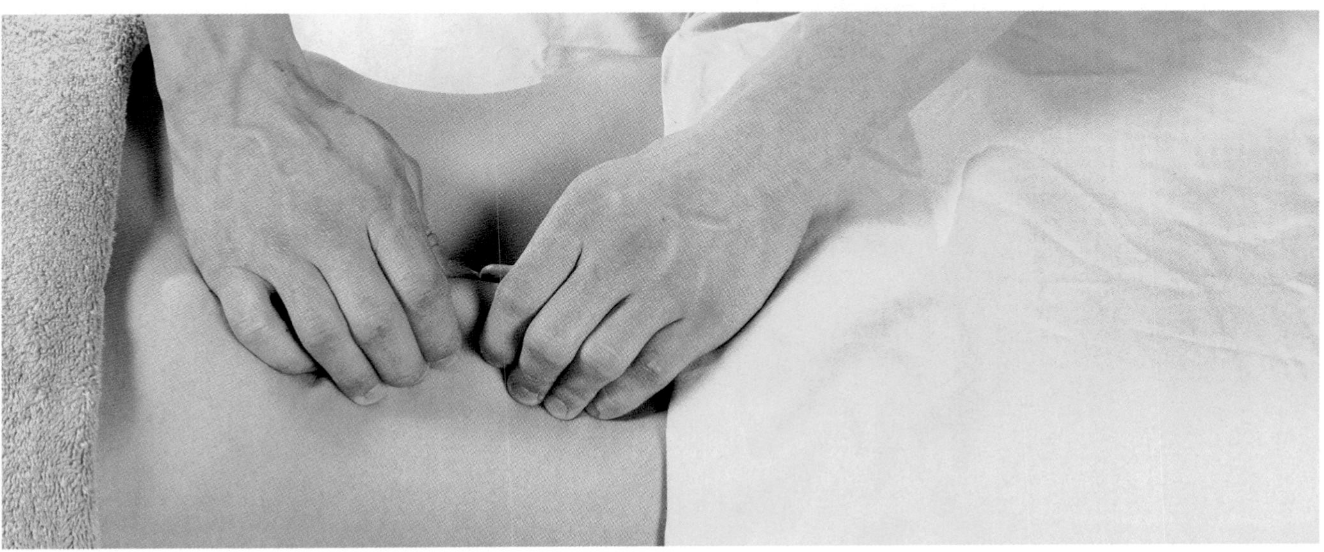

FIGURE 12-43D Apply a shaking movement. Grasp the skin of the abdomen and shake it gently. This movement stimulates the action of the large and small intestines.

7. Do alternate hand gliding strokes or shingles. Stand to one side of the client and reach over to the opposite side. Alternately pull your hands over the client's body toward you. As one hand nears completion of the stroke, the other begins a stroke. This movement begins just below the crest of the ilium (hip bone) and can continue all the way over the shoulder and up the neck. When working with breast draping, it is necessary to adjust the drape to continue this movement up to the axillary area and back down to the hip. When massaging the area of the ribs, flex your fingers slightly and rake gently between the ribs with your fingertips (Figure 12-43e-h).
8. Move to the other side of the table and repeat step #7 on the other side of the client's torso.
9. Move to the head of the table for the following stroke. This is referred to as the *caring stroke* and is a complete gliding stroke for the torso. This stroke can only be done when breast draping is not used. Begin by placing your fingers (pointing toward each other) with palms flat on the client's skin at the uppermost aspect of the chest. Stroke downward over the chest and abdomen to the pubic bone. Rotate your hands over the client's hipbone, around the gluteus medius, around the sides, and back up to the axillary area. Rotate your hands as you continue upward, around the shoulders, up the trapezius muscles to the back of the neck, ending at the occiput. Rotate your hands as you move them back down to the starting point. Repeat the movement several times. Beware of any residual tension that your hands might perceive, and spend a few extra moments to work on those areas. Then repeat the caring stroke (Figure 12-44a-d).

This completes the massage of the front of the body.

At this point, reposition the top cover or wrap to cover the client, secure the cover, and ask the client to turn over to a prone (face-down) position. Be sure to follow proper draping procedures. Make the client comfortable by supplying a face rest, a bolster under the ankles, and other supports for the chest or abdomen as needed.

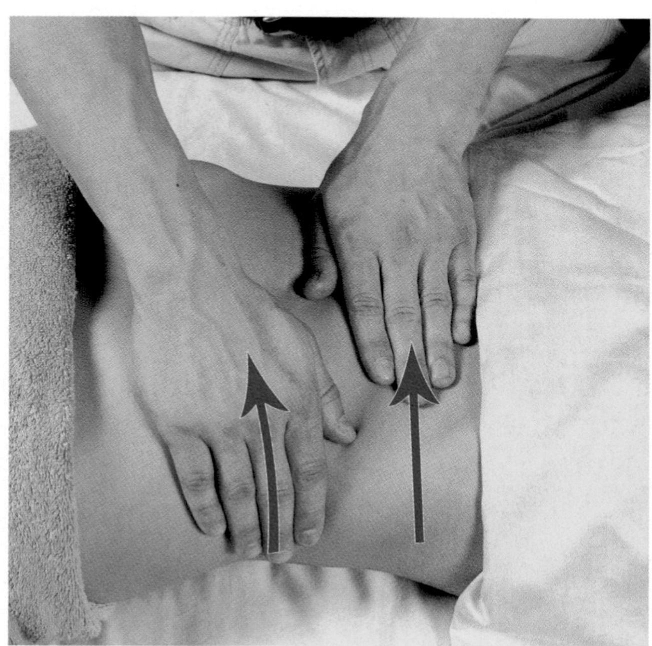

FIGURE 12-43E Apply alternate-hand stroking movements (shingles) from the trochanter to the axilla. Note: Shingles is the name often used to describe alternate-hand effleurage in which one hand repeats the stroke as the other hand is about to complete the stroke.

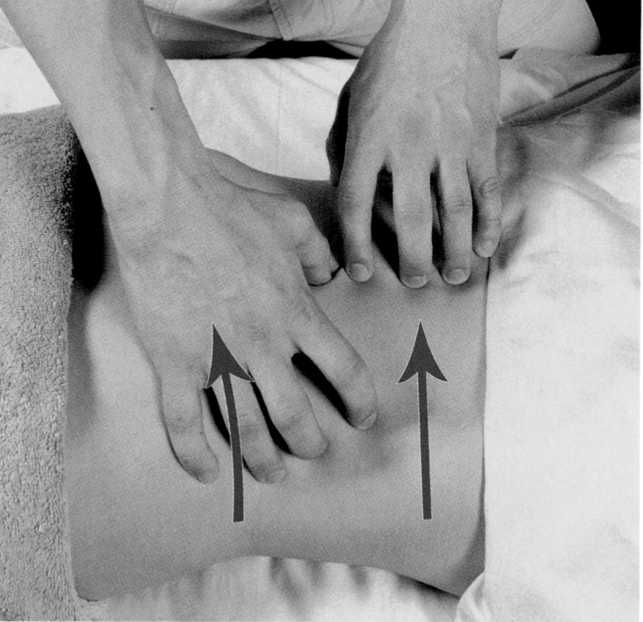

FIGURE 12-43F Apply a raking movement several times across the ribs and abdomen using the tips of the fingers.

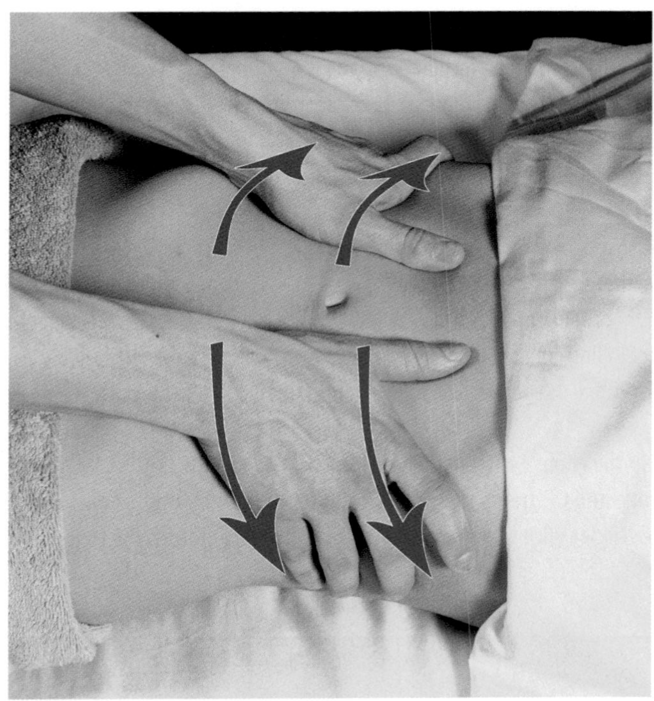

FIGURE 12-43G Stretch the muscles of the stomach area and the abdominal region outward.

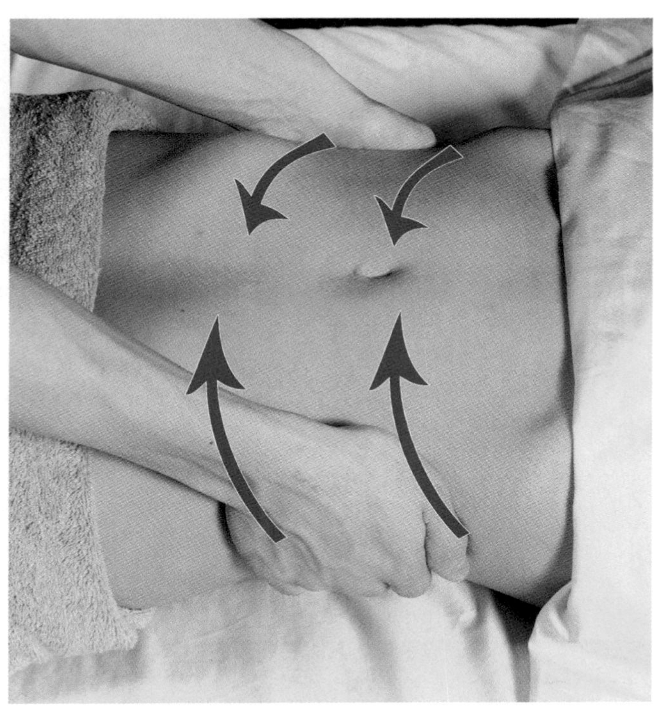

FIGURE 12-43H Stretch the muscles over the stomach area and abdominal region inward.

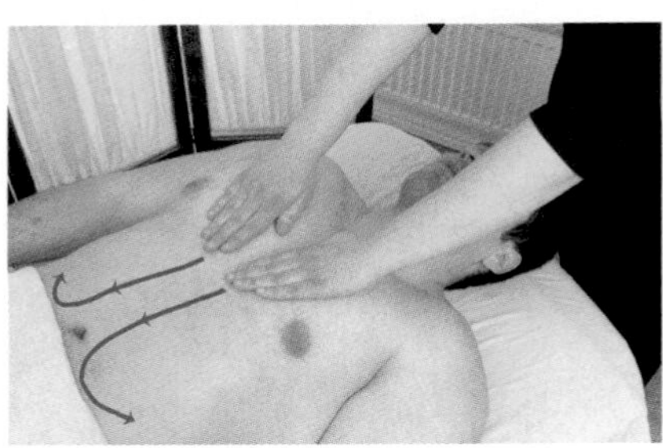

FIGURE 12-44A Using the caring stroke, cover the entire front of the body and the neck. It is not possible to do the full caring stroke on women when using breast draping.

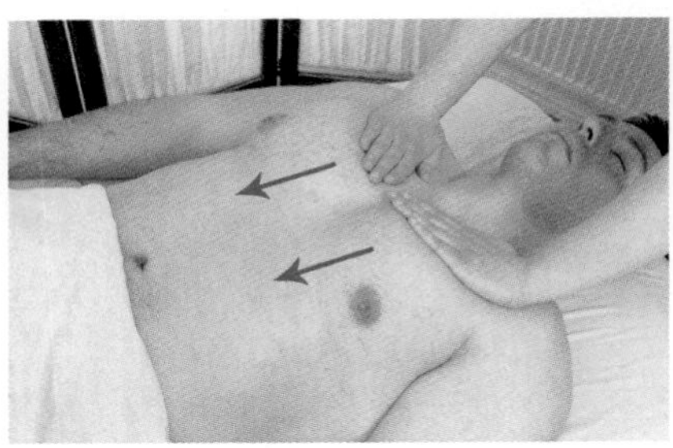

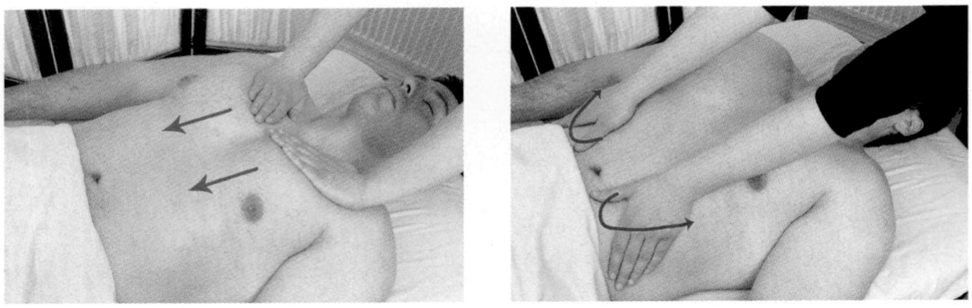

FIGURE 12-44B(1-2) Note that the caring stroke begins at the clavicle with a stroke down the front of the body to the pubic bone.

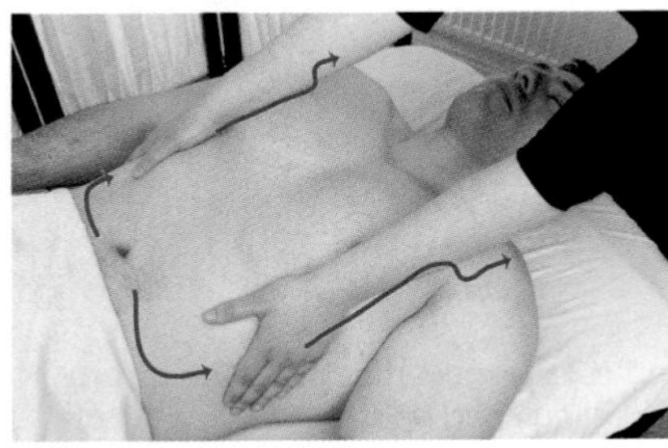

FIGURE 12-44C Without losing contact with the client, rotate your hands to the sides of the client's body and stroke up to the axillary area.

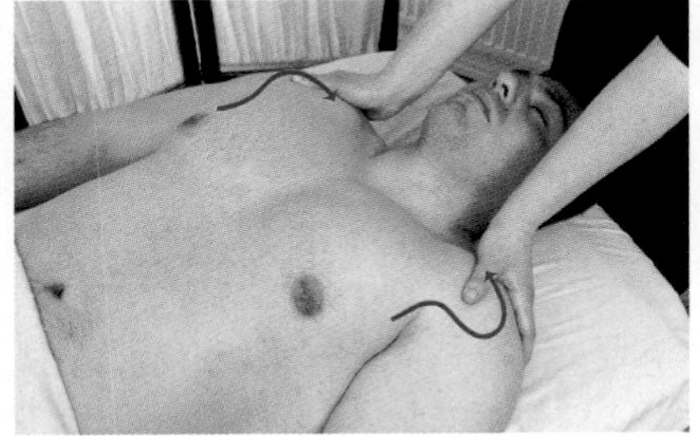

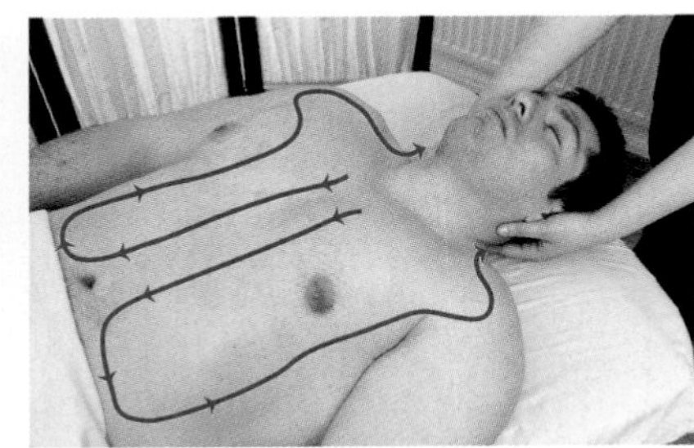

FIGURE 12-44D (1-2) Stroke up, over, and around the shoulders and up the neck. Repeat the stroke several times.

Massage the Back of the Legs

1. Undrape one leg. This massage is similar to the procedures for the front of the legs.
2. Make contact with the client's skin and apply the massage lubricant with light effleurage strokes.
3. Apply effleurage, leading with your lateral hand (medial hand following). Increase the pressure on the upward stroke with each pass. Maintain contact with much lighter pressure on the return stroke. Repeat three to five times.
4. Apply petrissage to the calf and thigh upward to the crest of the ilium (Figure 12-45a-g).
5. Repeat effleurage three to five times.
6. When there are particularly tight or tense areas, go over them with more specific friction movements such as compression, wringing, rolling, and deep friction. Using the heel of the hand or the elbow can be quite effective over the gluteal muscles and the hamstrings (Figure 12-46a-h).
7. Repeat effleurage.
8. Apply joint movements. Grasp the client's ankle and move the foot toward the buttocks with gentle pressure to flex the knee and to stretch the muscles on the front of the thigh. Continue by making increasingly larger circles with the ankle to rotate the hip joint. Return the foot to the table (Figure 12-47a-c).

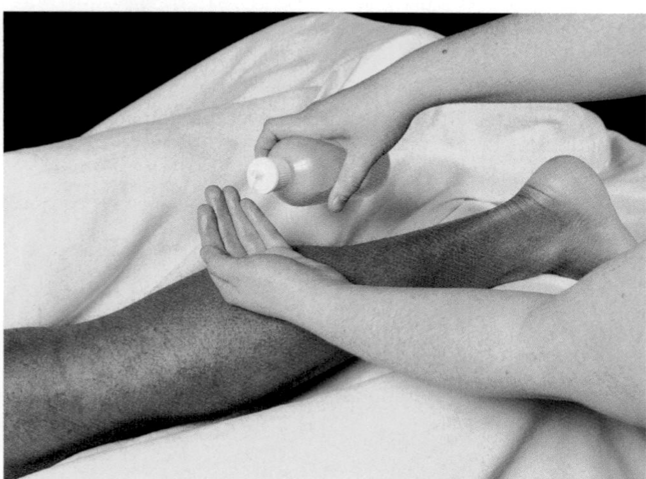

FIGURE 12-45A Before beginning massage movements, prepare the posterior leg by undraping and applying lubricant. Keep the back of your hand against the client's skin while pouring the lubricant into your hand.

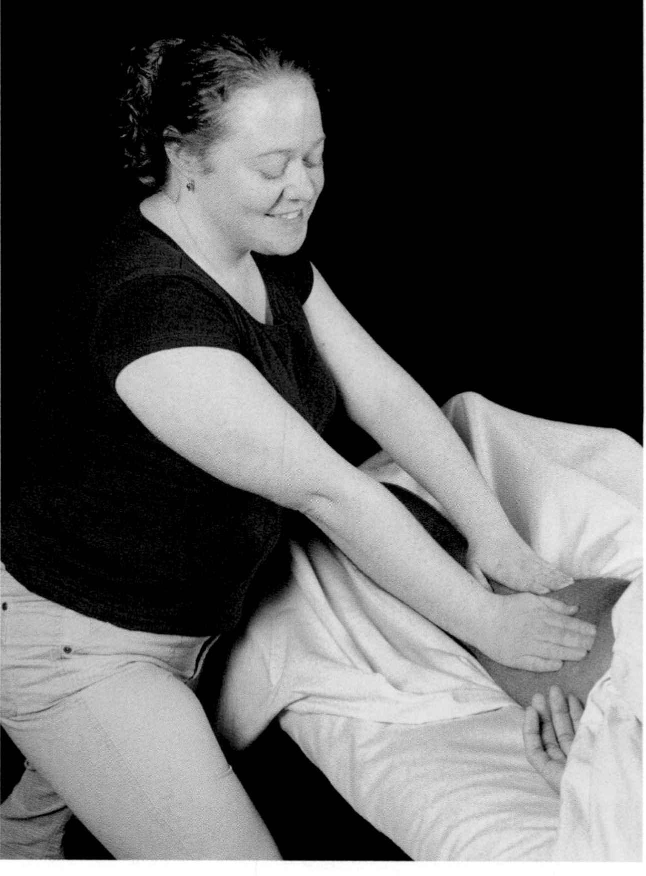

FIGURE 12-45B Apply effleurage movements. Stroke toward the heart. Note: Place the leading hand on the lateral aspect of the leg to travel up and over the gluteal muscles and the iliac crest and back down the lateral side of the leg. At the same time, the medial hand travels up to the gluteal crease and then lightly down the medial side of the leg. Return both hands to the starting point to repeat the stroke three or more times.

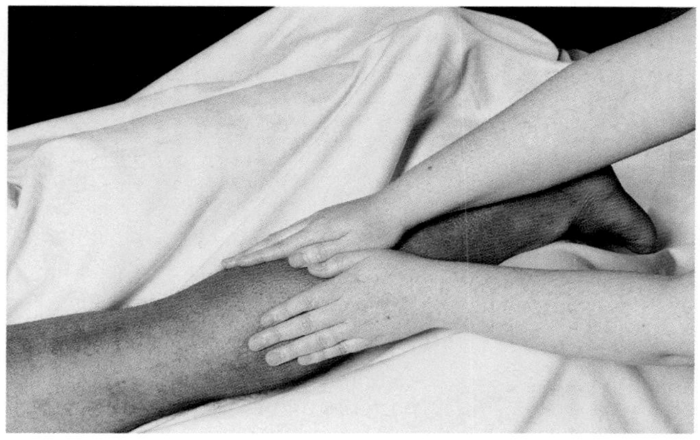

FIGURE 12-45C Stroke the leg upward with both hands.

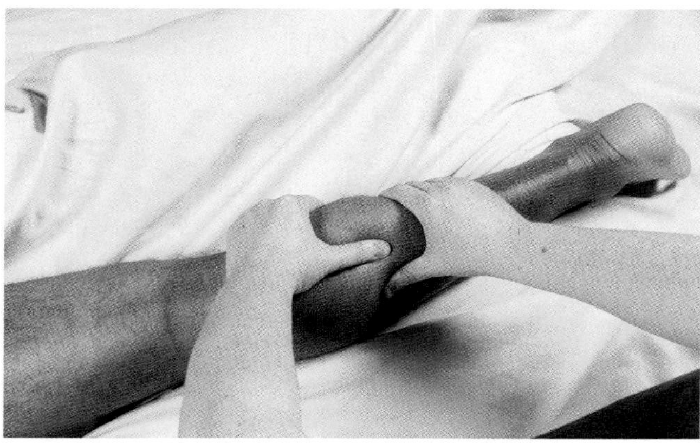

FIGURE 12-45D Knead the calf muscles.

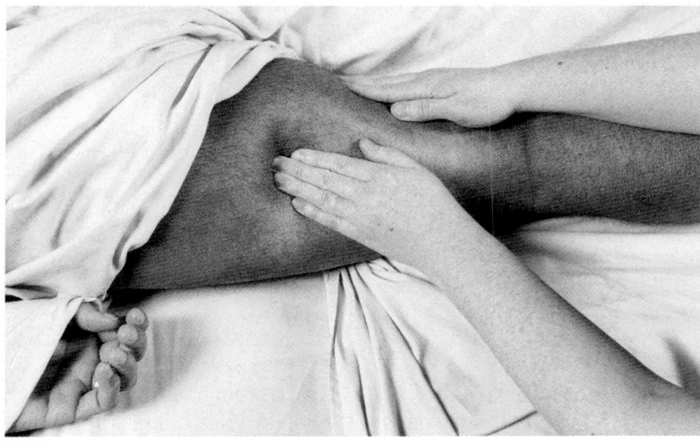

FIGURE 12-45E Knead the muscles of the leg and thigh in a circular motion.

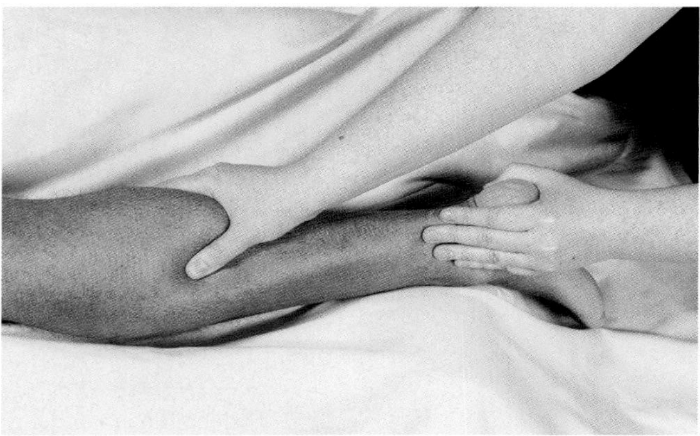

FIGURE 12-45F Apply the V-stroke for deep stroking of the posterior leg.

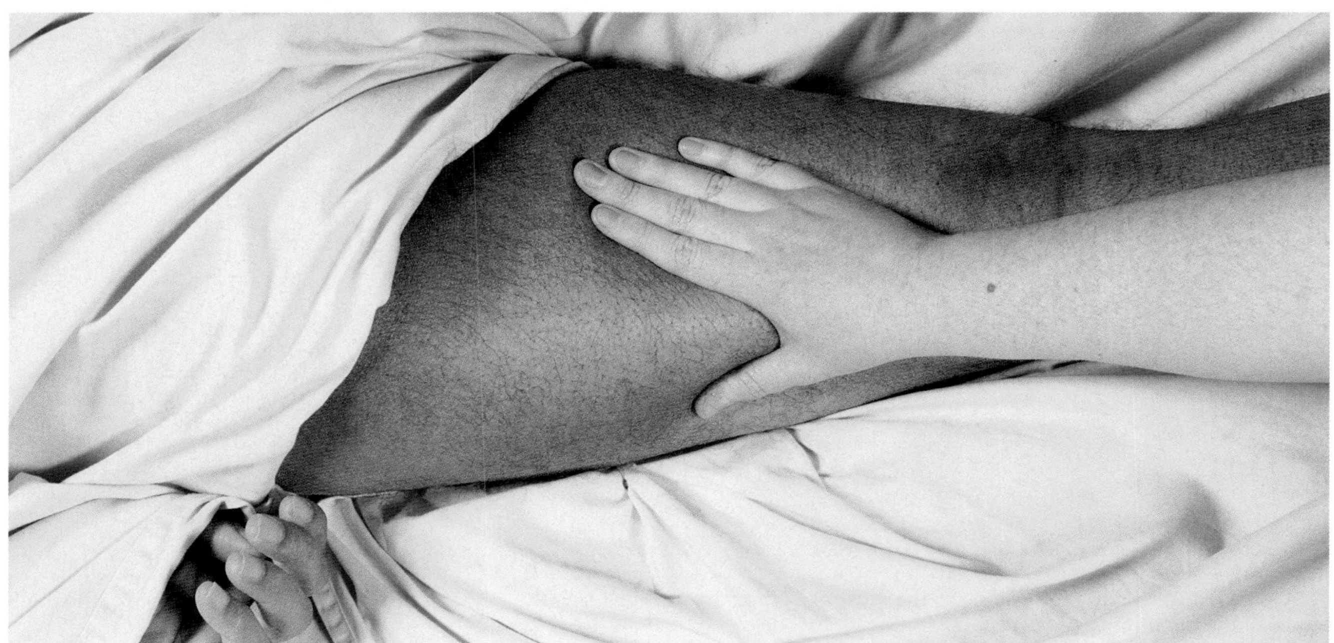

FIGURE 12-45G Continue the V-stroke up the back of the thigh.

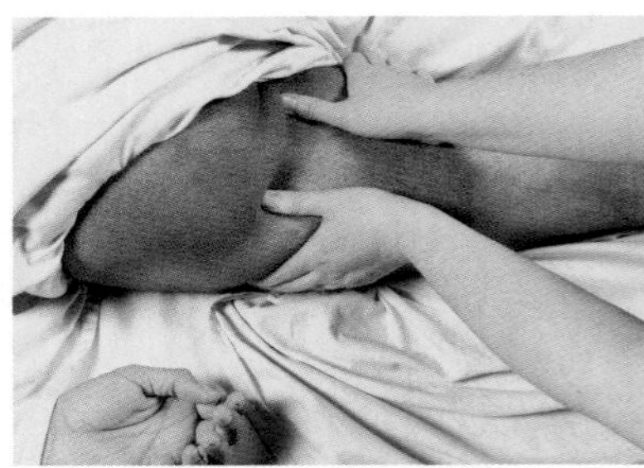
FIGURE 12-46A Apply fulling strokes to the entire leg.

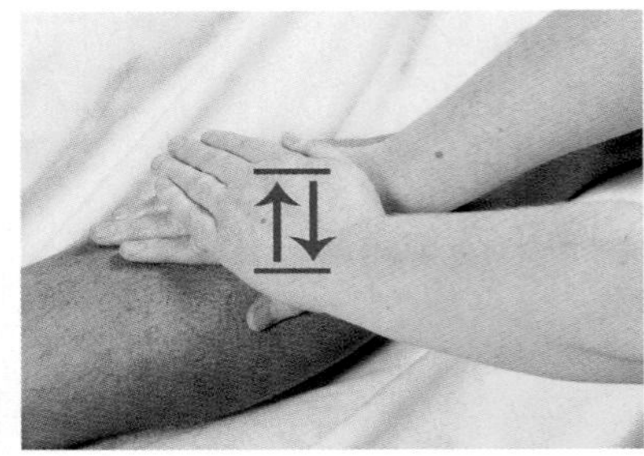
FIGURE 12-46B Apply compression movements to the leg.

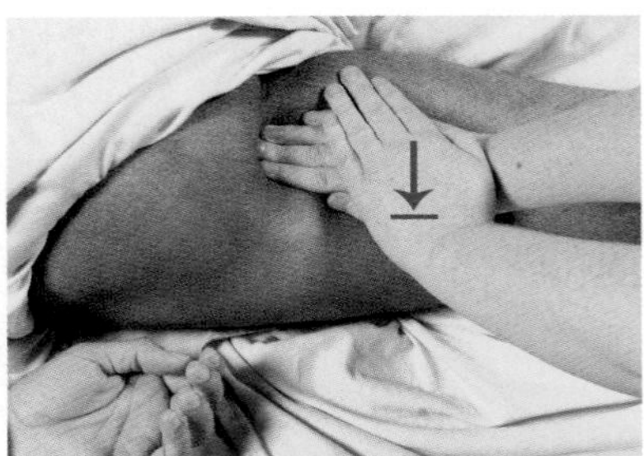
FIGURE 12-46C Apply compression to the posterior thigh.

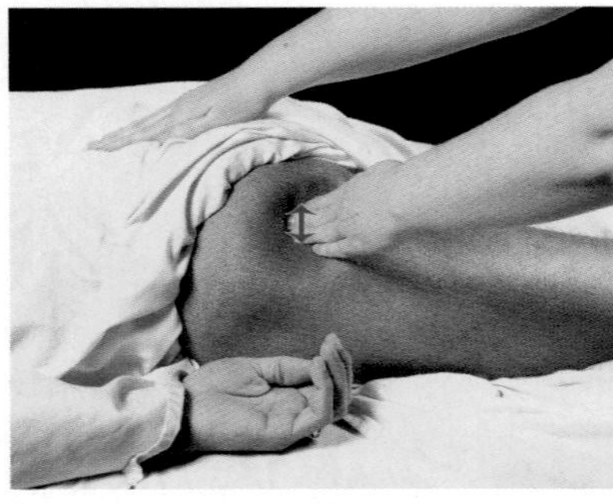
FIGURE 12-46D Apply digital friction to the gluteal area.

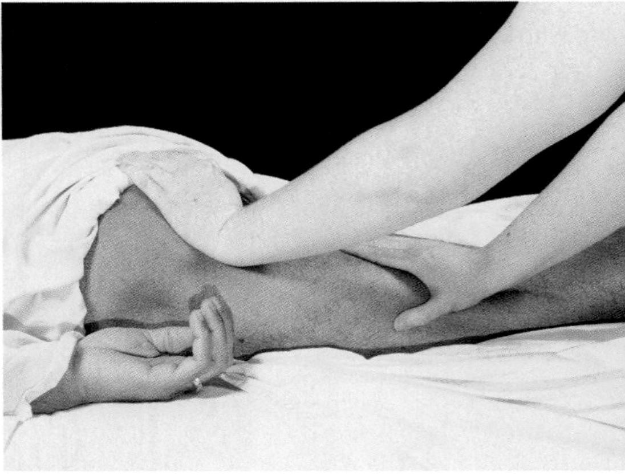
FIGURE 12-46E Using the heel of your hand, apply deep friction or deep pressure to the gluteal muscles.

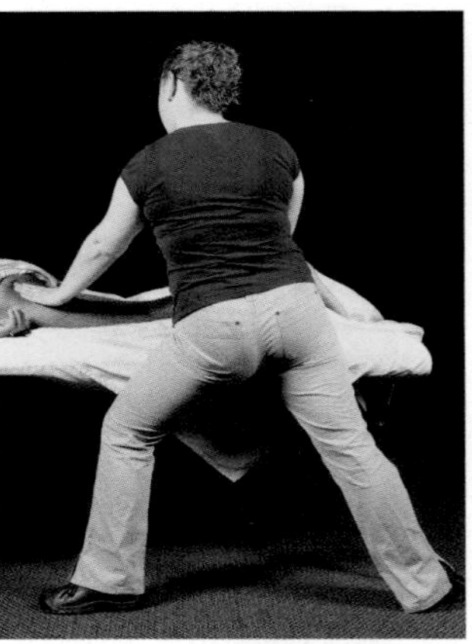
FIGURE 12-46F When applying deep pressure, always use proper body mechanics.

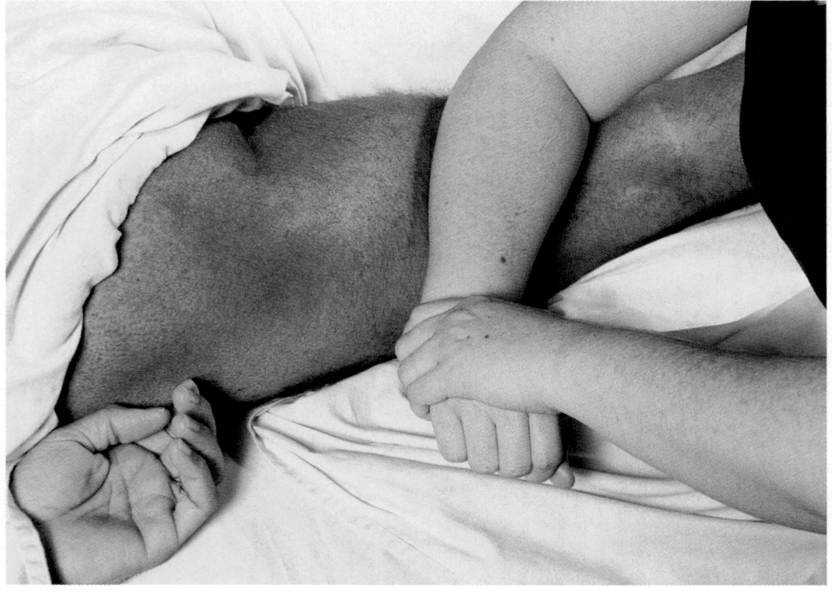
FIGURE 12-46G Apply deep gliding to the muscles of the posterior leg using the elbow of the forearm.

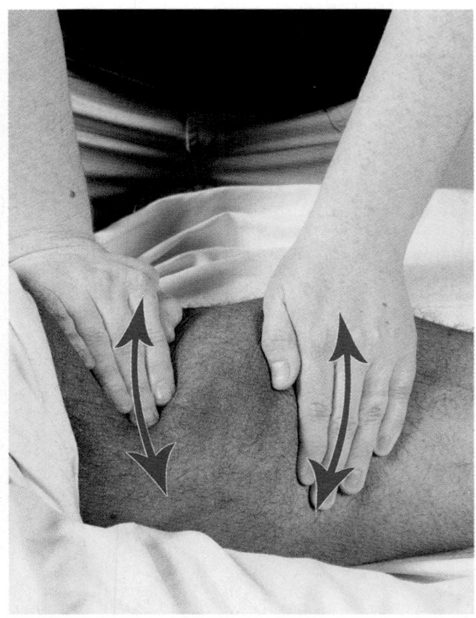
FIGURE 12-46H Wring the back of the thigh.

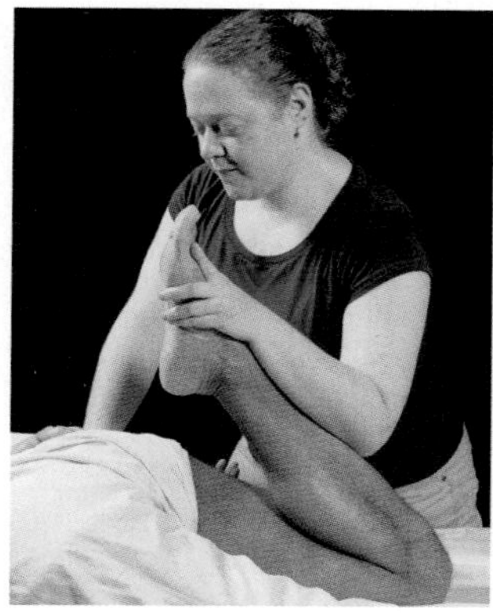

FIGURE 12-47A Flex the client's knee, pressing the heel against the gluteal muscles.

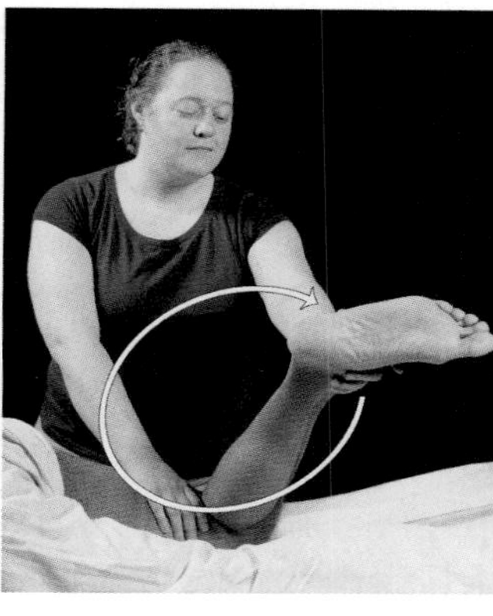

FIGURE 12-47B Support the knee, and circumduct the lower leg.

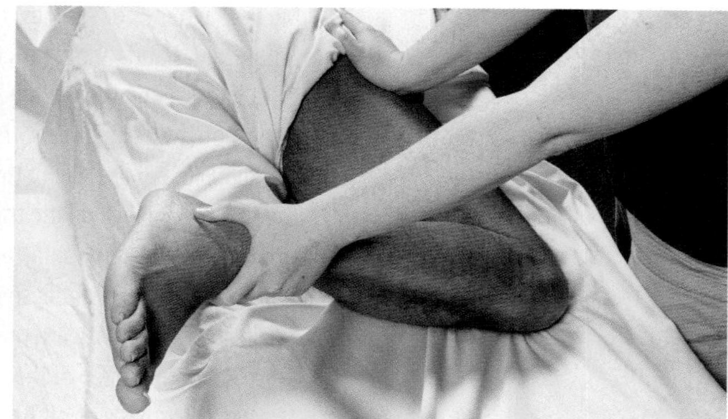

FIGURE 12-47C Apply joint movements to flex the knee and laterally rotate the hip.

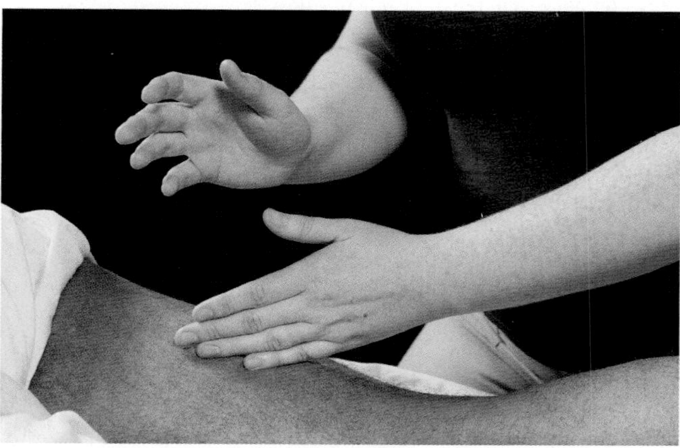

FIGURE 12-48A Apply percussion to the posterior leg. The ulnar side of the hand aligns with the direction of muscle fibers.

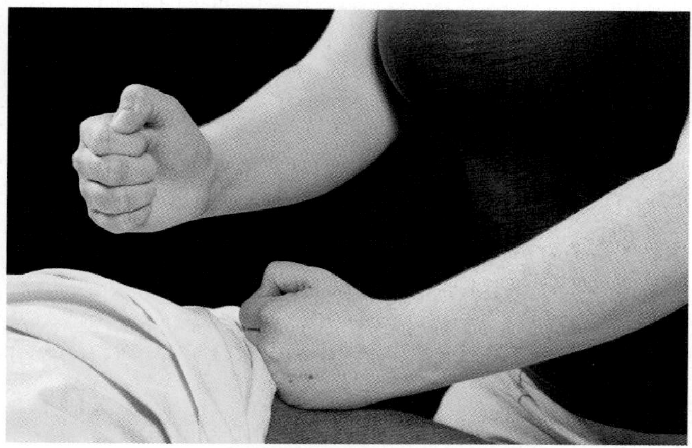

FIGURE 12-48B Apply percussion (beating) to the gluteal area.

9. Apply percussion (optional) over the leg (Figure 12-48a and b).
10. Repeat effleurage as a finishing stroke, gently changing to feather (nerve) strokes.
11. Re-drape the leg and repeat the entire procedure on the client's other leg.

Massage the Back

No massage is complete without a good back massage. It is important to give a good back massage because the client usually expects and looks forward to this part of the massage. Be sure to pace the massage so that you have ample time to devote to the back massage. There are hundreds of manipulations that can be performed on the back. They range from extremely superficial stroking to deep tissue work, using elbows and forearms when relieving tension around the spine, pelvis, and shoulders. The following is a basic soothing routine that is guaranteed to leave the recipient in a calm, relaxed state.

1. Follow proper draping procedures.
2. Stand to the side of the client. Apply massage lubricant with effleurage strokes.
3. Beginning at the top of the gluteal cleft, apply long effleurage strokes. Apply long gliding strokes up along the muscles on the sides of the spine to the nape of the neck.

4. Move your hands out and over the shoulders and down the sides of the torso and back down to the hips. Rotate your hands and return to the starting point. Repeat the gliding movement five to eight times. Use equal pressure on the pulling and pushing strokes (Figure 12-49a-c).
5. Apply petrissage. Begin with the gluteal region on the opposite side of the client from where you are standing. Knead the side of the body from below the ilium up into the axillary area. Continue over the shoulder to include the trapezius and neck. Move hands medially to a position nearer to the spine (midway between the spine and extreme side of the body), then knead back down to the gluteal area. Work along the side of the spine to include the sacrospinalis and erector spinea muscles.
6. Begin at the neck with alternate-hand strokes (shingles) from the side of the body to the spinal process. Move down to the top of the thigh and then back up to the top of the shoulder (Figure 12-50a-c).
7. Move to the other side of the table and repeat steps #2 through #6.
8. Flex the client's elbow (closest to you), and place the client's hand on the table about six inches from the armpit to elevate the medial border of the scapula. Some practitioners prefer to place the client's hand in the small of the back to abduct and elevate the scapula. In this position, several kneading and friction movements can easily be performed on all sides of the scapula. Special attention should be given to the teres major and minor, trapezius, the rhomboids, and the infraspinatus muscles.
9. Apply joint movement to the shoulder. With the client's hand still in position at the side, grasp the top of the shoulder with one hand. Place your fingers neatly into a notch near the coracoid process, and use this

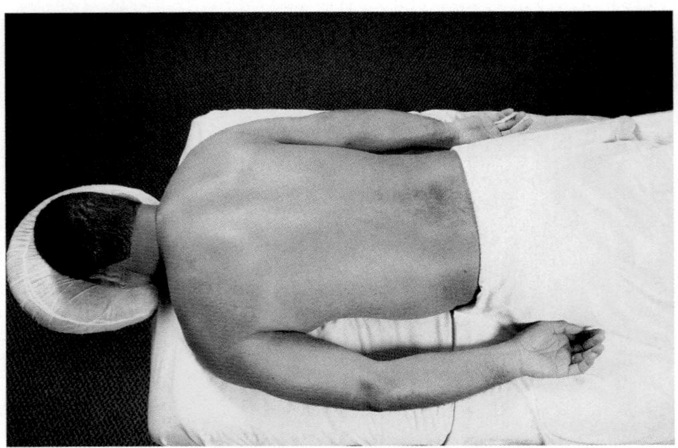

FIGURE 12-49A Prepare for the massage of the back by adjusting the draping and applying lubricant with a light effleurage stroke.

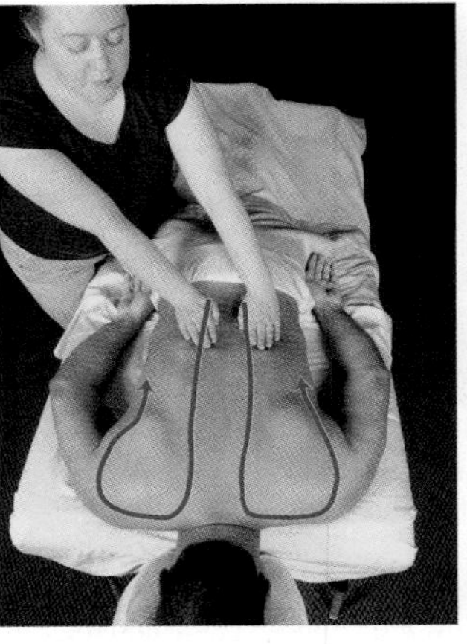

FIGURE 12-49B Apply long strokes up the back, beginning at the gluteal cleft. The ulnar side of the hand leads, with the fingers of one hand nearly touching the other at the midline of the back.

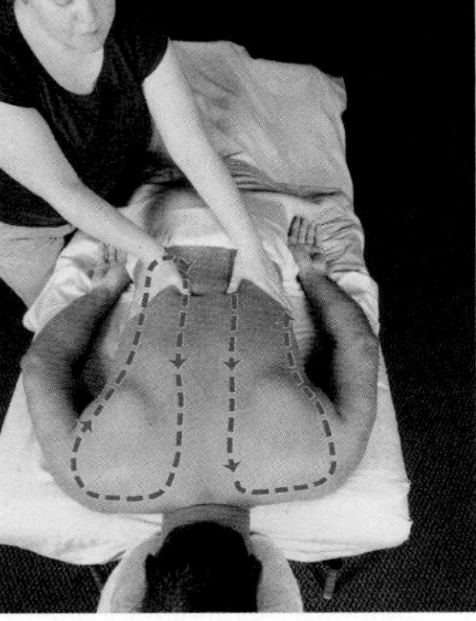

FIGURE 12-49C Continue with effleurage strokes back down the sides, returning to the starting point. Pressure is consistent throughout the entire stroke.

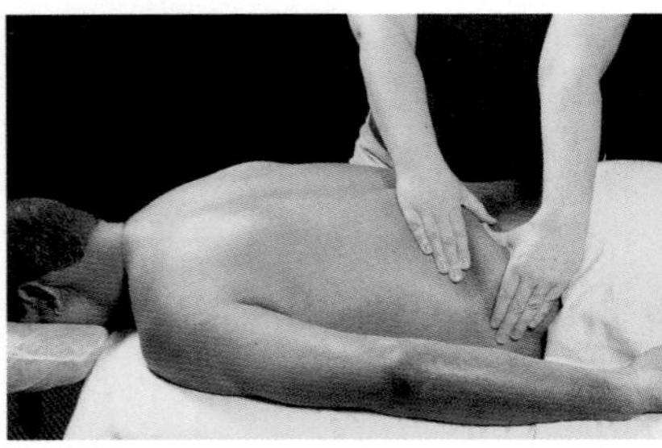

FIGURE 12-50A Apply petrissage to the entire side that is opposite to you. This takes several passes.

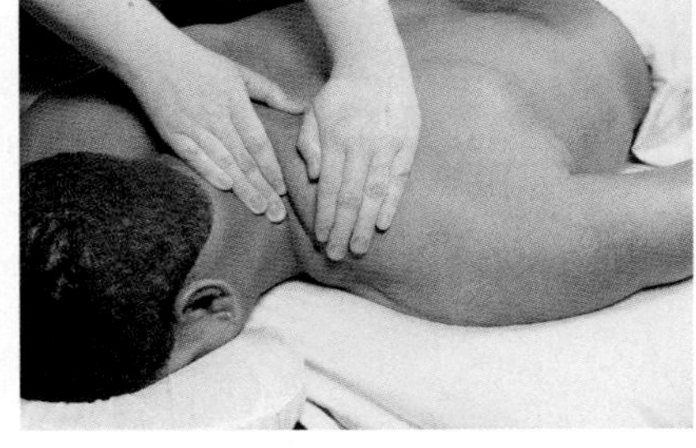

FIGURE 12-50B Note that petrissage includes the trapezius muscles.

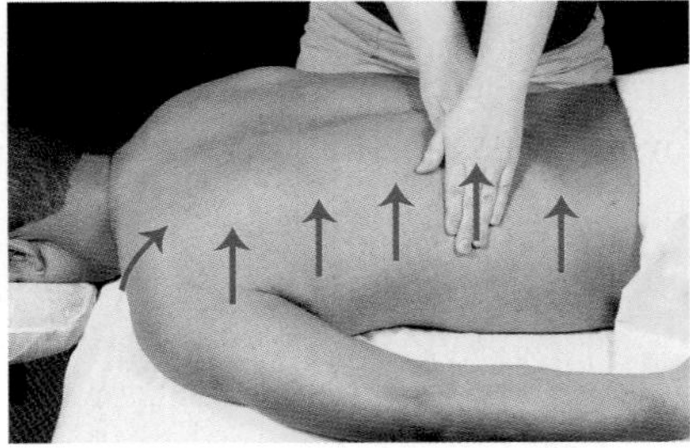

FIGURE 12-50C Apply alternate-hand stroking movements (shingles) up and down the entire side.

hold as a handle. Place the other hand just inferior to the scapula so that the inferior angle of the scapula fits neatly into the V formed between your thumb and index finger. Lift and rotate the scapula away from the rib cage. Although this might seem unnecessary, it is very effective in relieving several stress-related shoulder problems. Rotate the shoulder several times in both directions.

10. Abduct the elbow so that the upper arm is at a square angle from the body and the forearm is hanging down and relaxed at a square angle from the upper arm. Support the arm with both of your hands just proximal to the elbow, allowing the hand and forearm to gently swing the hand up and down, allowing the shoulder to rotate in a relaxed manner. Replace the hand and arm to the side of the body (Figure 12-51a-e).
11. Repeat all the movements, #8 through #10, on the other side of the back.
12. Apply deep kneading and friction to the gluteal area.
13. Repeat effleurage on the entire back area.
14. Apply wringing friction to the back, moving back and forth across the back and working all the way up the neck and back down.
15. Apply circular friction on each side of the spine on the erector spine muscles.
16. Do sacrospinalis vibration. Place the first two fingers of one hand to either side of the client's spine, about two inches apart. Bend your fingers slightly so that they apply deep pressure on the medial edge of the sacrospinalis muscle and along each side of the spinus process. Place your other hand on the top of the hand resting on the client's back, and press down firmly while vibrating slowly (about 120 vibrations per minute) from side to side along the client's body. Slowly glide both hands down along the spine, vibrating (jiggling) each portion of the sacrospinalis muscle back and forth about three to

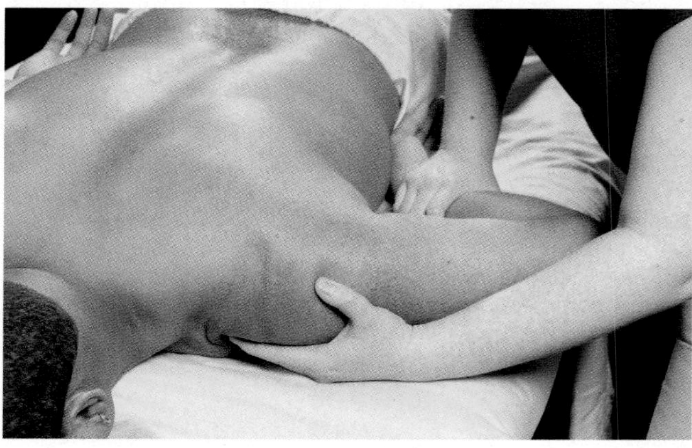

FIGURE 12-51A Position the arm to elevate the scapula.

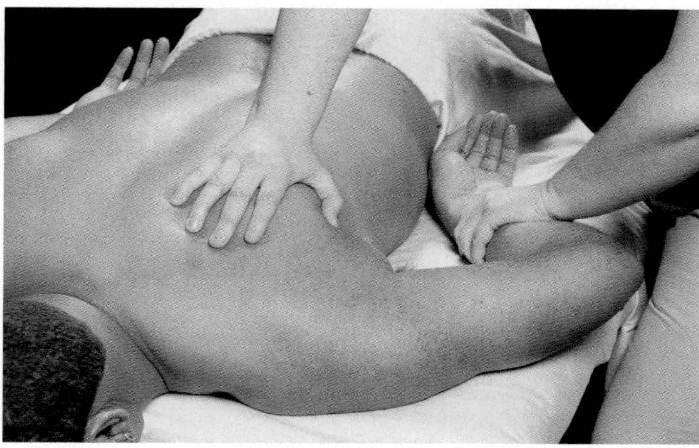

FIGURE 12-51B Apply friction and compression movements to the muscles of the scapula.

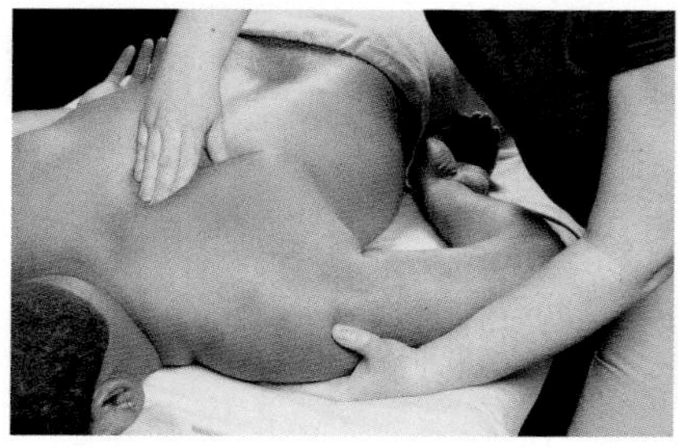

FIGURE 12-51C Elevate the scapula, and apply deep pressure and friction under the vertebral border.

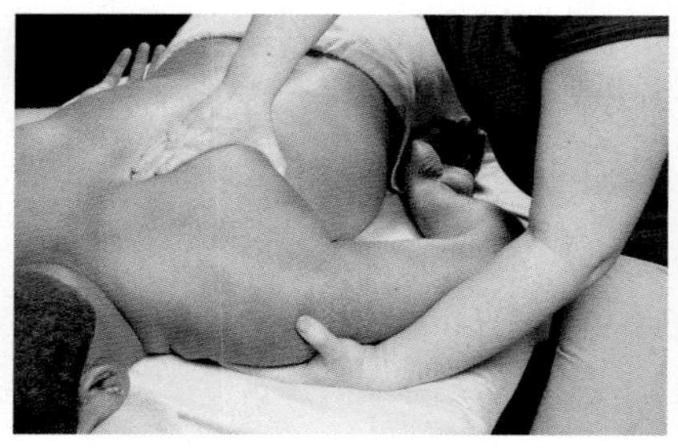

FIGURE 12-51D Rotation of the shoulder is followed by stretching.

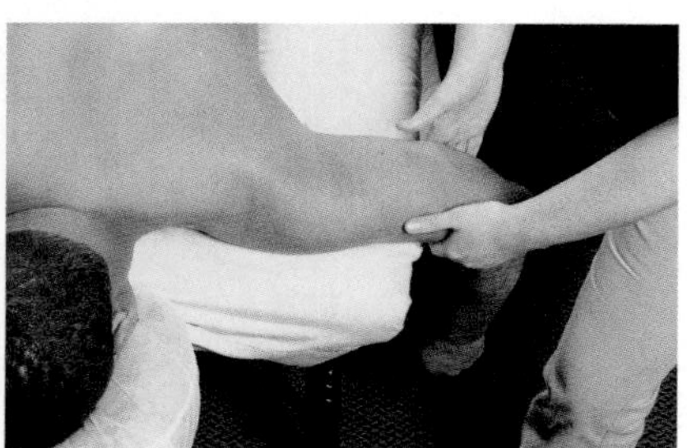

FIGURE 12-51E Hold the arm at the elbow and rotate the shoulder by swinging the forearm back and forth.

ten times. Pay attention to any area that seems especially tense, because these areas should be given extra attention. Work all the way down the spine from the seventh cervical vertebra in this manner. This technique can also be done from the top of the spine to the bottom (Figure 12-52a-h).

17. At this time, several percussion movements are optional. Hacking can be done lightly over the entire back. (Avoid percussion over the area of the kidneys, the popliteal fossa, or any bony areas.) Beating movements can be applied over the more muscular areas of the body, including the gluteals and the backs of the legs. To end a stimulating massage, light slapping can be applied over the entire body (Figure 12-53a-d).
18. A caring stroke completes the back massage. Remember that a caring stroke is an all-inclusive gliding stroke that is applied by standing at the head of the massage table. Place your hands on the upper back so that your fingers nearly touch in the area of the first and second thoracic vertebrae. Apply gliding strokes down the entire length of the spine. Your hands glide over the gluteals and return up the lateral portion of the torso to the axillary area, slide smoothly over the deltoids up the trapezius to the occiput, and return to the starting point. Repeat the movements several times (Figure 12-54a and b).

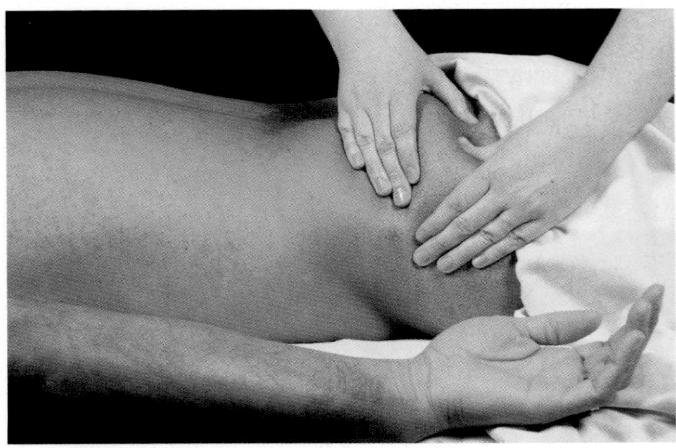

FIGURE 12-52A Apply deep kneading over the gluteal region.

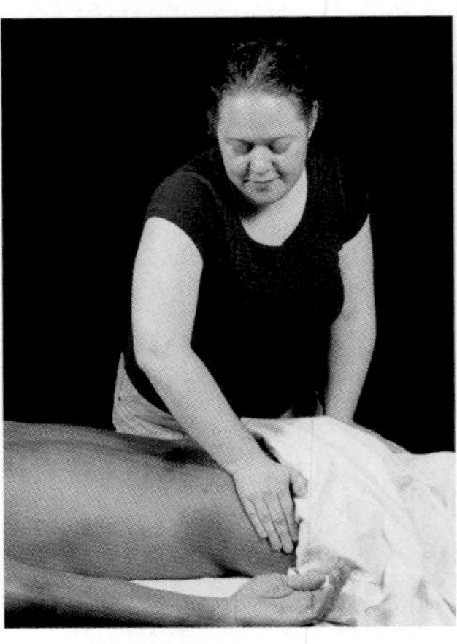

FIGURE 12-52B Apply friction (compression) to the gluteal muscles.

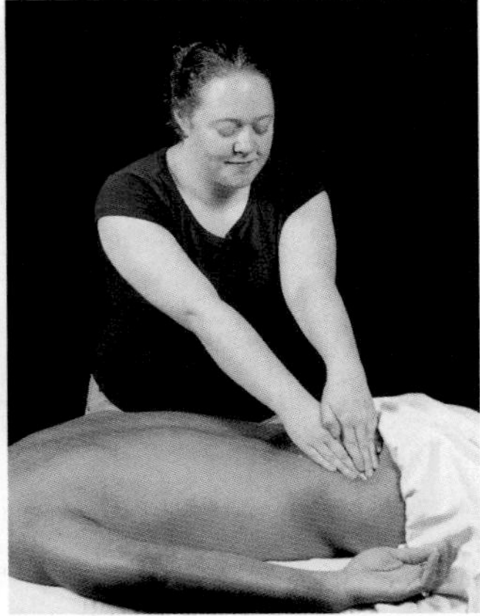

FIGURE 12-52C Apply digital friction to the gluteal muscles.

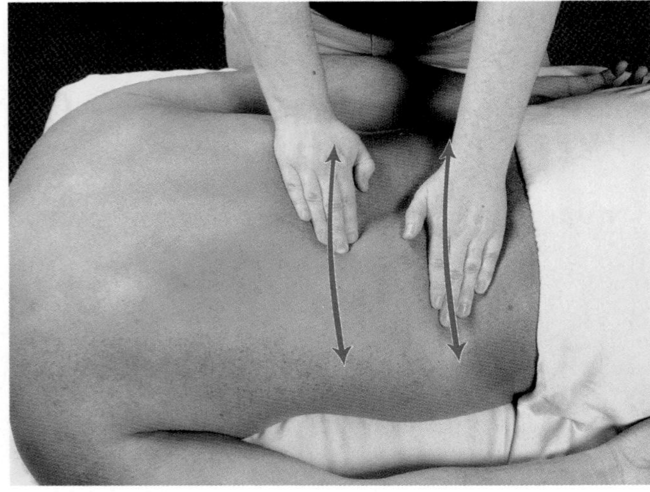

FIGURE 12-52D Apply wringing movements up and down the entire back.

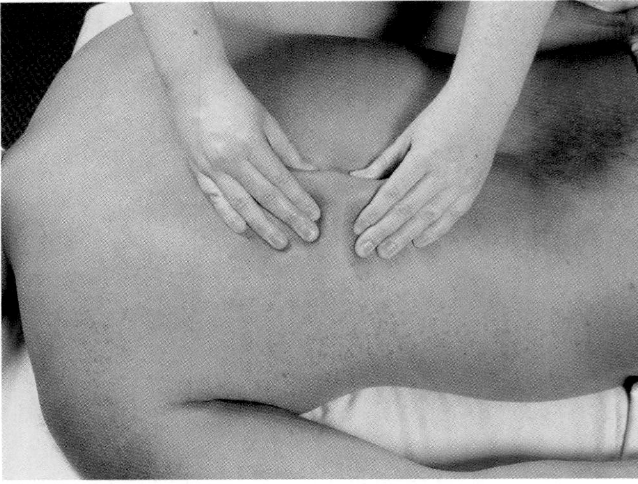

FIGURE 12-52E Knead around the spine.

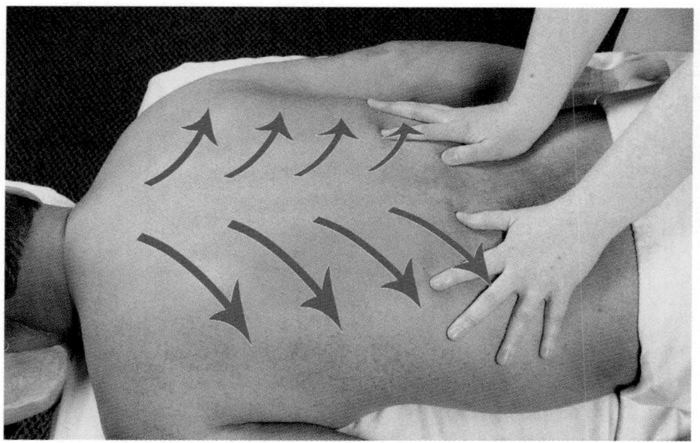

FIGURE 12-52F Fan stroke the back.

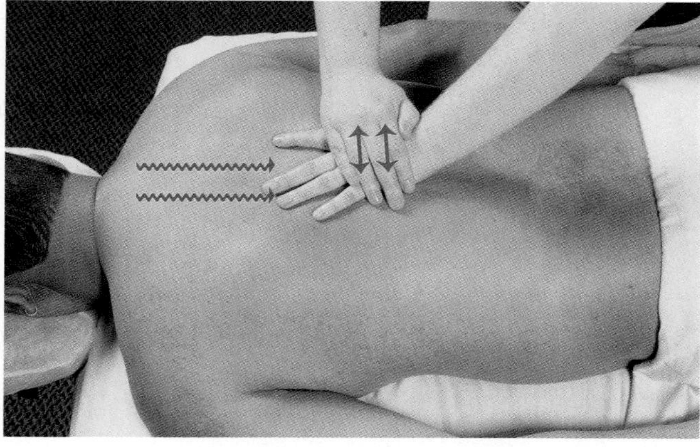

FIGURE 12-52G Vibrate along the sacrospinalis muscle.

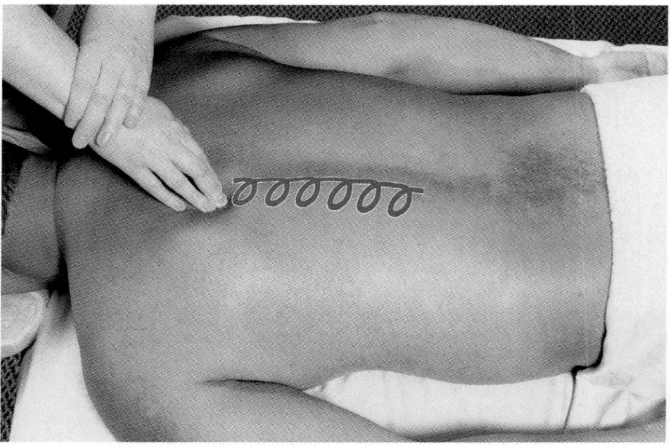

FIGURE 12-52H Apply friction movements to the muscles along the spine with the fingertips of one hand braced with the other hand. Apply movements along both sides of the spine.

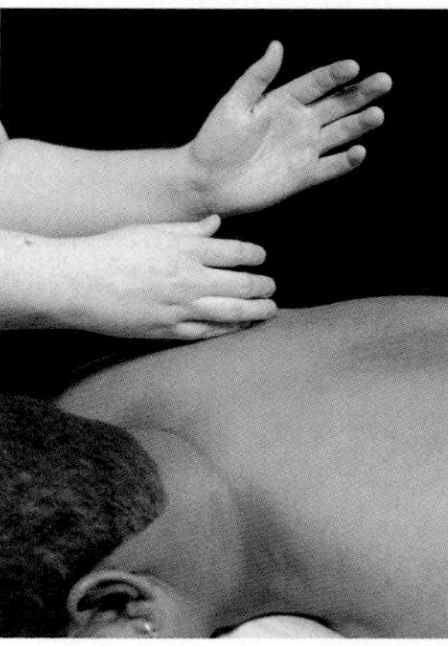

FIGURE 12-53A Hacking movements on the back.

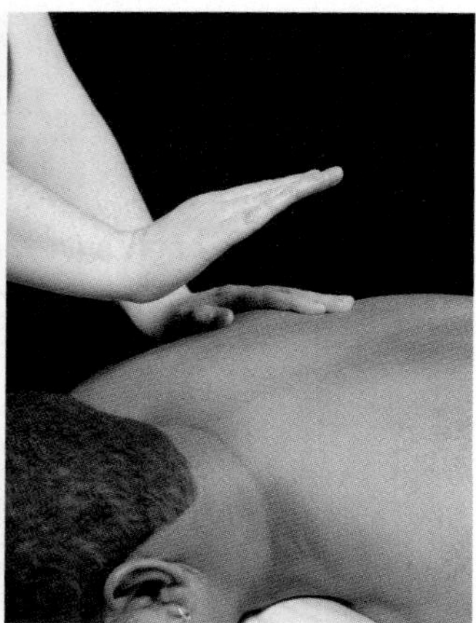

FIGURE 12-53B Slapping movements on the back.

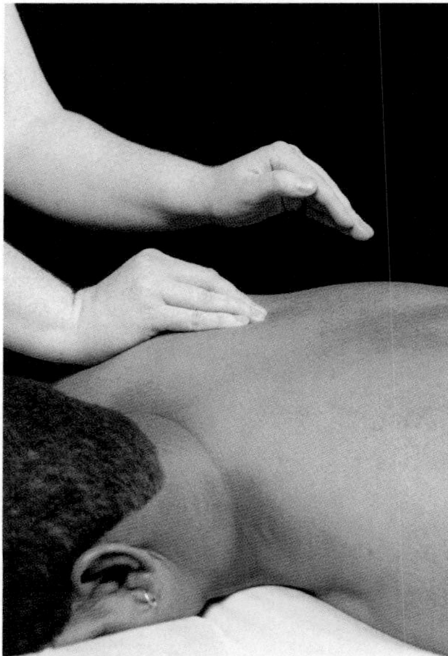

FIGURE 12-53C Cupping movements along the back.

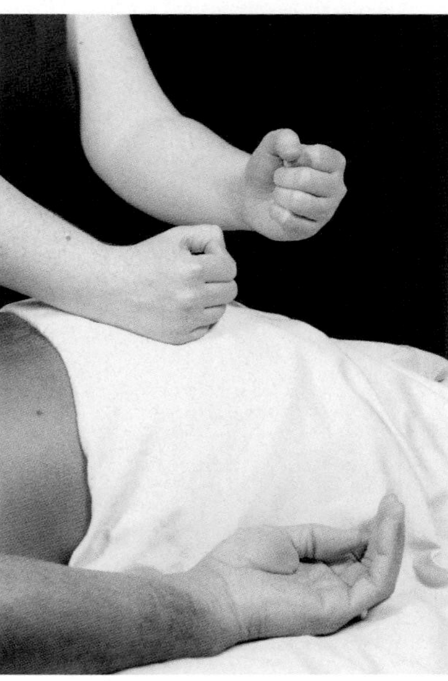

FIGURE 12-53D Apply percussion with beating movements to the gluteal muscles.

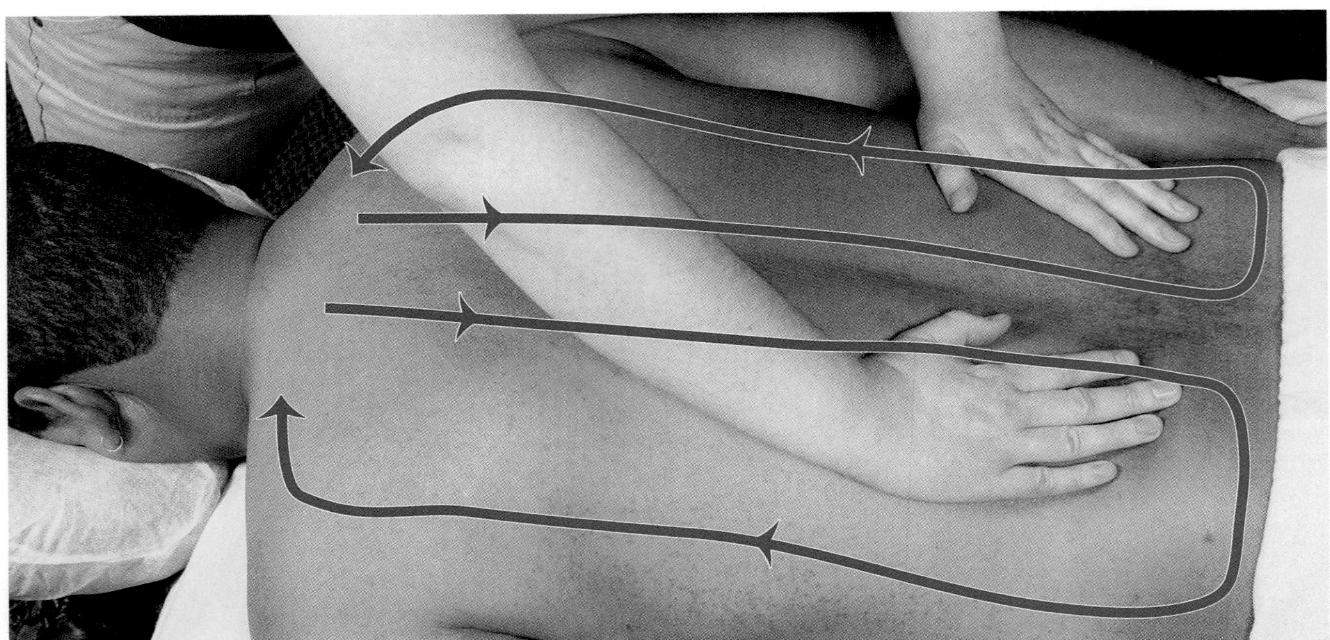

FIGURE 12-54A Apply effleurage movements (caring strokes) from a position at the head of the client, beginning at the nape of the neck.

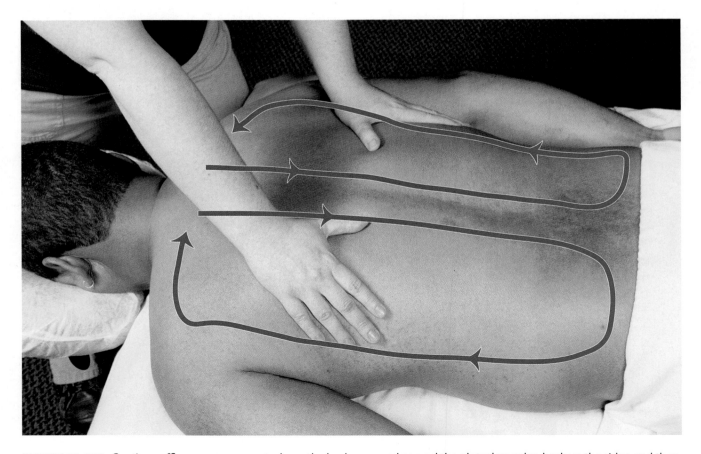

FIGURE 12-54B Continue effleurage movements down the back, over and around the gluteal muscles, back up the sides, and then over and around the shoulders to the nape of the neck.

A Finishing Touch

To complete the massage of the entire body, lightly place one hand on the sacrum and the other at the top of the spine and hold the position for several seconds. An option here is to apply a slight rocking motion (Figure 12-55).

The state of relaxation brought on by massage makes the client mentally receptive. When fully relaxed, the practitioner can guide the client through some mental or physical exercise to enhance or relieve a particular condition. For example, the practitioner can place both hands on the client and make suggestions such as "you feel rested, relaxed, and revitalized," or "you will sleep better tonight because you are free of tension," or "you feel more relaxed than you have for some time." This type of positive suggestion should be made just before the client is fully awake.

Allow the client to relax quietly without being disturbed for several minutes. Assist the client to a sitting position. Be sure that draping is properly placed, and assist the client from the massage table as necessary. Show the client to the dressing area. After the client is dressed, take time to answer any questions or make recommendations.

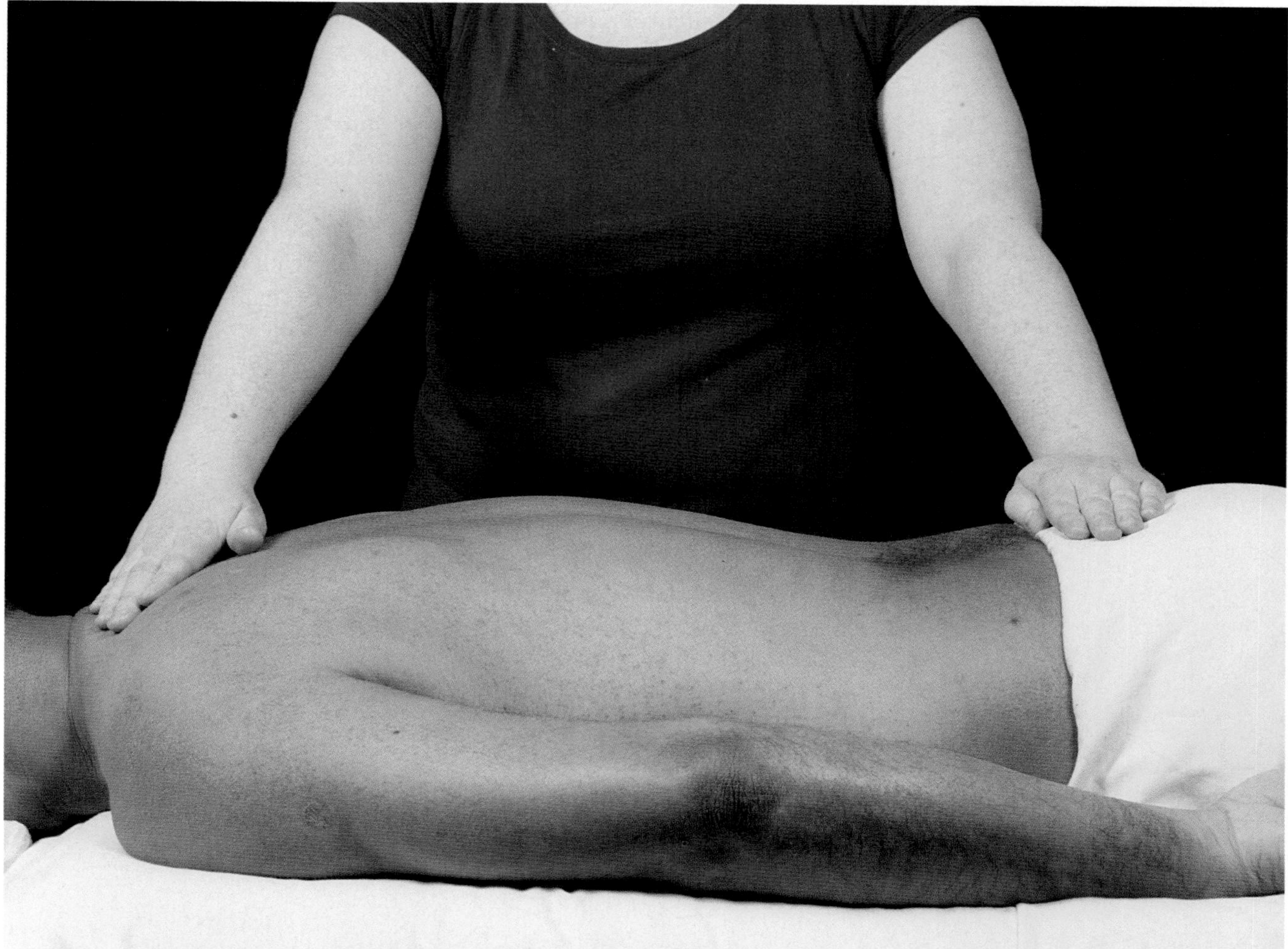

FIGURE 12-55 Say hello or good-bye to the client's body by applying a light touch to the base of the spine, the base of the neck, or the top of the head for a few moments.

Completion of the Massage

Following the massage, allow the client to rest for a short while before going out to face the world again. This rest period is beneficial especially if you have done bodywork to the extent that some changes have taken place in the client's physical structure. A few moments of relaxation helps to integrate these changes into the client's psychological and neurologic senses.

It is important to instruct the client in what to do and what to expect following the massage, especially clients who have come to you for the first time. For example, when suggesting that the client drink plenty of water to keep the system hydrated, explain that a massage, when done properly, can cause increased activity within the body tissues and that on the cellular level an increased rate of exchange of body fluids takes place. That increase means that some metabolic wastes have been expelled from the cells and have been put into the general systemic circulation. This waste material has to be processed because it puts an extra burden on the excretory system. An increase in the intake of water and other healthful fluids assists in the process of elimination by supplying more fluids for the kidneys, the colon, the lungs, and for perspiration.

Unless the practitioner is a nutritionist or physician, it is not proper to prescribe how much water a client should drink; however, you may suggest some guidelines as to the amount of water the client should drink. Some sources suggest that an average sized person should drink eight 8-ounce glasses of water a day, or 64 ounces (2 quarts). This does not take a person's size into account, however. Another popular formula for fluid intake that accommodates a person's size is to divide a person's weight (lbs) by two, and that equals the approximate amount of fluids in ounces that a person needs daily (i.e., a 150-lb person would need 150 ÷ 2 = 75 oz of water daily. In a 2004 report, the National Academy of Sciences Institute of Medicine set an official recommendation for the adequate daily intake of fluids. Based on this report, the average adequate daily intake of water (from all sources) for men is 3.7 quarts and for women is 2.7 quarts. These suggestions vary, but all agree that proper hydration is essential for good health.

Aftereffects of Massage

Some clients experience certain aftereffects following massage and should be told that this is no cause for alarm. Usually the effects are felt following the first or second massage. Some people complain of a slight headache, upset stomach and nausea, or the feeling of the onset of a cold. Such reactions are due to an increase in metabolic waste material in the circulatory system. The particular symptom that the client experiences depends on the organs that are overtaxed. The intensity of the massage movements should be limited until the client has built up more tolerance. The client will seldom have a symptom that lasts for any length of time; however, tell the client to call you if there is a problem.

SUMMARY

In this chapter, you were introduced to procedures to get a client on and off the massage table safely and to position the client with pillows and bolsters to provide maximum comfort. You were also taught two methods of draping to provide warmth, modesty, and access to the body to apply massage. You were introduced to employing sequences into a massage routine. Guidelines when sequencing strokes include working from general to specific and back to general, and working from superficial to deep and back to superficial. When performing a relaxing, full-body massage, similar sequences are used on each body part or area so that each area receives treatment that is equitable with other body areas. There is always latitude so that if a client indicates that there is extra tension or other related conditions in a particular part of the body, more attention and focus can be given to that area. In the overall massage, a sequence is used to ensure that every area of the body receives massage in a logical order, resulting in a relaxing, balanced, whole-body experience.

The effects of a massage movement vary according to the intention, duration, depth, speed, excursion, or length of the massage manipulation. The effects of the overall massage are also determined by the intention, duration, speed, depth, choice of massage strokes, and the sequence in which movements are applied.

The chapter contained two possible routines or guidelines for a relaxing, full-body massage. The routines are only a template for a nonspecific full-body massage. As a student, it is helpful to follow a routine and become comfortable performing a complete massage, but be careful not to become stuck in the routine. Pay close attention to the tissues that you are massaging, and ask your client for feedback. Adapt your techniques to best address your client's needs. As you gain experience, give yourself permission to experiment and improvise with combinations of techniques and massage strokes that you have learned. Create massage experiences that best suit your personal style but also meet the needs and desires of your clients. The possibilities for orchestrating a full-body massage are nearly endless. Have fun and remember to organize the massage into a logical order, using a sequence of strokes on each body area and then connecting the areas together, ensuring that each part of the body receives a thorough massage in a manner that integrates into a whole-body experience.

STUDENT ACTIVITY

Design a massage routine with the client beginning in a prone position. Conclude the massage by massaging the shoulders and neck.

QUESTIONS FOR DISCUSSION AND REVIEW

1. How often should the practitioner wash hands with soap and water?
2. Why is it advisable to assist a client on and off the table?
3. How can the practitioner prevent the client's body from becoming chilled?
4. Briefly describe two methods of draping.
5. Besides draping, how can the therapist ensure that the client stays warm?
6. How can the practitioner avoid scratching the client's body?
7. Which massage movements should be avoided because they convey fear of injury to the client?
8. Is it better to massage the body before or after the client has eaten a meal?
9. What is the average duration of a massage?
10. In which conditions should massage never be applied?
11. Which preliminaries require attention before body massage?
12. Which position does the client usually assume first for body massage?
13. What is the usual order of massage movements?
14. What are the final considerations after completing body massage?
15. What are some undesirable aftereffects of massage, and why do they occur?
16. Why should the client be advised to drink plenty of water?

CHAPTER

13 Hydrotherapy

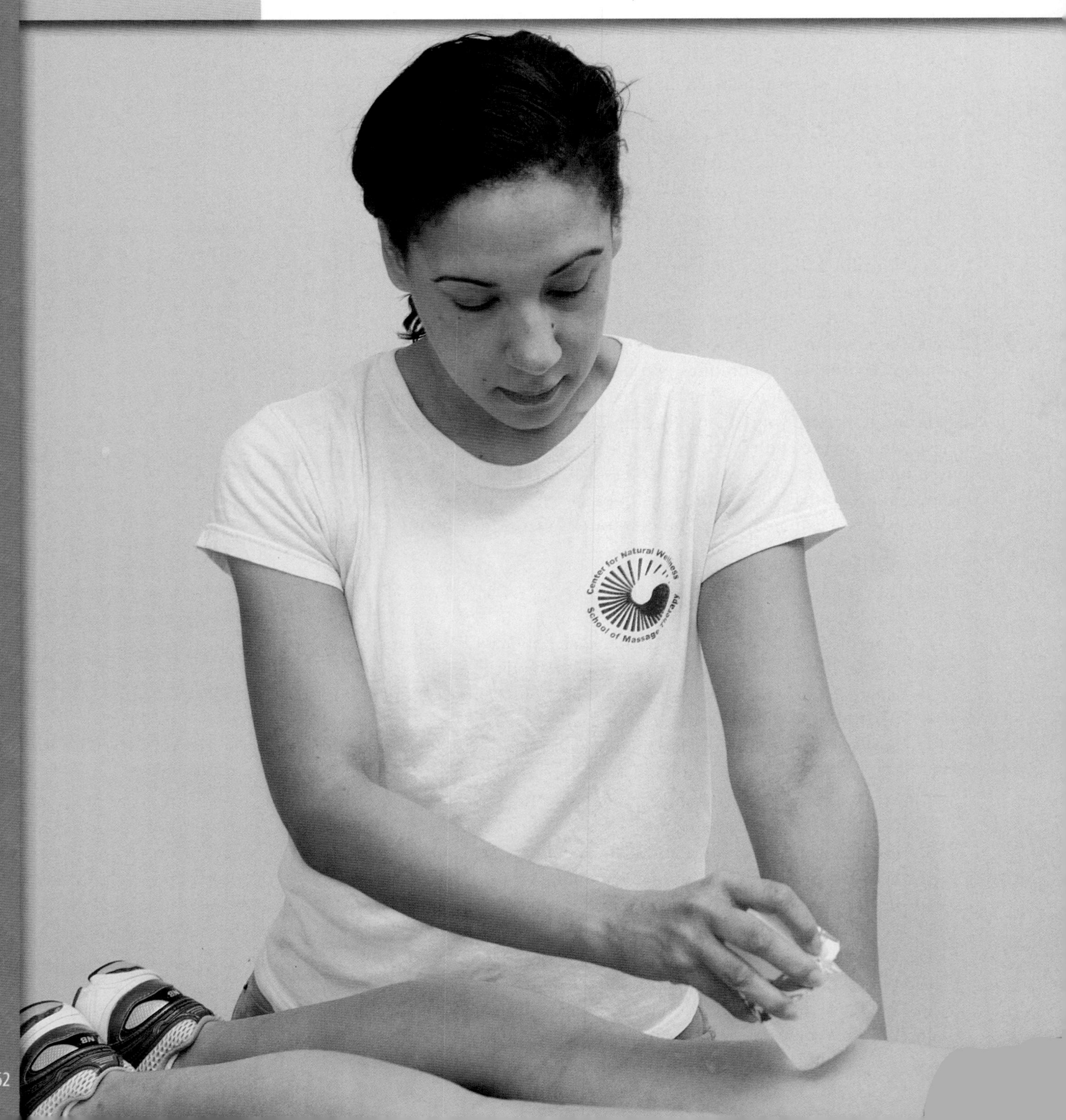

LEARNING OBJECTIVES

After you have mastered this chapter, you will be able to

1. **Explain hydrotherapy as a therapeutic aid.**
2. **Explain the effects of different water temperatures on the body.**
3. **Explain the use of heat and cold in body treatments.**
4. **Define cryotherapy and demonstrate at least three ways to apply it.**
5. **Describe at least five ways of applying heat to the body.**
6. **Describe the effects of various water treatments on the body.**
7. **Explain contraindications, safety rules, and time limits for various hydrotherapy treatments.**

INTRODUCTION

Although body massage is generally done by hand, there are many treatments that combine manual massage with various other modalities. Popular treatments that can be used in conjunction with massage use water in its various forms to warm or cool a part of or the whole body for therapeutic purposes. The therapeutic use of water is termed *hydrotherapy*. *Thermotherapy* is the use of heat for therapeutic purposes, and *cryotherapy* is the therapeutic process of cooling the body. These treatments are designed to encourage circulation, improve the body's efficiency in eliminating toxins, and promote relaxation.

The following chapter introduces several hydrotherapy techniques to augment the massage experience. Many hydrotherapy procedures, including wraps, baths, showers, frictions, and salt glows are popular offerings in spas and are discussed in the Chapter 14, Massage in the Spa Setting.

HYDROTHERAPY

Hydrotherapy (**HI**-dro-ther-uh-pee) is the application of water in any of its three forms (i.e., solid, liquid, vapor) to the body for therapeutic purposes. When properly used with body massage, hydrotherapy is an additional aid to the healthy functioning of the body.

hydrotherapy
is the application of water in any of its three forms to the body for therapeutic purposes.

Water has certain properties that make it a valuable therapeutic agent. Water is readily available and relatively inexpensive to use. It has the ability to absorb and conduct heat. It provides buoyancy and is considered to be the universal solvent. In its solid form as ice, it can be used as an effective cooling agent; in its vapor form, it can be used for facials and steam baths; and in its liquid state it can be used for compresses, showers, and immersion baths either to cool or warm the body, depending on the temperature of the water.

Changes in the body as a result of hydrotherapy are classified as thermal, mechanical, and chemical. Thermal effects are produced by the application of water at temperatures above or below that of the body. This is done by way of baths, wraps, and packs that raise or lower the temperature of the body. Mechanical effects are produced by the pressure exerted on the surface of the body by sprays, whirlpool baths, and friction. Buoyancy reduces the weight of an object immersed in water according to the volume of water displaced by the object. The total volume of a human body is approximately 5% heavier than the same volume of water so that body will sink in water. That body weighs only 5% of what it weighs out of the water. Buoyancy reduces the force of gravity and makes it possible to move, float, or exercise in a nearly gravity-free environment. Chemical effects are produced by any of a variety of products added to bath water or steam such as essential oils, herbal preparations, salt, Epsom salt, or baking soda.

Body Reactions to Water Treatments

Water treatments are based on the simple physical property of water; namely, that heat, cold, or pressure can be conveyed to many blood vessels and nerves in the skin. The effects of water on the body vary according to the temperature and duration of the treatment and whether the application is whole body or local in character. The circulation of the blood and the sensations produced by the many nerve endings in the skin can be greatly influenced by skillfully applied water treatments.

The temperature of water affects the body; therefore, understanding how water temperature relates to body temperature is important. The normal core temperature of the human body is 98.6°F or 37°C. The surface temperature of the skin is approximately 92°F. The boiling point of water is 212°F or 100°C. The freezing point of water is 32°F or 0°C. Obviously we must not use water of too high or too low a temperature because it would injure body tissues. Water temperatures above that of the body (98.6°F) are considered to be hot. Water that is slightly below normal body temperature is tepid to warm (approximately 92° to 96°F). Water that is in the temperature range of 70° to 90°F is considered cool, and at 70°F and lower, it is considered cold. Water approximating the temperature of the skin has no marked thermal effect on the body, although it does promote relaxation. If water at a temperature different from that of the skin is applied, the water either transfers or absorbs heat from the body. The difference in temperature has an effect on the vast network of connective tissue, blood vessels, and nerves. The greater the difference between the temperature of water and that of the skin, the more extreme the effect of the treatment will be.(See Box 13.1)

THE USE AND EFFECTS OF APPLICATIONS OF HEAT AND COLD

The normal core body temperature is 98.6°F. Physiologically, the body strives to maintain this temperature. When heat or cold is applied to the body, certain physiologic changes occur. If the temperature of the treatment is the same as the body temperature, there are no thermal effects. Treatments of short duration have different effects from longer treatments. For example, a short application of cold (2 to 5 seconds) has a stimulating effect, whereas an extended application (10 to 30 minutes) depresses metabolic activity. Local applications have specific local effects, whereas full body applications have systemic effects. Some thermal applications have both direct local effects and reflex effects. The physiologic effects from the application of heat and cold are predictable, which makes their use a powerful therapeutic agent.

Treatments using extreme temperatures of either short or long duration should be avoided or used under very close supervision. Using thermal treatments below freezing or above 115°F can damage tissues. Prolonged general treatments below 70°F can cause hypothermia. Prolonged general treatments above 104°F can cause hyperthermia. Either condition is potentially dangerous.

The application of heat causes a vasodilation and a circulation increase in an attempt to dissipate the heat. A whole-body application of heat raises the core body temperature, causing a fever-like reaction. There is profuse perspiration, the pulse rate increases, and the white and red blood cell count increases. A local application of heat causes local reddening (caused by vasodilation), increased metabolism and leukocyte migration to the area, relaxation of local musculature, and a slight analgesia.

The quick, short application of cold is stimulating, whereas prolonged application of cold depresses metabolic activity. A full-body application of cold reduces the body temperature (hypothermia). Although this has important therapeutic and medical advantages, it must be done only under strict medical supervision. Local applications of cold cause a reduction of nerve sensitivity,

Box 13.1

Water Temperatures and Body Sensations

Description	Temperature (F°)	Temperature (C°)	Sensation
Freezing	32°	0°	
Very cold	32–55°	0–13°	Painful
Cold	56–70°	13–20°	Uncomfortable
Cool	70–80°	20–27°	Can cause goosebumps
Tepid	80–92°	27–34°	Just below skin temp (92°)
Neutral	93–97°	34–36°	Comfortable
Hot	98–104°	37–41°	Tolerable
Very hot	105–110°	41–43°	Tolerable for short periods
Water temperatures above 110° F should not be used for hydrotherapy purposes.			
Water temperature for immersion baths and hydrotubs should not exceed 104°F			
Painfully hot	110–120°	43–46°	Intolerable
Dangerously hot	>125°	>50°	Can cause burns
Boiling	212°	100°	

Box 13.2

Effects of Heat and Cold

	Initial Cold	Prolonged Cold	Initial Hot	Prolonged Hot
Circulation	Reduced	Decreased	Increased	Increased
Heart rate	Increased	Decreased	Decreased	Increased
Respiration	Decreased	Decreased	Decreased	Increased
Metabolism	Increased	Decreased	Increased	Increased
Pain	Decreased	Decreased	Decreased	Decreased
Muscle tension/spasm	Increased	Decreased	Decreased	Decreased
Tissue Damage	Limited	Limited	N/A	N/A
Fascia	No Effect	Stiffens	Softens	Softens
Overall/General	Stimulates	Depresses	Stimulates	Relaxes

circulation, muscle spasms, and spasticity. They have a numbing, anesthetic, analgesic effect that makes them valuable in the relief of acute pain from bursitis, soft tissue injury, burns, and neuralgia.

Each water application initiates a series of predictable reactions that are the result of the body's accommodating itself to the new environment. The body reaction can be either stimulating or sedating to the circulatory system, the nervous system, and the eliminatory process. Any practitioner who uses hydrotherapy should be familiar with the specific effects of cold, cool, hot, and warm applications on the body.(See Box 13.2)

Contraindications for Hydrotherapy

Water treatments that involve hot or cold applications should not be given when the client has cardiac impairment, diabetes, lung disease, kidney infection, extremely high or low blood pressure, an infectious skin condition, or open wounds. The loss of the ability to feel hot or cold contradicts the application of treatments that could potentially burn or freeze the client's skin. Warm or neutral treatments are considered safe. Whole-body treatments that tend to raise the body's core temperature are contraindicated during pregnancy and for clients with multiple sclerosis. Treatments must be moderated for clients who have an aversion to either hot or cold. The client's physician should be consulted when any questionable condition exists.

CRYOTHERAPY

cryotherapy
is the application of cold agents for therapeutic purposes.

The application of cold agents for therapeutic purposes is known as **cryotherapy** (**KRIE**-o-ther-uh-pee). The primary goal of cryotherapy is to reduce the tissue temperature. As cold is applied to the body, heat is drawn from the tissues, causing cooling. The local application of cold is beneficial for painful, inflamed, and swollen areas. It acts as an analgesic to reduce pain and causes vasoconstriction to limit swelling.

The application of extreme cold should be of short duration to prevent tissue injury from freezing. The application of ice causes a series of sensations that can act as indicators of the duration of the application. The first sensation of the application of ice is naturally cold. Following the cold sensation comes burning, followed by aching. Next is numbness and the cessation of pain (the analgesic effect). When the fourth stage is reached, application should be temporarily suspended. The series of sensations is represented by the acronym **CBAN: C** = cold, **B** = burning, **A** = aching, and **N** = numbness. Treatment can be repeated as necessary, as often as once an hour.

Ice is first aid for traumatic soft tissue injuries. When a soft tissue injury such as a sprain or strain occurs, the standard first aid treatment is to apply **RICE**, an acronym in which **R** = rest, **I** = ice, **C** = compression, and **E** = elevation. This reduces swelling, pain, and the secondary tissue damage that results from excessive swelling. A recent addition to the acronym is **P** for *p*rotect the area, making the new acronym PRICE. After 48 to 72 hours and as soon as swelling has subsided, limited therapy including massage can proceed on the healing tissue.

Ice therapy can be used by itself or in conjunction with other modalities. In the case of swelling from local inflammation, ice offers tremendous relief from the swelling and accompanying pain. One of the best ways to increase circulation to an area to promote healing is the application of **contrast therapy**, which is the alternate application of heat and cold.

contrast therapy

the alternating application of heat and cold for therapeutic purposes.

Effects of Cold

The specific effects of cold applications on the body are an immediate and temporary effect or a secondary and more lasting effect. Cold applications are valuable in stimulating circulation, sedating the nerves, and slowing the metabolic activity of body cells. The prolonged use of cold applications has a depressing effect on the body and must be used cautiously under strict supervision.

The immediate effects of cold applications are manifested in the following ways:

1. The skin is chilled.
2. Surface blood vessels constrict, and blood is driven to the interior of the body.
3. Nerve sensitivity is reduced, reducing pain.
4. The metabolic activity of body cells slows.
5. Inflammation and swelling are reduced. Secondary tissue damage is minimized.

As soon as the cold application is discontinued, there is a secondary and more lasting effect on the area of the body being cooled.

1. The skin becomes warmed and relaxed.
2. The surface blood vessels dilate, bringing more blood to the skin.
3. Nerve sensitivity increases.
4. Adjacent body cells are stimulated in their functional activity

APPLICATION OF COLD

Sources for the local application of cold include:

- Cold compress
- Ice packs
  Chipped or crushed ice in a plastic bag or towel
  Commercial ice packs
- Ice massage
- Compressor units with thermal packs and controls
- Vasocoolant sprays
- Immersion baths

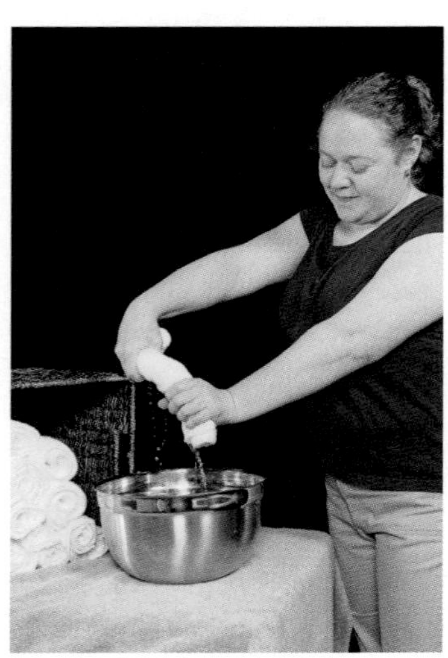

FIGURE 13-1A Prepare a cold compress by dipping a small towel or washcloth in cold or icy water, wringing it out, and folding it.

Cold Compress

A cold compress is a small towel, washcloth, or other material that is soaked in cold or icy water, wrung out, folded and placed directly on the client's skin (Figure 13-1a). The compress quickly draws heat from the body and so needs to be refreshed and recooled after two to five minutes. Cool compresses applied to the forehead, back, or the back of the neck help to maintain a client's comfort during thermotherapy treatments such as steam cabinet, steam canopy, or hot bath (Figure 13-1b).

Ice Pack

Ice packs are used for the local application of ice on a specific body part. They are effective in relieving pain, preventing swelling, and decreasing inflammation. They are indicated for the early treatment of sprains, strains, and other soft tissue injuries. They are effective in the treatment of acute joint and nerve inflammation.

A Ziploc bag or a plastic freezer bag filled with crushed ice makes an excellent ice pack (Figure 13-2). Be sure there are no leaks in the plastic bag. Fill it one third of the way with broken ice cubes or crushed ice, seal it closed, and apply it directly to the affected area. The ice bag can be held in place by an Ace bandage or towel wrap over the injured area for up to 30 minutes every 2 hours (Figure 13-3a to e).

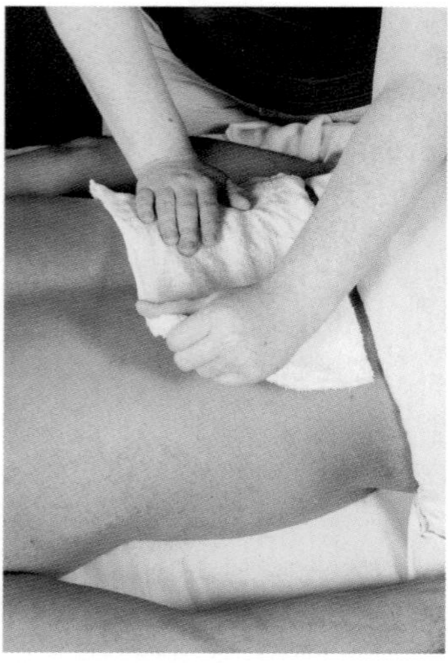

FIGURE 13-1B Place the folded compress on the body part to be cooled.
Option: Place a cool compress on the neck or forehead of a client receiving a hot treatment.

An inexpensive and convenient way to make a reusable ice pack is to combine one part rubbing alcohol (isopropyl alcohol) to four parts water in a sealable plastic bag and put it in the freezer until it is ready for use. Sealing the ice pack in a second plastic bag before using reduces the chance of the contents leaking. The alcohol prevents the contents from freezing solid, and the ice pack can be easily molded to the part of the body where it is applied. Owing to its extreme cold temperature, the ice pack must not be applied directly to the skin. A towel or other material is placed between the skin and pack.

Reusable commercial ice packs are available in a variety of types and sizes (Figure 13-4). These are usually a sealed plastic pack containing a chemical gel. The pack is stored in the freezer until needed. The pack is wrapped in a terry cloth to prevent direct contact with the skin. Direct contact is unsanitary and can also result in injury from freezing the tissue. The chemical gel in the pack stays pliable at freezing temperatures so that the pack can conform to the area

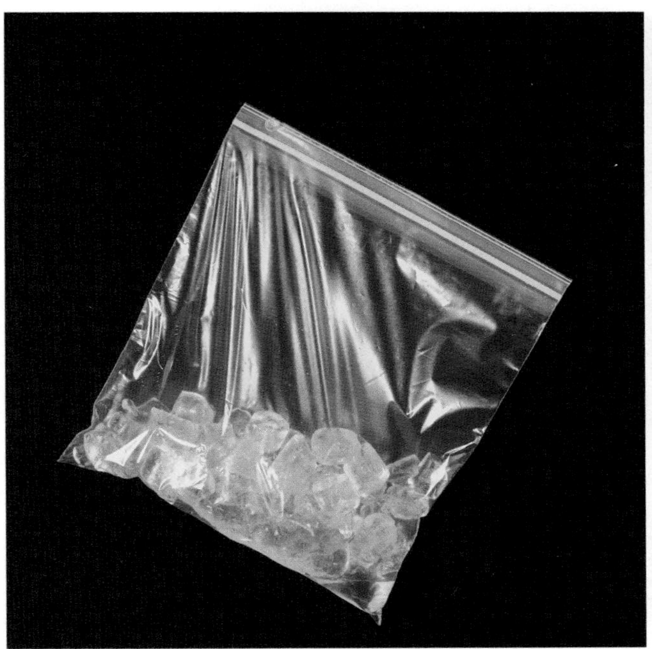

FIGURE 13-2 An inexpensive ice pack uses ice chips or cubes in a sealed plastic bag.

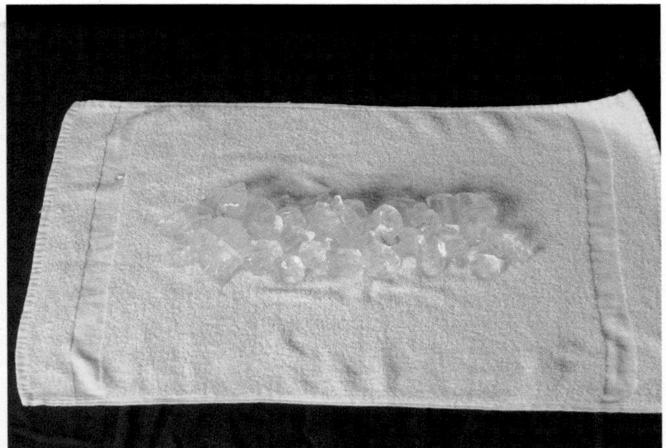

FIGURE 13-3A Another alternative is to wrap ice in a towel and apply it to the affected area. Put crushed ice in the center of a towel.

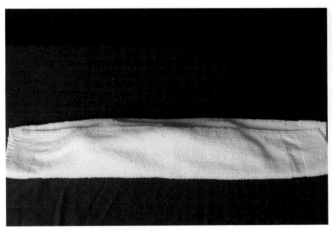

FIGURE 13-3B Fold the sides of the towel over the ice.

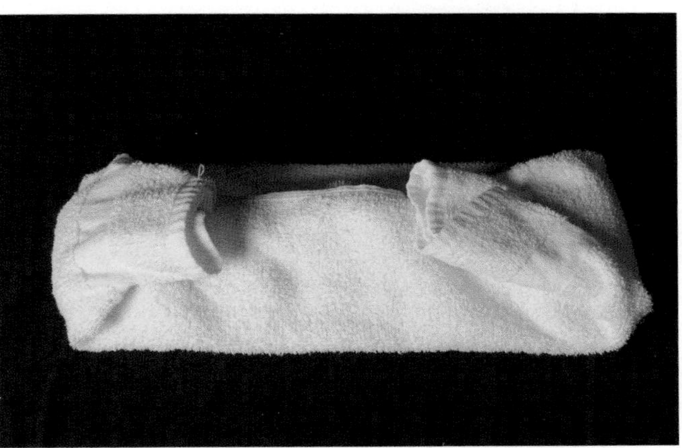

FIGURE 13-3C Fold the ends of the towel.

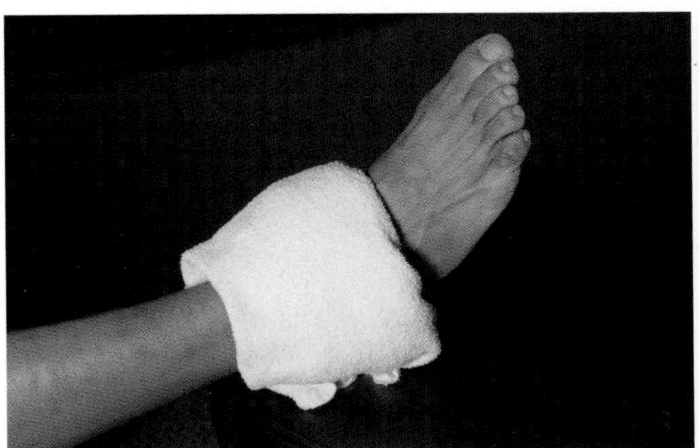

FIGURE 13-3D Wrap the ice towel around the affected body part.

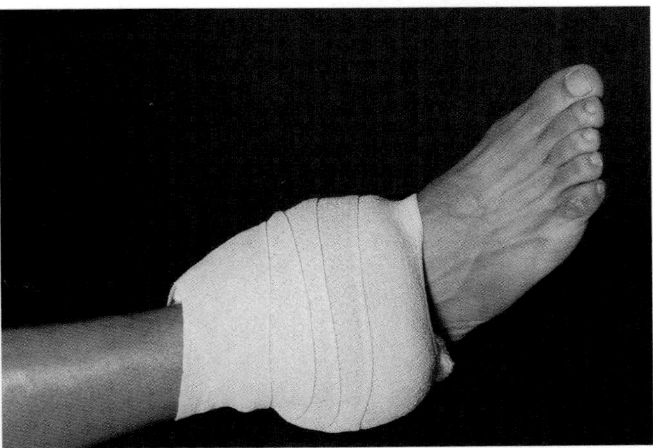

FIGURE 13-3E Wrap the towel with an Ace bandage to secure it, and then apply compression.

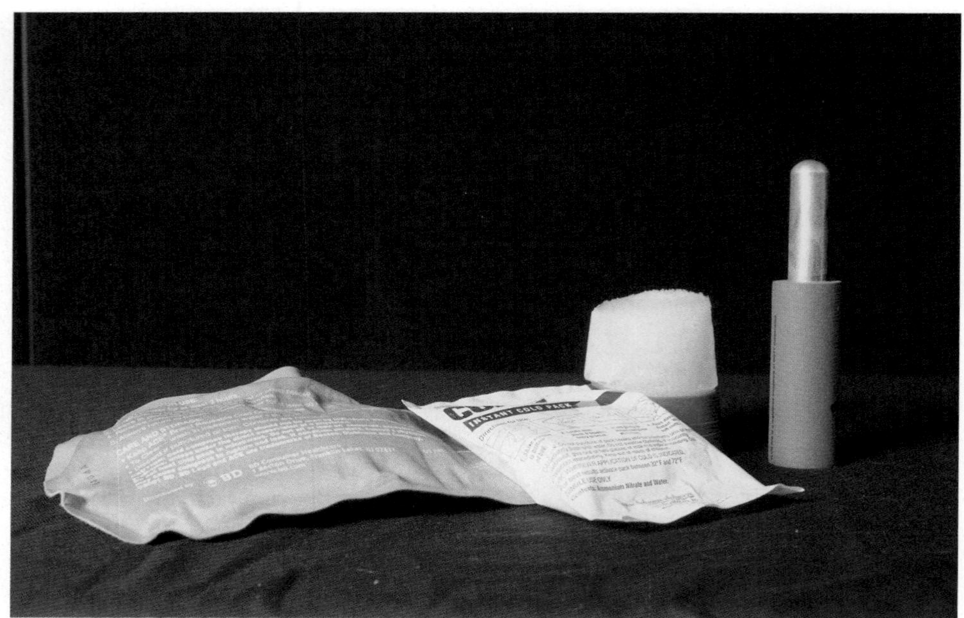

FIGURE 13-4 Commercially manufactured cold packs are available in a variety of shapes and sizes. They are stored in a freezer until needed.

of the body to which it is applied. When using gel or alcohol ice packs, lift the packs from the skin every few minutes and look to be sure the tissue is not being injured by the extreme cold. Crushed ice packs are safer, more economical, and cool the body more efficiently than either alcohol or chemical gel packs.

Ice Massage

ice massage

is a local application of cold achieved by massaging a cube of ice over a small area such as a bursa, tendon, or small muscle.

Another way in which cryotherapy can be applied is **ice massage.** Ice massage is a local application of cold achieved by massaging a cube of ice over a small area such as a bursa, tendon, or small muscle. Commercial ice cups are available that are filled with water and stored in the freezer until needed. They provide a mold for the ice cube that includes a handle frozen into the cube so that the therapist can perform the ice massage without freezing his or her hand (Figure 13-5a to c). Another way that this can be achieved is to freeze water in an eight-ounce Styrofoam or paper cup. Remove the frozen cup from the freezer and cut the top half of the cup away. Use the base of the cup as a handle (Figure 13-6a to c). An ice lollipop can be made by freezing a tongue depressor into a cup of water. The ice pop is removed from the cup and held by the stick for application. As the ice is rubbed over the surface of the body it has a cooling effect. Keep a towel handy to wipe up the water as the ice melts so that the table linens do not get wet and the client remains more comfortable. Ice massage is effective for reducing local pain, inflammation, and swelling and for stopping muscle spasms.

Compressor Units with Controls

Compressor units cool a fluid that is circulated through a pack that is applied to the body. The packs vary in size, and a mat can be used for a general application. (These are employed for the control of high fever.) A smaller pack can be used for local application to an extremity. The temperature can be controlled by adjusting the controls on the unit. These units are relatively expensive and most commonly found in medical institutions that treat a large number of traumatic injuries.

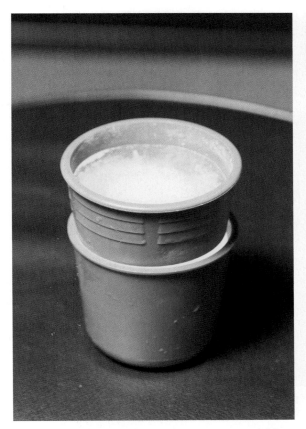

FIGURE 13-5A Commercial ice cups are available.

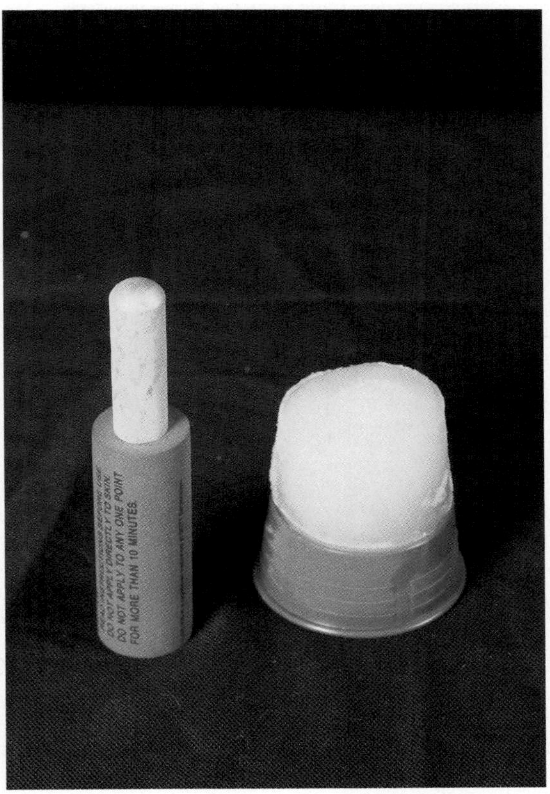

FIGURE 13-5B When the ice is removed from the mold, a handle frozen into the ice protects the therapist's hand from the cold.

Vapocoolant Sprays

Fluori-Methane is bottled under pressure and used as a vasocoolant spray. Unfortunately, Fluori-Methane contains fluorocarbons, which are environmentally damaging. The Gebauer Company has developed two products, *Instant Ice* and *Spray and Stretch,* that are safe, nonflammable and non-ozone depleting. When sprayed on the skin, these evaporate very quickly, causing rapid cooling of the skin. They are effective topical anesthetics used for trigger-point therapy and increasing the stretch in muscles. Caution must be used to avoid freezing the skin with these agents, however.

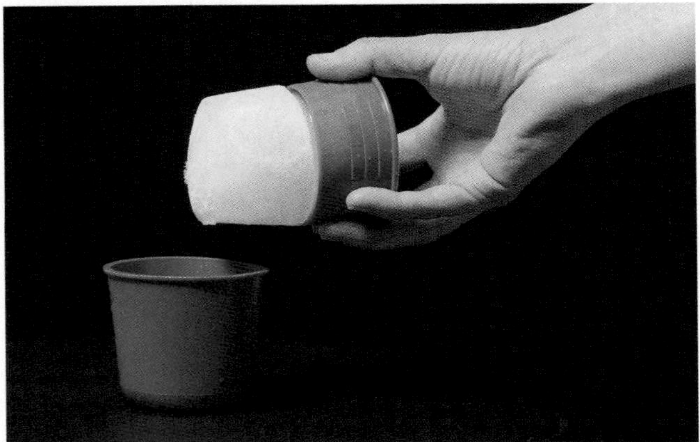

FIGURE 13-5C Hold the bottom portion of the cup and apply ice massage.

Immersion Baths

The entire body or a body part can be immersed in cool or cold water. Cold plunges are available at some spas and gyms where patrons can dip into a cool (about 70°) pool after a hot tub or sauna. When working with an extremity, such as a foot, ankle, hand, wrist, or elbow, an immersion ice water bath can be used

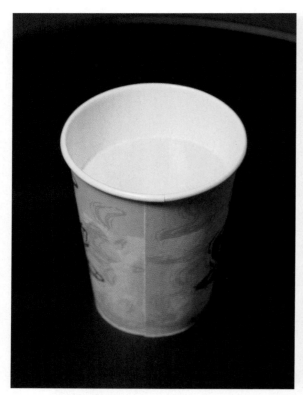

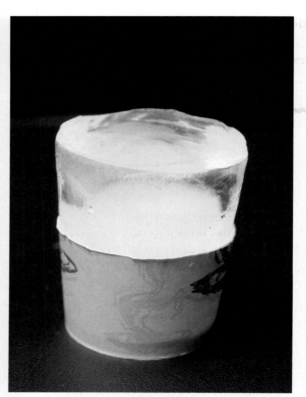

FIGURE 13-6A Water frozen in a Styrofoam or insulated paper cup works well for ice massage.

FIGURE 13-6B When the water is frozen, peel the top half of the Styrofoam or paper cup away to make an ice cup with an insulated handle.

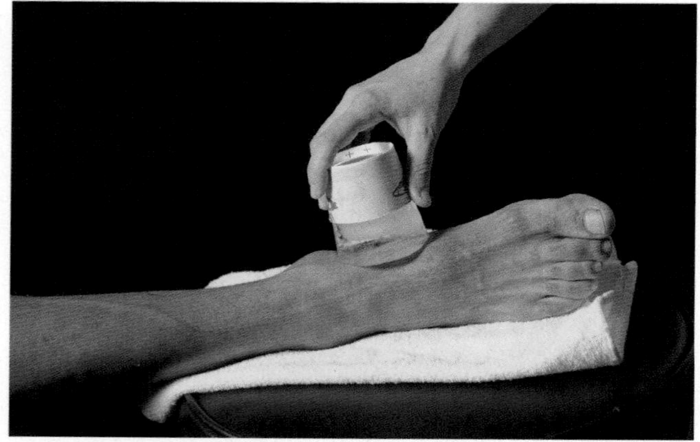

FIGURE 13-6C Hold the bottom portion of the cup and apply ice massage.

to reduce inflammation. Prepare a basin or tub of 40 percent ice and 60 percent water. Submerge the body part (e.g., foot, hand, forearm, or elbow) in the ice water until the feeling of cold or pain stops, then remove the body part from the bath.

THERMOTHERAPY–THE APPLICATION OF HEAT

thermotherapy

is the external application of heat to the body for therapeutic purposes.

Thermotherapy is the external application of heat to the body for therapeutic purposes. It is especially effective for relieving pain caused by muscle tension or spasm and to promote muscle relaxation. Heat is transferred to the body in one of four ways:

Conduction is the direct exchange of heat when the surface of the body is in direct contact with the thermal agent (heat pack, immersion bath).

Convection is the transfer of heat through the movement of the air (steam bath, sauna).

Radiation is the transfer of heat by way of rays contacting the body (the sun, infrared).

Conversion is the converting of an energy source into heat as it passes trough the body's tissue (diathermy, ultrasonography).

Effects of Heat Applications

The effect of the application of heat to the body depends on the temperature, the duration, and the area of the body contacted by the heating agent. The immediate effect of hot applications is to draw the blood away from the interior and bring it to the surface temporarily. Local blood vessels and capillaries dilate, increasing circulation and oxygen absorption. Long and continued hot applications increase all skin functions and cause profuse sweating. Pain and stiffness are reduced, and range of motion is increased. The superficial fascia is softened and the extensibility of collagen in connective tissue is increased. Moderately warm applications have a relaxing effect on the blood vessels, muscles, and nerves and promote the metabolic activity of body cells. The application of moist heat tends to penetrate deeper into the muscle tissues than dry heat.

Generally, the skin cannot tolerate hot water at a temperature in excess of 115°F. Above that temperature, water is injurious and can cause burns; however, the skin usually can tolerate steam vapor as high as 130°F. The recommended temperature for steam vapor is 105°–125°F. Whole body immersion baths exceeding 104°F can cause hyperthermia. It is important to consider the client's sensitivity and tolerance to heat or cold. A reliable bath thermometer is required to judge water temperature accurately. The temperature reading is obtained by moving the thermometer about in the water.

There are several sources for the application of heat. Many applications use hydrotherapy to provide moist heat, whereas other applications use various electrical apparatuses to transfer heat into the body. The choice of modality depends on the body part to be treated, its condition, and the objectives of the application. Modalities for the application of heat include

- Dry heat
    - Heating pad
    - Infrared radiation
    - Diathermy
    - Ultrasonography
- Moist heat
    - Packs and compresses
    - Wraps
    - Sprays and showers
    - Baths
        - Immersion baths
        - Air baths
        - Steam baths
        - Saunas

Heating Pads

Heating pads are plastic-covered pads that contain electric heating elements similar to those used in electric blankets. A heating pad supplies a local source of dry heat and is easy to apply. The heating pad is useful for local applications on one part of the body while the therapist works on another. There are usually three heat level settings. Some heating pads are manufactured for application of moist heat. Manufacturers' instructions must be followed to prevent injury from burns or electrical shock.

Rice Packs

A rice pack is a cloth bag that is partially filled with rice or another similar grain and heated in a microwave oven before being applied to an area of the body. Rice bags can be made in a variety of sizes and shapes, depending on the area of the body to be covered. Some microwave ovens do not heat the grain evenly, and therefore care must be taken to mix the heated grain in the bag and not to overheat the bag before applying to the skin. Heating the rice bag forces moisture from the grain, creating the effect of applying moist heat to the client.

Infrared Radiation

Infrared radiation can be produced from a bulb or an element. The warming effect of the sun is due to infrared radiation. As radiations are absorbed by the skin, heat is produced. The heat results in increased superficial circulation and sedation of sensory nerve endings. This results in the relaxation of tense or spasmed muscles, relief of pain, and increased availability of nutrients to the superficial tissues (Figure 13-7).

Diathermy

diathermy
is the application of oscillating electromagnetic fields to the tissue.

Diathermy (**DIE**-uh-thur-mee) is the application of oscillating electromagnetic fields to the tissue. The oscillating fields cause a distortion in the molecules and

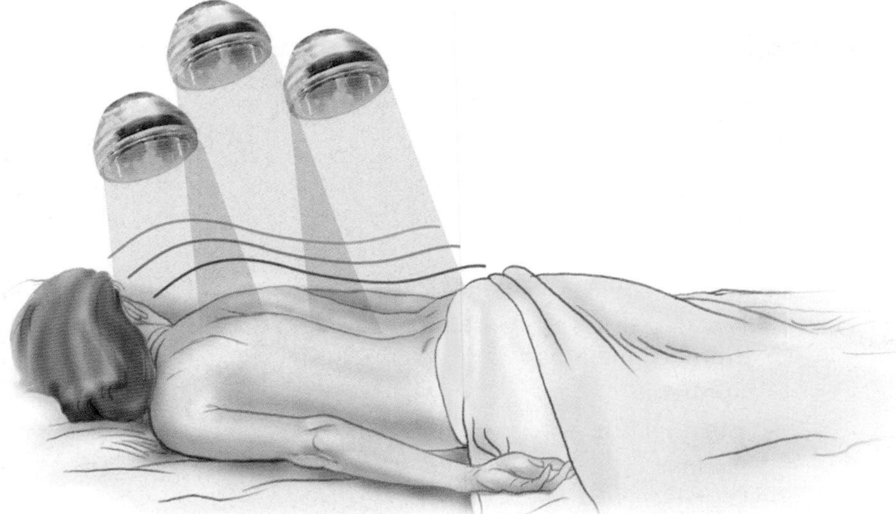

FIGURE 13-7 As infrared radiation is absorbed into the skin, heat is produced.

an ionic vibration that produces heat. A diathermy machine is designed to produce either shortwave or microwave radiation and transfer it into the tissues by cables and electrodes/applicators to the area of the body to be treated.

Ultrasound

Therapeutic ultrasonography is a type of diathermy that uses sound waves of a frequency between one and three megahertz (much higher frequency than can be heard by the human ear) that produces a deep heating in tissues such as muscles, tendons, joint capsules, and bone. Diathermy and ultrasound therapy require the use of specialized equipment and training and are beyond the scope of practice of massage therapy.

Paraffin Baths

A paraffin bath is one of the most effective methods of applying heat to relieve pain and stiffness. A warm paraffin bath relaxes muscles, relieves stiffness and muscle spasms, and stimulates circulation. The warm paraffin is also a moisturizer, producing healthier-looking, softer skin. Paraffin is a white or colorless waxy solid that is mixed with mineral oil and heated in a special paraffin bath appliance to between 115° and 134°F. The mineral oil lowers the melting point of paraffin and makes it easier to remove.

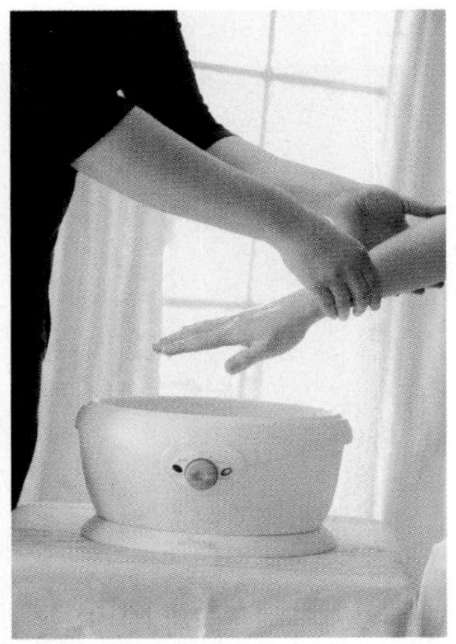

FIGURE 13-8 Paraffin baths provide warm relief for achy hands and feet.

Paraffin baths are usually applied to the hands, elbows, or feet by first covering them with a moisturizing lotion or oil and then dipping the extremity into the paraffin for a very short period several times to build up about a quarter-inch layer of the warming wax (Figure 13-8). The area is then covered with a protective plastic bag and wrapped in an insulating material such as a towel for 10 to 15 minutes or until it no longer feels warm. The paraffin is then removed and discarded. Gentle massage or other treatment can then proceed on the warmed tissue.

The application of moist heat generally involves various hydrotherapy treatments that are within a massage practitioner's scope of practice and can be used in conjunction with massage to enhance a client's experience.

Hot Compress

A hot compress is applied similarly to a cold compress, except that the water in which the compress is soaked is 110° to 115°F. A small towel is soaked in hot water, wrung out, folded, and placed on the area to be treated and then covered with a dry towel to provide insulation and hold the heat in (Figure 13-9a-c). Because the heat from the compress dissipates quite quickly, it works well to have a second compress that can be made hot and exchanged with the other every three to five minutes to keep warming the area.

Moist Heat Packs

Moist heat packs are generally chemical gel packs that are heated in a water bath, wrapped in a terry cloth cover, and placed on the body. A **hydrocollator** is used to heat and store the packs, which come in a variety of shapes, to conform to different areas of the body. The silica gel is formulated to retain heat

hydrocollator

an electrical appliance used to heat and store moist hot packs.

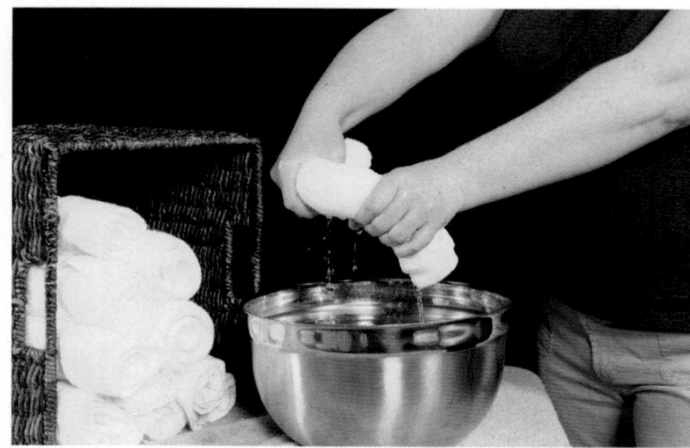

FIGURE 13-9A Prepare a warm compress by soaking a towel in hot water, wringing it out, and folding it.

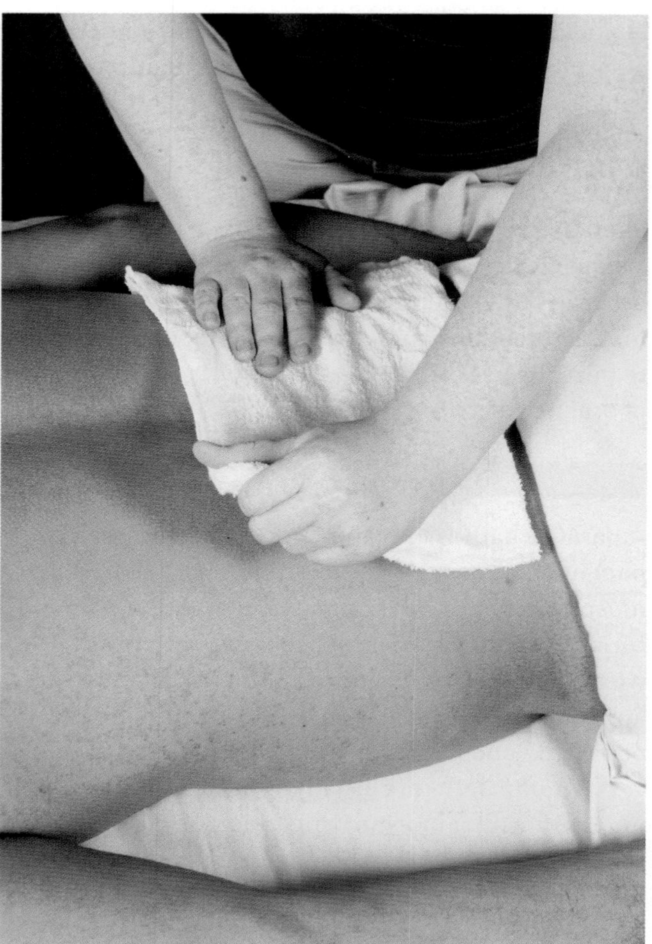

FIGURE 13-9B Place the folded warm compress on the area to be treated.

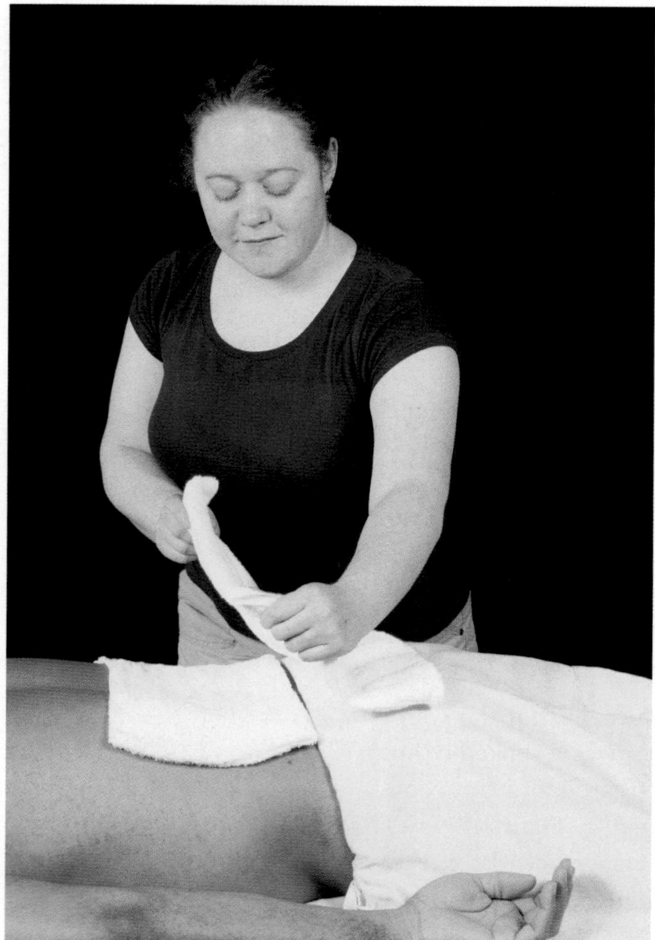

FIGURE 13-9C Cover the warm compress with a dry towel to hold in the heat.

and transfer it to the body part by means of conduction. Similar to heating pads, moist hot packs can be applied to one part of the body while the therapist works on another part (Figure 13-10).

Body Wraps

Body wraps use either wet or dry sheets and blankets to cover the entire body snugly (except the head) to warm the body, causing a false fever and profuse sweating. Wraps usually incorporate substances such as herbs or seaweed masks to nurture the body. Wraps are discussed in greater detail in Chapter 14, Massage in the Spa Setting.

Showers and Sprays

There are a variety of pulsating showerheads on the market today. The pulsating shower is an effective means of combining moist heat and mild compression.

This combination calms sensory nerves and increases peripheral circulation. Increased circulation restores nutrients as it clears away metabolic wastes. Sedated nerves mean reduction of pain, relaxation of tense or spasmed muscles, and reduced stress.

The Vichy shower, which originated in Vichy, France, is a multihead horizontal shower used in a wet room, where the client lies on a table under a soft, warm shower while receiving a massage or other spa treatment (Figure 13-11). The Swiss shower is a multiheaded shower stall found in some spas (Figure 14-8).

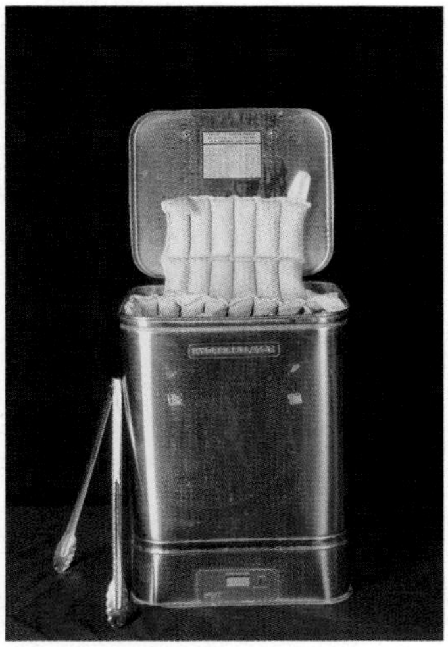

FIGURE 13-10 Moist heat packs are heated in water in a hydrocollator before being applied to the body.

Immersion Baths

Whenever the whole body or a body part is submerged in water, it is considered an immersion bath. Depending on the objective of the treatment, various areas can be treated and various temperatures used. Water is an effective medium for the application of thermal procedures (hot or cold) because it surrounds the body part and is an excellent conductor of heat or cold.

KINDS OF BATHS

The aim of all baths is the attainment of two objectives: external cleanliness and stimulation of bodily functions.

Depending on the temperature of water, the following kinds of baths are available for use:

1. Cold bath (55° to 70°F, equal to 12.8° to 21°C)
2. Cool bath (70° to 84°F, equal to 21° to 29°C)
3. Tepid bath (85° to 92°F, equal to 29.4° to 33.3°C)
4. Saline (salt) bath (90° to 98°F, equal to 32.2° to 36.6°C)

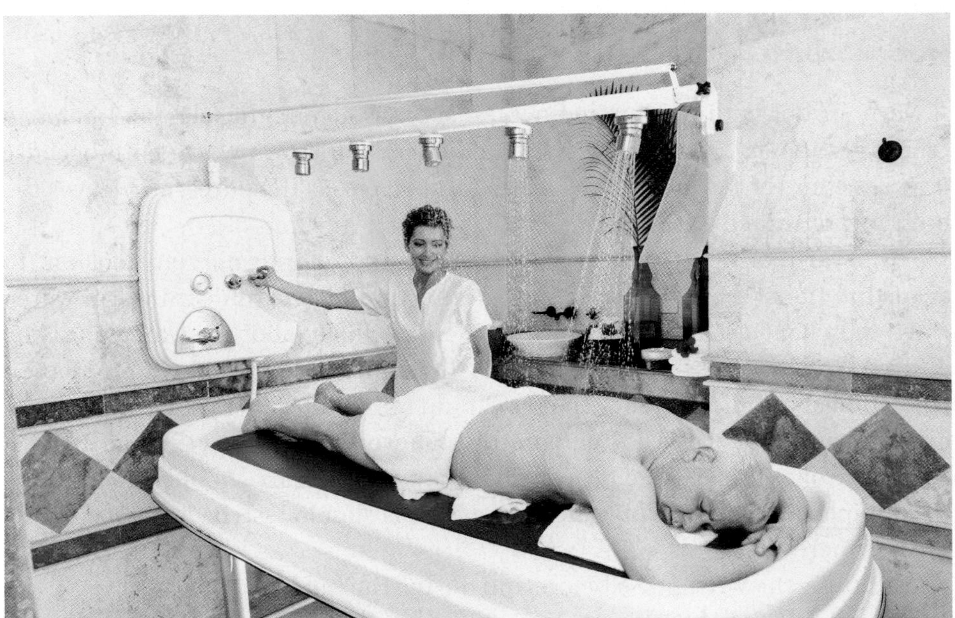

FIGURE 13-11 The Vichy shower is a multihead horizontal shower used in a wet room, where the client lies on a table under a soft, warm shower while receiving a massage or other spa treatment.

5. Warm bath (93° to 98°F, equal to 33.9° to 36.6°C)
6. Hot bath (99° to 104°F, equal to 37.2° to 40°C)
7. Sitz or hip bath (either hot or cold)

Cool Baths

Whether a cool bath is beneficial depends on its duration and the state of vitality and reserve strength of the client. If after a cool bath or shower the client comes out chilly, shivering, blue-lipped, or goose-fleshed, it indicates that his or her body reaction is not good. For the client who experiences a pleasant reaction and a feeling of warmth, the cool bath can be safely continued. A short cool bath or cold sponging of the body might be better tolerated if it is accompanied by friction and gentle rubbing with a rough towel.

The average duration for a cool bath or shower should be limited to between three and five minutes.

A tepid bath provides a satisfactory temperature for all-around bathing, particularly during warm weather.

Relaxing Neutral Tub Bath

The neutral tub bath exerts a soothing and relaxing effect on the body and is recommended for nervous and excitable people. The body is immersed in a tub of water at a neutral temperature (about 93° to 98°F) for about 15 to 25 minutes.

Saline (Salt) Bath

A saline (salt) bath, at a temperature of 90° to 98°F, produces a marked tonic effect on the body. The effect is similar to natural bathing in sea water. The amount of common salt to use is three to five pounds to a tub of water. The client is left in the saline bath for 10 to 20 minutes.

Hot or Warm Baths

A warm or hot bath quiets tired nerves, soothes aching muscles, and helps to relieve insomnia. A cool shower should generally follow a warm bath because it forces some of the blood away from the skin, closes the pores, and leaves the body in a refreshed condition.

The warm or hot bath induces relaxation and relieves nervous tension. To accustom the body to the high temperature, first fill the tub with warm water. Have the client get in the warm tub, then gradually add hot water until the desired temperature is reached. The U.S. Consumer Product Safety Commission has established guidelines for the maximum temperature for public hot tubs or baths to not exceed 104°F. Temperatures above that can cause hyperthermia or heat stroke. The average time for hot baths or showers should range from 5 to 20 minutes. The following safety precautions should also be observed by the practitioner:

- Take the wrist pulse before and during the hot bath.
- Give the client water to drink during the hot bath.
- If the client complains of unpleasant reactions, place cold compresses over the forehead or on the back of the neck.

Hot baths and very cold baths should be used only for clients who are in a healthy condition and who can withstand such treatments. For those clients whose health is not in the best condition, very hot or very cold baths can produce injurious effects. The hot bath or shower can cause undue stimulation to the body and overwork the heart. A cold bath or shower, on the other hand, can be a shock to the nervous system.

The following supplies and equipment are needed for various immersion baths:

1. Bathtub and bath thermometer
2. Bath towels and mat
3. Shower cap, robe, and slippers for client
4. Bath oil and lotion
5. Bath sheets
6. Compress cloth and basin of cool water
7. Air pillow and towel

IMMERSION BATH PROCEDURE

1. Check the room temperature to ensure that it is comfortable for the client.
2. Instruct the client regarding bathing and dressing procedures.
3. Fill the tub to the appropriate level.
4. Test the temperature of the water to ensure that it is at the recommended temperature range.
5. Assist the client into the tub, and place an air pillow or towel underneath his or her head.
6. Cover the client's body with a large towel or bath sheet.
7. Allow the client to relax for 5 to 25 minutes. Warm water can be added, if desired.
8. Assist the client out of the tub, and provide a towel for drying.
9. Supply the client with robe and slippers.
10. Allow the client time to rest.
11. Complete the client's records, noting benefits of the bath or any adverse reactions.
12. Be sure that the tub is sanitized thoroughly before the next bath.

Sitz or Hip Bath

The sitz or hip bath is applied only to the hips and pelvic region of the body, which is kept immersed in either hot, tepid, or cool water, or alternately hot and cool water. For a hot sitz bath, 5 to 10 minutes contact is usually sufficient. The time for a cool sitz bath varies from 3 to 5 minutes. The effects of a sitz bath depend primarily on the temperature of the water and its length of contact with the body. Generally, the sitz bath is given as a stimulant to the pelvic region. The temperature of the hot sitz is usually 100° to 104°F.

Besides being effective for treating chronic constipation, sitz baths are also beneficial for the kidneys, bladder, and sex organs.

A large basin or bathtub is suitable for a sitz bath. The bath is prepared by filling the basin or tub with water (of the correct temperature) to about a depth of 6 inches or enough to immerse the client's buttocks comfortably. When using a basin (the feet outside), a blanket should be placed around the feet for warmth and a towel can be placed under the knees for added comfort. The client sits in such a manner that the buttocks and upper thighs are immersed.

Whirlpool Bath

A whirlpool bath is a partial immersion bath in which the water is agitated to produce a slight pressure on the body. A whirlpool bath is beneficial to circulation, soothing to the muscles, and relaxing to the nerves. Physicians often order whirlpool baths as part of physical therapy for conditions such as arthritis, sprains, strained muscles, and relief of pain.

PROCEDURE

1. Fill the whirlpool tub to the recommended depth and test the temperature. Generally, the most desirable temperature is 104°F, but the bath can be cooler.
2. Add the recommended antiseptic agents to the water.
3. Instruct the client in how to enter the tub safely.
4. The treatment time is usually about 10 to 30 minutes.
5. Instruct the client about rest period, showers, and drying off.
6. Complete the client's records, noting benefits, reactions, effects, and the like.
7. Be sure that the tub is sanitized thoroughly before it is used again.

Air Baths

Steam and Sauna Baths

Heat in a steam bath is produced by a steam generator. Heat in a sauna is produced by a dry heat source. The temperature in a steam bath is 105° to 125°F, and the humidity is 100 percent, whereas the temperature in a sauna can be 180° to 190°F, with the humidity between 5 and 30 percent. A steam bath can be a cabinet where the head remains outside of the heat or a steam room. Because the heat in a steam bath is supplied by steam, the air is supersaturated. This greatly reduces the body's ability to cool itself with perspiration. Saunas are always a room heated by dry heat. Evaporation of the body's perspiration has a cooling effect, which is why the sauna can be so much hotter. Either type of bath causes profuse sweating. Caution must be used to avoid overheating and to replace body fluids. Those with heart conditions, diabetes, and other conditions must consult their physicians before using steam baths and saunas.

Cabinet Bath and Steam Canopy

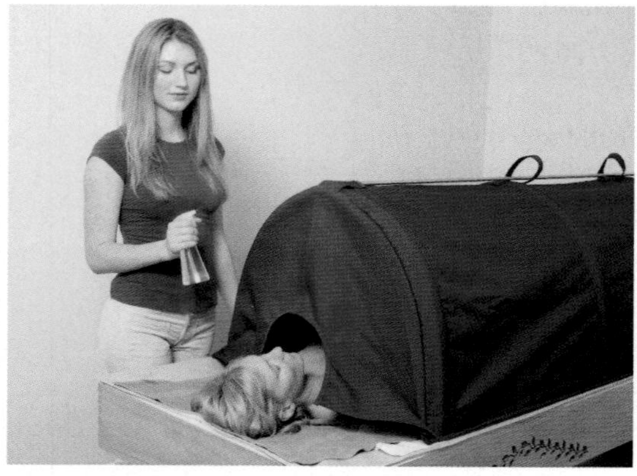

FIGURE 13-12 A Steamy Wonder steam canopy.

Bath cabinets are also known as vapor or steam cabinets. As used in body massage treatments, they are constructed in an upright or reclining position to accommodate the client's body while leaving the head exposed. A steam canopy is a lightweight tent that is placed over a client as he or she lies on a massage table so that only the head is outside the canopy (Figure 13-12). When the canopy is in operation, heat is generated, and warm, moist air surrounds the client's body. The heat, besides having a relaxing effect on the client, induces profuse perspiration. The intensity and duration of the heat can be controlled by a switch for low, medium, or high heat and by an automatic clock. The manufacturer's instructions are the most reliable guide for the proper use and care of the steam cabinet or canopy.

Not all clients react the same way to the steam bath. Knowing the condition and tolerance of the client is of assistance in controlling the temperature and duration of this treatment. A cool compress can be placed on a client's head or the back of the neck for added comfort during the hot treatment. A client in a weakened or nervous condition should be given gentle treatments of short duration until improvement is shown. Always consult a physician before administering cabinet baths for a client with a systemic disorder such as heart trouble or high blood pressure, or one having any severe illness.

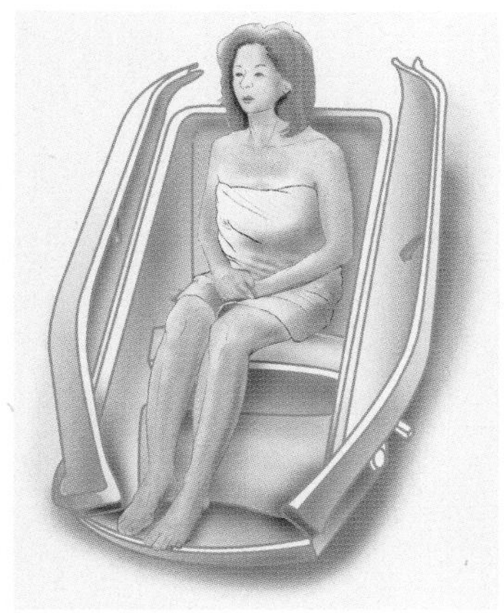

FIGURE 13-13 A client sitting in a vapor cabinet bath.

Length of Treatment

The exposure time in a cabinet bath or steam canopy ranges from 10 to 25 minutes. During this time, the practitioner should attend to the comfort and safety of the client and to his or her reactions to the heat treatment. The client's heat tolerance is greater if there is a gradual rise in the temperature of the bath cabinet. Postpone treatment if the client is ill, has an abnormal pulse or body temperature, or reacts unfavorably to the treatment.

The heat treatment induces profuse perspiration. To replace the fluids lost and to prevent body weakness, the practitioner should give the client water to drink periodically. If the client complains of a headache or a throbbing in the head, or of any adverse reactions during the treatment, discontinue the treatment.

After the cabinet bath, a mild tonic such as a tepid shower can be given. After this treatment, keep the client warmly wrapped to prevent chilling of the body (Figure 13-13).

CONTRAST THERAPY

Contrast therapy, or the alternating application of heat and cold, is one of the most effective methods of increasing local circulation. Contrasting hot and cold cause an alternating vasodilation and vasoconstriction of the blood vessels in an area. Increased local circulation relieves stiffness and pain from trauma and stimulates healing of injury and wounds.

Contrast baths require two tubs, one filled with hot water (104°F) and one with cold or ice water. First, immerse the body part in the hot water for three to five minutes or until the client becomes accustomed to the hot water (until the water no longer feels hot). Remove the limb from the hot water and place it in the cold water for 30 seconds to 2 minutes or until the client becomes accustomed to the cold water. While the client is in the cold bath, add hot water to the hot bath to bring it back up to temperature. Repeat the procedure three to six times, finishing with a cold application. Always complete the treatment with an immersion in the cold tub.

SUMMARY

Hydrotherapy is the application of water in any of its three forms to the body for therapeutic purposes. Water has certain properties that make it a valuable therapeutic agent. It is readily available and inexpensive. It provides buoyancy, is a universal solvent, and has the ability to absorb and conduct heat. As ice, it cools; as steam, it warms. As liquid it cleanses and can be used to heat or cool the body depending on the temperature of the water and how it is applied. The body's core temperature is 98.6°F, or 37°C. Applications of water approximating those temperatures are relaxing but have little thermal effect.

Temperatures above or below body temperatures either heat or cool the body. The nature and extent of those changes depend on the temperature and duration of the application, and the size of the body area and thermal conductivity of the body part involved. The greater the difference between the temperature of water and the temperature of the skin, the greater becomes the stimulating or sedating effect of the treatment.

Water treatments are generally safe; however, some contraindications do exist and must be considered, and extreme temperatures avoided.

Cryotherapy is the application of cold agents for therapeutic purposes. The primary goal of cryotherapy is to reduce tissue temperature. Ice is a common agent for the application of cold in the form of ice packs or ice massage. The application of ice causes a series of sensations represented by the acronym CBAN: C = cold, B = burning, A = aching, N = numbness. Cold applications are valuable in reducing swelling, sedating the nerves, and slowing the metabolic activity of body cells.

Thermotherapy is the external application of heat to the body for therapeutic purposes. It is especially effective for relieving pain from muscle tension or spasm and to promote muscle relaxation. The effects of thermotherapy depend on the temperature, duration and type of application. Circulation in the skin and perspiration increase. Muscles relax and connective tissue softens. Moist heat tends to penetrate deeper into the muscles. Thermotherapy can be applied with compresses, packs, showers, wraps, or a variety of baths. Non-hydrotherapy methods of heat application include hot pads, infrared lamps, and diathermy.

There are a wide variety of applications of hydrotherapy treatments. Only a few are discussed in this chapter. Many hydrotherapy treatments are part of spa treatments and are discussed in Chapter 14.

QUESTIONS FOR DISCUSSION AND REVIEW

1. Define hydrotherapy.
2. What are the qualities of water that make it a valuable therapeutic tool?
3. Describe the three classifications of the effects that hydrotherapy has on the body.
4. What are the contraindications for performing hydrotherapy?
5. Define cryotherapy.
6. What are the effects of the local application of ice?
7. What does the acronym PRICE stand for and how is it used?
8. What does the acronym CBAN stand for and what is its significance?
9. In which three ways are cold applications beneficial?
10. When are cold applications undesirable?

11. Name four convenient methods of applying cryotherapy.
12. What is thermotherapy?
13. What are the benefits of hot water applications?
14. How high a temperature can the skin safely tolerate?
15. What are the two objectives of baths?
16. What is the temperature of a warm bath? A hot bath?
17. What is the average duration of a cold bath, a cold shower, or a cold sitz bath?
18. What is the average duration of a hot saline or sitz bath?
19. What is the purpose of the cabinet bath?
20. List the safety precautions that should be observed during the operation of a bath cabinet.
21. What are the main benefits of a whirlpool bath?
22. What is contrast therapy?
23. What is the main effect of contrast therapy?

CHAPTER

14 Massage in the Spa Setting by Steve Capellini

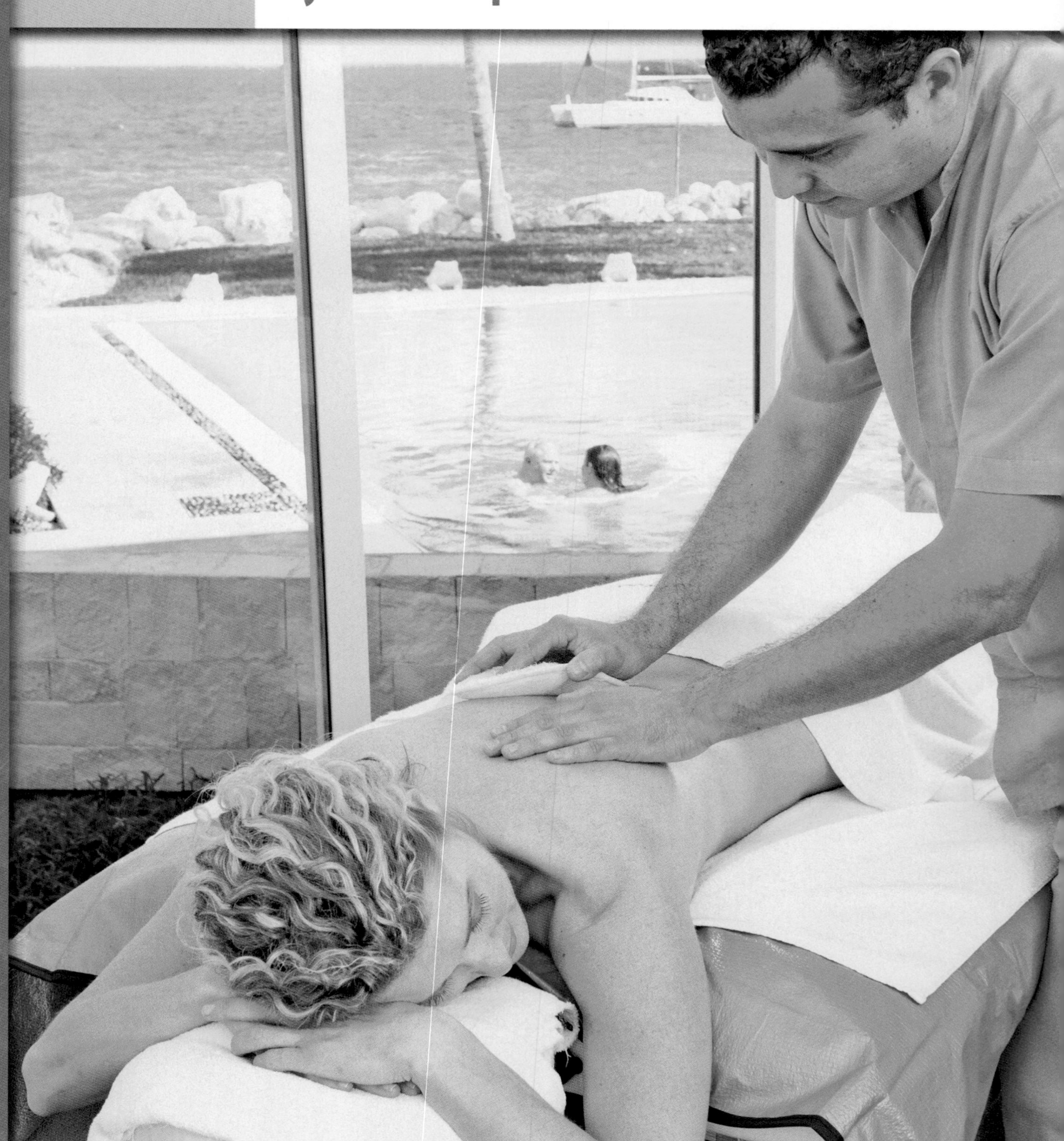

LEARNING OBJECTIVES

After you have mastered this chapter, you will be able to

1. **Describe the historical development of spas.**
2. **Describe the current state of the spa industry, including customer demographics and the various types of spas in which therapists work.**
3. **List and describe the most popular spa services performed by massage therapists.**
4. **Describe the most important attributes of an effective spa massage.**
5. **Demonstrate an ability to perform a spa exfoliation procedure and a spa body wrap procedure.**
6. **Describe the specialized hydrotherapy equipment and other apparatuses used in modern spas.**
7. **List and describe the qualities that make a massage therapist a good candidate for hiring by a spa, including customer service and other non–massage-related skills.**
8. **Describe the job potentials for massage therapists in spas, including possible career paths over time.**

International Spa Association (ISPA)

is a professional organization consisting of member spas, owners, directors, technicians, consultants, writers, marketers, and suppliers of products and equipment who meet at conventions and roundtables to create standards, share information, and chart directions for the development of the spa industry worldwide. (ISPA, 2365 Harrodsburg Road, Suite A325, Lexington, KY 40504, (888) 651-4772, www.experienceispa.com)

INTRODUCTION: WHAT IS SPA?

According to the **International Spa Association** (ISPA), a spa is a facility that is "devoted to enhancing overall well-being through a variety of professional services that encourage the renewal of mind, body and spirit." This official definition encapsulates much of what spa owners, operators, and employees attempt to do for their clients every day. Although some consumers continue to think of spas as places to indulge superficial pleasures and receive pampering services, and some spas continue to promote themselves as such, there is a growing trend toward recognizing the therapeutic and even life-changing value that spas can offer.

Spas are as diverse as the people who run them. Some are rustic retreats situated in nature, with a heavy emphasis on diet, internal cleansing, and physical fitness (Figure 14-1). Others are chic, modern facilities located in the heart of urban centers, offering the latest in high-tech skin care (Figure 14-2). There are large spas, with hundreds of employees, and tiny spas operated by just one person. Some spas have hundreds of thousands of dollars worth of hydrotherapy equipment; others have no such equipment at all. There are spas that offer psychological counseling, medical screening, shamanic vision-questing, Watsu, team building, Turkish bathing rituals, rock climbing, tennis clinics, cooking classes, weight loss, skiing, women's retreats, and much more.

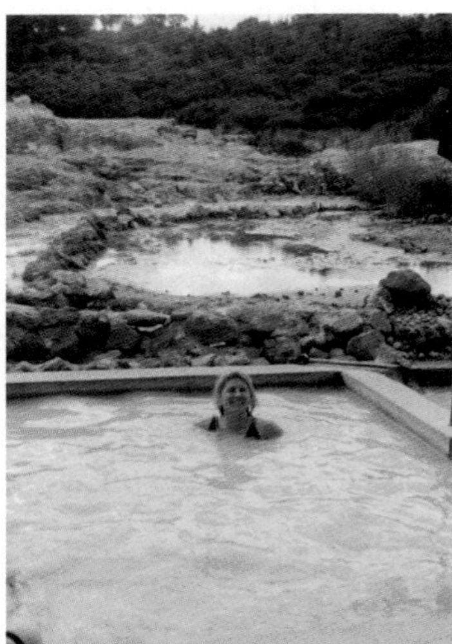

FIGURE 14-1 Some spas are rustic and natural, like this one in Rotorua, New Zealand. (Reprinted with permission from Spas Research Fellowship.)

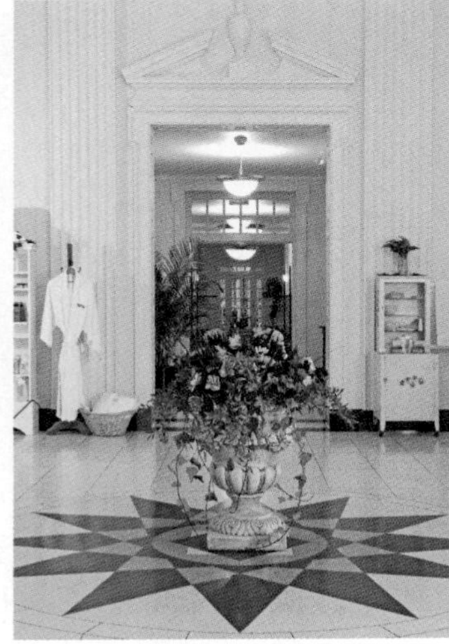

FIGURE 14-2 Some spas are modern and luxurious. (Courtesy of Roosevelt Baths, Saratoga Springs, New York.)

In recent years, spas have become specialized, with certain facilities featuring specific offerings and catering to specific audiences. These are explained in the section "The State of the Spa Industry Today." All of this specialization has made education a priority in the spa industry for two reasons. First, the public needs to be educated regarding spas to make the best choice for themselves when choosing a spa experience. Second, spa employees and potential employees need to be educated on the ever-growing number of modalities and special services available to perform them in a safe and effective manner.

The underlying factor that ties such a diverse group of facilities together can be discovered in that ISPA definition: spas (and the people who work in them) are devoted to enhancing overall well-being through a variety of professional services. It takes both devotion and skill to perform the professional services expected in a spa. This chapter explains these skills, and lets the reader discover what is expected when embarking on a career in the spa industry. What does a therapist need to know? Which services are they expected to perform? How many massages are expected in a day? Which non-massage skills are important to success? How difficult is it to get a job in a spa, and how realistic is it for therapists to open their own spa some day?

Spas represent the modern incarnation of a long line of healing and wellness facilities used by humans for millennia. A good place to start an exploration of the spa world, then, is in its historical roots.

A BRIEF HISTORY OF SPA

The origins of the word *spa* itself offer clues to a very important aspect of the spa experience—water. Water is the essence of many spa services. It is the environment in which much of the healing and rejuvenation at spas takes place. Archaeological studies and written accounts tell us that the earliest spas were often found at the source of a natural spring or, in the case of the ancient Romans, at sites to which such water was redirected by means of aqueducts. So what exactly does the word spa mean? By most accounts, it is an acronym, which is a word formed by putting together the first letters of other words. In this case, they are the Latin words *sanitas per aqua.* Several variations on the Latin have been cited, but they all mean the same thing, "health through water." This acronym, however, was tacked onto the word *spa* in recent years. The original derivation of the term is most likely from the Latin verb *spagere*, which means to sprinkle or flow, like a fountain or spring. That word was used to describe places where hot springs flowed, such as the town of Spa in what is present-day Belgium. A sixteenth century English physician was the first to use the word *spa* generically to refer to any such healing water source, and the moniker stuck.

Greek and Roman Roots

Both the ancient Greeks and Romans were, as a group, serious about bathing, and this is where much of the Western world's spa tradition began. During the height of the Roman Empire, for instance, the average citizen used 300 gallons of water per day, compared with just 50 gallons per day for the modern American. The baths were very important, not just for cleansing, but for health, fitness, and as a social gathering place. The larger baths could accommodate thousands of people (Figure 14-3). Poetry was read in the baths, political discussions took place, and, of course, there was massage. Patrons progressed through a series of rooms warmed to different temperatures by a great fire kept raging below the stone floors of the building in a furnace-like room called the *hypocaust.*

These early baths were expensive to construct and maintain, but the rulers of the day, the Roman emperors, looked on them as a way to impress the people with their generosity and greatness. The entry fee was kept very low, so that almost all citizens could attend the baths. The labor, and even the massage, was provided by slaves.

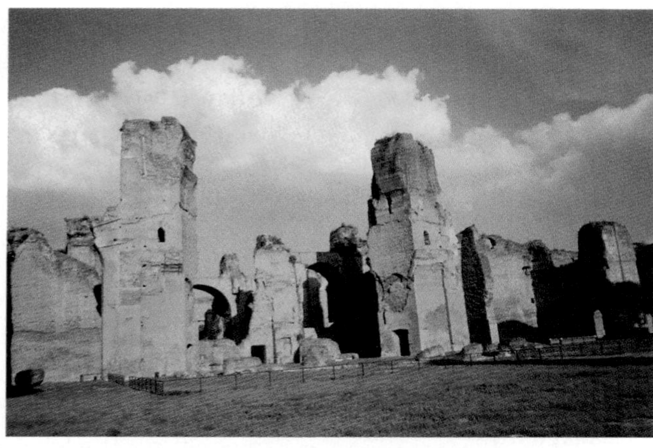

FIGURE 14-3 Ruins of the ancient Roman baths, or *thermae,* known as Caracalla. (Reprinted with permission from Spas Research Fellowship.)

As Roman civilization spread, so too did the use of the baths. Many Roman outposts were built at the site of a spring so that a bath could be constructed there, as occurred from northern Africa all the way to England. Many of these locations still feature spas today, and some, like Bath in England, have undergone extensive recent renovations.

Turkish Hammam

Descendants of the Roman *thermae,* **hammams** were a part of many mosques until they achieved an architectural and cultural significance of their own. Men and women bathe separately in the hammam, which, besides being a social center of the community, also holds spiritual significance. Often, the atmosphere inside the hot steamy main chamber where bathers are scrubbed and massaged seems more like a church than a spa, with diffused lighting and silence reigning. Arabic peoples for centuries have incorporated some form of the hammam into their lives. Mohammed himself, the founder of Islam, recommended sweat baths. He taught his followers that the heat in the hammam, which in Arabic means "spreader of warmth," improved fertility, and he wanted his flock to be fruitful and multiply.

hammam

(also spelled *hamam*), a Turkish steam bath with elaborate cleansing, exfoliation, and massage rituals passed down for centuries, played an important role in Ottoman culture.

Western nations, including England and the United States, have imported the concept of the hammam, which they called Turkish baths, with varying degrees of success. The concept has never become anywhere near as widespread as it is in Turkey and several other parts of the Islamic world, where it is interwoven with the daily lives of most people.

Asian Spa Roots

Through the centuries, people in Asia have given natural hot springs particular significance in their lives. Some cultures even considered them sacred, as in Japan, where the springs became known as *Onsen* and were used for communal bathing, personal renewal, and meditation. **Onsen** are always found in natural outdoor settings. They feature baths of varying temperature and treatments including massage and hydrotherapy. The Japanese treat them as more than a simple vacation; they regard them as spiritual retreats, where specific customs are to be observed.

Onsen

are Japanese hot springs at the site of natural volcanic spring water, usually with massage and other relaxing therapies available.

In other Asian cultures, such as in Thailand, massage and herbal therapies have been used through the ages, passed on from one generation to the next. Today in the Orient, traditional herbal spas exist side by side with modern European-inspired spas in resorts and hotels.

European Spas

bania

is a Russian-style communal steam bath.

sweat lodge

is a Native American enclosure for sweating, cleansing, and purification, in which participants pour water ceremonially over heated stones to create heat while praying and chanting.

kiva

is an underground chamber used by the Pueblo tribe of Indians for ceremonial sweats and other rituals.

Europe has a long tradition of spas and spa therapy, beginning with the expansion of Roman culture as previously mentioned. Baden Baden and Bad Wörishofen in Germany, Montecatini and Terme di Saturnia in Italy, Bath in England, and the town of Spa in Belgium are all examples of centuries-old spas. Czechoslovakia, Hungary, Bulgaria, and several other European countries also have a history of spa culture. The locales where these spas operate are still known today as "spa towns" (Figure 14-4). They owe their existence to the water source and the therapies that were applied there. In addition, the Finns are famous for their saunas and the Russians for their **banias**, but these are not full-fledged spa facilities as we have come to think of them.

For many years, Europeans have gone to spas to "take the cure." In fact, the German word *kur* came to be synonymous with spa in the 1800s when Sebastian Kneipp christened his new healing system by that name. His techniques centered on hydrotherapy, using heat, cold, and immersions, plus herbs, exercise, and proper diet, which has morphed over the years into some of our modern spa therapies and philosophies.

In Europe, spa philosophy always has been and continues to be more remedial and medically oriented than spa philosophy in the New World. Many European health plans pay for spa visits and spa treatments. Spa goers are likely to be prescribed a regimen by medical personnel on staff at the spa. This regimen can include multiple immersions in therapeutic waters and even the ingestion of mineral-laden spring waters in an attempt to improve physical conditions. More recently, some European spas have included the fitness and esthetic offerings of American spas, but at the same time, they have maintained their original dedication to medical treatments.

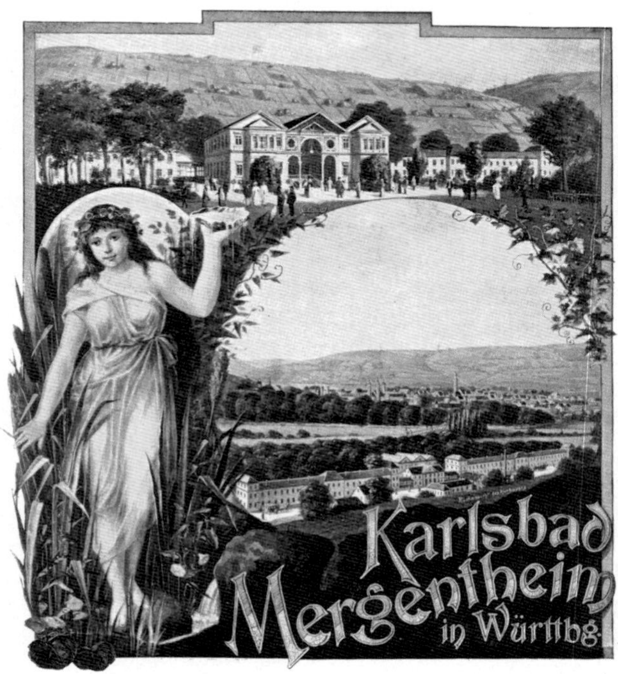

FIGURE 14-4 Advertisement for an early European spa in a typical spa town, Karlsbad, Germany. (Reprinted with permission from Spas Research Fellowship.)

Early America

On the North American continent, hot springs have been revered as sacred healing retreats for centuries. Native Americans often set these places apart and agreed not to fight or hunt there. Native Americans also created their own early spas by pouring water over heated stones in small enclosures known as **sweat lodges** or **kivas**.

During the nineteenth and early twentieth centuries, spalike health retreats were built in many areas, most notably Hot Springs, Arkansas (Figure 14-5); White Sulphur Springs, West Virginia; and Saratoga,

New York. John Harvey Kellogg also opened the Battle Creek Sanatorium in Michigan. Typical treatments administered at the early hot springs health spas always included a soak in the mineral pools (Figure 14-6), which became very popular. Saratoga Springs, for example, was first introduced in its natural state to white settlers by Native Americans in the 1700s, and by the early 1900s, it was accommodating thousands of visitors a day in extensive facilities.

Spa going underwent a decline in popularity in the early to mid-twentieth century when most such activity was confined to weight loss visits to "fat farms." As the 1900s progressed, however, these facilities gave way to more modern spa ventures that focused on holistic health, fitness, diet, and overall well-being. The first such spa was the Golden Door in California, which opened in the late 1950s. Since that time, spas have continued to expand and modernize their offerings and facilities.

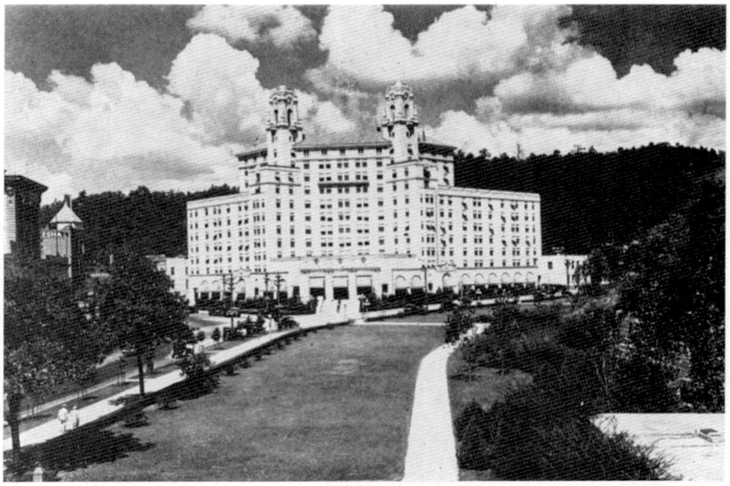

FIGURE 14-5 U.S. health spas or sanatoriums like the ones in Hot Springs, Arkansas, were popular early in the twentieth century and drew thousands of people to fancy new hotels like the Majestic. (Reprinted with permission from Spas Research Fellowship.)

The State of the Spa Industry Today

The spa industry today is a dynamic and ever-changing segment of the economy that has seen tremendous growth over the past 30 years. Officially part of the **hospitality industry**, spas provide extremely specialized services that set them apart from other choices when consumers are deciding where to spend their discretionary income. More and more people are seeing the benefit of these services, as evidenced by the rising tide in spas and spa going recently. The total number of U.S. spas more than quintupled from 1995 to 2007, rising from 2,674 to 14,600 (the statistics in this section are quoted from the ISPA's 2007 Spa Industry Report). People paid a total of 111 million visits to spas in 2006, spending $9.4 billion. Of the spa body services performed, massage therapy remains by far the most popular, with about 60 percent of all spa guests receiving a massage or body treatment.

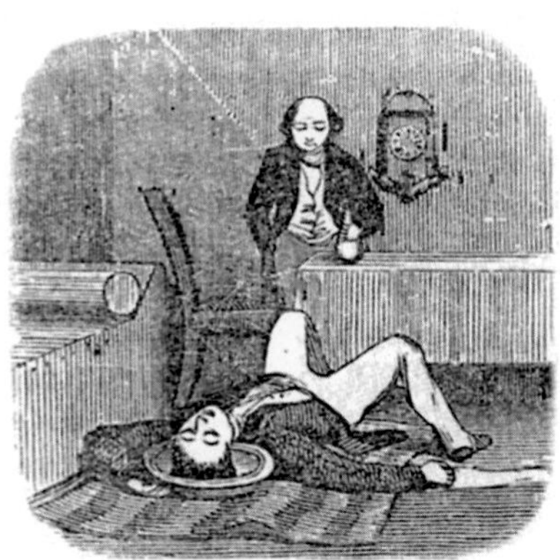

THE HEAD-BATH.

FIGURE 14-6 The head bath was used in sanatoriums to treat "all acute diseases about the head." (Reprinted with permission from Spas Research Fellowship.)

Since 2003, the spa industry has experienced a leveling out of this quick expansion, and many experts now think that it is entering a new phase of moderate growth. Although the number of facilities is still increasing, overall spa revenues and the total number of spa employees are not exploding any more and have even gone down in some cases. Spa owners and directors have begun to catch their collective breath and are now focusing on improving the quality of their workforce and their offerings for an increasingly experienced and demanding audience. Accordingly, the need for qualified, well-trained personnel continues to be strong.

hospitality industry is the combined hotel, resort, restaurant, and entertainment industries that rely especially on customer service and professional hospitality for their success.

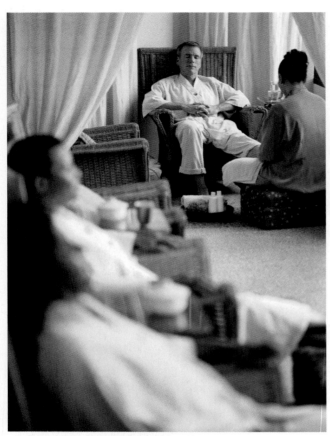

FIGURE 14-7 Spas are attracting an ever-growing number of male clients.

Although spa customers come from many different backgrounds, certain groups are more likely to visit a spa than others. More than 70 percent of visitors, for example, are female (figure 14-7). The average age is approximately 40, so the clientele tends to be mature and slightly older than the typical age for those who receive massage therapy outside the spa setting, which is approximately 30 years old. Income and education are also determining factors, with the average spa goer reporting an income of more than $70,000 and more than one half of them holding college degrees.

Several trends continue to shape the character of the spa landscape. According to Susie Ellis, president of Spa Finders, in 2009 these trends include

1. Energy Medicine: People are more open to alternative medicine, and there is more scientific evidence lending credibility to the field.
2. Medical and Spa Tourism: Traveling for health is happening for many different reasons and in many different ways, all over the globe.
3. Eco-embedded Spas: A Deeper Shade of Green: It's the most relaxing way for spa goers to enjoy and feel good about their spa experiences.
4. In-Transit Spa Going: The presence of de-stressing outlets during travel helps to make trips much more enjoyable.
5. Mindful Spending: Discounts, bargains, and added values are expected in almost every transaction, and spas are no exception.

Types of Modern Spas

Spas encompass a wide array of businesses, offering their customers many choices in much the same way that restaurants offer choices in price, menu, service, and ambience. Although each spa is unique, spas can be categorized into six major types: destination spas, hotel/resort spas, day spas, club spas, medical/dental spas, and mineral spring spas. (See Table 14.1 for more information about each type.)

Of course, spas in all of these categories are "devoted to enhancing overall well-being through a variety of professional services that encourage the renewal of mind, body, and spirit." This is their commonality, yet they attract a diverse clientele and present a wide range of philosophies and methods. The following two examples highlight the opposite ends of the broad spectrum of offerings.

Canyon Ranch Spa: Many therapists would consider it a dream job to work for Canyon Ranch, one of the best known destination spas in the world. The spa was founded in 1979 by Mel Zuckerman, a businessman in Tucson, Arizona. He was successful but overweight and unhealthy, like so many people who lead sedentary, high-stress lifestyles. A trip to a California spa offered him and his wife a

TABLE 14.1

TYPES OF SPAS				
TYPE OF SPA	APPROX. 2004 U.S. NO.	DESCRIPTION	LOCATION	CLIENTELE
Destination Spa	79	Facility with overnight accommodations catering exclusively to spa guests, often featuring advanced modalities and elaborate signature services in beautiful surroundings.	Usually a separate building or compound with several buildings set apart from neighboring businesses or residences.	High discretionary income individuals or couples willing to spend $2,500 to $6,000/week on health and wellness.
Hotel/Resort Spa	1,345	Spa facilities located within a larger encompassing hotel, or resort, or cruise ship. The spa can be a main feature of the property or simply an amenity for guests to use at their leisure, offering a wide array of treatments, some rivaling those at destination spas.	All major resorts and high-end hotels include spas with their new properties or add them to existing properties to compete effectively; spas rate high according to consumers on list of requested hotel features.	Families, couples; medium- to high-income range; either dedicated spa goers or casual vacationers; often one partner attends the spa while the other golfs, plays tennis, etc.
Day Spa	11,736	A spa where guests visit for a few hours or a day, with no sleepover accommodations available. These spas range from small one-person operations to full-blown centers offering treatments on a par with the large resorts.	Often situated within a hair salon; can be a storefront, stand-alone building, a single multipurpose room, part of a massage clinic, in a shopping mall, or even in airports.	Day spas cater to a wide array of people of many social classes, from low-medium to high-income levels who prize proximity, affordability, and personalized service.
Club Spa	428	Spas that are part of a larger physical fitness facility, ranging from a minor addition to a major focus of the business.	Many upscale urban fitness clubs consider it essential to include a spa, especially multi-purpose lifestyle clubs.	Physically active people who prize optimal performance and appearance; medium to medium-high income range.
Medical/ Dental Spa	976	Medical/dental spas are either dedicated spa facilities that operate in conjunction with a nearby medical practice or are incorporated into the actual practice, always under the supervision of a medical professional.	Can be located at a wellness retreat center, at a resort, in a stand-alone building, or as part of an existing medical/ dental practice.	Ranging from high-income people willing to pay extra for personalized medical services in a comfortable environment to everyday patients at medical/dental offices given extra attention with or without spa services in a spalike setting.
Mineral Springs Spa	51	Spas located at the actual source of mineral springs and incorporating these waters into their program and treatments.	Can be a stand-alone destination-style spa or can be located within a resort built on the mineral spring property, often in rural settings, ranging from rustic to high end.	A wide range, from weekend family vacationers at rustic spring sites to five-star hotel goers on gourmet retreats.

new vision, and they hoped to offer that same vision to guests at their new spa. The operation grew rapidly, expanded to a new location in Massachusetts in the 1980s, opened its first Spa Club at the Venetian Resort in Las Vegas in the 1990s, and continues to grow rapidly today. There is now a Canyon Ranch spa aboard the *Queen Mary II* cruise ship, a healthy lifestyle community in Miami, Florida, called Canyon Ranch Living, and another resort spa near Orlando, Florida. The Canyon Ranch Spa has become a global brand, attracting thousands of the most affluent and well-traveled people in the world. The staff of medical doctors, psychologists, fitness experts, nutritionists, bodyworkers, chefs, and hospitality specialists cater to people who pay thousands of dollars a week. This is definitely the high end of what spas represent today.

Joy Spring Day Spa: Spas need not be grand ventures backed by multimillionaire investors. Tiny spas can offer the same level of service and therapeutic value as the large spas like Canyon Ranch. One such spa was Joy Spring. Owned and operated by just one woman, Joy Spring was situated in a trendy California coastal town for many years. The owner has since sold her spa to eventually

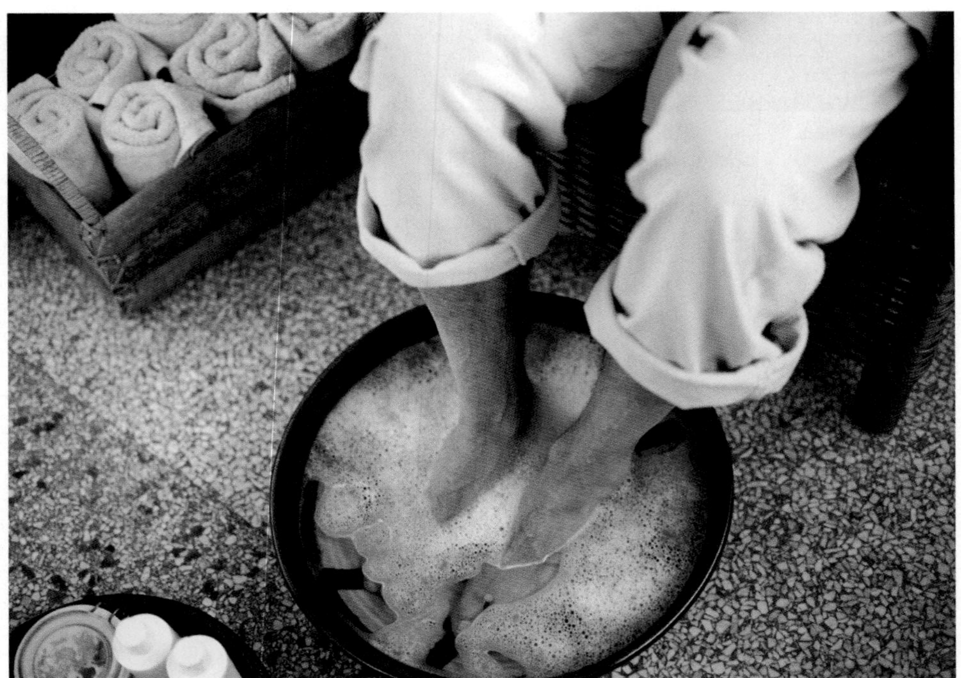

FIGURE 14-8 Even small spas can become luxurious by using simple items such as a basin to soak the feet.

open another location in Los Angeles, and her future is looking bright. The waiting room at Joy Spring consisted of two chairs and a single bookshelf in an area the size of a closet, but there was a little water fountain there and a sense of calm. The small selection of books and gift items on the shelf was carefully chosen and arranged in an appealing way. Inside the treatment area was a steam cabinet, a massage table, and not too much else. When clients spent time in that room, however, they felt as if the rest of the world had disappeared (Figure 14-8).

Both Canyon Ranch and Joy Spring have the right to call themselves spas, because spas can be so many things for so many people. Regardless of the size of the operation or the breadth of offerings found there, a spa's success or failure usually is determined by the quality of the therapeutic interaction between one guest and one therapist at a time. Canyon Ranch owner Mel Zuckerman was aware of this, and that is why he signed himself up for a massage and an herbal wrap every day during the first year of business, to keep the emphasis where it belonged—on the treatments.

MASSAGE IN THE SPA INDUSTRY: FORMING REALISTIC EXPECTATIONS

The prospect of working in a spa, large or small, can seem daunting at first because there are so many variables involved and so many questions to ask. Through the influence of the media, gossip, or sheer lack of information, some students and beginning therapists form incomplete or misguided perceptions about what it is like to work in a spa. These perceptions spread through the massage community, making it nearly impossible to tell myth from reality. Some of the most common misperceptions circulating about the spa industry are listed in the accompanying sidebar "Spa Myths versus Spa Reality."

It is important to have a realistic set of expectations about the role of massage therapists working in spas. The most relevant information that is needed in this regard can be categorized into three main topics:

1. What the therapist is expected to do
2. What the therapist is expected to know
3. How the therapist is expected to act

The following sections explore these three essentials of spa work to help therapists envision their potential role in the industry.

Spa Myths Versus Spa Reality

Myth: A therapist is expected to do ten massages in a row without a break.

Reality: Although a very small number of insensitive spa owners still try to force the maximum work out of their therapists, the trend today is to take care of therapists. A burned-out staff is not good for customer relations. Five or six services per day, often with a 10- to 15-minute break between sessions, is the normal maximum. In addition, spa modalities such as body scrubs and wraps are not as hard on therapists' bodies.

Myth: The only kind of massage done in spas is pampering massage.

Reality: Many spas offer advanced bodywork modalities on their menus, including craniosacral, neuromuscular, myofascial, and more. In some cases, training in these techniques is even provided and paid for by the spa.

Myth: Therapists are always poorly paid in spas.

Reality: Although it is true that spas have high overhead costs and must try to keep their expenses down, therapists still typically make $20 to $40/hour, with no overhead expenses of their own.

Myth: Only unmotivated or unskilled therapists work in spas.

Reality: Many highly motivated and skilled therapists work in spas. Some find it optimal to let the spa handle business while they focus on therapy, content to remain in that relationship for many years. Others quickly move up to become supervisors, trainers, lead therapists, and directors. Some therapists pursue other goals while working in the spa, using it as a career stepping-stone.

Myth: Therapists cannot perform in-depth work over time in spas because the clientele changes constantly.

Reality: Roughly three fourths of all locations are day spas or club spas with a local, repeat clientele. Even at resort and destination spas, therapists can work with clients several times during their stay or even during return visits.

MASSAGE PRACTICE IN THE SPA SETTING

First and foremost in the spa come the duties of a massage therapist. Massage is what therapists train for and are hired to do. It is therefore is natural for a newly hired therapist to think that all she needs do to successfully fulfill her duties is to get behind that closed door as quickly as possible and begin the massage. When practicing massage in a spa, however, therapists need to remain aware that they are operating within a larger structure that encompasses and helps to define what it is they are doing in the treatment room.

Each spa has developed its own particular protocols and standards when it comes to implementing massage on their premises. In addition to massage, therapists may be required to perform several other spa modalities including body wraps; body scrubs; specialized rituals and exotic services such as **ayurvedic** (eye-yur-**VEY**-dick), Indonesian, herbal detoxification treatments; and hydrotherapy baths and showers. It is up to the therapist to master these protocols and follow them while on the job. The following points are important to keep in mind when practicing in a spa setting: scope of practice, intake procedures, optimal number of massages per day, timing of services, guest greetings, preparation, and cleanup.

ayurveda

is an ancient system of Indian medicine and healing; it has been modified in recent years for use in spa treatments such as body scrubs, face treatments, and massages.

Scope of Practice

The massage therapist in a spa setting is of course subject to all the same limitations to scope of practice as are massage therapists in any professional setting. Additional points to consider in a spa are these:

- Many spa guests are receiving their very first massage, and it is important to be sensitive to this. Often, it is appropriate to use extremely light pressure over the entire body at first, until a level of comfort and rapport can be established. Even if the therapist specializes in deep bodywork and is willing to share it with spa guests, the guests are often unprepared for it and might react adversely. Therapists should limit massage strokes to basic Swedish unless the guest has requested otherwise or after clear communication.
- Because people are often on a quest for better health while visiting a spa, they are especially open to suggestions about diet, nutrition, and lifestyle. It must be remembered that these are not within massage therapists' scope of practice.
- Some people visit spas to address long-term physical conditions, ranging from addictions to obesity to heart disease, as well as many other conditions. It is tempting to want to help people with these conditions, showing them how a combination of massage, detoxification, improved diet, and lifestyle offered at the spa can help to heal many ills. It is important not to promise any benefits that cannot be substantiated or that are not sanctioned by the spa, however. In general, the benefits that therapists can rightfully claim for spa services include those created by heat; special products such as herbs, clays, and seaweeds; and massage therapy.
- Because so many spa treatments involve the use of hot water, therapists must be thoroughly familiar with all contraindications for the use of heat.

Intake Procedures

Each spa has its own unique intake procedures. Some employ an extensive screening process that can even involve a doctor's visit, a stress test, and a thorough physical examination. Some have well-trained **intake specialists** who spend a half hour or more molding the guests' experience, recommending treatments, and gleaning much important information that therapists can use in their sessions. These facilities usually fall into the destination spa, medical spa, or mineral spa categories. Some resort and club spas have an extensive intake procedure as well. Other spas, however, have a bare-bones intake form that asks only for emergency contact information and the guest's reason for requesting massage. Most day spas require little screening, and some require none at all.

intake specialists

also known as hospitality coordinators, spa concierges, and other titles, are spa employees who focus on pairing guests with appropriate treatments, therapists, services, and lifestyle choices during their stay at the spa.

As therapists study SOAP notes and charting during their massage education, they will no doubt see the value in these procedures, and the lack of such documentation in many spas might come as an unwelcome surprise. It is important, then, for therapists working in spas to use their own discretion when working with a guest for the first time. Whenever an intake form of any kind is available, it should be used to full advantage, and if the spa does not use one, it is permissible to ask the guest verbally about medical conditions and possible contraindications.

Some spas, especially hair and esthetics-based day spas, focus their intake questions on the skin rather than on overall health, because their main business consists of cosmetic procedures and the sale of cosmetic products. This paradigm works well for many spas. Some therapists new to the industry, however, perceive the lack of intake procedures at these spas as an insult to their therapeutic integrity, which can lead to tension between management and massage staff. If this is the case, it is permissible for the therapist to suggest an intake procedure to spa management, but if one is not implemented, it is best for the therapist to either accept this or seek employment elsewhere rather than create ill will among the staff and guests.

Number of Massages

Because massage therapy is the most popular service in spas, it is often necessary for therapists to perform several back-to-back sessions. What this means differs from spa to spa, however. Many spas maintain a strict break of at least 15 minutes between treatments, with some going as high as 30 minutes. Other spas offer very little break at all, as little as 5 minutes, but these are increasingly rare because spa owners are seeing the benefit of keeping their employees healthy. It is not good for business to have therapists out of work and receiving worker's compensation because of carpal tunnel syndrome.

For the same reason, it is customary for spas to limit their therapists' total number of massage treatments each day. The number varies, but the norm is five massages per day. Many factors contribute to altering this number in particular spas. For example, some spas have therapists perform only two or three massages in a row, with less-taxing spa treatments interspersed throughout the day. Thus, a therapist can perform eight total treatments, but three of them might be body scrubs, wraps, or specialty services.

On-call therapists not employed full time by the spa are often called on to perform more back-to-back services. When guest demand is at its peak, these therapists can sometimes perform eight massages or more. Attempting heroics by performing this number of full-hour sessions day after day is a sure way to cause injury. Although the lure of immediate income is strong, it is best to take a long-term point of view and pace oneself. Many therapists have enthusiastically entered the spa industry only to leave disillusioned a few short years later because of disability.

Spas that force therapists to perform too many massages, with no regard for their welfare, usually experience high turnover and lowered guest satisfaction. These spas are the least enjoyable to work for. There are many states that have no laws limiting the number of massages that a spa can ask employees to perform. Spas that overwork their therapists soon build a poor reputation in the industry.

Over an extended period of employment at a spa, therapists find a rhythm that both satisfies guest demand and preserves their own health. This rhythm is different for each therapist, with some choosing to perform only three or four services of any kind on a given day, or 20 in a given week. Others can perform several more as long as the massage services are interspersed with other spa treatments. There are a few therapists capable of performing many massages a day for weeks on end without experiencing injury or burnout.

Timing of Massage and Spa Services

Massage therapists sometimes find the strict time limitations imposed in the spa setting onerous. They think that constantly watching the clock drains value from the massage, and the same massage given over and over again within a certain number of minutes becomes stale and rote. Therapists who work in spas need to overcome this challenge and find ways to make their work fresh within the confines of the spa's necessary structure. Meeting this challenge is the essence of giving a good **spa massage**.

spa massage

is any massage given by a therapist within the structure and limitations of the spa setting, usually referring to the spa's basic Swedish massage, but also applicable to advanced modalities given in the spa.

Some therapists, wanting to give each guest the best service possible, habitually overrun the allotted time for each treatment, running in a perpetual state of slight delay. This can undermine the smooth running of the entire spa, from reservations to the front desk to the locker room—and, of course, it is not fair to the next guest who has arrived on time for an appointment. Some guests might have scheduled multiple treatments with different practitioners, and running overtime can affect other's schedules. It is necessary to end the massage at least 5 minutes before the next treatment is scheduled to begin. Certain services such as body wraps and scrubs require more time to prepare than massage, and this must be taken into consideration.

If a guest arrives late to an appointment, it is the therapist's responsibility to inform that guest that the treatment needs to end on time and will necessarily be curtailed. If the spa allows it and no appointment is scheduled afterward, the therapist might be able to adjust the schedule and perform the full service. Even if both therapist and client have free time directly after the scheduled service, it is usually not a good idea to run over or intentionally give a longer treatment, because guests given an extra long massage or spa service might tell other guests and cause jealousy. Another session also could be booked while that session in progress either for the therapist or another that needs to use that room.

Spas usually prescribe the length of each massage and spa service on their menu, and guests expect that this time does not include preparation and cleanup. Thus, a 75-minute massage is scheduled on the books in a 90-minute block, allowing for time before and after the actual hands-on treatment to prepare or clean up the space. The typical time frame for a full-body massage is 50 or 60 minutes at most spas, with a 75- or 80-minute extended option. It is rare for a spa to offer a 20- or 25-minute massage, unless it is localized and confined to one area, such as the neck and shoulders or the feet.

Most spas have a cancellation policy in effect and charge guests fully or partially for skipped services. In this case, the therapist might or might not be compensated, depending on the compensation structure and internal policies of the spa. If the therapist is paid for her time, it is her responsibility to find some productive work in the spa to fill the hour, such as stocking and tidying the treatment room, working on client notes, or cleaning.

Guest Greetings

Massage therapists generally greet their clients in a cordial manner, regardless of the setting, whether the massage takes place in a clinic, in an office, or in the client's home. Spa directors, however, expect extra cordiality from their therapists, above and beyond that rendered in other venues. Spas create high expectations among their guests, and therapists must be aware that their actions reflect on the entire operation. Some spas have a script for the greeting process, designating exactly what to say and do when meeting a guest, escorting him to the treatment room, explaining the treatment, especially draping, conversation during the treatment, and then saying good-bye. Therapists who work in one of these spas must memorize this script and adhere to it for the most part. More often, however, spas leave the details up to the therapist.

The following are general guidelines that apply in most spas when greeting guests:

- Shake hands firmly when first meeting, giving the guest confidence in your touch.
- Look the guest directly in the eyes for a moment to establish contact and trust.
- Speak slowly and clearly, introducing yourself with a sentence such as, "Hello, Mrs. Reed, my name is Elaine, and I will be performing your Balinese Ritual for you today."
- Lead the way to the treatment area, because the guest may be uncertain where to go.
- Explain the treatment clearly and thoroughly, including draping concerns, as many spa guests are modest and somewhat apprehensive at this stage of their spa experience.
- Do not solicit feedback from the client during the treatment other than asking about pressure and comfort.
- After the treatment, offer water, tea, or some other healthy refreshment, if the spa allows.
- Usher the guest back to the locker room or rest area, making sure he is reoriented.
- Do not solicit tips. Although tips may be accepted in most spas, therapists should never directly ask for them.

Preparation and Cleanup

Massage therapists in the spa setting do not have much time to clean their treatment room after each session and prepare it for the next. Therefore, it is necessary to learn effective planning and economy of movement. The room itself should be well stocked, using as much shelf space, under-table space, counter space, and cabinet space as possible to avoid unnecessary trips to the supply room down the hall. The limited time between treatments also must be used judiciously to attend to personal needs.

Therapists should make sure that all traces of the previous client have been cleaned up before ushering the next guest into the room. This can be difficult after certain spa treatments, which require the use of multiple towels and products. A hamper, bag, or other receptacle either in the room or nearby is helpful to deal with the quantity of soiled linens generated in the spa treatment room.

Therapists must arrive early enough beforehand to prepare for certain spa treatments that entail extensive lead time, such as the herbal wrap, for example, which requires five minutes for wringing the sheets.

Keep all surfaces and equipment sanitary before, between, and after all treatments, and especially at the end of the day. Some spas hire spa technicians, locker room attendants, and after-hours cleaning crews to do the bulk of this cleaning, but hygiene in the treatment room during the day is ultimately the therapist's responsibility, because it can directly impact the health of the client. Read more about sanitation in "Specialized Spa Equipment," later in this chapter.

Common Advanced Bodywork Techniques in Spas

There are certain advanced bodywork modalities that have found great favor in spas recently. They can be found on the treatment menus at large destination spas and small day spas alike. Many spa guests have become conversant in bodywork terminology and come to a spa seeking "deep work" or "Thai massage" or "craniosacral massage" Others, seeking adventure, will try something new as long as it is offered in the safe environment of the spa. Every advanced modality in existence is available in at least one spa, but there are several that are most popular. These modalities are listed in Table 14.2. Aromatherapy applications and stone massage are not listed in this table because they are so common in spas today. No longer considered advanced, aromatherapy and stone massage are almost essential for spas of any size to offer on their menus, and they are discussed later in this chapter.

Often, spa management will pay for the advanced education necessary for their therapists to become proficient in advanced techniques. Sometimes management invites instructors in to offer training at the spa itself. This creates loyalty among the staff and is sometimes extended to only those therapists who have been employed by the spa for a certain period, usually one year. It is one of the major benefits for working at an established spa with an emphasis on training.

SPA MASSAGE

Taking into account the wide variety of bodywork administered in spas, it is difficult to arrive at one simple definition for spa massage. When people use this term, however, they most often mean a spa's basic massage offering, which is commonly

TABLE 14.2

ADVANCED MASSAGE TECHNIQUES TYPICALLY OFFERED IN SPAS		
ADVANCED TECHNIQUE	**PURPOSE**	**POPULARITY**
Ayurveda	Meaning "knowledge of life," ayurveda is an ancient Indian system of medicine recently adapted for application in modern spas, where its main purpose is to rebalance the body's skin and internal organs through application of herbs, oils, creams, massage, and exfoliation.	Very popular in destination and resort spas, many spas have a menu of several Ayurvedic services available.
Craniosacral	Craniosacral therapy treats the bones and membranes surrounding the brain and spinal cord to free restrictions in the flow of cerebrospinal fluid, increasing overall health and relieving pain and stress.	One of the more popular advanced modalities in many spas, guests enjoy the delicacy of the touch as well as the effective therapy.
Deep tissue	Spas use this term to refer to a wide range of techniques, including connective tissue, neuromuscular, trigger-point, and even sports massage.	Quite popular among spa guests who like deep pressure but are unfamiliar or unconcerned with specific terms and techniques.
Lomilomi	A massage technique that originated in Hawaii that mostly uses the forearms to knead, rub, and weave like a dance. Aligns body, mind, and spirit.	Becoming more popular with seasoned spa guests who are looking for a different type of massage.
Manual lymph drainage	This gentle massage uses light, rhythmic, spiral-like movements to accelerate the movement of lymphatic fluids in the body.	Somewhat popular in spas, especially medical spas and spas with advanced esthetics programs.
Myofascial	A gentle stretching and elongation of the connective tissues in and around the muscles, especially at trigger points, this therapy restores balance, health, and elasticity while relieving pain.	Not as popular as craniosacral therapy in spas, this therapy is nonetheless prized for its gentle effectiveness.
Neuromuscular	A method for addressing soft-tissue abnormalities to reduce tightness, pain, and pathologic dysfunction.	Somewhat popular in spas, especially among guests with specific pains or complaints.
Reflexology	A system based on the theory that points on the hands and feet have a reflex effect on different parts of the body. Firm pressure is applied to points on the feet or hands has a balancing effect on the body.	A recognized and popular treatment in many spas.
Reiki	A system of treatment that channels universal healing energy through the practitioners' hands into and around the client's body, sometimes without direct hands-on application.	Although unproven scientifically, Reiki is quite popular in spas; some guests enjoy the esoteric and nonthreatening nature of the treatment.
Shiatsu	Focusing on a series of specific points along energy pathways or meridians, this technique from Japan uses finger pressure to invigorate the body and allow healing energies to flow more freely.	Many Asian therapies and themes are very popular in spas today, and shiatsu is one of the most popular of all.
Structural alignment	Any of several modalities that focus on realigning the body's connective tissues in a more balanced and healthy way.	Not very popular in spas because it features a series of treatments; guests prefer clinics or private practice settings for ongoing treatment series.
Thai massage	An ancient system of massage that includes stimulation of pressure points, energy work, and yoga-like stretching to improve health and well-being; several training programs exist in Thailand and the West, and some spas offer training on site.	Spa guests love the stretching in this technique, which is gaining rapidly in popularity; remaining clothed makes it more accessible for modest guests.
Watsu	Meaning "water-shiatsu," this treatment is given with both guest and therapist submerged in warm (90° to 98°F), chest-deep water; the therapist floats, stretches, and massages the guest to open joints, improve mobility, and open energy pathways to promote healing.	Becoming more and more popular in spas, it is only limited by the extensive infrastructure requirements (a special warm pool is needed to perform the treatments).

Swedish massage or relaxation massage (see the sidebar "The Real Meaning of 'Relaxation Massage'"). The term *spa massage* can have a negative connotation, as some people think that it is less effective compared with a therapeutic massage.

This distinction is both unnecessary and unhelpful. A massage session executed in a spa can be as therapeutic as one executed elsewhere.

It is challenging, however, for many therapists working in spas to give high-quality therapeutic massage sessions consistently. This is true for three main reasons:

1. Low expectations: Many spa guests arrive with no particular complaints or pains, and they do not expect much from the massage therapy session beyond simple relaxation.
2. Time constraints: It is difficult for therapists to retain enthusiasm and high energy levels when doing many massages each day or week, all within the same time guidelines.
3. Inexperienced clients: Many spa guests are first-time massage recipients or casual recipients who have not formed an appreciation for bodywork and have to be educated about its effects and benefits.

With these constraints in mind, it is still possible for spa therapists to make their massage sessions fresh and effective, giving each client a customized experience in spite of the fact that many of the massage moves and timing are the same from massage to massage. This requires discipline and enhanced skill on the part of the spa therapist. Far from being easier to perform than massage administered in other venues, spa massage in some ways can be more challenging, and therapists who master it can rightfully feel proud. To achieve this, therapists working in spas profit by paying particularly close attention to three special concerns while applying the massage techniques learned in this book: timing, transitions, and uniqueness.

Timing of the Spa Massage

One of the biggest challenges of a spa massage is to create a sense of timelessness within the very strict time structure imposed in the spa setting. There are three main ways to do this:

1. *Slow down.* Paradoxically, when therapists slow down movements during a massage and perform fewer maneuvers with greater concentration and focus, from the client's point of view, the massage actually seems longer and more luxurious. Rushing to include many massage moves actually makes the massage seem shorter. Therapists can choose three or four key techniques on each area, then focus on them slowly and methodically.
2. *Internalize timing.* A spa massage should be soothing and relaxing but at the same time retain specific therapeutic goals. To achieve this, spa therapists need to develop a heightened awareness of their own (as well as their clients') internal sense of rhythm. Instead of watching the clock constantly, feeling the deadline of the 50- or 60-minute time frame looming ever closer, it is possible to end the massage right on time yet rarely, if ever, glance at the clock. After performing hundreds of massages within the spa's tight time frame, the therapist's mind becomes accustomed to the time needed for each area and knows spontaneously when to move on. Learn to trust this inner clock.

3. *Focus on the moment.* Therapists should think about what they are doing at that moment, not about what they are going to be doing next. Once the spa massage routine becomes second nature, it is easy to think in terms of the next step instead of the step presently being performed. Several times throughout the massage, therapists should remind themselves to be in the moment and focus on the tissues beneath their fingers, and let that guide them to a new next step. By being present, therapists can become more in tune with the client, who will experience a more thorough massage with longer lasting results.

Transitions during Spa Massage

In the same way that the moments of silence between musical notes help to define the music, the movements between massage strokes, between segments, and between treatments are as important as the massage itself, especially when working within the limited parameters of a spa massage.

Between Strokes

Pay particular attention to and spend more time on maintaining physical contact with the client and developing a creative sequence during a spa massage. Focus on those movements that connect the separate strokes during a massage, making them flow and become part of a graceful whole rather than disjointed, which is especially important in the time-pressed environment of a spa.

Between Segments

By focusing on graceful transitions from one part of the body to the next, the therapist can avoid creating a hurried sensation while covering the entire body in a shorter time frame. Make the first stroke and the last on each area especially relaxing. Even while adjusting the drapes, use slow, deliberate movements to augment the client's sense of ease and timelessness.

Between Treatments

Between treatments is the one time when it is better to speed things up. Refresh yourself. Get the blood flowing. Move around, stretch, and take a few deep breaths. Rapidly clean the treatment room and set up for the next client so that there is no need to rush once it is time to start again.

Making a Spa Massage Unique

In the spa setting, remember that each client is unique, even though they all might have similar expectations, and even though the setting, protocols, and routine are the same for each. All clients on a given day might receive the same massage, yet each treatment should be slightly different and geared to that client's particular needs.

Target Problem Areas

A relaxing spa massage is made even better when the therapist applies targeted work to those areas holding tension. Using trigger-point and other

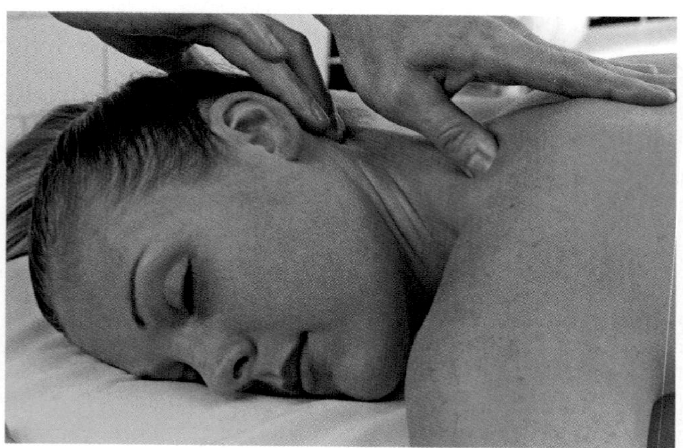

FIGURE 14-9 Spa massage can incorporate energy work along with other modalities and be every bit as therapeutic as therapeutic massage.

therapies (see Chapter 15) problem areas can be identified and techniques applied to relieve tension and holding patterns. These differ for each client. After focusing on such areas, move on seamlessly to the next step of the spa massage routine.

Focus on the Client's Breath

Therapists can use the client's breath as a guide to tune into each client's unique tension-release patterns. Do not make your own breath too conspicuous; instead, just focus on the client's breath. Observe and make subtle adjustments when a change in rhythm or depth is noticed.

Avoid Burnout

Therapists must take care of themselves physically and mentally so that they are fresh enough to offer each client a unique experience. This means receiving periodic bodywork themselves, getting adequate rest, taking time off, and practicing moderation.

The Real Meaning of Relaxation Massage

The literature at many spas refers to something known as a *relaxation massage*, which sounds relatively benign, if not bland, but what exactly is it? The standard response to this question is that a relaxation massage is a Swedish massage (as compared with one of the more advanced modalities), but as you are no doubt learning in school now, a Swedish massage can also be invigorating, stimulating, therapeutic, and downright intense (Figure 14-9). Is "relaxation" simply a code word for "fluffy spa-type with no therapeutic value"? Are spas doomed forever to suffer from this stigma as places where relaxation equals substandard?

Seen from another angle, all massage should be relaxation massage, should it not? Even deep structural integration, which can be intense in the moment, eventually leads to a relaxation of tissues and holding patterns in the body.

The problem is that we are looking at the terminology from a massage therapist's point of view. The real meaning of the term *relaxation* as it is used in terms of spa massage is correctly understood when seen from the *client's* point of view, because it probably has more to do with easing clients' fear than anything else. It is a way to let spa guests know that they are not going to be mauled by a rough Russian or Turkish character like the ones depicted in certain old movies. By default, over the years, the term has ended up applying to any massage that is nonthreatening, although unfairly so, because Swedish massage is actually much more than simply relaxing.

STONE MASSAGE

Stone massage has become extremely popular in spas (Figure 14-10). Displayed on the menu at many facilities, stone massage goes by many names, including *stone massage, hot rock therapy, hot stone massage*, and *LaStone therapy*; as well as many regionalized terms, such as *Hotter'n Texas Summer Rock Massage*, and terms personalized to particular spas, such as *Satori Wellness Spa Heated Stone Experience.*

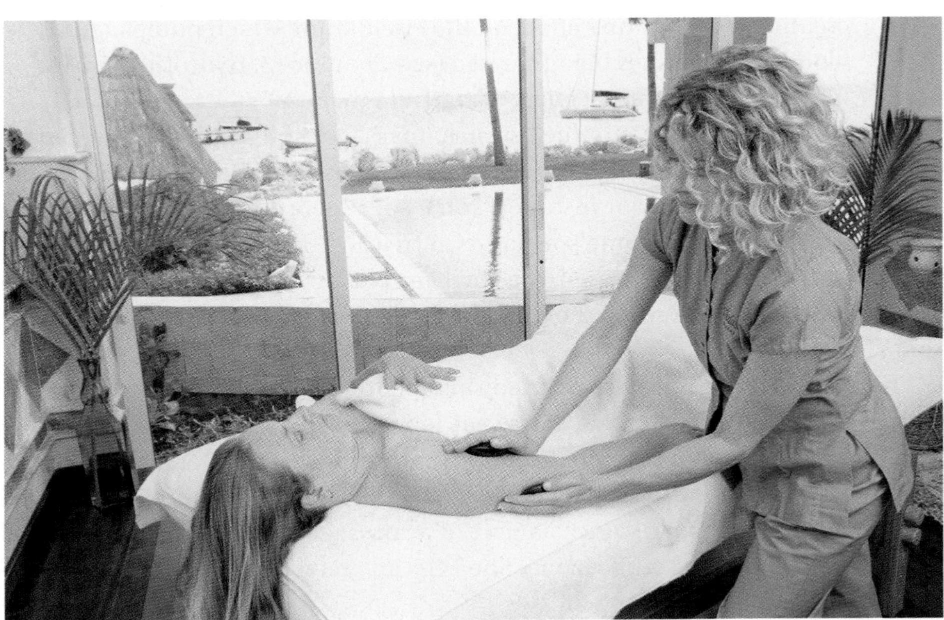

FIGURE 14-10 Many guests look forward to stone massage, which is one of the most popular modalities in spas.

Regardless of the name, these treatments all share certain common elements:

1. Stones: Several types of stone are used for treatments, the most common being basalt, which is volcanic in origin (Figure 14-11a). Typically, practitioners use smooth stones of several shapes and sizes appropriate to different parts of the body. These stones are heated in hot water, usually in a roaster, and then either placed on the body or used by the practitioner to apply massage techniques. Other types of stones, usually marble, are also cooled in a refrigerator, on ice, or in a freezer and applied to the skin to complement the effects of the heat (Figure 14-11b).
2. Massage: Although it can consist primarily of energy work and heat, stone massage is ultimately massage. The official definition of massage in most state and local laws includes the use of heat, cold, and therapeutic instruments in the treatment of soft tissue. Stones, in this sense, can be construed as therapeutic instruments.
3. Heat and cold: One of the most important effects of stone massage is its use of contrast therapy. Alternating hot and cold stones are applied,

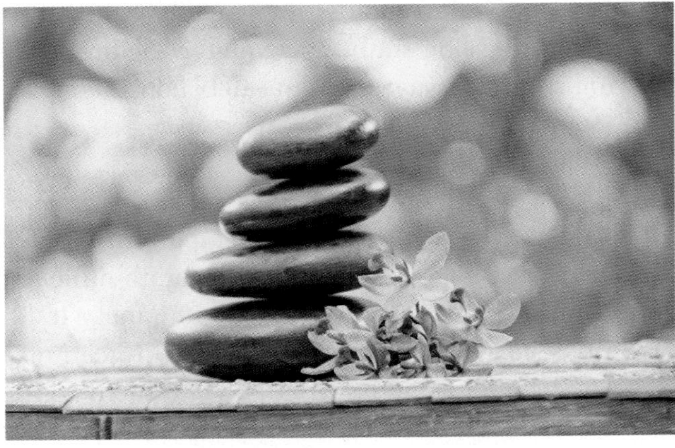

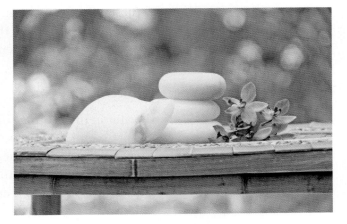

FIGURE 14-11A AND B Smooth basalt stones of various sizes are most popular for hot stones. Marble stones are used as cold stones.

creating a stimulating effect on the circulation, which pumps more blood to the tissues being treated (see Chapter 13, Hydrotherapy, for more on this pumping effect of contrast therapy).

These common elements (i.e., stones, massage, and temperature) can be modified with any number of specific techniques or products to make the stone treatment unique. For instance, some spas incorporate the use of essential oils with the stones, some specialize in treating the face with small stones, some spas use the stones primarily as instruments in deep tissue massage, and others create an entire stone theme for their spa, such as the Stone Spa in New York City.

Rocks and stones have been used therapeutically for hundreds of years by various cultures to create heat for sweat lodges, saunas, and ceremonies. The temperatures at which they are used for that purpose, however, are much too high for direct application to the body. In the 1990s, a new systemized method of applying hot and cold stones as part of a massage session was first devised by Mary Nelson of Tucson, Arizona. She is given credit for developing the technique called LaStone therapy.

One interesting aspect of ancient basalt is the fact that the rapidly cooling lava records the earth's magnetic field as it was at the time of formation. This means that a massage stone that is one billion years old contains the imprint of a different energy field than the one present on the planet today. Scientists theorize that the orientation of the magnetic poles has actually switched many times through the ages. The North Pole used to be the South Pole, and vice versa, over and over again. Thus, according to the precepts of **paleomagnetism**, this means that the massage stone held in one's hand and applied to the client's skin could contain energy patterns quite different than those experienced today and could therefore have a powerful energetic effect on the body.

Modern stone massage offers spas a simple way to add something exotic to the menu and put clients back in touch with a piece of the natural world. A stone massage program is easy to set up, requiring only a heating unit, a refrigerator or freezer, and the stones themselves. Caution must be exercised when practicing stone massage, however.

Safety and Sanitation

The application of hard, hot objects to the skin and tissues beneath is inherently hazardous. It follows that students must be trained adequately before using stones on clients. When applying stone massage, certain safety considerations must be kept in mind.

Water Temperature

Water in the heating container must be kept at the correct temperature, which is between 110° and 140°F. Temperatures below 110°F do not generate sufficient warmth for therapeutic application, and temperatures above 140°F make it difficult to handle the stones. Stones heated beyond this temperature can also cause discomfort for the client or even damage tissue if applied directly to the skin. As a general rule, stones that are too hot to be held by the practitioner are too hot to be placed on the client.

Client Protection

Stones can be placed directly on the skin, but the therapist must exercise caution when doing so. Often, it is preferable to place sheets, pillowcases, or towels between the rocks and the skin to protect the client from possible harm or discomfort. The thickness of these protective layers can be adjusted during the course of the treatment as the temperature of the stones changes.

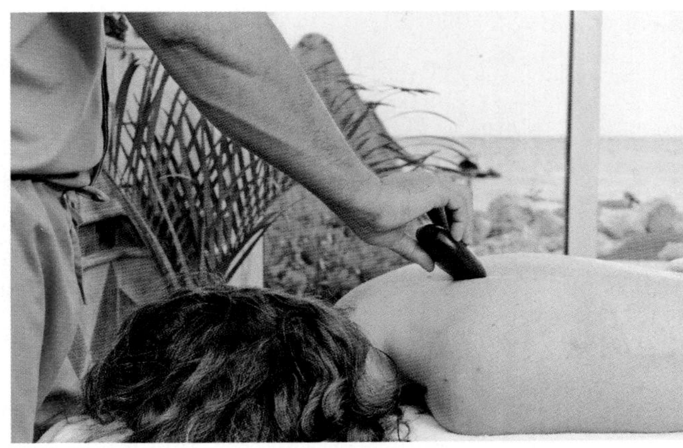

FIGURE 14-12 When using stones as massage tools, use caution to not use too much pressure.

Cleaning Stones and Implements

Proper sanitation is crucial to ensure a safe experience for the client. The stones should be cleansed with fresh water and antibacterial soap after each use and before being placed back in the heating unit. If the stones are sticky from lubricant, they can be cleansed with alcohol. The water in the heating unit should be changed daily. A sterilizing solution can be added to the heating unit each day to ensure a sanitary treatment.

Depth of Pressure with Stones

When using stones as tools during deep tissue massage, some therapists tend to apply excessive pressure as they strive for therapeutic effects. Stones penetrate the tissues much more forcefully than therapist's fingers or thumbs do (Figure 14-12). Extreme caution must be exercised to not cause damage.

Contraindications

Stone massage presents several contraindications, including the most obvious one for heat. Keep in mind, however, that stone massage does not create systemic effects in reaction to the heat application but only local effects. Even though a large area of the skin surface, such as the back, experiences a notable temperature increase, the core temperature of the body does not rise in reaction to a local external application. Clients with high blood pressure, for example, will therefore not be likely to experience the same adverse reactions to stone application as they do for a full-body heat immersion such as the herbal wrap or heated hydrotherapy bath. The heat of the stones can still cause harm, however, which makes it crucial for therapists to maintain continuous open communication with the client during a stone massage application regarding comfort and temperature.

The primary contraindications for stone massage are

- any condition for which general massage is contraindicated
- surgery in which nerves have been cut, causing loss of feeling
- nerve damage or neuropathy — avoid specific areas
- use of prescription medications that are adversely affected by heat applications
- infectious skin disease, rashes, lesions, or any skin conditions aggravated by heat

Several conditions warrant the use of caution, and clients with these conditions should receive a doctor's consent prior to the application of stone massage. These include

- pregnancy — except by practitioners certified in pregnancy massage; never in the first trimester
- heart disease and people prone to blood clots
- high blood pressure
- circulatory problems
- diabetic peripheral neuropathy — decreased skin sensitivity to temperature
- extreme obesity, which puts a strain on the heart
- metal implants – stones can heat these implants and cause discomfort
- cancer — immediately after chemotherapy or radiation
- Parkinson's disease

Finally, some conditions are not contraindicated outright for stone massage and do not require a doctor's consent, but people having these conditions should be handled with caution. These conditions include

- varicose veins – avoid hot stones directly to the area, but cold stones in moderation with light pressure are permissible
- older thin skin – use light pressure and lower heat
- open wounds, bruises, tumors, hernias, or recent fractures – avoid the areas
- acute inflammation – cold stone therapy can be used in these areas
- children – use cooler temperatures (110° to 120° maximum)

Placing Stones on the Body

1. Stones should be placed on the client's body on an exhalation so that the heat and weight of the stone can be more easily accepted. This is true for stones placed on the torso or limbs but not necessarily on the head or feet.
2. Stones should be lifted away from the torso and limbs on an inhalation so that it feels as if the body were helping to push the stones up and away.
3. Stones can be tucked beneath the client's body in strategic locations such as gluteals, occipital ridge, shoulder, and thigh.
4. Stones can be laid beneath the client, under a towel, in two rows along the area where the erector spinae will rest from sacrum to the cervical vertebrae. The client is then instructed to roll back onto the stones. The number of stones depends on the size of the client and the arch of the spine. Experiment until you become proficient in choosing and placing laid-out stones.
5. Stones can be placed on energy vortexes, or chakras, on top of the body (Figure 14-13).
6. Contour stones can be placed in the client's hand or on the sole of the foot.
7. Larger stones can be placed on top of the abdomen, beneath the abdomen, or on the sacrum.
8. Small flat stones can be placed between the toes (Figure 14-14).

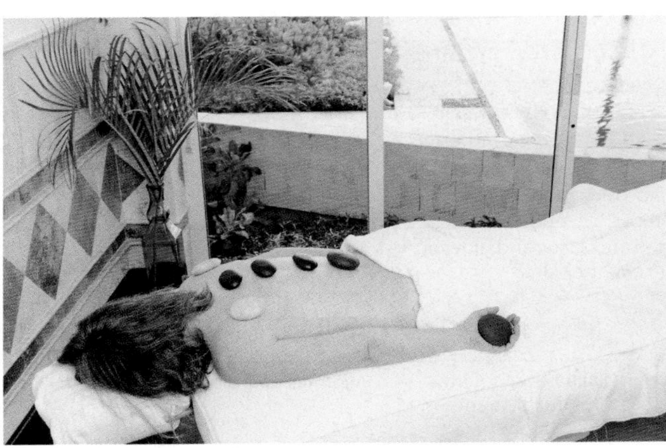

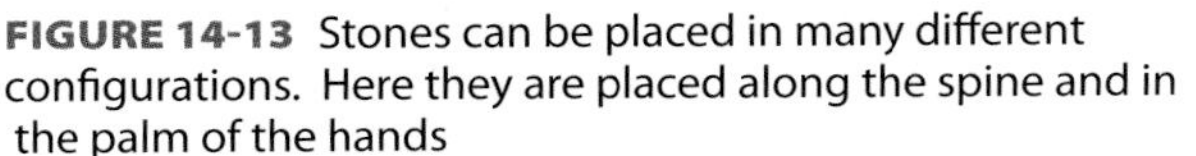
FIGURE 14-13 Stones can be placed in many different configurations. Here they are placed along the spine and in the palm of the hands

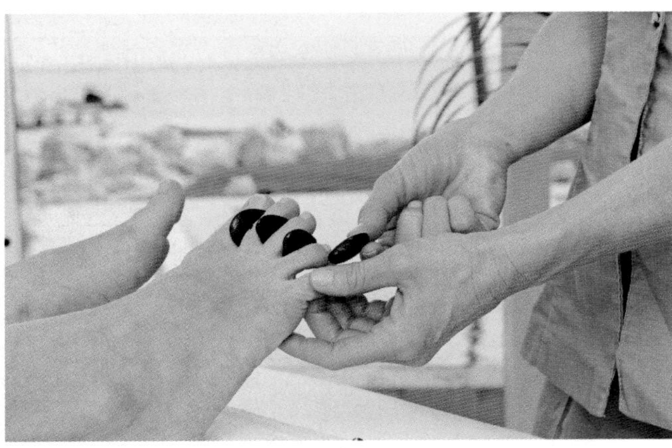
FIGURE 14-14 Small stones between the toes are relaxing.

9. Stones already placed on the body can be tapped with another stone to create the effects of piezoelectricity.
10. As stones cool, therapists can remove them or replace them with warmer stones.

exfoliation

is any of several spa treatments the primary purpose of which is to cleanse the body of dead skin cells, thus softening the skin, helping the body to eliminate better through the skin, preparing it for better absorption of other therapeutic products.

parafango

is a combination of paraffin wax and fango mud used in spa wraps and localized applications to soften, moisten, and purify the skin while warming and relaxing the muscles.

SPA MODALITIES

Therapists hired by a spa are often, although not always, required to perform other modalities in addition to their massage duties. These can include body wraps, **exfoliation**, foot treatments, back treatments, scalp treatments, face treatments, herbal detoxification treatments, hydrotherapy baths, therapeutic showers, cellulite treatments, aromatherapy, **parafango**, or clay, mud, and seaweed treatments (Figure 14-15). These modalities are listed in Table 14.3. Some spas also offer advanced treatments such as the *Rasul* and Balinese *Lulur* rituals that incorporate basic modalities but use specialized equipment and ingredients.

The therapists who stay busiest and therefore earn the most money are those who master as many of the spa's modalities as possible. It is therefore in the therapist's best interest to train extensively in general spa modalities before joining a spa team and then to continue training on specific modalities whenever the opportunity arises during employment. Therapists who do not wish to perform these modalities might lessen their chances for advancement and for getting preferred schedules. Sometimes practitioners acquire multiple certifications such as personal trainer or esthetician so they are qualified to perform more extensive spa treatments or activities. Spa directors appreciate those therapists who are proficient in a

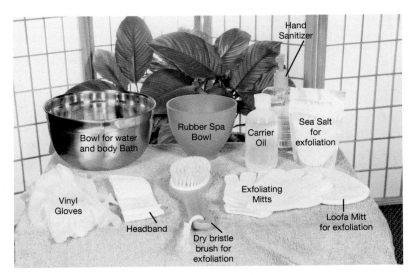

FIGURE 14-15 Popular items found in a spa therapist's treatment room:

TABLE 14.3

SPA MODALITIES THAT THERAPISTS TYPICALLY PERFORM			
SPA MODALITIES	DESCRIPTION	BENEFITS/USES	CONTRA-INDICATIONS
Back treatment	Also called a *back facial*, this treatment cleanses and draws impurities from the back area with mud and partial body wrapping.	Especially appropriate for modest clients who want a partial body wrap.	Sensitivity to heat; excessive open acne on the back.
Bust treatment	Not very popular except in some beauty-oriented day spas, this treatment uses creams and serums to firm the skin and subcutaneous tissues of the breast area.	Imparts a more elastic and glowing appearance to the skin.	Many clients are too modest for a bust treatment; local laws on draping and appropriate touch must be consulted and followed.
Cellulite treatment	Often including underwater massage in a hydrotherapy tub, this treatment features vigorous massage, wrapping, and special products (usually seaweed-based) to promote an improved appearance to affected areas.	Drains superficial tissues; noninvasive way to improve appearance in a comfortable spa setting.	Allergies to iodine; claustrophobia.
Exfoliation	Includes dry brushing, body polish, sea salt glow, and any number of procedures involving exfoliants (e.g., nutshell meal, seeds) to cleanse the skin	Prepares skin to absorb spa products, cleanses away dead cells, imparts healthy glow.	Open sores, cuts, abrasions; communicable skin conditions, psoriasis; aggravated acute acne.
Face treatment	A face treatment including cleansing, exfoliation, and nutritive mask that therapists can perform within their scope of practice in the spa setting.	Cleanses, balances, and imparts a glow to the skin of the face.	Open sores; cuts; communicable skin conditions; acute acne; and recent peels.
Foot treatment	Can include exfoliation, soaking, mud/seaweed application, wrapping, massage, and reflexology, in addition to pedicure if therapist is qualified.	Reflex benefits for the entire body, in addition to product benefits; softens tough feet; deeply relaxing.	Open sores, cuts or abrasions on feet, athlete's foot.
Herbal wrap	Hot herb-infused sheets are wrapped around the client to induce a false-fever state, promoting detoxification through the pores.	Spa guests often receive a series of herbal wraps to aid detoxification and cessation of smoking, caffeine, and so forth.	Heart disease, high or low blood pressure, pregnancy, diabetes, claustrophobia, allergies to specific herbs.
Mud/clay wrap	Most common types are black Baltic and fango (volcanic-based) muds, applied to skin prior to wrap.	Nourishes and exfoliates skin; humic acids also help draw out impurities.	None for non-heated mud; slight contraindications for warmed mud include high blood pressure, heart disease.
Mud immersions	Clients are completely immersed in warmed therapeutic mud, or they cover themselves head to foot in clay and then lie in the sun.	Deeply drawing and purifying of the entire body; nourishing for the skin.	Done only in specially equipped spas, usually near mud/clay source with proper sanitation.
Hydrotherapy bath (Figure 14-16)	The use of water's percussive, thermal, and chemical properties in a specialized tub; when the water's mineral and gas contents are used therapeutically, it is called **balneotherapy**.	To warm client prior to treatment, open pores, encourage detoxification, and soothe muscles.	Hypertension, dizziness, fever, communicable skin conditions.
Parafango	A blend of paraffin wax and fango (mud from a volcanic source) that is smoothed onto a part of or the whole body while warm; a wrap is then applied.	Effects created by heat penetrate to warm joints, relieve pain, and heal; softens skin.	Acute arthritis, blood clots, acute skin conditions; also high blood pressure (for full-body parafango).
Sauna/steam bath	Dry or steam heat is applied in a special chamber, usually in the spa's common area.	Excellent for relaxing muscles prior to treatment; cleansing; strengthens circulatory system.	High blood pressure, hypertension, heart disease, diabetes, pregnancy.
Scalp treatment	A cleansing of the scalp and hair, often with an oil or mud application and wrap, plus massage.	Promotes circulation to the scalp, cleanses, gives body and luster.	Extremely oily hair.
Scotch hose	A high-pressure hose that sprays the standing client (sometimes with seawater).	Highly invigorating, stimulates circulation.	More popular in European-style spas, less so in others; too stimulating for some clients. Spray should be aimed away from sensitive areas.

Table 14.3 (cont'd)

SPA MODALITIES	DESCRIPTION	BENEFITS/USES	CONTRA-INDICATIONS
Sea salt treatment	A specialized treatment that adds the benefits of the sea and seawater (remineralizing, rejuvenating) to those listed previously for general exfoliation.	Softens and smoothes skin, removes dead skin cells.	Open sores, cuts, abrasions; communicable skin conditions; aggravated acute acne; recently shaved legs.
Seaweed wrap (Figure 14-17)	A blend of reconstituted seaweed and essential oils is applied to the skin after exfoliation; the client is then wrapped and massage often follows.	Seaweed remineralizes the entire body as ingredients soak into pores; this rejuvenates skin.	Allergies to iodine, which is found in many seaweeds.
Swiss shower (Figure 14-18)	Multiple shower heads in stall aimed at client from all directions; water temperature is often adjusted by therapist/ technician for contrast therapy.	Used to effectively wash off spa products and stimulate circulation; invigorating.	Fine high-powered water stream can be too intense for some clients.
Thalassotherapy	The use of seawater or sea products (i.e., oils, extracts, powders, seaweeds) in baths or other spa treatments.	Remineralizes; promotes detoxification; supplies sea nutrients through pores.	Allergies to iodine.
Vichy shower	Multiple showerheads on a long arm suspended above the treatment table apply water pressure, sometimes including contrast therapy.	Relaxing; washes away spa products such as mud, salt, or seaweed.	None.

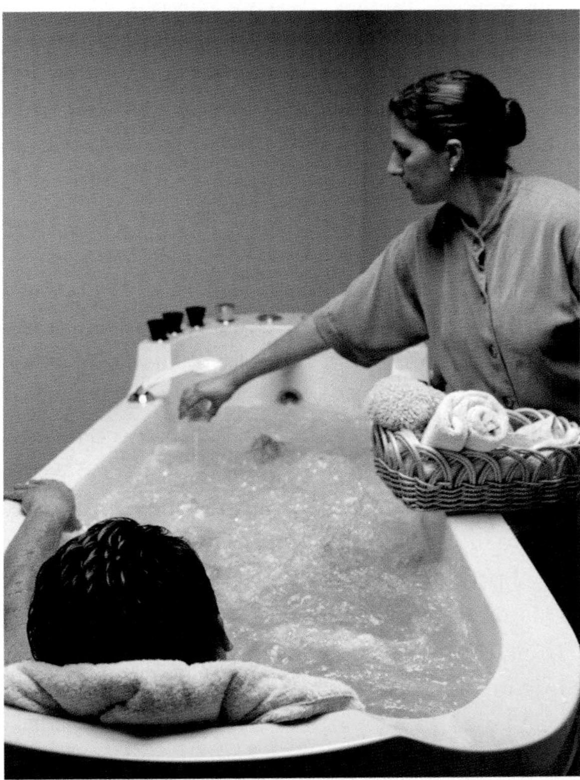

FIGURE 14-16 Hydrotherapy tubs, popular in larger spas, have multiple therapist-controlled jets and an underwater massage wand. They can also incorporate thalassotherapy and aromatherapy.

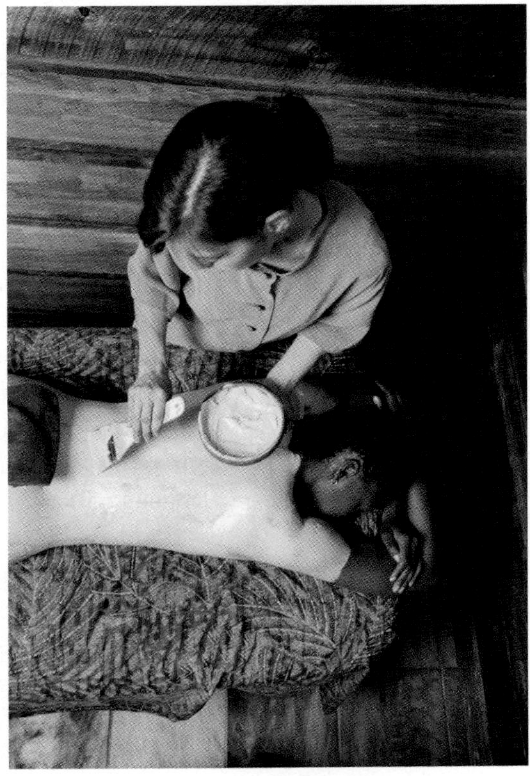

FIGURE 14-17 Body wraps employ the use of muds, seaweeds, clays, and other ingredients to nourish the skin and affect the entire body.

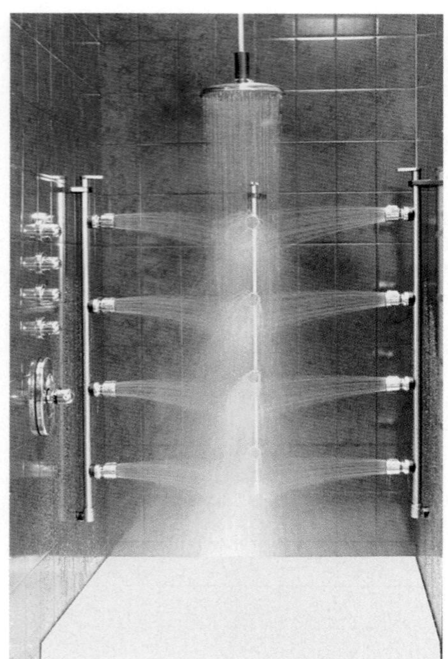

FIGURE 14-18 The Swiss shower, with its multiple heads, is a stimulating treatment that is also used to remove spa products after body wraps and exfoliation services. (Courtesy of HydroCo, USA: www.hydroco.com.)

wide range of treatments so that they can cover as many guest requests as possible.

AROMATHERAPY

Aromatherapy is commonly used in almost all spas in one form or another. In the spa industry, it can be defined as the use of essential oils processed from herbs, flowers, fruits, spices, stems, bark, and roots in massage, inhalation, or other modalities to affect mood and improve health and well-being. Some spas offer extensive aromatherapy treatment options on their menus, whereas others list just a basic aromatherapy massage, but it is rare for a spa to offer no aromatherapy treatments at all. At the very least, in small spas, aromatherapy candles or **diffusers** are used to impart some of the benefits of aromatherapy to guests even if no aromatherapy treatments are offered.

Essential oils and plant extracts have been used for many years in many lands, from the ancient Greek, Indian, and Egyptian cultures to the present day. They are used to treat ailments, promote beauty, and bolster well-being. The word *aromatherapy* itself was first used in the 1920s by Rene Gattefosse, a French perfumer.

When using essential oils, remember that they are powerfully concentrated substances, and as such should be treated with caution. When used improperly, some oils can overstimulate the body, and because very little of these substances (just a few drops) is needed to create an effect, it is usually recommended not to use them full strength or **neat**, but in combination with a **carrier oil** or other medium. Some common carrier oils are apricot kernel oil, avocado oil, grapeseed oil, jojoba oil, sesame oil, sweet almond oil, and wheat germ oil.

aromatherapy

is the use of essential oils processed from herbs, flowers, fruits, stems, spices, and roots in massage, inhalation, or other modalities to affect mood and improve health and well-being.

diffusers

are devices using fans, heat, or steam dispersion to release the aromas of essential oils into a room for therapeutic and/or esthetic purposes.

neat

refers to the application of an essential oil at its full, undiluted strength.

carrier oil

is massage lubricant into which essential oils are blended for aromatherapy applications.

A wide range of essential oils is available for use by the spa therapist, with an equally wide array of possible benefits. These include, but are certainly not limited to, mood uplifting or calming, accelerating wound healing, antibacterial and antifungal cleansing, hormonal balancing, pain reduction, easing of nasal and bronchial congestion, and enhancing circulation.

If they are kept out of direct sunlight in tightly capped, dark-colored bottles and stored in a cool dry place, essential oils can have a shelf life of several years. Dozens of companies offer hundreds of essential oils for use in spas, and many of them are high quality. Some oils are more expensive than others because they require a very large amount of initial product to produce a small amount of the oil. For example, 8,000 individual jasmine blossoms are needed to produce 1 gm of jasmine oil. It is only natural, then, that spas can charge a premium for massage and other services that include aromatherapy.

Common Essential Oils

Essential oils can be placed into one of three categories for easy description. *Top notes* are stimulating and uplifting, and their fragrance lasts just a few hours once it is out of the bottle. *Middle notes* last longer and are potent in their therapeutic effects on the body, but they do not have as strong a fragrance.

Base notes last the longest and are often sweet smelling and calming. Table 14.4 lists some of the popular oils used in many spas, with their effects.

TABLE 14.4

COMMON ESSENTIAL OILS USED IN SPAS					
ESSENTIAL OIL	DERIVATION	EFFECT	NOTE	USES	CONTRAINDICATIONS
Basil	Leaves/flowers	Uplifting, mental stimulant, eases congestion	Top/middle	Useful for headaches, depression, nausea, respiratory infections, mosquito bites	Can cause minor skin irritation, avoid during pregnancy
Bergamot	rind	relaxing, uplifting, cleansing, antiseptic	top/middle	useful for depression, stress, skin problems; balances oily or acne skin, acne, eczema, cold sores	avoid direct exposure to sunlight on the skin after application because bergamot causes photosensitivity
Chamomile	flowers	soothing, calming, anti-inflammatory	middle	useful for premenstrual pain, indigestion headache	may cause minor skin irritation
Clary sage	flowers/leaves	relaxing, calming, tonic	top/middle	useful against cramping, for balancing hormones and soothing anxiety	in large doses can generate headaches, avoid during pregnancy
Cypress	needles/twigs	grounding, calming, soothing, and toning	middle	useful in the treatment of excessive discharge of fluids and beneficial for the respiratory tract and as a vasoconstrictor	test small amount on skin prior to massage blend to test for sensitivity
Eucalyptus	leaves	stimulating, antiseptic	top	useful for coughs and colds, bronchitis, viral infections, muscular aches, cuts	can irritate skin in high doses, harmful if ingested
Frankincense	resin	relaxing, calming	base	soothes the respiratory tract, relieves muscular aches and pain, soothes rheumatism, rejuvenates and heals the skin	none
Geranium	flowers/leaves	mildly astringent, mildly diuretic, antidepressant	middle	useful for cuts, sores, fungal infections, as an insect repellant, and for soothing skin problems, eczema, bruises	may cause irritation to very sensitive skin
Grapefruit	rind	uplifting, cleansing	top	sometimes called the "joy oil" because it stimulates the lymphatic system and uplifts mood, stimulates the digestive system, cleanses congested oily skin and acne	can irritate the skin if exposed to strong sunlight after treatment
Jasmine	flowers	antidepressant, relaxing	base	useful for depression, postnatal depression, strengthening contractions during labor, aphrodisiac	may cause headaches in some people
Lavender	flowers	healing, calming, mildly analgesic, antiseptic	middle/top	useful for headaches, wounds, bruises, insect bites, oily skin, acne, swelling, insomnia, mild depression	none
Lemongrass	leaf	refreshing, antiseptic, diuretic	top/middle	useful to fight stress, fatigue, indigestion, muscle soreness, stimulates appetite, acts as an antidepressant	can be irritating to sensitive skin

Table 14.4 (cont'd)

ESSENTIAL OIL	DERIVATION	EFFECT	NOTE	USES	CONTRAINDICATIONS
Marjoram	flowers/leaves	warming, calming, relaxing	middle	useful for nervous tension, respiratory congestion, painful muscles and joints, digestive problems, sleep problems, and menstrual disorders	none
Neroli	rind	relaxing, mildly warming	top	useful for insomnia, anxiety, nervous depression, poor circulation, acne, premenstrual tension, backache	photosensitive, should not be applied before exposure to sun
Orange	rind	antiseptic, antidepressant, antispasmodic, anti-inflammatory	top	uplifts the mood while calming the nervous system and soothing digestive problems	can have a photo-sensitizing effect and should not be applied before going out into sunlight for prolonged periods
Patchouli	leaves	grounding, relaxing, diuretic, moistening for skin	base	repels insects, soothes dry or problem skin, fights water retention and uplifts mood	aroma can be irritating to some people and cause loss of appetite
Peppermint	whole plant	analgesic, cooling, increases alertness	top	relieves minor pains, sinus problems and nausea, uplifts mood and cools the skin	excess cooling and sensitization can occur because of menthol content
Rose	flowers	relaxing, emotional balance, skin healing	base	useful for sore throat and sinus, congestion, puffiness, mildly sedative, insomnia, premenstrual tension/pain, menopause	none
Rosemary	flowers/leaves	refreshing, stimulating, strengthening, detoxifying	middle	useful for physical and mental fatigue, forgetfulness, respiratory problems, asthma, rheumatic aches and pains	seizure disorders, high blood pressure
Sandalwood	inner wood	relaxing	base	useful for dry, cracked, or chapped skin; acne; calming relaxation during meditation; aphrodisiac	none
Tea Tree	leaves/twigs	antibacterial, anti-microbial, antiseptic, antiviral, antifungal	top/middle	useful for topical conditions such as acne, athlete's foot, cold sores, corns, cuts, insect bites, itching, warts; inhaling good for coughs and colds	can cause minor skin irritation in sensitive individuals
Vetiver	roots	centering, deeply calming	base	muscle and joint relief, known as "the oil of tranquility" because it is so calming	none
Ylang Ylang	flowers	relaxing	base	useful to instill confidence, reduce feelings of stress and anger, aphrodisiac	excessive use of it can lead to headaches and nausea

Aromatherapy Massage

Aromatherapy massage is the most popular aromatherapy modality used in spas. A few spas hire highly trained aromatherapy experts to administer these massages, but most spas require that all the massage therapists on staff, or at least a significant number, perform aromatherapy massage. The step-by-step procedure for an aromatherapy massage is similar to that for a typical Swedish spa massage, with a few notable distinctions.

- Before the treatment, the therapist must check the guest's intake form for sensitivities to aromas or, if no form is used, ask the guest.

- Before the treatment, the therapist should explain to the client the therapeutic outcomes desired through the choice of essential oils.
- The massage strokes are predominantly light and flowing, similar to an **Esalen massage** style. Lymph drainage, shiatsu and reflexology techniques are sometimes employed, however.
- Time is allowed for the client to experience the aromas. For example, at the beginning of a sequence over the face, the therapist cups her hands a few inches away from the client's face and asks the client to inhale the oil for its therapeutic benefits. This can be done through the face cradle when the client is prone.
- Make sure that blankets or an infrared heating lamp are in place to keep the client warm, if necessary, because spa guests often experience a chill during this treatment, either as an effect of certain oils or because the overall treatment is so calming and sedating.

Esalen massage

is a style of massage developed at Esalen Institute in northern California that features long, flowing strokes that connect all parts of the body into a whole.

Blending the Oils

Many spas offer standardized aromatherapy massage treatments on the menu. The essential oils for these treatments have been preblended into a carrier oil for ready use, and guests do not have a choice regarding the oil in their treatment. An example of this would be an "uplifting citrus aromatherapy treatment," using essential oils of orange, lemon, and neroli. For a customized aromatherapy massage, on the other hand, the therapist must consult with the client before the massage regarding any preferences and desired outcomes for the treatment. Then the essential oil drops are blended into the carrier oil in the presence of the guest directly prior to the treatment.

It is necessary to add the essential oils to the carrier oil drop by drop to achieve the correct strength. This process is facilitated by aromatherapy bottles themselves, most of which are outfitted with tops that allow one drop at a time to escape when upturned. The correct number of drops is 12 to 15 for each ounce of carrier oil. Thus, for a preblended mixture, a therapist could use approximately 96 to 120 drops for an 8-ounce bottle of carrier oil. Many companies sell preblended aromatherapy products, which eliminates the need for measuring and blending.

Essential oils can also be blended into massage lotions and creams. Certain of these do not readily absorb the oils and must be warmed appropriately to create an **emulsion** that works for massage. In all cases, stir or gently swirl the drops of essential oil into the medium rather than shaking.

emulsion

is a uniform mixture of two or more liquids, such as an essential oil and a massage lotion.

Aromatherapy Wrap

An aromatherapy wrap uses essential oils, a carrier oil or lotion, and wrapping layers like muslin sheets and blankets to create a cocoon experience for the client. Some spas prefer to use preblended products, whereas others customize the treatment, blending the oils according to the client's preference. The treatment is quite gentle and meditative, focusing on the client's mood and state of mind more than any musculoskeletal problems that are apparent. In fact, the therapist often foregoes massage entirely during an aromatherapy wrap and instead simply applies the product with long, superficial gliding strokes over the entire body. Some spas offer a choice between this simple application and a more comprehensive aromatherapy wrap with massage included.

To start the treatment, the therapist places a drop of essential oil blend on a fingertip, then touches it to several energy points, corresponding to shiatsu or acupressure points, along the body. After this, the blend is applied to the body in long strokes, and the client is covered immediately to ensure warmth. The client turns over, and the procedure is repeated on the front of the body before wrapping the client in layers of muslin and blankets. A bolster is placed beneath the knees, the lights are turned low, and the client is left wrapped for 20 minutes on average in most spas. During this time, the therapist often applies a light noninvasive therapy such as craniosacral to the head and neck area or pressure point massage to the face and scalp.

Aromatherapy Bath

Aromatherapy baths are popular in many spas. They can be defined as any bath that incorporates the use of aromatherapy essential oils. In this sense, many hydrotherapy baths on a spa's menu are in fact aromatherapy baths, although they are not labeled as such, because essential oils are routinely added to hydrotherapy tubs to enhance guests' experience. Popular essential oil choices for aromatherapy baths include chamomile, lavender, rose, and rosemary. Certain especially cooling or highly stimulating oils such as peppermint, ginger, or juniper should be avoided for aromatherapy baths.

Only five to ten drops of essential oil are added as the bath is filling. These drops can be blended with a carrier oil beforehand if a more silky texture is desired for the bath. The warm water, usually 100° to 104°F, helps to release the aroma of the oil, so that the benefits of inhalation are increased.

Aromatherapy Diffusers

Aromatherapy diffusers disperse the oils into the air of a room, spreading the beneficial effects over a wide area and enhancing the overall ambience of a space. They are used extensively in spas, especially those that specialize in aromatherapy. Often, they are used by smaller spas as a cost-effective way to add atmosphere and therapeutic value without a large investment.

Diffusers come in many forms:

- *Atomizers* are for the more advanced user. These turn the liquid oils into an extremely fine mist that fills the area with scent. They offer the highest concentration of oil in the air.
- *Fan diffusers* are extremely simple to operate and are inexpensive. Dabs of essential oil are placed on a piece of cotton or cloth and placed inside a small unit behind a fan that takes air in through the oils and disperses it into the room.
- *Clay/candle diffusers* come with a small tea candle or votive candle that warms essential oils placed in a clay or ceramic receptacle.
- *Light bulb rings* are small rings that are placed on top of light bulbs. When lit, the heat from the bulbs gradually burns away essential oils placed in the ring, filling the room with aroma.

EXFOLIATION

Exfoliation has been practiced in many cultures for thousands of years. In the days of the great Roman baths, or **thermae**, citizens would have their personal massage therapists (who were slaves) scour them with instruments known as **strigils** (a curved, metallic tool for scraping the skin) after taking their hot baths. Participants in athletic games would cover themselves with olive oil to protect their skin and then scrape it off with strigils, too.

thermae

are hot springs or baths, especially the baths of ancient Rome.

strigil

is a curved, usually metallic, instrument used in ancient Greece and Rome to scrape dead skin cells, oil, and dirt from bathers' skin.

The root of the word exfoliation comes from the Latin *ex* (to take away) and *folium* (leaf). So, exfoliation can be construed as meaning "taking away leaves," and you would see why if you were to look through a microscope at the upper layer of dead skin cells on your body, the stratum corneum, which looks like millions of tiny leaves. These leaves are sometimes visible floating in the air in enclosed spaces.

The main benefits of exfoliation include the following:

- It assists the skin's own regenerative processes.
- It aids in the absorption of spa products applied afterward.
- It thoroughly cleanses and promotes overall hygiene.
- It creates a healthy glow and gives radiant shine to the skin.

Although there are no contraindications for receiving exfoliation services more often, spa guests typically receive only one full exfoliation treatment per stay, but they can receive several shorter exfoliations as part of other spa services. For example, the skin is often exfoliated for 5 minutes before the application of a body mud or seaweed. Female guests should be warned not to shave their legs 24 hours before a salt-based exfoliation service, because it can cause discomfort and irritation. The room in which the exfoliation is given must be at least 80°F (and preferably 82°F, because clients cool down quickly when water is applied to their skin.

Exfoliation services go by many names in spas (Table 14.5), and many exotic scrubbing ingredients are used to lure clients into the exfoliation room.

TABLE 14.5

EXFOLIATION SERVICES OFFERED IN SPAS	
EXFOLIATION SERVICE	**DESCRIPTION**
Body scrub	This generic term refers to a wide range of exfoliation services and can even include salt rubs.
Body polish	This name usually refers to a more refined and gentler exfoliation service using smaller and perhaps softer particles of exfoliant; the polish is suitable for more sensitive skin types.
Sea salt glow	Sea salts are used to exfoliate the body thoroughly in this service, which is sometimes too abrasive for people with sensitive skin or those who have recently shaved their legs; the most popular salts for this service come from the Dead Sea in Israel, which are high in minerals.
Salt glow/salt rub/salt scrub	An abbreviated name for the sea salt glow, although the name can sometimes signify that the salts are NOT from the Dead Sea.
Body gommage	This term is popular, especially in European-inspired spas, and roughly translated it means a "gumming" of the skin using familiar exfoliating agents.
Dry brush massage	Using a dry bristle body brush, the therapist sweeps the skin clean for a full half-hour service; this is known to be especially therapeutic for the lymphatic system and is used during internal detoxification programs as well as to cleanse the skin.
Swedish shampoo	This term is used infrequently in spas today—it refers to a body scrub technique using a bath brush or mitt and soapy water; it is similar to a body polish or body scrub.
Loofah scrub	A somewhat rare spa service in which the therapist uses only a loofah to exfoliate the skin; it can be quite abrasive, depending on the texture of the loofah.

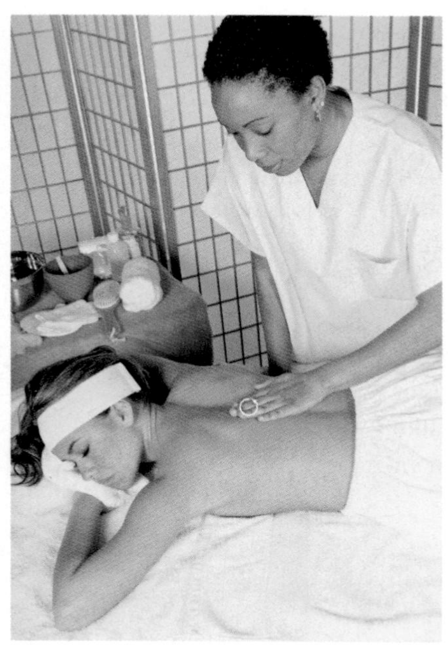

FIGURE 14-19 Exfoliation maneuvers are circular. Although they can involve pressure, the primary action is on the body's surface and not its inner structures.

Some common products used to scrub the body include: fruit seeds, crushed nut shells, cornmeal, salt (often from the Dead Sea), sugar, oatmeal, enzymes, jojoba wax beads, polyethylene balls, crushed pearls, pumice, and ground rice grains, among others. Additional products are added to the primary scrubbing agents to enhance the treatment or make it even more exotic. These can include, among many others, such ingredients as lime, lemon, orange, ginger, coconut, milk, honey, lavender, pomegranate, and chamomile.

The principal maneuver for all exfoliation techniques is a circular scrubbing action to avoid stretching the delicate connective tissues of the skin too far in any one direction. Massage therapists should remember that they are not giving a massage service during exfoliation. Exfoliation maneuvers are distinct and have different intents (Figure 14-19).

Wet Room versus Dry Room Exfoliation

In some spas, the client reclines on a **wet table**, which is a specially constructed waterproof treatment table with built-in drainage used for exfoliation and body wrap services. Products are washed from the body with a shower hose or a built-in **Vichy shower** above the table. This type of treatment area is called a **wet room**. In spas without the infrastructure or budget necessary for a room with plumbing and a wet table, a regular massage table can be used with a vinyl drape or thermal blanket over it for protection. This is called a **dry room** spa setup.

wet table

is a specially constructed waterproof treatment table with built-in drainage used in spas for exfoliation and body wrap services.

Vichy shower

is a multihead inline shower extending out over a treatment table, under which clients recline on a wet table to receive spa services.

wet room

is a tiled treatment room with plumbing that contains one or more of the following: wet table, shower, Vichy shower, hydrotherapy tub, Swiss shower.

dry room

is a massage room used for spa treatments performed without the use of showers and baths.

Regardless of the products used, the procedure for many body scrubs is the same. First, the client's skin is moistened, either with a hot wet towel in a dry room or a shower in a wet room; the exfoliant is then applied. The therapist works the exfoliant into the skin and then cleanses it off. Some exfoliations include washing with a body bath or soap. Finally, a moisturizer or massage oil is applied.

EXFOLIATION PROCEDURE

This procedure is for a dry room exfoliation using hot wet towels instead of a shower. The term *exfoliant* here refers to any chosen scrubbing agent, including salt. *Body bath* refers to any liquid type soap. In spas, the choice of liquid soaps for this purpose is usually aromatic, often with essential oils added.

Preparation

Rinse and wring out four hand towels and keep them hot in a towel cabinet or insulated container. Warm the exfoliant so that it does not shock the client during application. Fill a large bowl with hot water and place a loofah mitt or pad in the water. Prepare a massage table with a vinyl drape or a thermal blanket to protect the table from moisture. Then layer a large bath towel or bath sheet on top of this for the client to lie on (Figure 14-20a). Drape the client normally with a bath towel, or diaper drape. Keep in mind that this drape can become quite damp in a wet room but will remain mostly dry using the hot towel method in a dry room.

Exfoliating the Back and Back of Legs

1. First, moisten the back and back of the legs with the fabric side of the loofah pad or a sponge (Figure 14-20b).
2. Place a quarter-sized dab of exfoliant in the palm of one hand and rub into the back first, using the circular exfoliating movement (Figure 14-20c).
3. Apply more exfoliant as needed, move down to the right foot, and work up over the right leg to the buttock.
4. Repeat on the left leg.

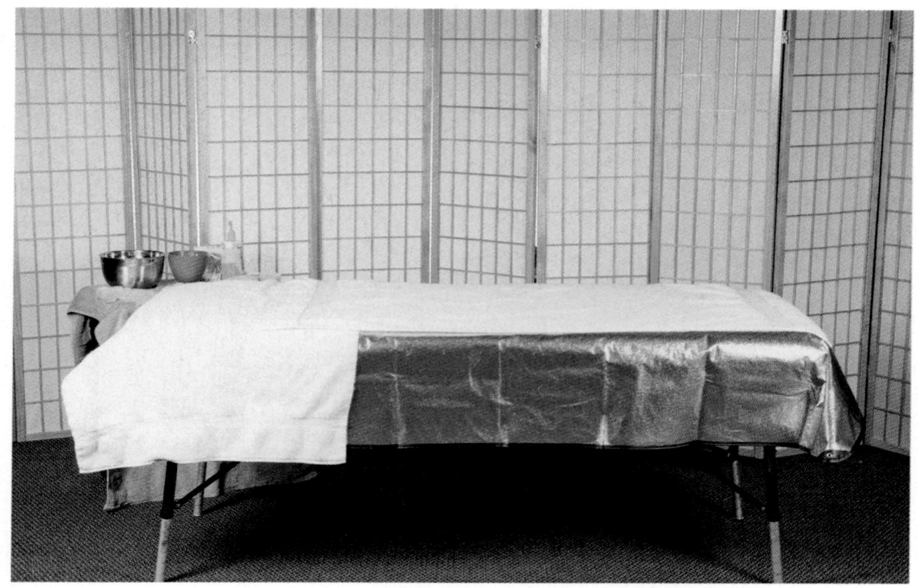

FIGURE 14-20A Prepare a massage table with a vinyl drape or a space blanket. Then layer a large bath towel or bath sheet on top of this for the client to lie on.

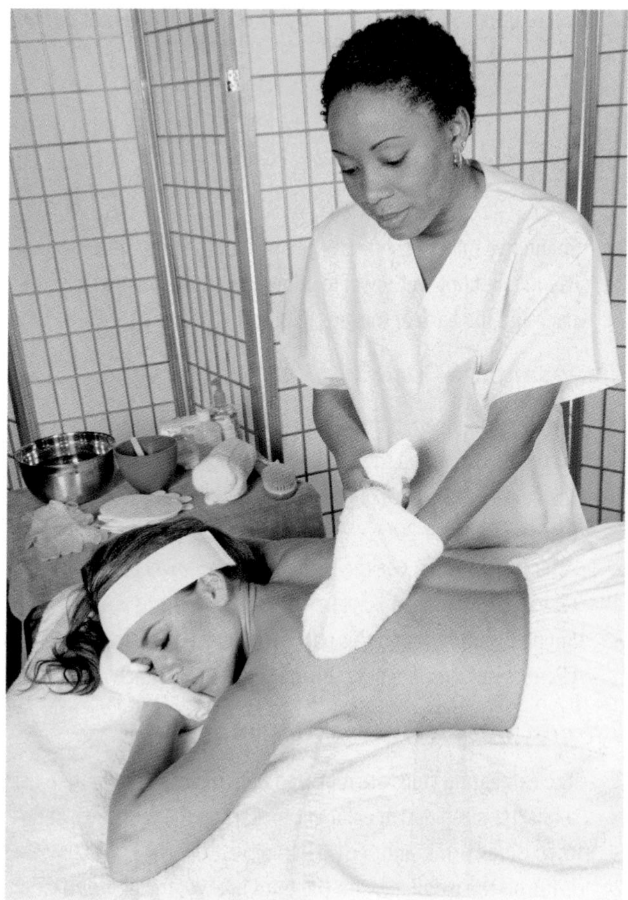

FIGURE 14-20B The first step in an exfoliation treatment is moistening the skin.

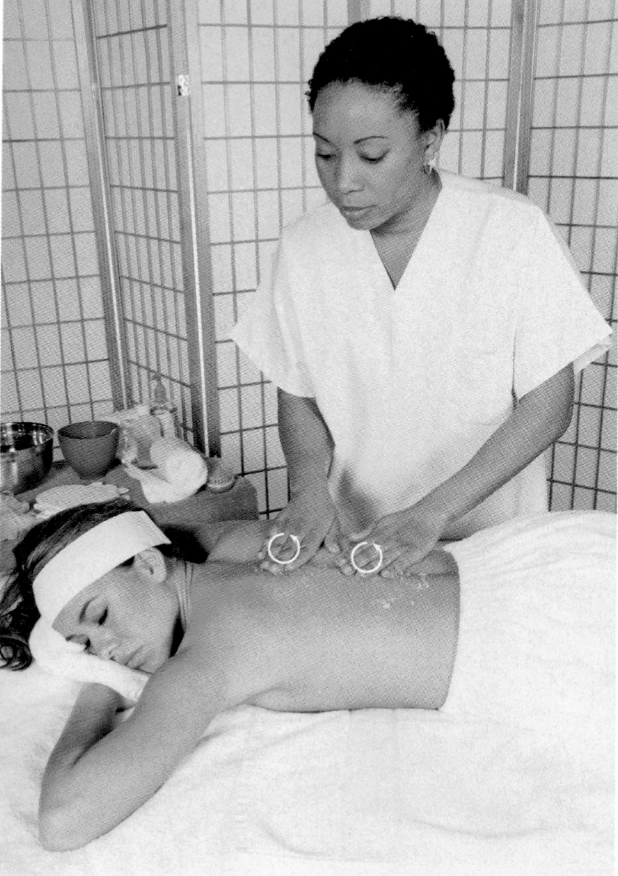

FIGURE 14-20C The therapist applies the exfoliant to one part of the body at a time, using circular movements, starting with the back and then continuing with the back of the legs.

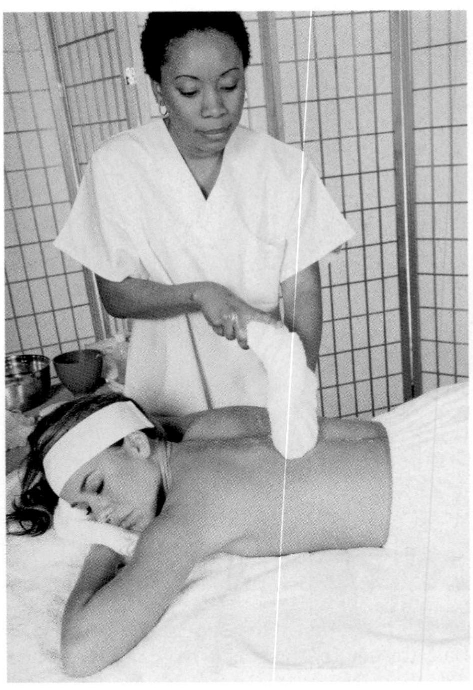

FIGURE 14-20D When the back is finished, the therapist wipes excess exfoliant away with hot, wet towels.

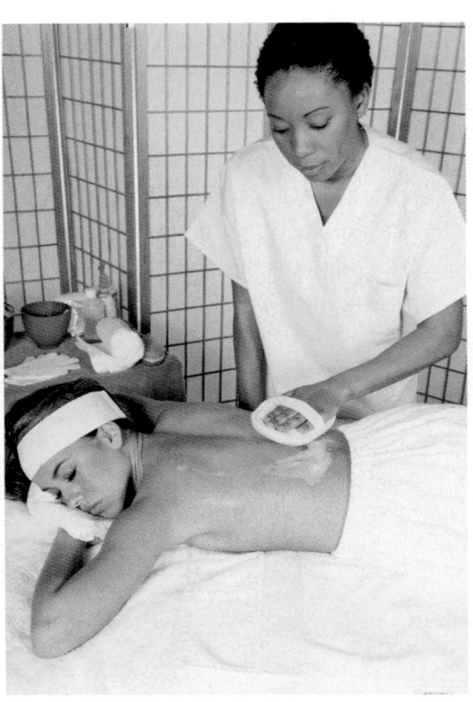

FIGURE 14-20E The therapist uses a sponge or loofah with body bath to cleanse the back and then the back of the legs.

décolletage

is the area of the upper chest above the breasts and onto the front of the neck.

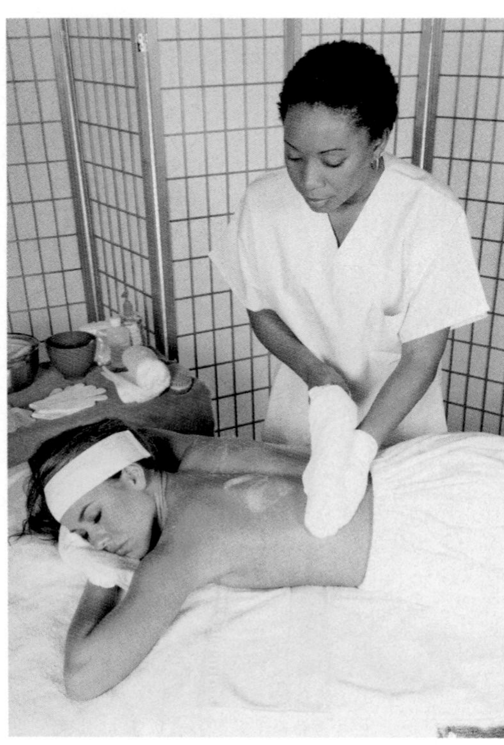

FIGURE 14-20F Then wipe soap off the body with another hot moist towel.

5. Spend five minutes on this entire part of the procedure, and then use the first hot wet towel to wipe away the exfoliant from the back and the back of the legs (Figure 14-20d).

Cleansing the Back and Back of the Legs

1. Dip the loofah pad in the bowl of hot water, place a quarter-sized dab of body bath on the scrubbing surface, and use it to cleanse the back and the back of the legs, using circular exfoliating movements (Figure 14-20e).
2. After five minutes, use the second hot wet towel to wipe off the excess soap (Figure 14-20f).
3. Spend five minutes on this part of the procedure, and then ask the client to roll over, keeping the drape covering intact.

Exfoliating the Front of the Body

1. The exfoliating steps are repeated here (Figure 14-20g to i), using a quarter-sized dab of exfoliant to start on the feet, legs, abdomen, sides, arms, and **décolletage**.
2. Wipe off the exfoliant with the third hot wet towel. This part of the procedure takes five minutes.

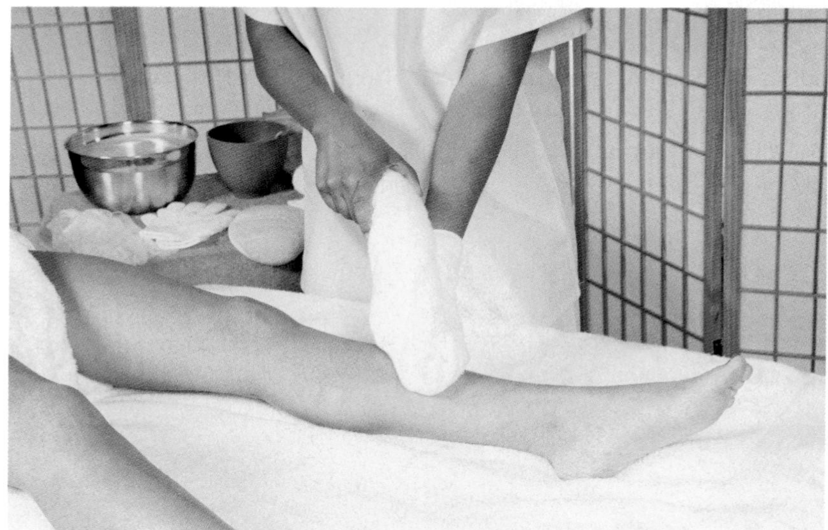

FIGURE 14-20G The client rolls over, and the process is repeated on the front of the body. First, the therapist moistens the skin.

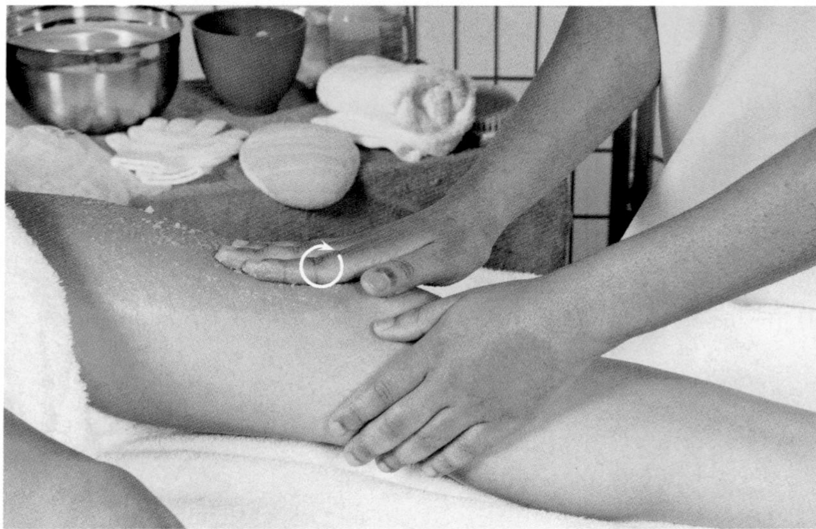

FIGURE 14-20H The therapist exfoliates the front of the legs, torso, arms, and chest. Female clients must be covered with a breast drape.

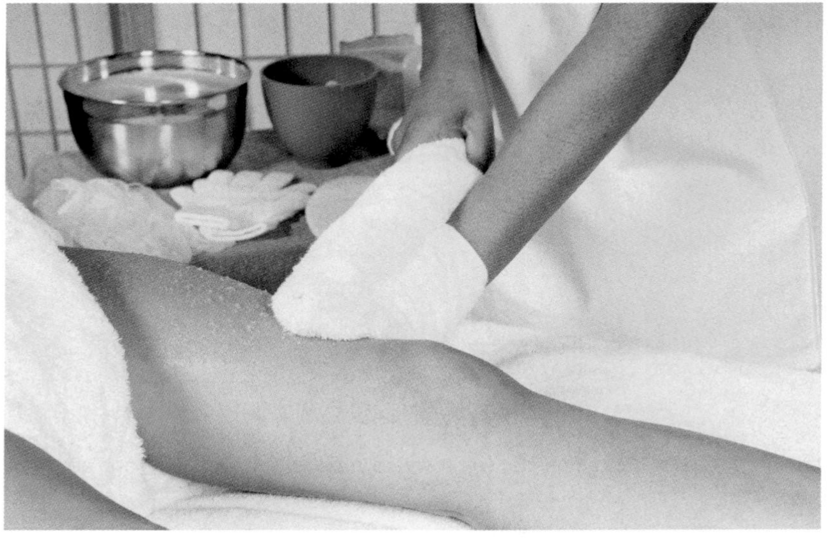

FIGURE 14-20I The exfoliant is wiped away with a hot wet towel.

Cleansing the Front of the Body

1. Apply body bath to the loofah pad soaked in hot water and use it to cleanse the front of the body (Figure 14-20j).
2. Wipe off soap with the last hot wet towel (Figure 14-20k).
3. Use a dry towel to wipe away any excess moisture. This part of the procedure also lasts five minutes.

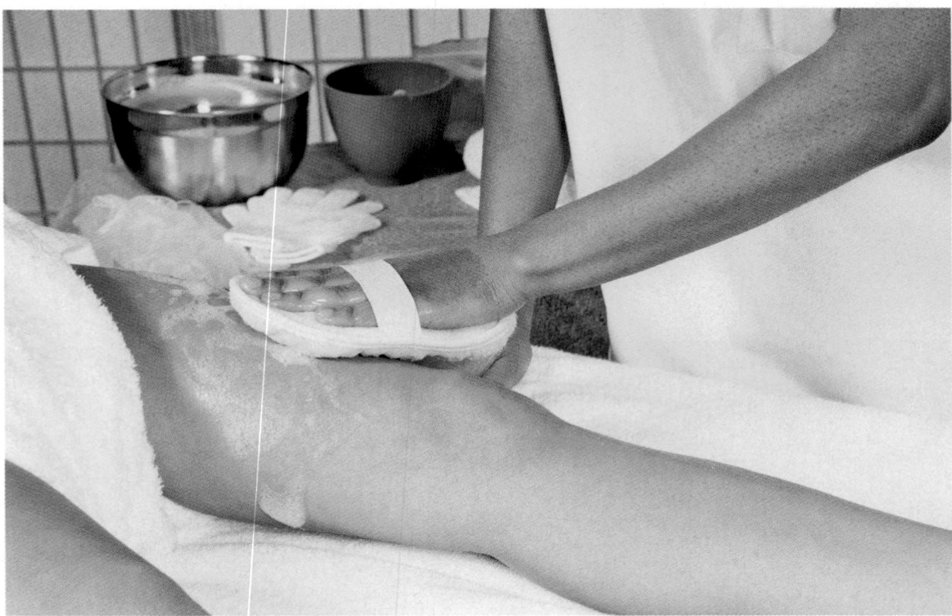

FIGURE 14-20J The therapist uses a sponge or loofah with body bath to cleanse the front of the body.

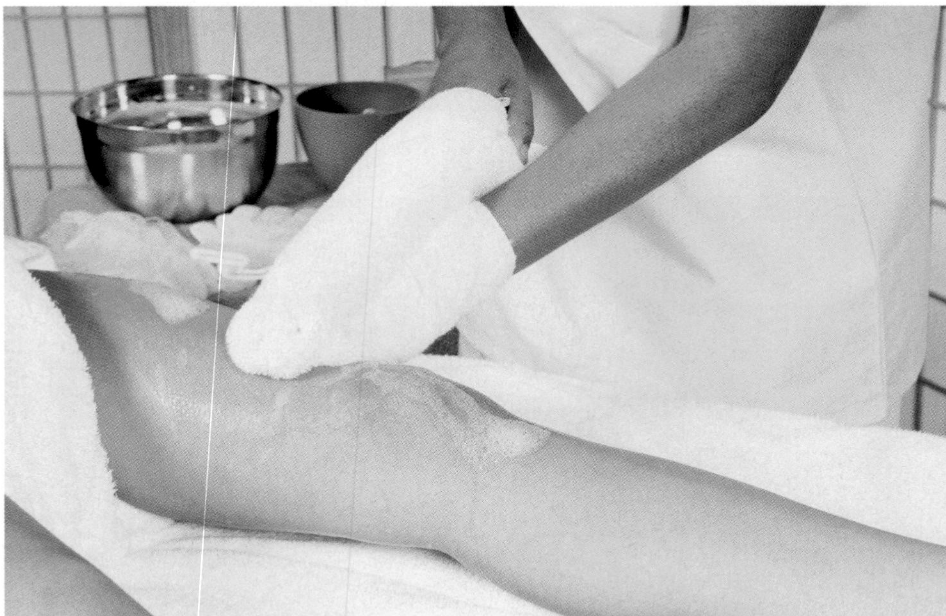

FIGURE 14-20K The therapist uses a final hot wet towel to wipe away excess soap and any leftover exfoliant.

Application of Moisturizer

1. Apply moisturizing lotion or massage oil to the front of the body. This can also be the start of a longer massage, creating a combination exfoliation/massage service (Figure 14-20l).

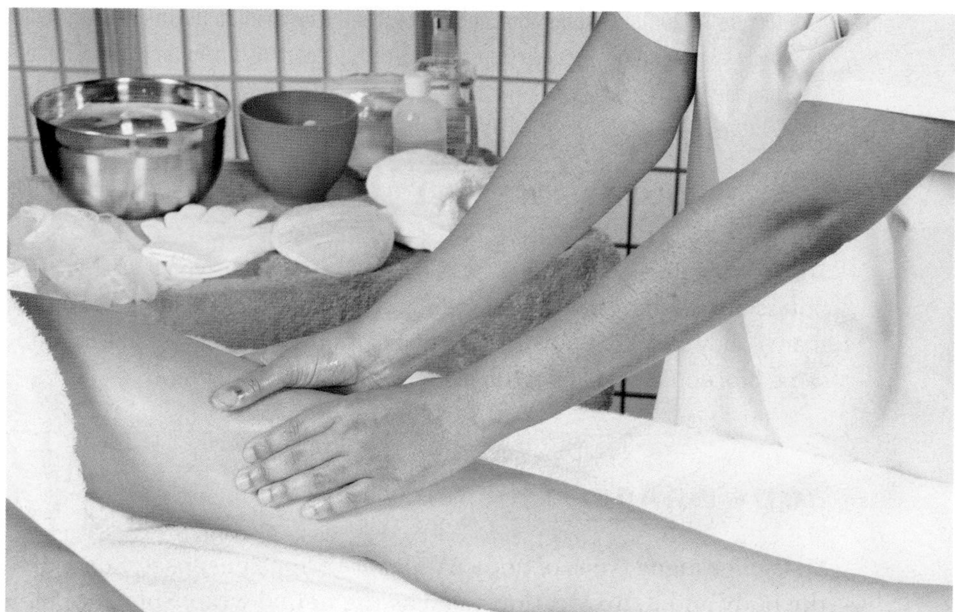

FIGURE 14-20L A lotion or oil is briefly applied to moisturize the skin. This can also serve as the beginning of a massage, extending the service to an hour or an hour and a half.

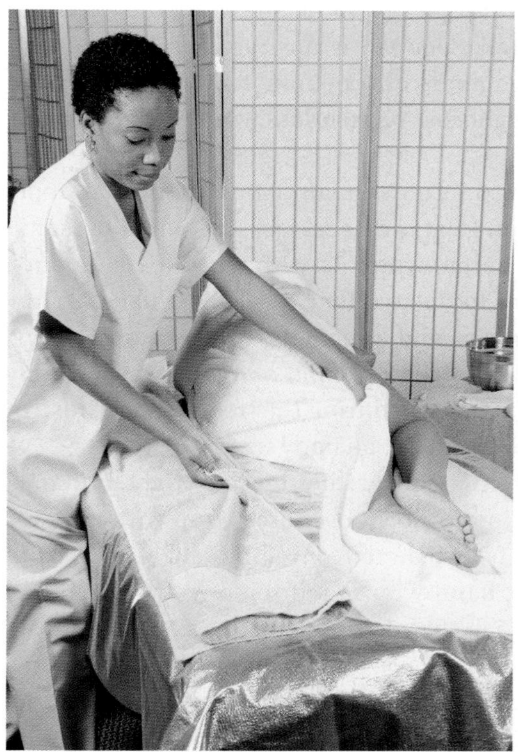

FIGURE 14-20M The client rolls over as the therapist changes the towel beneath her.

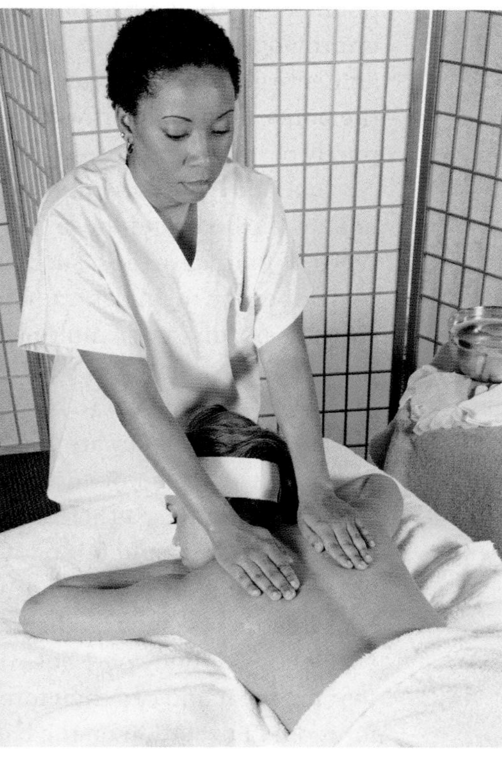

FIGURE 14-20N The treatment ends with an application of moisturizer to the back and the back of the legs.

2. Ask the client to roll over. Change the bottom towel while the client rolls, pushing it to one side, then slipping it out from beneath the client while sliding a new towel underneath (Figure 14-20m). This is so that the client does not lie in damp exfoliant and soap residue.
3. Finish the treatment with an application of moisturizing lotion or massage oil to the back (Figure 14-20n). The application and removal of the exfoliant to the front and the back of the body lasts 5 minutes for each step, for a 25-minute total treatment time with 5 minutes left to prepare for the next client.

SEA SALT GLOW PROCEDURE

The sea salt glow often utilizes salts from the Dead Sea, which are high in magnesium, potassium, calcium, bromine, and other minerals. The procedure is somewhat messier than a body scrub or body polish, but it can still be performed in a dry room, using the same procedure as that described for the exfoliation above.

BODY WRAPS

Spas offer many types of body wraps for various purposes. Some are for heating the body and detoxification, such as the herbal wrap. Some are meant primarily to relax and improve mood and well-being, such as the aromatherapy wrap. Some are meant to nourish, cleanse, and improve the superficial contour of the skin, such as cellulite wraps. Mud and clay wraps have multiple effects, such as purging and drawing impurities out through the pores, softening the skin, and improving joint elasticity when heated. Seaweed wraps remineralize the skin and entire body as the micronutrients and seaborne minerals soak in through the pores. Less frequently in spas, weight-loss or inch-loss wraps are applied for purely cosmetic purposes.

Spa body wraps can be categorized into two main types: those that apply heat to the body and those that do not. Heat is a necessary ingredient for some types of purging wraps, such as the herbal wrap. As with all heat treatments, remember the main contraindications for heated body wraps: high blood pressure, heart diseases, multiple sclerosis, and pregnancy. Non-heated wraps include the aromatherapy wrap and many seaweed and mud wraps, which rely on the body's own heat to keep the client warm during the treatment. Claustrophobia and pregnancy are contraindications for all body wraps.

Body wraps can be further differentiated as either loose or tight, and partial or whole. Thus, a therapist could perform a loose torso wrap with mud for purification, or a tight full-body wrap with seaweed for remineralization. Partial wraps include leg wraps, foot wraps, hand wraps, and torso wraps. There are also treatments, such as the back facial, that do not actually wrap around the entire body or body part but still involve the use of blankets or other coverings to retain heat and can therefore be considered a type of wrap (refer to Table 14.3 for more information on the back facial).

Although the purpose for each type of body wrap varies, they all have certain characteristics in common:

- *Comfort and security*: People generally experience a sense of safety and of being protected when they are wrapped up. It is a comforting sensation that is not generally available to adults except in the spa environment.
- *Warmth*: Whether applied externally or created as a process of body heat, warmth is an integral part of all body wraps, offering a sense of nurturing and engendering deep relaxation.
- *Enclosed environment*: The enclosed warm environment of body wraps offers ideal conditions for a wide variety of spa products to act on the body in an effective manner, absorbing through the pores rather than dissipating into the air.

General Body Wrap Protocols

All body wraps are similar in that they envelop the client inside various layers while products act on the skin. Each wrap is unique, however, in the particular manner in which it is applied. For example, some call for multiple layers of blankets, sheets, and towels to be wrapped around the client. Others, such as the aromatherapy wrap, call for only one blanket and one sheet. Still others, such as the drying clay wrap, require only a thin layer of gauze on the skin that is heated by an infrared lamp. Regardless of the wrap being performed, certain general protocols apply:

- *Exercise caution*: All wraps, especially heat wraps, can cause certain clients to feel claustrophobic. Therefore, the therapist should reassure the client about this issue, explaining that leaving the arms unwrapped over the head is usually more comfortable. With heat wraps, it is important not to apply any overly hot sheets or products, to avoid burning sensitive skin. The mouth and nose, of course, must remain unwrapped at all times. Always check for allergies or sensitivities to any products before applying a wrap.
- *Communicate*: Communicate verbally with the client about the nature of the wrap. Clients sometimes complain that they are unsure what to do while the wrap is being performed or while they are lying in the room wrapped up. Always let the client know that you are available. As a precaution, for the client's safety remain in the room to prevent the chance of the client having any sort of reaction. Inform clients how long the wrap will last and what they might expect to experience during it. Offer water, a cold compress for heat wraps, and anything else that can make the client more comfortable.
- *Always use a bolster*: Because of the extra weight on the legs created by most wraps, always place a bolster under the knees so that the client's lower back does not become hyperextended (Figure 14-21).

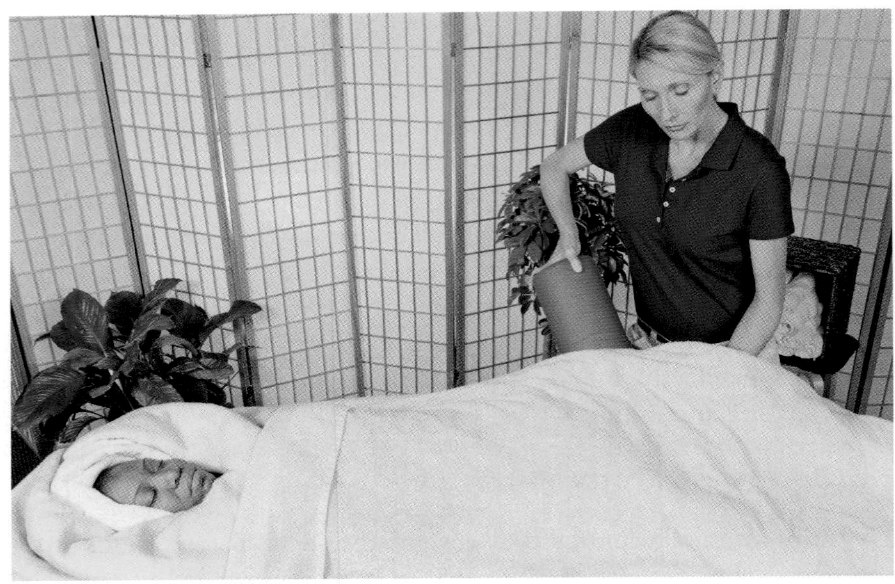

FIGURE 14-21 It is especially important to place a bolster under the knees of a wrapped client.

SEAWEED BODY WRAP PROCEDURE

Preparation

Prepare the table with the following layers: a double- or queen-size blanket on the table, a **thermal blanket** over that, a large bath towel or bath sheet, then a layer of **plastic body wrap** (Figure 14-22a). Another bath towel is used on top of the client for draping. Warm the seaweed mixture prior to use in a hydrocollator or other heating unit, avoiding microwaves. Seaweed products are usually mixed with an essential oil blend to improve effectiveness and aroma.

thermal blanket

also known as a space blanket. This type of blanket is a thin polyethylene and metallic-coated sheet that retains heat during spa body wraps and aromatherapy.

plastic body wrap

is a thin, transparent, disposable plastic sheet used to wrap directly around the client's skin during mud, clay, and seaweed body wraps.

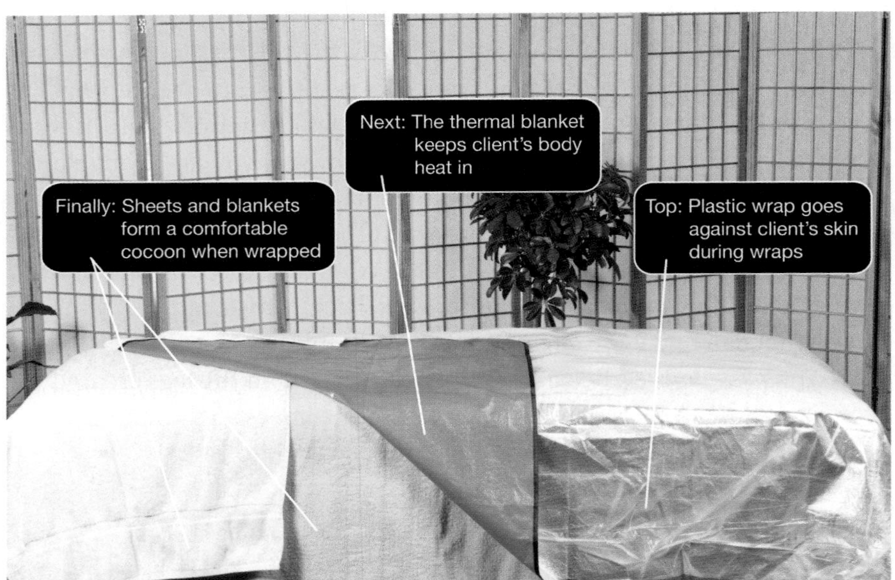
Finally: Sheets and blankets form a comfortable cocoon when wrapped
Next: The thermal blanket keeps client's body heat in
Top: Plastic wrap goes against client's skin during wraps

FIGURE 14-22A For a mud- or seaweed-based body wrap, the table is layered with a blanket, thermal blanket, towel, and plastic wrap.

If the treatment is given in a dry room, four hot moist hand towels are needed to remove the product. These can be stored in a roaster or insulated cooler.

The treatment is prefaced with an exfoliation of the skin. This can be a brief body-brushing or dry-loofah brushing, or a complete sea salt scrub or body polish added on as a separate treatment before the wrap.

Application

At the beginning of the treatment, the therapist should tell the client about the special benefits of the products being applied. This both educates the client and improves chances for sales of home care products from the spa after the treatment.

1. The client lays down supine under the drape. Fold the drape down and away from the client's upper body, inserting a breast and pelvic towel as appropriate (Figure 14-22b). Exfoliate the body for two minutes with a dry bristle brush or dry loofah.
2. Instruct the client to roll to one side while applying warmed seaweed to the back and the back of the upper leg and buttocks in a thin even layer with the hand or natural bristle brush (Figure 14-22c).
3. Help the client roll over to the other side and repeat the procedure.
4. Moving quickly to avoid the seaweed's cooling, apply in an even layer over the front of the client's body, starting with the legs. Wrap each area in plastic after the application, especially if the room is cool (Figure 14-22d). Avoid the feet if reflexology is to be applied during the wrap. Move to the abdomen, and the area around and between the breasts. Finish with the arms and décolletage.

Wrapping

1. When the client is completely covered with seaweed, wrap the body with plastic first, then a thermal blanket, then a blanket. Lay a bath sheet over this cocoon to seal in body heat and place an eye-pillow over the client's eyes (Figure 14-22e and f).
2. Place a bolster beneath the knees.
3. Allow the client to rest for 25 minutes.
4. Perform a gentle foot reflexology routine or scalp massage during this time. If the client prefers, you may leave the room to let her rest (Figure 14-22g).

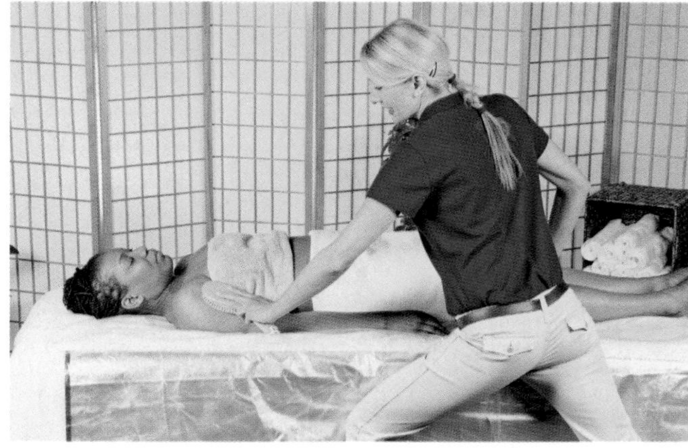

FIGURE 14-22B The client lies on the plastic and is draped appropriately. Preface the treatment with an exfoliation of the skin.

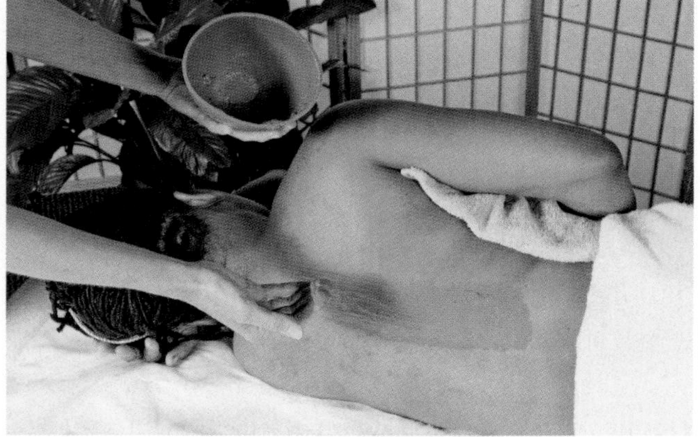

FIGURE 14-22C The application begins using hands or a natural bristle brush. The back can be reached as the client rolls slightly to one side.

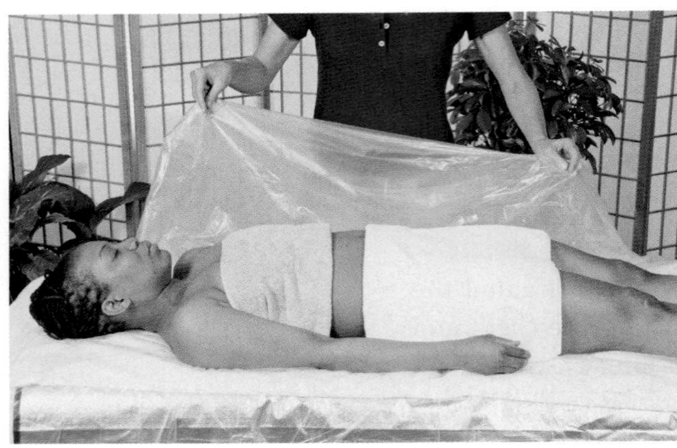

FIGURE 14-22D The therapist moves quickly to avoid cooling the client, and each part of the body can be covered with the plastic wrap as the application to that area is completed.

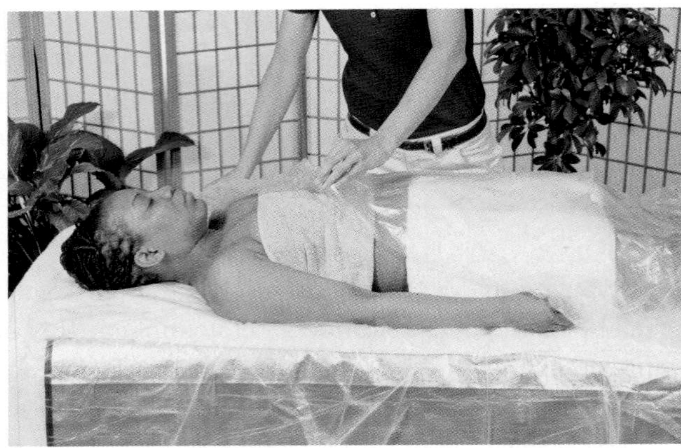

FIGURE 14-22 E1 When the client is completely covered with seaweed, wrap the body with plastic first, then a thermal blanket, and then a blanket.

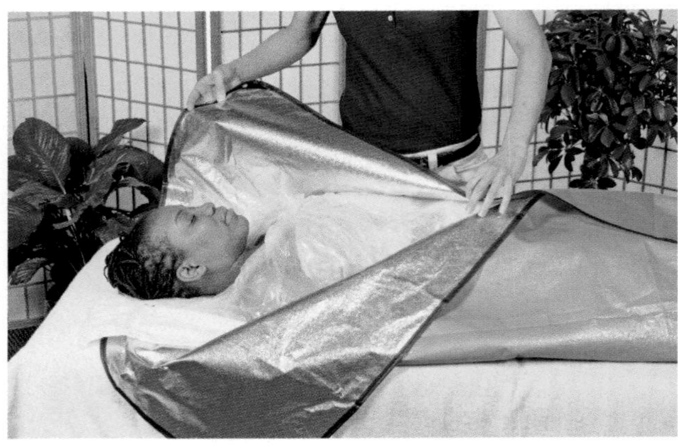

FIGURE 14-22 E2

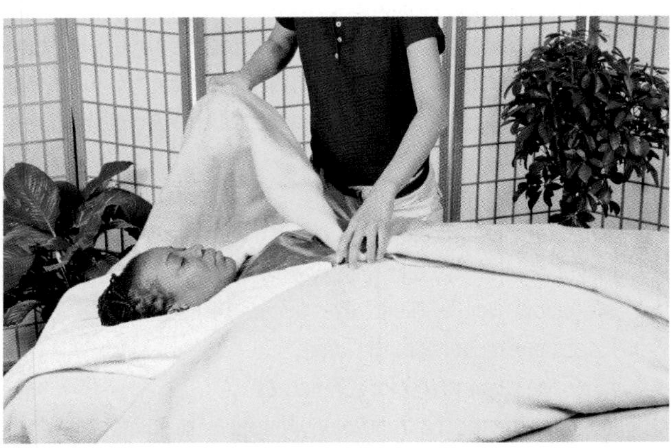

FIGURE 14-22 E3

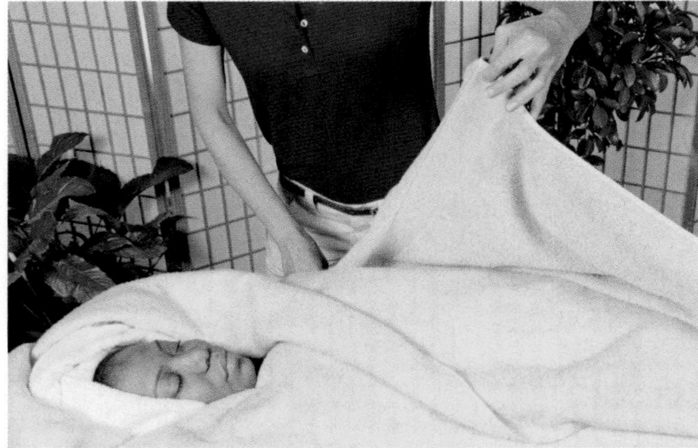

FIGURE 14-22 F1 Lay a bath sheet over the client to create a cocoon to seal in body heat; place an eye pillow over the eyes and a bolster beneath the knees. The client rests for 25 minutes.

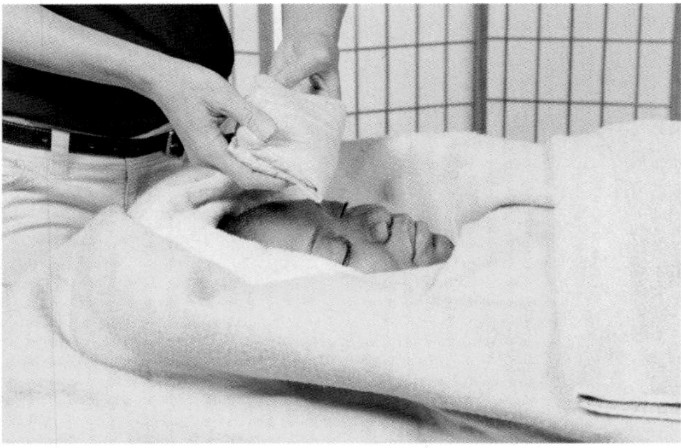

FIGURE 14-22 F2

Unwrapping/Cleaning

Note: This procedure is for a dry room body wrap. In a spa wet room, the client proceeds at this point into the shower while the therapist cleans and prepares the table.

1. Having a folded warm moist towel ready, peel away the plastic from the upper body while rolling the plastic down toward the table. Remove the seaweed from the stomach with the towel.
2. Remove the seaweed from the décolletage and arms (Figure 14-22h).
3. Assist the client in sitting up. With a fresh warm moist hand towel, press the towel lengthwise along the back to moisten the seaweed. Then remove the remaining seaweed from the back.
4. Prior to the client's lying back down, roll the plastic and thermal blanket toward the buttocks. Have the client lie down and cover the upper body with a bath sheet.

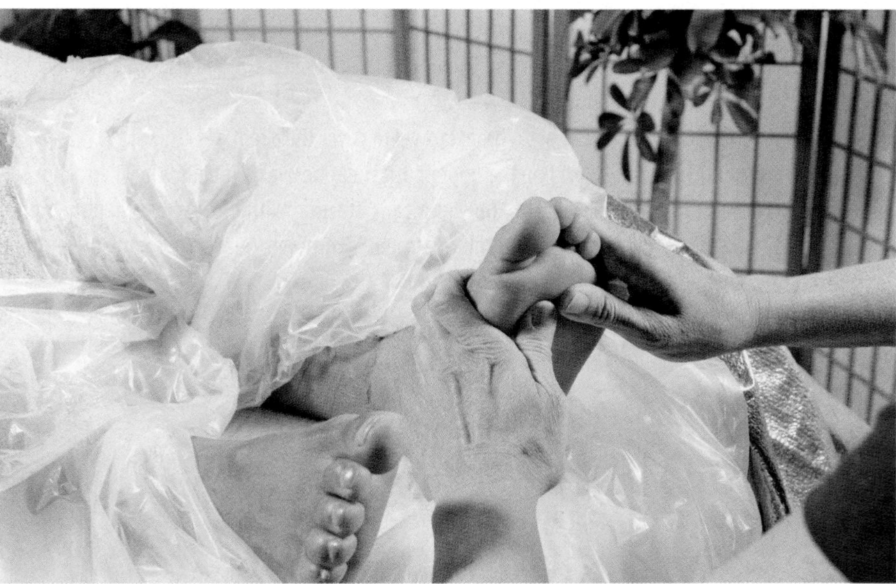

FIGURE 14-22G Perform a gentle foot reflexology routine or scalp massage during this time.

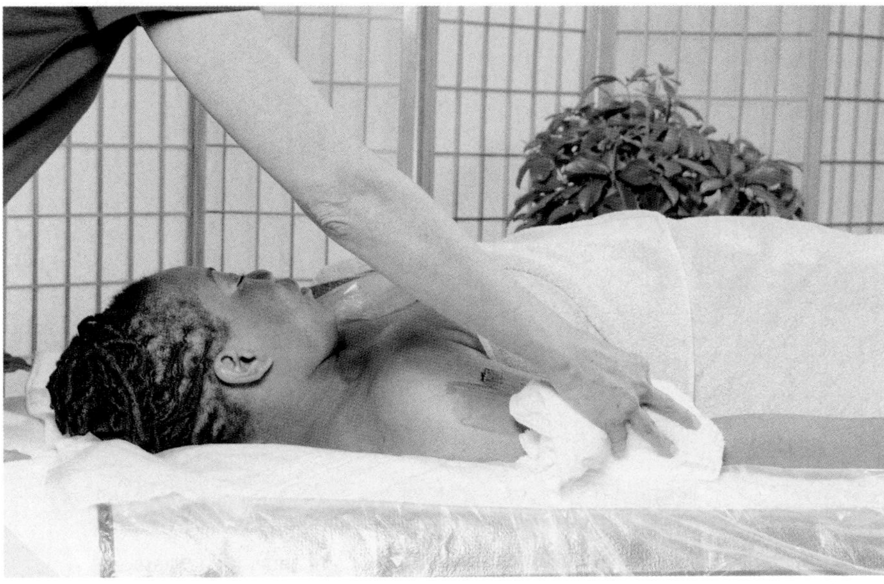

FIGURE 14-22H Unwrap the client, and remove the seaweed with four hot wet towels, peeling away layers one area at a time.

5. Peel back the plastic from the client's right leg, and remove the seaweed with a separate, fresh, moist hand towel. As the leg is cleansed, have the client lift her hip and roll/fold the plastic and thermal blanket from under the body.
6. Repeat on the client's left leg. Remove the plastic/thermal blanket from the table entirely. Cover the client with a bath sheet to prevent chilling.

Finishing

1. At this point in the treatment, you can finish with a five- to ten-minute application of a hydrating lotion or proceed with a particular massage therapy service.
2. If proceeding with a massage, instruct the client to lie face up on top of a fitted sheet. Drape appropriately. Incorporate a massage to expand the procedure, making it a full one-and-a-half-hour treatment.
3. For a simple application, undrape and redrape the client as appropriate while a finishing lotion or body butter is applied. Start with the right leg, then the left leg, then move to the stomach and décolletage, left arm, then right (Figure 14-22i).
4. When applying lotion to the stomach, use a breast towel to cover the client.
5. When finished with the front side, hold up the upper bath sheet between you and the client and have the client turn over onto her stomach. Apply lubricant, starting with the left leg, then the right leg, and finishing with the upper back. When the treatment is complete, leave the room and let the client rest until she is ready to get dressed.

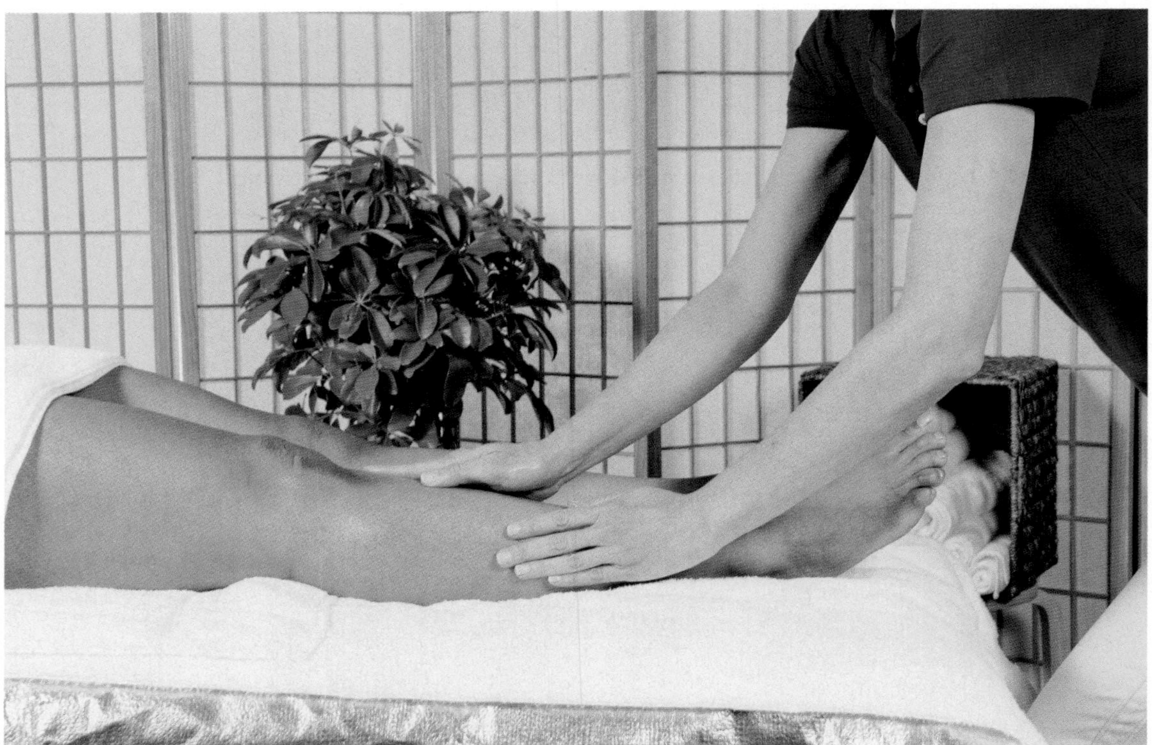

FIGURE 14-22I Finish with a 5- to 10-minute application of a hydrating lotion or proceed with a massage therapy service.

SPA COMPANY POLICIES AND PHILOSOPHY

In addition to performing massage and other modalities, spa therapists also need to interact with fellow employees and learn to thrive within the larger structure of the spa. Some therapists find that working for a company is the most challenging aspect of spa work because it means that they are not as independent as they would perhaps like to be. To work successfully at a spa, however, therapists need to know, accept, and adhere to company policies. These policies cover a range of employee issues, including time concerns, appearance, attitude, professional development, and physical attributes.

- *Time concerns*: punctuality; amount of time per service; amount of time between services; time spent on tasks other than massage; time spent charting, logging, and filling out intake forms
- *Appearance*: uniform, hair length, facial hair, body piercings, visible tattoos, makeup, weight, cigarette smoking, neatness
- *Attitude*: team player, responsible, mature, communicative, positive, calm under pressure, trustworthy, humble, attentive, able to follow instructions
- *Professional development*: desire for continuous improvement, ongoing skill building through advanced education, passion for the work, development of customer service skills, development of sales skills, longevity in spa positions
- *Physical attributes*: healthy lifestyle, endurance, strength

Before accepting a position in a spa, therapists should ask themselves whether they are willing to accept an employer's guidelines regarding these issues. It is important to read a copy of the spa's employment policies thoroughly (usually found in a company employee manual or handbook), prior to beginning work. Any spa policies that seem unacceptable should be discussed with spa management.

Professional Career Management

Perhaps the most common issue that causes tension between therapists and spa management is compensation. Some therapists resent working in spas because the spa takes a large percentage of the income from each treatment. This resentment is unproductive for all involved. It reduces the quality of the guests' experience, poisons the atmosphere of the spa, frustrates spa management, and could result in the dismissal of the therapist.

The percentage of total treatment cost kept by the spa is not the most important issue. Rather, remember that the spa is performing a valuable service for the therapist. This service can be called "professional career management." The spa, in exchange for a percentage of the price of each treatment, offers therapists many benefits, including a built-in clientele, marketing, advertising, appointment booking, billing, payroll, supplies, equipment, training, support staff, and a clean facility. Everything down to laundry services is taken care of for the therapist, and the high cost of this support must be taken into account.

Product and Treatment Knowledge

In addition to knowing the spa's policies and procedures, therapists must also possess a thorough knowledge of spa products and treatments. Often, this information is provided by the vendors who manufacture and sell the products to the spa. These vendors naturally have a bias in favor of their own products and procedures, and therefore it is beneficial for the therapist to seek additional information beyond what the vendors provide. The spa might offer a treatment guidebook, which should be studied diligently. In case the spa does not offer such a guidebook, the therapist should take the time to study on her own. The following are the main topics to study regarding spa product and treatment knowledge:

- *Benefits/effects*: What are the benefits of the product or service? Which systems of the body do they work on? Is the procedure effective used just once, or are repeated applications required?
- *Contraindications*: Which conditions should not be treated with the products or procedure? How might they adversely affect people with specific conditions?
- *Background*: What is the history of the product or treatment in spas? Is there any folklore associated with it? Which information is scientific and which is anecdotal? Is the treatment performed differently in different spas or different areas of the world? Were the products or treatment originally developed as part of any indigenous culture?
- *Integration*: Can spa guests integrate the benefits of the treatment into their lives by means of a home care regime? If so, how? Which retail products are associated with the treatment? Can the guest adopt certain lifestyle activities to help to integrate the intended outcomes of the treatment?

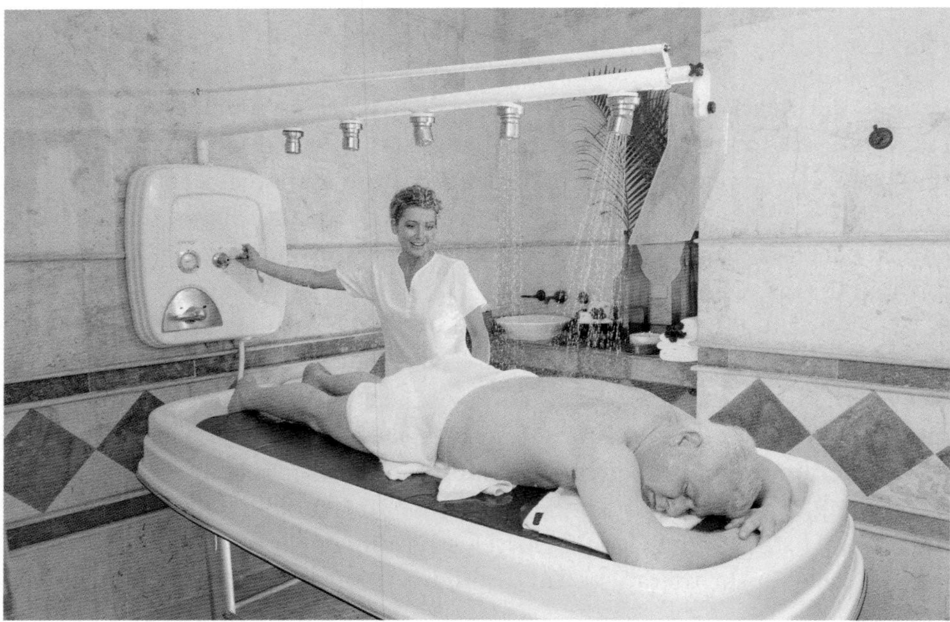

FIGURE 14-23 Vichy shower with wet table.

SPECIALIZED SPA EQUIPMENT

Modern spas use many specialized pieces of equipment to create their advanced services (Figure 14-23). Each spa offers some degree of training on this equipment, but it is important to have a grasp of general equipment knowledge before arriving for work at a spa. It is also important to be familiar with the precautions and sanitation requirements for each item. The equipment in Table 14.6 can be found in many spas throughout the world.

CUSTOMER SERVICE

Spa customers expect a high level of customer service, and it is vital that the spa therapist learn those techniques and skills that add to the spa's ability to provide it. To excel in this area, therapists must first of all understand precisely what

TABLE 14.6

SPECIALIZED SPA EQUIPMENT					
EQUIPMENT	DESCRIPTION	USES	WHERE FOUND	PRECAUTIONS	COST
Endermologie	Computerized massage device using rollers and suction to stretch and tone superficial subcutaneous connective tissue	Used in spas mainly as an anticellulite treatment, although also used for sports and therapeutic applications for athletes, burn victims, and others	Somewhat popular in U.S. spas, although more so in Europe and Asia; has spawned numerous competing devices for similar use	On strongest settings can be overstimulating to skin	$30,000 to $35,000
Hydrotherapy tub	One-person tub with multiple therapist-controlled jets aimed at specific body zones; most also have a "wand" for high-powered underwater massage	Used for baths, immersions, soaks, cellulite treatments, and other modalities, often in combination with a massage or body scrub; relaxes muscles, opens pores, relieves tension	Popular in larger spas with extensive menus; often underused in smaller spas, where these tubs can become a financial drain and are often sold at a loss	Care taken when clients enter/exit tub; heat can cause dizziness; must be cleaned with disinfectant after every use; many tubs have a built-in cleaning cycle	$9,000 to $20,000+
Scotch hose	A high-pressure spray (sometimes using sea water) aimed at a standing client	Extremely invigorating; stimulates circulation; used for bracing and toning effects, especially if cold/hot contrast therapy used	Most popular in older European-style spas and spas modeled after that style	Clients must be forewarned about intensity of spray; area needs to be cleaned and disinfected after use	$500 to $5,000
Swiss shower	A shower stall with heads aimed at the client from all sides and above, usually controlled by a therapist outside of stall	Used for washing off muds, seaweeds, and exfoliants and for stimulating percussive and thermal effects, often with contrasting hot and cold	Usually constructed only in larger spas; popularity is waning as newer spas opt for Vichy showers over Swiss	Same as regular shower stall; some clients find the spray too intense (it is called a "needle shower" by some)	$1,500 to $5,000
Vichy shower	A long horizontally aligned pipe with multiple heads aimed down to spray a client's body while she reclines on a wet table	Used primarily for exfoliations and wrap services to wash off product; also adds luxurious feel to specialty massages beneath heavy spray; provides hot/cold benefits	Very popular, although somewhat expensive to install	Table beneath shower must be cleaned after use; pooled water should be wiped away; spray must be directed away from the client's face	$3,000 to $6,000

customer service entails. *Customer service* can be defined as the ability of an organization or individual employee to take care of the needs, wishes, questions, requests, and complaints of its clientele. Excellent customer service consists of doing these things consistently, to a very high standard of satisfaction, and in a largely transparent manner, which means that customers often do not even notice the efforts being made on their behalf.

Therapists new to the spa industry often make the mistake of thinking that it is their hands-on skills alone that determines their value in the workplace. Spa directors and owners, however, think otherwise. They consistently rank customer service skills at the top of the list and often omit massage skills entirely when speaking about what they seek in new employees. A certain level of technical skill is taken for granted; customer service skills are cherished. Two of the main customer service skills that therapists need in the spa setting are retail skills and teamwork skills.

Retail Skills

Therapists employed in spas sometimes complain if they are expected to recommend products for spa guests to buy or to perform any sales-related activities whatsoever. It is important to realize, however, the importance of retail sales for the success of the spa. Most spas depend on retail profits to keep the business operational. Without these profits, many spas would close and many therapists would be out of a job. It is therefore in spa therapists' best interests to help with retail sales, as long as these sales are executed with integrity, honesty and skill.

Sales Integrity

When selling products in the spa, therapists must believe in their hearts that the products involved will make a real difference in clients' lives. It is preferable, in fact, that the therapist has actually used the products at home and can vouch personally for their effectiveness. There is no need to become a professional salesperson. Sales flow naturally from a discussion about the benefits of the treatment. Products simply extend those benefits into the home. For this reason, it is important to look at spa products as part of a home care regime, not as just an indulgence.

Some spas offer their therapists a commission on the products sold. Even if this commission is of no interest to the therapist, the sale is still important for the success of the spa and the satisfaction of the client. If therapists feel uncomfortable taking commissions for sales, they can offer this extra money to the front desk staff or even donate it to a charity.

Therapists should know that selling products to a client is not against the ethical code of any massage association. Selling is not against the law; it is not against the rules. What it does run counter to is some therapists' view of themselves as quasi-medical practitioners. Medically oriented massage usually does not involve retail sales, although some practitioners of this modality offer their clients medicinal herbs, exercise equipment, stretching devices, and other associated items for sale. Remember that spa massage is not medical massage, and it is completely permissible to offer spa clients the opportunity to take home the benefits of the products that they have had applied in the spa. Therapists should know that this is a normal, acceptable part of their duties at many spas. In fact, therapists who are comfortable with selling are highly regarded by spa owners and directors.

Sales Honesty

Therapists should never make false or misleading claims about the effectiveness of the products for sale in the spa. Instead, they should state only that which has been verified through long experience. Vague, general claims should be avoided. The spa world has been the subject of much scrutiny from the media and the public regarding false claims, and to counter this, the best policy is to assert only that which can be proved. Exfoliating products do indeed rid the body of dead cells. Seaweed does indeed penetrate the pores and add minerals to the body. Hot herbal wraps do indeed help the pores to leach impurities out. If no fantastic promises are made, and clients are given realistic expectations regarding the use of spa products, sales in the spa can benefit everyone—the spa, the client, and the therapist.

Therapists should always let clients know before the treatment begins that they will be recommending home care products for purchase after the service is over. This is so that clients do not feel unfairly taken advantage of when they are relaxed and their guards are lowered after the treatment. The fact that products are available should be stated before, during, and after the treatment. The statement should be matter-of-fact and informational.

Sales Skill

For therapists to sell skillfully, they must possess a thorough knowledge of the product (see "Product and Treatment Knowledge," earlier in this chapter), a certain level of enthusiasm about the results to be gained from using the product, and at least some degree of comfort with the act of selling itself. It is helpful, in this regard, to observe the skill and ease with which many estheticians offer products to their clientele. They expect the client to want to purchase products to continue the effects of the treatment at home. They are confident that clients will be happy with the results, and so they are not squeamish about suggesting that the client make the purchase.

When the therapist is comfortable in a selling situation, certain skills come easily, making the transaction a natural part of the therapeutic offering (Figure 14-24). Three basic techniques can help the therapist to sell spa products tactfully and successfully:

- *Self-observation*: When attempting to sell something in the spa, therapists need to gauge their own feelings and reactions to the process. Often, clients react more to the nonverbal message and body language of the spa employee, rather than the words spoken. The most important thing is to be comfortable, not slick.
- *Closing*: At the same time, it is also important to actually ask for the sale. Some therapists who find selling uncomfortable beat around the bush and never state outright their request that the client buy something. A simple "Would you like to purchase this product and make it part of your home care routine?" is sufficient.

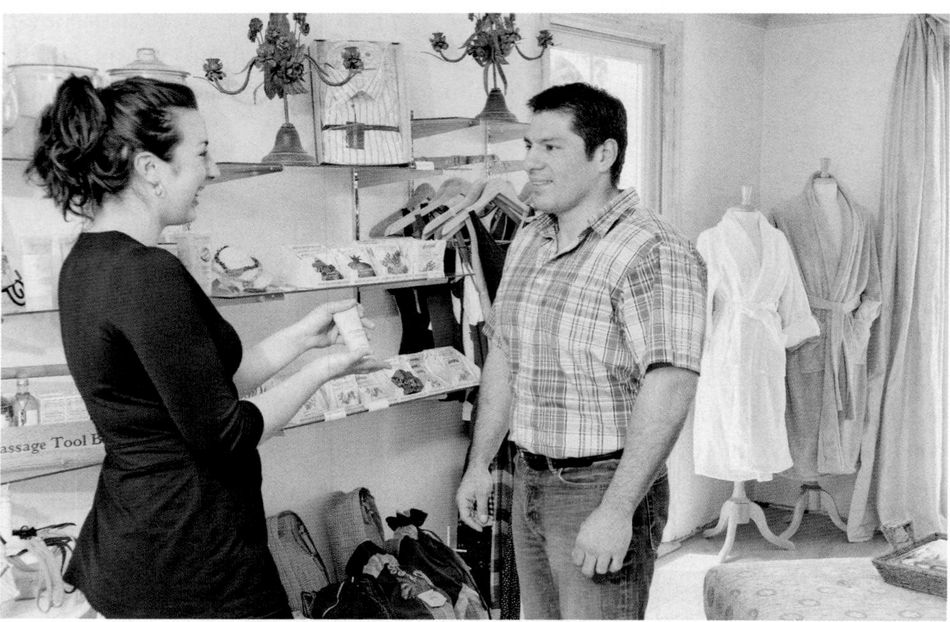

FIGURE 14-24 This therapist is assisting a guest in choosing products in a spa store. Although selling is not a spa therapist's primary responsibility, retail sales are an important part of the job description.

- *Detachment*: No matter the response from the client, therapists should not take it personally. In fact, the more detached and serene about the transaction the therapist is, the more comfortable the client feels, and the better the chance is for a sale.

Teamwork Skills

Massage therapists, unlike most other professionals, have the ability to work for the most part independently and free of support. The moment that a therapist walks through the door of a spa for the first day on the job, however, that independence is taken away. Therapists who work in the spa industry are irrevocably part of a team, sometimes a large team, and it is important to remember this.

As anyone who works at the front desk or in management at a spa knows, a team-oriented attitude on the part of the massage and spa treatment staff is absolutely essential for the overall functioning of the spa. Everything that therapists do and say behind closed doors during that vast amount of quality time spent with the guests reflects mightily on the perception that guests have of the spa. Spa therapists are in a real sense setting the underlying tone of the entire operation.

The main teamwork skills required to work successfully in a spa include

- *Ability to follow direction*: Spa therapists must follow the guidance handed down from spa management. Although this can prove difficult for independent-minded practitioners, it is absolutely essential for the team to work together as a unit. All teams have a leader, and spas are no exception.

- *Anticipating others' needs*: Spa therapists should constantly be looking out for ways that they can help guests before the guests even know they need help. Offer directions to other areas of the spa. Bring water or tea before it is requested. Suggest ways to improve guests' experience.
- *Presenting a united front*: Therapists should refrain from speaking to guests about the internal operations of the spa, especially problems with management or other employees. Every business operation has its share of conflicts. Therapists should leave these conflicts outside the treatment room, or the level of service of the entire spa suffers.
- *Pitching in*: Even if a particular task, such as picking up dirty towels or cleaning a bathroom counter, is not on a massage therapist's job description, it should still be executed diligently and with a positive attitude to ensure the smooth, seamless running of the spa. If no one else is available at the moment, the rule is "pitch in."

EMPLOYMENT OPPORTUNITIES IN THE SPA INDUSTRY

The contact between service providers and customers is perhaps greater in spas than in any other industry, thus making the hiring and training of quality personnel especially important as owners and directors continue to seek well-qualified therapists with the proper attitudes to fill many positions in spas all over the world. Spas employ nearly a quarter million people in the United States alone, and by far, the largest percentage of pay goes to the hands-on staff. Therapists and estheticians are the backbone of the industry. On the other hand, spas are currently the largest source of jobs for therapists and the single largest employer of new massage school graduates. Spas need therapists; therapists need spas. This synergy creates a most promising job market in a wide range of possible workspaces.

Today, therapists can find work not only in the traditional spa settings described in Table 14.1 but also in many unique environments. Many therapists seek the adventure of working aboard a cruise ship, for example. Spas can be found in airport terminals, and some airlines have begun offering massage and spa services to passengers on transatlantic flights. Safari spas can be found in the wilds of Africa, soul-stirring spas in the Himalayan highlands, thermal spas in outback Chile, adventure spas in Australian rain forests, exotic spas in Thai jungles, wine-themed spas in Napa Valley, and thousands of local spas right around the corner in every city and in most towns.

So how exactly does one go about finding and securing the right job in this vast industry? Therapists are understandably confused when first setting out to seek a position. Should they just walk in the front door and ask for a job? Should they get a recommendation from somebody first? To whom should they present it? Is a résumé important? Which spas are more likely to be hiring? When is the best time to apply?

Realistic Expectations

Therapists should follow certain practical steps as they begin to carve out a career for themselves in the spa industry. First, create a résumé that includes vital statistics, school history and training, job experience, and personal achievements. Even therapists new to the job market present themselves more professionally if they have a well-prepared résumé, with proper spelling, full dates, previous work history, and schools attended.

Recommendations are not necessary to obtain an interview at a spa; however, a therapist's chances at landing the job will not be hurt if she comes to the interview highly recommended by somebody who knows the spa director or owner personally. Written recommendations are best, but a phone call can help too.

Timing is important when applying for a spa job. Many spas operate on a seasonal basis, meaning that they have busy times of the year and slow times. Therapists will be more successful in their job searches if they time applications to coincide with the beginning of the busy season, when spas are looking for personnel. These times vary widely according to location. Spas in ski resort towns will be looking to hire in November, for example, whereas beach resort spas will hire more therapists in May. It is also important to time any job application to occur at a quiet time during the spa's daily operations. Mornings, when the spa first opens, are usually the best time.

Spas advertise their need for therapists in several ways: through magazines, mailings, classifieds, job postings in massage schools, and word of mouth. Therapists seeking their first spa position should be prepared to work "on call," which means they are not a part of the spa's permanent staff at first. This position is usually temporary, and as the therapist shows responsibility and skill, she can move to a full-time position. The key to success in a spa position is to be willing to do whatever is necessary for the overall success of the spa. To do this, therapists must think of the business as their own, even if they work part time. Those therapists who maintain an outsider's attitude and do not help to co-create success for the spa business as a whole stand a much lower chance of progressing in the industry, no matter how skilled they are in the treatment room.

Interviewing for Spa Positions

In the larger spas, especially in the resort sector, it is usually necessary to pass through the human resources department on the way to a therapist position. In smaller facilities, interviews are conducted directly with the spa director or manager. Some spas also use peer interviews, which means that members of the massage staff screen any prospective therapists.

When interviewing with any of these gatekeepers, therapists should emphasize the customer service and teamwork skills discussed in previous sections in this chapter. Spas are wary of therapists who present themselves as "job junkies" who move quickly from position to position, leaving because of poor relationships with management. They watch for patterns of past injury on the job, because this can point to improper work habits. They also pay attention to the reputation of the therapist's massage school. One other important point is flexibility in scheduling. Therapists who can work any shift, including evenings, weekends, and holidays, are given preference because the spa industry requires these hours of its employees.

Therapists should come to the interview prepared to talk about how they chose massage as a career, past work situations, attitude toward clients, and how they would handle problems on the job. In addition, they should have some knowledge of the spa at which they are applying and be able to explain why they want to work at that particular facility. Research helps with this question.

Top Behavioral Characteristics of a Successful Spa Therapist

A group of 12 spa directors from top U.S. spas were gathered at a symposium and asked what were the top characteristics on which they judged massage therapy job candidates. These directors had their own views on the importance of various qualities, so none could be ranked as more important than another. These, in random order, were their responses:

- Team player
- Responsible
- Caring and open-hearted
- Open-minded
- Mature
- Good communicator
- Positive
- Calm under pressure
- Honest/trustworthy
- Able to follow instructions
- Passionate about doing spa work and massage
- Healthy/leading a healthy lifestyle
- Customer-service oriented
- Sales-oriented
- Common sense
- Ability to accept change
- Humility
- Desire for continuous improvement (how many classes have they taken?)
- History of success/longevity in previous positions
- Neatness/tidiness

The Interview Massage

Perhaps one of the most feared hurdles that therapists must leap on the way to a spa position is that of the interview massage. For many people, it is nerve-racking to perform under such conditions, but it is usually a necessary step if the spa is going to get a good idea of a candidate's skill. The interview massage involves giving a full treatment to somebody on the spa's staff, most often a supervisor, manager, owner, or director. Both participants in this process know that the therapist is being judged, which does not make for a relaxing treatment much of the time.

Therapists can overcome some of the anxiety that attends these interview massages by practicing on as many people as possible before applying for the position, ideally with several of these practice treatments given back-to-back, as this is the way many spas are now operating interview massage interviews. To simulate the real-world conditions of a spa, applicants are often asked to give two or three massages in a row to see how well they hold up under the pressure and the strain.

Remember, the interview massage is not just about massage. Applicants are also being screened for certain invisible, yet crucial, attributes that can make or break a therapist's chances at getting a job. (See the accompanying sidebar, "Top Behavioral Characteristics of a Successful Spa Therapist".) Although newly graduated therapists are rightfully proud of their technical skills, it is not massage talent alone that can get them that coveted position at an exciting spa, but rather character, personality, presence, and attitude.

ADVANCING YOUR SPA CAREER

Because the spa industry has grown so quickly, it has afforded many opportunities for employees to move up through the ranks. Often these employees are massage therapists. There are no precise statistics on this matter, but therapists now hold a large number of upper management spa positions, including supervisor, trainer, manager, director, and even owner.

Moving up the corporate ladder has advantages and disadvantages. On the one hand, therapists who move up can achieve more security and make higher salaries; however, some therapists who move up find that the money does not compensate for the increased paperwork and managerial responsibilities. In fact, the per-hour wage for performing massage in a spa is often higher than that received by many managers because managers have to work so many more hours. In this sense, therefore, professional advancement within the spa industry is a trade-off. Therapists trade their hands-on work and extensive interactions with clients for more involvement in spa operations, more prestige perhaps, more opportunities for travel, and sometimes more compensation. Therapists who work in other capacities within the spa industry also find that they can save their bodies from the symptoms of overuse that plague some practitioners.

If, after careful consideration, a therapist decides to move up within the spa industry, there are several points to keep in mind:

- *Laying a foundation*: Some therapists jump the gun when it comes to promoting themselves in the industry. It is important to learn the job from the ground up, becoming thoroughly familiar with all aspects of daily operations before moving on to supervising others. This is a particular strength of massage therapists, compared with managers who come to the industry from outside. Those who take their time to climb the ladder often do better once they have scaled it rung by rung.
- *Becoming active*: Therapists who expect to move into higher positions need to get involved with the overall operations of the spa at an early stage, even before making a career advancement. There are always opportunities for volunteer work, assisting the manager, learning the

Spa Resources for the Beginning Practitioner

There are many resources available for massage therapists who are interested in pursuing a career in the spa industry. Familiarize yourself with these resources prior to making a final decision about a career path. The resources included here are spa magazines, spa books, spa associations, spa trade shows, and spa Web sites.

Spa Magazines

- *American Spa*: a "pro-sumer" (targeting both professionals and consumers) magazine with industry information and spa profiles; www.americanspamag.com
- *Day Spa Magazine*: a trade magazine dealing with day spa issues; www.dayspamag.com
- *PULSE*: the official magazine of the ISPA; www.experienceispa.com
- *Luxury SpaFinder*: An interactive online magazine offering a huge amount of information on spas worldwide, plus much industry information; www.spafinder.com
- *Spa Magazine*: a consumer magazine focusing on the benefits of the spa lifestyle; www.spamagazine.com
- *Spa Management Magazine*: A magazine focusing on issues pertinent to spa managers, directors , and staff; www.spamanagement.com

systems, and more. This must be done in unobtrusive and helpful ways. Therapists can also show a willingness to help in other departments outside their own, because this is expected of managers as well.

- *Learning from others*: Therapists should watch how managers and supervisors conduct business, learning the protocols and routines of the spa.

Spa Resources for the Beginning Practitioner

Books on Spas

- *100 Best Spas of the World*, by Bernard Burt (Globe Pequot Press): top spas reviewed
- *Day Spa Techniques*, by Erica Miller (Milady): hands-on information for the spa therapist on several popular techniques
- *Day Spa Operations*, by Erica Miller (Milady): instructions and insight into opening and operating a day spa
- *Fodor's Healthy Escapes*, by Bernard Burt: a travel guide to spas around the world, with information about program, price, orientation, and other topics.
- *The Complete Spa Book for Massage Therapists*, by Steve Capellini (Cengage): all facets of spa work discussed and clarified

Spa Associations

- International Spa Association (ISPA): the most comprehensive, worldwide spa association, originated in 1991; great networking and educational opportunities; www.experienceispa.com
- Day Spa Association: works in conjunction with the Medical Spa Association; focused primarily on smaller facilities; www.dayspaassociation.com
- Medical Spa Association: works in conjunction with the Day Spa Association, focused on medical/wellness spas; www.medicalspaassociation.org
- Spa Canada: the latest information about the growing spa industry in Canada; www.spacanada.com

They should ask questions of people in other departments, even those considered below the rank of therapist, such as locker-room attendants. Everyone who knows the spa has a key to some area of the operation that can be useful.

Therapists can also find opportunities to become trainers or consultants in the spa industry. Much room for growth exists in this sector, and to pursue it, therapists should focus on learning as much as they can about the business of spas as well as the treatments. This can be achieved by attending spa conferences and taking advantage of the educational offerings provided there. Therapists also should learn as many modalities as possible to attain a broad understanding of all spa offerings. This, and plenty of on-the-job experience in the spa, will prepare therapists to make the leap to training and consulting. Often, this leap is facilitated through extensive networking in the industry, and this only happens over an extended period.

Opening Your Own Spa

The ultimate dream of many therapists who enter the spa sector is to one day open their own spa facility. Plenty of therapists have done so, some with more success than others. One important point to keep in mind is that spas are first and foremost a business. Although spas are often run by professional therapists, estheticians, doctors, and other professionals who are passionate about what they do and treat their spas as very personal projects, spas must also be run as businesses—by the numbers—and someone involved with the operation must be willing to take a dispassionate look at the enterprise.

Spa Resources for the Beginning Practitioner

Spa Trade Shows

- American Spa Expo: held in New York City in the spring, with much emphasis on medical spas, cosmetic applications, and business building ideas; www.americanspaexpo.com
- Esthétique SPA International: with shows in Vancouver, Halifax, and Toronto; for more information, see www.spa-show.com
- International Congress of Esthetics: a focus on esthetics, with shows in Long Beach, Philadelphia, Dallas, and Miami; www.dermascope.com
- International Cosmetics, Esthetics, and Spa Show (ICESS): held in Las Vegas each spring and Orlando each fall, this show draws attendees from the salon, day spa, and resort spa industries. Las Vegas is the more well-attended show; www.magda.com
- International Spa Association (ISPA) Annual Convention: alternating between Dallas and Las Vegas, in the fall, a gathering of industry leaders from around the world; the most spa-intensive of all the trade shows; www.experienceispa.com
- Spa & Resort Expo & Conference/Medical Spa Expo & Conference: Held in Los Angeles, this conference draws practitioners from many regions but especially those based on the West coast; www.spaandresortexpo.com

Each therapist is familiar with her own strengths and weaknesses. If, as is often the case, the therapist who is passionate about opening a spa is not strong in business or accounting, it is appropriate to partner with someone who is. Therapists can also learn about business through books, seminars, and school programs. If, after considering the challenges, a therapist decides to pursue opening a spa, certain initial steps should be taken to maximize the potential for success:

- *Start slowly*: Therapists often feel rushed as they pursue their spa goals. They want to move forward quickly because they perceive competition moving in and windows of opportunity closing. In addition, their enthusiasm propels them forward, sometimes too quickly. It is best to take an ordered, measured approach to any plans that are being made and not rush into a project that might fail later owing to lack of foresight.
- *Assess limitations*: Therapists should stay within their own limits. Undercapitalization is the number one reason that new spas fail, and this simply means that not enough funds have been put aside to start and sustain the new business through its early phases, before the clientele builds and income increases. It is best to start out small, even if it means simply adding spa services to a one-room massage therapy practice.
- *Enlist allies*: Most spa projects larger than a one-room operation require the skills and energies of more than one person to materialize. Therapists should not be shy about asking for help and creating ways to share responsibilities and profits in a new venture.
- *Keep learning*: Running a spa business requires extensive knowledge of many areas of expertise, including bookkeeping, management, retail, housekeeping, human resources, equipment maintenance, and customer relations, and this list does not even include the main reason that most therapists want to open their own spa in the first place,

Spa Resources for the Beginning Practitioner

WEB SITES

- www.royaltreatment.com: the Web site of spa trainer and author Steve Capellini
- www.spafinder.com: a spa-specific travel and education site to make bookings and discover new information, along with much industry news and updates
- www.spagoer.com: the insider's guide to the spa industry, with people, names, places, jobs, gossip, and more, by the author of *100 Best Spas of the World*
- www.spamailinglist.com: an extensive review of many spas with contact information, plus much information for the professional
- www.discoverspas.com: a clearinghouse of every type of information about the spa industry, for both consumers and professionals
- www.wynnebusiness.com: a successful spa owner and business developer has created multiple-day trainings for therapists and others who are serious about starting their own spa businesses, including information on hiring, compensation, budgets, demographics, and customer service

which is to create a space where they can use their skills to help to improve their clients' lives.

Keeping all of the previous warnings in mind, therapists should still know that it is entirely possible to start a successful spa business. Many therapists have, and many will continue to do so. A large segment of the public is open to receiving massage in the spa setting, and it is a powerful way to reach out to a wider audience than ever before, allowing people to experience the benefits of touch therapy and natural therapeutic spa products.

CONCLUSION

The conclusion to a recent ISPA spa industry study stated

> The rapid growth of the industry has created significant competition for scarce qualified resources at all levels. The problem in the industry has shifted away from the size of the labor pool to the quality of the labor pool. In a one-on-one service industry, the image of a business is a direct reflection of the image of its staff. It is critical that spa industry human resources be properly trained and developed into qualified professionals to uphold a sterling image for the industry.

This quote highlights how important it is for therapists to become well trained and highly qualified if they are to fulfill their role in the booming spa market. Massage therapists truly are the most vital resources in spas, the key to any spa's success, and a growing force in the ongoing development of the industry as a whole. Through education, diligence, and good working relations with professional people from allied fields, therapists will continue to find their opportunities for success in the spa world expanding exponentially.

QUESTIONS FOR DISCUSSION AND REVIEW

1. What are the origins of the word *spa*?
2. What were the names of the early spas or baths developed in Rome, Turkey, and Japan?
3. How big was the U.S. spa market in 2007?
4. Name the major categories of spas.
5. Name some of the spa modalities in addition to massage that therapists might be required to perform.
6. Which points are most important to keep in mind when practicing massage in a spa setting?
7. What are the major challenges to giving high-quality therapeutic massage consistently in the spa setting, and to which three aspects of a spa massage should therapists pay attention to overcome them?
8. By law, can only massage therapists perform body wraps and scrubs in a spa setting?
9. What is the definition of a spa cellulite treatment?
10. What is the definition of a spa parafango treatment?

11. How can aromatherapy be defined in the spa industry?
12. What are some carrier oils commonly used for aromatherapy massage?
13. What are some distinctions that make an aromatherapy massage different from a Swedish massage?
14. What are some of the purposes body wraps are used for in the spa?
15. What are the main benefits of exfoliation?
16. What is the principle maneuver for all exfoliation techniques?
17. Which employee issues, defined in a spa's company policies, should be known, accepted, and adhered to by spa therapists?
18. Define professional career management as it applies to massage therapists working in a spa setting.
19. What is a Vichy shower and what is it used for?
20. What is a wet table?
21. Define customer service as it can be applied in the spa.
22. Why are retail sales important in the spa?
23. What are the main teamwork skills required to work successfully in a spa?
24. What should therapists be prepared to talk about when going on a spa job interview?
25. Which steps should therapists take if they are considering opening a spa?

CHAPTER

15 Clinical Massage Techniques

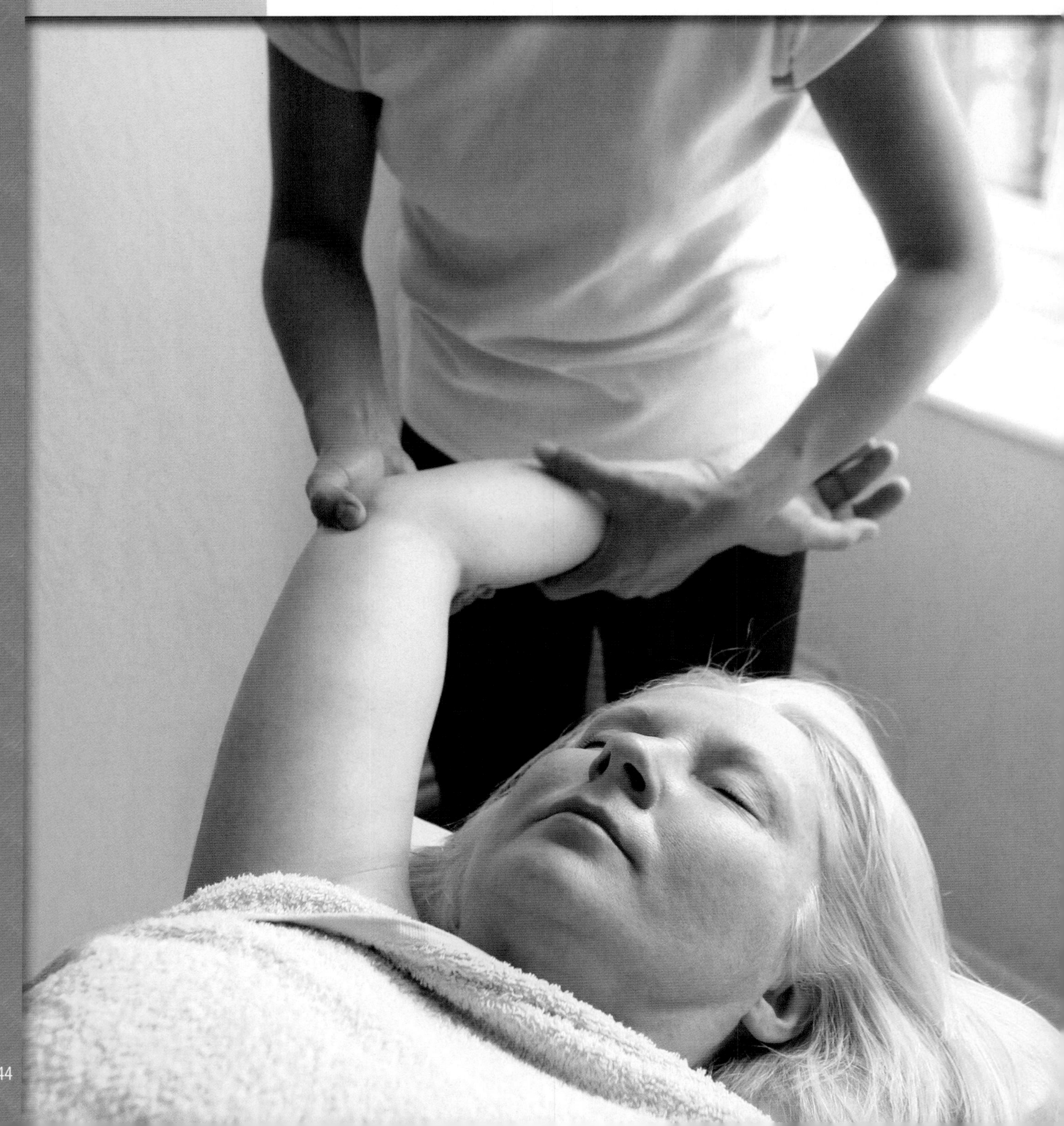

LEARNING OBJECTIVES

After you have mastered this chapter, you will be able to:

1. **Describe the techniques used in neuromuscular therapy.**
2. **Define a trigger point and describe its location.**
3. **Differentiate between central trigger points and attachment trigger points.**
4. **Describe how to treat trigger points.**
5. **Describe the techniques used in muscle energy technique.**
6. **Differentiate between post-isometric relaxation and reciprocal inhibition.**
7. **Define passive positioning and list the bodywork styles that incorporate passive positioning.**
8. **Demonstrate how to determine a position of ease when performing position release technique.**
9. **Differentiate superficial fascia and deep fascia.**
10. **Describe and demonstrate three myofascial techniques.**
11. **Describe the craniosacral system.**

INTRODUCTION

This chapter introduces those therapeutic massage techniques that address specific conditions and complaints that clients might present. Techniques introduced in this chapter include neuromuscular techniques, muscle energy techniques, position release techniques, and myofascial techniques. Lymph massage techniques are discussed in the following chapter. These techniques, with the Western massage techniques covered in the previous chapters, form the foundation of a clinical massage practice. These techniques are invaluable when addressing soft tissue pain, injury, and dysfunction in clients.

The essential elements required for the successful application of neuromuscular and myofascial techniques are a working knowledge of the physical structures being addressed (anatomy), how they function (physiology and kinesiology), a clear idea of what you are trying to accomplish (intent), and how to accomplish the task (technique). A clear understanding of the structure and function of the soft tissues of the body is essential to apply the clinical massage techniques described in this chapter effectively. The student is encouraged to review the anatomy of the soft tissues, the interrelationships of the various body systems, especially the myofascial network, including the muscles, fascia, and nervous system.

To apply many of these therapeutic techniques successfully requires an understanding of the structure and function of the soft tissues of the body. Assessment and critical thinking skills to determine when to use which techniques on which part of the body are essential. The following chapters offer an introduction to these valuable skills and techniques. To become more fully proficient, students are encouraged to continue their education with ongoing instruction from qualified instructors in the form of advanced studies and continuing education.

NEUROPHYSIOLOGIC THERAPIES

Several therapy systems are emerging that are directed toward neurophysiologic processes that affect the musculoskeletal system. These systems recognize the importance of neurologic feedback between the nervous system and the musculoskeletal system in maintaining proper tone and function. Alterations or disturbances in the neuromuscular relationship often result in dysfunction and pain. Neurophysiologic therapies use methods of assessing tissues and delivering soft tissue manipulative techniques to normalize the tissues and reprogram the neurologic loop to reduce pain and improve function. These neurophysiologic therapies include trigger point therapy, neuromuscular therapy (NMT), muscle energy techniques (MET), passive positioning therapies or position release technique (PRT), and myofascial techniques.

NEUROMUSCULAR THERAPY

Neuromuscular therapy (NMT) was originally developed in the 1930s and 1940s by Dr. Stanley Leif in England. Leif was born in Latvia, one of the Baltic States, and was raised in South Africa. He received training as a chiropractor and naturopath in the United States before World War I. He established Champneys, a healing resort in Hertfordshire, England and there, with his cousin Boris Chaitow, developed the system of soft tissue manipulation called *neuromuscular therapy*.

In the 1950s in the United States, chiropractors Raymond Nimmo and James Vannerson developed and published the first papers on what they called *receptor tonus technique,* which treated "noxious nodules" in hypertonic muscles using repeated ischemic compression techniques. Also in the 1950s, Janet Travell, MD, came to be noted for her successful treatment of soft tissue pain conditions by injecting procaine into what she called *myofascial trigger points*. Travell continued her research into soft tissue pain and published along with David Simons the definitive *Myofascial Pain and Dysfunction: A Trigger Point Manual, Vol. I, The Upper Body* in 1983, followed by *Vol. II, The Lower Body* in 1992. Volume I was extensively revised in 1999.

In the 1970s, Paul St. John, a student of Nimmo, began teaching NMT seminars in which he incorporated many of Nimmo's theories and methodologies. In 1984, Judith Walker (later to become Judith DeLany) became an instructor for St. John, and for the next five years they worked together to develop effective neuromuscular protocols for use by soft tissue therapists. In 1989 the two parted ways. Paul St. John continued to develop and teach NMT using the St. John Method, later Neurosomatic Therapy. Judith Delany continued to study, teach, and develop NMT, the American version. Leon Chaitow, DO, Boris Chaitow's nephew, has carried on with the scientific development of European neuromuscular techniques. He continues to research, lecture, teach, and write, including more than 50 books on NMT and related subjects. In 1996, Chaitow published *Modern Neuromuscular Techniques,* in which, for the first time, European and American NMT appeared in the same text owing to the considerable input of Judith DeLany. A recent collaboration between Chaitow and Delany produced *Clinical Applications of Neuromuscular Techniques* (Vols. 1 and 2). These two texts contain comprehensive descriptions of neuromuscular techniques from both the United States and Europe to address every area of the human body.

The body continuously endures stresses from trauma, improper body mechanics, poor posture, and improper nutrition, as well as tensions of a psychological or emotional nature. Regardless of the nature of the stress—be it mechanical, postural, chemical, or emotional—the adaptive tendencies of the body attempt to compensate for the stress by producing neuromuscular changes. Many of the changes result in reduced mobility, pain, fatigue, and depression. Conditions arising from one or a combination of these influences many times manifest as soft tissue pain and dysfunction and can appear as:

- inflammation
- ischemia
- trigger points
- muscle tension or muscle weakness (or both)
- nerve entrapment or compression

Neuromuscular dysfunction is self-perpetuating. When an area of the body is restricted because of pain or mobility impairments, other areas of the body compensate, resulting in further physiologic dysfunction.

NMT identifies soft tissue abnormalities and at the same time manipulates the soft tissue to normalize its function. In so doing, the perpetuating cycle is broken, much of the referred pathologic activity is reversed, and overall function is improved.

NMT depends on anatomic knowledge and palpatory skills to assess the tissue condition and treat neuromuscular lesions. Careful and systematic examination of the muscle and associated soft tissue identifies abnormal signs, including:

- Postural and biomechanical deviation
- Congestion in the tissues
- Contracted tissue or taut, fibrous bands
- Nodules or lumps
- Trigger points
- Restrictions between the skin and underlying tissues
- Variations in temperature (warmer or cooler than surrounding tissues)
- Swelling or edema
- General tenderness

Neuromuscular lesions are always hypersensitive to pressure and often associated with trigger points. NMT recognizes the importance of trigger points and their relation to local and referred dysfunction and pain. Beside trigger points, NMT also takes into account other natural and physiologic laws that account for hypersensitive or painful areas on the body. For example, acupuncture points and neurolymphatic reflexes not associated with trigger points are often tender. Tenderness usually means some degree of dysfunction in the associated tissues or organs. NMT treatment often stimulates the reflex improvement of the associated or referred function.

NMT treatment involves assessment and soft tissue manipulation. Postural assessment is important to determine any postural distortion. Postural distortion indicates an imbalance in the tone of structural muscles and is an indicator of chronic stress patterns. Assessment also includes palpating the tissues with initial light strokes and progressively deeper strokes revealing areas of tension, hypersensitivity, contracted tissue, and trigger points.

NMT is not appropriate for soft tissue pain from injury in its acute inflammatory phase. This phase of healing can last 48 to 96 hours or more, depending on the nature of the injury. Appropriate cryotherapy, lymph drainage massage, and possibly position release techniques can be employed during the acute stage. First aid for acute soft tissue injury is described by the acronym, PRICE:

- **Protect** the tissues
- **Rest** the area
- **Ice** the area to arrest the swelling and reduce pain
- **Compress** the area with a compression bandage if appropriate
- **Elevate** the injured area to help reduce swelling and pain.

When more chronic pain conditions are presented, DeLany (2002) suggests a four-step therapy protocol:

1. Decrease ischemia and trigger points in the soft tissue.
2. Restore flexibility with joint mobilization and passive and active stretching.
3. Rebuild strength with exercise and weight training.
4. Restore endurance with conditioning exercises

Experience has shown the importance of applying these interventions in the order listed. Failure to do so can result in aggravating the condition, increased pain, or re-injuring the tissue. Although NMT is very effective at reducing or eliminating soft tissue pain, it is ultimately up to the client to incorporate an ongoing self-care program and make any necessary lifestyle adjustments to eliminate or alter activities and habits that perpetuate the condition to attain long-lasting relief and healing.

Box 15.1

Neurologic Laws and Theories

Several theories or principles have been developed to describe the nature of reflexes or predictable responses of cutaneous nerve receptors. These theories support the rationale for many neuromuscular and myofascial massage techniques.

- Arndt-Schultz Law - *weak stimuli activate physiologic processes whereas strong stimuli inhibit them.* Steady, low levels of pressure stimulate a neurologic response, whereas intense, high levels of pressure or stimulation can actually be counterproductive and inhibit positive responses.
- Law of Facilitation – *After a nerve impulse has traveled a pathway through a certain set of neurons, future impulses will tend to travel the same pathway.* This explains the tendency of repeated pain patterns in the same area and explains why trigger points tend to return to the same areas.
- Hilton's law – *The nerve that innervates a joint also innervates the muscles of that joint and the skin over the insertions of those muscles.* When a joint is injured, the muscles surrounding the joint contract to immobilize and protect the joint.
- Bell's law – *A law stating that the anterior or ventral roots of the spinal nerves are motor and the posterior or dorsal roots are sensory.* Spinal cord reflexes can be initiated by pressure along the spine.
- Gate control theory for pain – *Activation of nerves that do not transmit pain signals can interfere with signals from pain fibers and inhibit a person's perception of pain.* The gate control theory thus explains how a stimulus that activates only non-nociceptive nerves can inhibit pain. The pain seems to be lessened when the area is massaged because activation of non-nociceptive fibers inhibits the firing of nociceptive nerve fibers in the dorsal root of the spinal cord.

NMT treatment techniques are similar to the gliding and pressure techniques used to palpate and assess the tissue. Many NMT treatment techniques are incorporated from other modalities. They include but are not limited to:

- **Gliding**: The primary technique of NMT generally uses the thumb to move across, along, and through the tissues. Gliding strokes can be superficial or deep, depending on the intention with which they are preformed. Superficial gliding strokes are soothing techniques that introduce an area of the body to the therapist's touch, distribute massage lubricant, enhance local circulation, and prepare the area for deeper, more direct techniques. Superficial gliding is used to gather information about the quality of the tissue and identify palpable irregularities in tissue texture, density, and temperature. Light pressure assesses the superficial tissues and stimulates circulation of lymph and blood.

Deeper stroking assesses deeper structures and stretches the fascia, releasing fibrotic adhesions. Deep gliding strokes are usually applied with the thumb, knuckles of a loose fist, or the forearm, and they are applied in the direction of the underlying muscle fibers (Figure 15-1 a-d). A minimal amount of lubricant is used to allow the movement to glide smoothly over the skin. The amount of pressure varies to engage, assess, and treat incrementally deeper layers of tissue, beginning with lighter pressure on the skin and continuing with increased pressure as the movement is directed toward the deeper fascia and muscle tissue. The pressure is always within the tolerance of the client. The rate of motion or speed of the gliding stroke can vary according to the depth and intention for which the stroke is being applied. Sometimes referred to as *muscle stripping*, deep gliding follows the direction of the muscle fibers from one attachment to the other, usually distal to proximal. Occasionally, the direction is reversed, and sometimes it is applied across the muscle. Gliding strokes are used for both assessment and treatment of soft tissues. Gliding strokes warm the tissues, increase circulation, and reduce ischemia at the same time as the sensitive thumbs assess the tissues for edema, tension, tenderness, or the taut bands that indicate the presence of trigger points. When these taut bands are encountered, gliding longitudinally along the taut fibers can locate tender nodules, indicating central trigger points near the middle of the fibers or attachment trigger points near myotendonous or tendinoperiosteal junction.

- **Ischemic compression or trigger point pressure release:** When painful spots and trigger points are located, pressure is held directly on these points (Figure 15-2 a and b). The depth of the pressure is determined by the tolerance of the client. The pressure should be deep enough to elicit a mild amount of discomfort in the client. Pressure that is too deep causes the client to tense up and is counterproductive, and pressure that is too light is usually ineffective. Duration of the pressure, according to St. John, is from 8 to 12 seconds and is repeated.

ischemic compression involves digital pressure directly into a trigger point.

- **Stretching:** After hypersensitive spots have been quieted and trigger points inactivated, the involved muscle and connective tissue must be stretched to achieve normal resting length. This is accomplished with passive and active stretching. Slow, sustained passive stretching is encouraged to regain and maintain length of the connective and

stretching is passive and active stretching of muscle and connective tissue to achieve normal resting length.

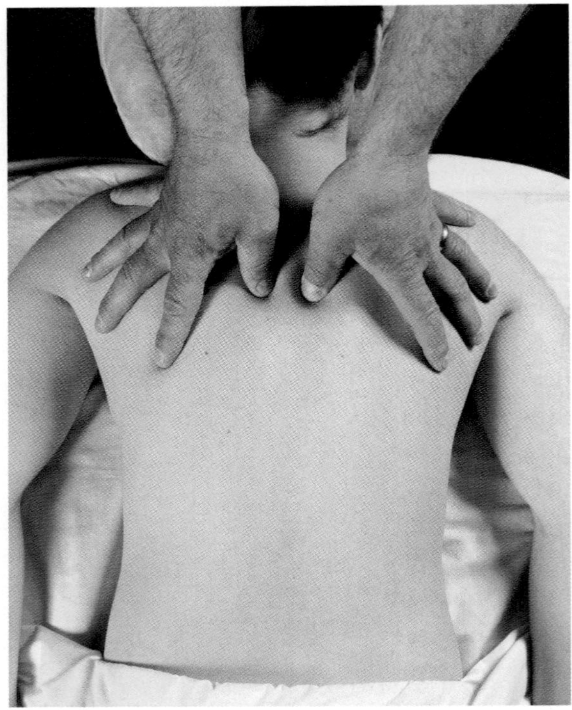

FIGURE 15-1A Thumbs apply gliding strokes and pressure as the fingers support weight and stabilize the hands.

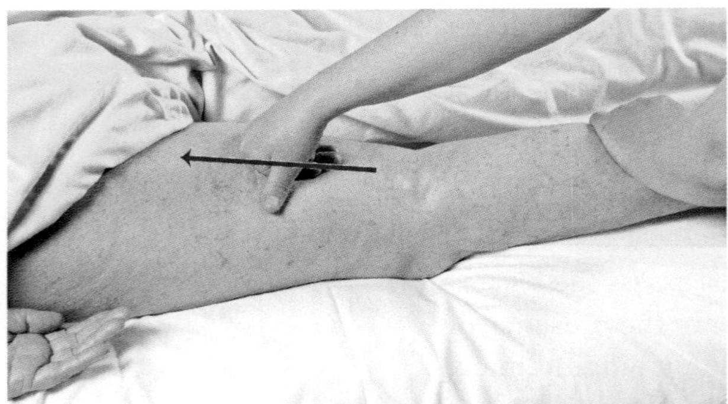

FIGURE 15-1C Deep gliding applied with the knuckles of a soft fist.

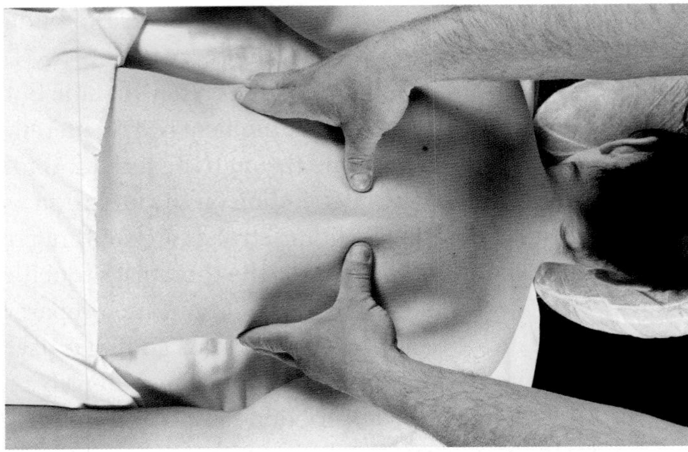

FIGURE 15-1B Improper application of gliding technique stresses the thumb joints and can result in inflammation and injury.

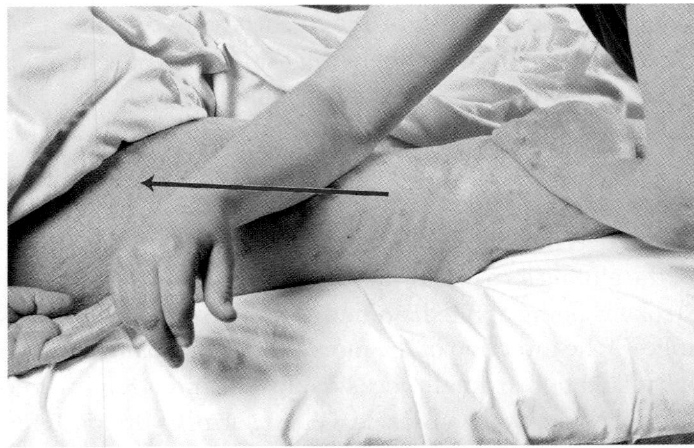

FIGURE 15-1D Deep gliding applied with the forearm.

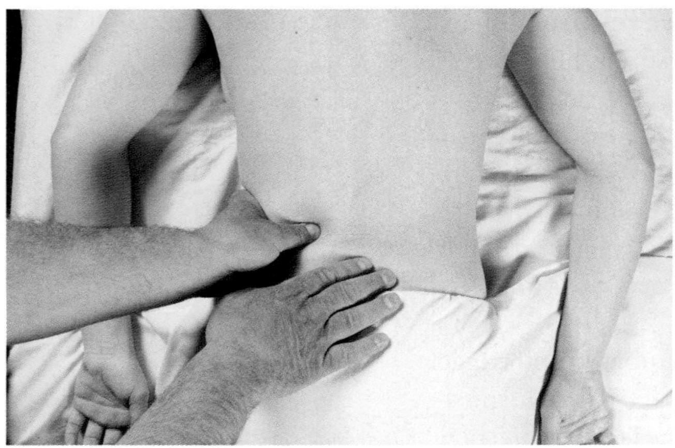

FIGURE 15-2A Trigger point pressure release or ischemic compression is usually applied with the thumb.

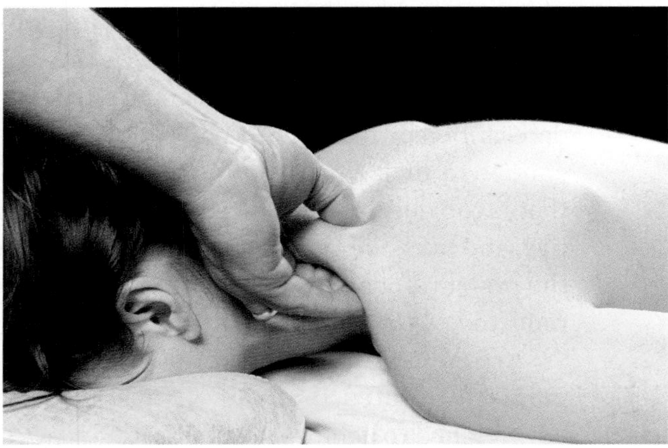

FIGURE 15-2B In some areas, such as the upper trapezius, pincer palpation can be used to deactivate trigger points.

muscle tissues. Active stretching is valuable in overcoming contractions and neuromuscular programming that restricts mobility. Active stretching, also known as *muscle energy technique* (MET), is discussed later in this chapter.

The order in which NMT is applied is from superficial to deep. Palpation and techniques that do not use lubricant are performed first, followed by gliding strokes to improve circulation and probe deeper tissues. Trigger points are addressed last.

NMT of trigger points is described in the following section on the treatment of trigger points. Successful application of trigger point therapy is key to neuromuscular therapy.

Neuromuscular techniques also include muscle energy technique, position release techniques, and myofascial techniques to address soft tissue pain and dysfunction.

To maintain improvements achieved with NMT, the stresses that precipitated the soft tissue dysfunctions must be addressed and, if possible, eliminated. It is also helpful to monitor the areas of dysfunction with follow-up NMT sessions and incorporate a program of regular exercise to improve strength, endurance, posture, and stamina.

TRIGGER POINT THERAPY

Musculoskeletal dysfunctions that can include restrictions in joint mobility, myofascial pain, and constricted muscles commonly involve contractile tissues that house myofascial trigger points. In most cases, deactivating the trigger points reduces pain and improves musculoskeletal function.

Trigger points are hyperirritable nodules associated with dysfunctional contractile tissue that illicit a pain response when digital pressure is applied. There are several different classifications of trigger points depending on where they are located and whether they refer pain when palpated. Trigger points are classified by Travell and Simons (*Myofascial Pain and Dysfunction, Second Edition,* 1998) according to their response to pressure and their location.

trigger point

is a hyperirritable nodule associated with dysfunctional contractile tissue that elicits a pain response when digital pressure is applied.

An *active myofascial trigger point* is a hypersensitive spot associated with a palpable nodule located in a taut band of muscle that prevents full lengthening of the muscle and refers pain or other definable sensations to referral areas when digitally compressed.

A *latent myofascial trigger point* is tender when compressed but does not refer pain to other areas. Latent trigger points can become active trigger points with continued stresses.

A *central trigger point* is an active or latent trigger point that is located near the center of the muscle body and is closely associated with the motor endplate that activates the muscle.

An *attachment trigger point* is located at the musculotendinous junction or at the osseous attachment of the muscle and is thought to be caused by the continuous tension of the taut band caused by a central trigger point. Attachment trigger points are often inactivated when the central trigger point is inactivated.

A *primary or key trigger point* in one muscle can activate a *satellite trigger point* in another muscle. When the key trigger point is inactivated, the satellite trigger point also inactivates.

A *satellite trigger point* forms as a direct result of the dysfunction of the primary myofascial trigger point. The satellite trigger point can appear in the pain referral area or in the antagonist or synergist muscles to the muscle housing the primary trigger point. Many times, deactivating the primary trigger point also inactivates the satellite trigger points.

An *associate trigger point* is located in another muscle and forms concurrently and because of the same overload or abuse that is the source of the primary trigger point. Deactivating the primary trigger usually does not inactivate an associate trigger point.

Trigger points can also be located in the skin, scars, ligaments, joint capsules, and fascia. Nearly 70 percent of common trigger points are located at the site of known acupuncture points. A trigger point is commonly palpated as a nodule in a taut band of muscle tissue. When pressure is applied, a sensation of pain, tingling, numbness, or some other sensation radiates from the point to another area of the body that is usually not associated by nerve or dermatomal segment. If this happens, that point is defined as an active trigger point. The pattern of referred pain is generally characteristic of a specific point. Active trigger point referral areas are very predictable and have been mapped by Travell and Simons in *Myofascial Pain and Dysfunction.* A client might experience pain in an area of the body that can be directly correlated to referral areas of a specific trigger point. Deactivating that trigger point often relieves the related pain (Figure 15-3a-r).

When a suspicious nodule or point is palpated and only local pain is experienced with no referred sensation, it is considered to be a latent trigger point. Latent trigger points might (or might not) radiate pain around the point. Latent trigger points can become active under conditions of continued or exaggerated stress. Active trigger points can also become latent trigger points if aggravating circumstances are reduced.

Trigger points can become active because of many factors, including acute or extended overload, trauma, joint dysfunction, arthritic conditions, visceral disease, and emotional stress. The presence of trigger points is often associated with the report of poorly localized pain, aching, or even numbness in muscles, joints, or subcutaneous tissues. This pain and discomfort can be distant from the trigger point but in the common referral area of the trigger point, which differentiates it from numbness or prickling pain often associated with nerve entrapment.

Trigger points, whether latent or active, result in dysfunction. Muscles containing trigger points are prevented from reaching their full stretch length and are therefore restricted in strength and endurance. Muscles containing trigger points tend to fatigue more quickly and are more likely to be painful when stressed.

physiopathologic reflex arc

is a self-perpetuating dysfunctional neurologic circuit.

Trigger points are associated with dysfunctional neurologic reflex circuits. A **physiopathologic reflex arc** is a self-perpetuating neurologic phenomenon that not only affects the muscle where the trigger point is located but also has referred effects on tissues supplied by associated nerves of both the peripheral

MAJOR TRIGGER POINTS AND THEIR REFERRAL AREAS OF THE NECK AND UPPER BACK

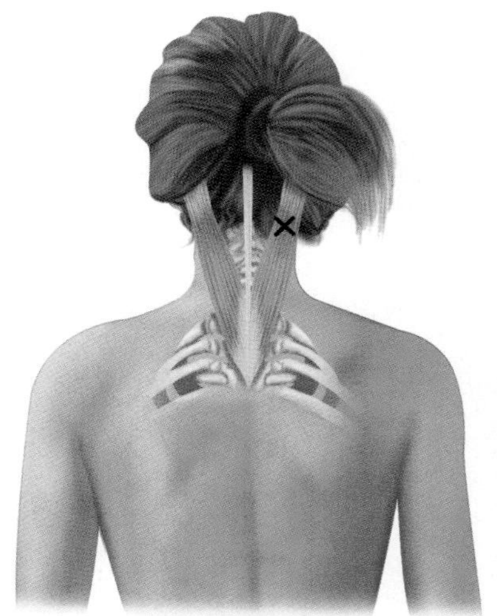

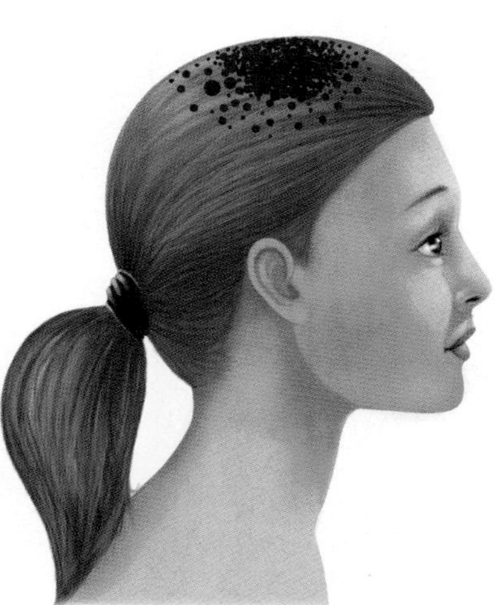

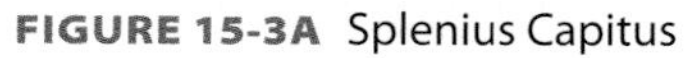

FIGURE 15-3A Splenius Capitus

FIGURE 15-3C Levator Scapulae

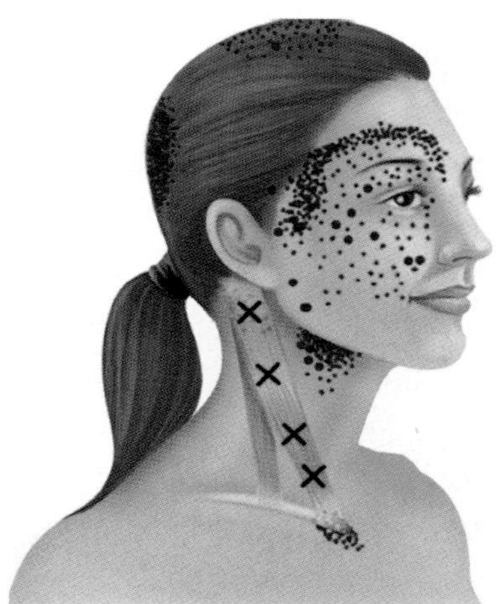

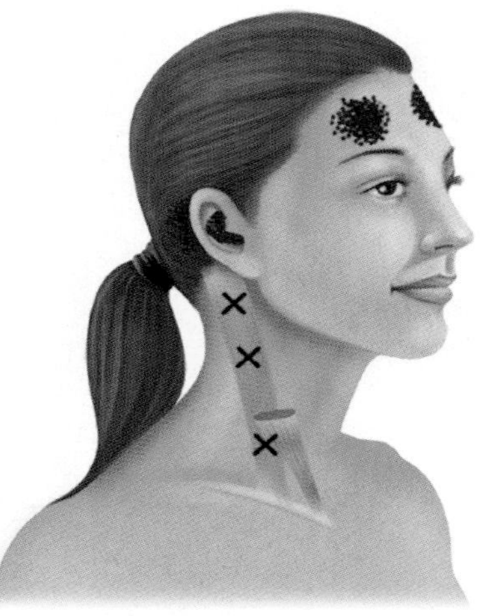

FIGURE 15-3B Sternocleidomasoid 1 and 2

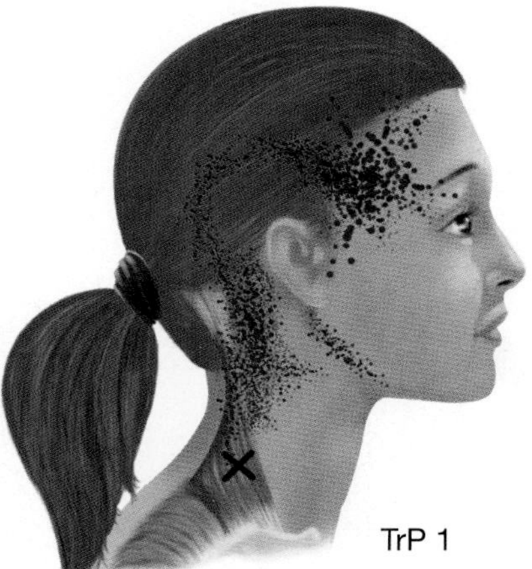

FIGURE 15-3D Trapezius 1

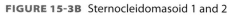

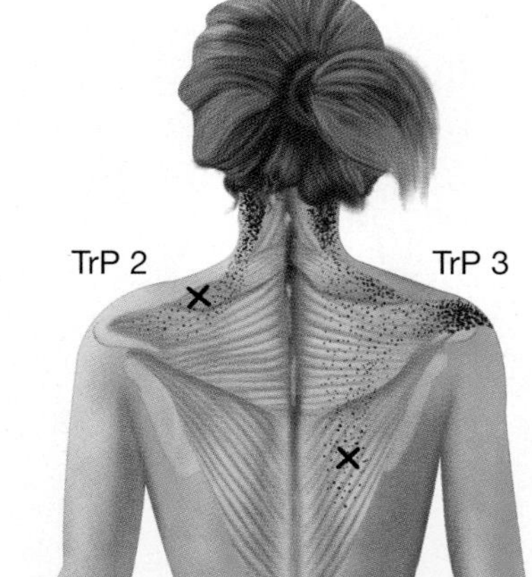

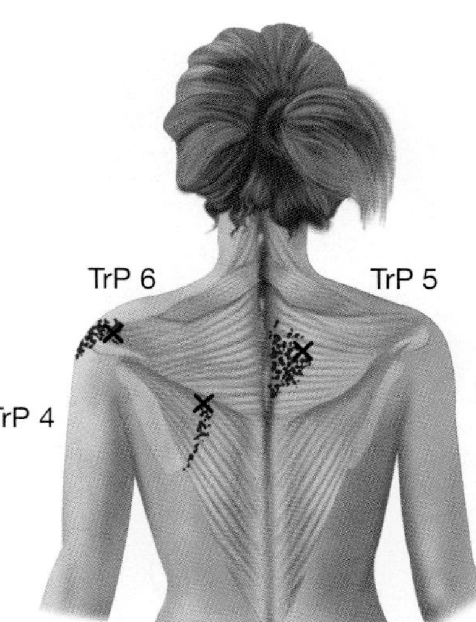

FIGURE 15-3E Trapezius 2

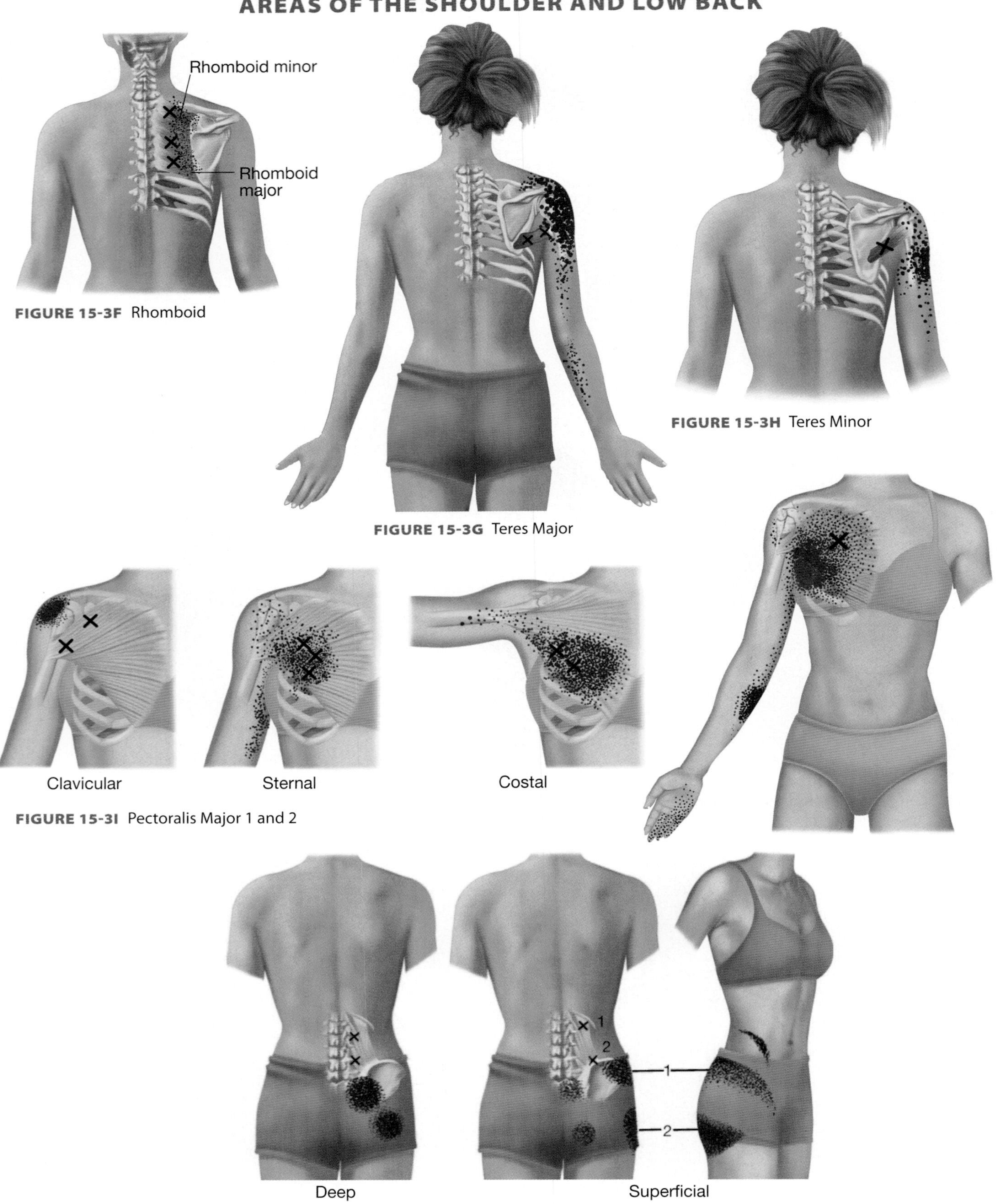

FIGURE 15-3F Rhomboid

FIGURE 15-3G Teres Major

FIGURE 15-3H Teres Minor

FIGURE 15-3I Pectoralis Major 1 and 2

FIGURE 15-3J Quadratus Lumborum

MAJOR TRIGGER POINTS AND THEIR REFERRAL AREAS OF THE PELVIS

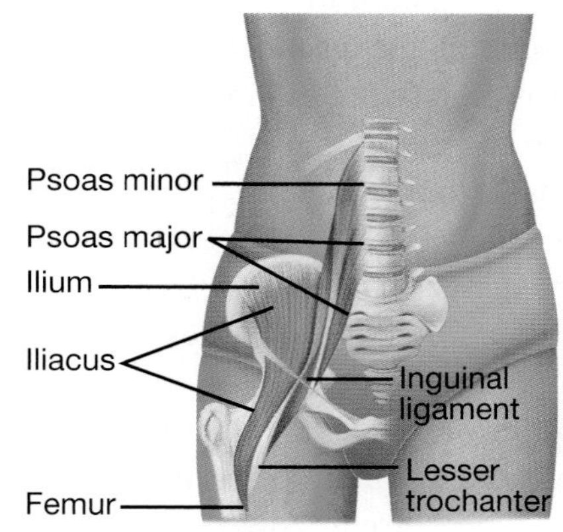

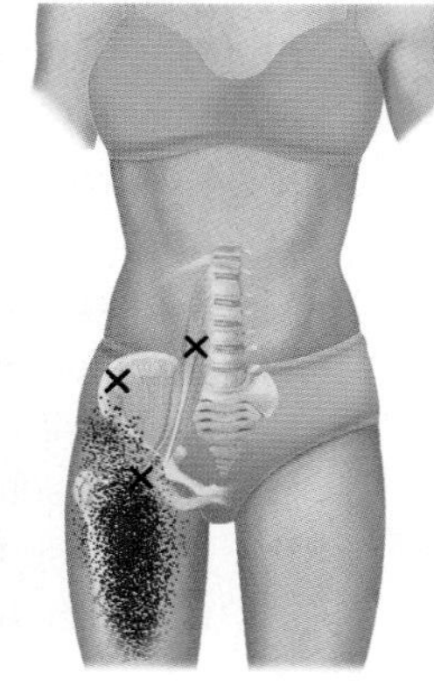
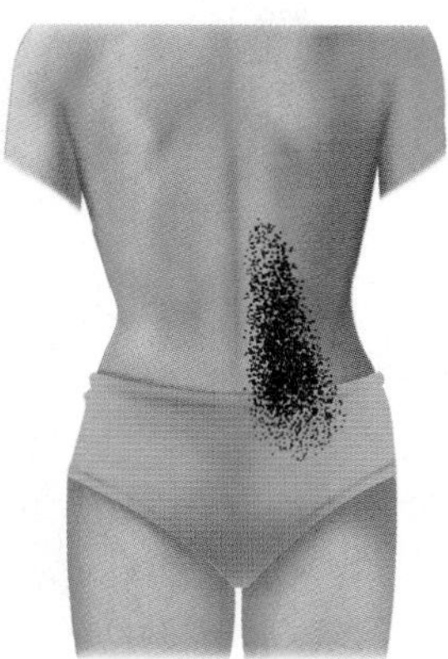

FIGURE 15-3K Iliopsoas

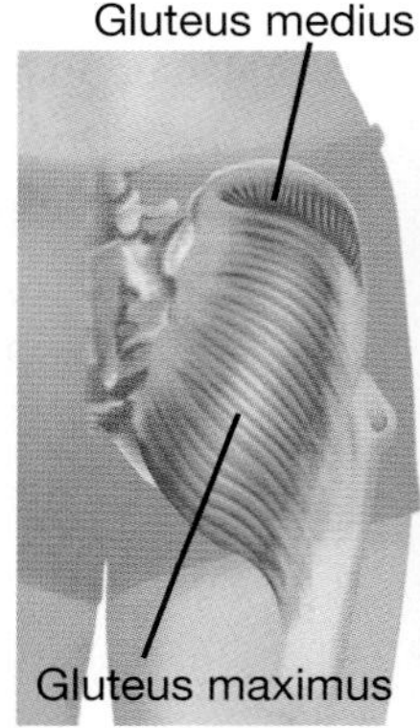

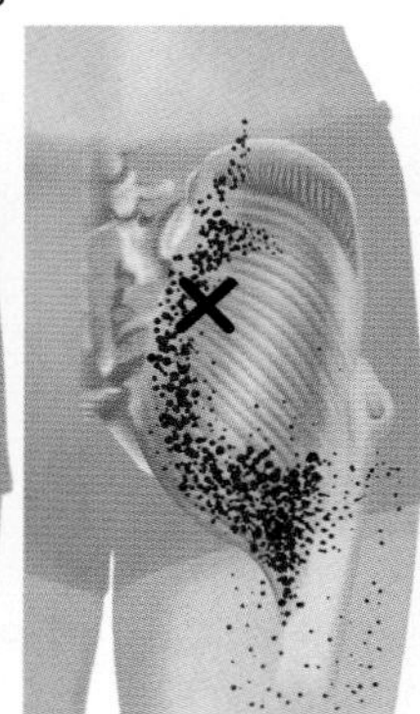
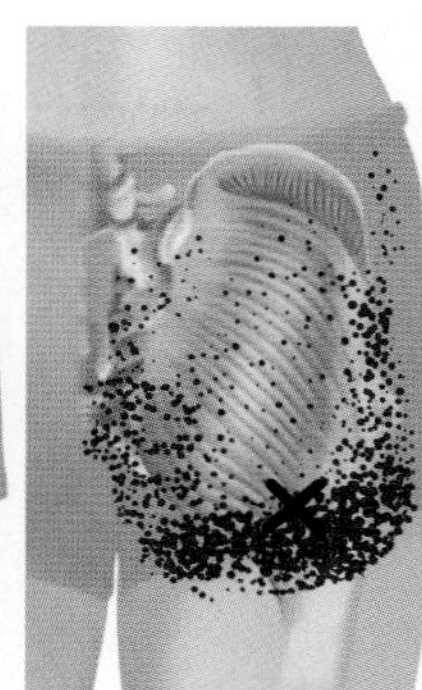
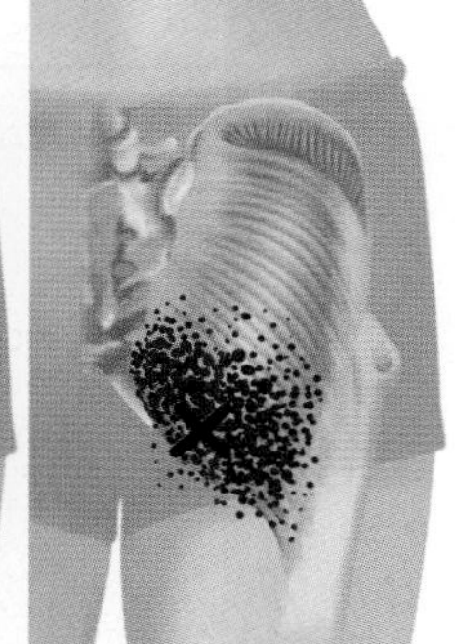

FIGURE 15-3L Gluteus Maximus

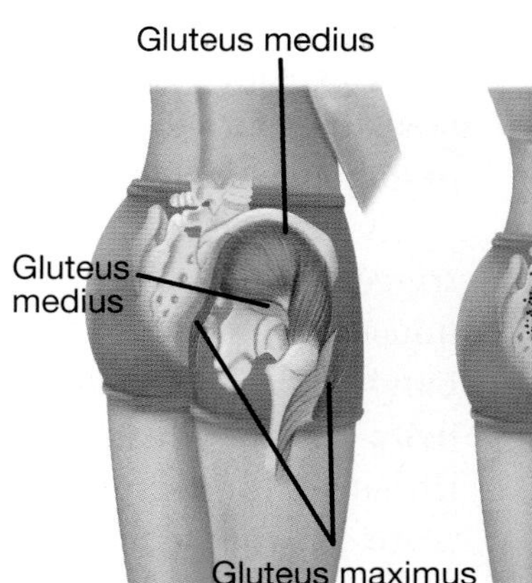

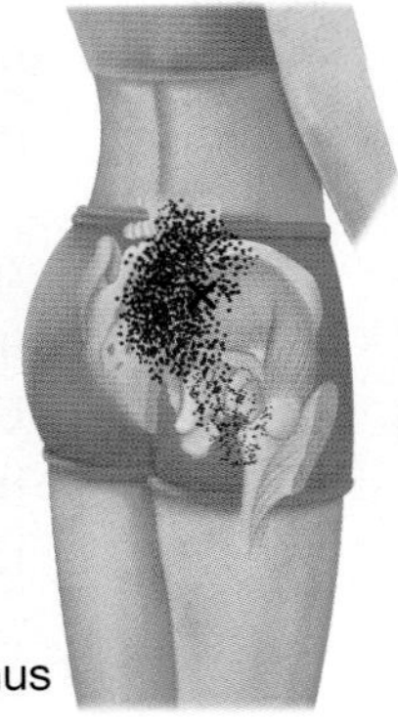

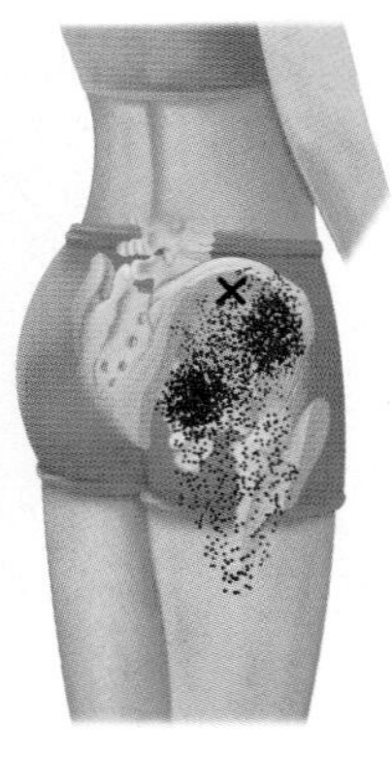

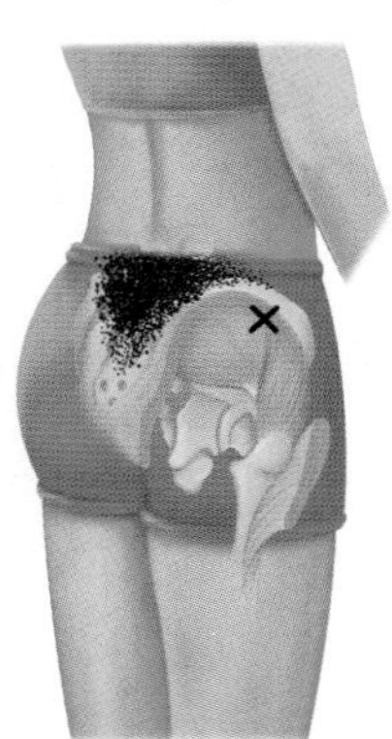

FIGURE 15-3M Gluteus Medius

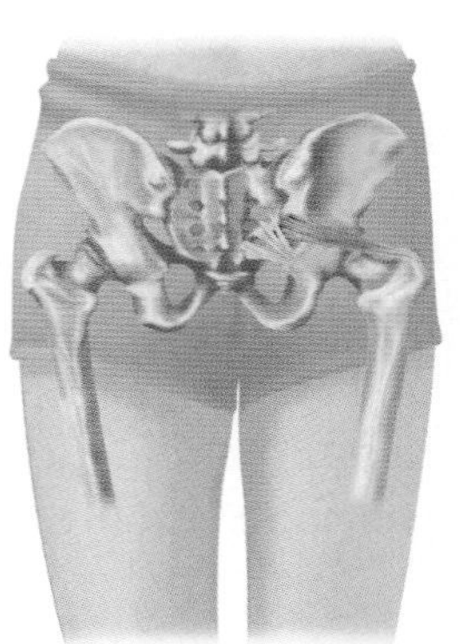
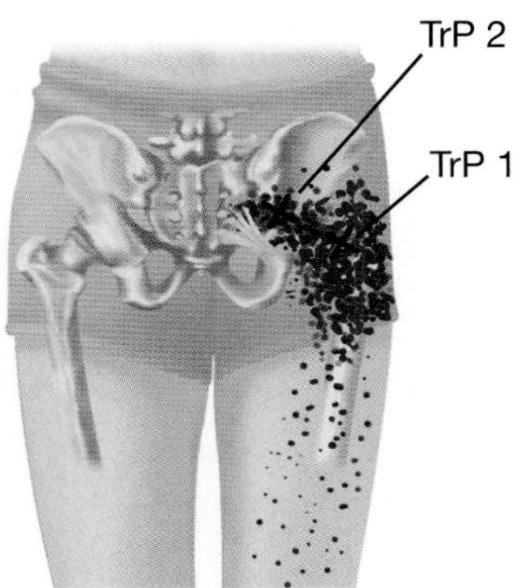

FIGURE 15-3N Piriformis

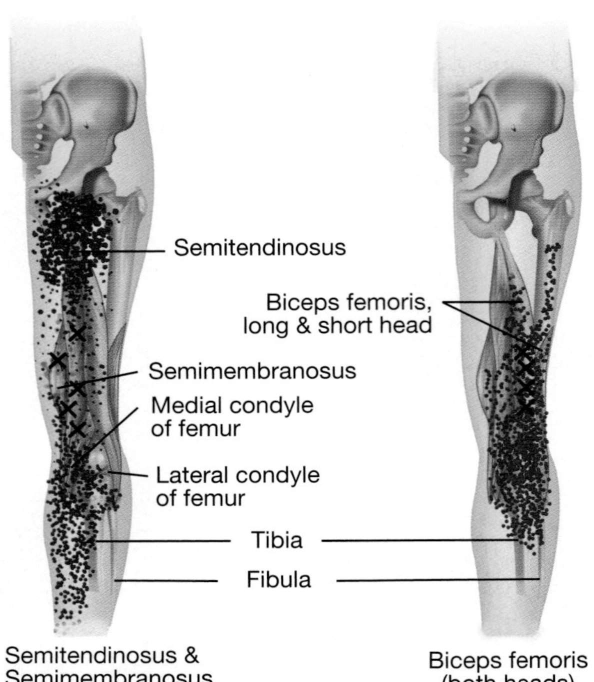

FIGURE 15-3O Hamstrings

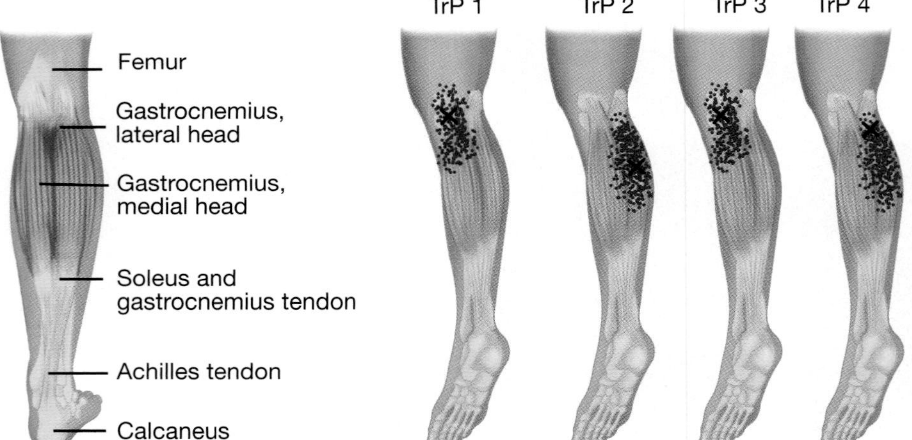

FIGURE 15-3P Gastrocnemius

and autonomic nervous system. In other words, a trigger point is more than a tender nodule: a trigger point is an indication of physiologic dysfunction. The trigger point can be reflexively related to any of the following:

- Contracture in the muscle
- Increased muscle tonus
- Constriction and hypersensitivity in the skin in local or referred areas
- Increased pressure in the joints associated with the muscle
- Decreased activity in visceral organs associated through depressed autonomic nerve activity
- Constriction in local circulation resulting from hypertonus and constriction in the muscle
- Vasoconstriction in referred areas from effects in the autonomic nervous system
- Development of satellite and associated trigger points owing to compensation from the effects of the primary trigger point

Research and practice indicate that deactivating the trigger point reflexively improves the function of the associated referred phenomena. When an active trigger point is successfully quieted, the referred pain and dysfunction decrease.

A central myofascial trigger point is centrally housed in a palpable taut band of myofibrils in the belly of the muscle, at the site of the motor endplate of the associated nerve. According to Travell and Simons, dysfunction at the motor endplate sets the conditions for continued contraction of the section of the muscle fiber close to the endplate, forming the nodule. Contraction of the sarcomeres in the area of the endplate causes tension throughout the muscle fibers, resulting in the palpable taut band. Continuous tension of the taut band on the connective tissue attachment sites sets up conditions to produce attachment trigger points at the musculotendinous or tendinoperiosteal junction of the muscle. Releasing the central trigger point usually results in release or reduction of the attachment trigger points. Locating and deactivating trigger points are valuable for reducing pain and improving function in the location of the trigger point and in the referral areas.

Trigger point Endplate Theory

Because of strain, overuse, or trauma, calcium is released from the nerve endplate at the neuromuscular junction, initiating the release of the neurotransmitter acetylcholine (ACH). ACH causes the actin and myosin filaments to slide together at the site of the motor nerve endplate, causing a contracture. (It is considered a *contracture* rather than a *contraction* because there is no impulse from the nervous system.) The contracture interferes with local circulation, causing ischemia and a reduction in the available adenosine triphosphate (ATP), which is needed to remove the calcium, creating a local energy crisis and a perpetuating cycle. The actin and myosin slide together (which is a weakened state) at the site of the motor nerve endplate, forming a palpable nodule characteristic of trigger points. The motor endplate is generally located in the middle of the muscle fiber. As the sacromeres in the middle of the fiber contract, forming the nodule, the remaining sacromeres of the fiber are stretched forming a taut band, also a characteristic of trigger points.

Central trigger points form at the center of the muscle fiber and are usually associated with the motor nerve endplate. Attachment trigger points form at the myotendonous or the tendinoperiosteal junction of the fibers that house the central trigger point owing to the tension created by the stretched muscle fibers that provokes inflammation and fibrosis. Deactivation of the central trigger points usually quiets or eliminates the attachment trigger points.

By definition, when pressure is applied to them, trigger points exhibit referred pain or other sensations to a target zone that are often recognized by the client. Both central and attachment trigger points have this capability. Target zones or referral areas for many common trigger points are quite predictable and have been documented by various researchers. There are various charts available

Criteria for Recognizing Trigger Points

1. A taut, palpable band in the muscle
2. An exquisitely tender nodule located in the taut band
3. Pressure applied to the nodule provokes pain, numbness, tingling, or other sensations to be referred in a pattern recognized by the client.
4. There is a reduced limit to the range of motion of the tissue housing the trigger point.

that show referral areas for many of the common trigger points. (Figure 15-3a-r) These are helpful if a client presents with a particular pain pattern to help locate the associated trigger point. (Travell & Simons *Myofascial Pain and Dysfunction*, Vols. I and II). Trigger points can form in any muscle and have also been noted in other tissues such as fascia, ligaments, and the skin. They can exhibit varying referral patterns. Regardless of where they are found, effectively deactivating the trigger points reduces the associated pain and improves the function of the tissue in which they reside.

Trigger points usually become active either after a clearly identifiable event or movement or as the result of prolonged and repetitive activity. To treat trigger points effectively, it is necessary to deactivate the point and change or eliminate the activity that activated it.

In the case of an acute, single-incident onset, the client usually can describe the activity that initiated the pain: an accident, a fall, or injury such as a fracture, sprain, or trauma to the tissue. After the initial healing of the tissues, the deactivation of the related trigger points should be fairly straightforward. Because the trigger points were a result of a single incident, the chance of their recurrence is quite small.

Trigger points with a gradual onset are often the result of chronic overload to a muscle, and identifying the cause might be more difficult. If the activity or conditions that initiated the trigger point are not identified and altered, treatment of the symptoms provides only temporary relief. Trigger points with a gradual onset can result from poor postural habits, improper ergonomic positions at work, emotional issues, visceral conditions, or other hidden causes. The client is encouraged to pay close attention to situations that aggravate or intensify the pain to try to identify and modify any perpetuating activities. Without eliminating or altering the perpetuating factors creating the trigger point activity, any attempt to inactivate the trigger point will be short-lived and rather futile.

Palpating for Trigger Points

Palpation skills are essential when working with trigger points and trigger point release techniques. Through palpation, the therapist recognizes variations in tissue texture and can differentiate between normal soft tissue; constricted, hypertonic tissue; fibrotic tissue; taut bands in muscle; and the congested, hyperirritable nodules associated with myofascial trigger points (Figure 15-4a). Palpatory skills also come into play when monitoring the tender points during and after position release or trigger point pressure treatment.

When assessment findings indicate a limitation in range of motion, constricted movement, or myofascial pain in a referral area, trigger point activity can be verified by palpating the suspect muscle tissue. Palpation is done with the fingertips or thumb. **Flat palpation** is done either in line with or perpendicularly across the fibers of the muscle tissue (Figure 15-4b). Enough pressure is applied to engage and feel the muscle tissue through the skin and either glide along or across the fibers. The skin and subcutaneous tissue are moved over the fibrous muscle tissue to detect ropey, fibrous, or flaccid conditions beneath. A hypersensitive nodule might be encountered while gliding along parallel to the muscle fibers.

flat palpation
is done with the fingertips or thumb either in line with or perpendicularly across the fibers of the muscle tissue.

Pincer palpation can be employed in areas where the muscle tissue can be picked up between the thumb and fingers of the same hand (e.g., sternocleidomastoid muscle). The belly of the muscle is rolled between the thumb and fingers in search of taut bands, fibrotic tissue, or sensitive nodules (Figure 15-4c).

Palpation is done with the suspect muscle in a slightly elongated position. In this position, the muscle fibers are not stretched, but any taut bands can be more easily identified. The taut band is located by palpating across the muscle. A palpable band is apparent to the sensitive fingers. When a taut band is identified, the therapist explores the length of it to locate a nodule or hypersensitive spot, which identifies the trigger point. If the client reports pain, discomfort, or other sensations referred to another area when the point is compressed, it is confirmed as an active trigger point. The area of referred pain might be a recognized reproduction of the client's symptomatic pain. If a hypersensitive nodule is found that does not produce a referral pattern on mild compression (deeper compression might produce a referral pattern), it is considered a latent trigger point. Central trigger points are generally palpated near the middle of the taut band. There can also be trigger points near the ends of the taut band or at the attachment of the muscle to the bone. Attachment trigger points form as a result of continuous tension because of the contraction of the fibers in the taut band associated with the central trigger point. These attachment trigger points often disappear when the central trigger point is deactivated. Active trigger points become a priority for inactivating, but latent trigger points and attachment trigger points should still be addressed during the treatment.

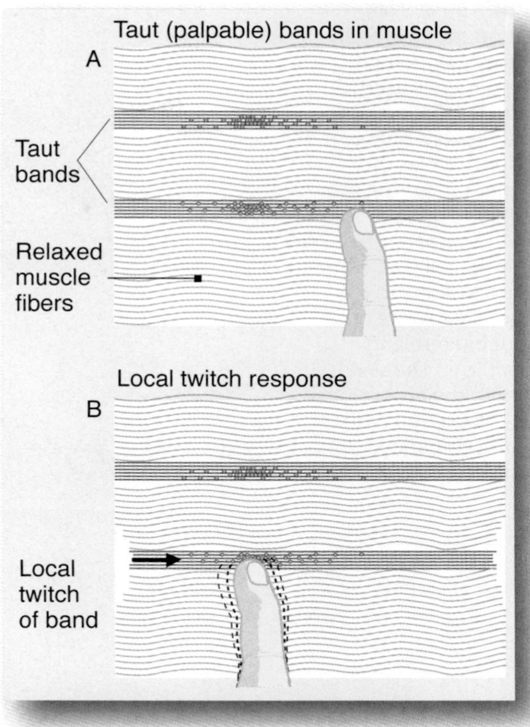

FIGURE 15-4A Taut bands, myofascial trigger points, and a local twitch response seen in a longitudinal view of the muscle. (a) Palpation of a taut band (*straight lines*) among normally slack, relaxed muscle fibers (*wavy lines*). The density of stippling corresponds to the degree of tenderness of the taut band pressure. The trigger point is the most tender spot in the band. (b) Rolling the band quickly under the fingertip (snapping palpation) at the trigger point often produces a local twitch response that is most clearly seen toward the end of the muscle, close to its attachment.

pincer palpation

is employed in areas where the muscle tissue can be picked up between the thumb and fingers of the same hand (e.g., sternocleidomastoid muscle), where the belly of the muscle is rolled between the thumb and fingers.

Deactivating Trigger Points

According to Travell and Simons, there are several ways to address and deactivate trigger points and by so doing reduce myofascial pain and increase the neuromusculoskeletal function of the client. Although several of these methods are outside the scope of practice of massage therapy, other very effective treatment modalities are well within the scope of soft tissue manipulation. The following section lists possible modalities that are divided as in or out of the scope of a massage therapist.

TP Deactivation Techniques That Are Outside the Scope of Practice of Massage Therapy

Injection of an agent into the trigger point. Common agents including procaine, lidocaine, or a saline solution are injected into the trigger point with a syringe.

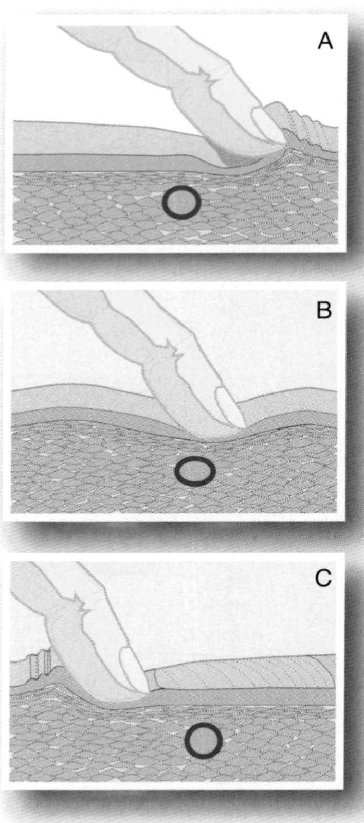

FIGURE 15-4B Flat palpation of a taut band and its trigger point. Flat palpation is used for muscles that are accessible from only one direction, such as the infraspinatus. (a) The skin is pushed to one side to begin the palpation. (b) A fingertip is slid across the muscle fibers to feel the cordlike texture of the taut band rolling beneath it. (c) The skin is pushed to the other side at the completion of the snapping palpation.

This practice falls outside the scope of practice of the massage therapist.

Dry needling or acupuncture into the trigger point is done with an acupuncture needle. This practice also falls outside the scope of practice of the massage therapist.

TP Deactivation Techniques That Are Within the Scope of Practice of Massage Therapy

Spray-and-stretch techniques use a vapocoolant spray applied over the trigger point and associated muscle, followed by stretching the involved muscle. Cool-and-stretch techniques use ice applied with a stroking movement over the trigger point and muscle, followed by stretching the involved muscle.

Travell and Simons found spray-and-stretch techniques to be some of the most effective at relieving trigger point activity (p. 128, Vol. 1). Unfortunately, the products originally used to spray as a vapocoolant either contained environmentally damaging fluorocarbons, in the case of Fluori-Methane, or are unavailable or are too volatile for safe use, as in the case of ethyl chloride. More recently, two new products have emerged on the market, which are non-ozone depleting and nonflammable. *Spray and Stretch* by Gebauer and *Instant Ice* are vapocoolants that can be safely used for spray-and-stretch techniques. Ice has been used as a substitute but with somewhat less effective results.

The coolant is applied in parallel lines over the muscle in the direction toward the referral area. The coolant is applied at the rate of about 4 cm/sec in parallel lines that barely overlap. As the coolant is applied, the underlying muscle is

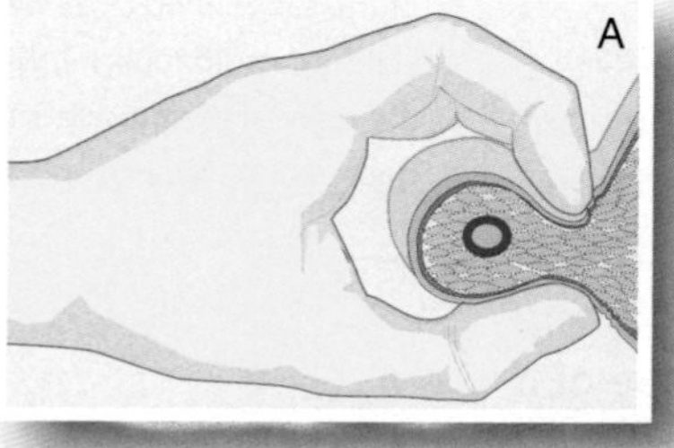

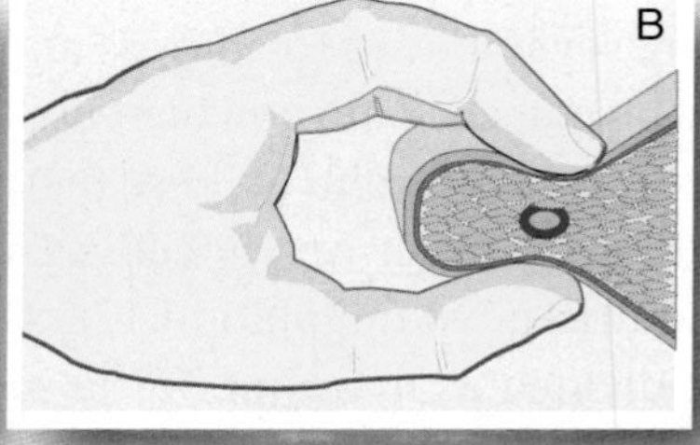

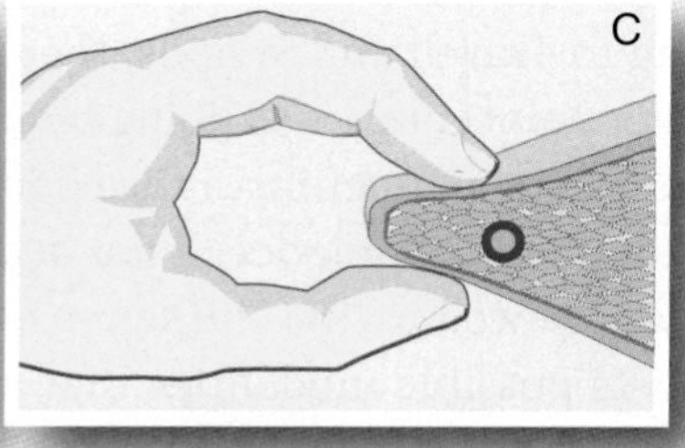

FIGURE 15-4C Pincer palpation of a taut band at a trigger point. Pincer palpation is used for muscles that can be picked up between the digits, such as the sternocleidomastoid, pectoralis major, and latissimus dorsi. (a) The muscle fibers surrounded by the thumb and fingers are shown in a pincer grip. (b) The hardness of a taut band is felt clearly as it is rolled between the digits. The change in the angle of the distal phalanges produces a rocky motion that improves discrimination of the fine detail. (c) The edge of the taut band is sharply defined as it escapes from between the fingertips, often with a local twitch response.

passively stretched to take up any slack. A maximum of two to three passes over each area is enough to cool the surface but not the underlying muscle. Cooling the surface acts as a distraction, suppresses the pain, and allows for a relaxation and gentle stretching of the affected muscle fibers. (For more detailed discussion, refer to *Myofascial Pain and Dysfunction,* Vols. 1 and 2.)

Ischemic compression or **trigger point pressure release** with gentle stretching, **position release**, and **muscle energy technique** are three therapeutic modalities available to the massage therapist to reduce trigger point activity and restore muscle and fascia to a more normal, pain-free, functional length. These three methods can be combined to address and release trigger points very effectively.

ischemic compression involves digital pressure directly into a trigger point.

position release is a method of passively moving the body or body part toward the body's preference and away from pain, seeking the tissue's preferred position. Movements are toward ease and away from bind, away from any restrictive barrier and toward comfort.

muscle energy technique uses active muscle contraction, relaxation and passive stretching to reduce constrictions in muscle and increase ROM of associated joints.

Trigger Point Pressure Release

Trigger point pressure release or ischemic compression involves digital pressure directly into the trigger point. Ischemic compression was popularized by Bonnie Prudden and is used extensively in the practice of Myotherapy and NMT. The idea is that pressure on a point causes hypoxia or a lack of oxygen, therefore the term *ischemic.* When the pressure is released, fluids return to the area. Deep pressure is usually applied with the thumb, or sometimes with the elbow, to a specific trigger point. The pressure must be deep enough and held long enough to deactivate the trigger point. Too much pressure causes the client to react by tightening muscles in a protective response that defeats the purpose of the treatment. Pressure on a trigger point will cause pain, and the deeper the pressure, the more intense the pain. The amount of pressure must be regulated to stay within the tolerance of the individual client. Pressure is increased until the client begins to elicit a pain reaction. As the pressure is maintained, the pain intensity usually decreases. As this happens, the pressure can be increased to maintain the level of intensity. When the point has been inactivated, the pain level is greatly reduced.

Paul St. John, in the St. John Method of NMT, suggests applying enough pressure to a hypersensitive nodule to cause mild discomfort for 8 to 12 seconds, during which time the discomfort should diminish.

Travell and Simons suggest applying digital pressure to a trigger point until a restrictive barrier is approached. The pressure is enough to cause a noticeable discomfort, but not pain. The pressure is maintained until the therapist notices a release of tension in the tissues (5 to 30 seconds), at which time the pressure is released and repeated at a somewhat deeper pressure, again deep enough to engage the restrictive barrier. If there is no noticeable change after about 30 seconds, the therapist reassesses the area for trigger point activity.

Neuromuscular Therapy to Release Trigger Points

Neuromuscular treatment of trigger points varies for central and attachment trigger points. To locate and treat central and attachment trigger points, the practitioner must have a clear understanding of muscle anatomy, including muscle fiber arrangement, attachment sites, and tendon arrangement of the target tissues (Figure 15-5). Because central trigger points are located in the middle of the muscle fiber, knowing fiber arrangement is essential for determining how and where effective treatment is conducted.

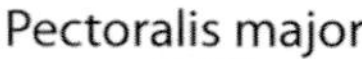
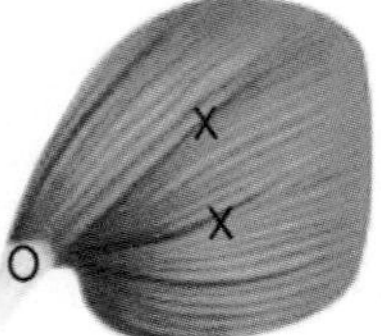

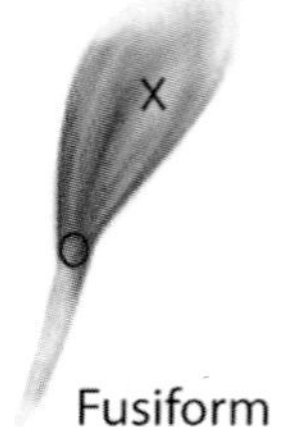

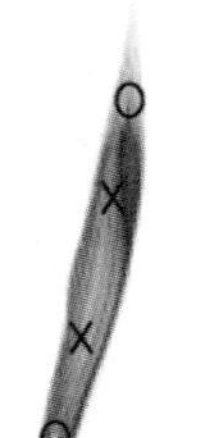

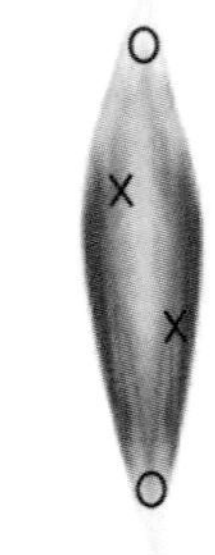

FIGURE 15-5 The location of central trigger points (X) is in the middle of the muscle fiber, which is determined by the muscle type. Attachment triggerpoints (O) are located at the myotendonous junction.

Ischemia around central trigger points is addressed with repeated effleurage or gliding strokes to increase circulation to and flush out the area. Trigger point pressure release is applied to the site of the central trigger point repeatedly. Pressure is held on the point for 8 to 12 seconds, then released for 3 to 5 seconds, and then repeated. Trigger point pressure release is followed by short gliding strokes or J-strokes applied from the center of the fiber toward the attachment or the myotendonous junction to elongate the fiber gently, lengthening the shortened sacromeres at the center of the fiber and reducing the tension in the taut band without putting any added tension on the muscle attachment. Passive or active stretching (muscle energy technique) can also be used in an attempt to return the muscle to its normal resting length. Failure to return the muscle to a relaxed, full resting length increases the chance that the trigger point will reactivate.

When trigger point pressure release or ischemic compression techniques are used to deactivate trigger points, the appropriate amount of pressure varies according to the sensitivity of the client, the area of the body, and the condition of the trigger point. It is essential to communicate clearly with the client to determine the appropriate pressure. Create a subjective pain scale so that the client can give instant feedback and be actively involved in the process. Using a 1-to-10 scale of discomfort, in which 1 is no discomfort and 10 is extremely painful, 5-6-7 is optimal for attaining good results. When the trigger point is located, gently apply pressure into the point until the client indicates a mild to moderate discomfort (5-7 on the pain scale). Maintain the pressure for 8 to 12 seconds or until the point dissipates, then release the pressure for 3 to 5 seconds and reapply the pressure to a depth that the client indicates is a discomfort rating of 5 to 7. Many times the amount of pressure tolerated by the client increases on subsequent applications of pressure as the trigger point deactivates. Repeating the application of pressure for 8 to 12 seconds several times is more effective that sustaining the pressure for 60 seconds or more, because every time the pressure is released, blood and other fluids flood into the area, nourishing the tissues, resolving the energy crisis, and providing oxygen and ATP to release the contracture.

Position Release to Inactivate Trigger Points

Position release techniques are very effective for inactivating trigger points and releasing the taut bands that house them. (Read more about position release techniques on pages 571-578.) Both central trigger points and attachment trigger points respond well to position release and can be used effectively as monitor points to find a preferred position. A working knowledge of muscle action and attachments is crucial to use position release techniques effectively when addressing trigger points. When a trigger point is identified, knowing which muscle it is in, the orientation of the muscle fibers, and attachment sites and action of the muscle all play an important role in successfully positioning the muscle and deactivating the trigger point.

Finding the release position involves passively moving the joint in the same direction that the involved muscle would if it were to contract. In effect, this moves the ends of the taut band toward the trigger point. The precise position can include dynamic movement in all planes (i.e., flexion or extension, adduction or abduction, side bending, and internal or external rotation). Usually the preferred position is in the midrange of the muscle's range of motion.

The indicator for the correct position is a change in the trigger point. Trigger points can be palpated as nodules that are hypersensitive; they are especially sensitive when digital pressure is applied to them. When a position for release is achieved, the sensitivity in the associated trigger point diminishes by 70 to 100 percent, and the palpable nodule softens and often disappears.

Besides monitoring palpable changes in the trigger point, feedback from the client is essential when finding the preferred position. Chaitow suggests using a pain scale in which an amount of pressure is applied to the trigger point and the client is instructed to rate that amount of discomfort as a 10 on the scale. The therapist maintains the same amount of pressure on the point and begins moving the joint in positions to approximate the ends of the muscle's fibers while asking the client to rate the discomfort at the palpated point. When the client reports a discomfort level of 3, 2, or less, and the palpable point has diminished, that is a good indication that a preferred position has been found.

After the preferred position is achieved, Jones and Chaitow suggest holding the position for 60 to 90 seconds and then very slowly and passively returning the joint to a neutral position, rechecking the trigger point, and looking for other associated points.

It is the author's experience after years of practice that after the preferred position is achieved, a slight compression into the joint from the approximate muscle attachments should be incorporated. The compression is only enough to engage the nerve receptors in the joint, approximately 5 to 7 lbs of pressure. It is theorized that feedback from these receptors as well as the proprioceptors of the muscle activate, reorganize, and normalize after the muscle fibers are shortened and stress is removed.

While the position is held, the therapist is encouraged to continue monitoring the trigger point area with a light touch to note any changes. Common palpable signs are what feels like an unraveling at the point, and very often a pulse is noted, an indication that circulation is flowing back into the area. After holding the position for up to 90 seconds, or for 10 seconds after a pulse is noted in the monitor point, gently release the compression, and passively and very slowly, without any help from the client, return the body part to a neutral resting position. Again, it is important to release the position slowly and to return the joint to a neutral position slowly. Recheck the alarm point and other related points, such as synergist and antagonist muscles.

Restoring the Muscle to Its Resting Length

Regardless of the technique used, after the trigger point is inactivated, the muscle that housed the trigger point must be restored to a normal resting length. If the muscle is not restored to its normal resting length, its function will be reduced, and the chance of the trigger points returning is increased. Gentle stretching can be used to restore the muscle to its functional length; however, there is a chance of re-traumatizing the tissue. A preferred technique would be MET using the antagonist. (Read more about MET later in this chapter.) When applying MET using the antagonist, move the joint that the muscle containing the trigger point acts on so that the muscle is lengthened until it approaches its resistive barrier. The practitioner supports the joint or limb in that position and instructs the client to inhale as she continues the movement with about a 20 percent effort. The practitioner matches the client's effort, thereby allowing no movement for about 7 to 10 seconds, at which time the client is instructed to relax and exhale. As the client exhales, the joint is moved, and the muscle is lengthened to its new resistive barrier. This process is repeated until there is no increase in muscle length. Caution must be exercised not to overstretch the muscle and possibly re-traumatize the sensitive muscle tissues.

Combining Techniques to Inactivate Trigger Points

Trigger points are effectively inactivated by combining these various techniques:

1. A trigger point is identified through assessment and palpation.
2. Trigger point pressure release is applied for 8 to 10 seconds, left off for 3 to 5 seconds, and repeated several times.
3. Pressure is applied to the point to elicit a pain response from the client. The client is asked to rate the pain as a 10, and position release is applied, positioning the joint so that the ends of the taut band move into closer approximation until the pain sensation has reduced to a 2 or less. The position is held for 60 to 90 seconds, then slowly returned to a neutral position.
4. MET using the antagonist is employed to help to restore the muscle to its normal resting length.

MUSCLE ENERGY TECHNIQUE

Muscle energy technique (MET) is a soft tissue mobilization technique that was developed in the osteopathic profession. Elements of MET have been documented and described for many years using different terminology. Kabat, Knott, and Voss developed techniques in the 1940s and 1950s called *proprioceptive neuromuscular facilitation* that used many of the same physiologic mechanisms. Dr. T. J. Ruddy developed a technique he called *resistive duction,* in which the therapist resisted multiple rapid small muscle contractions of the client, which was meant to increase blood flow and strengthen muscles. Fred Mitchell Sr., DO, is given credit for the development of modern muscle energy technique. He developed the techniques in the 1940s and 1950s, publishing his work in the yearbook of the American Academy of Osteopathy in 1958.

MET is a valuable tool when addressing soft tissue conditions that involve tense or shortened muscles. Muscle spasms are effectively quieted, and joint mobility can be improved and lengthened, or weak antagonistic muscles can be toned. MET can be applied in several different ways, depending on the condition of the tissue and the intended response. It can be used to increase joint mobility where constricted contractile tissue restricts movement, to release hypertonic muscles, and to reduce fibrosis in chronically shortened muscles.

MET involves the active participation of the client, who is instructed to contract isolated muscles against a counterforce provided by the therapist. MET uses active muscle contraction, followed by relaxation and subsequent passive stretching, to reduce constrictions in the muscle and increase range of motion of the related joints. MET uses neurophysiologic muscle reflexes to improve functional mobility of the joints. By employing active joint movements, muscle activity that restricts movement is inhibited, allowing for better mobility.

There are two basic inhibitory reflexes that are incorporated during MET manipulations:

- **Postisometric relaxation:** Following an isometric contraction, there is a brief period of relaxation during which impulses to the muscle are inhibited.
- **Reciprocal inhibition:** When a muscle acting on a joint is contracted, the muscle responsible for the opposite action on that joint is inhibited.

postisometric relaxation

means that following an isometric contraction, there is a period of relaxation during which muscle impulses are inhibited.

reciprocal inhibition

occurs when a muscle acting on a joint contracts and the opposing muscle is reflexively inhibited.

MET involves the contraction of a muscle by the client against the resistance provided by a therapist. The direction of the contraction and the position of the muscle and the limb previous to the contraction are determined by the condition and movement restrictions of the joint and target muscle or muscle groups. Range of motion and palpation assessment techniques are used to determine the nature of the restriction and the direction of maximum limitation. Depending on the intended outcome of the treatment, the force applied by the therapist can be equal to that of the client, allowing no movement; it can be less than that of the client, allowing movement in the range of motion; or it can overcome the force of the client. Various outcomes include relaxing and lengthening hypertonic muscles, stimulating and strengthening weakened muscles, and lengthening chronically shortened fibrotic muscles.

METs have many variations, depending on the condition of the target tissue, the condition of the client, and the intended outcome of the treatment. Some variations include the following:

- The starting position
- The direction of the client's effort
- The amount of effort applied by the client
- The length of the effort
- Whether the therapist's force matches, overcomes, or is less than the client's force
- How the breath is incorporated
- Whether there is a passive, active, or no stretch after the contraction
- Whether to stretch through the barrier after a contraction
- Whether to repeat the sequence
- Whether to use MET with other techniques

MET Applications for Hypertonic Muscles

Hypertonic muscles are usually shortened, many times containing trigger points and taut bands of muscle tissue, and are often involved in joint constriction.

They can be painful and also can be the site of an acute or chronic injury. These conditions are determined during the assessment procedures. Results are improved if trigger points in the target muscles are deactivated before MET is applied.

There are three main variations of muscle energy technique that are effective in lengthening tense and shortened muscles:

- Contract relax or agonist contract
- Antagonist contract
- Contract-relax-contract the opposite

Contract Relax or Agonist Contract

contract-relax technique incorporates postisometric relaxation theory, which states that as soon as an isometric muscle contraction releases, the muscle relaxes.

The most common MET procedure used to relax constricted and hypertonic muscle involves contracting and then relaxing and lengthening the target muscle. The **contract-relax technique** incorporates the *postisometric relaxation* theory, which states that as soon as an isometric muscle contraction releases, the muscle is inhibited and relaxes.

To perform the contract-relax or agonist-contract technique (Figure 15-6 a and b):

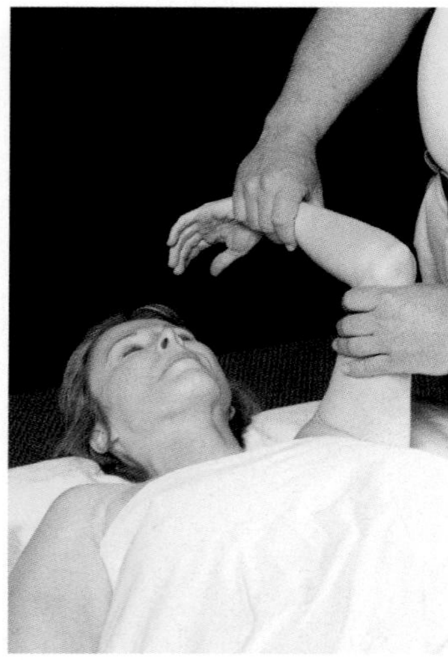

FIGURE 15-6A To perform contrast-relax or agonist-contract MET on the triceps, move the arm until the muscle approaches its resistive barrier and support it while the client contracts the muscle.

1. Position the limb so that the target muscle is in a lengthened but comfortable position. This can be done by moving the limb until the resistive barrier is engaged or to the point of resistance and then backing off slightly. (In the performance of MET, the *resistive barrier* in a joint movement is when the first resistance is met when moving a limb or joint through its normal range of motion. This resistive barrier is usually encountered before the physiologic limit of the possible joint movement. The resistive barrier is the beginning of the soft tissue constriction to the joint's flexibility.)
2. Support the limb in that position securely, ask the client to inhale, and have the client contract the target muscle isometrically against the resistance for 5 to 10 seconds. It is not necessary for the client to perform a maximal contraction. A contraction of 20 percent is adequate for this procedure. The contraction should not cause acute pain. If the contraction is painful, try the antagonist-contraction procedure discussed next.
3. After about 7 to 10 seconds, ask the client to exhale and slowly relax the contraction.
4. Ask the client to inhale and exhale again, and as she exhales, move the limb until a new resistive barrier is felt. The range of motion should increase slightly.
5. Repeat steps 1 to 4 two to five times or until there is no more increase of ROM when moving to a new barrier.

Alternatives include increasing the client's effort to up to 50 percent, and/or increasing the time of the contraction up to 20 seconds.

Antagonist Contraction

reciprocal inhibition occurs when a muscle acting on a joint contracts and the opposing muscle is reflexively inhibited.

If muscle tissues are in a subacute stage of healing, if a trigger point has just been treated, or if there is any pain when the target muscle contracts, the preferred MET technique would involve the antagonist. Antagonist contraction takes advantage of a physiologic process known as **reciprocal inhibition**. When a muscle acting on a joint contracts, the muscle that causes the opposite action is reflexively inhibited. This is the preferred MET to use after deactivating trigger points to reduce hypertonia and return shortened muscle fibers to a more normal resting length. Remember, if the procedure causes pain, *stop*. To perform the antagonist-contract technique (Figure 15-7a and b):

1. Position the limb so that the target muscle is in a lengthened but comfortable position. This can be done by moving the limb either to the middle of the range of motion or until the resistive barrier is approached, then backing off several degrees.
2. Support the limb securely in that position and instruct the client to attempt to continue the movement with only a 20 percent effort. Resist the movement for a couple of seconds, and then allow the movement to continue slowly. The contraction should not cause acute pain. If there is acute pain on both contract-relax and antagonist-contract techniques, pathologies might be present that contraindicate MET.
3. After 7 to 10 seconds, instruct the client to exhale and relax (hold the limb in the same position).
4. Ask the client to inhale and exhale again, and as she exhales, passively move the limb to its new barrier and again back off several degrees.
5. Repeat steps 2 to 4 two or three times or until there is no more improvement in the lengthening muscle and therefore no more increase in ROM before the barrier is encountered.

The amount of effort can be increased up to about 50 percent, and the length of the contractions can be increased to as much as 20 seconds.

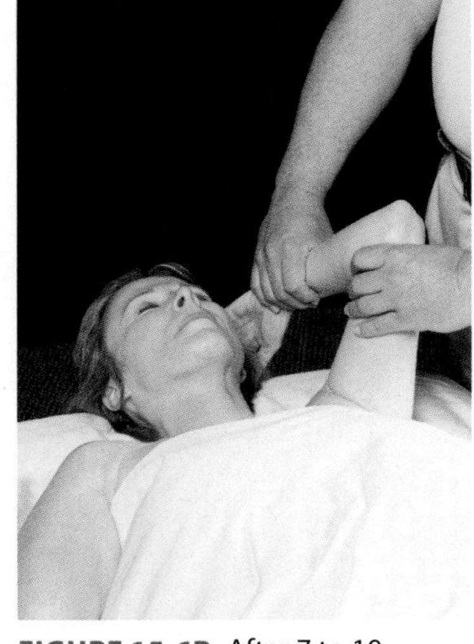

FIGURE 15-6B After 7 to 10 seconds, the client relaxes and takes a breath, and as she exhales, the therapist moves the arm to a new barrier and repeats the procedure.

Contract-Relax-Antagonist-Contract

This technique, sometimes called *contract-relax-contract the opposite*, essentially combines the two previous techniques. To perform the contract-relax-antagonist-contract technique (CRAC; Figure 15-8a-d)

1. Position the limb so that the target muscle is in a lengthened but comfortable position. This can be done by moving the limb until the resistive barrier is engaged or to the point of resistance or pain and then backing off slightly.

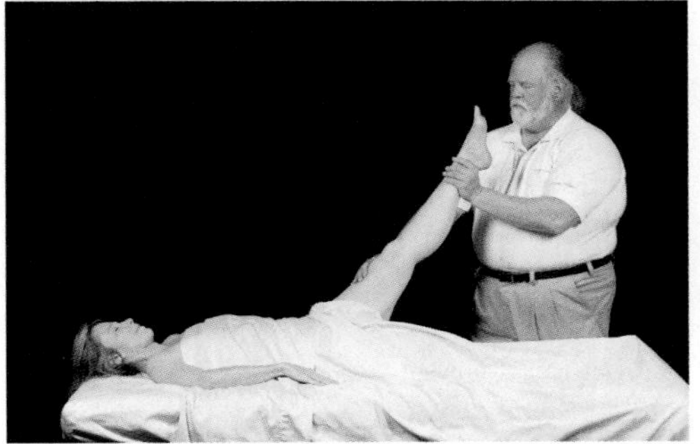

FIGURE 15-7A To perform antagonist-contract MET on the hamstrings, flex the hip with the leg extended until the restrictive barrier is felt, and then back off a few degrees. Hold the leg in that position and instruct the client to continue the movement.

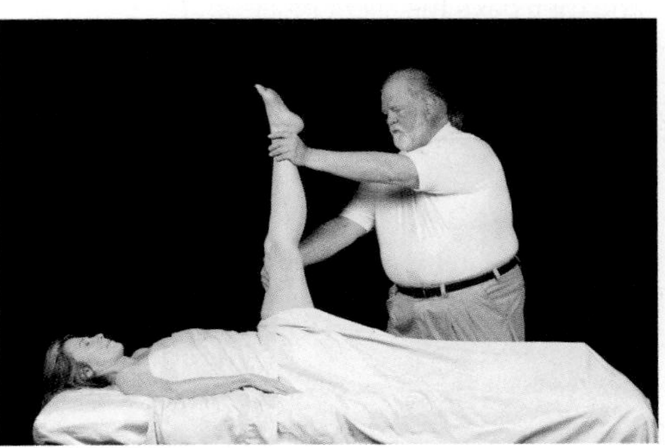

FIGURE 15-7B After 7 to 10 seconds, instruct the client to relax the contraction and inhale, and as she exhales, move the leg to a new resistive barrier. Back off from the barrier, support the leg, and repeat the procedure.

2. Support the limb in that position securely and have the client inhale and contract the target muscle isometrically against the resistance for 5 to 10 seconds.
3. Instruct the client to exhale and relax the muscle, and then contract the muscle opposite the tight muscle (the antagonist). In so doing, the client actively moves the limb in the direction of the intended stretch. The therapist can assist in the final stretch or not.
4. After a short rest, repeat the procedure.

Pulsed Contractions of the Antagonist

During the 1940s and 1950s, T. J. Ruddy, DO, developed a system of rapidly pulsed contractions against a resistance that he called *rapid rhythmic resistive duction technique*. A more simplistic, modern term is *pulsed muscle energy technique (PMET)*. Many times, when joint constriction involves a hypertonic muscle often containing trigger points, the antagonist is found to be hypotonic and inhibited. Pulsed MET is directed at the inhibited muscle to facilitate proprioceptive reeducation, increase circulation, stimulate the weakened muscle, and further inhibit the opposing hypertonic muscle (RI). According to Ruddy, the technique produces more oxygenation and better lymph and venous flow to the muscle. To practice PMET

1. Move the limb so that the hypertonic tissue is lengthened to its resistive barrier and support the body part in that position.

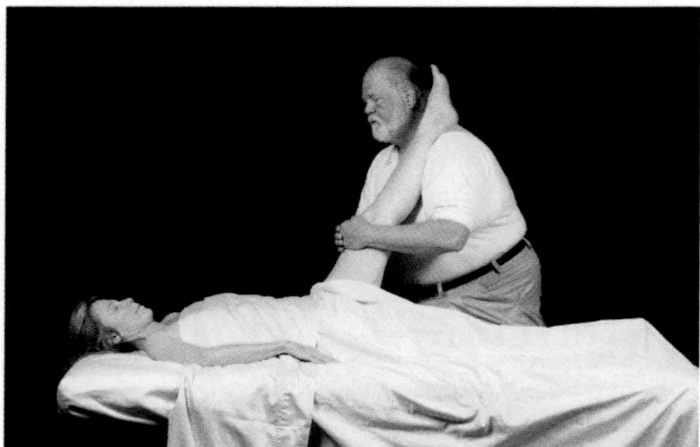

FIGURE 15-8A To perform contract-relax, contract the opposite for the hamstrings, flex the hip with the leg extended until the resistive barrier is approached, and support the leg in that position. Hold the leg in that position, and then have the client inhale and contract the target muscle for 7 to 10 seconds.

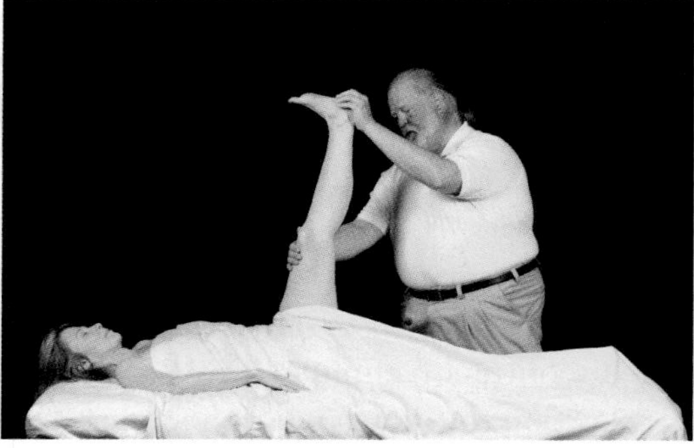

FIGURE 15-8B After 7 to 10 seconds, instruct the client to relax, exhale, and then inhale again and actively contract the quadriceps to move the leg farther toward the barrier.

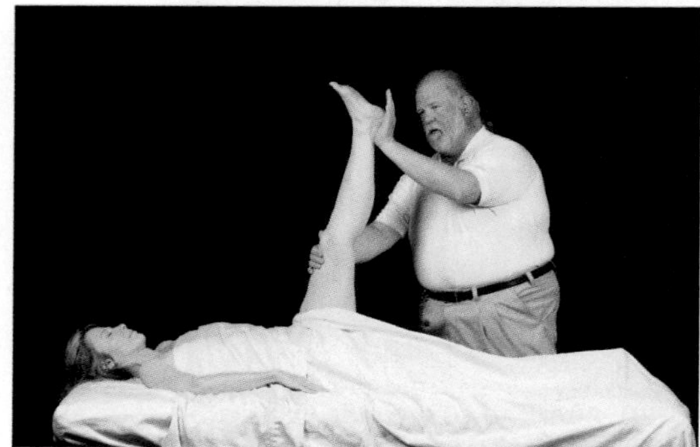

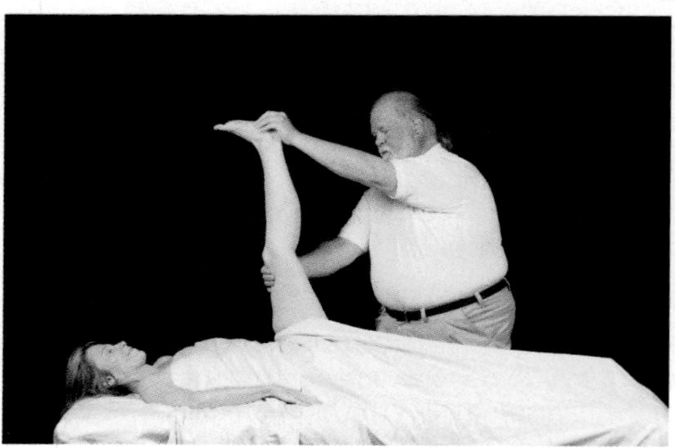

FIGURE 15-8C, D Hold the leg in the newly achieved position and repeat the procedure two to five times or until there is no more increase in range of movement.

2. Ask the client to begin a series of rapid, minute contractions toward the barrier (contracting the antagonist). The contractions are small and at a rate of about two per second. The effort is small, and in Ruddy's words, creates "no wobble or bounce."
3. Continue for about 20 contractions, rest for 10 seconds, and then repeat.

PMET is a valuable adjunct therapy to use after the constricted, hypertonic muscles have been treated directly by methods such as stretching. After the hypertonic muscles have been lengthened, stimulating and facilitating the hypotonic or weakened antagonists improves the overall function of the joint.

Essential Factors for MET Success

Several factors determine the effectiveness of MET. It is essential to identify the contractile tissue involved in the movement limitation and direct the resistance to the contraction directly toward or away from those restrictions. Generally, pathologic changes to structures of the joint other than contractile tissues do not respond to MET. The success of MET depends on the skill of the therapist in performing the following:

- Assessing the muscles involved
- Determining the direction of maximum limitation
- Determining when the joint movement is approaching its limitation
- Choosing the most appropriate, postisometric relaxation or reciprocal inhibition technique
- Instructing the client in the direction, duration, and intensity of the contraction

METs are contraindicated for acute soft tissue injuries, such as muscle strains, for at least the first 72 hours after the injury is sustained. During the acute period, the preferred treatment is designated by the acronym PRICE—protect, rest, ice, compression, and elevation.

After the initial acute period is a subacute period, when appropriate therapeutic interventions can accelerate the healing process, reduce scarring and adhesions, and apply therapeutic stresses to return the tissues to optimal function. Appropriate therapeutic interventions apply gentle stresses and cause no pain to the injured area. METs using the antagonist with other appropriate techniques such as position release techniques and cross-fiber massage are invaluable when rehabilitating soft tissue injuries.

A naturally occurring neuromuscular process known as *splinting* causes muscle fibers closely associated to the injured fibers to shorten to protect the injured area. This splinting and the associated hypertonic tissue often persist beyond the time needed for the injured tissue to heal. MET is a method that encourages those tissues to return to their normal resting length.

MET for Improving Strength

There are two other variations of MET that are valuable for toning weak muscles or reducing fibrosis in the muscle fascia.

During the course of treatment, it can be beneficial to stimulate a hypotonic muscle, tone a weakened muscle, or reeducate an injured or habitually misused muscle. There are many reasons why a muscle or muscle group might be underused, resulting in postural distortion or joint dysfunction. A form of MET that employs an isokinetic contraction helps to awaken, stimulate, and tone the muscle.

To improve tone or strengthen a weakened muscle, the client is instructed to move the limb through the full available range of motion as the therapist provides resistance directed against the target muscle. For maximum effect, movement through the full range of motion should take about 3 to 4 seconds. During the first repetition, the client uses approximately 20 percent effort, resisted by the practitioner. On subsequent repetitions, the resistance is increased until maximum resistance is achieved. The resistance is continuous during concentric and eccentric contractions. The resistance from the therapist is continuous during the entire movement. When a muscle is identified to be hypotonic, deficient, or in a weakened state, the procedure is as follows:

1. The therapist moves the target muscle and related joint passively through its range of motion to demonstrate the intended movement to the client.
2. The therapist instructs the client to move the joint through the described range of motion using about a 20 percent effort as the therapist resists the movement with a gentle resistance throughout the full range of the movement. (*Note:* The therapist's hands should be placed to isolate the target muscle during the entire range of motion. For instance, for movements of the shoulder, one of the therapist's hands should contact the distal portion of the humerus near the elbow to resist the movement while the other hand supports the client's hand during the movement or supports the shoulder to isolate the movement.)
3. The client is instructed to repeat the movement several times. Each time, the therapist increases the resistance until maximum resistance is achieved or the muscle begins to fatigue.

Rapid gains in strength are experienced with this type of exercise. The use of this technique is limited, depending on the strength of the therapist relative to the strength of the target muscle. The therapist might not be able to provide enough resistance for large muscles or muscle groups such as the hip flexors. The therapist must be aware of positioning and body mechanics to avoid injury to self or to the client.

MET for Reducing Fibrosis

Fibrosis in the muscle fascia can be the result of trauma, inflammation, strain, or aging. Fibrosis causes contractures and loss of mobility. Constriction in contractile tissues can be due to fascial sheaths gluing together with collagenous cross-hatching. NMT gliding techniques and myofascial release stretching are helpful in these conditions, as are MET isolytic techniques. A MET manipulation that can be effective in reducing fibrosis involves a resistance that overpowers a muscle contraction. As the client contracts the target muscle, the therapist provides a resistance greater than the force of the contraction and forces the muscle to lengthen (Figure 15-9a-c).

To perform isolytic MET

1. The therapist positions the associated body part so that the target muscle is in a mild stretch, near its resistive barrier.
2. The therapist supports the joint in that position and instructs the client to inhale and gradually contract the muscle to a near-maximum effort.

3. When at a maximum effort, the client is instructed to exhale and maintain the contraction as the therapist overpowers the contraction and moves the joint farther toward (but not beyond) the physiologic barrier.
4. The client is instructed to relax as the therapist releases the stretch.
5. Repeat steps 1 to 4, two or three times.

Isolytic MET can cause mild discomfort or burning, but it should not cause acute pain. When using this technique, a maximum contraction is most effective, but the client must be instructed to contract the muscle to the extent that is within the comfort level. The therapist must not use ballistic movements against the contractions. The resistance must be steady and forceful enough to overcome the client effort. The therapist must remember to use extreme caution to avoid further injury to the muscle tissue.

POSITION RELEASE

Position release techniques, also known as *passive positioning techniques*, are perhaps the gentlest of soft tissue manipulations when addressing mobility restrictions caused by pain and soft tissue dysfunction. As the name implies, passive positioning involves the gentle, passive movement of a joint into a position of maximum comfort, holding it there for an appropriate time and then very slowly returning it to its normal resting position. Position release is an indirect method of treatment, meaning the body part is moved away from the resistance barrier and toward a position of ease and comfort.

Three bodywork systems that incorporate this technique are strain-counterstrain, Ortho-Bionomy, and structural muscular balancing. Although each system uses passive positioning, each determines the appropriate position for maximum release differently and is discussed individually.

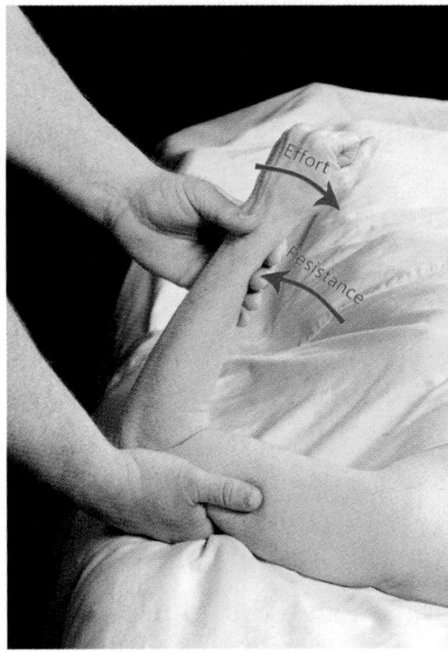

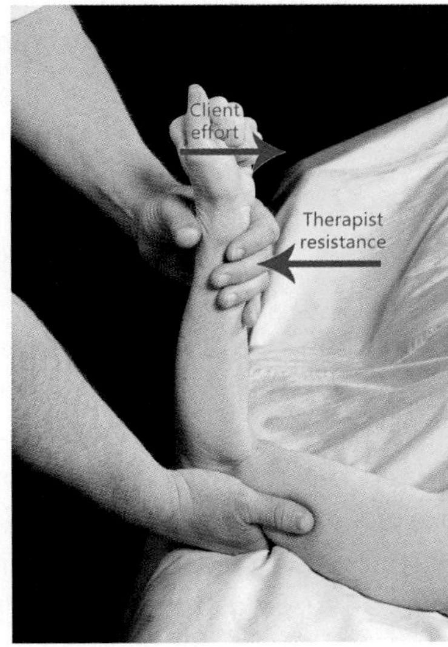

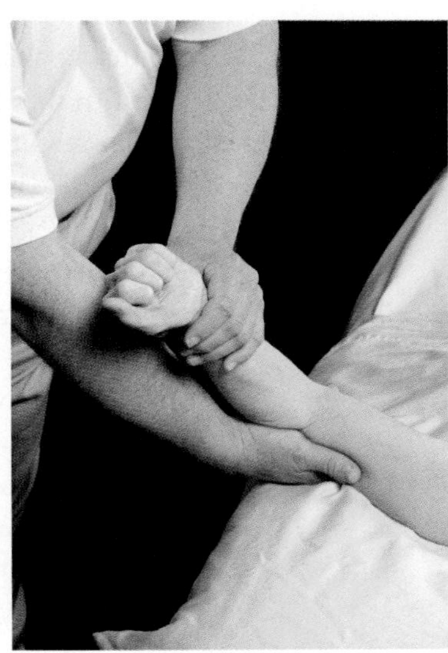

FIGURE 15-9A-C To help reduce fibrotic conditions of the subscapularis muscle, as the client contracts the muscle, the therapist gently overpowers the contraction to lengthen the muscle.

Strain-Counterstrain

The strain-counterstrain (tender point) technique was developed by Lawrence Jones, D.C. Jones happened on the basis of the technique by accident, when a patient came into his office in a great deal of pain. At the time, Jones was very busy and was unable to treat the patient immediately. He instructed his assistant to take the person into the next room, tell him to lie on the table, and make him as comfortable as possible. The assistant did as instructed. He had the patient lie down, and using various cushions and pillows, the assistant positioned the patient's body so that he was virtually out of pain and then left him there until the doctor was able to see him. When the doctor finally came in, he carefully removed the pillows and gently positioned the client flat on the table and asked where the pain was. The patient then realized that the pain had disappeared.

Jones was able to produce similar results with other patients by positioning and supporting them in pain-free comfortable positions. Through his own research, he developed the technique that he calls *strain-counterstrain.*

Jones postulated that impaired joint mobility is often caused by protective proprioceptive reflexes that fire when the muscle is shorter than its resting length. In other words, as the body attempts to move through its normal range of motion, a premature myotatic reflex (stretch reflex) causes the muscle to contract, thereby limiting movement. Often, the contraction is accompanied by spasm and pain. Jones theorized that this pathologic reflex might have been initiated when the joint was in a stretched position, and a panic reaction to return to a normal position caused the muscles opposite the stretched muscles to spasm. For example, a woman bends over for a short time. When she attempts to stand up, there is a sharp pain and she is unable to stand up without pain. There is a position, however, somewhere between the bent-over position and an erect position that is pain free. An overcontraction of the antagonist of the stretched muscle resists any attempt to return to a normal position.

Jones thought that a quick stretch of the shortened antagonist muscle caused the spindle cells to report to the central nervous system (CNS) that the muscle was being strained. A physiopathologic reflex circuit is created that maintains the antagonist muscle in a hypertonic state. This phenomenon can also result from muscle splinting after trauma. Once the reflex has been initiated, the body has no way to reset it.

Jones found that by positioning the joint in a position of comfort, which was usually close to the position where the spasm occurred, the pain ceases. By holding that position for a short time, which is usually a more exaggerated angle than the painful posture, then very slowly and passively returning the joint to a normal position, the muscle shortening and the pain and spasm are eliminated.

Jones also noted that most joint problems have associated tender points. Tender points are usually located in tissues that were in a shortened state at the time when the strain took place, rather than in the tissues that were stretched. Tender points that are used as monitors are generally located in muscles that are antagonists to those that are working at the time the pain or restriction are noted. When movement of a joint is restricted, pressure on the associated myofascial tender point is painful. As the joint is moved into the position of maximum comfort, the pain in the tender point diminishes. The position of ease usually involves folding or crowding the tissue around the tender point. By monitoring the sensitivity of the associated tender points while positioning the joint, the ideal angle for maximum benefit can be determined. When the client indicates that the pain in the point is reduced and there is a noticeable "letting go" in the palpated tissues, the pain or discomfort in the joint is also reduced, and the client is in a comfortable position. That position is then held for about a minute and a half (90 seconds), and then the body is slowly returned to a neutral position. The pain and restriction are often eliminated, and the pain in the associated tender spot has disappeared.

When multiple points are going to be treated, choose those closest to the head and to the center of the body first. Of those, begin with those that are most tender. It is a good idea to treat no more than five points in any one session to not overwhelm the body and allow the body time to adapt. When points have been defined, use the minimal force and pressure to achieve maximal comfort, ease, and relaxation while producing no additional pain anywhere else in the body.

Ortho-Bionomy

Ortho-Bionomy was developed by an English osteopath named Arthur Lincoln Pauls. After reading of the work of Lawrence Jones, Pauls began to develop a healing system based on the body's self-correcting reflexes. *Ortho-* means to correct or to straighten. *Bionomy* is the study of life processes. Pauls defines the term **Ortho-bionomy** as the correct application of the natural laws of life.

Ortho-Bionomy
is a healing system based on the body's self-correcting reflexes.

Pauls thought that disease and injury are often the result of the body's inappropriate response or reaction to some stimulus or situation. The inappropriate reaction is a misinterpretation or a misunderstanding brought on by fear or habit. Ortho-Bionomy works to restore the body's natural understanding by safely and slowly moving the body into and through those places where fear or habit is holding it in patterns that block vital energy, restrict movement, or cause pain.

Techniques include both methods that use physical contact and those that address energy systems of the body (i.e., chi, aura, etheric energy). The hands-on manipulations used in Ortho-Bionomy are passive positioning methods that relax tense ligaments and muscles by moving them into their position of greatest comfort and gently supporting them there. Techniques combine contact of trigger points with passive movement of the joint to produce the release of pain and tension in the related muscles. There are movements to release every joint of the body that also increase circulation and relaxation throughout the body. The client experiences movement through a wider range of motion with less pain and tension.

Because of the gentle, caring, and loving way in which Ortho-Bionomy is done, the release of muscular tension is often accompanied by mental and emotional release. As areas of the body begin to unwind, especially in areas where there has been trauma (physical or emotional), the stored body memories also release. The release of physical and emotional restrictions and the restoration of circulation and energy flow provide an environment in which the self-healing powers of the person can function.

To learn more about Ortho-Bionomy or more training, check online at www.ortho-bionomy.org.

Structural/Muscular Balancing

Structural/muscular balancing integrates techniques from several bodywork systems including those of Drs. Lawrence Jones and Arthur Pauls. Dr. Ray Lichtman incorporated the passive positioning techniques of Pauls and Jones with precision muscle testing into a system he called *positional release.* Mark Beck and Marcia Hart further adapted the techniques of positional release to include tools to identify and balance the body-mind or psychophysical aspects that are intimately related to physical dysfunction.

Structural/muscular balancing (SMB) is a method of:

- Gently moving the body away from pain and toward more comfort
- Improving neuromuscular communication in the body
- Rebalancing the energy flow in the muscles
- Releasing tension that limits the body's range of motion

SMB provides an extremely gentle, noninvasive method of working with a client's unique self-knowledge to locate and release constricted tissues that cause pain and rigidness. SMB uses a variety of techniques to address the physical, neuromuscular, and energetic aspects of a person's dysfunctional patterns. The main physical techniques used in SMB include precision muscle testing, passive positioning, directional massage, and deep pressure. The aim of SMB is to release tension in the structural muscles and reset the neuromuscular reflexes that perpetuate tension, spasms, and the associated pain.

Position Release Techniques

Position release is a very noninvasive system of soft tissue manipulation that originated in osteopathic practices. It is a gentle technique that affects the deepest neuromuscular mechanisms to relieve pain and dysfunction and restore normal function. The benefits of position release are increased local circulation and a neurologic resetting of the proprioceptive mechanisms that maintained the dysfunctional state. Position release affects the neuromuscular mechanisms and the proprioceptive system by passively relieving the shortened, constricted tissue, allowing circulation into the area to nourish the tissues and flush out toxins. Position release addresses muscle tissue that is tense, hypertonic, overcontracted, or in spasm. Muscles in a hypertonic state generally are ischemic, contain trigger points, have a high level of nerve activity, and can be painful. The presence of tight muscles in one area of the body usually is an indication of muscle imbalance in other areas as well. This is especially true with structural muscles of the pelvis and trunk.

The tense muscle is attempting in vain to bring its ends closer together. The tension can be the result of a protective reflex, muscle splinting, or strain. Tension is often self-perpetuating. The static tension of tight muscles restricts the flow of blood and fluids in those tissues. Tension causes increased metabolic activity, requiring more nutrients and producing more metabolic wastes. This ischemia and congestion impede the function of the muscle and can cause pain. Pain causes spasm, muscle splinting, and protective posturing, which further perpetuate the dysfunction.

Neuromuscular activity is increased. Proprioceptive feedback maintains the local tension and facilitates imbalances in the immediate area and in other related areas of the body. A vicious cycle of tension-pain-dysfunction builds to a point that activity becomes restricted or stopped.

Positional release breaks the tension cycle by gently allowing the body to achieve the exaggerated positions it has been attempting without straining or initiating protective reflexes. Position release is accomplished by placing the target tissues in their ideal position of comfort.

Contracted tissues are gently moved into their direction of contraction (*preferred position*). The body part is slowly and passively positioned so that the ends of the hypertonic muscle tissue are brought closer together. When the right position for release is achieved, a slight compression into the joint is applied. The proprioceptive information created during the positioning resets the pathophysiologic reflex circuits that have held the joint and associated tissues in a state of tension. The feedback at the annulospiral ends of the spindle cells has a chance to reset to a more normal state, and the gamma feedback to the Golgi tendon organs is reduced. After holding the position for 30 to 90 seconds, the body part is slowly and passively returned to its normal position. Muscle tension is reduced, and associated trigger points are inactivated.

The beneficial results achieved with position release techniques seem to be due to the circulatory and neurologic changes that happen in distressed tissue when it is placed in its most comfortable, pain-free position of ease. Hypertonic tissues impede local circulation, resulting in local ischemia and a reduction of local oxygen that can be a factor in the perception of pain and a precursor to the development of myofascial trigger points. Position release puts the strained, ischemic tissue into a position of ease and reduced tension, in which circulation is restored. When a joint is held in position by shortened muscles in spasm, attempting to move that joint toward its "correct" or normal position will be resisted and possibly painful. Moving the joint farther in the direction of the constricted tissue (direction of ease or preferred position), however, softens the spasm and relaxes the hypertonic tissue. Proprioceptors sending conflicting messages because of previous strain or injury have the opportunity to reset when placed in a position of ease. Maintaining the position for an adequate time allows neurologic reflexes and proprioceptors to resolve in a state of comfort. Returning the tissues and joint very slowly to a normal resting length is then achieved without the dysfunctional guarding, tension, and pain.

INCORPORATING POSITION RELEASE TECHNIQUES IN THE MASSAGE PRACTICE

Position release techniques can easily be incorporated into a massage practice. Whenever tight, constricted tissue is encountered, position release techniques can be employed to release the constriction gently and restore the tissues to an improved functioning state. Position release is less effective on tissues with chronic fibrosis than on areas of hypertonicity and spasm.

Applying Position Release Techniques

There are several different methodologies for practicing position release, but they all involve the passive positioning of the body or a body part to reduce the tone in restricted contractile tissue (Figures 15-10a-g). Position release is done by passively moving the body or body part toward the body's preference and away from pain, seeking the tissue's preferred position. Movements are toward ease and away from bind, away from any restrictive barrier and toward comfort. Positioning is done slowly, in such a way as to not cause any increase in pain. Positions are held for a period of usually 60 to 90 seconds. After the correct position for release is achieved and held for an appropriate period, it is essential that as the position is released, the body part is passively and slowly returned to a neutral position.

When a painful or dysfunctional area has been identified, one method to find the position for release involves simply and passively moving the body part or joint associated with the painful condition into its preferred position. To find the preferred position, first flex and extend the joint. Choose the direction that is away from pain and toward comfort. Next, abduct and adduct the joint, again choosing the direction away from discomfort and toward comfort. Finally, rotate the joint first clockwise, then counterclockwise. Once again, choose the direction toward the most comfort. Now, combine the three movements that were toward comfort. For instance, flex, adduct, and rotate the joint clockwise into the middle of the range of movement until a resistive barrier is encountered. The position should be very comfortable. After the body part is in position, add a slight compression into the joint and hold the position for 30 to 90 seconds. After holding the position for about 90 seconds, release the position and slowly and passively return the limb to a neutral position. Reassess the area for improvement and continue the massage or apply position release to another area.

Joint and neuromuscular dysfunctions usually have one or more associated hyperactive myofascial tender points that respond favorably to position release techniques and therefore are effective monitors for finding the correct position for release. These hypersensitive points can be trigger points in the target muscle, or occasionally the points are located in the antagonist or a synergist to the target muscle. Position release techniques create an environment in which the hypersensitive points deactivate and the dysfunctional tissues are restored.

Releasing Muscles with Trigger Points

Position release has been found to be very effective in relieving constricted muscles with central trigger points in taut bands of muscle or attachment trigger points in hypertonic muscle. Trigger points in myofascial tissue are excellent monitors when performing position release. Identifying the muscles that contain trigger points and knowing the actions that those muscles perform help to determine the preferred direction in which to move the body part to achieve the correct position for release. The body is positioned to bring the attachments of the affected muscle closer, passively mimicking the action of the muscle. Monitoring the myofascial

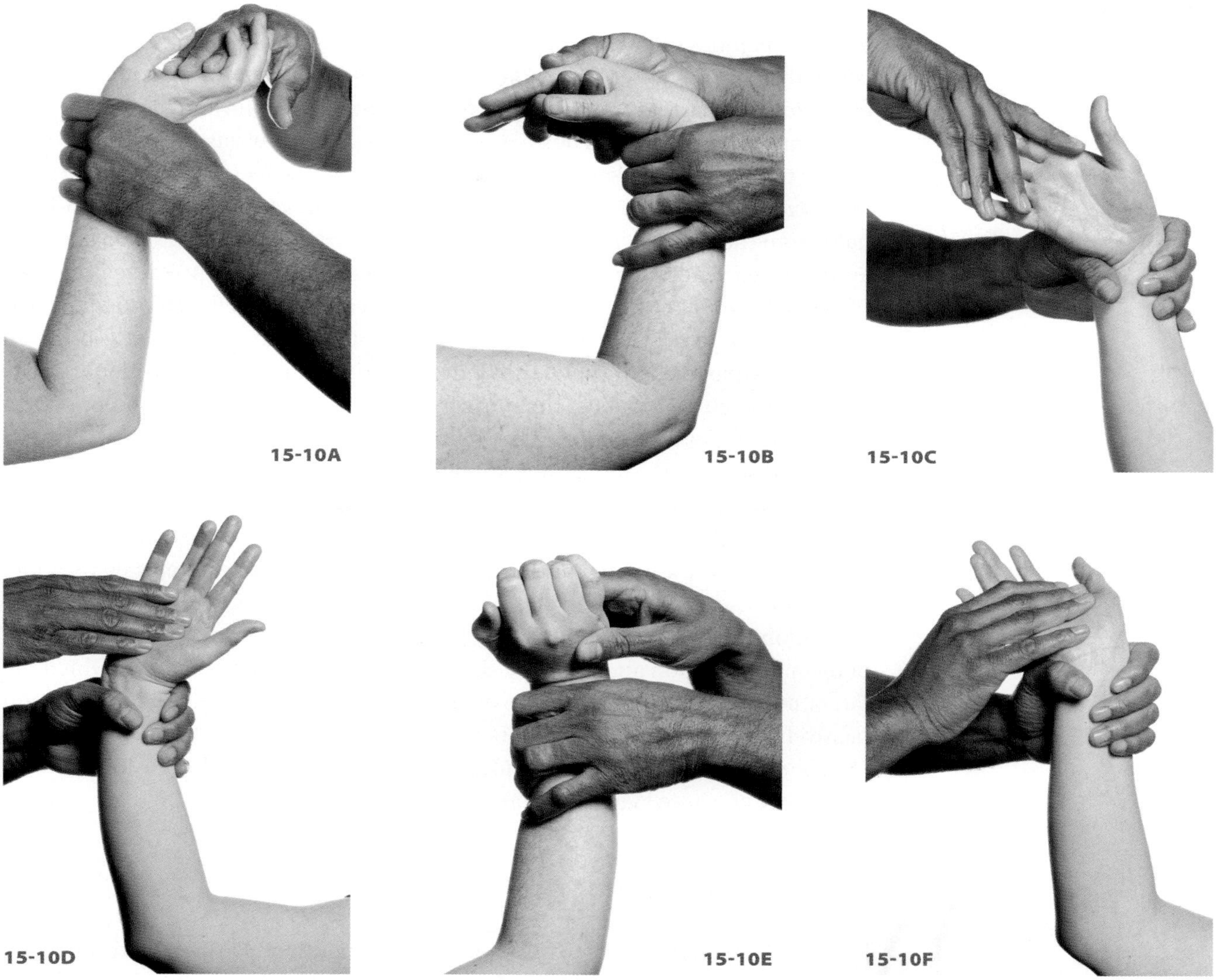

15-10A 15-10B 15-10C

15-10D 15-10E 15-10F

FIGURE 15-10A–F To determine the preferred position or position of ease for position release technique, the therapist moves the affected joint through each component of motion and selects the direction that is away from pain and toward comfort. (a) Wrist extension has some discomfort; (b) wrist flexion, no pain; (c) abduction produces no discomfort; (d) adduction causes pain; (e) medial rotation produces discomfort; and (f) lateral rotation is comfortable.

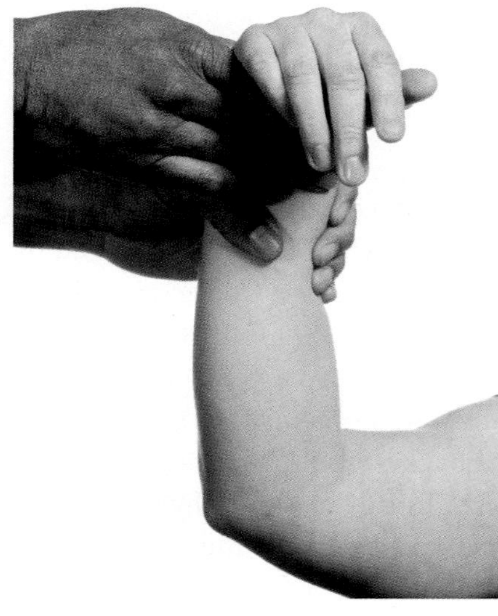

FIGURE 15-10G The therapist combines the three movements that are toward comfort to move the joint into a position of ease, lightly presses into the joint and holds the position for up to 90 seconds.

tender point while fine-tuning the position ensures the most appropriate position for release. Jones (1980) has demonstrated that tender points on the anterior of the body respond better to flexion, and those on the posterior respond better to extension. The farther the points are from the midline of the body, the more side-bending and/or rotation is needed to achieve a position of ease.

In his books *Position Release Techniques* and *Clinical Applications of Neuromuscular Techniques,* Dr. Leon Chaitow incorporates a pain scale to elicit feedback from the client to help in finding the preferred position. Contact is made on an identified tender point or trigger point, and an amount of pressure is applied to the point of manageable discomfort. The client is instructed to gauge the discomfort as a 10 on the pain scale. The therapist maintains the same pressure and begins passively to move the body part into its preferred position, usually bringing the attachments of the muscle closer together. All three components of movement are used to achieve the preferred position. First flexion or extension is applied to shorten the target muscle passively. Then side-bending and finally rotation are applied until the sensitivity at the tender point is reduced by at least 70 percent. The client is asked to report the discomfort level at the contact point as the therapist continues to adjust the body toward the muscle's preferred position. When the discomfort at the point is reduced to a response of 3, 2, or less, this is the indication that affected tissue is in a position of ease. The practitioner holds the body in this position and applies a slight compression into the joint on which the target muscle acts. The position is held for 60 to 90 seconds, and then slowly and passively the limb is returned to its neutral position. The practitioner reassesses the area for improvement and continues the massage or applies position release to another area (see Figure 15-11a-c).

MYOFASCIAL MASSAGE

Myofascial massage refers to bodywork techniques that are directed toward and have the goal of maintaining or restoring the functional capacity of the myofascial system. Myofascial techniques are intended to loosen, broaden, or stretch fascia and release fascial adhesions, whether site-specific or general, superficial or deep. The intension of myofascial massage is to restore mobility and function to the body and to release fascial restrictions that cause postural distortion, pain, poor cellular nutrition, and myriad other dysfunctions.

History of Myofascial Massage

Many myofascial massage techniques have their historical roots in osteopathy. Myofascial techniques were originated by Andrew Taylor Still and advanced by William Neidner in the early years of the twentieth century. Connective tissue massage (*Bindegewebsmassage*) was developed in the 1920s in Germany by physiotherapist Elizabeth Dicke. It involved stretching the myofascia with skin rolling and other techniques to promote health. Robert Ward, DO, coined the term *myofascial release* in the 1960s to describe a system of techniques that he used to address the body's myofascial anatomy. In the 1980s, a physical therapist named John F. Barnes gave the term *myofascial release* to methods that he systemized for freeing the myofascial system of restrictions and dysfunction.

Craniosacral techniques, which also use myofascial release-type manipulations, were developed by William Sutherland and advanced by John Upledger and associates of The Upledger Institute. Myofascial therapies rely on three osteopathic principles: (1) given the correct conditions, the body can heal itself; (2) body structure and function are interrelated; and (3) the body is a whole interconnected by fascia.

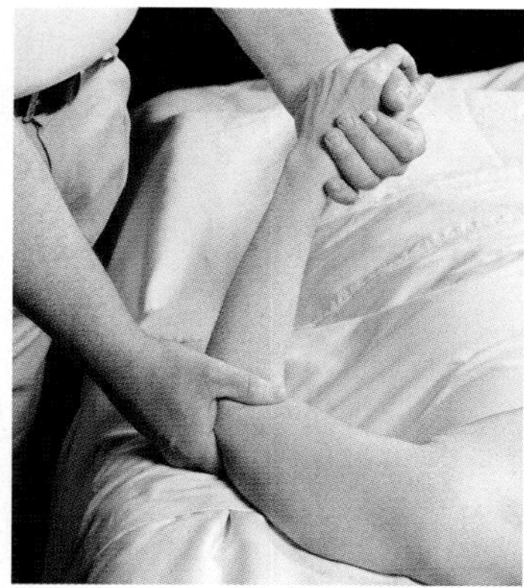

FIGURE 15-11A Apply position release to the forearm extensors by first locating the trigger point in the muscle belly near the elbow.

Fascia

Fascia is connective tissue and is composed of fibers and cells suspended in a matrix of ground substance. Collagen fibers are strong yet flexible and resistant to injury. They are the most abundant fibers in most connective tissue. Reticular fibers are weblike and provide structural support. As the name implies, elastic fibers have the ability to stretch and then return to their original shape.

Fibroblasts are the most abundant cells in connective tissue. They produce a wide variety of substances and elements that make up connective tissue. The most common are a variety of collagen fibers. Collagen fibers are composed of amino acids that are formed in the Golgi complex and endoplasmic reticulum of the fibroblast and spewed out into the intracellular spaces to become the connective structure of a variety of structures, including ligaments, tendons, the covering of the brain and nerves, and the spongy tissue of the lungs and myofascia, to name just a few. Fibroblasts have the ability to migrate to any place in the body and produce the specific type of connective tissue required to heal or repair the local tissues. Fibroblasts synthesize connective tissue and are the key cells for regeneration and repair throughout the body.

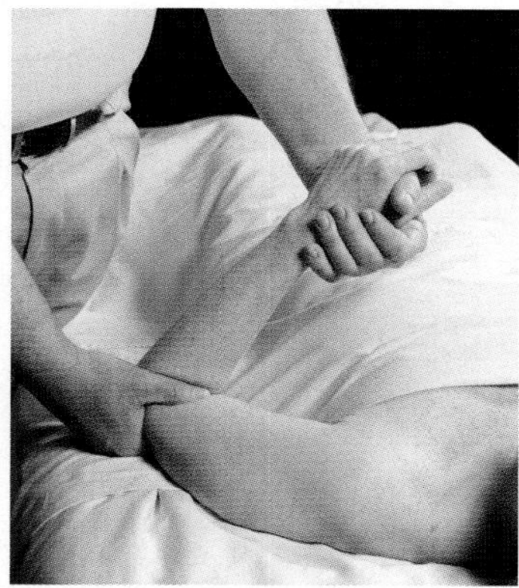

FIGURE 15-11B Press on the trigger point to elicit a pain response from the client and position the arm by passively flexing the elbow, extending the wrist, and rotating the forearm in one direction and then the other. Experiment with different positions until the pain response at the point greatly diminishes or disappears.

The fibroblasts and the mast cells produce the ground substance that is composed of various polysaccharides including heparin sulfate, chondroitin sulfate, keratin sulfate, and hyaluronic acid. These colloids form a gluelike gel that both hold cells together and provides an environment for the movement and exchange of the many nutrients and substances required for cells to thrive. Mast cells produce histamines and bradykinin, which play an important part the inflammatory process when tissues are damaged. When tissues are damaged or stressed, a release of histamines causes blood vessels to dilate and become more permeable, allowing fluids and repair cells into the area as part of the inflammatory process that is vital to the healing process.

Plasma cells produce antibodies that attack pathogens. Macrophages are white blood cells that migrate into an area and then engulf dead cells and destroy pathogens.

The collagen fibers in fascia are responsible for the strength and stability of the tissue. *Collagen* is composed of three polypeptide chains twisted around one another, forming a triple helix that are arranged in a parallel pattern and held together by hydrogen bonds. The patterns in which collagen and elastin are distributed depend on the role of the connective tissue and the stresses applied to it. In tendons, fibers are parallel, providing strength under unidirectional loads. Ligaments exhibit a dense but more multidirectional arrangement, to provide strength and stability to the joint as it moves in different directions. In myofascia, collagen and elastin fibers are not as dense and allow for the normal stretch

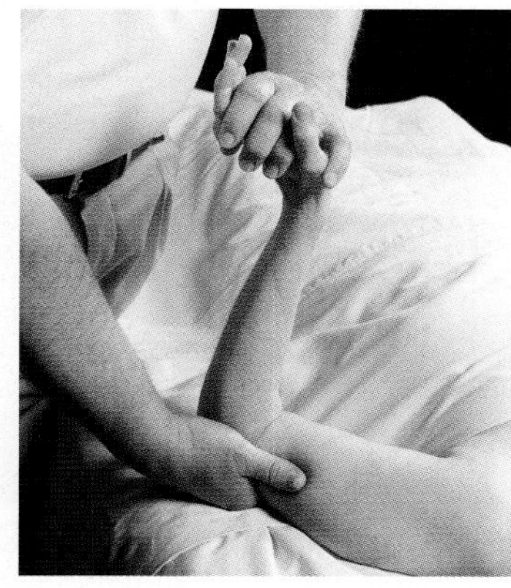

FIGURE 15-11C Hold this position and compress gently into the wrist and elbow for 60 to 90 seconds, then release the compression and passively return the forearm to the table.

Box 15.2

Position Release Protocol

1. Contact the alarm point in muscle tissue. It is felt as a nodule and is tender to the touch. Apply pressure to the contact point to elicit a pain response.
2. Passively articulate the joint to bring the end points of the target muscle closer together (mimic the action of the muscle). It might be necessary to use all components of movement to find the preferred position of the muscle (i.e., flexion/extension, adduction/abduction, and rotation). The tenderness in the point should diminish by 70 percent, or the point might disappear as the correct position is achieved.
3. When the preferred position is achieved, maintain that position and gently and lightly compress into the joint on which the muscle acts. Continue to lightly monitor the alarm point. Often, a release and a gentle pulse can be felt at the point.

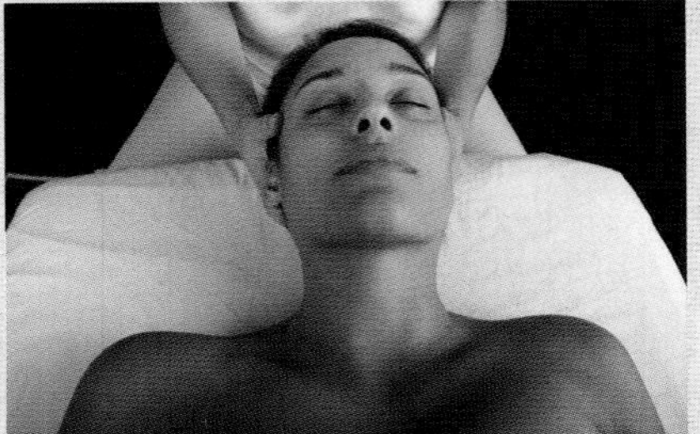

FIGURE 15-12A To perform position release on the posterior neck muscles, locate the tender point just posterior to the transverse process of C-2 or C-3. Use that point as a fulcrum point and shift the head laterally away from the point. Avoid laterally flexing, twisting, or turning the head.

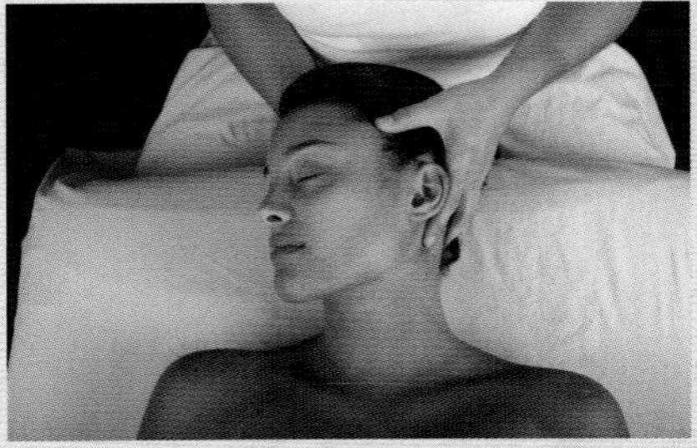

FIGURE 15-12B Palpate the tender point or nodule and roll the head medially toward the point until there is a softening of the point and a reduction in tenderness.

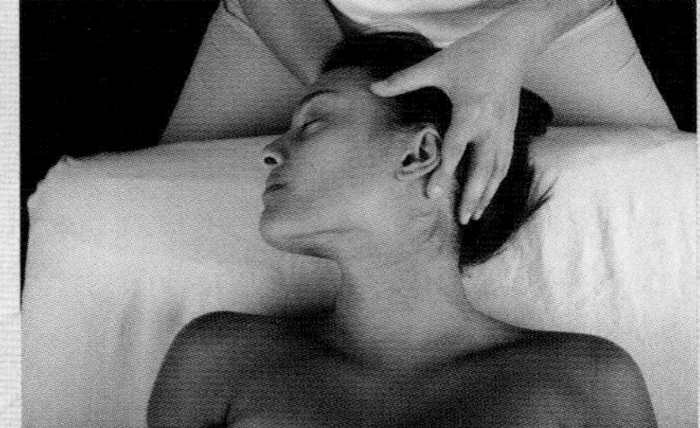

FIGURE 15-12C Again, use the tender point as a fulcrum to extend the neck at the tender point then rotate the head very slightly. When the position is correct, there will be a release of tension and pain at the tender point.

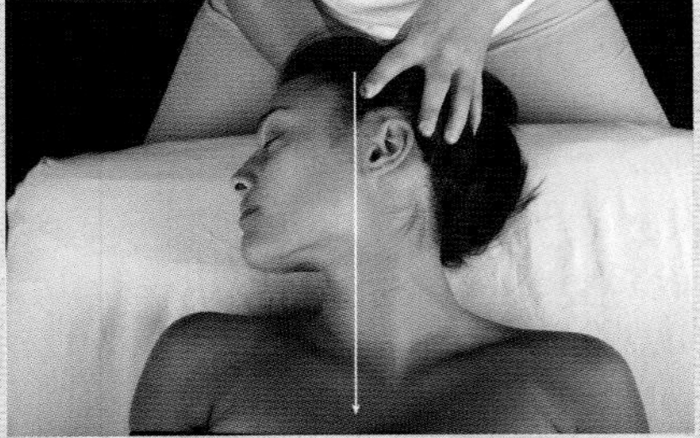

FIGURE 15-12D Without changing position, gently add compression on a line from the top of the head directly toward the feet. Hold for 30 to 60 seconds. Release and very slowly, without any assistance from the client, return the head to a neutral position. For best results, repeat position release at the same level on the opposite side of the neck and then on other points lower on the neck.

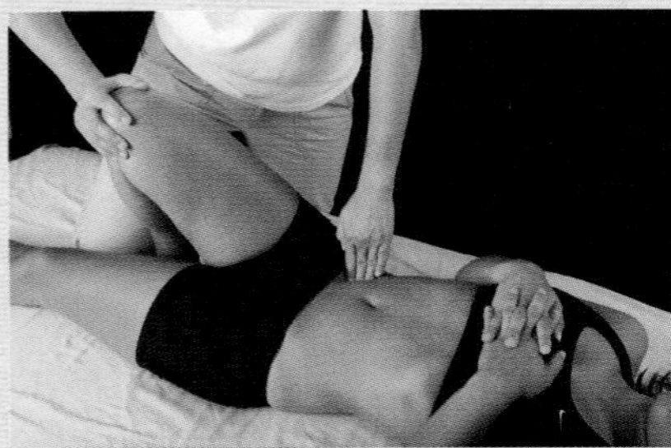

FIGURE 15-13A Position release of the psoas is performed with the client supine. Flex the hip and place the client's foot on the table. Locate the tender point in the psoas muscle, deep in the abdomen. Position the leg to reduce the sensitivity in the tender point.

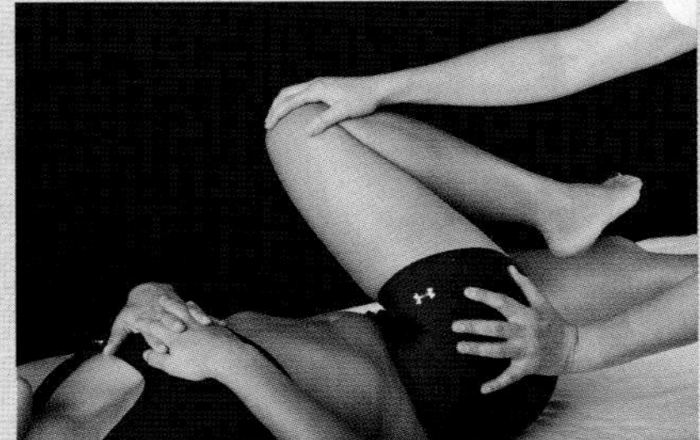

FIGURE 15-13B When the leg is in position, add compression to the greater trochanter directed toward the umbilicus and hold for 30 to 60 seconds.

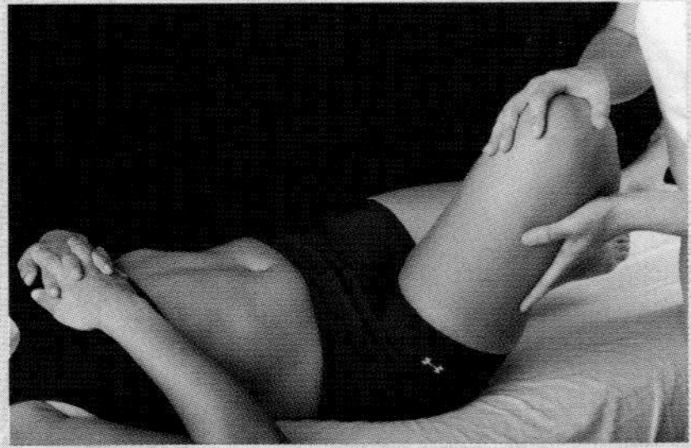

FIGURE 15-13C Release the compression and slowly abduct the knee and extend the leg to a neutral position.

Box 15.2 (Cont'd)

Position Release Protocol

4. Hold the position for 30 to 90 seconds, or until a pulse is felt at the point, plus another 10 seconds.
5. Gently release the compression, and passively and slowly, without any help from the client, return the body part to a neutral resting position.
6. Recheck the alarm point and other related points such as synergist and antagonist muscles. For instance, on the neck, after releasing one side, it is a good idea to release the other side at the same level (figures 15-12a-d, 15-13a-c, 15-14a-c).

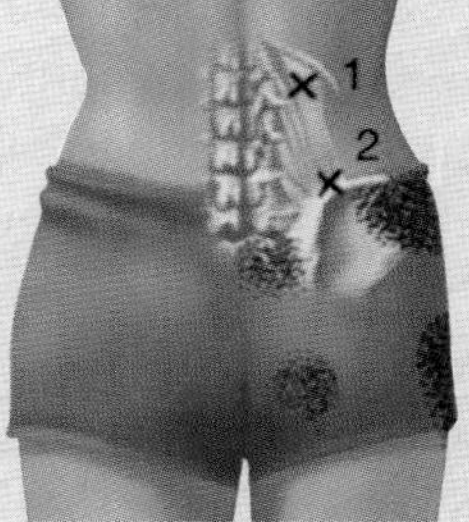

FIGURE 15-14A Tender points for the quatratus lumborum muscle are located 2 to 3 inches lateral to the spinous processes of L-1, L-2, and L-3.

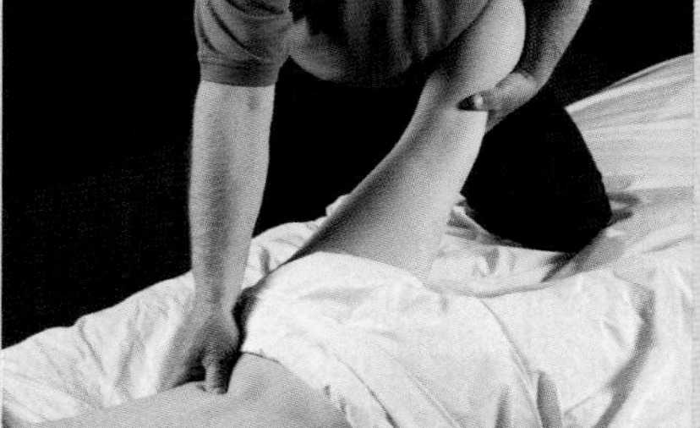

FIGURE 15-14B Position release of the quadratus lumborum is performed with the client prone. The practitioner stands at the side of the table with one knee on the table and lifts the client's leg onto his or her thigh. The client's leg on the same side as the muscle is located is extended and abducted until the tenderness in the point is reduced by 70 percent.

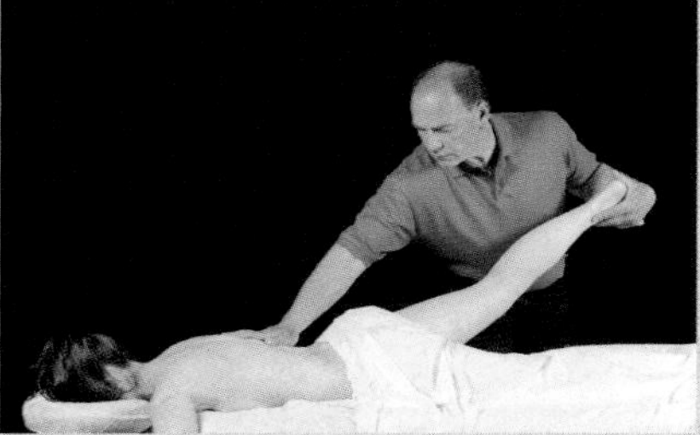

FIGURE 15-14C When the position of ease is achieved, compress into the release position: Wrap one hand around the client's foot. Place the thumb of the other hand between the eleventh and twelfth ribs, resting the rest of the hand on the rib cage, and block with that hand. Gently add compression from the client's foot through a straight leg toward the blocking hand for about 30 to 60 seconds. Reposition the leg back toward the midline without assistance from the client.

and contraction of the muscle fibers. Superficial fascia presents a latticework of fibers and cells to hold skin, vessels, and nerves in place.

The elastin fibers in fascia give it an elastic quality that allows fascia to deform when a force or pressure is applied, with the potential to recover and return to more of its original shape when the force is removed. If the elastic quality is stretched beyond the limit of the collagen fibers or the force is maintained over time, the fascia responds in a more plastic manner, resulting in a deformation of the tissue. Heavy pressure suddenly applied can result in micro tears or complete rupture of the tissues. Rapidly applied forces lead to a defensive tightening of the tissues, whereas slowly applied forces allow fascia to lengthen and release. Continuous or extreme stresses applied to fascia result in fibrosis, a build up of collagen fibers, excessive cross-linking (gluing), or scar tissue.

Fascia is colloidal, meaning it is composed of solids (fibers and cells) suspended in a liquid (ground substance). Colloids are not rigid and tend to assume the shape of their container. Colloids respond to pressure and stress in such a manner that the more rapidly the force is applied, the more resistant the response. This is why the slow, sustained pressure of myofascial techniques is effective when working on soft tissue.

Whereas the collagen and elastin fibers provide the structural component of fascia, *ground substance* is the fluid component that provides the space or cushion between the fibers and the immediate environment for every cell in the body. Ground substance is the medium for transport of nutrients, cellular wastes, hormones, antibodies, and gases between the bloodstream and the cells. The condition of the ground substance therefore affects the rate of diffusion and the ultimate condition of the fibers and the health of the cells that it surrounds. Owing to its colloidal nature, ground substance in fascia and other connective tissue becomes more gel like and less hydrated from lack of movement, disuse, or under chronic stress. The gel state is less conducive to movement and the free transport of elements to and from the cells. Energy applied to the tissue by means of muscle movement (exercise, passive or active stretching), soft tissue manipulation and pressure (as provided by massage), or heat transform the gel into a more sol or watery substance. This is a characteristic known as *thixotrophy*. This sol state is more conducive to transport of nutrients, metabolic wastes, and other elements necessary for cellular health and regeneration.

Fascia is pervasive throughout the body and is involved in numerous functions pertaining to structure, support, locomotion, fluid transport of nutrients and cellular wastes, protection against bacterial invasion, tissue repair, and many others. Restrictions or dysfunction of the fascial network can adversely affect any of these functions.

Box 15.3

Components of Connective Tissue

- Ground substance - a viscous gel made up of as much as 70 percent water that provides the medium for connective tissue fibers and cells. Acts as a spacer between and lubricant for collagen. Also provides for the diffusion of nutrients and waste products between the cells and blood stream.
- Fibers
  Collagen – has high tensile strength and provides primary structure of connective tissue. Collagen is categorized into different types depending on its location and function.
  Elastin – smaller and more stretchy than collagen. Has the ability to stretch and return to its resting length. Found in arterial walls, the subcutaneous fascia, and lungs.
  Reticular – similar to collagen but thinner and more delicate. Forms the framework of some organs and glands and provides support around smooth muscle and nerves.
- Cells
  Fibroblasts – synthesize components of connective tissue, including collagen, elastin, reticular fibers, and ground substance.
  Mast cells – secrete histamine (a vasodilator) and heparin (an anticocoagulant)
  Macrophages – responsible for phagocytosing damaged cells, foreign matter, and invading microorganisms.
  Plasma cells – part of the immune system and responsible for synthesizing antibodies.

The Fascial System

The fascial system is an integrated three-dimensional connective tissue network that is continuous throughout the body from the top of the head to the tip of the toes.

Fascia surrounds, supports, separates, and connects every cell, muscle, bone, nerve, blood vessel, and organ of the body so that if every structure that was not fascia were removed, what remained would maintain the form of every part of the body. Fascia provides support, form, and cohesion as well as separation and movement. Its purpose and function is to provide form for the body as a whole, to bind and separate certain structures, and to provide a framework for the passage of nerves, blood vessels, and lymph. The fascial system is continuous throughout the entire body; therefore, distortions in one part of the system can affect other parts throughout the body. The *myofascial system* refers to all the connective tissue associated with the skeletal muscles of the body, including the tendons, ligaments, and the attachments of muscle to bone and other structures. The myofascial system also includes the muscle tissue, neuromuscular connections, and the superficial fascia.

Muscle and fascia are anatomically inseparable. Muscle tissue is composed of long contractile muscle cells or fibers that are organized by fascia, more specifically termed **myofascia.** Every muscle cell is surrounded by **endomysium** and arranged parallel to other muscle cells in bundles or *fascicles* that are surrounded by **perimysium.** Fascicles are arranged along side of one another to form muscles and held in place by the **epimysium.** The endomysium and perimysium extend beyond the ends of the contractile muscle fibers to form tendons or flat sheets called **aponeuroses,** which attach the muscle tissue to bones or other tissues so that when the muscle tissue contracts, the tendon transfers that contraction to the bones or other tissues to produce movement. Complex muscular contractions regulated through neural activity apply forces through the tendons, bones, joints, and ligaments, creating the potential for movement, upright posture, and locomotion. Tom Meyers, an instructor of structural integration, describes in his book *Anatomy Trains* how muscle tissue, fascia, tendons, ligaments, and bones function together. According to his description, fascial chains link the contractile muscle tissue imbedded in fascia to rigid skeletal structures in a way that creates meridians of dynamic forces that provide the possibility of erect posture and coordinated movement. The book defines eleven basic *anatomy trains*; however, every movement incorporates fascial chains where muscles, skeletal structures, and the neural network coordinate creating movement.

Myofascial restrictions can reduce the functional length of muscles, reducing strength and flexibility or creating strain patterns that pull the related skeletal structures out of alignment. Fascial restrictions can entrap nerves or blood vessels, resulting in ischemia, pain, and loss of function. According to DeLany (2002), the development of myofascial restrictions can be due to a variety of factors, including misuse, disuse, abuse, or overuse. Disuse and immobilization result in dehydration (a loss of water content) and a change from sol to gel and a loss of ground substance. Less ground substance means the fibers are closer together, impeding their ability to move, creating more cross-linking between fibers and more adhesions, resulting in less mobility and flexibility.

Misuse or abuse can result in injury, causing an inflammatory response and the development of adhesions and scar tissue. Besides scar tissue at the site of the injury, exudates from the inflammatory process from the swelling around the injury cause contractures in the surrounding contractile tissues (*splinting*) and *fibrosis* in the connective tissue (random cross-linking between the myofascial sheaths).

Therapeutic methods to address myofascial restrictions hydrate the tissues, restoring the ground substance from a gel to a more sol state, and gently release cross-links to elongate and soften the fascia. Manual therapies such as gentle pressure, stretching, and myofascial and neuromuscular techniques accommodate these changes.

Myofascial Techniques

Myofascial techniques stretch, broaden, and soften fascia with the intention of reducing the collagen bonds that cause the different layers of connective tissue to adhere and to make the ground substance more fluid. Relieving myofascial constrictions that confine or compress nerves, blood, and lymph vessels reduces pain and improves circulation and lymph flow. Myofascial techniques are applied with the goal of restoring or maintaining the integrated function of the myofascial system.

Myofascial techniques are directed toward two types of fascia: loose connective tissue (superficial fascia) and dense connective tissue (deep fascia). *Superficial fascia* is located just below the surface of the skin and is continuous over the entire body, connecting the skin to the deeper fascia. Dense or deep fascia surrounds, penetrates, and infuses the muscles and includes the tendons that connect the muscles to bones and other tissues, and the ligaments that connect bone to bone. Muscle tissue and fascia are inseparable. Myofascial massage focuses on superficial fascia, dense fascia, and skeletal muscle and its innervating tissues (sensory, motor, and proprioceptive nerves). Thomas Meyers and John Barnes have noted that the body is made up of one muscle with over 600 myofascial pockets. When considering myofascial

Box 15.4

Definition (from Fascia 2007: From the Introduction by Thomas Findley and Robert Schleip of 2007 Fascia Research Congress Report).

Fascia is the soft tissue component of the connective tissue system that permeates the human body. It forms a whole-body, continuous three-dimensional matrix of structural support. Fascia interpenetrates and surrounds all organs, muscles, bones, and nerve fibers, creating a unique environment for body systems to function. Fascia includes all fibrous connective tissues, including aponeuroses, ligaments, tendons, retinaculae, joint capsules, organ and vessel tunics, the meninges, the periosteum, and all the endomysial and intermuscular fibers of the myofascia (Fascia 2007).

techniques, the practitioner must use a system-wide approach and view the body as a whole.

Assessment of Myofascial Restrictions

Because of the pervasive nature of the myofascial system and body tensegrity, a restriction in a particular area can have far-reaching effects. A pull in one area of the fascial net is communicated throughout the fascial network, similar to the way that a pull on one part of a sweater affects the whole garment. It is helpful to observe the whole person when a client complains of pain in a particular area of the body to determine which myofascial chains might be affected and how best to plan the session. Because the fascia is three-dimensional throughout the whole body, it is important to look at the entire structure as a client is standing, moving, and lying down at rest.

Postural/visual inspection of tissue

Observing posture provides clues to restriction in tissue. Imbalances in body posture such as tilted pelvis, stooped or rotated shoulder, protracted head, or an elevated ilium or shoulder are indications of restricted myofascia. The myofascia, in an attempt to stabilize a faulty posture, begins to create pressure on pain-sensitive neurons, causing spasm, fatigue, and pain.

- Observe the client standing, beginning with the position of the feet. Are they positioned at similar angles? Is there any pronation, and is the body weight distributed evenly on both feet? Is there any uneven rotation of the feet, ankles, legs, or knees?
- Check the position of the pelvis to note if it is tilted or torsioned. This can be done by palpating both anterior superior iliac spines (ASIS) simultaneously with the thumbs and noting any imbalance. Likewise, the posterior superior iliac spines (PSIS) can be palpated bilaterally to note if they are even. By palpating the ASIS and the PSIS unilaterally, the tilt of the pelvis can be easily observed.
- Note the rib cage, shoulders, scapulae, and clavicles for any rotation or imbalance.
- If the head is tilted or in a forward-tilted position, the posterior neck muscles and the back and lumbar myofascia experience added tension and strain to maintain an erect posture, which can result in fatigue, fascial restriction, and pain in the posterior musculature.

Postural asymmetry can direct the therapist to more specific areas of concern, where further assessment with palpation, skin rolling, range of motion, and tissue excursion can identify the restricted area.

Palpation, Skin Rolling, and Tissue Excursion

Restrictions in the fascia can be palpated by skin rolling, checking tissue excursion with fascial glide or positional testing. By slowly rolling the skin and superficial fascia between the thumbs and fingers, resistance or thickening in the superficial fascia can be noted (Figure 15-15). The therapist evaluates the thixotropic condition of the fascia, especially considering the texture,

Box 15.5

Properties of Fascia

Tensegrity – is an architectural term coined by the late Buckminster Fuller that refers to the integrity of structures as being based in a synergy between balanced tension and compression components. It described a structure that continuously maintains its integrity by continuously adjusting tension and compression. Biologic structures such as muscles and bones, or rigid and elastic cell membranes, are made strong by the unison of tensioned and compressed parts. The musculoskeletal system is a tensegrity of muscle, connective tissue, and bone; the muscle and the related fascia provides continuous pull while the bones provide discontinuous push. The bones are held together by ligaments and act as compression struts that are held and supported by the tension created by myofascia. The forces between the bones and myofascia are held in constant balance that provide for upright posture and form the basis for all physical mobility.

Thixotrophy is the ability of a substance to soften as a result of warmth, pressure, or manipulation, and to harden in the absence of the same. The hyaluronic acid in connective tissue's ground substance enables it to shift from a more gel state to a more fluid state. This process is called *thixotrophy*. Thixotrophy, the shape-shifting quality of connective tissue, makes connective tissue more fluid, pliable, and resilient when it is warmed or experiences movement, and makes it more solid and inflexible when it "sits without being disturbed." With disuse, the connective tissue surrounding muscles becomes a little colder, less energized, and more sluggish, and losing its full quality and ability to soften, stretch, and flex.

Physical activity, exercise, stretching, and massage can all provide the warmth, pressure, and movement needed to keep connective tissue encased muscles pliable. In massage, the practitioner's hands contribute heat (thermal energy). Far more significantly, the pressure, motion, and friction created by deep manipulation raise thermal and thixotropic levels far beneath the surface. This pressure (lengthening, separating, and differentiating) carefully applied at specific points and in specific directions results in a softening and lengthening of the connective tissue, helping connective tissue to be more fluid and less gelled.

Piezoelectricity is the characteristic of certain materials to create and conduct an electrical current under pressure or stress. Certain inorganic and organic substances with a crystalline structure have the ability to produce a mild current when pressure is applied. When the material is deformed, either by stress or pressure, the bonds between the molecules create a slight electric current known as *piezo* (pressure) electricity. Collagen fibers in connective tissue generate piezoelectricity, which is conducted through the connective tissue. This weak current is thought to communicate changes in forces on and movement of the body. The connective tissue responds by either augmenting, reducing, or adjusting the patterns of collagen in the connective tissue in relation to the forces placed on the body. When an area is under consistent strain, fibroblasts are stimulated to lay down more collagen fibers that become polarized and oriented along the piezoelectric charge that is aligned with the line of tension. In this way, the connective tissue is strengthened to adapt to the added tension.

mobility, adherence to adjacent tissue, and tenderness. Many times, fascial restrictions in deeper fascia are apparent in the superficial fascia in the same area. When performing skin rolling, the intention is first directed toward the more superficial layers, gradually increasing the intention and perception to the deeper tissues. The most appropriate areas for skin rolling are the lumbosacral area, along the erector spinae, the abdomen, over the iliotibial band, and the forearm.

To perform **fascial glide,** or *tissue excursion,* the therapist's hand contacts the client's skin and gently moves the skin over the deeper structures in the cardinal planes (i.e., superior, inferior, lateral, and medial) to stretch the

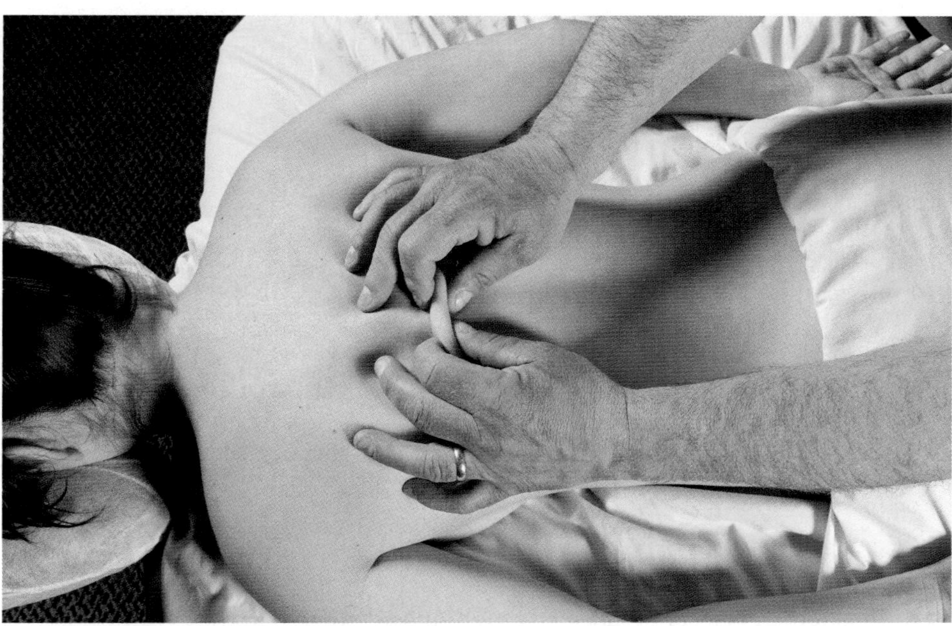

FIGURE 15-15 Skin rolling is used for assessment and release of the subcutaneous fascia.

tissue to its limit in all directions (Figure 15-16a). A restriction can be observed in the superficial fascia by contacting the skin with the pads of the fingers and gently stretching it in all directions, noting if a resistance if felt in any one direction (Figure 15-16b). The therapist's hand and the client's skin must move as a unit and the hand should not slide over the skin. The pressure and direction of the glide determine the fascia being assessed. Lighter pressure is used to contact more superficial fascia, deeper pressure for deeper fascia. The areas of the body and the direction of greatest restriction to movement are noted. Tension or resistance can indicate fascial restrictions that could be the result of fibrous cross-linking, ischemia, or dehydration of the ground substance.

Positional testing is done by passively moving a body part or limb through its normal ROM and noting any restriction or barrier to "normal" motion. Restrictions in the fascia can affect the direction or quality of movement. If there is a fascial restriction, it will be encountered before the normal capsular end-feel of the joint.

Direct Myofascial Techniques

The goal of myofascial techniques is to release or reduce the collagenous cross-links that cause restrictions and encourage the ground substance to change from a solid to a more viscous state. Direct myofascial techniques can target the superficial or deep fascia and are generally applied at the site of the myofascial restriction. Direct myofascial techniques move into the fascial restrictions, engage the soft tissue barrier, and gently move through and beyond the barrier. This tends to break down the fibrous adhesions between connective tissue layers. Because of thixotrophy, the application of pressure and heat cause the colloidal properties of the ground substance to change from gel to sol quite quickly.

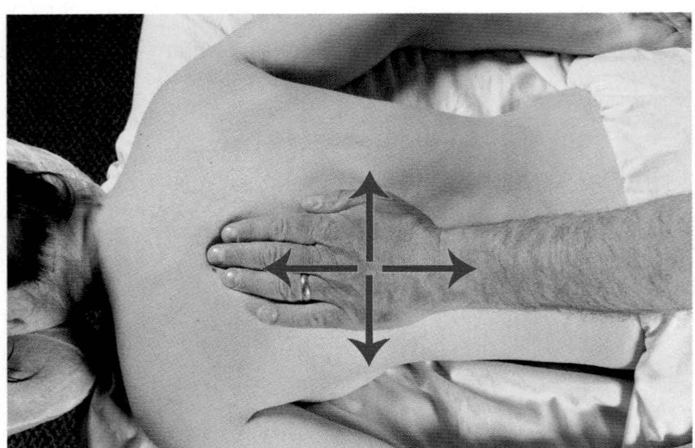

FIGURE 15-16A Tissue excursion is used to assess broad areas of superficial fascia. Multiple layers of fascia should slide easily in any direction. Tension or resistance in one or more directions usually indicates a fascial restriction.

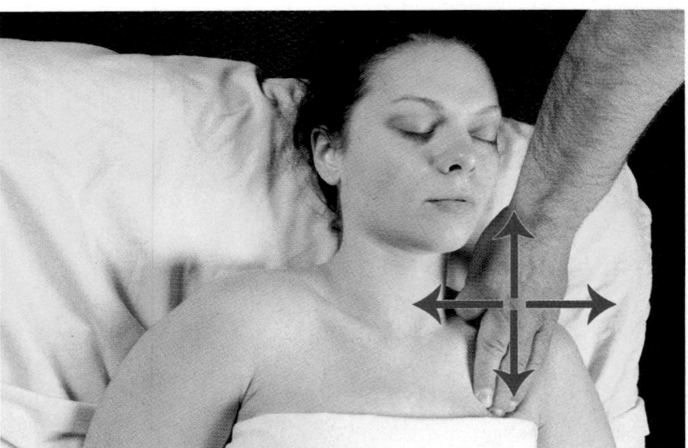

FIGURE 15-16B In smaller, more confined areas, tissue excursion can be done with the fingers.

The effectiveness of myofascial techniques depends on the drag or pull created by the therapist's hands moving the client's skin and superficial tissues over deeper structures; therefore no lubricant is used.

Fascia is three-dimensional. The superficial fascia, which lies just beneath the skin, is continuous from head to toe. Fiber orientation in superficial fascia is multidirectional and not determined by the underlying muscle fiber direction. The direction of the myofascial strokes directed to the superficial fascia therefore is determined by the tissue restriction rather that the orientation of the underlying muscle.

Deep fascia is contiguous with the superficial fascia and penetrates to the bone, surrounding and supporting every muscle, nerve, blood vessel, and organ down to the cellular level. Many myofascial techniques engage the skin and the underlying superficial fascia and then use that connection as a handle to affect the deeper fascia. The amount of pressure used determines the level of fascia addressed. Heat, hyperemia, and a lengthening or softening in the tissue are indications that a release has happened.

The intent of direct myofascial techniques to the superficial fascia is to soften and loosen the tissue and prepare the area for deeper work. Skin rolling and two-handed stretching are myofascial techniques used to do this. Cross-fiber friction and J-strokes are also employed to address site-specific adhesions in deeper fascia. Broad-plane techniques include cross-hand stretching, traction, and transverse releases to reach all levels of the myofascia.

Skin Rolling

Skin rolling is used both to assess the condition and quality of the superficial fascia and to loosen and release constricted tissue. Skin rolling is performed by picking up the skin and underlying superficial fascia between the thumb and fingers and slowly gathering up more tissue with the fingers as it slips out from under the thumbs. Both hands are held close together and work together. The speed of the stroke is slow and determined by how quickly the tissue releases as it is drawn up between the fingers and thumbs (see Figure 15-15).

Muscle Rolling

Muscle rolling is a deeper form of skin rolling used in specific areas where the therapist can pick up an entire section of muscle or muscle group and roll it between the thumb and fingers. The intension is to sift through the fibers to find any tension or restrictions and gently broaden and separate the fibers, releasing adhesions. Muscle rolling is also effective for identifying taut bands of muscle fibers and their embedded trigger points. Sites appropriate for muscle rolling include the sternocleidomastoid muscle, the upper trapezius, the biceps, the gastrocnemius, and others where the therapist is able to lift and grasp the muscle (Figure 15-17a–c).

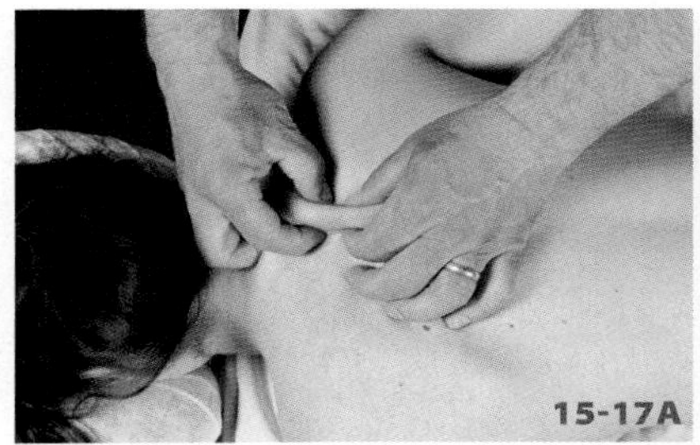

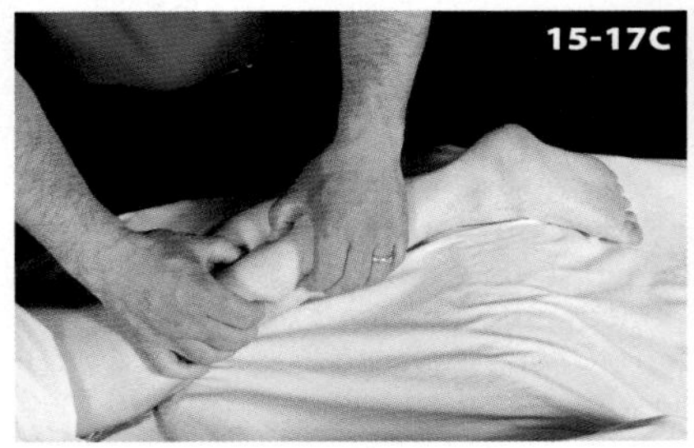

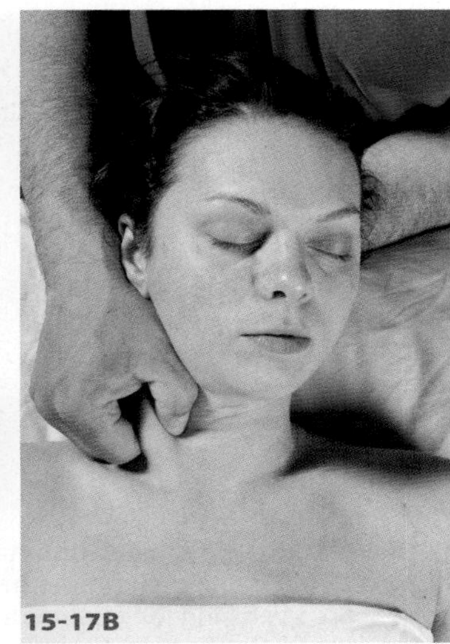

FIGURE 15-17A-C Muscle rolling of the (a) trapezius, (b) sternocleidomastoid, and (c) gastrocnemius

Cross-handed Stretch

As the name implies, two-handed stretching manually stretches the fascia and underlying muscle. It is applied by the therapist crossing the wrists and placing both hands on the targeted tissue, then leaning into the tissue and, without gliding over the skin, spreading the hands apart, gently stretching and lengthening the fascia between the hands (Figures 15-18a–d). With practice and tissue awareness, the therapist will be able to sense restrictions in the fascia and determine a direction to apply the stretch. When applying the stretch, the therapist senses a line of resistance and moves into it, just meeting that barrier until it releases and then following the movement. Once the fascia is engaged, a stretch is applied to take the slack out of the tissue and a barrier is encountered. The stretch is held for a sufficient amount of time for bonds in the tissue to release, and then the stretch is continued into the next barrier. An increase in warmth and a pulsing or fluttering feeling in the tissue under the hands can occur before the release. The key is a steady, sustained pressure, maintaining the tissue stretch for an extended, adequate amount of time. There is an elongation that happens in the fascial tissue that takes time to occur. It may take 90 to 120 seconds to begin the process. The therapist applies a consistent pressure into the direction of ease, connecting with the barrier, feeling the shift or release, and then moving with the tissue to the next barrier, sometimes encountering numerous barriers and taking four or five minutes per release. A lasting release of the fascia takes time and patience. Become quiet and allow intuition and proprioceptive sense of touch to guide the movement. As you reach a barrier, your hands will stop. Then the tissue will soften and shift, allowing your hands to approach the next barrier. There might be multiple barriers. Be gentle, not forceful, and do not let the hands slide

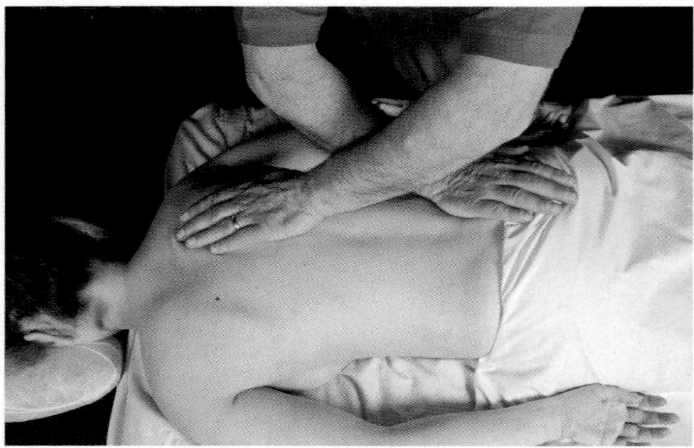

FIGURE 15-18A Cross-handed stretch applies pressure to engage the fascia and then slowly the therapist moves the hands apart, stretching the elastic component until a barrier is encountered. On the lumbosacral area, one hand is placed on the lower thoracic/upper lumbar area with pressure toward the head. The other hand is placed just above the sacrum with pressure toward the feet.

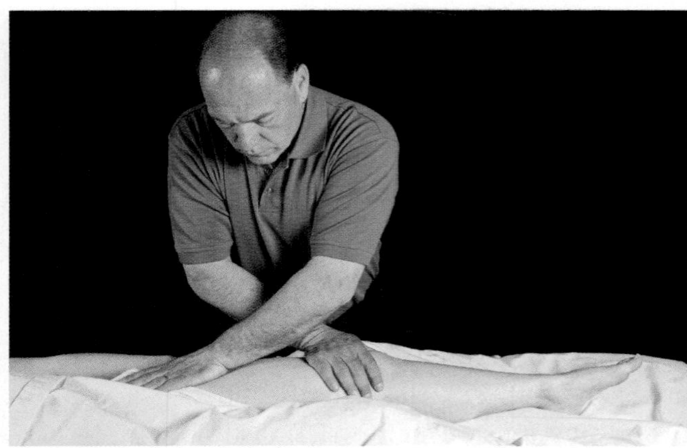

FIGURE 15-18B Maintain the gentle sustained pressure/stretch, and as the barrier releases, follow the motion three-dimensionally until the next barrier is met. Continue barrier to barrier until there is no more release. This technique can be performed centrally or unilaterally.

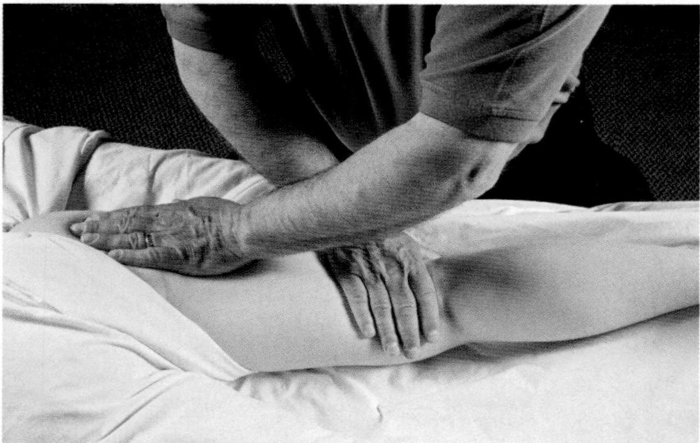

FIGURE 15-18C Cross-handed release can be applied in any direction in which there is a restriction, but usually it aligns with muscle fiber orientation. On the quadriceps and hamstrings, cross-handed stretch lengthens and releases the fascia.

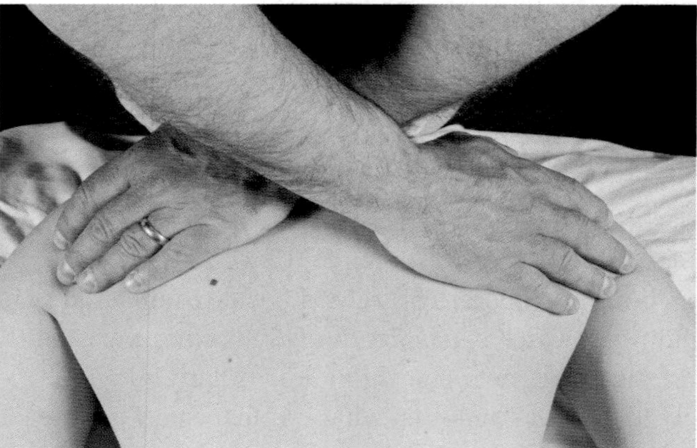

FIGURE 15-18D Release of the middle trapezius and rhomboids engages the medial borders of the scapulas and gently spreads them apart, releasing barrier after barrier.

across the skin. When a final softening is sensed and that the release in the area is complete, slowly relax the pressure and move to the next area of restriction.

The J-stroke

The J-stroke applies stresses to the fascia and is often directed toward the Golgi tendon apparatus or spindle cells. This stroke can also be used to elongate contracted muscles or to stretch, separate, and align constricted fascia.

The J-stroke is usually applied with one or both thumbs but can also be done with the fingertips (Figures 15-19a–c and 15-20a–c). It is a friction stroke that moves the superficial layers of tissue over the deeper layers. The side of the tip of the thumb makes light contact with the skin and pulls it slightly back in the opposite direction of the intended stroke and then moves deeper into the tissue to contact the fibrous tissue beneath. The thumb hooks and rotates as a

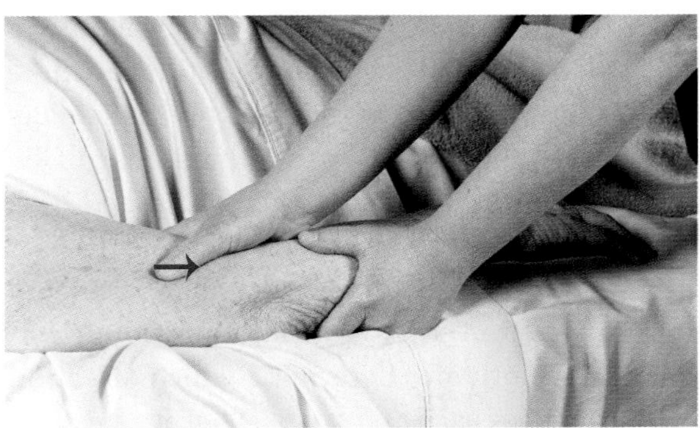

FIGURE 15-19A The J-stroke begins by making contact with the skin and slightly pulling the superficial tissues in the opposite direction of the stroke.

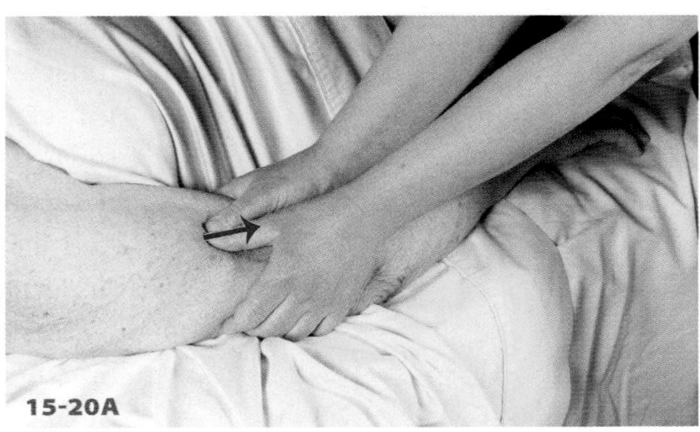

15-20A

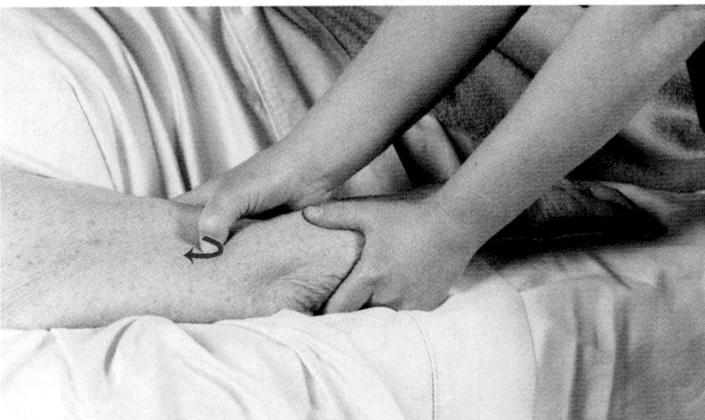

FIGURE 15-19B Continue the J-stroke by pressing deeper into the tissues with a hooking movement into the direction of the stroke.

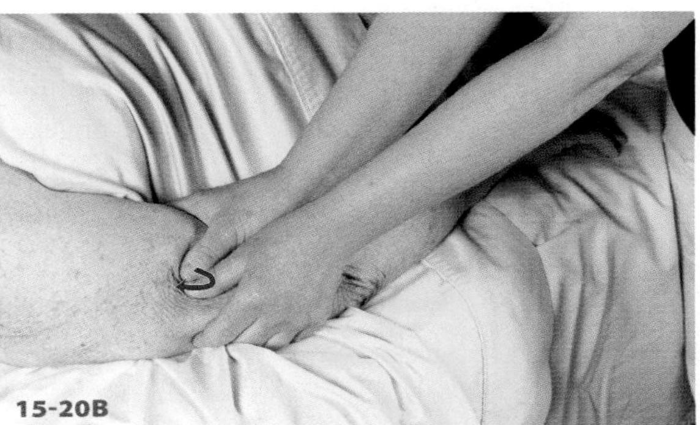

15-20B

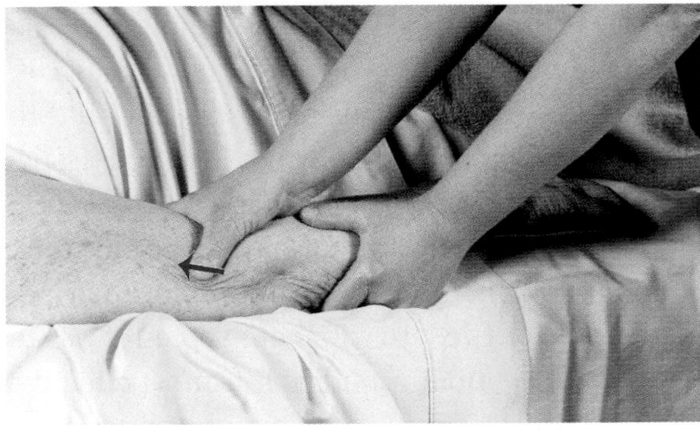

FIGURE 15-19C Complete the J-stroke by moving in the direction of the stroke as far as possible without sliding over the skin.

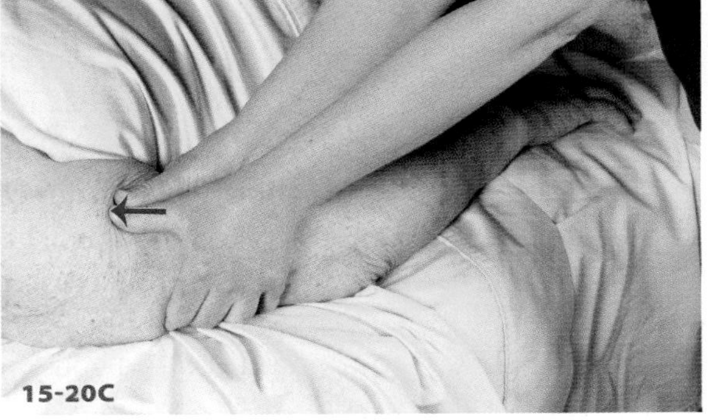

15-20C

15-20A–C The J-stroke, using two thumbs, covers a wider area on the muscle.

deep stroke is then given in the intended direction, which is usually in line with the direction of the fibers of the underlying muscle or tendon. The stroke is as long as the superficial tissue movement allows without the thumb gliding over the skin. The J-stroke can be repeated three to five times on the same spot or progress backward (in the direction that of the stroke) along the muscle being massaged.

To apply the J-stroke to a muscle, begin near the muscle attachment and do three to five strokes from the muscle toward the tendinoperiosteal attachment site, move toward the muscle body, and repeat two or three strokes so that they

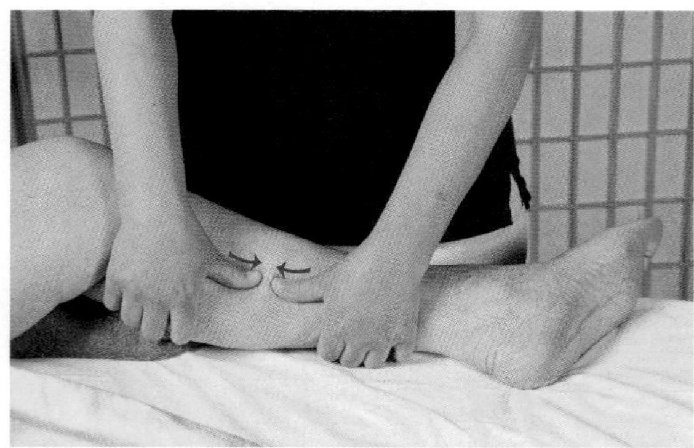

FIGURE 15-21A To sedate a hypertonic or spasmed muscle, simultaneously apply J-strokes toward the center of the muscle.

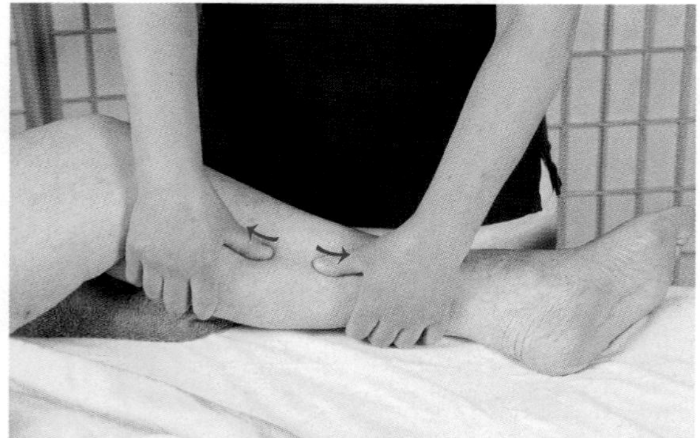

FIGURE 15-21B To stimulate a hypotonic muscle, simultaneously apply J-strokes away from the center of the muscle.

just barely overlap the previous position. Move back along the muscle and repeat the procedure; continue until the whole muscle has been covered. Although the direction is usually toward the insertion, it can be reversed. Direction can be determined by palpating fascial preference of bind and ease and using the J-stroke to reduce fascial restrictions. Fascial preference can be determined by applying a slight pressure with the thumb or fingers into the tissue and moving first in one direction and then another to determine which direction moves the farthest the most easily.

A J-stroke can be used to stimulate or sedate a muscle, depending on the muscle condition. To calm or sedate hypertonic muscle, directional massage should be directed toward the center of the muscle on the muscle body's contractile tissues ("unloading the spindles"). On the body of the muscle, both hands engage the muscle to shorten the muscle fibers and crowd the spindle cells (Figure 15-21a). To stimulate a hypotonic muscle, the directions would reverse, massaging the muscle body away from the center, stretching the muscle fibers, activating the spindle cells, and encouraging the muscle to contract (Figure 15-21b).

Cross-fiber friction

Cross-fiber friction (also termed *transverse friction*) techniques were first described by James Cyriax, MD, and are intended to break down existing adhesions or prevent their formation in muscles, tendons, and ligaments. As the name implies, cross-fiber or transverse friction massage is applied at a 90-degree angle to the fiber direction. When applied with light pressure, it is used as an assessment aid to locate taut bands associated with trigger points and constricted fibrous tissue. Cross-fiber friction, directed more specifically at deeper tissues, is a therapeutic modality to reduce fibrosis and separate fascial layers that have become stuck as a result of connective tissue gluing following local injury and inflammation. Cross-fiber techniques are used in chronic or the late subacute stages of tissue healing to break down adhesions that might hinder mobility. It is most effective when directed precisely toward a lesion in the muscle where adhesions interfere with the muscle's ability to contract and broaden painlessly or efficiently. Lesions can be in the muscle belly, the musculotendinous junction, or in the tendon — wherever trauma, microtrauma, or injury occurs. Initially, the fibers that form at the site of a trauma are disorganized and form cross-links between layers of fascia. Cross-fiber friction tends to release these cross-links and restore mobility to the tissues. Cross-fiber friction helps to reduce adhesions between fascial sheaths while at the same time encouraging the formation of a strong, pliable scar tissue at the site of the injury.

This is a site-specific technique, in which the therapist's thumb or braced finger is placed on the skin over the lesion and the skin and superficial tissues are moved over the site of the adhesion perpendicular to the direction of the affected fibers, whether they are in a ligament, tendon, or muscle (Figure 15-22a-b).

The length of the stroke is long enough to tease, roll, and separate the deeper fibers and short enough to not snap back and forth over the fibrous or taut bands. The pressure used is enough to compress and engage the deeper fibers while staying well within the client's pain tolerance, and the length of the stroke is just enough to move across the tissues without sliding over the skin.

Because cross-fiber friction is applied directly to the soft tissue lesion and with relatively deep pressure, the technique has the tendency to be somewhat painful. Specific consent is therefore required before applying the technique, and continuous communication with the client about comfort levels should continue throughout treatment. Initially, the pressure used is to the client's tolerance. After a short while, because of an analgesic effect, the client might report a lessening of pain, at which time the pressure can be increased slightly. If the intensity of the pain does not subside or increases, the technique should be discontinued.

Broad cross-fiber strokes are less-specific compression strokes, usually done with the palm of the hand (Figure 15-23). Pressure is applied against the muscle body toward the underlying bone structure, with movements transverse to the fiber direction of the muscle. This is done with the intention of spreading and broadening the muscle tissue. Close attention is paid to the quality of the fibrous tissue as it moves under the hands for indications of taut bands or fibrosities that require more specific work.

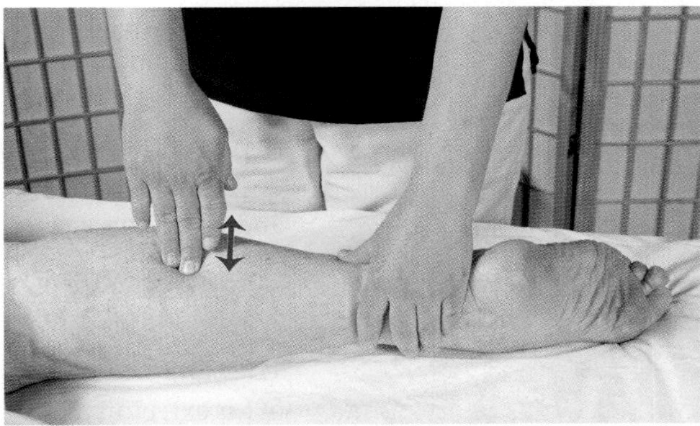

FIGURE 15-22A Cross-fiber friction applied with the fingers.

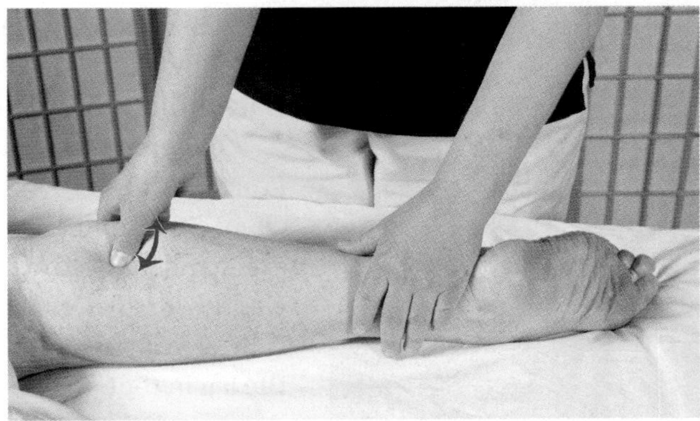

FIGURE 15-22B Cross-fiber friction applied with the thumb.

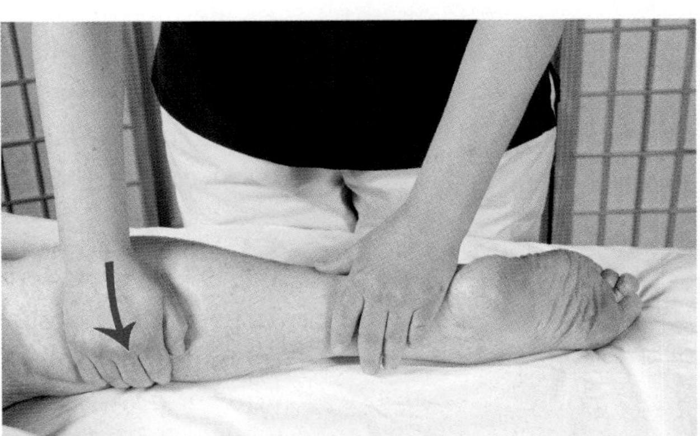

FIGURE 15-23 Broad cross-fiber friction is applied with the hand.

Deep Tissue Technique

Deep fascia is addressed by a technique that combines two directional strokes that can be applied by braced fingers, a braced thumb, the knuckles, or the elbow. The first component is vertical pressure descending through the muscle and fascia toward the bone. The pressure is not invasive but increases gently as the fascia opens and allows penetration as deeply as is comfortable. The second component is a movement perpendicular to the first and in the direction of the myofascia that is targeted for release (Figure 15-24a). A thorough anatomic knowledge of muscle fiber orientation is invaluable when applying these techniques. The myofascial structure and fiber orientation provide a channel, but the direction of the movement is determined to a large extent by the way that the tissue moves most easily. With experience and patience, the therapist will sense the "direction of ease" and follow the movement in the direction that the tissues want to move and the direction that leads out of the restriction. As the tissue releases, there is softening, lengthening, and a feeling that the body is guiding the direction and movement. If there is no apparent direction after holding the vertical pressure for a minute, release and change the placement of the contact slightly and reapply the technique.

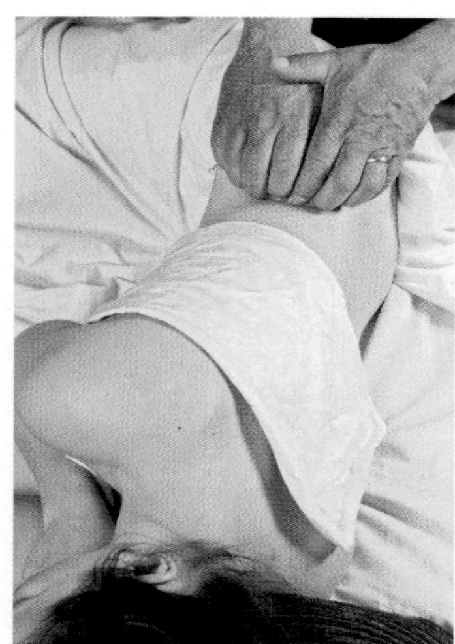

FIGURE 15-24A Deep tissue techniques applied with braced fingers along the iliac crest. Pressure is first applied to engage the restriction; a perpendicular movement then follows the tissue preference.

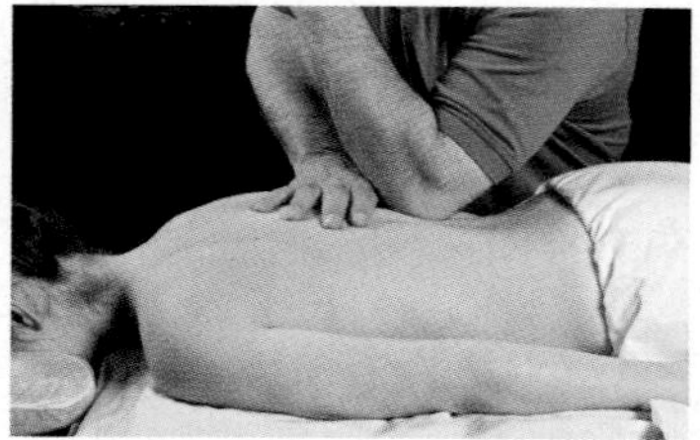

FIGURE 15-24B Deep tissue massage using the elbow along the erector muscles of the back to soften and elongate the tissues.

The pressure needed to apply these deep techniques is supplied by the therapist's making contact and then leaning into the client, and not from muscle strength. Proper body mechanics are essential. Face the direction of the stroke with the feet, hips, shoulders, and head in alignment. By leaning into the pressure, remaining relaxed and at ease, the therapist can monitor the minute changes that take place in the tissues and adjust the "lean" to follow the tissues as they release and elongate (Figure 15-24b).

Traction

Traction, when used as a myofascial technique, is a longitudinal stretch, usually of an extremity, to stretch and release fascial restrictions gently throughout the limb. By engaging all of the fascial components of the limb, any restriction can be gently stretched and released. Traction techniques are usually used after more specific releases have been completed. All traction releases are done slowly and carefully, tuning into each subtle resistance and simply holding the gentle traction until the barrier releases, before moving on to the next point of resistance.

To apply a traction release to the lower extremity, the client is supine on the table and the therapist stands at the foot of the table. The therapist grasps the client's heel and ankle with the medial hand and the ball of the foot with the lateral hand and gently leans back to apply traction to the entire leg (Figure 15-25a). Gently dorsiflex the foot and laterally rotate the leg. Closely monitor for any tension or restriction in any of the movements. When a restriction is sensed, hold the leg in that position until the barrier releases, then continue the traction while moving the leg farther into abduction and then into hip flexion. After completing the full ROM, return the leg to its neutral position on the table (Figure 15-25b).

Resume the traction and dorsiflexion and move the leg into an internal rotation and adduction. Continue adduction, crossing the leg over the opposite leg, causing the hip to roll forward, rotating the lower trunk (Figure 15-26). Maintain the traction throughout the movement, tuning in to the tissue and pausing anytime a restriction is sensed until the barrier releases. Slowly return the foot to its neutral position.

Traction Release of the Arm

To perform a traction release of the arm, the client is supine on the table and the therapist is at the side of the table. The therapist externally rotates the client's arm and grasps the hand just distal to the wrist with both hands and gently leans back to apply traction to the entire arm and shoulder. Traction is maintained as the arm is abducted through a full ROM, finishing with the hand and arm above the client's head (Figures 15-27a-c). Continue the traction while returning the arm through the full arc of motion to the client's side. As with other releases, anytime a restriction is sensed, stop the movement, maintain the traction, and wait until the barrier releases before continuing the movement.

To continue the release of the arm and shoulder, move to the opposite side of the table and lift the client's opposite hand toward the ceiling, flexing and adducting the shoulder. Apply traction to the arm by lifting the hand toward the ceiling and continue adducting (horizontal flexing) the arm. This will cause the shoulder to roll up off of the table. Continue traction at the wrist with one hand. Place the other hand over the scapula of the raised shoulder to assist with the traction and continued rotation of the upper torso. Whenever any resistance is noticed, stop the movement, maintaining the traction until the barrier releases and then continue the stretch through the full ROM. This stretch provides a release of the triceps, posterior deltoids, teres, rhomboids, and latissimus dorsi (Figure 15-28a-b).

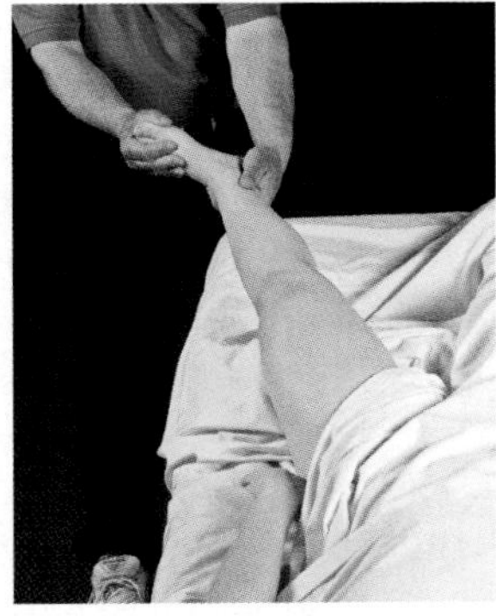

FIGURE 15-25A To apply traction to the lower extremity, grasp the heel and the ball of the foot. Apply dorsiflexion, external rotation, and traction through the length of the leg, and then slowly abduct the leg, feeling for any slight resistance at which point movement is stopped until the barrier releases before continuing.

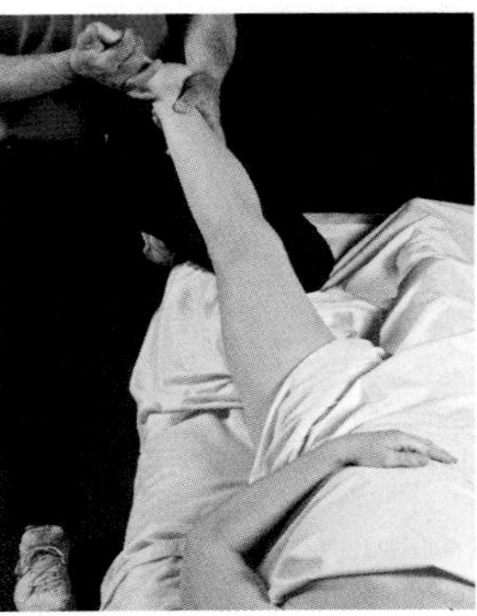

FIGURE 15-25B Traction and dorsiflexion are maintained as the leg is moved into hip flexion to stretch the posterior aspect of the leg.

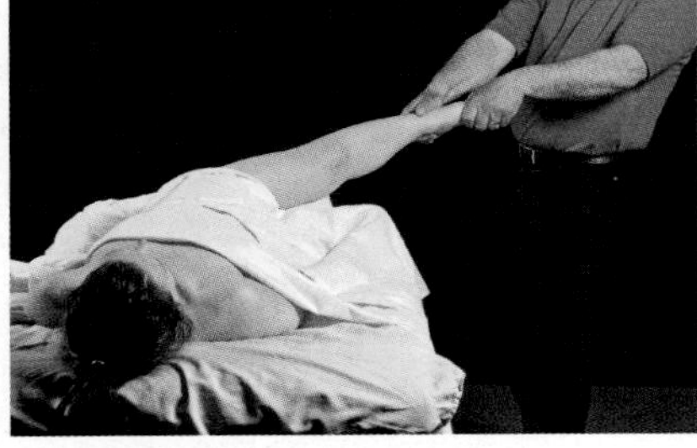

FIGURE 15-26 Dorsiflexion and traction on the leg are continued as it is moved into internal rotation and adduction. This causes a lower trunk rotation to release the hip, sacroiliac, and lumbar fascia.

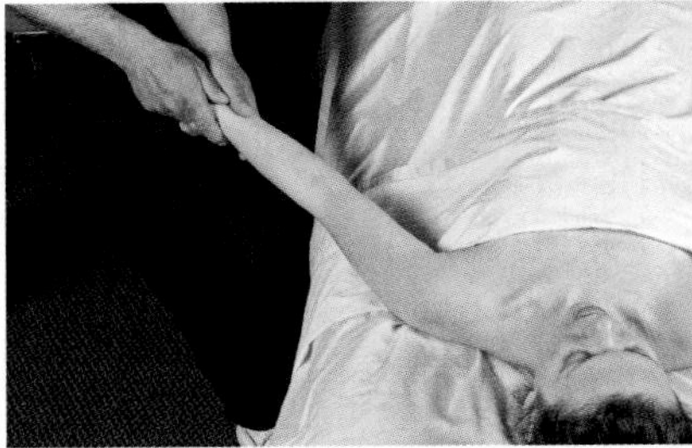

FIGURE 15-27A Apply external rotation (supination) and gentle traction through the length of the arm and shoulder.

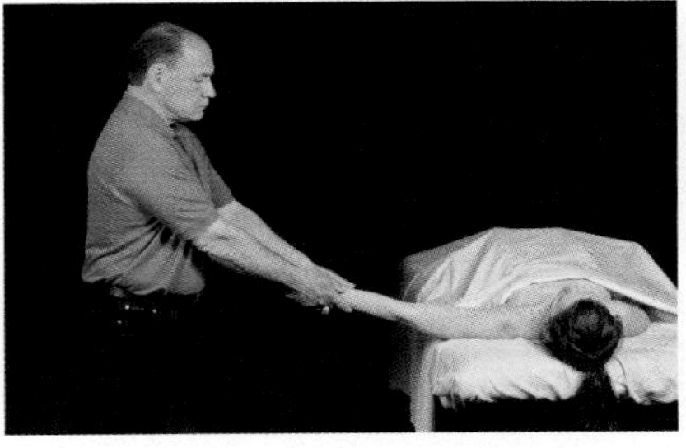

FIGURE 15-27B Slowly abduct the arm and tune in to any barriers felt as slight resistance, and maintain traction in that position until the barrier releases.

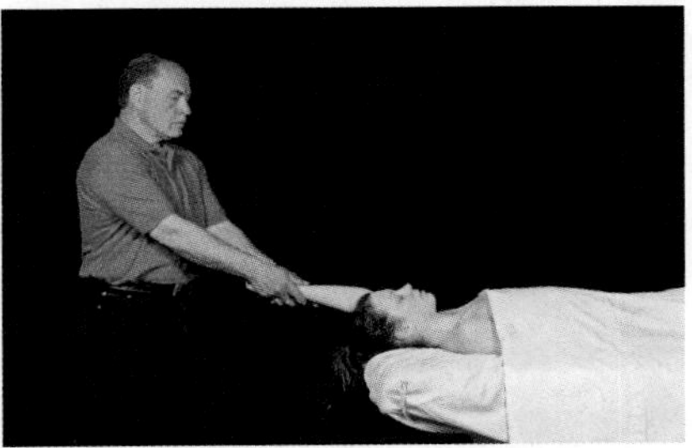

FIGURE 15-27C Continue abducting through the full ROM.

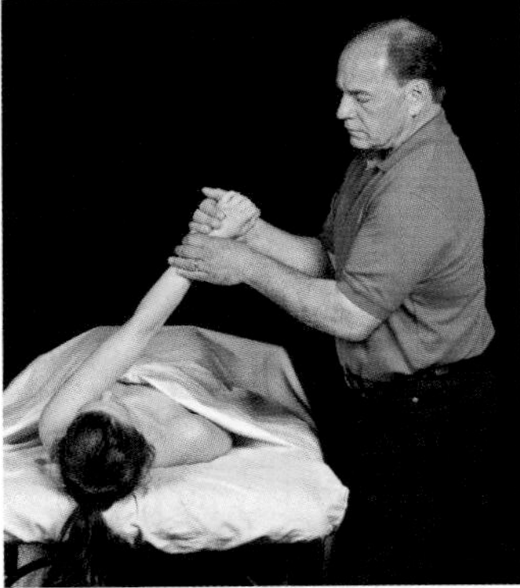

FIGURE 15-28A Continue ROM of the shoulder into adduction and shoulder flexion; this will cause the upper torso to rotate. Pause any time that a restriction is sensed, and allow time for the barrier to release.

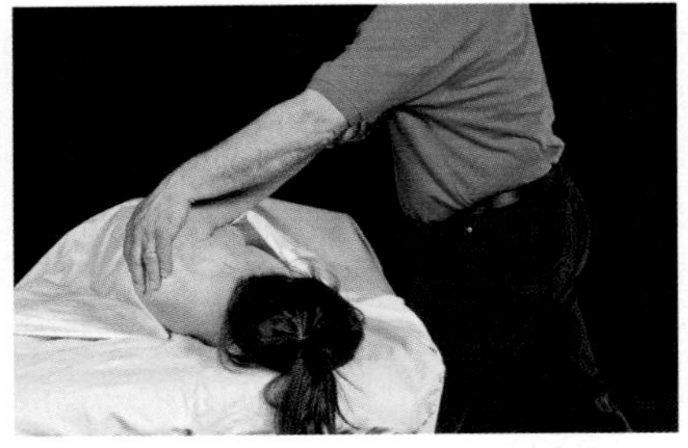

FIGURE 15-28B Maintain the traction and rotation of the arm and shoulder with one hand, and apply a lateral pull to the medial border of the scapula with the other. Reverse the direction, maintain the traction, and return the arm to the starting point.

Indirect techniques

Indirect myofascial techniques use similar techniques to assess and address fascia. The intention is to unlock the restrictions. The therapist applies enough pressure to contact the fascia and moves the tissue in the direction that it moves most freely, the *direction of ease*, until the slack in the tissue is taken up. The direction of ease is usually away from the restriction or barrier. This position is held as the tissue attempts to return to its original position. Eventually the tissue stops resisting and becomes quiet, and more slack will then develop in the tissue. The therapist takes up the slack and the routine is repeated several times until the release is complete and no more slack develops.

Transverse Plane Releases

Even though fascia in the body is three dimensional, most fascia releases tend to be longitudinal; that is to say, most myofascial stretches are directed to lengthen the tissue toward the head or the feet. The exception to this is the thoracic inlet, the respiratory diaphragm, and the pelvic floor. These are three areas where fascia transverses the body cavities. The myofascial releases for these three fascial planes are similar. The client lies supine on the treatment table, with the therapist seated at the side of the table. The hand placement varies for each release, but the process is essentially the same.

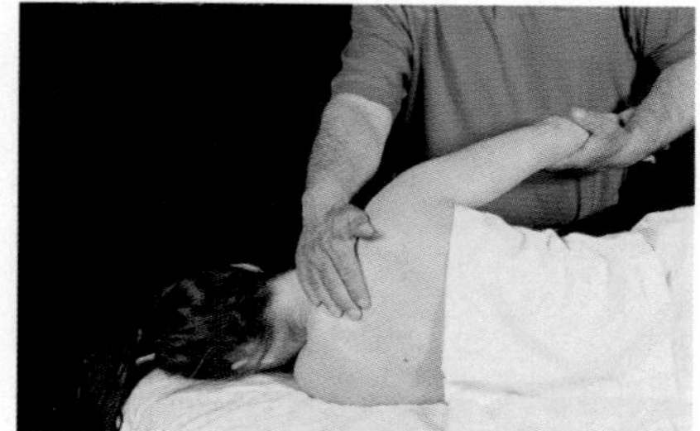

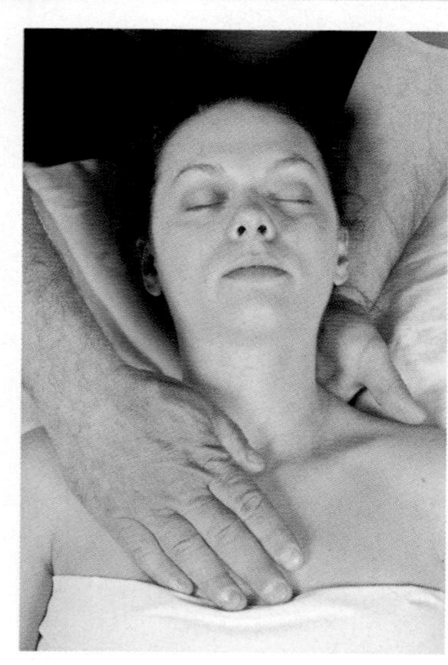

FIGURE 15-29 A,B Release the horizontal fascia for the thoracic inlet. (a) The posterior hand is placed under the client at the cervicothoracic junction. (b) The anterior hand is placed just inferior to the sternal notch.

The therapist positions one hand under the client as a foundation and the other on the front of the client with a slight compression toward the foundation hand. The pressure used is very light and gentle, not much more than an intentional contacting of the tissue. The therapist eases the compression and tunes in to the three-dimensional fascia by sensing tissue resistance in various planes (up-down, side-to-side, superficial-deep). Quietly maintain a very light pressure, and an inherent tendency of motion can be sensed. The motion can be directional, rotational, or a little of both. Follow the movement into the direction of ease, maintaining a slight compression until a resistance or barrier is encountered, and hold the position until the barrier releases. Follow the ease of movement to the next barrier until it releases. Continue the process until there is no more release or a quietness is sensed, and then slowly release the stretch and compression and remove the hand. It might take 30 to 90 seconds for the fascia to begin to release. As the fascia releases, successive barriers are encountered and released until there is no more movement. The entire release might take three to five minutes or more to complete.

To perform the release for the thoracic inlet, the foundation hand is place under the cervicothoracic junction, covering C-7 to T-2. The hand is placed transverse of the spine so that the spinous processes of the vertebrae are in the palm of the hand. The upper hand is placed over the upper sternum, the sternoclavicular joints, and the supraclavicular notch (Figure 15-29a–b). The foundation hand lightly lifts the torso very slightly while the top hand applies a slight compression and a gentle stretch, usually toward the feet to the point of tissue resistance. The position is held until a release is sensed, and then the stretch is continued to the next barrier. The process is repeated through successive barriers until there is no more movement or release. When the release is complete, the therapist first reduces the stretch, then the compression, and slowly removes her hands from the client's body.

The release of the respiratory diaphragm is similar. The foundation hand is placed under the thoracolumbar junction of the spine so that the spinous processes of T-11 to L-1 are resting in the palm of the hand. The top hand is placed over the epigastrium so the thumb is just inferior of the xiphoid process (Figure 15-30a–b). The foundation hand stabilizes the thorax and provides a very slight lift, while the top hand applies a slight compression and a gentle stretch into the direction of ease until a resistance is felt. With practice, the therapist can sense the barrier in a particular direction or possibly a clockwise or counterclockwise torsion. The compression and stretch is directed into the barrier and maintained until a release is sensed and then adjusted and continued through successive barriers until all have released. When the release is complete, first the stretch and then the compression is relieved, and the hands are slowly removed from the client.

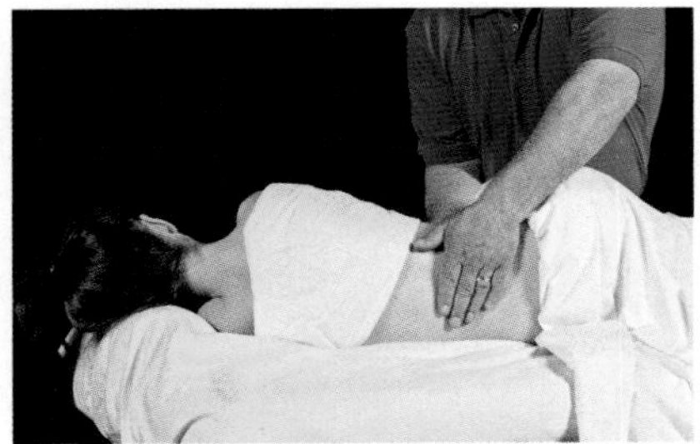

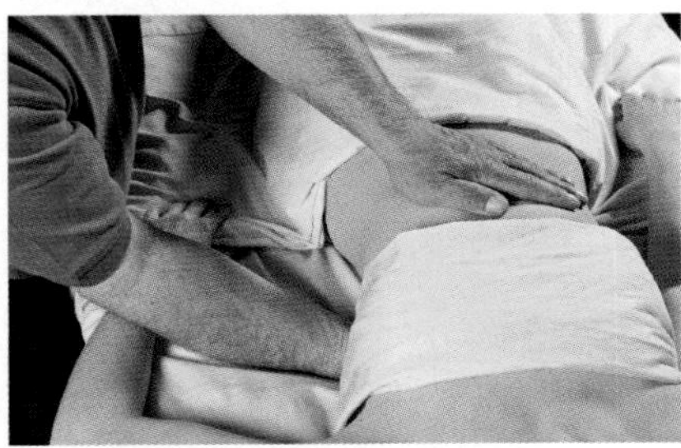

FIGURE 15-30 A,B The transverse release of the diaphragm. (a) The posterior hand is placed under the thoracolumbar junction of the spine. (b) the anterior hand is placed on the epigastrium, just inferior to the xiphoid process.

Releasing the thoracic inlet and the respiratory diaphragm can help to improve breathing, relieve strain and pain in the middle and upper back, and help to relieve protracted shoulders and kyphosis.

For the pelvic floor release, the foundation hand is placed horizontally under the spine at the level of the lumbosacral junction. The top hand is place on the lower abdomen so that the ulnar border of the hand is just superior to the pubic bone (Figure 15-31a–b). The foundation hand provides stability while the top hand applies a very slight compression and stretch to perceive a direction of ease and then moving to a point of restriction. The primary direction of the stretch is usually towards the head, although it can be lateral or torsioned. As with the two previous releases, the therapist moves into tissue resistance until the barrier releases then moves to the next successive barrier. When no more resistance is sensed, first the stretch and then the compression are released, the hands are slowly removed and the therapist proceeds to the next release.

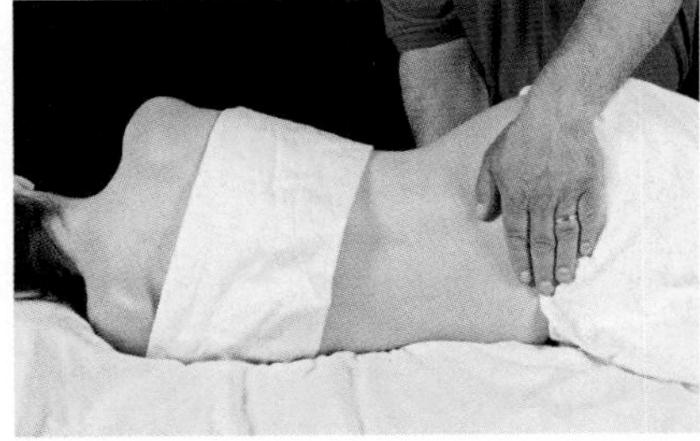

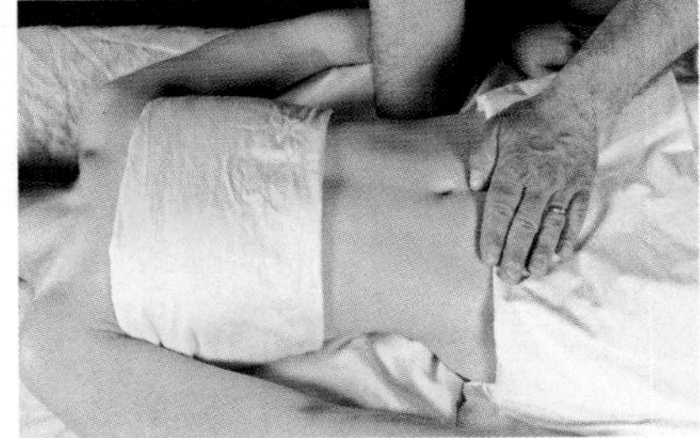

FIGURE 15-31 A,B The pelvic floor release. (a) The posterior hand is placed horizontally under the spine at the level of the lumbrosacral junction. (b) The top hand is place on the lower abdomen so that the ulnar border of the hand is just superior to the pubic bone.

CRANIOSACRAL THERAPY

Craniosacral therapy has been developed largely by John Upledger, DO. In 1970, while assisting in surgery to remove plaque from the spinal cord of a patient, Upledger observed a rhythmic movement of the cord that was independent of the patient's heartbeat or respiration. The phenomenon intrigued him because he could not find an explanation for it from colleagues or in textbooks. He did learn of the work of fellow osteopath, Dr. William Sutherland, who since early in the twentieth century had contended that the bones of the cranium were structured to allow movement and, in the 1930s, had developed a system of cranial osteopathy. The common belief of the scientific and medical community was that the sutures of the skull held the cranial bones in a solid, immovable structure. Dr. Upledger surmised,

craniosacral therapy is a gentle, hands-on method of evaluating and enhancing the functioning of the craniosacral system.

however, that if there were indeed movement of the cranial bones, there would be a feasible explanation for the rhythmic movement he had observed in the spinal cord during surgery.

While serving as a clinical researcher and professor of biomechanics at Michigan State University from 1975 to 1983, Upledger had the opportunity to lead a research team made up of anatomists, bioengineers, physiologists, and biophysicists to explore the existence of cranial bone motion. The research confirmed Sutherland's theory and provided a better understanding of the actual mechanisms creating the movement—that is, the craniosacral system—which led Upledger into the development of craniosacral therapy. In 1985, Upledger established the Upledger Institute in Palm Beach Gardens, Florida, as a facility to do further research, train practitioners, and provide a state-of- the-art treatment center for craniosacral therapy. Since then, more than 60,000 practitioners have been trained in craniosacral therapy, including osteopaths, medical doctors, chiropractors, psychologists, dentists, physical therapists, acupuncturists, and massage therapists.

The Craniosacral System

Craniosacral therapy is a gentle, hands-on method of evaluating and enhancing the functioning of a physiologic body system called the *craniosacral system*. The craniosacral system is a semiclosed hydraulic system comprising the meninges, the cerebrospinal fluid that surrounds and protects the brain and spinal cord, the physiologic structures that control fluid input and outflow, and related bones. The meninges consist of three layers of connective tissue that surround and protect the structures of the central nervous system. The pia mater is the innermost layer, closely associated with the brain and spinal cord tissue; it is highly vascularized, providing nutrients to nervous tissue. The middle layer, the arachnoid membrane, is a thin layer separated from the pia mater and dura mater by a fluid-filled space, allowing relatively independent motion between the three layers as the spine turns, bends, and twists. The outer layer of the meninges, the dura mater, is made of a tough, rather inelastic connective tissue that surrounds the central nervous system, contains the cerebrospinal fluid, and therefore encloses the hydraulic craniosacral system. The dura mater is closely associated with the cranial bones of the skull, the sacrum, and the fascia surrounding the spinal column, so that the craniosacral rhythm is palpable on many parts on the body.

During craniosacral therapy, trained practitioners use a light touch, equivalent to a nickel's weight, to feel the rhythmic motion theoretically created by the movement of the cerebrospinal fluid within the craniosacral system. Practitioners check the rate, amplitude, symmetry, and quality of this wavelike motion in places where the craniosacral membrane barrier attaches to bones such as the skull, sacrum, and tailbone. The craniosacral rhythmic motion is most readily palpated on the cranial bones of the head, but because of the close association of the dura mater with the body's fascial system, with practice, the craniosacral rhythm can be perceived almost anywhere on the body. The craniosacral system normally moves through a flexion and extension phase at a rate of six to twelve cycles per minute. On the cranium, flexion is palpated as a transverse widening and a front-to-back shortening of the skull. Conversely, extension is sensed as a transverse narrowing and a front-to-back lengthening of the cranium. Craniosacral motion is transmitted throughout the fascia of the body with flexion noted as a gentle external rotation and widening of the body, and an extension palpated as an internal rotation and a very slight narrowing of the body. The cranial motion is most easily perceived at the ankles, thighs, pelvis, thorax, and head.

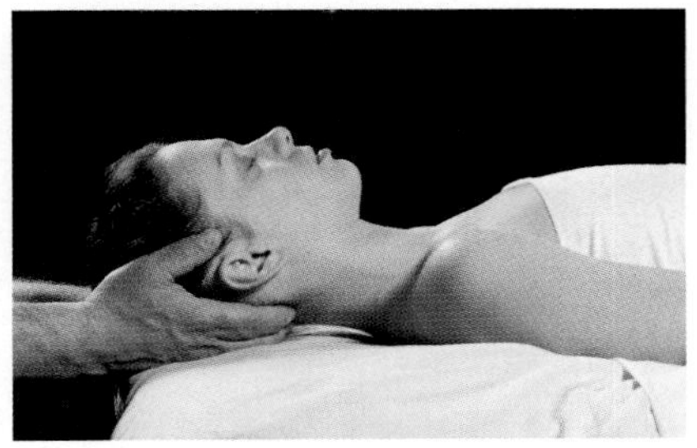

FIGURE 15-32 The pulse of the craniosacral motion can be monitored by gently cradling the head between the palms of both hands and sensing the minute flexion and extension of the cranium.

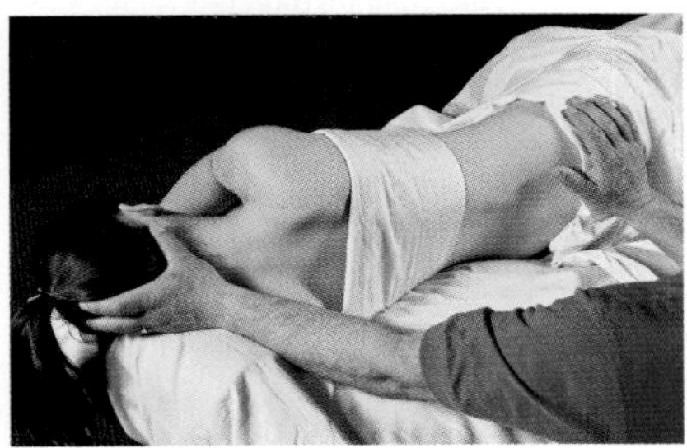

FIGURE 15-33 The craniosacral pulse can be felt with the client in a side-lying position. Place one hand on the occiput and the other on the sacrum, with a gentle pressure separating your hands. The occiput and sacrum move very slightly from flexion to extension and back to flexion in a rhythm different from the blood pulse or respiratory pulse.

With practice, the pulse of the craniosacral motion can be easily differentiated from the cardiovascular pulse and respiration. Craniosacral motion is palpated and monitored by lightly touching the client with as much of the surface of the hand as possible and noting the extent and quality of the motion (Figures 15-32 and 15-33). It is necessary for the client and therapist to be in a relaxed and quiet space. With the client lying quietly and face up on a massage table, the therapist sits at the head of the table and lightly places his hands so that the thumbs are near the temple and the palms and fingers lightly contact the back of the head. With eyes closed, the therapist allows his hands to meld with the client's head yet maintains the lightest pressure possible to maintain contact. The therapist becomes aware of the proprioceptive information of his arms. Soon the slight narrowing and lengthening, followed by pause, and then a widening and shortening of the cranium are sensed.

Craniosacral therapy treatment techniques are noninvasive, usually indirect, approaches intended to resolve restrictive barriers and restore symmetrical, smooth craniosacral motion. When an abnormal motion or restrictive barrier to motion is palpated, indirect technique would attempt to release the restriction by encouraging movement away from the restriction and toward ease. When monitoring the motion, the practitioner quietly follows the movement. To apply indirect technique, the practitioner should follow the movement in the direction that it moves most freely. At the farthest extent of the movement, the practitioner simply becomes immovable, holding against the cyclic return as the craniosacral movement continues through its cycle. As the motion progresses through another cycle, it moves farther into its direction of ease, at which time the practitioner simply takes up the slack and again becomes immovable, holding the tissue in the farthest extent of its cycle. This is repeated through several cycles until there is no further movement into the direction of ease or until the craniosacral system becomes quiet and still. This is referred to as a *still point.* The stillness might continue for a matter of seconds to several minutes. After a still point has been induced, the practitioner releases the hold and returns to monitoring the motion. As the still point subsides, craniosacral motion will resume, usually in a more symmetrical manner with less or no restriction.

A restriction in one part of the craniosacral system can affect the entire system, so that treatment might involve working at a point distant from an overt symptom. Any restrictions or blockages are treated with light-touch adjustments.

Craniosacral therapy is effective for a wide range of physiologic conditions associated with pain and dysfunction and is used as a preventive health practice because of its ability to improve the function of the central nervous system and bolster the body's resistance to disease.

Students interested in learning craniosacral therapy can contact the Upledger Institute to locate seminars in their area on the Web site, www.upledger.com.

DEEP TISSUE MASSAGE

deep tissue massage refers to various regimens or massage styles that are directed toward the deeper tissue structures of the muscle and fascia.

The term **deep tissue massage** refers to various regimens or massage styles that are directed toward the deeper tissue structures of the muscle and fascia. Some of the techniques focus just on the physiologic release of tension or bonds in the tissues, whereas others use bodywork in conjunction with or as a means of psychological or emotional release. In most deep tissue massage techniques, the aim is to affect the various layers of fascia that support muscle tissues and loosen bonds between the layers of connective tissues. Some deep tissue massage techniques are named after the person who developed or specialized them: Rolfing after Ida Rolf, Trager after Milton Trager, Hellerwork after Joseph Heller, and Feldenkrais after Moshe Feldenkrais. The following are brief explanations of some of these techniques.

Structural Integration

As the name implies, structural integration attempts to bring the physical structure of the body into alignment around a central axis. This is done by manipulating the fascia of the structural muscles. After structural integration sessions, physical and psychological balance is often experienced by the client.

Throughout life, traumas, both physical and emotional, can cause a reduction of movement that results in a shortening or binding together of the connective tissue that surrounds muscles. Restriction can affect fibers, bundles, and whole muscles. This condition can also come about as a result of habitual postures while sitting, walking, and standing. Poor posture can be learned by imitating parents, from environmental factors, or as a reaction to some forms of punishment and emotionally charged situations. Structural integration can be beneficial when given by a practitioner who knows the methods and understands how to achieve the desired results.

Rolfing

Rolfing, a brand of structural integration, is a deep connective tissue treatment system originated by Dr. Ida Rolf, a biochemist. Rolf discovered that in a normal, healthy body, the spine and body segments are correctly aligned, allowing the organs to function properly. During childhood and in early adult formative years, however, poor posture habits are often formed, throwing the body off center or out of its normal, healthy alignment. This in turn causes structural problems. Incorrect body alignment can also cause tension in muscles and connective tissues that can interfere with normal functioning of internal organs. Rolf originated a series of treatments called *Rolfing* to bring the body into proper structural alignment.

The goal of Rolfing treatments is to reshape the body's physical posture and to realign the muscular and connective tissue. The benefits of Rolfing also include increased suppleness of the muscles, improved appearance, and a renewed sense of well-being.

Rolfing techniques involve the use of heavy pressure applied carefully to the client's body with the fingers, a knuckle, a fist, or sometimes an elbow. Rolfing is usually done in a series of ten treatments of one-hour duration each. During this time, the practitioner (Rolfer) works on various portions of the body.

Contraindications for Rolfing are the same as for any other type of bodywork. When in doubt about the use of this type of treatment, consult the client's physician. The practitioner who wishes to pursue Rolfing techniques should study under the supervision of a qualified instructor (www.rolf.org).

SUMMARY

A wide variety of massage styles and therapeutic modalities are practiced that provide many approaches to enhance a person's health and well-being. This chapter provides an introduction to several therapeutic soft tissue interventions that are invaluable when addressing soft tissue pain and dysfunction. Neuromuscular techniques to recognize and deactivate trigger points, muscle energy techniques, position release techniques, and myofascial massage techniques are powerful tools for working with clients who are recovering from injury or who are suffering from soft tissue pain. These techniques and the classical massage skills of the previous chapters provide a solid foundation for a clinical massage practice.

To apply the neuromuscular and myofascial techniques described in this chapter effectively requires a thorough understanding of the anatomic structures that are being treated. By practicing these techniques, the student can continue to develop important palpation skills and a sensitivity of the soft tissues to recognize and address areas of pain and dysfunction. Continued study of the structure and function of the human body, as well as the modalities introduced in this chapter, will ensure success in the application of the techniques and the satisfaction of the client. Successful application of these techniques also requires an accurate assessment to determine which areas of the body to work on and which techniques to apply. A more thorough discussion of assessment techniques is discussed in Chapter 17.

QUESTIONS FOR DISCUSSION AND REVIEW

1. What is the basis for neurophysiologic massage therapies?
2. Who developed the system known as neuromuscular therapy?
3. What are the abnormal tissue signs that indicate neuromuscular lesions?
4. What is the four-step protocol for treating neuromuscular dysfunction?
5. What are the primary treatment techniques used in neuromuscular therapy?
6. What is a trigger point?
7. Where are myofascial trigger points located?
8. Explain the differences between central and attachment trigger points.
9. What are the criteria for recognizing active trigger points?
10. Which techniques deactivate trigger points?
11. Name the two inhibitory reflexes used in MET.
12. What are the three primary active joint movements used in MET when addressing hypertonic muscles?
13. What are passive positioning techniques?
14. What are three important considerations when using passive positioning techniques?
15. Who developed the technique known as strain-counterstrain?
16. How is the preferred position determined in strain-counterstrain?
17. What are the primary tools used in structural/muscular balancing?
18. What does the term *preferred position* pertain to and how is it attained?
19. What composes myofascia?
20. Where is superficial fascia located?
21. What are three techniques for assessing myofascial restrictions?
22. What are three hands-on techniques used for myofascial massage?
23. What is the craniosacral system?
24. What is deep tissue massage?
25. What is the purpose of structural integration?

CHAPTER

16 Lymph Massage

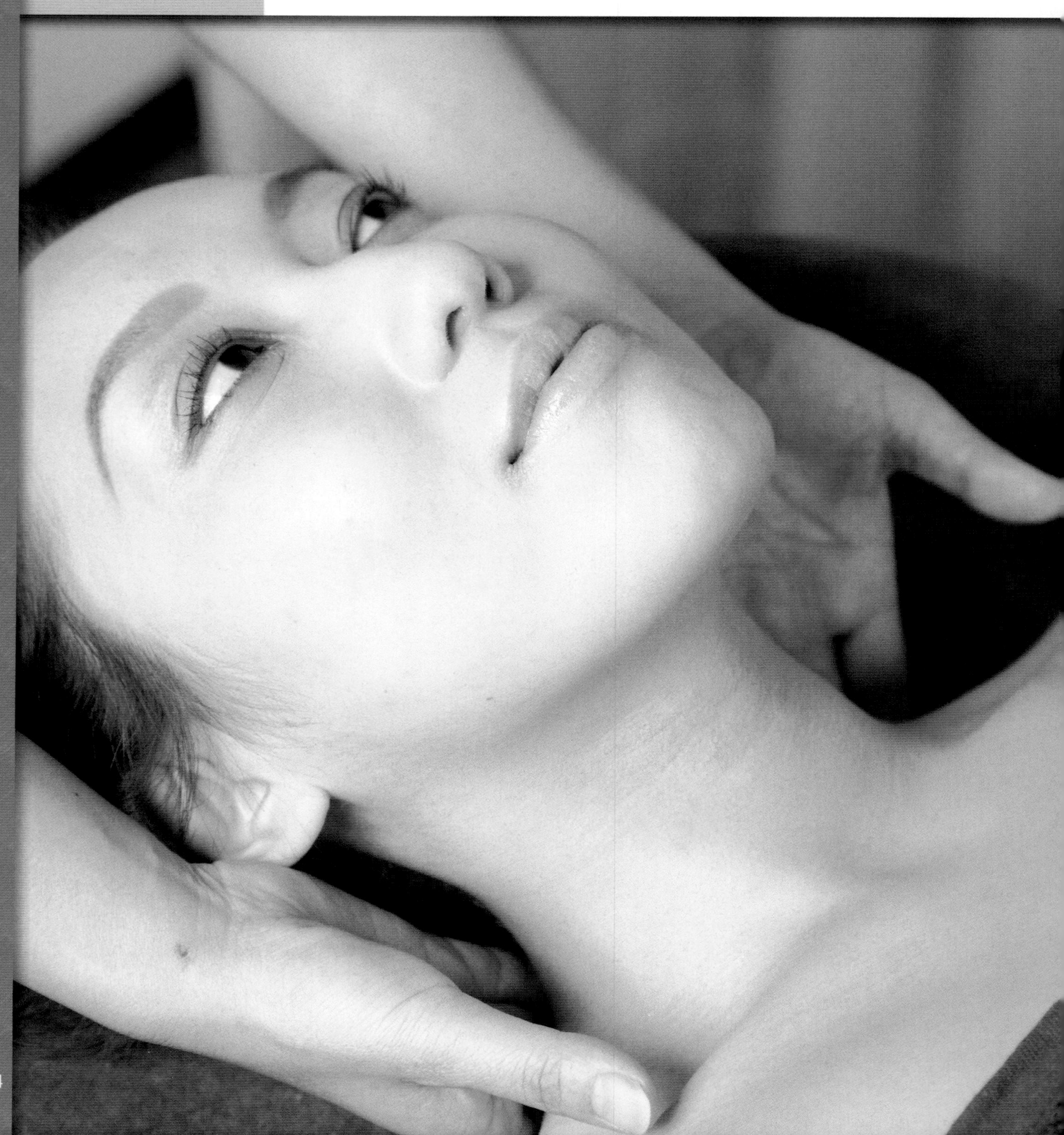

LEARNING OBJECTIVES

After you have mastered this chapter, you will be able to:

1. **Name three people who have been influential in the development of lymph massage.**
2. **Describe lymph circulation and differentiate between blood and lymph circulation.**
3. **Describe the function and location of lymph nodes.**
4. **List the major contraindications to lymph massage.**
5. **Describe and demonstrate the primary technique used in lymph massage.**
6. **Describe and demonstrate the sequence of movements for lymph massage on an area of the body.**

INTRODUCTION

Lymph massage is a systematic, gentle massage directed toward the superficial tissues, with the intent of enhancing lymph circulation. The successful application of lymph massage requires a fundamental understanding of the structure and function of the lymph system and the sensitivity and skill of applying the gentle rhythmic massage movements of lymph massage. This chapter provides a review of the lymph system, an introduction to the primary manipulations used for lymph massage and a description of a basic lymph massage. Lymph massage as it is described in this chapter is a simplified version of lymph drainage therapy and is useful when providing massage to generally healthy clientele. Practitioners who wish to work with clients with more serious lymphatic conditions are encouraged to seek out further training in manual lymph drainage therapy or decongestive therapy under the guidance of qualified instructors.

LYMPH MASSAGE

Lymph or *lymphatic massage* is a descendant of Swedish massage. Dr. Emil Vodder, of Copenhagen, Denmark, pioneered the practice of manual lymph drainage massage in the 1930s. Because he was not a physician, however, the therapeutic value of his techniques was not really recognized until the 1960s (see Chapter 1). He is credited with having discovered the benefits of lymphatic massage and for the development of massage techniques widely used today. Dr. Vodder's method of manual lymph drainage massage uses light, rhythmical, spiral-like movements to accelerate the movement of lymphatic fluids in the body.

In 1967, a German physician, Johannes Asdonk, conducted a scientific study of more than 20,000 patients and published a report on the effects, indications, and contraindications for lymph drainage massage. Currently, in many parts of Europe, doctors recommend lymph drainage massage for the management of lymphedema. More recently, Dr. Bruno Chikly of France developed methods to recognize the rhythm and flow of both superficial and deep lymph movement and techniques to map lymph flow to better assist its movement with lymph drainage therapy.

Before beginning the study of lymph massage, the practitioner or student must have a thorough knowledge of anatomy, particularly of the lymphatic system. Lymph drainage massage requires careful training procedures. Vodder's manual lymph drainage massage and Chikly's lymph drainage therapy are taught in the United States, Canada, and Europe. Students and therapists interested in practicing these techniques are urged to enroll in training under the guidance of qualified instructors.

The following overview is intended to help you, the practitioner, understand the basic functions of the lymphatic system and the principles of the lymph massage.

The Lymphatic System

angulus venosus

is the juncture of the jugular and subclavian veins.

The lymphatic system is a system of vessels and nodes supplementary to the blood vascular system and provides another pathway for fluids of the circulatory system to return to the heart. In contrast to blood circulation, which is a closed loop, lymph circulation is one way, beginning when interstitial fluid enters the closed-end lymph capillary and ending when lymph reenters the venous blood flow in the subclavian vein at the junction of the internal jugular vein in an area called the **angulus venosus**, just before the blood returns to the heart. The lymphatic system consists of lymph, lymph vessels, and lymph nodes. Lymph vessels include initial lymphatics or lymph capillaries, precollectors, collectors, and lymph ducts or trunks.

Lymph Vessels

The walls of lymph capillaries are composed of a single layer of flat, endothelial cells. The outer surface of these cells have has fine anchoring filaments that connect the capillaries to the surrounding tissue (Figure 16-1). Movement of the tissue or fluid pressure in the connective tissue pulls on the filaments, thereby opening the space between the cells of the capillary walls and allowing the tissue fluid to enter the lymphatic capillary. These anchoring filaments play an important role in lymph drainage massage in that the gentle movements of the massage tug on the filaments, encouraging fluid into the lymph system. The spaces created between the cells in the walls of the lymphatic capillaries act as tiny valves that allow fluid from the interstitial spaces to enter the capillaries. Once inside the capillaries, the fluid is considered lymph. Lymph is carried from the capillaries into slightly larger pre-collectors containing bicuspid valves that prevent backflow and direct the lymph into even larger collector vessels. *Collectors* are the main transporting vessels that carry the lymph toward the lymph nodes and then on to the larger trunks or ducts. The walls of the collector vessels are several cells thick and contain smooth muscle that helps to propel lymph through the system. Smooth muscle in the lymph collector vessels is under the control of the autonomic nervous system and is most active when activated by the parasympathetic impulses. Trunks or ducts are the largest lymph vessels that carry lymph to the deep veins at the base of the neck where the lymph is reunited with the blood just before it reenters the heart.

chyle

is a cloudy liquid, consisting mostly of fats, that passes from the small intestines, through the lacteals, and into the lymph system.

Specialized lymph vessels in the walls of the small intestine, called *lacteals*, carry away fat that is absorbed in the digestive tract. The milky fluid that collects in the lacteals is called **chyle**.

Lymph

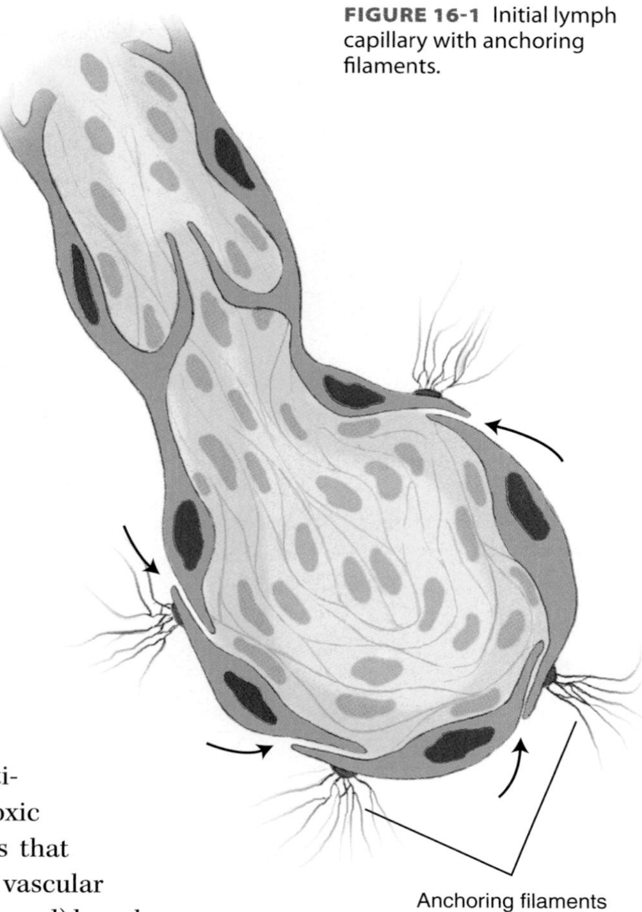

FIGURE 16-1 Initial lymph capillary with anchoring filaments.

Lymph is interstitial fluid that is absorbed into the lymphatic system. Interstitial fluid is derived from blood plasma and continuously bathes the cells and connective tissues. Tissues receive nourishment and building materials from this interstitial fluid and also release waste products and toxins into the fluid. Without it, tissues would soon dry out and degenerate. Between 80 and 98 percent of this fluid, containing dissolved gases, waste products of metabolism, and water, is reabsorbed into the blood vessels. Between 2 and 20 percent of the fluid is absorbed into the lymphatic system to become lymph.

Lymph is composed of approximately 96 percent water and can contain proteins, fats, hormones, enzymes, lymphocytes, phagocytes, tissue debris, cell parts, bacteria, viruses, or other toxins, including cancerous tissue. The reabsorption spaces in the lymphatics are four to five times larger than those in the venous capillaries. This allows the lymphatic capillaries to absorb larger proteins, antigens, and other waste elements that are too large or toxic to be absorbed into the venous system. Contaminants that could be harmful if left to circulate freely through the vascular system are carried in the lymph by way of the afferent (inward) lymph vessels and deposited in the lymph nodes. Here, antigens, damaged cells, and toxins are acted on, broken down, or devoured by the lymphocytes. They are turned into harmless substances and passed out of the lymph nodes through efferent (outward) vessels. Eventually, they pass through the lymph ducts and back into the blood system to be eliminated through the liver, kidneys, lungs, or digestive system.

Lymph generally flows toward the heart. Superficial lymph flow in a mostly healthy, nonobstructed system is toward the nearest lymph nodes that are responsible for draining the area. Lymph flows from lymphatic capillaries to pre-collectors and then to larger collectors that carry the fluid toward the lymph nodes. Lymph travels from the lymph nodes into deeper collecting vessels toward the thoracic duct from the lower extremities and toward the venous reentry site at the base of the neck from the upper extremities. Lymph from the right side of the head and neck, the right upper extremity, and the right side of the torso above the belt line flows into the right lymphatic duct before reentering the venous blood system near the junction of the right subclavian vein and right jugular vein (Figure16-2). Lymph from the lower extremities flows toward the inguinal lymph nodes and then toward and into the cisterna chyli at the base of the thoracic duct. The lymph is joined by chyle from the lacteals. Lymph from the left side of the head and neck and the left upper extremities flows toward and into the left thoracic duct before it

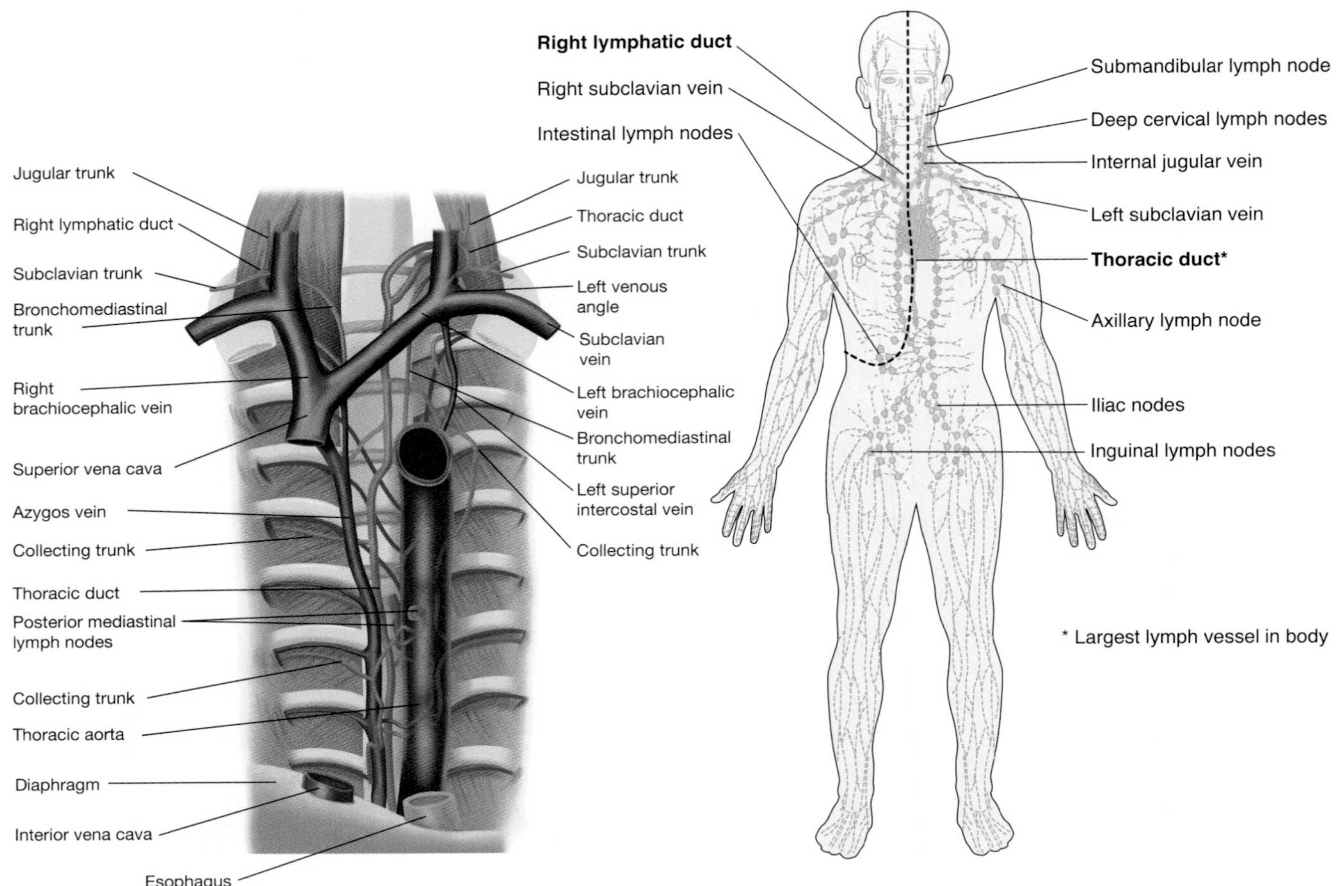

FIGURE 16-2 Areas of the body drained by the right lymphatic duct and the thoracic duct. Lymph massage movements contact the skin and first move transverse to the flow of lymph and then in the direction toward the nearest lymph nodes. a. Massage movements on the neck. b. Movements on the arm are toward the axillary nodes. c. Movements on the leg are toward the inguinal nodes.

reenters the venous blood flow at the left subclavian vein near the junction of the left jugular vein.

Lymph flow can become inhibited for many reasons, including lack of physical activity, stress, fatigue, or emotional trauma. Surgical procedures sometimes remove lymph nodes or create scar tissue that obstructs lymph flow.

Lymph circulation is vital to life: When it slows down, waste products can accumulate and stagnate. Body tissues often become puffy and show signs of edema. The movement of lymph is maintained by the actions of the smooth muscles in the larger lymph vessels, by normal respiration, and by muscular movements of the body in general.

Lymph Nodes

Lymph nodes are small masses of lymphoid tissue. They vary in size and shape but are usually less than 1 inch (2.5 cm) in length. They are often beadlike or bean-shaped compact structures that lie in groups along the course of lymphatic vessels. There are an estimated 400 to 1,000 lymph nodes in the body. Superficial lymph nodes are located in areas where the body folds, except the wrists. Major areas of nodes that drain the flow of superficial lymph are the sides of the neck, the axillary area, and the inguinal crease. Nearly one half of the lymph nodes in the body are located deep in the abdomen, and they collect lymph from intestines and other organs of the body. When inflamed and swollen, lymph nodes can be felt beneath the skin.

Functions of the lymph nodes include the following:

- The filtration of toxins and other elements from the lymph.
- The breakdown or destruction of harmful substances by the action of lymphocytes and phagocytes.
- Concentration of lymph by reabsorbing fluid back into the venous system.
- Production of monocytes and lymphocytes.

Lymph nodes are usually distributed in groups. Regional lymph nodes include the following:

- Submaxillary nodes are located beneath the mandible.
- Preauricular nodes are located in front of the ear.
- Postauricular nodes are located behind the ear in the region of the mastoid process.
- Occipital nodes are located at the base of the skull.
- Superficial cervical nodes are located at the side of and over the sternocleidomastoid muscle.
- Deep cervical nodes are located along the carotid artery and internal jugular vein.
- Axillary nodes are located in the axilla (armpit). Constituting the main group of the upper extremity, axillary nodes receive lymph from vessels that drain the wall of the thorax, mammary glands, upper wall of the abdomen, and the arm.
- Supratrochlear nodes are located in the elbows.
- Inguinal nodes, located in the groin and constituting the most important group of the lower extremity, receive lymph from the leg, external genitalia, and lower abdominal wall.
- Popliteal nodes are located behind the knee.
- Abdominal and pelvic cavities also contain numerous lymph nodes.

Lymph nodes are part of the lymphoid system and the immune system. The immune system produces lymphocytes and other cells in response to the presence of inflammation, antigens, bacteria, viruses, and other cellular debris in the body. Lymphocytes are active in the immune responses of the body and play a major role in wound healing and fighting infections. The primary lymphoid organs are the bone marrow and the thymus gland, where most of the lymphocytes are produced. B-lymphocytes are produced and mature in the bone marrow. Lymphocytes produced in the bone marrow that migrate and mature in the thymus are termed T-lymphocytes. When an antigen enters the body, B-lymphocytes produce antibodies that counteract the antigen and produce an immune response that protects the body from future exposures. When an antigen enters the body, T-lymphocytes activate and destroy the foreign invader.

Secondary lymphoid organs include the spleen, tonsils, adenoids, appendix, and the lymph nodes. Lymphocytes reside in the secondary lymphoid organs in high concentrations, ready to actively counter any problematic substances they encounter. Lymphocytes also penetrate all tissues and are abundant in blood, mucous membranes, connective tissue, skin, and all body organs except the central nervous system. (For more information on the lymph system, see Chapter 5, page **202**)

Influence of Massage on Body Fluids

It is important to understand the influence of massage on the circulation of fluids in the human body. Both the lymphatic and venous circulation systems are accelerated by massage movements. Lymph massage activates the movement of lymph into and through the lymph system. Lymph massage stimulates the activity of the lymph nodes, increases the production of lymphocytes, and improves the body's metabolism. Lymph massage helps to drain stagnant interstitial fluids, toxins, and proteins from the interstitial fluid, helping to rid the body of toxins and waste materials. Lymph massage stimulates the immune system by bringing more antigens in closer contact with lymphocytes in the lymph nodes. The slow rhythmic pace of lymph massage is very relaxing and stimulates the parasympathetic nervous system, which in turn is helpful in relieving stress, depression, and some types of insomnia.

Lymph massage promotes the balance of the body's internal chemistry, purifies and regenerates tissues, helps to normalize the functions of organs, and enhances the function of the immune system.

Contraindications for Lymph Massage

Contraindications for lymph massage are generally the same as for general Swedish massage. If there is any question about a condition, refer the client to a doctor and work under the guidance or supervision of a physician or other qualified health practitioner.

Contraindications for lymph massage include the following:

- Acute infections and fever.
- Inflammation (e.g., heat, redness, swelling, pain).
- Cardiac problems; congestive heart failure, uncontrolled high blood pressure, cardiac insufficiency.
- Kidney dysfunctions.
- Acute tuberculosis.
- Venous obstructions (e.g., phlebitis, thrombosis).
- Bleeding, hemorrhage, or weeping sores.
- Malignant illness, cancer when the tumor is still present, or lymphomas. Lymph massage has proven beneficial as a postsurgical treatment to manage secondary lymphedema resulting from the surgical removal of regional lymph nodes. This should be done only by experienced therapists trained in lymph drainage massage, under the supervision of a physician, and with the informed consent of the client after having signed a release form.
- Edemas of unknown origin: Avoid work on edemas caused by kidney, heart, or liver dysfunction. Always consult the client's physician if there is any doubt.
- Any condition that could be made worse by increasing fluid circulation.

Techniques of Lymph Massage

The techniques of lymph massage are gentle, rhythmic, slow, and somewhat circular movements. Lymph massage encourages the flow of lymph into and through the lymphatic capillaries and toward the lymph nodes that drain the area being massaged. Light circular movements create a wavelike action that encourages the movement of lymph through the lymph vessels.

The practitioner's hand lightly contacts the client's skin and gently and slowly moves the skin over the subdermal layers. The pressure is between 1 and 8 ounces per square inch (1 to 8 oz/in^2). The more delicate the tissues or severe the edema, the lighter the pressure. The maneuvers are somewhat circular or elliptical, with the hand in contact with the skin as it moves first across the natural direction of lymph flow and then in the intended direction of the lymph flow. The practitioner applies only enough pressure to contact the skin and create movement of the superficial tissues. First the superficial tissue is stretched very slightly transverse to the direction of the lymph flow, which pulls on the filaments. This action opens the initial lymphatics, allowing the uptake of lymph from the interstitial spaces. This is immediately followed by stretching the tissues in the direction of the lymph flow, which moves the fluid through the superficial vessels toward the appropriate lymph nodes and deeper collecting vessels. After a slight stretch, the skin is released so that it snaps back, closing the lymphatics. The circular movement is continued to the point where contact is reestablished and the circle is repeated. Each circular stroke slightly stretches the skin and underlying tissues in an inverted L-shaped pattern and then releases the contact, returning the skin to its original position. The process is then repeated. The rhythm is slow, with five to ten repetitions per minute depending on the natural, personal rhythm of the client. The movement is repeated in the same area several times before the practitioner moves to an adjacent area. With some practice and awareness, the practitioner can become attuned to the rhythm of the lymph movement.

The target of lymph massage is the superficial lymphatic capillaries located just a few millimeters below the skin surface in the dermis. It is estimated that superficial lymph circulation accounts for approximately 70 percent of the lymph in the body. When lymph massage is performed, the hand pressure against the skin is therefore very light. If the practitioner can feel any of the deeper structures or tissues, the pressure is probably too heavy. The pressure should be just enough to feel the fluid nature of the subdermal tissue. The pressure is lightest on the delicate tissues of the face and only slightly more on the thicker tissues of the arms or legs. Pressure may be increased a bit more where lymph nodes are located in the axial and inguinal areas.

Touch and Pressure

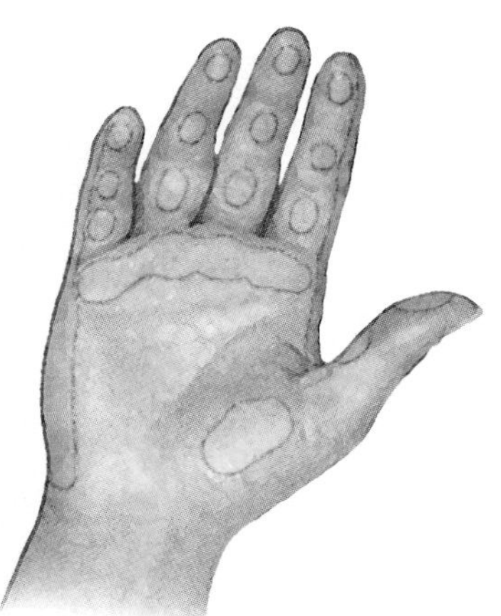

FIGURE 16-3 The soft pads on the palm of the hand make contact during lymph massage.

The touch is very light, using the soft pads of the fingers, thumb, and palm of the hand (Figure 16-3). Just enough pressure is used to encourage fluid into the delicate lymph capillaries. Too much pressure tends to collapse the lymphatics and increase the volume of fluids filtrating from the blood capillaries, which is directly counterproductive to the intention of lymph massage. The very light circular movements of lymph massage are gentle, rhythmic, and in harmony with the natural body rhythms of the client.

Direction

The direction of the movement is first transverse to the flow of lymph, to encourage the uptake of fluid, and then toward the closest concentration of lymph nodes.

Rhythm

The rhythm is slow. The practitioner moves according to the client's natural rhythm. Each pulsation of the circular movement is between 4 and 10 seconds. The practitioner should quietly tune into and enhance the unique wave of fluid movement.

Frequency

The movement is repeated in the same area five to ten times, sometimes more, before moving to the next adjacent area. There is a discernable softening or warming of the tissues as the fluid begins to move.

Successful lymph drainage massage depends on the expertise and sensitivity of the practitioner. Practitioners must consider the effects to be achieved by various movements. For example, body fluids can be displaced intravascularly (within vessels) or extravascularly (in the interstitial spaces). This displacement of fluid is achieved by manual strokes.

Sequence of Movements

The sequence of movements generally begins and ends at the site of the collecting lymph nodes draining the area being massaged or at the reentry site where lymph rejoins the venous blood at the angulus venosus. Lymph massage on the neck and head begins and ends inferior and superior to the clavicles near the sternal notch. Lymph massage on the extremities begins and ends at the site of the lymph nodes in the axilla or inguinal crease respectively. The lymph massage sequence begins proximally, to clear out the lymph channels, and then works distally and then again from distal to proximal, finishing by once again helping to clear the area of the lymph nodes.

Movements are first directed toward the regional lymph nodes. Successive movements then progress away from the nodes while directing the movements to encourage lymph flow toward the nodes. On the arms, the movements begin in the axillary area and progress down the arm to the hand. The slow rhythmic movements encourage lymph flow toward the medial aspect of the arm and toward the lymph nodes in the axillary area. Similarly, on the legs, the movements begin in the inguinal crease to clear the inguinal nodes and progress down the leg to the foot. Movements direct the lymph flow toward the inguinal area. After massaging all the way to the foot, the therapist works back up the leg, finishing by once again clearing the inguinal nodes. On the back of the thigh, movements are directed toward the inguinal area on the medial aspect of the thigh or around the lateral aspect to the front leg and then on toward the inguinal nodes. On the back of the lower leg, movements are directed toward the popliteal space behind the knee, the location of some minor nodes.

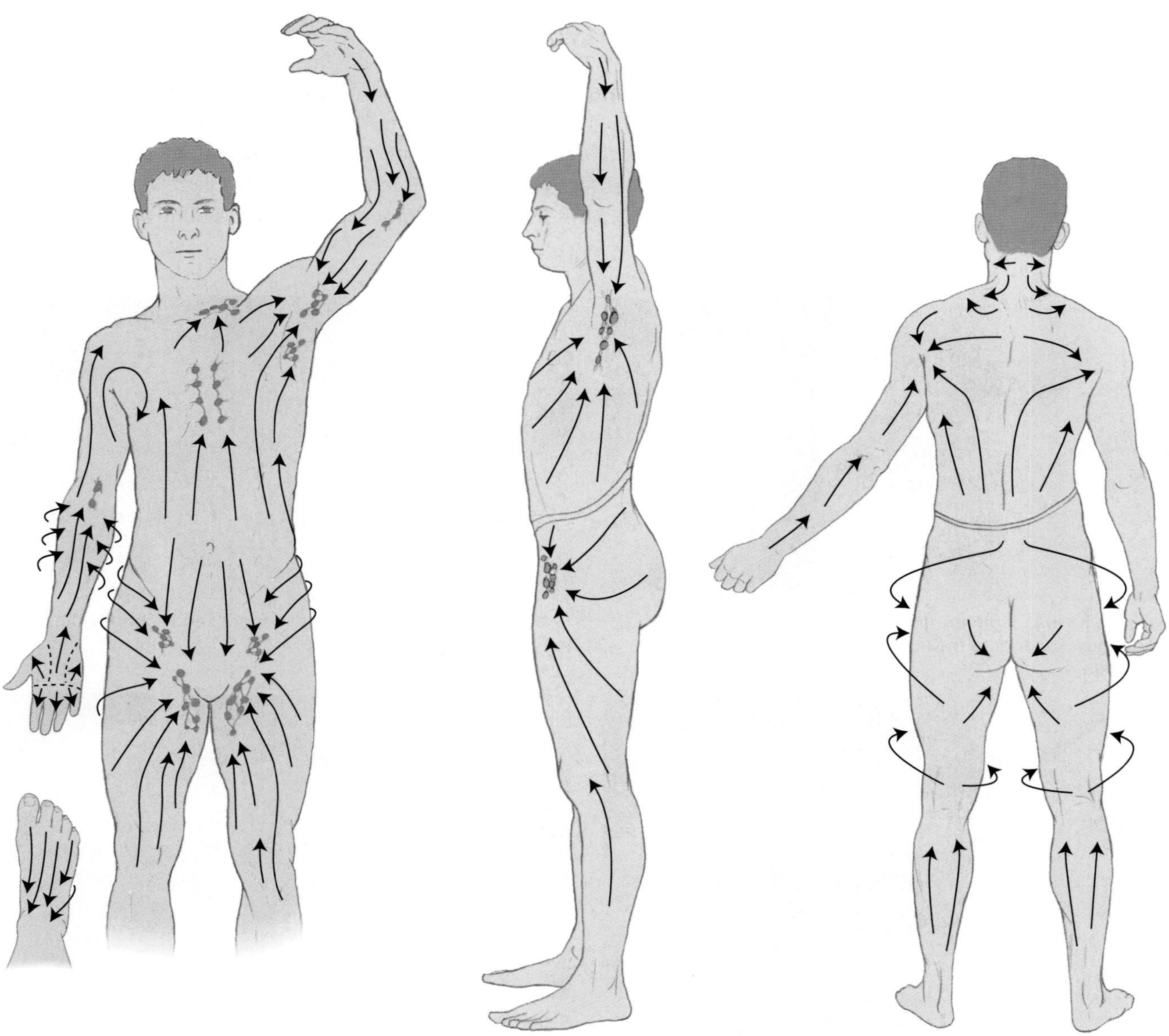

FIGURE 16-4A Direction of superficial lymph flow on the anterior of the body.

FIGURE 16-4B Direction of lymph flow on the lateral and posterior aspects of the body.

Superficial lymph flow in the torso is generally directed toward the closest concentration of lymph nodes. Above the belt line, approximately at the level of the umbilicus, lymph flow is toward the axillary nodes of the same side of the body. Below the belt line, lymph moves inferiorly toward the inguinal nodes on the same side of the body (Figure 16-4a and b).

Before attempting lymph massage, the practitioner should be thoroughly familiar with the functions of the lymphatic system. Lymph massage is done to enhance, but not force, the movement of lymph through the lymphatic system. The procedure begins at the junction of the right thoracic lymph ducts and the subclavian vein adjacent to the junction of the jugular veins, and just behind the clavicle near its articulation with the sternum. This is where the lymph system empties into the venous blood.

PROCEDURE FOR A LYMPH MASSAGE

The massage described in this chapter targets the lymph system in general and is appropriate for clients who might have a somewhat sluggish lymph flow because of inactivity, overactivity, or local trauma but otherwise are generally healthy. Additional training is recommended for therapists who intend to work with clients who have more serious lymphatic conditions. The following procedure should be done only under the supervision of a qualified instructor.

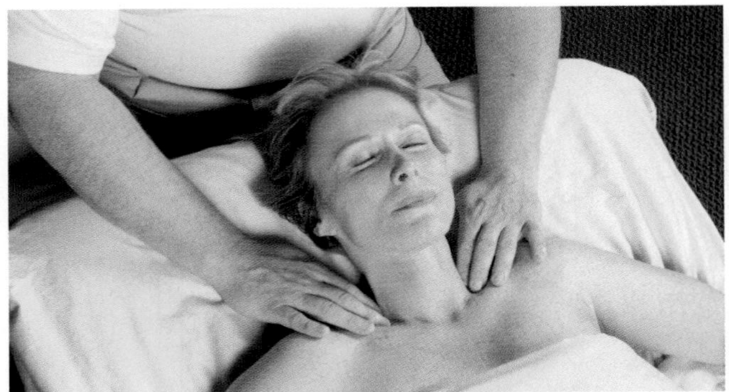

FIGURE 16-5A Begin the lymph massage with the therapist's fingers just superior to the medial clavicle near the angulus venosus.

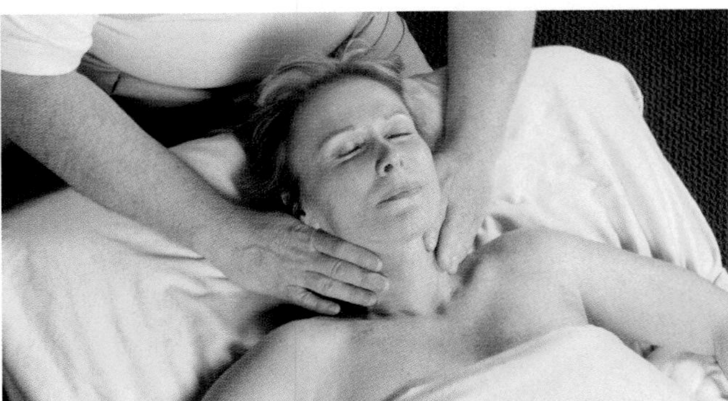

FIGURE 16-5B Move the hands superior and continue the slow movements of lymph massage.

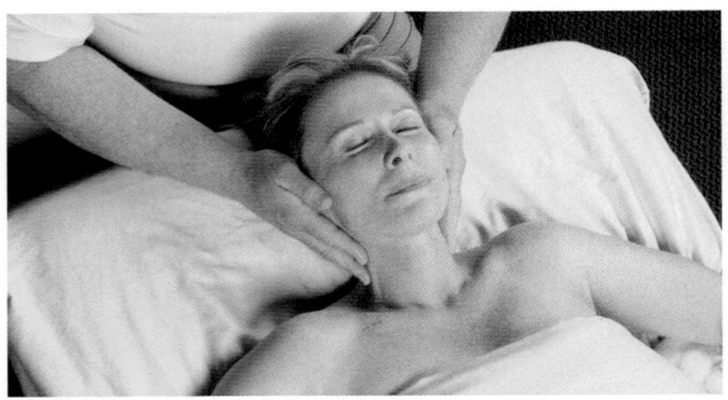

FIGURE 16-5C Continue with the lymph massage movements, directing the lymph flow downward while working up the neck.

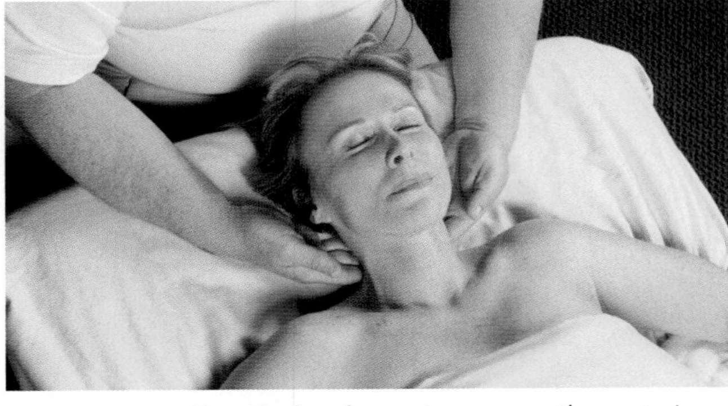

FIGURE 16-5D Turn the hands over to massage the posterior aspect of the side of the neck from the bottom to the top.

1. *Neck:* The high concentration of lymph nodes in the neck protects the organism from infectious invasion through the mouth, nose, eyes, and ears. Methodically encouraging lymph movement through and out of this area is a valuable practice. Lymph massage begins where lymph circulation ends, at the base of the neck, just superior to the clavicles, close to their sternal attachment. The client is positioned supine on the massage table, and the practitioner is preferably seated above the client's head (Figure 16-5a). The pads of all four fingers are used to contact the area just superior to the medial clavicle on both sides of the neck. Small, light, circular or elliptical movements encourage lymph movement toward the angulus venosus, which is the junction of the subclavian and the jugular veins. The movements are slow, approximately six to ten rotations per minute, and repeated several times in the same spot. The practitioner's hands then move slightly superiorly and posteriorly (Figure 16-5b) and continue the light, circular movements with the soft pads of the fingers, directing the flow toward the base of the neck. After five to ten repetitions or revolutions, move the fingers up to the next adjacent area (Figure 16-5c) and continue the slow, gentle, wavelike movements, directing the lymph flow down the neck. Methodically proceed to massage the entire lateral aspect of the neck, from the anterior border of the sternocleidomastoid muscle to the lateral aspect of the splenius capitis or the trapezius and from the base of the neck to the base of the ear and the occiput at the top of the neck (Figure 16-5d). Finish with superficial effleurage in a downward direction on the entire side of the head and neck.

2. *Pectoral and axillary area:* Superficial lymph from the central, upper chest flows toward the clavicles and the angulus venosus. Light circular strokes along the sternal and subclavicular borders are therefore directed toward the angulus venosus. Massage can continue just inferior to the clavicle all the way to the axillary fold, directing the flow toward the angulus venosus.

   Lymph from the axillary lymph nodes flows into deeper collector vessels and toward the midclavicular region and the angulus venosus. Initial massage to the axillary lymph nodes can begin bilaterally by gently placing the fingers deep into the axillary fold and directing the movements in a midclavicular direction (Figure 16-6a and b). Access to the axillary nodes can be increased by abducting and laterally rotating the client's arm (Figure 16-7a to c). Continue the gentle, circular, wavelike movements in different aspects of the axillary area that can be easily accessed from this position. Remember, slow movements should be repeated several times in the same area. Continue to direct the lymph deep toward the midclavicular direction. Complete this area of massage by again clearing the subclavicular and supraclavicular areas near the lymphatic trunks and the angulus venosus.

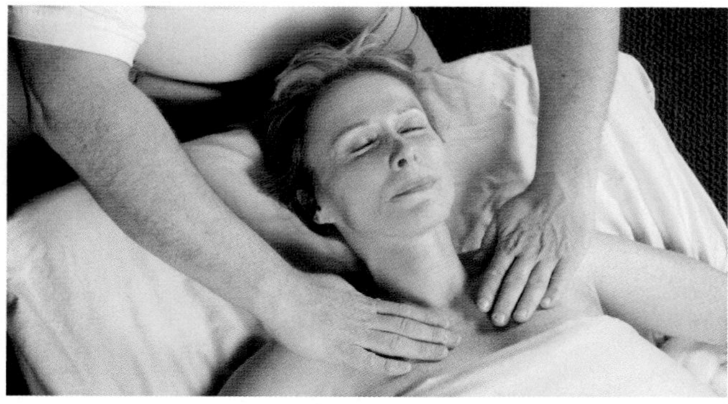

FIGURE 16-6A Lymph flow is directed toward the angulus venosus from the subclavicular areas.

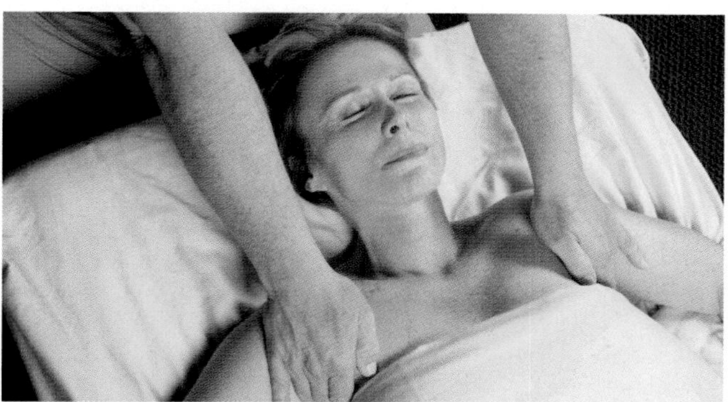

FIGURE 16-6B Lymph in the axilla is directed toward the midclavicular area.

The preceding massage maneuvers are performed with the practitioner seated above the client's head. The following movements are done with the practitioner standing on the same side of the client being massaged.

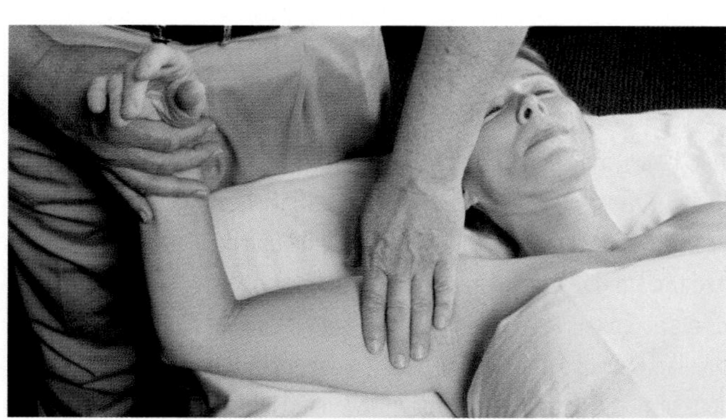

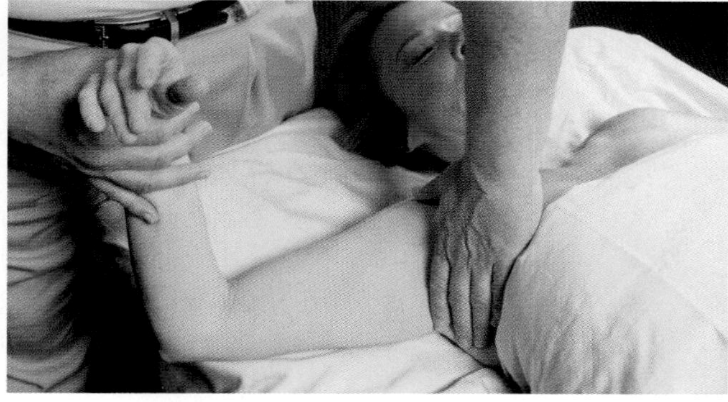

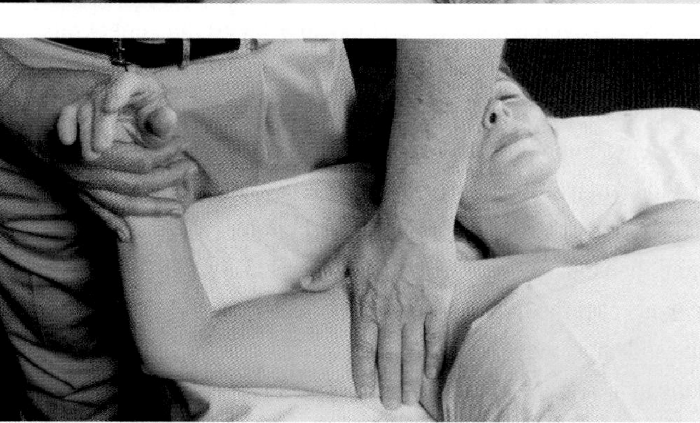

FIGURE 16-7A, B, AND C More of the axilla can be massaged by abducting and laterally rotating the arm.

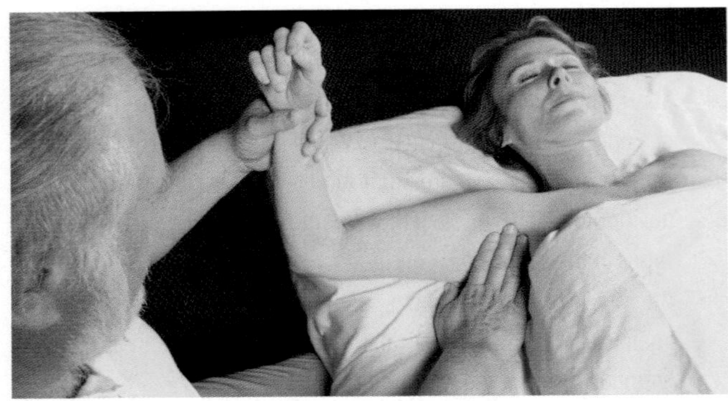

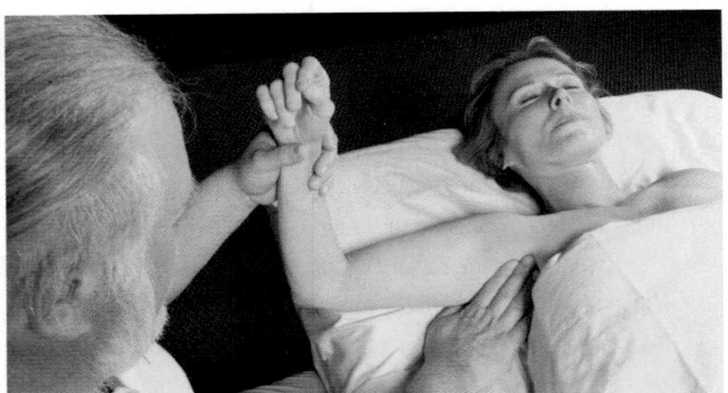

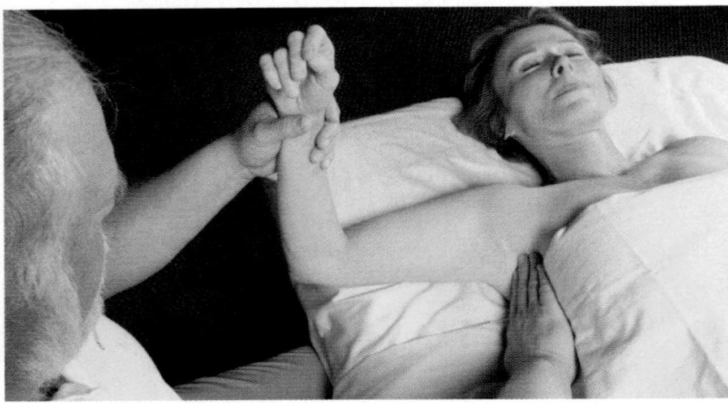

FIGURE 16-8A, B, AND C While the client's arm is abducted, the therapist can massage the (a) anterior and pectoral, (b) posterior, and (c) inferior nodes of the axilla.

Massage of the upper quadrant can continue by repeating the lymph massage to the axillary nodes or by proceeding to the arm.

The Upper Quadrant

3. *Axillary area* (*continued*): Superficial lymph from the upper quadrant generally flows to the axillary nodes on the same side of the body. (An exception is when axillary nodes have been surgically removed or otherwise damaged; lymph can then adopt other pathways into neighboring quadrants.)

   Continue massage directed toward the axillary area from a standing position at the client's side. Gently place the soft pads of the fingers onto areas of the axilla that were not addressed previously. Apply slow, rhythmic, circular, wavelike movements directed deeper into the axilla. Approach the area from different directions until the entire area has been covered (Figure 16-8a to c).
4. *Upper quadrant of the torso:* Superficial lymph from the pectoral area, breast, and upper torso flows toward the lymph nodes in the axillary area of the same side. Lymph massage in this area begins proximal to the axillary fold (Figure 16-9a and b). Movements can be applied with the entire hand or even both hands when appropriate (Figure 16-9c and d). Place the hand close to the axilla, with as much of the hand making contact as possible. Apply gentle, circular, wavelike movements directed toward the axillary nodes. Repeat the slow, rhythmic movements five to ten times in the same place and then move the hands to an adjacent area just distal and repeat the movements. Apply movements over the lateral and anterior rib cage, and work in sections. Begin just inferior to the axilla and apply movements with the intention of moving lymph toward the axilla while working in increments to the bottom of the rib cage, then repeat the movements moving closer to the axilla. Massage the pectoral area in the same way, beginning

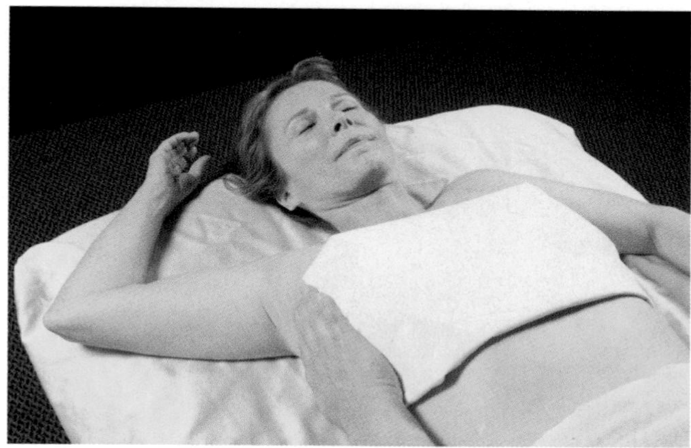

FIGURE 16-9A Lymph massage on the lateral torso begins near the axilla.

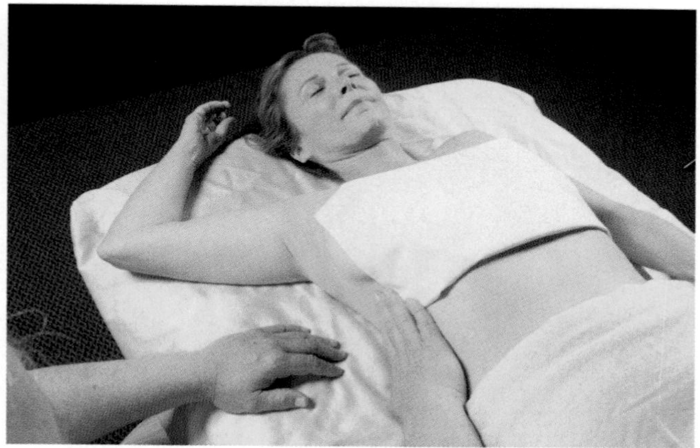

FIGURE 16-9B Lymph massage continues down the side. directing lymph toward the axilla. Two hands can be used.

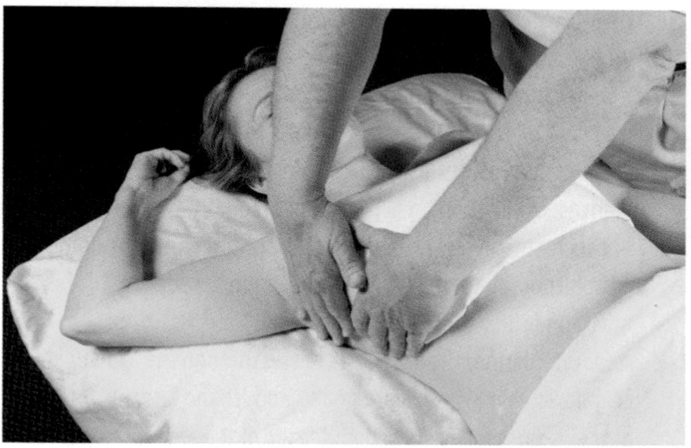

FIGURE 16-9C The therapist can stand on the opposite side of the table while applying lymph massage to the torso.

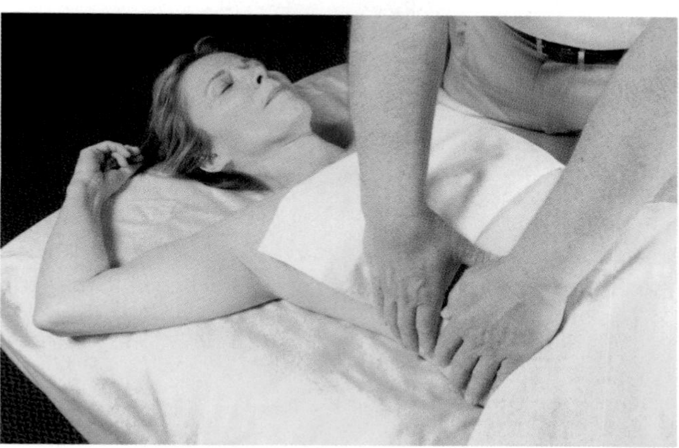

FIGURE 16-9D Continue working down the side of the torso while directing lymph flow toward the axilla.

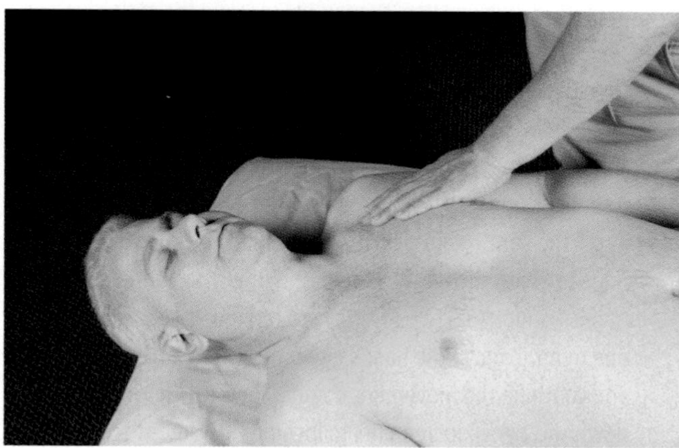

FIGURE 16-10A Lymph is directed from the pectoral region to the axilla.

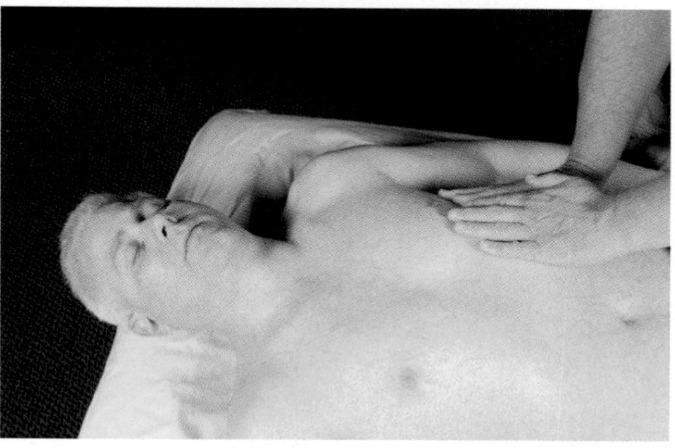

FIGURE 16-10B Two hands can be used in some areas.

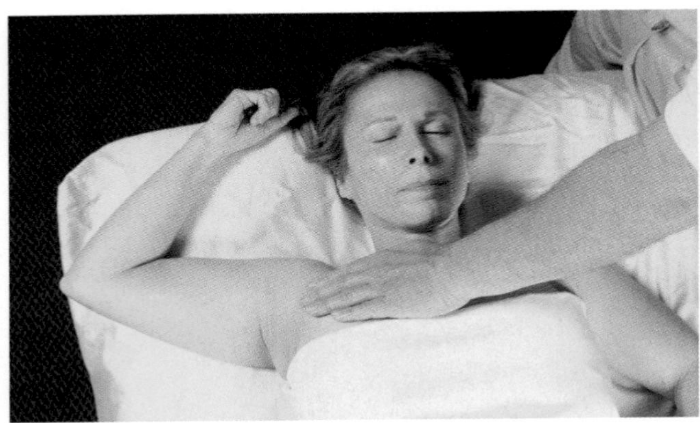

FIGURE 16-11A Proper draping is used on female clients. Apply lymph massage on the upper pectoral area.

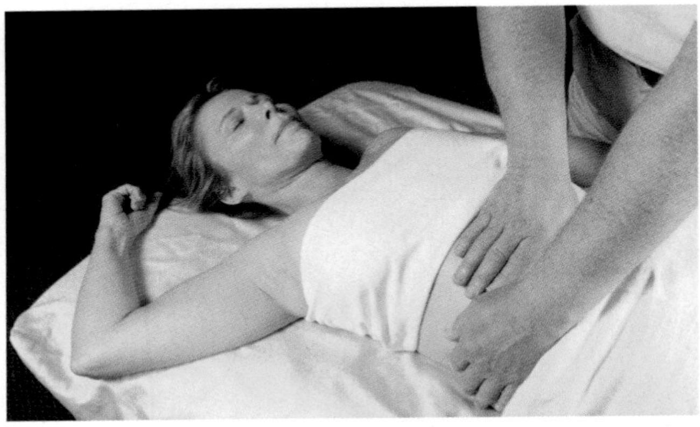

FIGURE 16-11B Apply massage below the breast, avoiding the breast tissue.

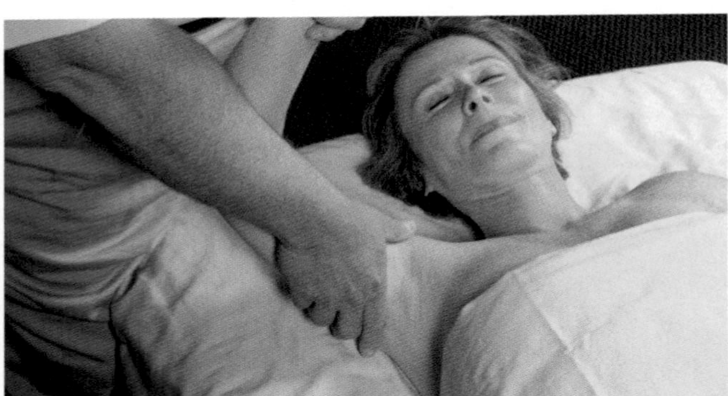

FIGURE 16-12A Lymph massage of the arm begins at the axilla.

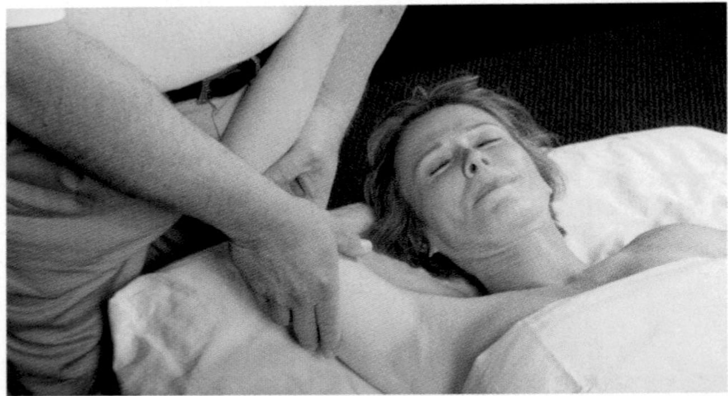

FIGURE 16-12B Massage continues down the brachial aspect of the arm, directing the flow toward the axilla.

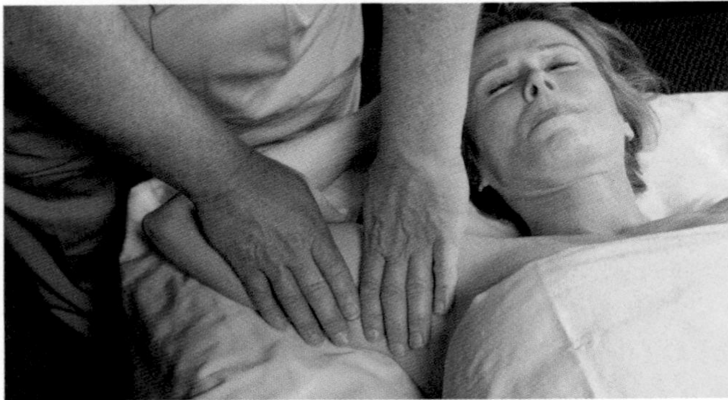

FIGURE 16-12C One or two hands can be used on the inner arm.

close to the axilla, moving incrementally away to cover the pectoral area and then back to the axilla, all the time directing lymph flow toward the axillary nodes. On male clients, begin near the axilla and apply movements first below the nipple line and then above the nipple line (Figure 16-10a and b). On female clients, apply movements above and below, but avoid massage of the breast tissue (Figure 16-11a and b). Although lymph massage of the breast is a benefit in some circumstances, instruction on this methodology is beyond the scope of this text. The serious student can seek advanced training in lymph therapy to offer this highly beneficial service. (Breast massage is also illegal in some jurisdictions.)

5. *Arm:* Lymph from the arm flows to and through the axillary nodes. To gain access to the axillary nodes, abduct and laterally rotate the arm to expose the axilla and underside of the arm and support it in this position. Begin lymph massage of the arm in the axillary fold, directing the lymph flow toward the angulus venosus. Using the soft pads of the fingers of both hands, apply the gentle rhythmic movements of lymph massage to the posterior, medial, and anterior aspects of the axilla (Figure 16-12a to c). Spend a minute or more in each position, thoroughly covering the entire axillary space. Continue movements down the brachial aspect of the arm from the axilla to the elbow and then from the elbow to the axilla. Replace the arm by the client's side on the table.

   Continue lymph massage of the arm by placing one or both hands near the shoulder, over the deltoid muscle, and apply the gentle, slow, circular, wavelike movements of lymph massage with the entire palmar and finger pad surface of the hands (Figure 16-13a). After five to ten revolutions, or about one minute, move the hands down the arm to an adjacent area and continue the movement (Figure 16-13b). Continue moving down the arm in increments to include the forearm, hands, and fingers, all this time directing the lymph flow up the arm toward

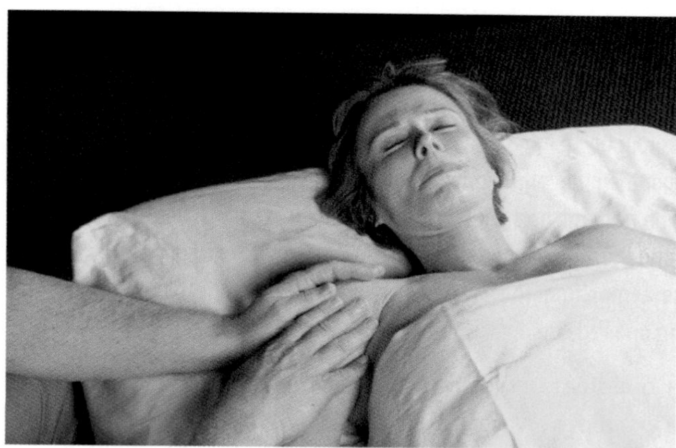

FIGURE 16-13A Arm massage continues on the shoulder; the therapist can use one or two hands.

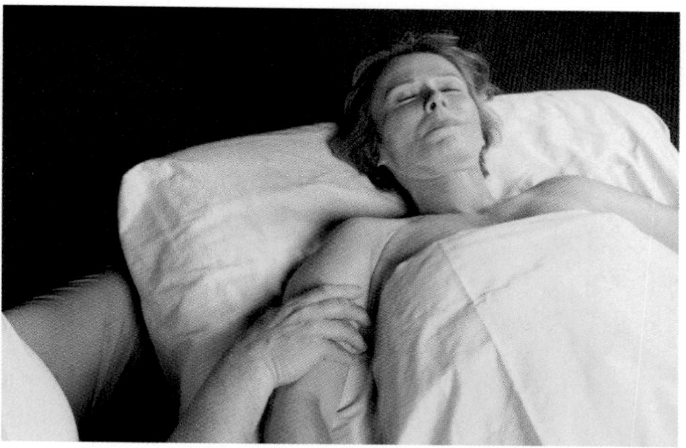

FIGURE 16-13B Lymph massage continues down the arm with the intention of directing lymph toward the axillary nodes.

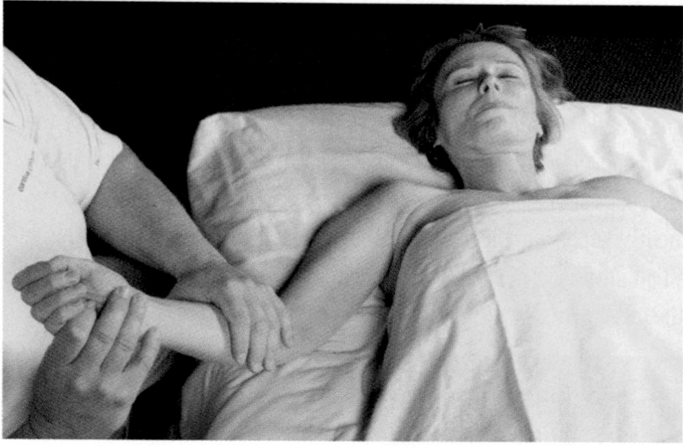

FIGURE 16-13C On the lower arm, lymph flows up and around to the soft side of the arm and continues up to the axillary nodes.

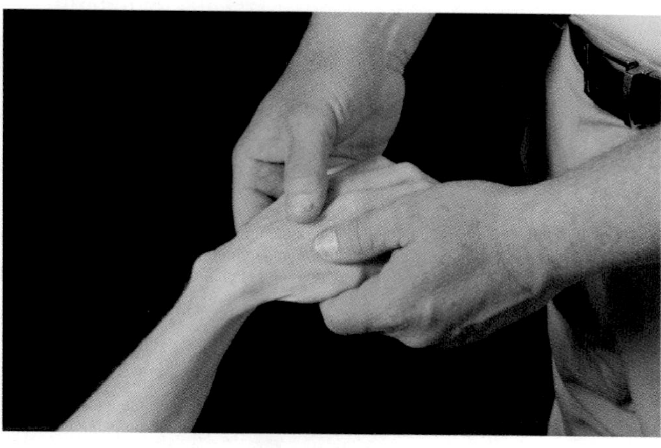

FIGURE 16-13D Massage the back of the hand and the palm with light pressure with the thumb and fingers.

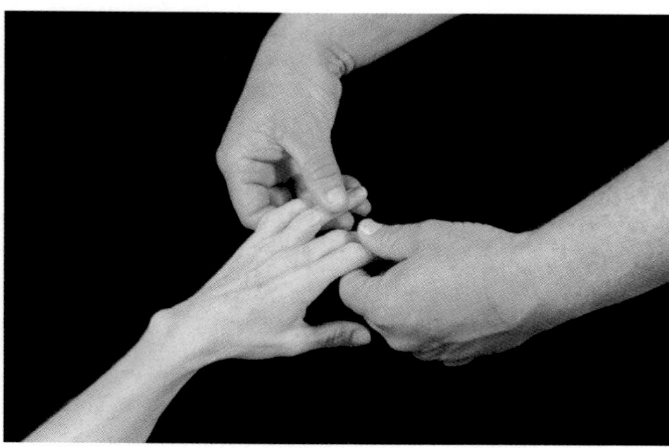

FIGURE 16-13E Apply light circular pressure to each finger and the thumb.

the axilla (Figure 16-13c to e). Briefly repeat the movements from the fingers to the shoulder. Spend extra time in any areas that seem to be congested, again clearing proximal vessels to allow movement from the area. Signal the end of the arm massage with very light effleurage from the hand to the shoulder.

In lymph massage, this procedure illustrates the process of beginning at the site of the central lymph nodes, working from proximal to distal, and then back to proximal again. This regimen can be applied to any area of the body.

Conclude lymph massage of both upper quadrants by moving to the head of the table and again applying massage to the axillary nodes, along the inferior and superior aspects of the clavicles, and finally at the base of the neck near the angulus venosus.

FIGURE 16-14 Major lymph nodes and superficial lymph flow of the lower quadrant.

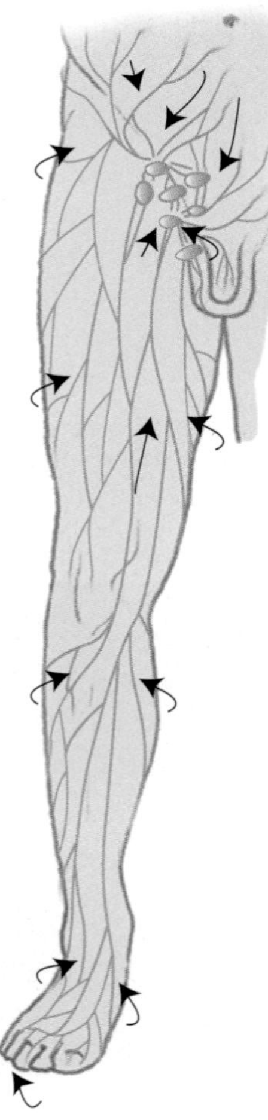

6. *Lower quadrant:* Superficial lymph from the lower quadrant generally flows toward lymph nodes just inferior to the inguinal ligament, and then into deeper iliac nodes and to the cisterna chyli at the inferior end of the thoracic duct, deep in the abdominal cavity. *Note*: The upper boundary of the lower quadrants of the body is roughly defined by a belt line about the level of the umbilicus. Superficial lymph from the lower abdomen flows inferiorly toward the inguinal nodes on the same side of the abdomen. Superficial lymph from the hips, gluteals, and lower back tends to flow more laterally toward the front of the body and the inguinal nodes. Lymph from the lower extremity flows up the leg toward the inguinal crease. Lymph from the lateral aspect of the thigh tends to flow around toward the front of the leg and on to the inguinal nodes (Figure 16-14).

Lymph massage of the lower quadrant begins in the area of the inguinal lymph nodes. The inguinal lymph nodes are located in an area that is quite vulnerable, being touchy and even ticklish, with the lower nodes located very near the genital area. Discuss the lymph massage of the inguinal area with your client before the session and obtain informed consent to work in this area. As you begin massage in this area, alert the client about how you will proceed and explain the placement and movement of your hand. Be extremely discreet and gentle with your hand placement, being careful to employ proper draping skills.

7. *Anterior Legs:* Massage of the leg and lower quadrant begins at the site of the inguinal lymph nodes, which are located along a line just inferior to the inguinal ligament. Begin the massage of the anterior leg by slightly flexing and laterally rotating and abducting the hip. The flexed knee can be supported with either the practitioner's body or a pillow (Figure 16-15a). First contact the lateral, more superior area just below the inguinal ligament with the soft pads of the fingers and begin to apply gentle, slow, rhythmic movements, encouraging the movement of lymph into the deeper vessels. Repeat the wavelike movements ten to twenty times and then reposition the fingers medially and inferiorly until the lower hand borders on the gracilis muscle. Then continue the movements (Figure 16-15b).

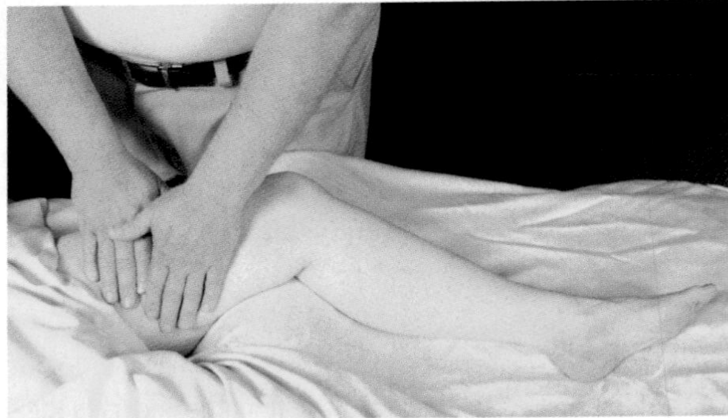

FIGURE 16-15A Lymph massage begins at the site of the inguinal lymph nodes. Flexing and abducting the thigh slightly provides easy access to the inguinal nodes.

FIGURE 16-15B Lymph massage progresses down the medial aspect of the leg.

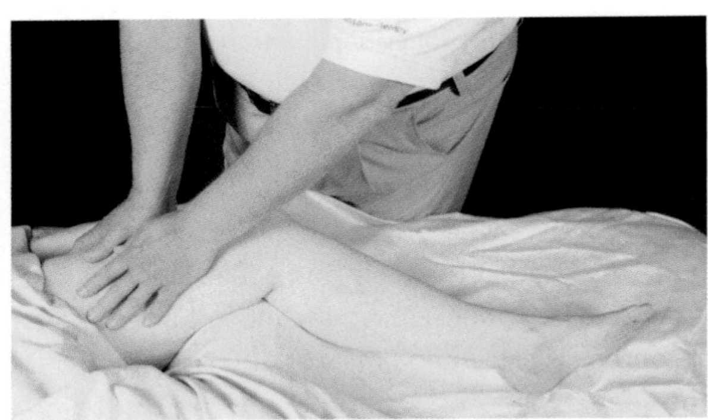

FIGURE 16-15C Two hands can be used to cover a larger area of the leg.

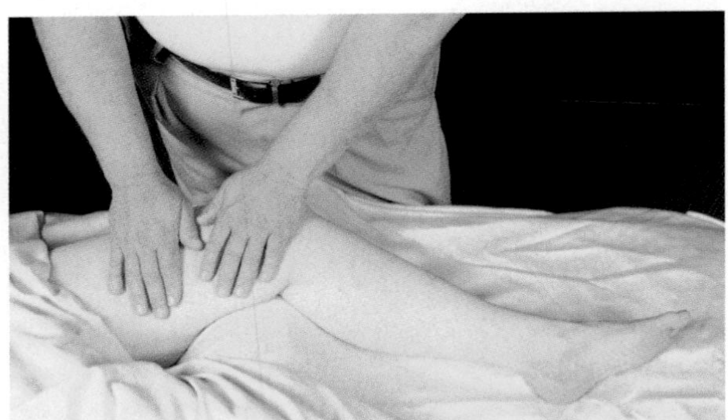

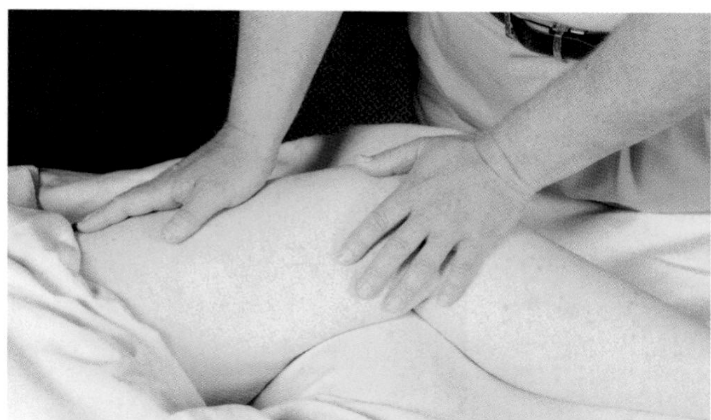

FIGURE 16-16A Lymph massage on the upper lateral thigh is directed toward the inguinal nodes.

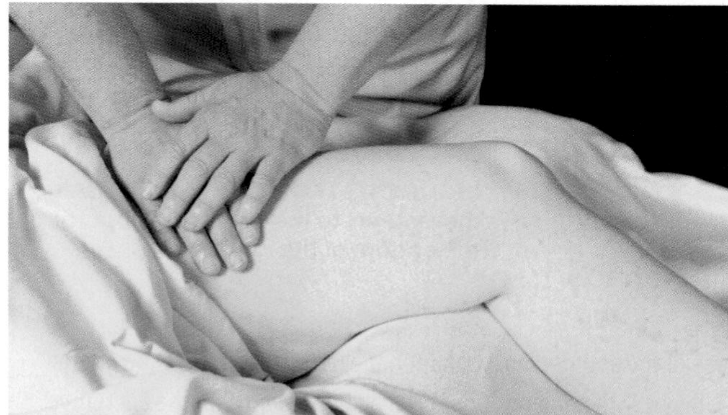

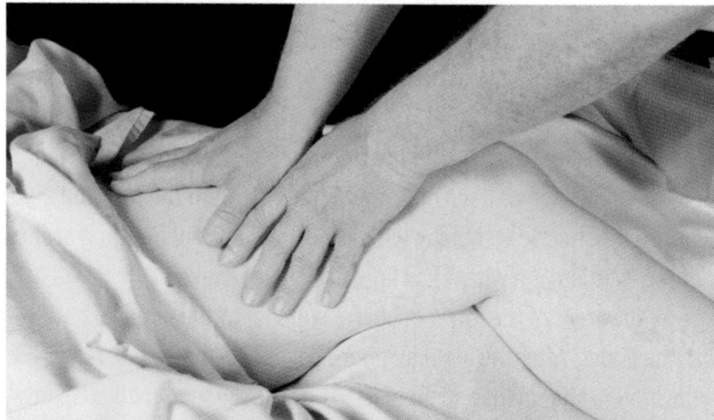

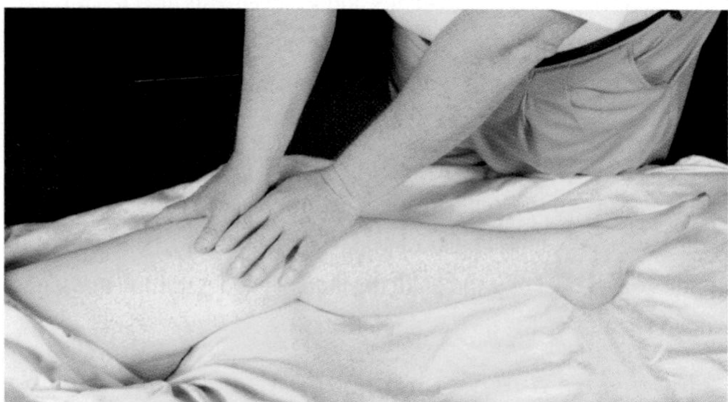

FIGURE 16-16B, 1, 2, AND 3 Two hands can be used on larger areas of the thigh. Begin near the inguinal nodes and progress down the leg, directing the movements toward the inguinal nodes.

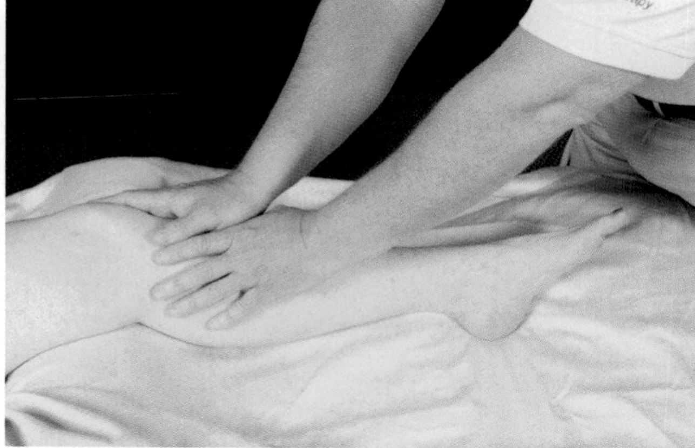

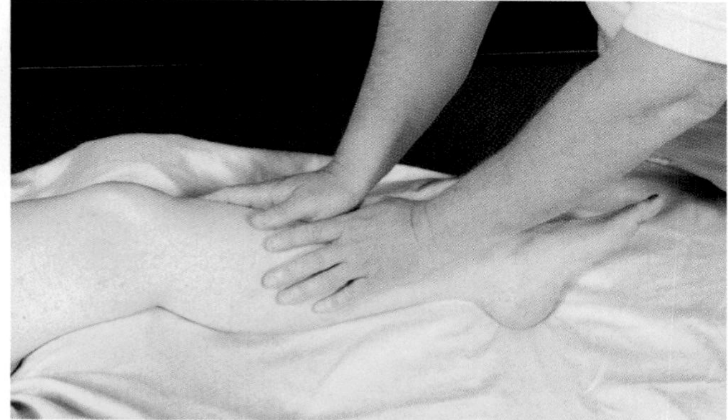

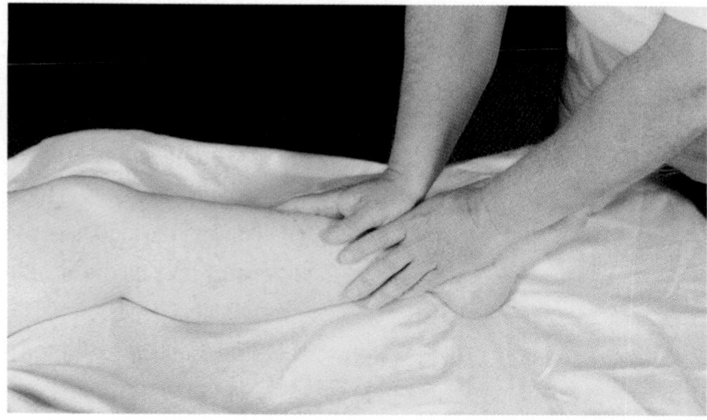

FIGURE 16-16C, 1, 2, AND 3 Continue massage down the lower leg, directing lymph flow up the leg.

With the leg in the same position, lymph massage can easily be applied to the medial aspect of the thigh from the inguinal crease to the knee. Begin with hand positions proximal to the inguinal nodes, applying five to ten slow repetitions, and move incrementally toward the knee (using two hands if so desired) until the medial thigh has been massaged (Figure 16-15c). At this point, light effleurage can be applied from the knee to the hip, or for a more thorough treatment, the lymph massage steps can be reversed. Beginning at the medial aspect of the knee, apply the lymph massage movements, working up the leg and finishing on the inguinal nodes. These return movements can be of a shorter duration.

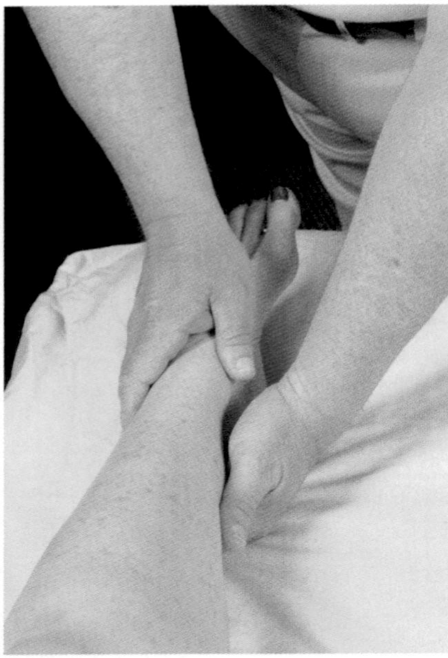

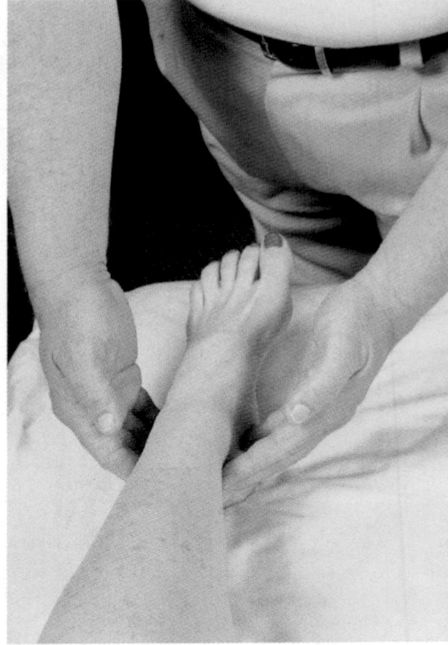

FIGURE 16-16D, 1 AND 2 Beginning with the ankle, apply lymph massage to the foot.

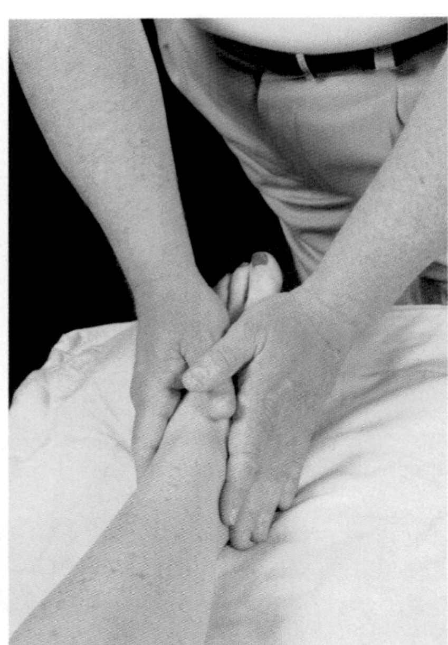

FIGURE 16-16E Apply lymph massage movements to the top while supporting the bottom of the foot.

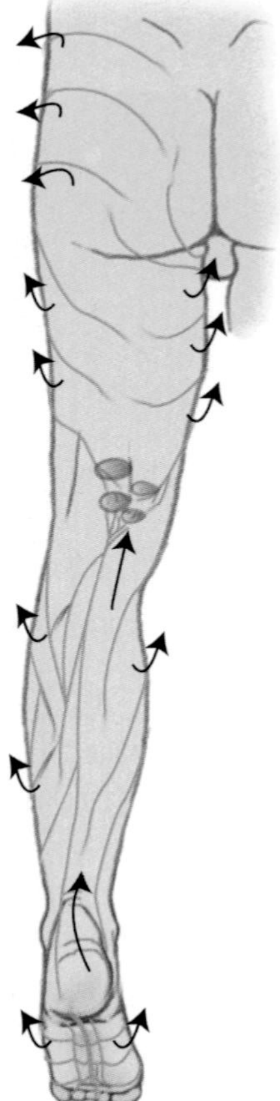

FIGURE 16-17 Superficial lymph flow on the posterior lower quadrant on the body.

To continue lymph massage of the anterior leg, straighten the leg so that it is resting on the massage table (Figure 16-16a). Begin with hand positions on the upper thigh near the ilium. Two hands can be used on much of the legs to cover a larger area in less time. Apply the gentle, slow, circular, wavelike movements of lymph massage with the entire palmar and finger pad surface of both hands. After five to ten revolutions, or about one minute, move the hands down the leg to an adjacent area and continue the movement (Figure 16-16b, 1, 2, and 3). Continue moving down the leg in increments to include the foot (Figure 16-16c to e), all the time directing the flow up the leg toward the inguinal nodes. When the entire leg has been massaged, continue from the foot and work back up the leg using the same slow, gentle technique with a shorter duration, finishing at the inguinal nodes. Signal the end of the leg massage with a few light effleurage strokes.

8. *Lower abdomen:* Lymph massage on the areas of the lower quadrant superior to the inguinal nodes directs the flow inferiorly toward the nodes. After the inguinal nodes have been massaged, massage continues just superior to the inguinal ligament and medial to the anterior superior iliac spine (ASIS). Use the pads of the fingers of one or both hands to gently apply movements directed toward the inguinal nodes for five to ten repetitions. Reposition the hands just superior on to the abdomen and repeat the rotations. Continue new hand placements until the abdomen below the umbilicus has been massaged.
9. *Posterior legs:* The client assumes a prone position on the table. Superficial lymph in the posterior aspect of the lower quadrant still flows toward the inguinal nodes (Figure 16-17). In the upper portion of the quadrant, including the lower back, hips, and most of the gluteal muscles, lymph tends to flow laterally around to the anterior part of the body and on to the inguinal nodes. Lymph massage on these areas therefore is intended to enhance the flow in this direction.

Lymph flow in the posterior thigh divides with lymph from the medial aspect moving directly toward the inguinal nodes, whereas lymph from the lateral aspect finds its way around to the anterior thigh toward the inguinal nodes. This creates w hat is termed a

watershed somewhere near the center of the posterior thigh where the lymph flow splits. A therapist practicing lymph massage movements on the posterior thigh must take this into consideration.

watershed

is the separation of flow of lymph into different drainage territories..

Lymph massage on the lateral aspect of the posterior leg begins in the neighborhood of the greater trochanter. Movements are made with the intention of enhancing lymph flow toward the front of the body. Movements can then progress either up over the gluteal area or down along the lateral aspect of the leg to the knee.

Lymph massage on the medial half of the posterior thigh begins at the gluteal crease near the ischial tuberosity and directs the lymph flow anteriorly toward the inguinal nodes. Massage on the medial portion progresses down toward the knee and then back up the medial thigh, always directing lymph flow toward the inguinal nodes.

On the posterior aspect of the lower leg, superficial lymph flows toward lymph nodes located in the popliteal space behind the knee. Lymph from these nodes often bypasses the inguinal nodes and flows into deeper nodes in the pelvic cavity. Massage on the lower leg begins by addressing these popliteal nodes. Bend the knee slightly and apply gentle lymph massage movements with the soft pads of the fingers to the soft area just superior to the crease behind the knee. Apply ten to twenty repetitions to this area and then move down to the back of the knee and continue with ten to twenty more repetitions. Lower the foot to the table and proceed with lymph massage movements, working down the back of the leg to the heel.

After applying lymph massage to the entire back of the leg from the hip to the heel, begin at the heel and apply the movements, in an abbreviated form but still slowly back up the leg to the hip. Complete the leg massage with light effleurage movements.

10. *Upper posterior quadrant:* Superficial lymph of the back generally flows toward the closest lymph nodes. Above the umbilical belt line, which is at approximately the level of the first lumbar vertebrae, lymph flows toward the axilla on the same side of the body. Below the belt line, lymph flows around to the anterior of the body toward the inguinal lymph nodes. Lymph massage on the back of the body therefore is directed to enhance lymph movement toward these areas.

Begin lymph massage on the upper back near the axilla, directing movements toward the axillary nodes. Movements proceed medially to the spine and inferiorly to cover the posterior and lateral aspects of the rib cage.

While the client is in the prone position, you can also apply lymph massage can also be applied to the posterior aspects of the shoulder and the upper arm. Movements in these areas are also directed toward the axillary lymph nodes.

Conclude the lymph massage by asking and then assisting the client him or to turn over to a supine position. Once again, clear the axillary lymph nodes, the infra- and supraclavicular spaces, and the area of the angulus venosus. Finish with a gentle, relaxing neck and shoulder massage.

Lymph massage is very soothing and relaxing. Allow your client to relax and assimilate the effects of the massage for a few moments and then assist the client to first roll onto the side and then sit up on the side of the table. Allow the client to sit on the table for a moment to reorient, and make sure that any dizziness has passed. Discuss any homework and possibly demonstrate self-massage techniques or exercises that the client might use. Assist the client off the table, toward the dressing area.

SUMMARY

Lymph massage was developed in the 1930s by Dr. Emil Vodder in Denmark, and many of the techniques that he developed are still used today. Dr. Bruno Chikly of France more recently developed methods to recognize the rhythm and flow of both superficial and deep lymph movement and to map lymph flow so that lymph drainage therapy can be much more effective.

The lymph vascular system consists of lymph capillaries, vessels, trunks, and nodes and provides a supplementary pathway for tissue fluids to reenter the circulatory system. Interstitial fluid that contains proteins, bacteria, or cell debris that cannot be reabsorbed into the blood vascular system enters lymph capillaries, becomes lymph, and is transported through lymph vessels to lymph nodes, where lymphocytes and macrophages destroy or neutralize harmful elements before the fluid reenters the bloodstream at the subclavian vein, just before the blood enters the heart.

The gentle movements of lymph massage stimulate the movement of lymph into and through the lymph system. Lymph massage helps to drain stagnant interstitial fluids, toxins, and proteins from the interstitial fluid, stimulates the activity of the lymph nodes, increases the production of lymphocytes, and stimulates the immune system. Lymph massage tends to be very relaxing and stimulates the parasympathetic nervous system, reducing stress depression and some types of insomnia.

The primary movement used for lymph massage is a semicircular movement that lightly contacts the skin and moves it over the subdermal tissues in an inverted L pattern. The first part of the movement is transverse to the intended flow of lymph, to gently open the initial lymphatics and encourage the uptake of fluids. The second phase of the movement slightly stretches in the direction of flow, toward the nearest lymph nodes. The contact with the skin is then released so the skin snaps back as the hand continues the circular motion back to the original contact point and the movement is repeated. The movements are slow, about five to ten repetitions per minute, and the movement is repeated seven to ten or more times in the same area before moving to the next area. The sequence of movements is proximal to distal and back to proximal. Massage begins at the reentry site, where lymph rejoins the venous blood at the angulus venosus. The lymph massage sequence begins proximally to clear out the lymph channels and works distally and then again from distal to proximal, finishing by once again helping to clear the area of the lymph nodes. Lymph massage is done to *enhance* but not *force* the movement of lymph through the lymphatic system.

This chapter provides an introduction to lymph massage techniques to enhance lymph circulation for clients who are generally healthy but might be experiencing minor lymph congestion from inactivity or local trauma. Students who wish to work with clients with more serious lymphatic conditions are encouraged to seek additional training with qualified instructors and can check the following resources:

Dr. Vodder Method of Manual Lymph Drainage (http://vodderschool.com)
Dr. Bruno Chikly, Lymph Drainage Therapy (www.upledger.com, click on the "therapies" tab across the top of the main page)
The Academy of Lymphatic Studies in Sebastian, FL (http://acols.com)

QUESTIONS FOR DISCUSSION AND REVIEW

1. Name three people who have had a major influence on the development of lymph massage.
2. Describe lymph circulation.
3. What are four functions of the lymph nodes?
4. What are lymphocytes?
5. What is lymph?
6. What are the major benefits of lymph massage?
7. What is the sequence of lymph massage movements on an area of the body.

CHAPTER

17 Therapeutic Procedure

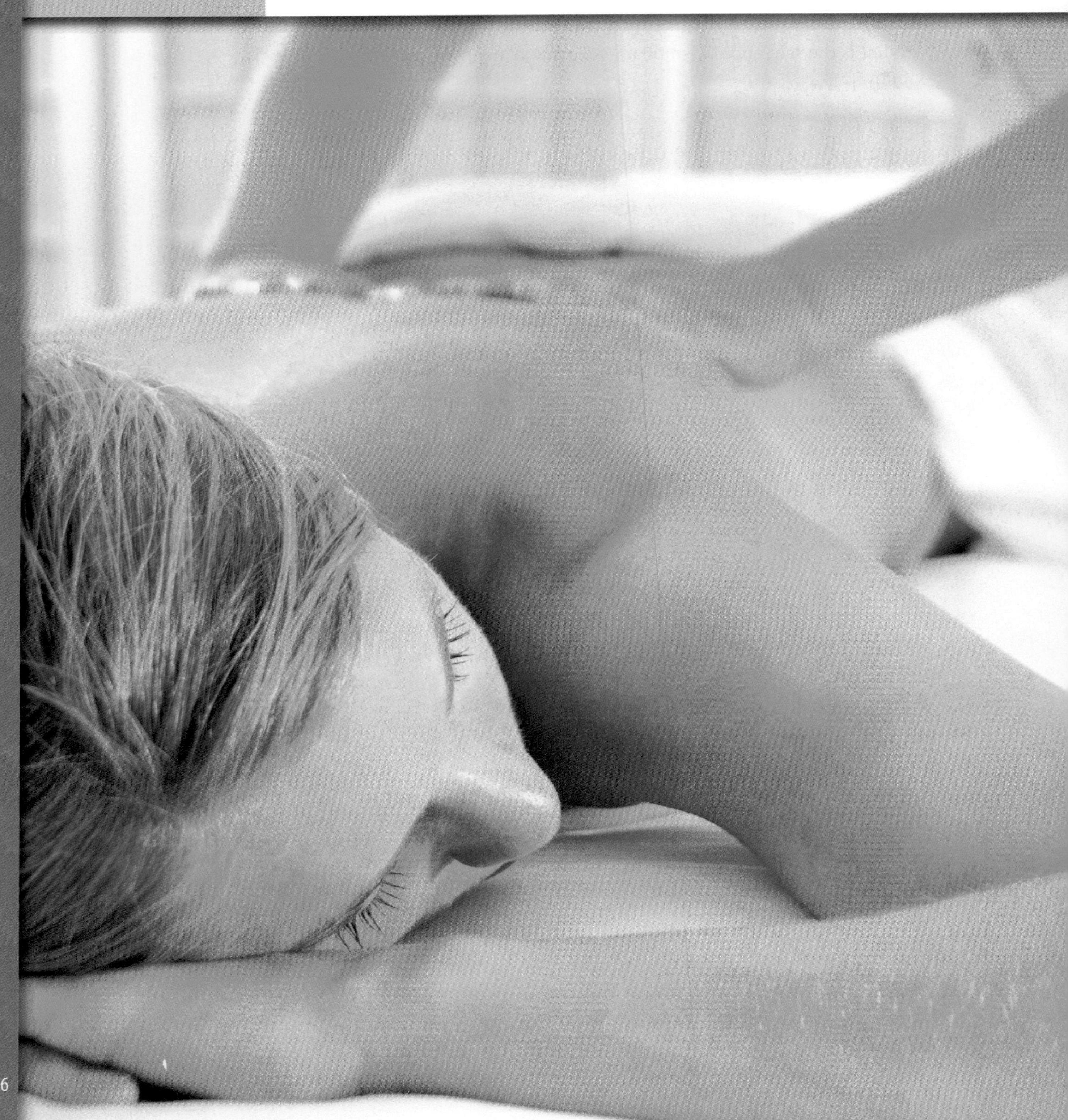

LEARNING OBJECTIVES

After you have mastered this chapter, you will be able to

1. **Describe the four parts of the therapeutic procedure.**
2. **Demonstrate a client intake procedure for a therapeutic massage session.**
3. **Perform posture and gait assessment.**
4. **Demonstrate assessment by passive, active, and resisted movement.**
5. **Identify soft tissue barriers.**
6. **Palpate and differentiate tissue layers and textures.**
7. **Explain how assessment findings are used to develop session strategies.**
8. **Determine performance strategies that are specific to a client's needs.**
9. **Demonstrate how to identify and release constrictions in hypertonic tissue.**
10. **Explain the importance of evaluation.**

INTRODUCTION

Chapter 12 described possible full-body massage routines. The therapist can choose from an endless number of possible routines for a full-body massage, or the massage can focus on a particular body area according to the client's request. People seeking massage for relaxation and stress relief benefit from relaxing full-body massages; however, when seeking relief from painful conditions or recovering from injury, more specific treatment regimes are better suited. The previous chapters discussed hydrotherapy, neuromuscular and myofascial techniques, and lymph massage. These therapeutic modalities and classical massage techniques can be combined in many ways to best fit the needs and desires of a client. Becoming competent in more sophisticated therapeutic applications requires ongoing training, practice, and expertise on the part of the therapist to determine — through assessment — where and what soft tissue components or body functions are involved and then provide appropriate therapeutic interventions. Chapter 17 introduces therapeutic methodology to identify more specifically those soft tissue conditions that respond to therapeutic soft tissue interventions. **Therapeutic procedure**, which includes acquiring a concise medical history, assessment procedures to determine constricted and painful conditions, developing treatment plans, performing appropriate treatment practices to address the conditions more specifically, and then evaluating the results, is discussed here.

therapeutic procedure is the process of acquiring a concise medical history, assessment procedures to determine constricted and painful conditions, developing treatment plans, performing appropriate treatment practices to address the conditions more specifically, and evaluating the results.

Therapeutic procedure involves four basic steps:

1. Assessment
2. Planning
3. Performance
4. Evaluation

Assessment involves reviewing any information available at the onset of the process to understand the present conditions. During the *planning* stage, the information gained from the assessment is used to set treatment goals, determine strategies, and select therapeutic techniques to address the specific conditions found during the assessment. The *performance* is the actual application of the selected techniques. The *evaluation* examines the outcome of the session in regard to the effectiveness of the selected procedure for the condition.

All information must be carefully documented in the client's files. Subjective, objective, assessment, and plan (SOAP) charts are well suited to recording information gained in each segment of the therapeutic procedure. (See Chapter 9 for information about SOAP charts.)

The therapeutic process can be implemented in many ways in the course of a massage therapy program. The process is valuable for long-range goal setting, short-range planning, and during an actual massage session. In long-range goal setting, the assessment might be extensive, and the planning could encompass several sessions (six to ten). After the treatment strategy has been formulated and discussed and the treatments given, an evaluation is performed to determine the progress that has been made and what further therapy is needed.

Short-range planning can involve a single session. In this case, the assessment process might not be as extensive, but it can focus more on a specific complaint. The client's needs are considered, indications and contraindications are determined, and a treatment strategy is chosen. The session is performed, and at the conclusion, the outcome is evaluated as to the effectiveness of the session.

During the application of a therapeutic massage, the therapeutic procedure is constantly being applied. As the therapist proceeds through the massage, the hands are continuously assessing the condition of the tissues. The quality and constrictions in the tissue, or the movement of the limbs and the response from the client as different massage movements are being performed, continuously provide information that the therapist uses to plan the next movements. The evaluation process is also continuous because the therapist elicits feedback about the effectiveness throughout the treatment.

CLIENT INTAKE FOR THERAPEUTIC MASSAGE

Reasons for receiving massage vary widely. According to a 2007 survey conducted by the Caravan Opinion Research Corporation, 22 percent of the respondents who received massage did so to relax or reduce stress, 30 percent sought massage to improve some health concern, and 13 percent did so to pamper themselves. Primary concerns included pain management, injury recovery, muscle soreness/stiffness, and other soft tissue dysfunction.

The preliminary client consultation is discussed in Chapter 9. A preliminary consultation for a therapeutic massage contains all the same elements as discussed earlier, but more extensive assessment techniques and planning strategies are included to better determine which services can be provided to address the particular concerns of the client. A primary focus of the preliminary interview is to establish rapport between the therapist and client. The therapist must be receptive and show genuine interest for the client and at the same time be professional and confident. Mirroring the client with a similar voice tone and posture help to establish rapport. Establishing a good rapport enhances mutual respect, which strengthens the therapeutic relationship. It is essential to establish an environment for open communication. Clear communication is paramount, especially for determining the client's needs and concerns. Practicing good listening skills and maintaining eye contact when conversing are also important. The therapist can paraphrase and repeat back to the client what has been explained to be sure that what is being said is understood. Encouraging feedback anytime—before, during, and after the session — ensures that the client's needs are being met and boundaries not encroached upon.

The extent of the intake process depends on the purpose of the client visit and the intent of the massage treatment. The client intake process for a therapeutic massage is more extensive than that for a wellness/relaxing massage. The intake process begins when the client calls or makes the appointment and continues until there is agreement between the client and therapist to proceed and the massage treatment commences. The intake involves an exchange of information to determine the best course of action for the therapeutic relationship. Client intake includes several segments that can vary according to the individual situation. Some segments are

- Setting the appointment—This might include an initial screening to determine the primary reason for the client visit and whether the practitioner's services match the client's needs.
- Initial greeting and consultation—Extra time can be scheduled for the first consultation to fill out intake forms (Figure 17-1) and exchange information such as reasons for the visit, policies, and procedures.
- Assessment—The assessment process consists of a client interview, health history, observation, palpation, and special tests such as range of motion.
- Treatment plan—When the relevant information has been collected during the assessment, client and therapist can determine a plan for the session or a number of sessions.
- Informed consent—After the therapist and client discuss the assessment findings and agree on a treatment plan, the client gives informed consent and the session commences.

ASSESSMENT TECHNIQUES

The successful practice of therapeutic massage depends on an accurate and thorough assessment. The therapist must understand as much about the client and the condition as possible to determine which massage procedures to perform or whether it is advisable to refer this client to another health professional. The extent of the examination depends on the intended therapy to be given. If a relaxing massage is the intent of the visit, only enough information needs to be exchanged to determine that there are no contraindications. Informed consent is then obtained, and the session can commence. If the intent of the visit is to respond to specific concerns that the client has or to address some soft tissue dysfunction, however, a more extensive assessment can provide information to determine the nature of the dysfunction or pathology to help to determine the best course of treatment. The assessment tools used can vary according to the

FIGURE 17-1 Client intake form.

Client Intake Form

Name ______________________ Today's date ______________________
Address ______________________ Phone ______________________
City-State-ZIP ______________________ Email Address ______________________
Date of birth __________ Age _____ Sex _____ Social Security # ______________
Occupation ______________________ Employer ______________________
Employer address ______________________ Business phone ______________
Marital status __________ Spouse/partner's name ______________________
Children's name(s) and age(s) ______________________
Have you had massages before? _____ By whom? ______________________
How did you find out about our services? ______________________

Primary Health Care Provider ______________ Phone # ______________
Provider address ______________ City __________ State ___ ZIP _____
May I have permission to consult your health provider? No ___ Yes ___ _____ (initial if yes)
List other health providers you use on the back of this page.

Insurance Company ______________________ Policy # ______________
Name of policyholder ______________________
ID # __________ Group # ______________ Claim # ______________
Adjuster's Name ______________________
Adjuster's Address ______________ City __________ ST ___ ZIP _____
Phone # ______________________ Time and date of verification ______________

In case of emergency notify ______________________ Phone ______________
Relationship ______________________

I understand that the massage services are designed to be a health aid and are in no way to take the place of a doctor's care when indicated. I am aware that the massage therapist does not diagnose disease nor prescribe medications. Information exchanged during any massage session is educational in nature and is intended to help me become more aware and conscious of my own health status and is to be used at my own discretion.
Client signature ______________________ Date ______________

preferred modality. A common assessment protocol includes client and medical history, close observation, palpation of the suspected structures and any number of functional or orthopedic assessments. The goal of the assessment is to, as specifically as possible, identify the dysfunctional tissues and, if possible, the conditions that caused the problem.

FIGURE 17-2A Client health history form. (front)

Client Health History

Name ______________________ Today's date ____________________
Address ____________ Home phone ___________ Other phone __________
City-State-ZIP ___________________ Email address __________________
Date of Birth _______________ Age _____ Occupation _______________
Who were you referred by or how did you find out about our services? __________
What is the reason for your visit to our office? ______________________
____
What results would you like to achieve with our work? __________________
Have you seen a doctor or another health practitioner regarding this or similar conditions? _____________________________
List their names and phone numbers. Do I have your permission to contact them? _____
____
When did you first notice the condition and what started it? _________________
What makes it worse? / better? ______________________________
Please indicate any of the following conditions that apply to you. Mark any current conditions with an "X" and past conditions with an "O."

__ Chronic pain, where __________
__ Joint pain, where __________
__ Muscle pain, where __________
__ Other pain, where __________
__ Headache
__ Numbness, where __________
__ Broken bones, where, when __________
__ Sprains/strains, where __________
__ Arthritis
__ Osteoporosis
__ Bursitis
__ Tendonitis
__ Scoliosis
__ Bone disease
__ Dizziness
__ Difficulty breathing
__ Sinus conditions

__ Asthma
__ Fatigue
__ Frequent respiratory illness
__ Lung or respiratory condition
__ Cold hands or feet
__ Swollen ankles
__ Varicose veins
__ High blood pressure
__ Low blood pressure
__ Lymphedema
__ Heart condition
__ Indigestion
__ Loss of appetite
__ Diarrhea
__ Constipation
__ Gas/bloating
__ Ulcers
__ Digestive condition
__ Bowel condition
__ Eating disorders
__ Panic attacks/anxiety
__ Hyperactivity

__ Learning difficulties
__ Depression
__ Trouble sleeping
__ Trouble concentrating
__ Memory loss
__ Hearing problems
__ Vision problems
__ Contacts
__ Paralysis
__ Nervous system conditions
__ Allergies
__ Rashes
__ Skin conditions
__ Tumors/cancer
__ Shingles/herpes
__ Pregnancies
__ PMS
__ Hysterectomy
__ Menopause
__ Birth control
__ Prostate
__ Reproductive concerns

Explain any conditions noted above. ______________________________
____

FIGURE 17-2B Client health history form. (back)

Infectious and childhood diseases (list what and when) ______________________
Congenital or acquired disability (describe) ______________________________
Surgeries (list what and when) _______________________________________
Injuries or accidents causing injury ____________________________________
List any other medical or health condition not listed ______________________
____
List, including frequency of use, all medications, remedies, herbs, and supplements you use. ____
____
____
Do you use any of the following? List frequency and amount.
Caffeine ________________ Nicotine ________________ Alcohol ________________
Sugar __________________ Recreational drugs ________________
List stress-relieving activities you participate in. Include type and frequency; that is, exercise, massage, hobbies, sports, etc. ____
____
____
List any other concerns or comments regarding you health status or well-being. _______
____

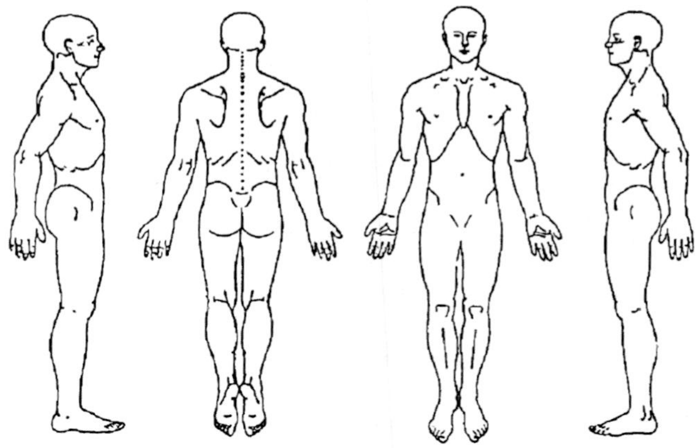

On the above diagram, indicate any areas in which you experience pain with an *X* and circle any other areas of concern.
To the best of my knowledge, I have disclosed all of my past and current health conditions. I will inform the therapist of any changes in my health status.

Client signature ___________________________________ Date __________________

A concise client history provides a wealth of background information about social, physiologic, and psychological elements related to the complaints of the client. Client information and medical history forms are filled out on the client's first visit (Figures 17-1 and 17-2). A client information form can include questions about the client's age, occupation, hobbies, and the reason for seeking your services. These forms can be designed to provide extensive and vital information about the client's past and current physical condition, and the client's expectations and concerns. The medical history form provides information about the client's past medical conditions, including major illnesses, medications, surgical procedures, traumas, and allergies. The form should include contact information for doctors or other health care practitioners whom the client is seeing for any current conditions and a written request for permission to contact those health care practitioners. The form should also include questions about particular conditions that the client has and the history of those conditions, as well as a diagram of the body so that the client can illustrate areas of concern. The client must sign a separate "Release of Medical Information" form

Release of Medical Information Form

Client's name ______________________ Phone ______________________
Address ______________________ City ______________ State ___ ZIP __________
I hereby authorize ______(Practitioner's Name)______ to release to any physician or health care practitioner directly involved in my care any medical records or other personal health information necessary for the purpose of receiving physician's recommendations and approval, or sharing concerns regarding my health and well-being.
This authorization remains valid for the period of ____________ to ____________ or for the time period that I am seeing the above-named practitioner.

Signed ______________________________ Date ____________________

FIGURE 17-3 Release of medical information form.

for you to share any of personal information with other health professionals (Figure 17-3).

After the client has had an opportunity to fill out the intake and medical history forms and the practitioner has had a chance to review the forms, a consultation or interview between the client and practitioner provides an opportunity to clarify any information on the forms and set the intentions for the session. This is the opportunity for the client to tell the story.

Information from the forms combined with a client interview clarifies the client's concerns, needs, and expectations. Reviewing the completed forms and questioning the client to clarify any information on the forms provides the therapist with preliminary information to make decisions on how to proceed, whether the client should be referred to another health professional, or whether the client's doctor should be contacted before going further. If in doubt, remain on the cautious side. Refer the client to an appropriate health professional for more clarification about questionable conditions. Confer with or work under the supervision of a medical doctor or other therapist in difficult or questionable situations.

Data from the forms and interview provide information about the nature of the complaint, which part or parts of the body are affected, whether the condition is chronic or acute, and what makes it worse or better. Find out when and how the condition started, what the client has done about it to date, which treatments that the client has received and by whom, what has helped, what has made it worse, and so on. Was there some incident that started the condition? Was the onset sudden, or did it come on gradually? What has been the progression of the condition? Where in the body did the client first notice it? Is this the first time that the client has experienced this condition? If not, how often, when was the last time, when was the first time the client had this condition? Questions should also ascertain how long the condition has persisted and whether it is constant or intermittent.

If it is a painful condition, determine the location of the pain. Can the client put a finger or hand on it? Does it radiate, or has it traveled from its original location? What affects it? What makes it worse or better? Does the time of day or activity affect it? What is the intensity, duration, and frequency of the pain? Does it come and go? How often does it recur and what instigates its return?

Box 17.1

Health History Question Examples

1. What is the client's current overall health condition?
2. What are the current symptoms, and how long have they been present?
3. How did the condition start? What has been the progression of the condition?
4. What has the client done about it? Has the client received other treatment? Which type(s)? What have the results been?
5. Has it been diagnosed by a doctor?

If it is an injury-related condition

6. When did the injury occur?
7. Can the client describe what was injured?
8. What was done at the time of the injury? First aid?
9. Which types of treatments has the client had for the injury?
10. Which symptoms is the client experiencing currently? Pain? Swelling?

If it is a painful condition

11. Where is the pain? Is it localized? Radiating? Over an extensive area?
12. Describe how/why the pain started.
13. Describe the pain. Is it sharp? Dull? Throbbing? Radiating? Constant? Intermittent?
14. What makes it worse? What makes it better?
15. Does it affect daily activities? How?
16. Is the client using medication for the pain? Which medications?

Describe the pain. Is it sharp? Dull? Radiating? Does the pain interfere with daily activities?

Question the client about tolerance of the condition and what the client has done to cope with and correct the problem. Learn about the client and that person's willingness to do something about the condition. Take notes on the answers and include them in the client files for future evaluations.

By this time, the therapist knows what the client's primary concerns are and whether the services can be of benefit. The therapist also now has a better idea of further assessments that can identify the involved structures, patterns, or causative factors related to the complaint.

After the interview, the intake process can continue with various assessments that include observation or visual assessment, a variety of functional assessments, palpation, and specialized tests specific to the suspected condition or selected modalities. Information from the various assessments is gathered and analyzed to determine the best course of treatment. Both client and therapist discuss the results of the assessments and options for possible interventions or treatment modalities, and a treatment plan or care plan is created and mutually agreed on. The client again provides informed consent by signing the care plan. This marks the end of the intake process, and the performance or application portion of the therapeutic procedure begins.

Subjective and Objective Findings

Information gained during the interview and assessment portion of the session is both subjective and objective in nature. Subjective information will come as the client describes the personal experience of the situation. The client should answer questions about what and where the client feels the condition. When did it start? Is it constant or intermittent? What affects it, makes it better, or makes it worse? During various tests, the client can describe the experience or how it feels.

The therapist, or another observer, determines objective information through observation, palpation, and specialized tests in which the findings are quantifiable and usually measurable.

Pain Scale

A **subjective pain scale** is a useful tool to assess the relative discomfort that a client is experiencing. The client is able to rate pain as the client describes the condition, guides the therapist during a therapeutic technique, or assesses any improvement in the condition following a session. The pain scale provides the client the opportunity to describe the discomfort or pain being experienced on a scale of 0 to 10 (or 1 to 5) where 0 (or 1) is no discomfort and 10 (or 5) is unbearable, excruciating pain.

The pain scale can be used when a person is describing discomfort during a preliminary assessment. At the end of the session, clients can again rate discomfort to help determine the session's effectiveness.

A pain scale is also used to determine appropriate amounts of pressure to be used during certain treatment modalities such as trigger-point release or positional release. For instance, when applying pressure to a trigger point, ask the client to rate the discomfort and tell you when the rating is between 6 and 7. This is the ideal amount of pressure to have the greatest therapeutic value. If the discomfort rises above this level—that is, between 8 and 10—the client becomes defensive, and any therapeutic gains plus the trust of the client could be lost. Therapeutic use of the pain scale is discussed more in the trigger-point release and position release section of Chapter 15.

The Arndt-Schultz Law

The **Arndt-Schultz law** states that weak stimuli activate physiologic processes, and strong stimuli inhibit them. If the therapeutic intervention (pressure on the muscle) is too strong, the nervous system will not respond to the intervention and will not shift its message from the spinal cord to the muscle. If there is too little pressure, the nervous system will not respond. At the level of 6 or 7 on a 10-point scale, the nervous system *will* respond to the intervention and shift the message that goes out the reflex arc to the muscle. Clients have to be trained that the old "grin and bear it" method is not the best way to shift pain patterns.

OBSERVATION

Observation plays a major role in the assessment process. The observation portion of a client assessment should begin when the client walks in the door and continue until the client leaves. The client's body language—that is, how the client holds posture, stands, moves, and sits—gives clues to where pain and tension are being held. Observing body language can also give some insight to the client's emotional makeup and self-esteem. Watch for guarded movements that the client uses to avoid or mask any pain.

Through visual observation, the therapist can assess structural alignment and balance, bilateral discrepancies, and variations in skin color and integrity. Look for bilateral symmetry both structurally and in the way the client moves. Throughout the assessment, it is helpful to compare one side of the body with the other. When doing many of the comparisons, look at the good or unaffected side first to get an idea of the personal norm for that person, and then look at the affected side to assess the deviation from that norm. Note in how a person moves whether that person holds one side of the body tighter or higher. Is the gait (walking) balanced and normal? Does the client stand erect, list to one side, or stoop? Observation comes into play more formally when assessing posture and gait.

Posture Assessment

Assessing posture is observing how a person maintains an upright position in relation to gravitational forces. Posture is considered to be ideal when the body's mass is evenly distributed around its central axis, which passes through the body's center of gravity (Figures 17-4 and 17-5). When a client exhibits optimal posture, the postural muscles maintain a state of normal tonus. When postural balance becomes less than optimal, however, postural muscles must actively contract to redistribute the body mass in relation to the center of gravity and maintain that contraction, putting stress on joints and other connective tissue.

Observing posture gives many indications of muscular imbalance and structural deviation. Many postural discrepancies are due to agonist/antagonist imbalances. Posture is best observed from all four sides when the client is standing comfortably erect. Assess from bottom to top, noting the symmetry of the body's bony landmarks, including the ankles, fibular heads, greater trochantor, iliac crests, scapulas, acromioclavicular (AC), joints, and ears. Beginning at the feet, notice whether they are evenly angled and placed equal distance from the midline, and whether the arches support the ankles. From the back, is the Achilles' tendon aligned perpendicular to the floor? Are the patellae pointing forward? Is the pelvis rotated or tilted, either side to side or front to back? The angle from the posterior superior iliac spine (PSIS) to the anterior superior iliac spine (ASIS) should be no more than 10° from the horizontal for women and 5° for men. If a person has good posture, a plumb line perfectly bisects the body when it is viewed from the front or back. From the side, the line would go through the ear, shoulder, elbow, acetabulum (as-e-**TAB**-yoo-lum), knee, and just in front of the ankle. By extending the vertical plumb line forward, ideally the symphysis pubis, manubrium, and front of the zygomatic arch would be vertically aligned. When observing a person, notice whether one side of the body is held higher than the other. Notice the hips, the shoulders at the AC joint, the hands, the ears, and the eyes to check whether they are level and even. Notice any rotation: is there any rotation in the torso? Is either arm

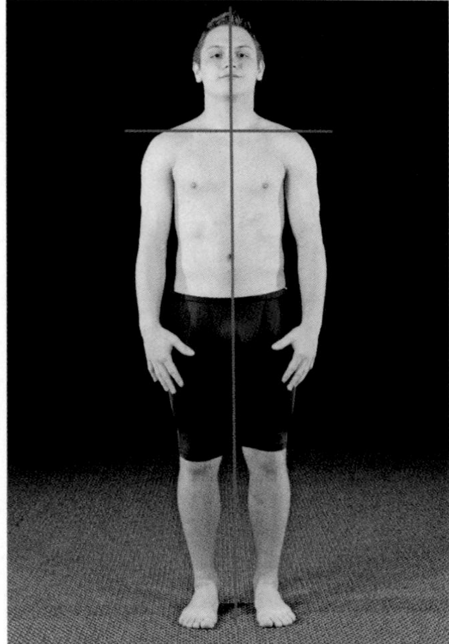

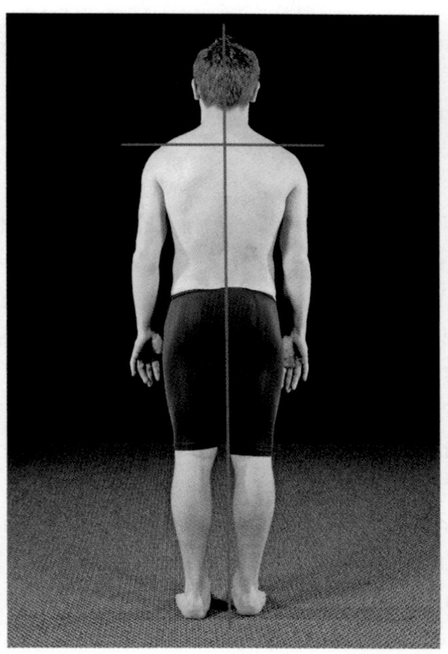

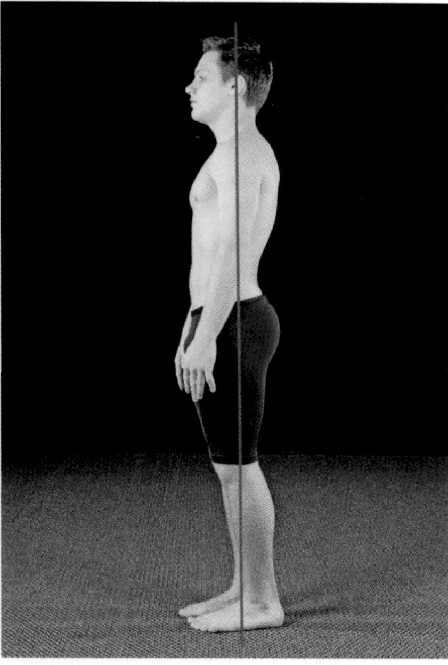

FIGURE 17-4A, B, and C Posture is observed from the (a) front, (b) back, and (c) side. A plumb line or grid is helpful to determine deviations in the posture.

or leg rotated? Is the head rotated or tilted? Assess for relative muscle bulk, symmetric skin folds, and scars. Any deviation suggests muscle imbalance or fascial constriction. The farther out of balance the body is, the more strain is placed on the postural muscles. As the body ages, the pull of gravity tends to increase the deviations.

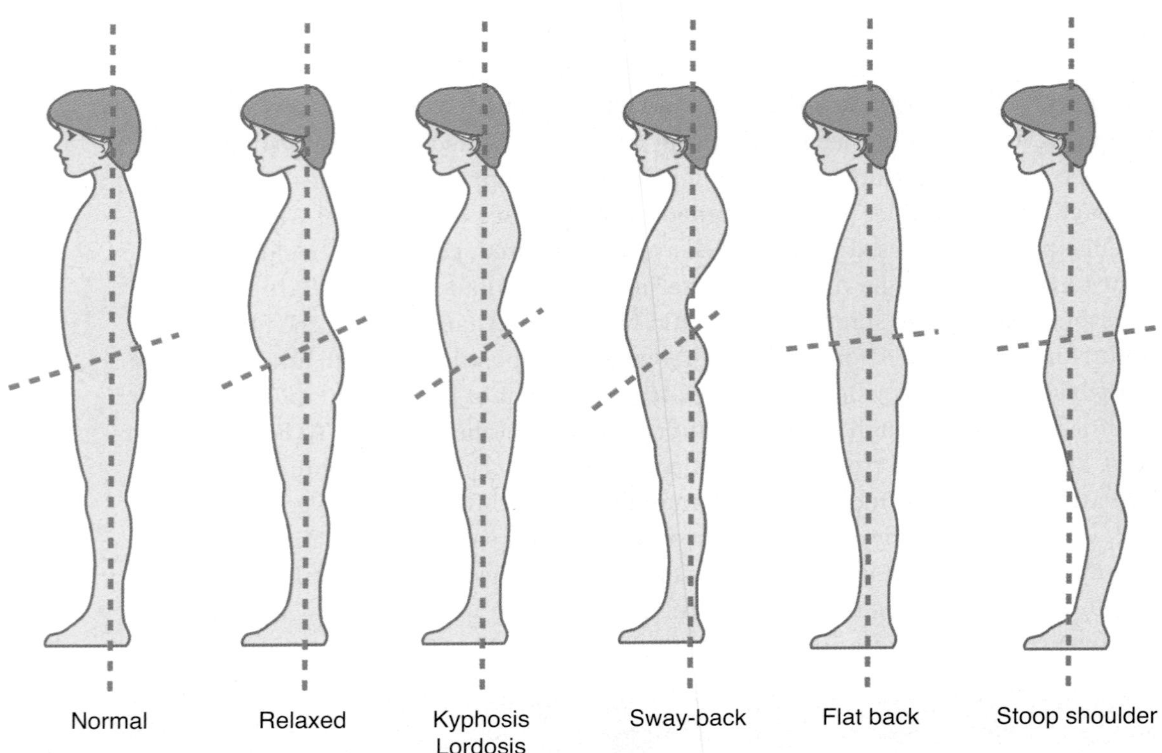

FIGURE 17-5 A variety of common postural deviations (with plumb line).

When assessing posture, the therapist notes spinal curves, deviations from the coronal or sagittal plane, differences in elevation or rotation of postural (bony) landmarks, and any asymmetric anatomic position. These findings are combined with information from other assessments to identify areas of possible somatic dysfunction.

When the client lies supine on the table and is comfortable, again notice any deviations from bilateral symmetry. Observe the contour of the body as well as structural and skeletal symmetry. Is the client straight? Is the head tilted or turned? Is one leg rotated at a different angle? Are the hips level? Most minor postural deviations are caused by muscular imbalance. There is either muscle weakness (flaccidity), muscle tension, or both. There is often an agonist/antagonist imbalance, in which one muscle is hypertonic and constricted whereas the opposing muscle is hypotonic and weak. There can be fascial constrictions or adhesions. Some forms of massage and soft tissue techniques can be very effective for relieving these imbalances.

Make note of abnormal marks, discoloration, varicosities, differences in skin texture, and scars. Check for skin conditions, redness, areas of increased heat, or swelling (i.e., signs of inflammation). Be aware of anything that might be a sign of former trauma or conditions that could indicate or contraindicate massage.

Postural distortion can result from a wide range of influences, including physical or emotional trauma, poor work habits, pathologic conditions, or age. Through the process of compensation, a deviation in one area of the body can cause a shift in another in an attempt to reestablish an overall balance. Compensation usually results in increased tension on connective tissue and postural muscle. The farther out of balance the body is, the more the postural muscles are strained, resulting in increased pain and dysfunction.

Gait Assessment

Assessing **gait** is similar to assessing posture, except that the body is in motion. Methods of **gait assessment** have advanced with the use of computers, video cameras, and sophisticated measuring devices. For the purposes of massage therapy, the monitoring devices are the therapist's eyes. The client's gait should be viewed from the front, back, and both sides to gain as much information as possible. The gait assessment is performed as the client walks in a comfortable relaxed manner for several paces, back and forth in front of the therapist.

gait

is a pattern or manner of walking.

gait assessment

is observing the manner in which a person walks to determine constrictions or related conditions.

When a person is walking, the steps should be even and smooth, with the heel of one foot making contact with the floor as the weight on the other foot transfers smoothly to the ball of the foot. The movement of the legs is in the direction of the line of motion with the knees and feet pointing in that direction. The steps are smooth and even. The torso is balanced above the body's center of gravity, and the pelvis shifts slightly at each step. The arms swing easily at the sides, opposite the legs. As the right foot moves forward, the left arm swings forward and vice versa. The hands are relaxed with the thumb forward, and the hands swing straight, forward and back. The head is balanced on the top of the spine, and the motion is fluid and smooth.

There are other considerations to observe. Is the gait initiated without undue pelvic tilt? Do the feet clear the ground with each step? Does the foot strike the ground in a heel-to-toe fashion? Is the step length symmetric? Is the width of the stride symmetric? Is there a straight alignment of the hip, knee, and ankle through the entire stride cycle? Is there ample extension in the hip to allow the step to roll off the ball of the foot and toe?

When assessing gait, the therapist notes any asymmetry, crossover, or rotation of the feet or arms, or any restrictions of free movement. Is there pain anywhere? The information gained during gait assessment can indicate body structures that are constricted. This information is combined with findings from other assessments to help to determine areas of the body to focus on and to determine which interventions to use.

Assess Range of Motion

Observation is also important in tests such as **range of motion** to notice any restrictions in joint mobility, the quality of movement, and the client's reaction

range of motion

is the movement of a joint from one extreme of the articulation to the other.

to the tests. *Range of motion* is the action of a joint through the entire extent of its movement. Assessing the extent and quality of that movement by testing the active, passive, and resisted (isometric) movement provides information about the tissues associated with the joint.

Dr. James Cyriax, an osteopath from England, developed an extensive system of testing all the joints to isolate lesions in the hard and soft tissues. Cyriax clarified and defined some terms and concepts that are invaluable when assessing range of motion. Those concepts include contractile tissue, inert tissue, end feel, and capsular patterns.

contractile tissues

are the fibrous tissues that have tensions placed on them during muscular contractions.

inert tissues

are the tissues that are not contractile such as bone, ligament, or nerves.

end feel

is the change in the quality of the movement as the end of a movement is achieved.

capsular pattern

refers to the proportional limitation of any joint that is controlled by muscular contractions.

- **Contractile tissues** are the fibrous tissues that have tensions placed on them during muscular contractions and include muscle tissue, tendons, and the muscle attachments.
- **Inert tissues** are the tissues that are not contractile, such as bone, ligament, bursa, blood vessels, nerves, nerve coverings, and cartilage.
- **End feel** refers to the quality of the sensation the therapist feels by passively moving a joint to the full extent of its possible range.
- **Capsular pattern** refers to the proportional limitation of any joint that is controlled by muscular contractions.

When assessing range of motion, the good or unaffected side is tested first to help to determine that person's norm. First the active movements are tested, then the passive, and finally the resisted movements. When testing, observe and record objective and subjective findings. *Objective findings* are things that the therapist sees or feels, such as muscle strength and degree of joint movement. *Subjective findings* include the amount of pain or discomfort the client feels and how the client reacts to the pain. Objective findings generally can be measured, whereas subjective findings are usually felt or perceived.

Assess Active Movements

Assessing active movement indicates the client's ability and willingness to move a body part through a range of motion that is normal for the joint. The client is instructed to move through a particular range of motion (Figure 17-6 a–c). The client makes the movement totally unassisted. If the entire movement can be made smoothly and painlessly, there is probably no problem with that joint or the associated soft tissue. Both contractile and inert tissues are involved during active movement, so if there is an obvious limitation, pain, or hesitation during the movement, a closer assessment is needed.

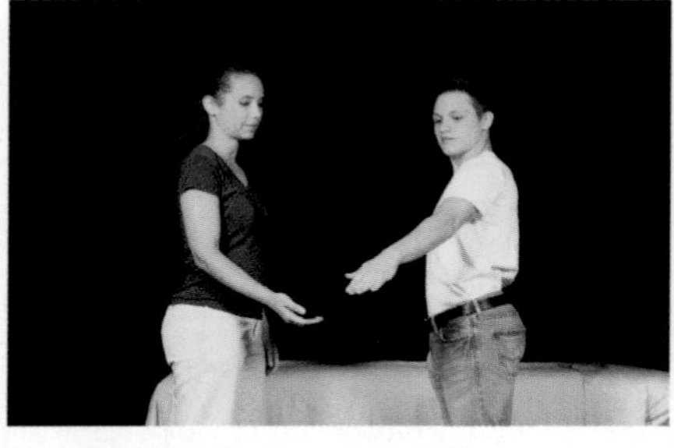
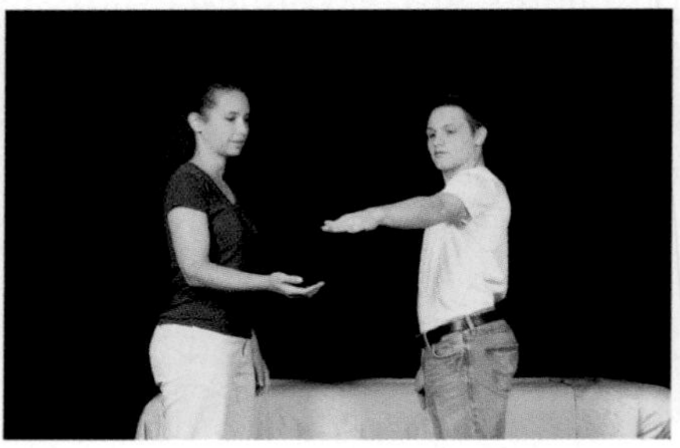
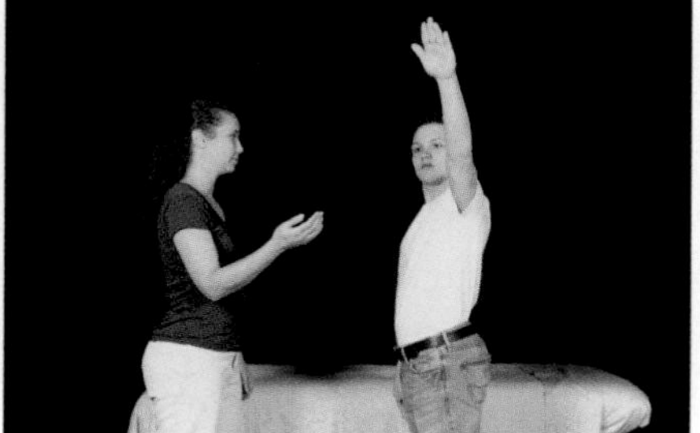

FIGURE 17-6A, B and C Active movements are made by the client, and the therapist observes and notes any restrictions or pain.

If there was any pain during the movement, the therapist should note at which point in the movement the pain occurred, the location of the pain on the client's body, the intensity and quality of the pain, and the client's reaction to the pain. If there is limitation to the movement, note where the limitation occurred and whether it was accompanied by pain.

Assess Passive Movement

When assessing passive movement, the practitioner moves the client's joint through the full range of motion that is normal for that joint while the client remains relaxed (Figure 17-7 a–d). During passive movement, the practitioner determines the degree and quality of movement in a joint. The practitioner can sense whether the joint is hypermobile or hypomobile. The therapist also notes whether there are any catches, crepitus, or pain involved. The reactions of the client must also be observed. Any apprehensiveness or unwillingness must be considered and respected.

End feel plays a very important part in assessing passive movement. End feel is the feeling that the therapist senses by passively moving a limb to the limit of its range of motion. The quality of the end feel indicates the presence, type, and severity of lesions in the tissues associated with the joint.

There are three types of end feel that are considered normal: hard, soft, and springy.

- *Hard end feel* is a bone-against-bone feeling. This is an abrupt, painless limitation to further movement that happens at the normal end of the range of motion, such as knee or elbow extension.
- *Soft end feel* is a painless, cushioned limitation in which soft tissue prevents further movement, such as knee or elbow flexion.
- *Springy end feel* is the most common. Limitation is caused by the stretch of fibrous tissue as the joint reaches the extent of its range of motion, such as hip flexion or extension.

Normal end feel happens when the range of motion is stopped by the anatomy of the joint and, unless carried to extremes, is painless. Pain or an observable limitation of movement indicates that some abnormal condition or lesion is present. If there is pain before reaching the end of the movement and there is no muscular resistance or spasm, bursitis or capsulitis might be involved. If the movement causes a sudden painful muscle reaction or spasm, the body might be protecting an injury in the area. Cyriax calls this an *empty end feel.* The more acute and severe the injury is, the more severe the pain and spasm. A medical referral and diagnosis should be recommended in these cases. Other abnormal patterns are similar to normal end feel, except that there is reduced movement or associated pain.

Passive movement assessment indicates the condition of the inert (noncontractile) tissues. Limitation of movement and pain are the indicators of dysfunction. Full, painless range of motion indicates that the joint and associated structures are healthy. Reduced range of motion that is limited with a painless, hard (bone-to-bone) end feel indicates osteoarthritis. Pain and limitation in all directions generally involve the whole joint and indicate capsulitis or arthritis. Pain or limitation in one direction and not another is usually caused by stretching

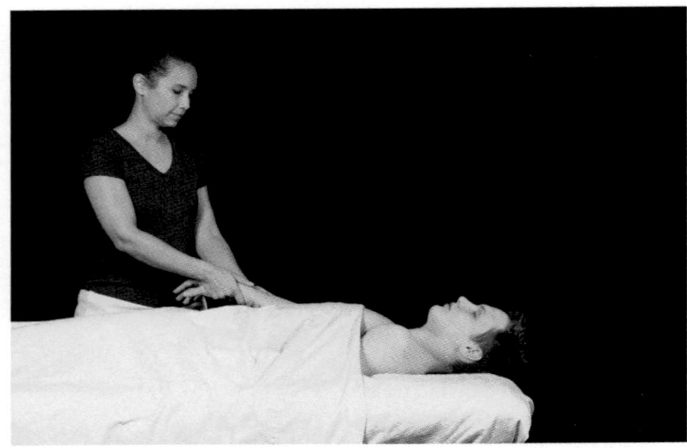

FIGURE 17-7A To assess passive movement, the therapist moves the client's joint through its range of motion while the client remains relaxed.

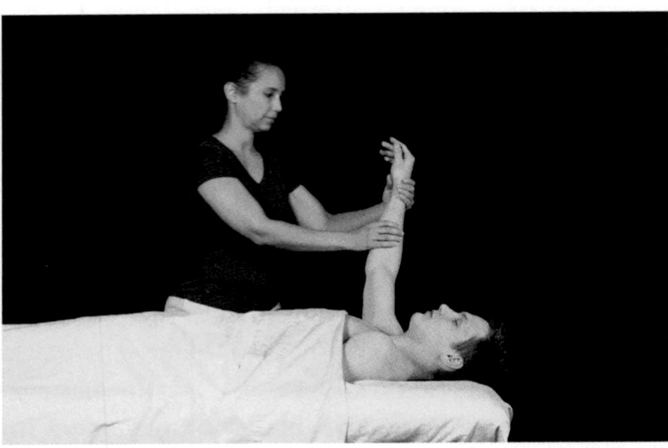

FIGURE 17-7B The practitioner notes the client's willingness to move the limb and the degree and quality of the movement.

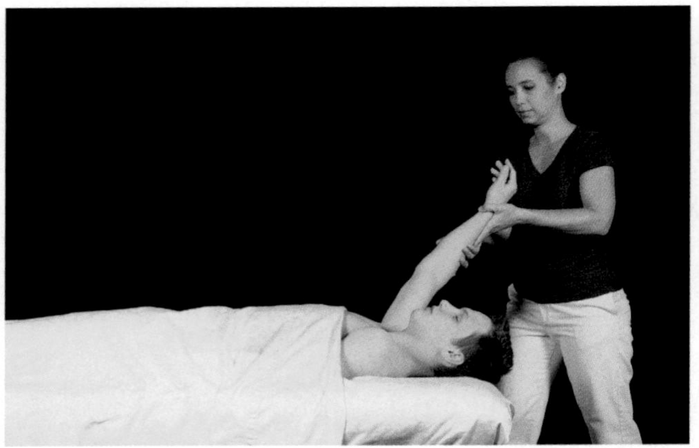

FIGURE 17-7C The practitioner also notes any catches, crepitul or pain during the movement.

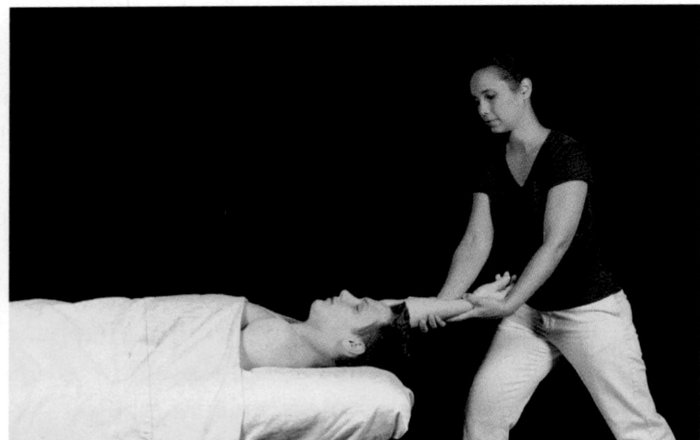

FIGURE 17-7D The practitioner determines the type of end feel as the movement approaches the end of the ROM.

or compressing the involved tissue. More specific assessment must be performed to isolate the involved tissue.

Assess Active Resisted Movement

Active resisted movement assesses the relative strength of muscles. Resisted or isometric movement is used to assess the condition of the contractile tissues (i.e., muscles, tendons, and attachments). This method is also known as *muscle testing.*

Indicators of lesions in the contractile tissue are weakness and pain. To perform active resisted movement assessment or muscle testing, the therapist stabilizes a body part in a neutral position near the midrange of the joint and instructs the client to move that body part in a specific direction. As the client contracts the muscle required to move in that direction, the therapist applies

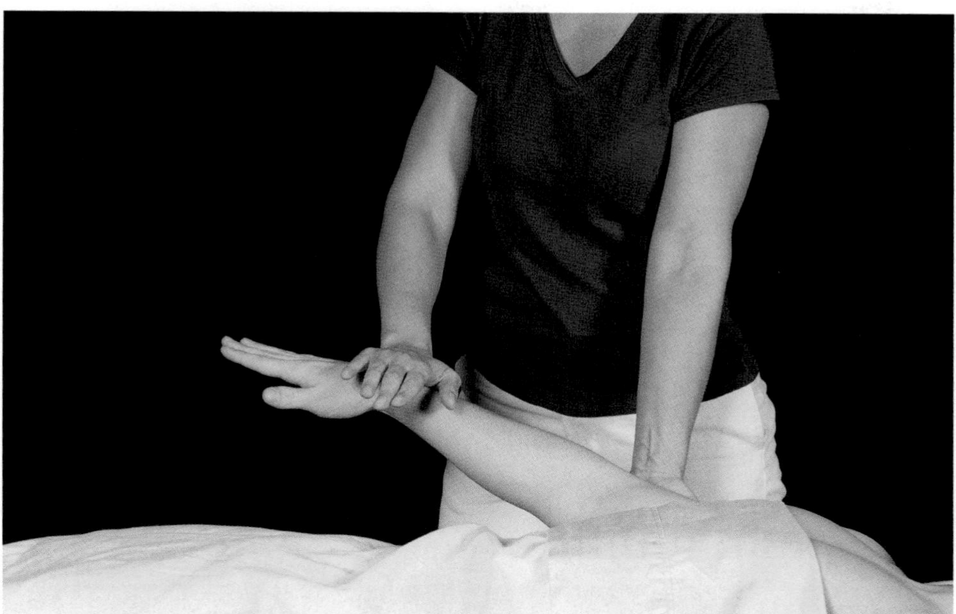

FIGURE 17-8 To perform muscle testing or assess resisted movement, the client is instructed to hold a limb in a neutral position while the therapist attempts to move the limb.

pressure to move the body part in the opposite direction so that the limb does not move. Eliminating any joint movement minimizes reactions of the inert tissues and indicates the relative strength and condition of the targeted contractile tissues. Positioning the body part and instructing the client to make a specific movement isolates specific muscles to be tested (Figure 17-8).

When contractile tissues are involved, active movement and resisted movement both give positive results. Passive movement shows nothing except at the end of the movement, where the contractile tissue is stretched and which then reacts with pain or spasm.

Muscle testing provides information about the condition of the muscles involved in a specific movement. As with the other physical assessment tools, it is important to compare one side of the body with the other. Test the good side first for comparison. A muscle test that is strong and pain free indicates healthy muscle tissue. A strong and painful muscle test indicates a lesion in the contractile tissue such as a minor (first- or second-degree) muscle strain. A weak and painless muscle test indicates interference with the nerve supply, circulation, or energy to the muscle. No strength in the muscle could be caused by a severed muscle or tendon (third-degree strain) or a loss of innervation. A very weak and painful muscle test indicates a severe lesion, possibly a torn ligament or fracture that should be referred to a doctor.

In general, the more severe the condition is, the more severe the pain.

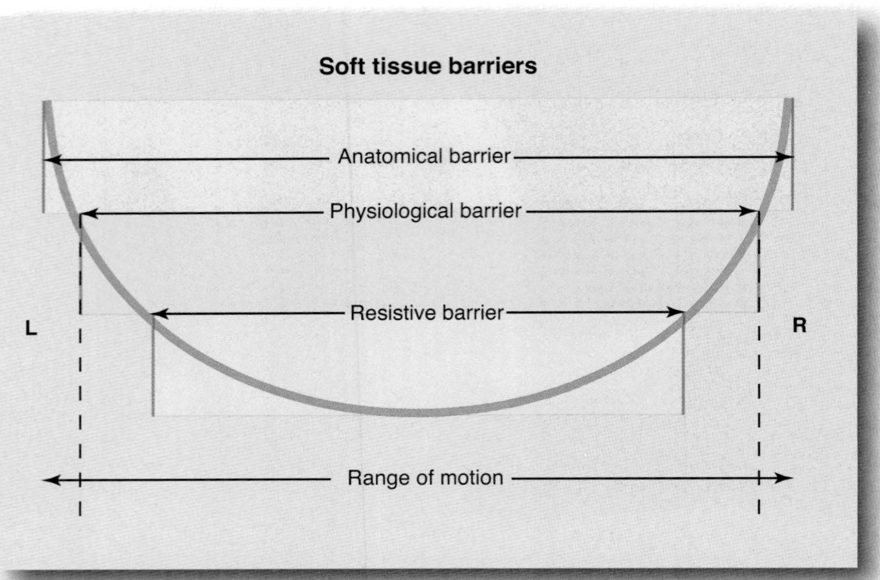

FIGURE 17-9 Soft tissue barriers.

OTHER ORTHOPEDIC TESTS

There are many special orthopedic tests and assessments that isolate certain structures or provoke specific symptoms to identify conditions or pathologies that a client might be experiencing. These assessments are often named according to the area of the body being tested or after the name of the person who devised the test (e.g., Adson's test, Phalen's test, Ober's test). There are orthopedic tests for most of the body's structures, but discussion of these tests is beyond the scope of this text. Students interested in clinical and orthopedic massage skills are encouraged to seek advanced study and continuing education in orthopedic assessment.

SOFT TISSUE BARRIERS

soft tissue barriers are notable physiologic changes in the quality of movement in soft tissue that represent the limits within which the tissues can be effectively manipulated.

resistive barrier also known as the pathologic barrier, is the first sign of resistance to a movement as tissue is moved and manipulated through its range of motion.

When assessing and treating soft tissue conditions, the therapist must recognize **soft tissue barriers.** These barriers represent the limits within which the tissues can be effectively manipulated (Figure 17-9). In developing sensitivity to soft tissue barriers, the therapist can better adjust the amount of pressure used to generate a therapeutic response from the tissues. Soft tissue barriers come under consideration when compressing the tissues, stretching the tissues, or mobilizing joints. For instance, when a therapist is passively moving a healthy limb through its normal range of motion, the limb moves freely, without any resistance through the middle of the range. As the end of the range is approached, the therapist will notice the slightest resistance as the slack is taken out of the tissues and they begin to stretch. This is the beginning of the resistive barrier. The client might or might not sense the beginning of the **resistive barrier.** As the stretch is continued toward the end of the movement, more force is necessary until the tissues are stretched and the client feels like "that is about as far as it goes," which represents the **physiologic barrier**. With more force but possible discomfort to the client, the **anatomic barrier** is approached at which the tissues would be maximally stretched; going any farther might cause damage to the tissue.

physiologic barrier

represents the extent of easy movement allowed during passive or active movements.

anatomic barrier

refers to the anatomic limit of motion of particular tissue. To move beyond the anatomic barrier would cause injury and disruption of tissues and supportive structures.

Soft tissue barriers vary according to the condition of the tissues. In healthy tissue, for instance, free and relatively painless movement can continue easily well into the physiologic barrier and approach the anatomic barrier before any resistance is encountered. In damaged tissue or tissues that house latent or active trigger points, scar tissue, or other injuries, restrictive and physiologic barriers might be encountered early in the movement.

Barriers are also taken into consideration when performing compression and fascial stretching manipulations. When using ischemic compression over a trigger point, the first contact with the nodule might be considered the resistive barrier. The client might realize that you are on a tender spot, but there is no discomfort. As pressure is increased, the physiologic barrier is approached, and the client might express a response of discomfort, often accompanied by pain in referral areas. The anatomic barrier should never be approached or passed, because doing so could cause damage to the tissues, injuring the motor endplates, bruising the tissue, or possibly activating latent trigger points.

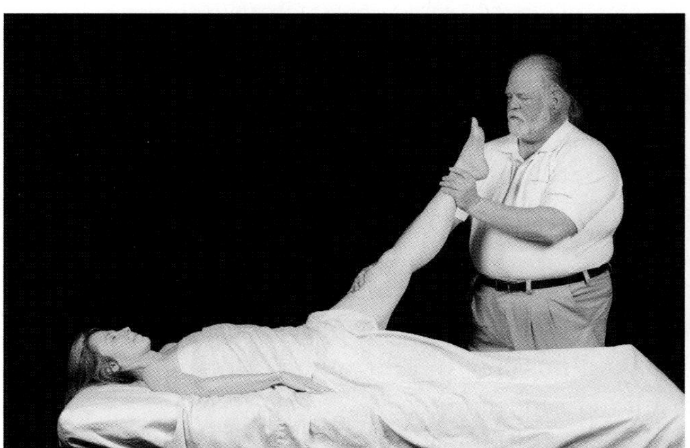

FIGURE 17-10A The resistive barrier is the first sense of resistance.

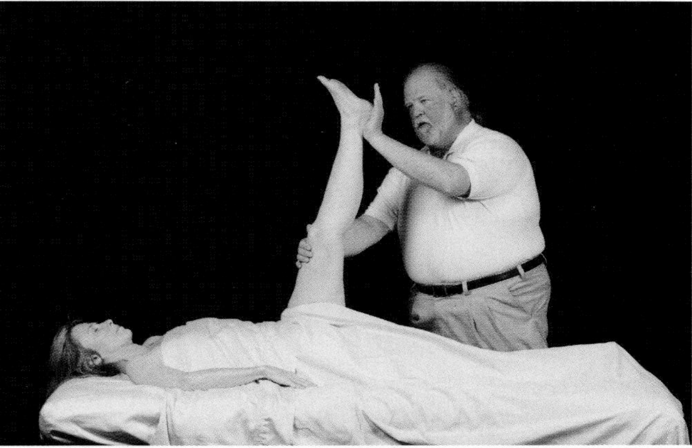

FIGURE 17-10B The physiologic barrier is as far as the joint can move before the client experiences discomfort.

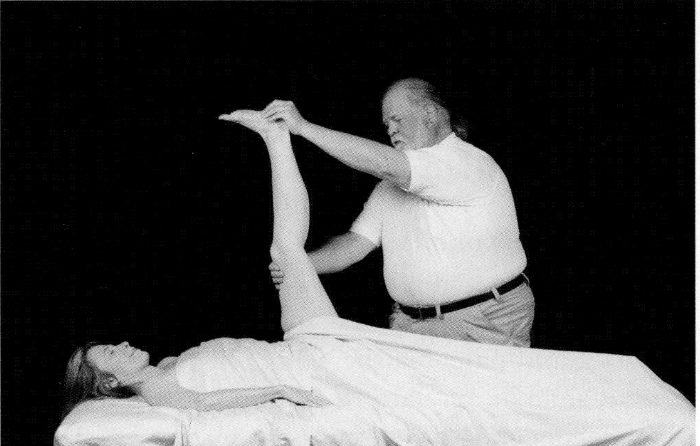

FIGURE 17-10C The anatomic barrier is the anatomic limit of the joint. To move beyond this would injure the tissues around the joint.

freely flexible range of movement

refers to the pliable and easily movable range of the tissue.

As tissue is moved and manipulated through its range of motion, three types of barriers can be considered:

- The **freely flexible range of movement** refers to the pliable and easily movable range of the tissue.
- The *resistive barrier* or pathologic barrier is the first sign of resistance to a movement and is important when assessing and treating soft tissue conditions (Figure 17-10a).
- The *physiologic barrier* represents the extent of easy movement allowed during passive or active movements (Figure 17-10b). The physiologic barrier is within the anatomic barrier and represents the comfortable end of soft tissue stretch in the range of motion.
- The *anatomic barrier* refers to the anatomic limit of motion of particular tissue (Figure 17-10c). To move beyond the anatomic barrier would cause injury and disruption of tissues and supportive structures.

Physiologic and resistive barriers are well within the anatomic limits of movement of the involved tissues. Approaching barriers that are abnormally restricted or painful but that are within the normal range of motion might reflect a pathologic condition in the tissues. Resistive and physiologic barriers reflect conditions of **bind** and **ease** related to contractile muscle tissue and fascia. When healthy tissue is manipulated or moved through its possible range, an ease of movement is sensed throughout the movement. As the tissue approaches the outer limits of possible movement, the first sense of bind is felt. The first encounter of bind represents contact with the resistive barrier in that direction. By using incrementally more force, movement can continue through the resistive barrier into increased bind and resistance until the physiologic barrier is encountered. When contractile tissue is constricted or injured, the physiologic barrier is encountered before the end of the normal range of motion and well before the anatomic barrier. If more force were applied, movement could continue through the physiologic barrier into more bind, until the anatomic barrier is approached. Movement beyond the physiologic barrier usually causes excessive discomfort and possibly more trauma. Moving beyond the anatomic barrier would result in tissue damage.

When addressing soft tissue conditions with less-than-healthy tissues, the amount of force used to approach barriers varies greatly and requires a developed sensitivity on the part of the therapist. The best therapeutic response is achieved by applying forces that elicit responses between the resistive and physiologic barriers.

PALPATION SKILLS

Many forms of bodywork disciplines require skill in sensing, through touch, the conditions and subtle changes that take place in the body's soft tissues. Acupuncture diagnosis reads the subtle differences in the deep and superficial pulses and palpates the exact locations of the acupuncture points. Acupressure, shiatsu, Jin Shin Do, and other touch modalities derived from the Asian model depend on the sense of touch to identify points on the body and monitor subtle changes in those points as they are treated. Craniosacral therapists monitor cranial rhythms and other subtle changes in the tissue as they palpate and treat body structures. In myofascial release, fascial preference and changes are monitored through palpation.

The sense of touch is one of the massage therapist's most powerful tools. It is what puts the therapist in close contact with the client. It is the means of communication between the therapist and the client's body. Developing palpation skills, sensing the difference in tissue quality and integrity, and responding with appropriate therapy techniques are marks of a good massage therapist.

Palpation is a skill and an art developed by the therapist that is a primary assessment tool allowing the therapist to listen to the client's body through the therapist's hands (Figure 17-11). Palpation skills are learned through experience. Palpation is an effective assessment tool because of the extreme sensitivity of the practitioner's hands and the ability to differentiate between subtle variations of temperature, texture, moisture, and density of the target tissues. The successful massage therapist develops skills to differentiate between the feel of normal and abnormal soft tissue. By palpation, the therapist should be able to identify bony structures, skeletal alignment, individual muscles, and various conditions of the soft tissue such as tight/loose conditions, tenderness, adhesions, constrictions, spasms, fibrosis, taut bands, and nodules or trigger points within the muscle.

palpation
is a skill and an art developed by the therapist that is a primary assessment tool allowing the therapist to listen to the client's body through the therapist's hands.

Palpation is an assessment tool used during the preliminary assessment to identify and localize areas of concern, and it is also used extensively during the treatment phase to identify target tissues and monitor changes continuously in soft tissue as the session progresses. The hands are the main vehicles to deliver manipulations to soft tissue, and yet at the same time the hands carefully monitor the underlying tissues for changes in response to the manipulations.

Although many massage therapists use palpation as the primary form of assessment, it is most accurate when used in conjunction with and after the aforementioned ROM and orthopedic assessment skills. Especially in pain conditions where there is radiating or referred pain, observation and examination can isolate the cause of the pain and then palpation pinpoints the source.

As with the other assessment techniques, the therapist should make bilateral comparisons palpating the unaffected or good side first. Although many conditions affect both sides of the body, bilateral comparison helps to establish what is normal for that person and to determine whether the tissue in question is involved in the dysfunctional condition.

Assessment by palpation is both objective and subjective. As the therapist's hands palpate the body's tissues, the therapist must pay close attention not only to the qualities of the tissue but also to the reactions of the client. The therapist begins lightly and proceeds to probe deeper into the tissues, noting any signs of tension, lesions, or pain.

Assessment using palpation can be done at many levels, from superficial to deep. The most superficial level is just above the body, not quite touching the skin. Variations in temperature can be sensed. Warm areas can indicate increased activity or inflammation. Cooler areas can indicate congestion or reduced circulation. A subtle energy field also can be sensed at this level as a slight pressure against the palm of the hand, possibly indicating a highly active area, or as an empty feeling, indicating a depleted condition.

Box 17.2

Descriptive terms for Layer Palpatory Examination

The texture and condition of the various tissues felt during palpatory examination can fall within one or more of following continuua of opposites:

superficial ~ deep	dry ~ moist
nonpainful ~ painful	soft ~ hard
cold ~ hot	compressible ~ rigid
hypomobile ~ hypermobile	flexible ~ stiff
smooth ~ rough	acute ~ chronic
thin ~ thick	circumscribed ~ diffuse

The next level of palpation is the skin surface. Note the temperature, texture, color, and moistness of the skin are noted. Increased temperature or surface moisture is indicative of conditions in deeper tissues. Remember, inflammation is a contraindication for local massage. The signs of inflammation are heat, redness, pain, and swelling. Palpation also detects abnormal sensations that the client might be experiencing, such as lack of sensation or increased or diminished sensation.

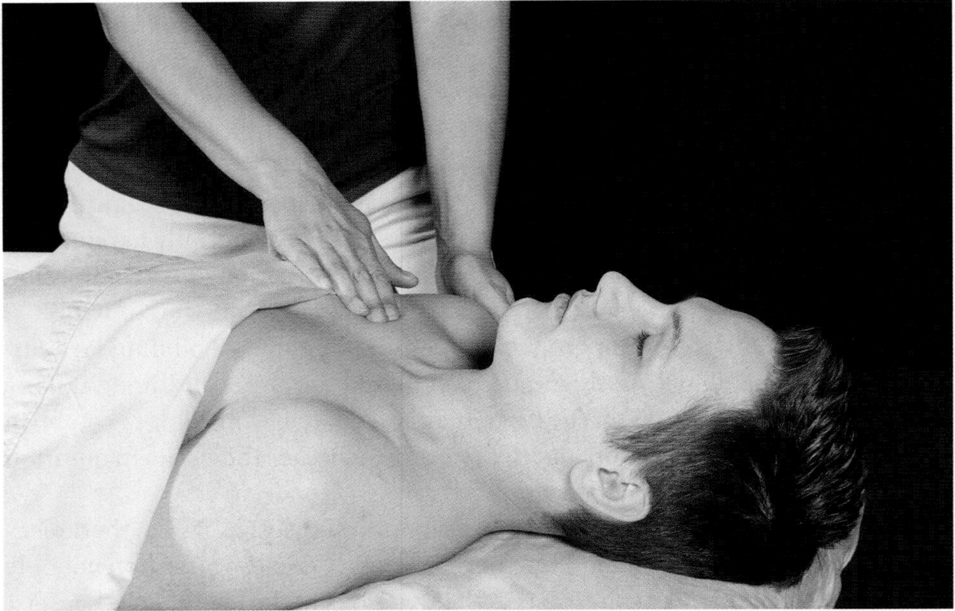

FIGURE 17-11 Flat palpation is done with the flat portion of the fingers or palm of the hand.

The quality of the subcutaneous tissue or superficial fascia is the next level to be assessed by palpation. The superficial fascia connects the skin to the underlying muscle and other tissues while at the same time allowing independent movement between them. Skin rolling is an important part of layer palpation; it gives the clinician information about the extensibility of the subcutaneous

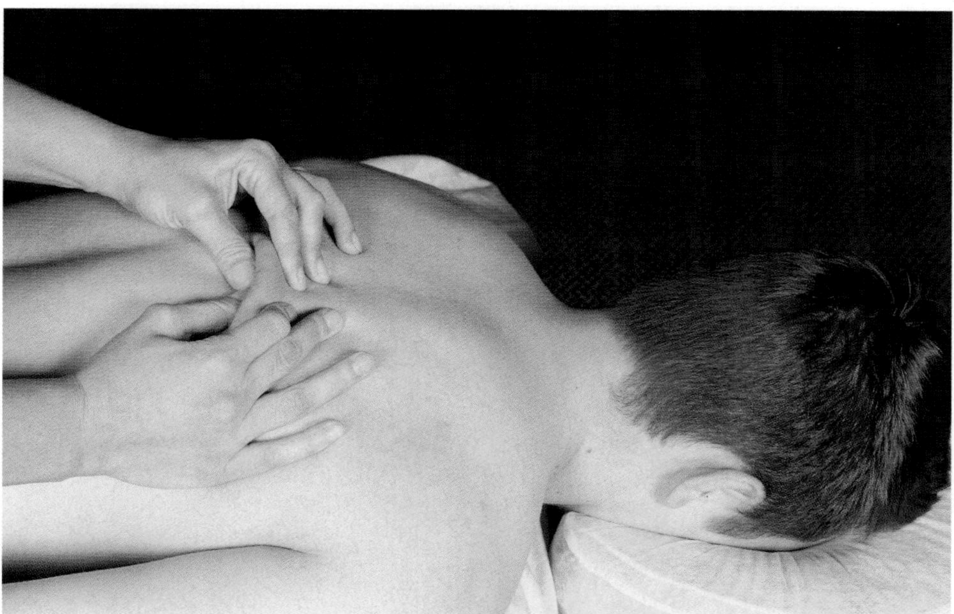

FIGURE 17-12 Skin rolling is valuable when palpating the superficial tissues.

connective tissue. In skin rolling, the skin and superficial connective tissue are lifted up, away from the deeper tissues (Figure 17-12). The extensibility of the tissues, as well as their integrity, can be palpated. A slight compression with the palm side of the fingers or hand should give the sense of a springy cushion between the skin and the deeper tissues. The skin should also glide over the underlying tissues a short distance in every direction, although it tends to have a preference to move one direction more freely that any of the others. Fascia that tend to be tight or stuck might indicate a deeper dysfunction.

The superficial fascia is also the site of superficial lymph nodes and blood vessels. The blood pulse can be felt by palpating superficial arteries. Lymph nodes feel like small nodules between the size of a small pea and a kidney bean. They can often be palpated along the side of the neck, in the axillary area, or along the inguinal area. Enlarged lymph nodes should be brought to the attention of your client and the client referred to a doctor so that the cause of the swollen nodules can be properly diagnosed.

The next level of palpation is that of the skeletal muscles and their related textures and structures. The deep palpatory examination includes compression and shear. **Compression** is palpation through layers of tissue perpendicular to the surface of the tissue. **Shear** is movement of tissues between layers, moving parallel to the tissue. Muscle is composed of contractile fibers that are organized and held in place by layers of connective tissues to form distinctive patterns that can be easily palpated. When palpating muscles, the therapist observes tissue consistency and texture. In a relaxed state, muscle is somewhat pliable and evenly grained, with the fiber orientation easily identified. Normal qualities when palpating over a muscle would allow a moderate movement of

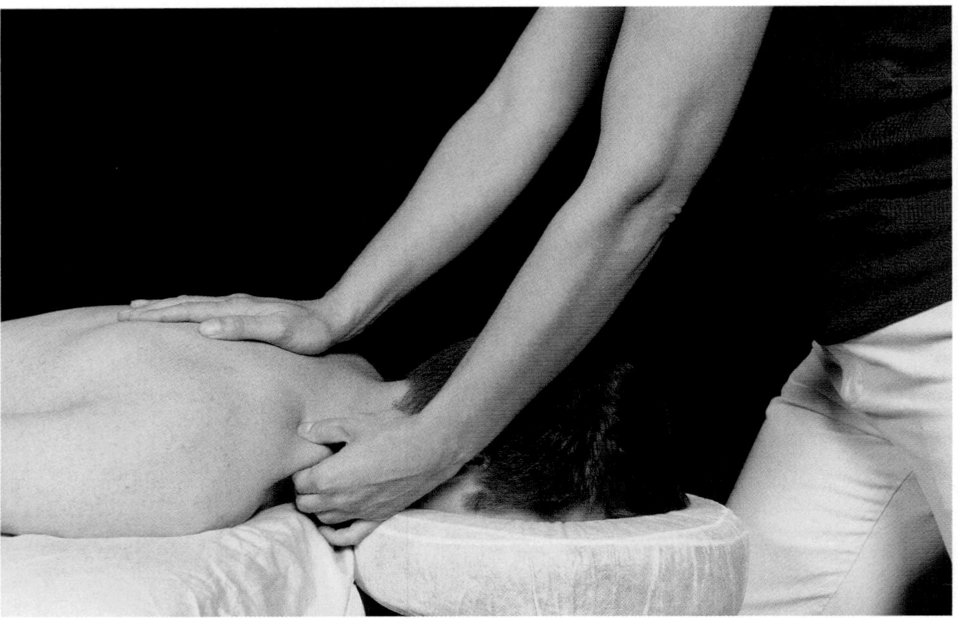

FIGURE 17-13 Pincer palpation can be useful when assessing muscle tissue.

the skin and subcutaneous tissue over the muscle tissue in all directions; an even, smooth grain when moving across the muscle fibers; and a soft, yielding, painless firmness when pressing into the muscle. Abnormal qualities include a restriction in the movement of the skin over the muscle sheaths and underlying structures, ropey or fibrous muscle tissue, tense or spasmed muscle tissue that is painful to the touch, or hypersensitive nodules that are painful when compressed. Constricted muscle feels denser or tighter, more restricted, more fibrous, and less pliable. A common palpable condition found in muscle that is usually associated with a lesion is a fibrous or taut band. Taut bands usually

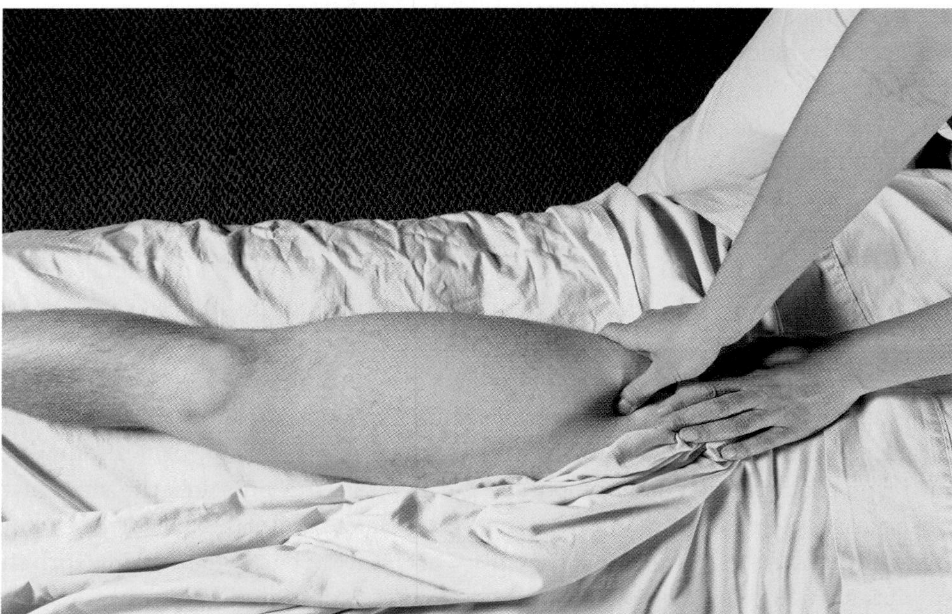

FIGURE 17-14 The thumbs are valuable tools when palpating deeper structures such as muscle attachments and tendons.

run the length of a muscle and feel like a hardened, fibrous bundle that you can actually pluck. Taut bands are usually associated with a previous injury, a strained muscle, or a habitually overstressed area. Often a taut band harbors one or more hypersensitive points that can be latent or active trigger points. Finding and reducing taut bands and trigger points is one of the most effective ways of treating soft tissue pain and dysfunction (Figure 17-13).

Toward the end of the muscle body, the connective tissue that separates and organizes the muscle fibers continues beyond the ends of the muscle fibers and becomes the muscle attachments in the form of ropelike tendons or wider tendon sheaths. This area, known as the **musculotendinous junction**, is a common area to palpate hypersensitive spots that indicate trigger points or microtrauma from overexertion.

Tendons can be palpated from the ends of the muscle to the attachment to the bone, also known as the **tendinoperiosteal junction**, where some tenderness can be noted if the muscle has been under excessive stress (Figure 17-14).

The massage therapist palpates bones as landmarks to identify muscle attachments or structural alignment. Palpating bony landmarks helps when observing structural discrepancies such as a tilted or rotated pelvis. Palpating the bony tissue around joints can indicate abnormal development or calcification. The position and regularity of the skeletal structure are also noted.

The next level to be palpated is that of the joints and the related ligaments. A joint is where two bones join together. Ligaments are tough, somewhat flexible connective tissue that connects the bones at the joints. They are slightly elastic and just flexible enough to allow an appropriate amount of movement and at the same time are resilient enough to stabilize the joint. Excessive play in the joint or a painful response when palpating a ligament usually indicates a dysfunction.

Joints are usually palpated during active or passive joint movements. The quality of movement is assessed, noting smooth, unrestricted, and painless movement through the range of motion. The end feel as the joint approaches the end of its range is also noted.

Another application of palpation is the visceral organs of the abdominal cavity. The liver and large intestine can be palpated easily. The body of the psoas muscle can be palpated and massaged through the abdominal muscles and viscera.

Structures that can be palpated

skin
subcutaneous fascia
blood vessels
lymph nodes
muscle sheaths
muscle bellies
musculotendinous junctions
tendons
deep fascia
ligaments
bone
joint spaces
abdominal viscera and structures

FIGURE 17-15 Structures that can be palpated.

The therapist should be able to identify and differentiate the location of the various structures during the palpatory examination (Figure 17-15). Is only the skin being palpated, or is the subcutaneous fascia also being palpated? Is the muscle sheath being palpated or has the muscle belly been penetrated? Is the clinician palpating the musculotendinous junction or the tendon itself? Perfecting layer palpation requires development of tactile skills and includes the ability to detect tissue texture abnormalities. How is the tissue at that level different from surrounding tissues at the same level of depth or the tissue on the contralateral side? Palpating the soft tissues helps the therapist to determine

Box 17.3

Tart

An assessment protocol that incorporates palpation and is used when addressing soft tissue dysfunction is represented by the acronym **TART**.

T = Texture of the superficial and deep tissues. Variations from normal include taut bands, adherent tissue, and hypertonic or flaccid tissues.

A = Asymmetry in body structure as observed by a rotation, a curvature, or a bilateral inconsistency in the body structure. Asymmetry is also noted as bilateral difference in motion, tone, temperature, and the like.

R = Range of motion of a single or a number of related joints in an area of the body. Quality of movement, end feel, and restricted or excessive range are all noted.

T = Tenderness or pain in an area or in specific tissues. Pain can be evident in an area, or excessive tenderness can be provoked when an area is palpated. Referred pain when pressure is applied to a point is an indication of an active myofascial trigger point.

the feel of the individual client's normal soft tissue, detect anatomic anomalies, and detect soft tissue lesions or pathology.

Developing the skills of assessing the texture and condition of the tissues takes time and practice. The ability to accurately sense the tissues, with the knowledge and skill to apply the appropriate therapeutic intervention to positively affect those tissues, provides the beneficial outcome to the client and is the hallmark of a good therapist.

ACUTE AND CHRONIC CONDITIONS

acute

refers to a condition with a sudden onset and relatively short duration.

chronic

refers to a lingering or ongoing condition.

Acute and **chronic** are terms used to describe a condition, pain, or illness. Acute refers to a condition with a sudden onset and relatively short duration. Chronic refers to a lingering or ongoing condition. Acute pain is sharp, the symptom of an identifiable incident or illness, a warning to take action, but it is usually temporary. Chronic pain is persistent or intermittent over a long period, often dull, diffused, and many times without an identifiable cause or source.

An acute illness has a rapid onset and is relatively short lived. A chronic illness progresses slowly, is difficult or impossible to remedy, and can last weeks, months, years, or can even be lifelong.

Acute Soft Tissue Injury

inflammatory response

is a natural process of healing and repair when soft tissue is injured.

An acute injury is usually due to trauma or abuse resulting in damage to the hard or soft tissue. When soft tissue is injured, whether at a cellular level or there is gross tissue damage, a natural process of healing and repair takes place. The process, known as the **inflammatory response**, is fairly predictable, with the focus being repair and reorganization of the damaged tissues. The stages of inflammation include the acute phase and the subacute phase, including the regenerative phase and the remodeling phase.

When tissue is injured, histamines are released that cause local vasodilation and increased vasopermeability, resulting in swelling, heat, and increased tenderness at the site of the injury. During this early phase, local and systemic activity involves many biologic processes that are working to reestablish homeostasis. Locally, the tissue is flooded with interstitial fluid as dead and damaged tissue is carried away while fibroblasts begin to lay down a random network of fibrin to secure the damaged tissue. During this initial period, which lasts anywhere from a matter of hours to a week depending on the nature of the injury and the condition of the client, any treatment that might disrupt these delicate fibrin structures, including massage, is contraindicated. During this time, proper treatment would include protecting the area, rest, ice, compression, and elevation (PRICE). An important benefit of PRICE is that it reduces some of the swelling that would otherwise separate the ends of the injured tissue as well as the layers of fascia related to the injured tissue. Another advantage is that pain is greatly reduced. Lymph massage proximal to the injury site helps to further reduce swelling.

During the regenerative phase, fibroblasts generate collagen fibers that rather randomly create bridges to bind the tissues together, thereby creating not only scarring of the damaged tissue but also fibrous cross-linking between fascial sheaths. Stability of the tissue improves; however, if left unchecked, cross-linking in the fascia and scarring can negatively affect functionality. At this stage, tissues are very delicate, but gentle techniques can be employed that encourage alignment of the collagen network to restore stability as well as function. Techniques include mild tensioning or lengthening with passive, pain-free range of motion and light cross-fiber manipulations. Non–weight-bearing, active range of motion helps to restore mobility and produce strong, pliable scar tissue. Techniques are applied to the surrounding tissues to help to reduce spasms and splinting and to promote circulation, reducing ischemia and encouraging drainage.

Collagen production and cross-linking continue during the remodeling phase. Tensile strength of the tissue increases; however, pliability and functionality can be reduced because of the scarring and collagen cross-hatching that effectively glue the involved layers of fascia together. Manipulations that slowly and deliberately lengthen the injured tissue to its full functional length, such as pain-free range of motion, muscle energy technique (MET; using the antagonist), and gentle stretching exercises help to reduce fibrosis and restore the tissue to full functionality. Gentle cross-fiber massage helps reduce and prevent cross-linking and aligns fibrous connective tissue to form functional scar tissue. Ice massage or an ice pack applied to the area helps to reduce inflammation. As flexibility is restored, gentle exercises can be initiated to help the client to regain strength and tone in the tissues.

A common physiologic response to an acute injury is for spasms to occur in neighboring tissues, effectively splinting the injured tissue. It is not uncommon, however, for these spasms to linger long after the injury has healed. Trigger points and ischemia develop, and what started as an acute injury becomes a long-standing chronic condition long after the injured tissue heals.

Treatment strategies for acute and chronic conditions are very different. Most acute conditions and injuries are a contraindication for most forms of massage and bodywork. Acute illnesses are often accompanied by fever and are contraindications for massage. Acute injury with tissue disruption is a contraindication for massage until the tissues have stabilized and infiltration and swelling have subsided. In the subacute stage of soft tissue injury, gentle lengthening and gentle cross-fiber techniques can be employed. The sessions are rather short and quite frequent, sometimes daily or even twice a day. Sessions for more chronic conditions are usually of a longer duration and not as frequent.

USE ASSESSMENT INFORMATION TO PLAN SESSIONS

When the assessment has been completed, the therapist should have a clearer understanding of the client's reason for making the appointment. Information from the medical history, intake form, interview, observation, and various tests is combined and analyzed to better understand the conditions and concerns of the client. Information from movement assessments notes restrictions from pain and constriction and helps to determine which tissues and structures are involved. Careful palpation further identifies affected tissues. Using the assessment information, the therapist is better able to develop a *treatment plan* to best suit the needs of the client.

Part of developing a *treatment plan* is establishing goals for the session or a series of sessions (Figure 17-16). Goals must be realistic and attainable. The client's concerns and needs and the assessment findings are considered when setting goals. Session strategies and therapeutic interventions are then chosen to work toward those goals. After the implementation of those strategies, evaluation of the session helps to determine whether those goals have been met or whether modification to the treatment plan is necessary to achieve those goals in future sessions. Depending on the findings of the assessment and the chosen goals, a *treatment plan* can include the following:

- Referral to another health professional for further assessment
- Referral to another health professional for treatment in lieu of or in conjunction with massage
- The initial number and frequency of sessions to be given
- The estimated length of the treatments and whether they are full body or specific to the condition
- The use of other modalities such as heat, ice, or hydrotherapy
- Which massage techniques will be used and avoided
- Areas of the body to be addressed or avoided
- Recommendations for home self-care
- Which results are expected and by when

Accurate assessment allows the therapist to design treatments with modalities and massage techniques and regimes that best benefit the client. The modalities and techniques used depend on the skills and knowledge of the therapist and techniques that the therapist is qualified for and able to perform.

The assessment findings and treatment plan are discussed with the client so that one can be actively involved in the therapy process. Clients who actively participate in the therapy generally reap more benefits, respond to the therapy faster, and tend to follow through for a more lasting remedy. Discussing the assessment findings with clients teaches people about the functions of the body and the nature of the condition so that clients can make educated choices as to which changes can be made to help correct the causes of the condition.

Goals for the performance of therapeutic massage

- Help the body function more efficiently
- Help increase client's self-awareness, balance, and fluidity
- Relieve pain
- Increase circulation
  - Reduce ischemia
  - Flush out toxins
- Normalize soft tissue
  - Release hypertonic muscle tissue
  - Facilitate/strengthen hypotonic muscle tissue
  - Lengthen constricted fascia
- Improve flexibility and ROM
- Reintegrate function into the whole
- Relaxation/stress relief

FIGURE 17-16 Goals for the performance of therapeutic massage.

Discussing optional therapy strategies enables clients to be involved and make choices about what to do about a condition. Discussing therapy strategies with clients gives them a clear idea of what the therapy will consist of and what might be expected during the actual sessions. The goal of the treatment plan is to inform the client of what will happen during the session so the client can be more relaxed and receptive to the treatment.

When discussing assessment findings and treatment plans with clients, use terminology that clients can understand. Some clients are more interested than others. Be clear in describing assessment findings. Use diagrams and charts to illustrate physical conditions when possible. Describe the techniques that you have chosen to use, as well as the expected benefits and the possible risks. Give enough information to inform clients without saturating them with unnecessary technicalities. Answer any questions that the client might have about your findings and the chosen interventions. When the assessment findings and proposed treatment plan are understood and agreed upon, once again obtain informed consent and proceed with the session. Always respect the client's right to modify or withdraw consent at any time while the session is in progress.

THE ROLE OF CONTINUING EDUCATION

In the current massage and bodywork profession, there are numerous modalities or systems of bodywork. (See Chapter 21 for a partial list of modalities.) Each modality has a different way of viewing the organism, assessing deviations from the optimum, and treating the body to encourage a return toward normalcy and balance. Some modalities work on different levels, such as the physical, mental, emotional, energetic, or spiritual. The serious student is encouraged to explore other modalities. Continuing education is the key to advanced learning, deeper understanding, additional skills, and greater appreciation of the human condition.

PERFORMANCE

In the performance portion of the therapeutic procedure, the therapist applies techniques and modalities to meet the goals of the treatment plan and address the needs, concerns, and conditions discovered during the assessment, with the intention of restoring normalcy, balance, and function.

When the preliminary assessment has been done and a treatment plan has been developed, the actual therapy can begin. Depending on the chosen strategy, several modalities can proceed or follow the actual massage. Hot packs, ice packs, ice massage, hot baths, or hot showers can be used before the massage therapy to enhance the desired therapeutic effects. Used with other therapy modalities, various types of stretching and exercise can be incorporated to produce excellent results.

The assessment and planning stages of the therapeutic process provide a blueprint for the procedures performed during the actual therapeutic massage. By the time the therapist begins the massage portion of the session, you know what the general conditions are and which approach and modalities to use. It is not until the therapist begins to massage the client and the hands make contact and begin to manipulate the soft tissues that a continuous flow of information directs the intricate flow of the session, however. Even though a proposed outline for the massage session is followed, there is always room to alter the treatment according to the specific conditions encountered in the tissues during the actual session. Throughout the massage, the therapist continues the assessment by working on each part of the body. As the therapist approaches an area of the body during the performance of a massage, a visual assessment notes body position, symmetry, and the color of the area. The first contact notes temperature, texture of the skin, and surface moisture. Deeper contact provides information about the connective and muscle tissue. These assessments during the performance of the massage help to continually formulate the session. Throughout the session, close attention is paid to the response of the client. Responses can be verbal, subtle movements, or changes in the actual tissue that is being manipulated. Many times nonverbal cues from the client such as facial expressions, sounds, or grimaces indicate pleasure or discomfort. The therapist continuously elicits feedback from the client and modifies the session to obtain the ultimate results. The assessment and evaluation continue to intermingle throughout the actual performance of the massage, and although the plan for the massage is followed, adjustments and modifications to the plan can occur during the actual massage according to new information gained during the session.

Therapeutic massage is like an intense conversation. The therapist listens to, observes, and examines the client to get an idea of the condition. Then the therapist's hands listen to the client's body and respond with manipulative touch. The body listens to the manipulations and responds. Hearing and feeling these responses, the therapist chooses the next delivery. Thus goes the close interaction of a therapeutic massage.

Massage Therapy for Soft Tissue Dysfunction

Musculoskeletal dysfunction is often characterized by postural deviation or movement restriction and is often accompanied by pain. Constrictions in soft tissue usually result from overuse, underuse, misuse, abuse, or trauma to the body. Soft tissue–related pain, myofascial pain, muscle pain or spasm, and ischemia all respond well to soft tissue interventions and therapeutic massage techniques. Tension, restricted movement, asymmetry, localized or referred pain, and stress are also indications for therapeutic massage. The intention of soft tissue intervention is reducing pain; restoring circulation; oxygenating tissue; releasing hypertonicity, trigger points, and fascial restrictions or adhesions; improving functional range of motion; and integrating the restored area back into the whole.

To restore the muscles successfully to a healthier state when there has been dysfunction, pain, trauma, or compensation to an area of the body, requires proper rehabilitative steps to ensure a longer-lasting recovery. After careful assessment to determine which tissues are involved and that there are no contraindications to treatment, the first step is to restore circulation and neuromuscular response to the tissues. The second step is to release any trigger points and fascial restrictions in the muscle tissue and restore flexibility. Follow that by rebuilding strength and endurance to the muscle. The first steps can be accomplished in the treatment room. Strength and endurance is included in a self-care plan and is done through exercise. It is also important to, as far as possible, identify and try to remove the causative factors that initiated the dysfunction. In the case of acute, single-event onset conditions, this is fairly simple. In the case of chronic conditions, however, isolating the causative factors is more difficult, and eliminating them can mean changing habitual patterns or modifying workspaces. In either case, treatment does not begin and end in the office during the session and usually involves homework, such as exercises or modifying some aspect of daily activity to alter the conditions that initiated the dysfunction.

Box 17.4

Conditions that respond to Soft Tissue Intervention:

soft tissue pain
tension
asymmetry
restricted movement because of pain
restricted movement because of constricted muscle
muscle strain
hypertonic muscle
hypotonic muscle
fibrosis
scar tissue
old injury sites
hypersensitive points or areas
trigger points
taut bands in muscle
fibromyalgia
stress

Postural versus Phasic Muscles

Skeletal muscles can be categorized into groups according to function, fiber type, and reaction to stress. Skeletal muscles are composed of two types of muscle fibers: type I (slow twitch) and type II (fast twitch) fibers. (Review Chapter 5 page 132). Most muscles contain both types of fibers. The proportion of slow and fast twitch fibers depends on the primary function of the muscle. Postural muscles primarily maintain upright posture, require endurance, and have a higher proportion of slow twitch, type I fibers. They are slower to respond to stimulation and resist fatigue. Muscles with a higher proportion of slow twitch fibers respond to stress or disuse by shortening and becoming hypertonic, developing trigger points and fibrosis. Under continuous strain, the connective tissue of postural muscles thickens to help to support the body.

Phasic muscles are the movers of the body and respond quickly and forcefully when stimulated. Phasic muscles contain a higher proportion of type II, fast twitch fibers that react quickly but also fatigue quickly and tend to respond to disuse and stress by weakening. Because of the quick, forceful actions of phasic muscles, common problems include strain, tendonitis, and microtrauma at the musculotendinous and tenoperiosteal junction.

Hypertonic and Hypotonic Muscles

Common structural body and postural imbalances generally involve muscles or groups of muscles that are constricted or hypertonic—that is, they seem tight or result in a postural deviation or constriction in joint movement, or both. Constricted tissues could be the result of hypertonic musculature or, in cases of chronic conditions, constrictions or fibrosis in the fascia supporting the muscles. Examining the involved tissues with range of motion and palpation can reveal which tissues are involved. When examining and treating an area of the body, look beyond the specific site and include associated muscles in the treatment. When a muscle is constricted and overactive, it is common for the antagonist (the muscle responsible for the opposite movement) to be flaccid, weak, or hypotonic. By the same token, when a weak muscle is found, often the opposing muscle or possibly the synergistic muscles are found to be overactive, tight, or hypertonic. In this type of circumstance, releasing the hypertonic or constricted tissues is often the primary focus; however, stimulating and strengthening the hypotonic antagonist is also a major consideration in the treatment plan. If the target (constricted) muscle contains trigger points, relieving those and encouraging the muscle to reestablish a normal resting length is important. At the same time, stimulating and strengthening the antagonist has an inhibitory and balancing effect on its hypertonic partner. The overall result is a more balanced structure.

MASSAGE TECHNIQUES TO ADDRESS SOFT TISSUE DYSFUNCTION

Abnormal and dysfunctional soft tissue conditions respond exceptionally well to systematically applied massage techniques directed specifically toward the affected tissues (Figure 17-17). Massage techniques affect the dysfunctional tissues either directly by manipulating the tissues or indirectly by influencing the neuromuscular mechanism in an attempt to restore more normal function. Many effective techniques are similar to those used in wellness/relaxation massage, including effleurage, petrissage, friction, joint movements, and stretching, but are directed toward the dysfunctional tissues. Therapeutic techniques are modified or combined for the specific effects that they produce when applied to the body. Neuromuscular, myofascial, and lymph massage techniques are valuable tools when addressing many soft tissue conditions. Massage techniques are used to identify abnormal tissues, normalize and restore function, and finally to reconnect and integrate the area with the whole.

FIGURE 17-17 Effective techniques to address soft tissue conditions.

EFFECTIVE TECHNIQUES TO ADDRESS SOFT TISSUE CONDITIONS	
Classic Swedish techniques	
Effleurage, Petrissage, Friction, Percussion, Joint Movements	Refer to Chapter 10
Hydrotherapy	
Cold packs and ice therapy	Helps to reduce pain and swelling from inflammation
Hot packs	Promotes relaxation. Softens connective tissue and fascia
Contrast Therapy	Increases local circulation
Lymph Massage	Increases lymph circulation. Reduces edema and swelling
Neuromuscular Therapies	
Gliding techniques	
Superficial gliding	Introduces area to touch. Applies lubricant. Assesses superficial tissue quality. Stimulates parasympathetic nervous system. Increases local circulation. Soothes and relaxes
Deep gliding (stripping)	Assesses superficial and deeper tissue quality. Increases local circulation. Softens connective tissue. Separates adhesions
Cross-fiber techniques	
Digital or point specific	Assesses connective and contractile tissue Reduces adhesions and scar tissue
Broad cross-fiber massage	Assesses connective and contractile tissue. Broadens fibrous tissue. Softens and reduces adhesions
Position Release Techniques	Releases hypertonic contractile tissues and resets pathophysiologic neuromuscular circuits
Muscle Energy Techniques	
Postisometric Relaxation (PIR)	Helps muscles to regain their normal resting length. Increases ROM
Reciprocal Inhibition (RI)	Helps muscles to regain their normal resting length
Contract-Relax-Antagonist Contract (CRAC)	Restores flexibility and ROM
Active Resisted Range of Motion	Stimulates weak or hypotonic muscles
Trigger-point Techniques	Locates, assesses, and reduces trigger-point activity
Trigger-point Pressure Release (Ischemic Compression)	Reduces trigger points
Position Release Techniques	Releases trigger points in taut bands and resets neuromuscular feedback circuits
Muscle Energy Techniques (MET)	Restores muscles to their normal resting length
Myofascial Techniques	
Skin Rolling	Assesses superficial and deep connective tissues. Releases superficial fascia
J-strokes	Stretches, separates and aligns constricted fascia
Cross-handed stretches	Releases restricted fascia
Traction	Stretches superficial and deep connective tissue. Improves ROM

Determine the suspected areas of the body to be addressed during the assessment and planning stages of the session. During the performance of the massage, the actual physical contact allows the therapist to identify the specific tissues involved. The therapist is able to palpate and identify the abnormal tissues with superficial gliding and light cross-fiber strokes. Massage techniques are then chosen to normalize the tissues (Figure 17-18). Trigger points are quieted with position release, ischemic compression, and muscle energy technique. Fascial constriction is reduced with deep gliding, J-strokes, cross-fiber friction, and myofascial stretching. Hypotonic muscles are tonified with muscle energy technique, J-strokes, and exercise. Finally, passive joint movements and superficial gliding help to integrate and reconnect the tissues to the surrounding area and to the whole.

FIGURE 17-18 Treatment goals and suggested techniques to address those goals.

TREATMENT GOALS	TECHNIQUES TO ADDRESS TREATMENT GOALS
Relaxation/Stress Relief	Deep Breathing, Classic Swedish massage: Effleurage, Petrissage, Friction, Passive Joint Movements
Accustom client to therapist's touch	Light touch, effleurage, encourage open communication, deep breathing. Before addressing specific conditions or injury site, apply relaxing techniques to unaffected body parts, including the contralateral uninjured limb, to obtain an idea of tissue normalcy.
Acute soft tissue conditions	Massage techniques that would disrupt the delicate injured/healing tissues are contraindicated for 48–96 hours
Reduce inflammation	Hydrotherapy - PRICE (Protect-Rest-Ice-Compression-Elevation)
Reduce inflammation/swelling	Lymph massage proximal to the injury (not on the injury site, not distal to the injury site.) Begin nodal pumping on lymph nodes proximal to the injury followed by stationary, slow circles on tissues proximal to the injury site. Light directional effleurage
Subacute soft tissue conditions	
Reduce swelling/edema	Lymph massage proximal to the injury. Begin with nodal pumping on lymph nodes proximal to injury followed by stationary, slow circles on tissues proximal to the injury site. Light directional effleurage
Increase local circulation	Hydrotherapy – contrast therapy; alternating hot and cold packs or baths Massage – Effleurage and petrissage
Reduce adhesions and realign connective tissue to form functional scar tissue	Gentle, short cross-fiber massage, gentle, pain-free, passive range of motion of related joints. Follow with ice massage to reduce inflammation.
Maintain range-of-motion	Pain-free passive joint movements and active free range-of-motion exercises
Address any compensating structures	Assess any compensating structures for hyper or hypotonicity, trigger points, adhesions, or fibrosis and treat accordingly
Chronic soft tissue conditions	
Increase local circulation	Hydrotherapy – contrast therapy;alternating hot and cold packs Massage - Effleurage, petrissage,
Reduce chronic edema	Tissue fluid could be trapped within layers of fascia and connective tissue. Check for restrictions in fascia with tissue excursion (fascial glide); then use myofascial techniques (skin rolling, cross-handed stretch) followed by proximal lymph massage
Reduce ischemia	Superficial and deep gliding (stripping), petrissage
Check for adhesions and fascial constrictions	Effleurage, petrissage, deep gliding, skin rolling
Reduce adhesions and fascial constrictions	Myofascial techniques – skin rolling, cross-fiber techniques, J-strokes, cross-handed stretches. Longitudinal muscle stripping. Follow with ice massage to minimize inflammation
Reduce hypertonicity	Position release techniques, deep gliding (stripping)
Relieve trigger-points	Trigger-point pressure release, position release techniques followed by MET/RI to restore muscle length.
Restore range of motion	Passive joint movements, traction
Increase range of motion	Muscle energy techniques, PIR, CRAC
Address any compensating conditions and structures.	Check for hypertonicity, trigger points, ischemia, hypotonicity or other conditions in adjacent muscles, contra-lateral limbs, or other areas of the body and treat accordingly

Self-care/Homework	
Educate client about condition	Avoid activities that would stress or aggravate the condition. Change daily activities/habits that perpetuate the condition.
Maintain/increase circulation	Proper hydrotherapy
Maintain/increase range of motion	Pain-free active range-of-motion exercises (both sides), stretching exercises
Maintain/increase strength	Active resisted isometric and isotonic exercises
Refer	Refer the client to another health practitioner for alternative therapies when appropriate

How Much Pressure Is Enough?

The right amount of pressure to use when doing bodywork varies greatly depending on the type of bodywork, the technique being applied, the condition of the client, and the condition of the target tissues. For example, in lymph massage the pressure is very light, whereas in deep connective tissue therapies, such as deep gliding, cross-fiber friction, or ischemic compression, the pressure is considerably deeper. The right amount of pressure to achieve the optimal therapeutic response is therefore relative to the technique being used, the location and condition of the target tissue, and the intention of the manipulation. In most soft tissue techniques, the pressure is enough to engage the target tissues without causing an alarm response or damaging the target or surrounding tissues. Pressure is applied gradually manner where contact is made, and pressure is increased the same way so as not to invade the tissues or startle the client. When working deeply into an area, enter slowly and occasionally pause and allow the tissues to open as they become more receptive to the pressure being applied. The amount of pressure varies from one client to another and from one part of the body to another. Pressure can vary according to the texture and sensitivity of the target tissue; the goal is to achieve a therapeutic response from the tissue.

The optimal therapeutic pressure is that which would elicit the maximal therapeutic response without triggering an autonomic defensive reaction from the client. If the pressure is too abrupt or too intense, the client will respond with defense mechanisms that will negate any therapeutic gain, erode trust in the therapist/client relationship, and possibly cause injury to the tissues.

Dr. Arthur Pauls, the British osteopath who developed Ortho-Bionomy, described *rebound* as a palpable tissue response to therapeutically applied pressure. *Rebound* refers to a springy, responsive, active feedback when a tissue is compressed or stretched just enough to engage the neuromuscular and proprioceptive reflexes. When compressing a point, as in ischemic compression, rebound is encountered between the resistive barrier and the anatomic barrier. To find it, make contact and slowly press into the point nearly to the level to elicit an "ouch" response from the client, and then back off slightly. The pressure is enough to engage the point, to sort of float on the point, and to sense the dynamic changes in the tissue as the body responds to the therapeutic input. Likewise, when doing a joint movement, move the limb to the extent of possible movement, and back off slightly and hold that position. Engaging the tissues in the rebound space is an optimal therapy zone where the body is most receptive to integrating the therapeutic input.

Trigger Points and Fibrosis

Trigger points are hypersensitive nodules that are usually located in hypertonic, dysfunctional, and often painful muscle tissue, although similar hypersensitive points are occasionally found in fascia, tendons, and even ligaments. Eliminating troublesome trigger points and restoring muscles to their normal resting length usually result in restoring pain-free function to the associated body area. Reducing fibrosis, eliminating trigger points, and restoring contractile muscle tissue to a normal resting length are three goals of therapeutic massage. Massage techniques that are effective at accomplishing these goals are passive positioning, myofascial, and muscle energy techniques. Trigger points, trigger-point release techniques, position release, myofascial techniques, and muscle energy techniques are discussed in Chapter 15.

REVIEW OUTCOME IN RELATION TO INTENT OF SESSION

Evaluation involves examining the outcome of the process in relation to the expected goals and objectives. Evaluation is important because the client and therapist can gauge the effectiveness of the selected course of therapy according to the success in attaining the goals. Examining the outcome is important when deciding ongoing therapy, and it provides a rationale for applying similar therapies for similar conditions in the future. Evaluation identifies the grounds for altering parts or all of the process to achieve desired results more effectively. Finally, evaluation helps to determine whether goals have been met and whether referral to another professional is warranted.

Evaluation is both subjective and objective. Much of the evaluation is based on how the client feels as a result of the therapy. Levels of posture, mobility, pain, and function can be reassessed to indicate the success of the treatment.

Evaluation is performed at various times during the therapeutic process. After the assessment, an evaluation is performed to decide how or whether to proceed. Evaluation occurs after a single session and during the performance of a session to determine the effectiveness of the chosen modalities and techniques. If the decision is made to continue with several sessions, evaluations after each session help to determine the continued course of therapy. The evaluation can carry over to the beginning of the following massage session to note more long-term improvements and effects of the chosen treatment and make adjustments to any follow-up sessions. An evaluation at the end of the series helps to determine the course into the future.

SUMMARY

There are numerous massage techniques and modalities that can enhance a person's health and well-being. Determining which techniques are best suited to a particular situation or condition requires training and experience. *Therapeutic procedure* is a process of acquiring a concise medical history, assessment procedures to determine constricted and painful conditions, developing treatment plans, performing appropriate treatment practices to address the conditions more specifically, and evaluating the results to ensure that the client is receiving effective treatment to address current health concerns. Four steps of therapeutic procedure include assessment, planning, performance or treatment, and evaluation. A common assessment protocol includes a concise medical history, a consultation (including close observation of body language), posture and gait assessments, palpation of tissues, and various functional and orthopedic tests. The medical history provides vital information about the client's past and current health that could relate to current concerns and your choice of treatment. During the consultation or interview, information from all written forms is clarified, and questions are asked to further determine the client's concerns. The assessment continues with observation, palpation, and a variety of functional tests. Subjective and objective information from the various assessments is analyzed, and appropriate modalities are chosen to address the conditions found during the assessment. Assessment findings and modality choices are discussed with the client, and some treatment goals are agreed on. Both therapist and client create a treatment plan or care plan to address the treatment goals. With the treatment plan as a blueprint, the therapist begins the performance portion of the therapy session, applying modalities and techniques to address the soft tissue conditions. Flexibility is built into the plan so that the therapist can continually assess the client's body and tissues and make minor adjustments to the treatment, with the client's permission. At the conclusion of the session or after several sessions, an evaluation is performed to determine the effectiveness of the chosen techniques in addressing the goals of the session(s). Examining the outcome provides a rationale for continuing or changing the chosen therapy or for applying similar techniques for similar conditions in the future.

Therapeutic procedure provides a process that the therapist can follow to ensure that the client receives services to address health conditions in a manner that is safe and effective.

QUESTIONS FOR DISCUSSION AND REVIEW

1. What are the four steps of a therapeutic procedure?
2. What is the purpose of each step of the therapeutic procedure?
3. How can the therapeutic procedure be implemented in therapeutic massage?
4. Name five important parts of the assessment process.
5. What is a pain scale, and how is it used in the therapeutic process?
6. Name three types of movements tested when assessing range of motion.
7. Differentiate between the resistive barrier, the physiologic barrier, and the anatomic barrier.
8. List at least seven levels at which soft tissue can be palpated.
9. According to Dr. James Cyriax, what is contractile tissue? Inert tissue? End feel?
10. Name three classifications of end feel considered to be normal.
11. What are the characteristics of abnormal end feel?
12. Differentiate between a chronic and an acute soft tissue condition.
13. What is the appropriate therapy in the initial stage of an acute soft tissue injury?
14. What information is used to develop a treatment plan?
15. Why are the assessment findings and treatment plan discussed with the client?
16. How is a therapeutic massage like an intense conversation?
17. Differentiate how postural and phasic muscles respond to stress.
18. What are the important advantages of using the evaluation portion of the therapeutic process?

CHAPTER

18

Athletic/ Sports Massage

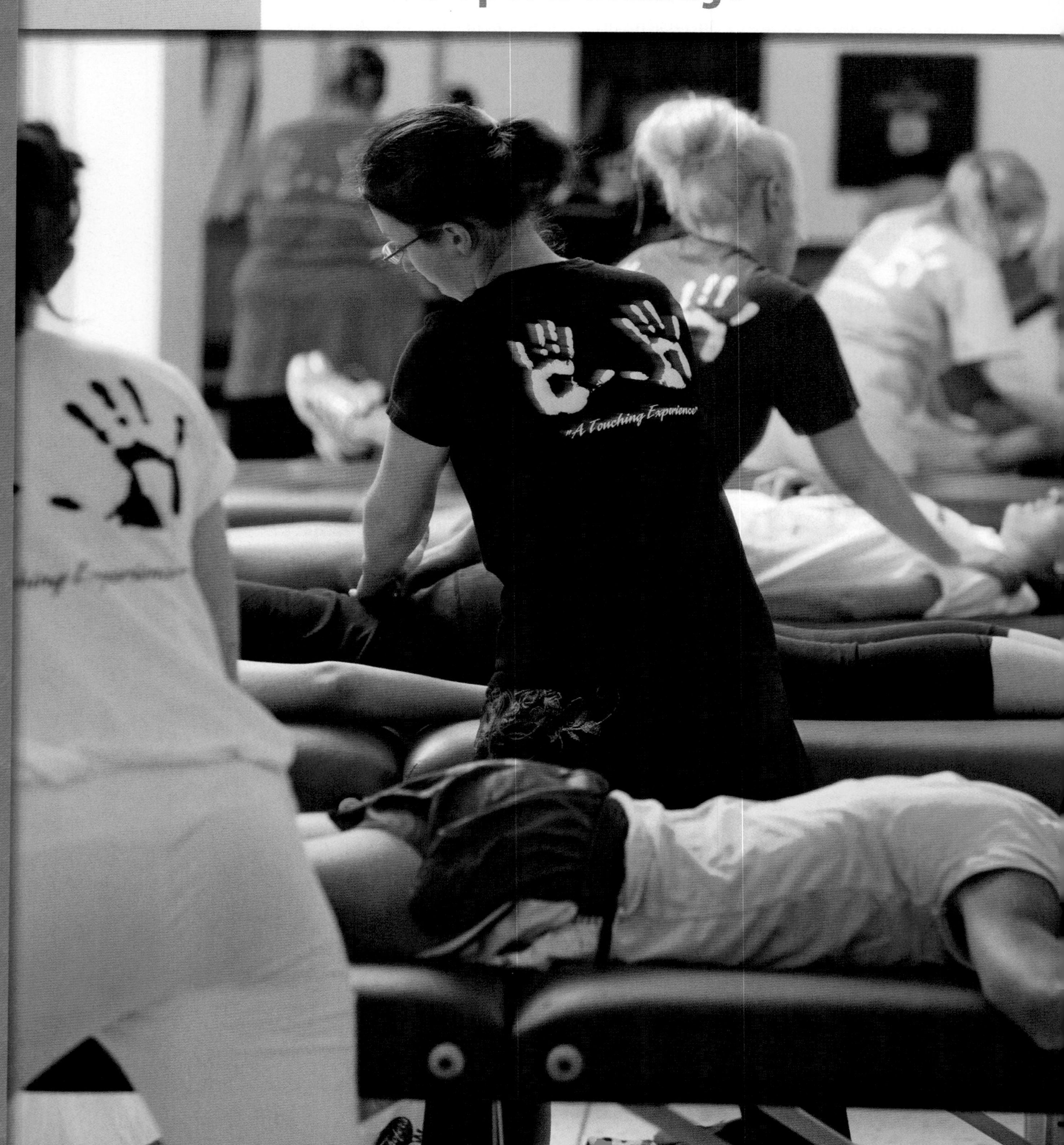

LEARNING OBJECTIVES

After you have mastered this chapter, you will be able to

1. **Define athletic/sports massage.**
2. **Explain the purposes of athletic massage.**
3. **Explain the causes of muscle fatigue.**
4. **Explain the major benefits of athletic massage.**
5. **Explain contraindications for athletic massage.**
6. **Describe the three basic applications of athletic massage and the goals of each.**
7. **Demonstrate massage techniques commonly used in pre- and post-event athletic massage.**
8. **Explain the importance of warm-up exercises and massage to the athlete's performance.**
9. **List the therapeutic modalities used in restorative massage.**
10. **Demonstrate how to locate the stress points of the body.**
11. **List the therapeutic modalities used in rehabilitative athletic massage.**
12. **Explain the relationship of certain athletic or sports activities to possible injuries.**
13. **Differentiate between acute, subacute, and chronic athletic injuries and the treatment choices for each stage of injury.**

INTRODUCTION

As far back as antiquity, massage was used to restore and to rejuvenate war-torn and weary soldiers as they returned to Rome. The Roman athletes also enjoyed the benefits of restorative massage and baths.

For many years, the great athletes of the European and Soviet countries have included massage as part of their intensive and continuous training schedules. In 1972, Lasse Viren, nicknamed the Flying Finn, credited daily deep friction massage with his ability to train hard enough to win gold medals in the 5,000 and 10,000 meters at the Olympic games. In 1980, Jack Meagher and Pat Boughton published the first book in the United States on the subject, entitled *Sportsmassage.*

In the United States, massage is recognized as a valuable asset to improve the athlete's ability to perform better with fewer physical ill effects from maximum effort. In 1984, for the first time, massage was made available for all athletes competing in the Summer Olympic Games in Los Angeles. Since then, massage areas have become a common sight at many athletic events across the country. Many athletes participate in regular massage as part of their training regimen. Many professional athletic teams, including baseball, basketball, football, and hockey, employ professional massage therapists as part of their training staff. For many athletes and trainers, massage has become the therapy of choice in the rehabilitation of minor sports injuries.

Throughout the 1980s, sports massage was instrumental in opening the door for the recognition of massage as a viable treatment for soft tissue injury, dysfunction, and pain. Many massage techniques used and developed for sports massage are just as applicable for soft tissue lesions and injuries suffered in the practices of day-to-day living.

PURPOSE OF ATHLETIC MASSAGE

Athletic massage, also called *sports massage*, is the application of massage techniques that combine sound anatomic and physiologic knowledge, an understanding of strength training and conditioning, and specific massage skills to enhance athletic performance. Athletic massage enables athletes to attain their highest potential by accelerating the body's natural restorative processes, enabling the athlete to participate more often in rigorous physical training and conditioning. Massage helps to reduce the chance of injury by identifying and eliminating conditions in the soft tissue that are at potential risk of injury. When injury has occurred, massage helps to restore mobility and flexibility to injured muscle tissue, while reducing recovery time. Athletic massage, when performed correctly, can improve the athlete's ability to perform while reducing the incidence of lost time from injury and fatigue. Receiving sports massage on a regular basis can extend the athlete's career.

Adaptive sports massage (or sports massage for athletes with disabilities) is a specialty that requires additional knowledge and training in the disabilities that these athletes have. These might include mental disabilities (e.g., experienced by Special Olympians) or physical disabilities (e.g., experienced by athletes with amputated limbs, in wheelchairs, or who are sight or hearing impaired). Although athletes with disabilities do not get the recognition and media attention they deserve, their need for massage therapy and athletic training is just as important as for any other athlete.

The sports massage techniques are the same for athletes with disabilities, although they might be used at different times. For instance, a pre-event massage done on a sprinter with cerebral palsy would be very relaxing instead of invigorating. Although most athletes are very agile at getting around, at times lifting or using a transfer board is necessary. As with all people, however, the person who knows what is needed to give peak performance is the person living in the body.

Athletic massage is not reserved just for the highly competitive athlete. The same techniques are effective on any active person for assessing and working on soft tissue conditions.

The Athletic/Sports Massage Therapist

To be an effective athletic (sports) massage therapist, a person should have a thorough understanding of anatomy, physiology, kinesiology, biomechanics, and massage technique. The massage therapist should have a sound knowledge of anatomy and be familiar with the various structures of the body. Of particular interest are the skeletal system, the muscular system, and the system of connective tissue and fascia that integrates them. It is important also to understand the circulatory system and the nervous system, especially the neuromuscular functions. An understanding of *kinesiology*, which is the study of body movement, helps the therapist to recognize which structures are involved in the movements of particular sports, especially when pain is present. The therapist must also understand which muscles and muscle groups that the athlete uses the most in a particular sport.

Biomechanics refers to the integrated movement of the entire body. For instance, the manner in which the foot is placed affects what the knees, hip, back, shoulders, and head do. Tension in a particular body area also indicates tension or misalignment in other areas of the body. Because the body is used in a particular way, specific areas are going to be stressed. A deviation in the structure of one area of the body is then reflected throughout the body. Deviations often appear as patterns of structural imbalance. These deviations, when stressed, often result in injury. The more severe the deviation, the sooner an injury might occur.

Physiology is important in understanding the role that each system plays in supporting the others so that they function as a whole organism. The better the therapist understands the body's response to exercise, strain, and injury, the better she can offer massage services that will benefit the athlete.

An accepted principle in sports physiology is that to improve either strength or **endurance**, appropriate stresses must be applied to **overload** the system, forcing the body to adapt to the heavier load. Proper conditioning involves overloading the system an acceptable amount, and then allowing the system time to recuperate and adapt to a new level of ability. If the intensity of the training exceeds the body's ability to recuperate, injury or breakdown probably will result.

endurance

is the act, quality, or power of withstanding hardship or stress.

overload

the principle of applying stresses that are greater than what the body is accustomed to, thereby forcing it to adapt to the heavier load by increasing strength or endurance.

During intense training, competition, and sometimes in everyday life, muscle strength and endurance are pushed to the beyond their limits. The result can include:

- Increased metabolic waste buildup in the tissues.
- Strains in the muscle or connective tissue. These range from microscopic trauma to major injury.
- Inflammation and associated fibrosis.
- Spasms and pain that restrict movement.

These are negative effects of exercise. Skillfully applied athletic massage effectively counteracts each of these conditions. It normally takes a muscle that has been stressed to a point of fatigue 48 to 72 hours to rest, adapt, and recuperate. Athletic massage can reduce the recuperation time by as much as 50 percent.

Beneficial Effects of Athletic Massage

The goal of athletic massage is to enhance the athlete's performance. Performance is regulated by the efficiency, precision, and freedom with which the athlete is able to move. Efficiency depends on training and conditioning, and athletic massage allows for more intense training. Restrictions from pain, spasms, and tension inhibit freedom of movement. Without freedom of movement, precision is adversely affected. Athletic massage reduces many of the restrictions.

The following are the beneficial effects of athletic massage:

1. It causes hyperemia, making more oxygen and nutrients necessary for growth and repair available to the body area being massaged.
2. It stimulates venous circulation and lymph drainage to flush out the metabolic wastes of exertion quickly.
3. It stretches and broadens muscles, tendons, and ligaments.
4. It reduces muscle spasm.
5. It identifies possible trouble areas and helps to eliminate them.
6. It breaks down adhesions between fascial sheaths.
7. It separates fibrosis and breaks down adhesions that result from inflammation and trauma.
8. It helps to realign collagen fibers that are formed as a result of injury to produce a strong, flexible scar.

For more serious or competitive athletes, there are additional benefits of sports massage when used on a regular basis. Athletic massage accomplishes the following:

1. Encourages better performance and reduces the chance of injury.
2. Allows the athlete to reach peak performance sooner and sustain it longer.
3. Improves muscle flexibility, allowing muscles to respond more quickly and powerfully.
4. Identifies and eliminates possible trouble spots, thereby preventing injury.
5. Greatly reduces muscle stiffness from excess metabolite buildup, rejuvenating muscles quicker after intense workouts or events.
6. Reduces ischemic pain and pain from spasms, splinting, and tension.
7. Assists injuries in healing quicker and stronger without loss of power from transverse fibrosis.
8. Offers the athlete a chance to relax and recuperate more quickly.
9. Extends the overall span of the athlete's career.

Techniques of Athletic Massage

A thorough knowledge of the various massage techniques and their proper application makes the difference between an effective or ineffective sports massage therapist. Many of the techniques of athletic massage are identical with those of classical Swedish massage such as effleurage, petrissage, kneading, passive and active joint movements, percussion, vibration, and friction. Neuromuscular techniques are useful to identify and relieve trigger points and stress points and reduce tension and hypertonicity in muscles. Myofascial techniques effectively address constricted fascia and adhesions. Lymph massage enhances fluid movement and reduces swelling. Some therapeutic techniques in sports massage bear special consideration and are discussed here.

Compression Strokes

hyperemia

is an increased amount of blood in the muscle.

Compression is applied with a rhythmic pumping action to the belly of the muscle. Compression strokes cause increased amounts of blood to remain in the muscle over an extended period. This **hyperemia** is of value in pre-event, restorative, and rehabilitative massage.

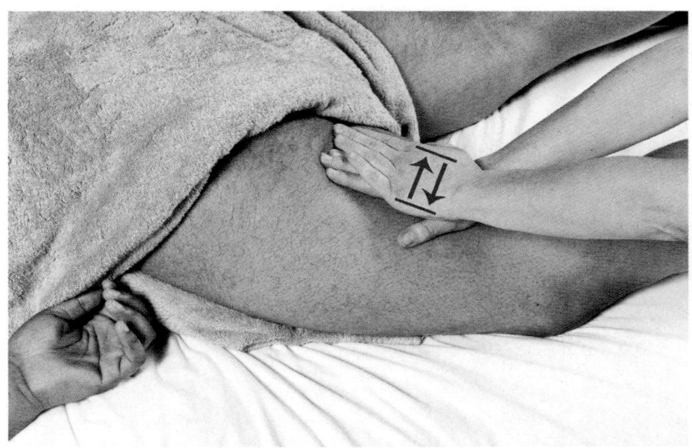
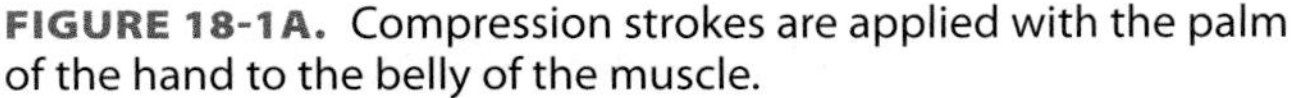

FIGURE 18-1A. Compression strokes are applied with the palm of the hand to the belly of the muscle.

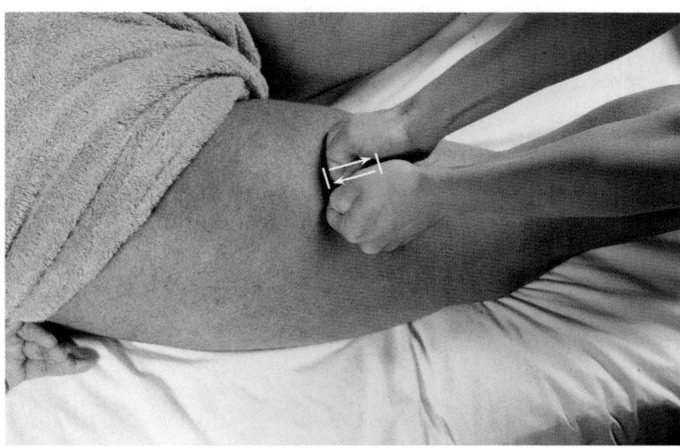

FIGURE 18-1B One or both soft fists can be used to apply compression strokes.

Compression strokes for athletic massage use the palm of the hand or a soft fist to repeatedly press the muscle against the bone. The depth of pressure begins as a light touch and gradually deepens as the muscle relaxes. This procedure can be repeated three or more times along each part of the muscle, with special attention given to the body of the muscle. Large, broad muscles require several passes to cover the entire muscle.

Compression promotes increased circulation deep in the muscle at the same time that the muscle is broadened and the fibers are separated. When the compression movement is applied with a short transverse motion at the deepest pressure of the compression, it also acts to stretch and broaden the muscle to separate adhesions in the muscle fascia that result from postedemic fibrosis in the muscle fibers and fascicles.

Usually in the process of applying compressions, specific areas of the muscle are identified that contain fibrous bands, knots, or stress points. The stroke can be changed to a cross-fiber movement to tease and separate the muscle fibers. When done correctly, this stroke mashes the tissue and slightly stretches it, causing a broadening of the muscle and a loosening of the binding fascia surrounding the fibers. This stroke also enhances fluid movement at the intercellular level.

The most important goal of compression is to create hyperemia in the muscle tissue. Deep compressions stretch, broaden, and separate muscle fibers and in the process release histamines (**HIS**-tah-meens) and acetylcholine (as-ee-til-**KOH**-leen). This causes the blood vessels throughout the massaged area to dilate and become more permeable, to produce a lasting hyperemia (Figure 18-1a and b).

Deep Pressure

Deep pressure is usually applied with a braced thumb, a braced finger, the forearm, or the elbow. Deep pressure is also referred to as *ischemic compression* or *trigger-point pressure release technique.* The amount of pressure used varies according to the person's pain threshold and the condition of the tissue. Deep pressure is used effectively to treat tender points that might be found in muscle, fascia, tendon, ligaments, joint capsules, or periosteum. If pressure on a point causes pain to radiate or refer to another area, that point is considered to be

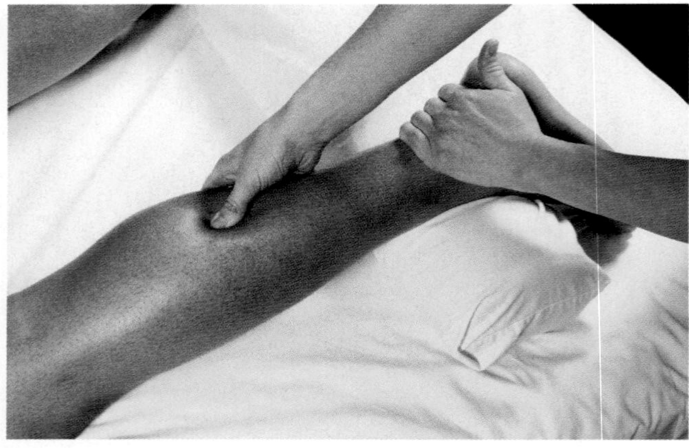
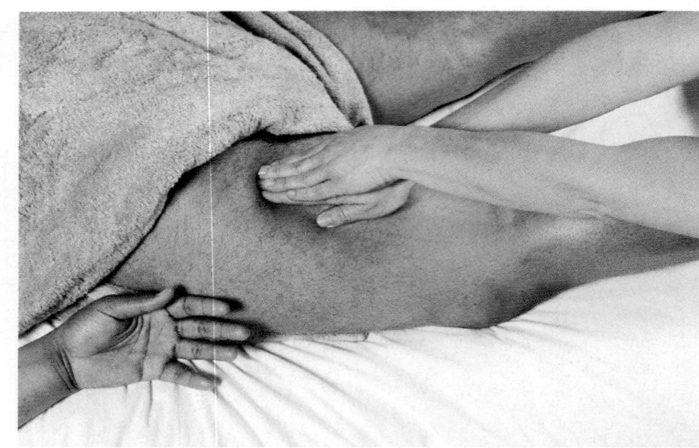
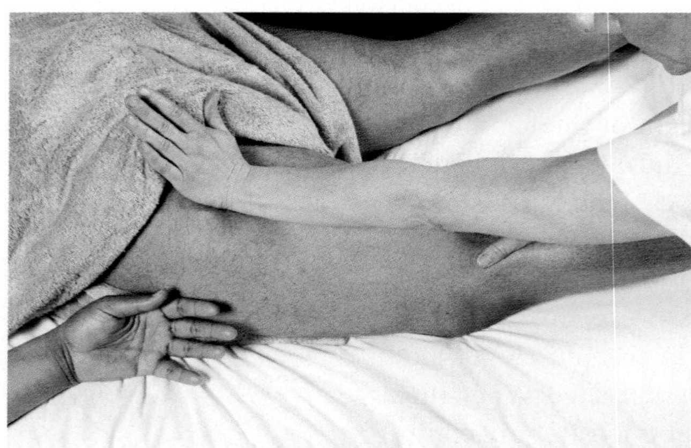
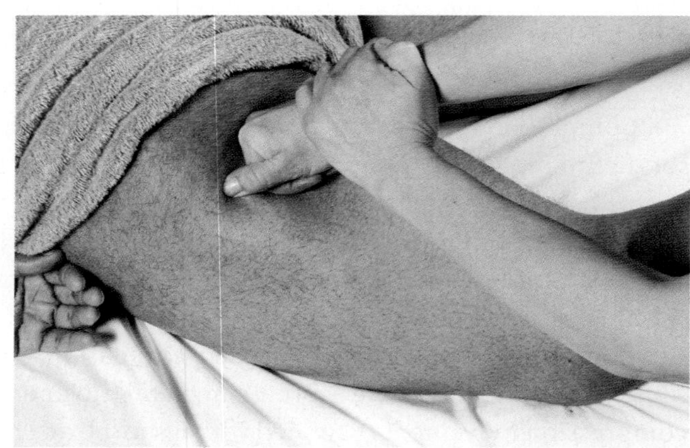
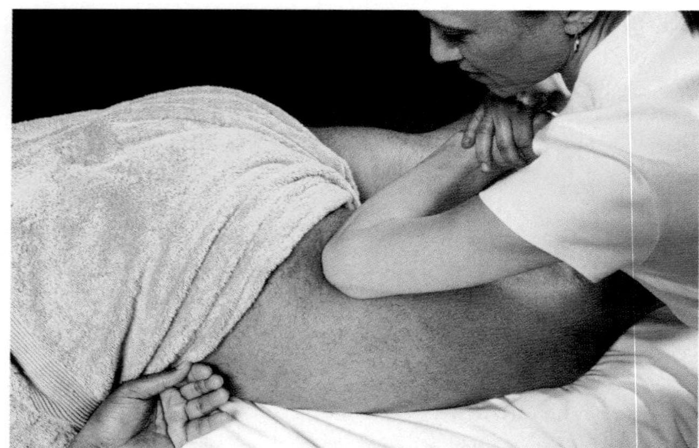

FIGURE 18-2A-E Deep pressure can be applied with the thumb, fingers, hand, or elbow. Pressure should never be so extreme as to injure the client. Proper body mechanics ensure better effects with minimal stress to the therapist.

an active trigger point. Trigger points are found in taut bands of muscle tissue and can be active (i.e., produce and refer pain during daily activities) or latent (i.e., producing pain only when pressure is applied). Pressure is used on trigger points to deactivate them and increase function to the referred area. Left untreated, they can cause restricted and painful movement.

When a trigger point is located, pressure is applied directly into that point. The amount of pressure is determined by the tolerance of the athlete and the condition of the tissue. The pressure must not be so great as to cause the athlete to tense the muscles in a protective response. If the athlete were to rate the intensity of the discomfort on a scale of 1 to 10 (1 being very little discomfort and 10 being excruciating), the discomfort level should be about 5 or 6. After the therapist maintains the same amount of pressure for a short time, the intensity rating will decrease to about 2. This is an indication that the point has been deactivated, and the therapist continues with the treatment by returning the muscle to its normal resting length with gentle stretching

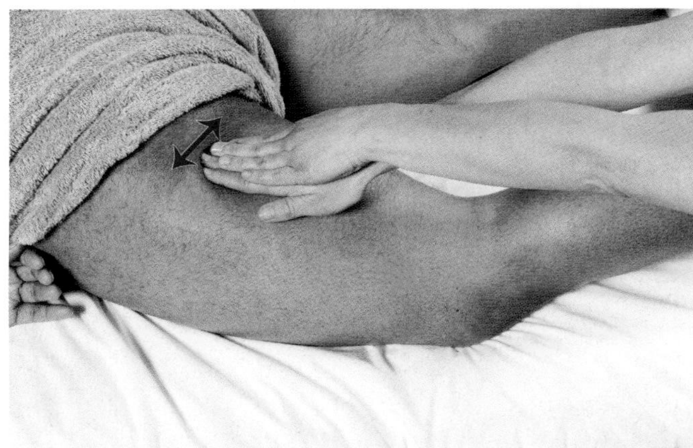

FIGURE 18-3A Cross-fiber or transverse friction is applied to the hamstring attachment on the ischial tuberosity. The stroke must be broad enough to cover the area and deep enough to reach the lesion.

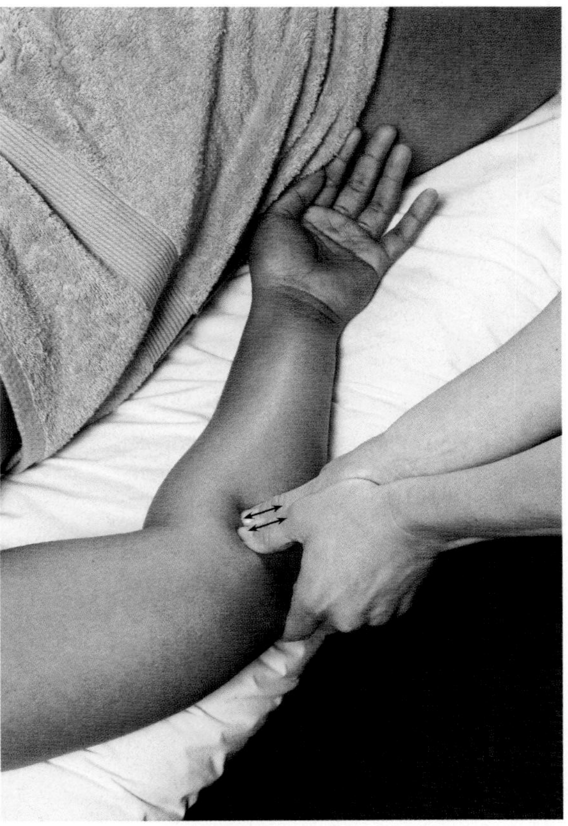

FIGURE 18-3B Cross-fiber friction applied with the thumb on the attachment site of the wrist flexors.

or active joint movements. See Chapter 15 for more information on trigger point release techniques (Figure 18-2a-e).

Transverse or Cross-fiber Friction

Transverse or *cross-fiber friction* is a deep myofascial technique that is applied by rubbing across the fibers of the tendon, muscle, or ligament at a 90-degree angle to the fibers. The use of transverse friction massage for treatment of soft tissue lesions was popularized by the British osteopath Dr. James Cyriax. Cross-fiber friction effectively reduces fibrosis and encourages collagen proliferation to promote the formation of strong, pliable scar tissue at the site of healing injuries. Cross-fiber friction is effective at reducing the fibrosis that forms between tendons and the surrounding paratenon that sometimes accompanies painful tendonosis. Cross-fiber friction can prevent or soften adhesions in fibrous tissue. Cross-fiber massage also promotes collagen production in fibrous tissue.

Cross-fiber massage is used during the subacute and chronic stages of strains, sprains, and contractures, or in any situations in which scar tissue and adhesions are present. Cross-fiber techniques or any other massage techniques that would disturb the fragile healing tissues are contraindicated during the acute stages of healing and inflammation.

Cross-fiber massage is generally applied with braced fingers or the thumb and performed perpendicular to the target fibers. As with other types of friction, the fingers, the skin, and superficial tissues move as a unit against the deeper tissues. The pressure used in cross-fiber friction is deep enough to reach the target tissue but stays within the pain tolerance of the athlete. The stroke must be broad enough to cover the targeted fibrotic tissues without bouncing over or plucking the fibers.

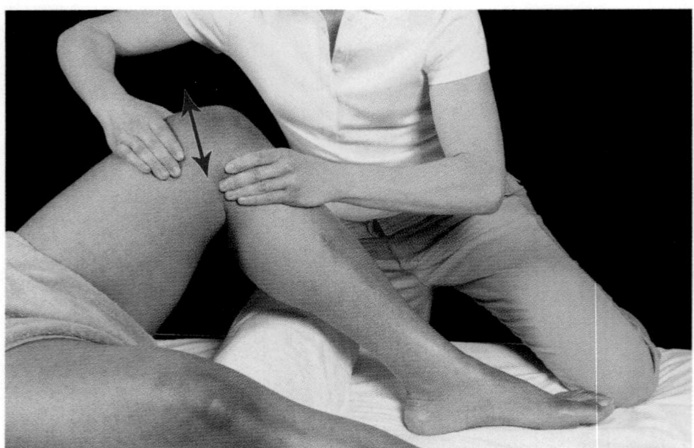

FIGURE 18-4A Shaking the calf and thigh by rapidly moving the bent knee side to side.

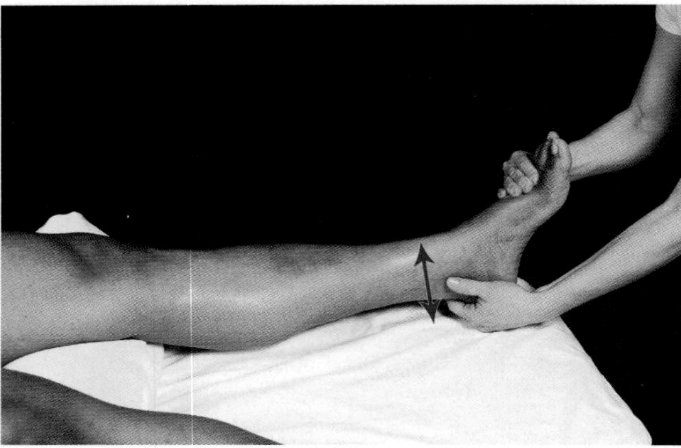

FIGURE 18-4B To shake a leg, grasp the ankle as shown, apply traction, and bounce the entire leg vigorously up and down on the table. Be careful not to hyperextend the knee.

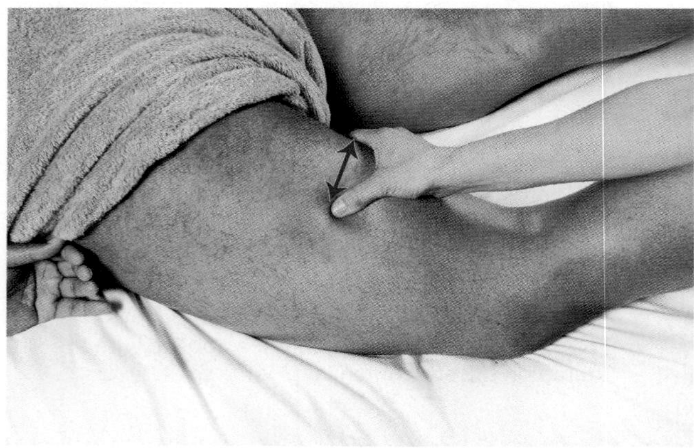

FIGURE 18-4C Jostling the hamstrings. Lightly grasp the muscle and jostle it back and forth.

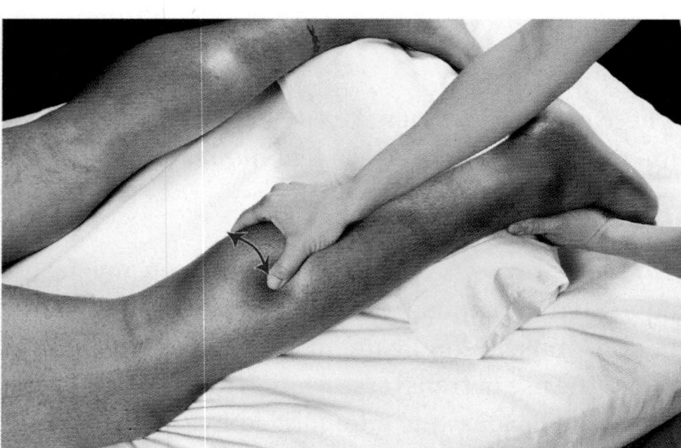

FIGURE 18-4D Jostling the calf muscles.

Broad cross-fiber friction can be performed with the thumb, fingers, heel of the hand, knuckles, or soft fist, and depending on the location, can engage more than one muscle group at a time. It is used to stretch muscles and separate fibers.

Local cross-fiber friction must be applied directly at the site of the lesion, with a goal of creating smooth fibrous tissue (Figure 18-3a and b).

Shaking and Jostling

A good way to relieve the intensity of deep work on the muscle is to shake or jostle the entire muscle mass or limb vigorously. This not only releases the tension that can result from the manipulations but also works to loosen fascia and improve lymph movement.

Shaking is done by grasping the body part and vigorously moving it up and down or back and forth so that the relaxed flesh flops around the bone. For example, with the client in the supine position with the knee bent and the foot flat on the table, grasp the knee and vigorously move it laterally back and forth so that the muscles of the thigh and calf are shaken. Or, grasp the wrist with both hands, apply a slight traction to the arm and vigorously shake the entire arm and shoulder up and down. When shaking a limb, it is important not to hyperextend any joint, especially the elbow or knee.

To jostle a muscle, place the massaging hand across the muscle belly, and then lightly grasp and vigorously move the muscle laterally across the axis.

Shaking and jostling require that the muscle be relaxed as it is moved quickly back and forth (Figure 18-4a-d).

Active Joint Movements

In the early 1950s, Dr. Herman Kabat developed several active movement exercises to be used in the rehabilitation of conditions such as orthopedic disabilities, spinal cord injuries, cerebral palsy, and polio. The exercises used therapist-assisted active and resisted movement in specific patterns. Kabat based the therapy on Sherington's physiologic principles of reciprocal enervation, reciprocal inhibition, postisometric relaxation, and the process of irradiation. Following Kabat's retirement, the development of the technique was continued by physical therapists Margaret Knott and Dorothy E. Voss. In 1954, this therapy system adopted the name Proprioceptive Neuromuscular Facilitation (better known by the acronym PNF). Today, PNF is still a widely used and effective therapy for the rehabilitation of neurologic and soft tissue disorders.

Active stretching movements used in athletic massage borrow from the principles of PNF. A form of active joint movements, originally developed by an osteopathic physician named Dr Fred Mitchell, is called Muscle Energy Technique (MET). MET is based on reciprocal inhibition and postisometric relaxation. (MET is discussed in more detail in Chapter 15.) MET helps to counteract muscle spasm, improve flexibility, and restore muscle strength. MET is performed by moving a body part involving the affected muscle into an extended or stretched position to a point of pain or discomfort, then moving it back out of that position to a point at which there is no discomfort. The therapist then supports the body part in this position while the client contracts the agonist or antagonist muscle for 5 to 30 seconds and then relaxes. The therapist then moves the athlete's limb toward the barrier just to the point of discomfort and backs off slightly. The process is then repeated several times as the range of motion (ROM) of the affected muscle or articulation increases until flexibility is restored and spasm reduced.

Caution: The extent of these techniques is regulated by the level of pain experienced by the client. If any movement causes the client to tense due to pain, that movement is contraindicated.

APPLICATIONS FOR ATHLETIC MASSAGE

There are three basic applications for athletic massage. Each has a different goal and requires a different approach. The basic applications are:

1. Event massage – massage that is delivered at the site of the athletic event and designed to help athletes either to prepare for or recover from participation in the event. There are three applications of event massage.

   a. Pre-event massage – massage prior to an event to prepare the athlete for the exertion of all-out competition.
   b. Intra-event massage – massage between events to assist athlete in recovering from one athletic activity and preparing for an upcoming event.
   c. Post-event massage – massage after an event to normalize the tissues and relax the athlete after competition.
2. Restorative or training massage – massage during training to allow the athlete to train harder with fewer injuries.
3. Rehabilitation massage – massage during rehabilitation to recover from injury more quickly with less chance of reinjury.

Pre-event Massage

Pre-event massage, given 15 minutes to 2 hours prior to an event, prepares the body for intense activity. The massage is short (10 to 30 minutes), stimulating, and directed toward the parts of the body that will be involved in the exertion. The main goal of the pre-event massage is to increase circulation and flexibility in the areas of the body about to be used. This is a time to decrease muscle tension and to soften and loosen fascia and connective tissue to increase ROM and power. Pre-event massage is fast paced and invigorating. Except for athletes who are extremely hyperactive, or with some adaptive sports athletes, this is not the time for relaxing movements. Pre-event massage warms and loosens the muscles, causing increased blood supply (hyperemia) in the muscle groups specific to the athletic event. This enables the athlete to reach peak performance earlier in the event and maintain that performance longer. Increased flexibility allows the athlete more power, speed, and endurance, with less possibility of injury.

Pre-event massage is not a replacement for proper warm-up before a performance but is an adjunct to it and an aid in preparing the athlete for the all-out competition. Ideally, pre-event massage is given near the end of the athlete's warm-up routine. This is not a good time for the athlete to receive his first massage, because the effects of the massage could adversely affect an athlete's timing and performance. Pre-event massage is not the time to work too deeply, break down adhesions, or work on muscle spasms.

Pre-event massage uses no lubricant and is usually given through the clothing. Specific techniques are compression, light cross-fiber friction, shaking, jostling, rolling, kneading, ROM, and stretching.

Intra-Event Massage

Intra-event athletic massage is provided at sporting events where the athlete can participate in multiple events on the same day with periods of rest or "down time" in between, such as tennis or gymnastic tournaments, or swimming or track meets.

The main goals of intra-event massage is to encourage a quick recovery from the previous activity, address any areas of tension or concern that might have developed during the activity and help the tissues to prepare for the upcoming event. The athlete can usually direct the therapist to any areas of concern.

The therapist can quickly assess the tissues with effleurage and petrissage, quiet any tension or spasm, and enhance circulation to and from the area. Position release and METs are valuable tools to quiet hypertonicity. Intra-event massage is generally shorter that pre- or post-event massage, usually no more that 10 to 15 minutes in duration. It is intended to augment the athlete's regular intra-event routine and not replace it. As with the pre-event massage, the intra-event massage is fast paced and intended to avoid sedating the athlete.

Post-Event Massage

Post-event massage is given within the first hour or two after participation in an event and can be 15 to 30 minutes in length. The goal of post-event massage is to increase circulation, clear out metabolic wastes, reduce muscle tension and spasms, and quiet the nervous system. The focus is on the large muscle groups and tissues that were stressed during the activity. These techniques enhance the movement of blood and lymph out of the most intensely worked muscles and back toward the heart and center of the body. Lactic and pyruvic acids formed as a result of oxygen depletion are flushed from the muscles. This prevents delayed onset muscle soreness and reduces the time that it takes the body to recover from exertion.

Post-event massage is given after the athlete has had a chance to cool down from the exertion of the competition or exercise. The post-event massage is performed at a slower pace and should increase circulation while calming the nervous system. It is a relaxing massage that reduces the physical and mental intensity of competition.

The most effective techniques for post-event massage are light and deep effleurage, petrissage, kneading, compression, jostling, generalized friction movements, and light stretching. All movements are aimed at "flushing out" the areas of the body that have been used during the event. The general massage rule of working from general to specific and back to general, and from superficial to deep and back to superficial, is observed.

Many serious athletes or teams have a massage therapist on staff to provide pre- and post-event massage. Often, sports massage therapists are available at the site of a competition. It is common for massage areas to be set up at major athletic events such as running, cycling, swimming, and skiing competitions, as well as the Olympic and Paralympic Games.

After an exhaustive competition, the athlete cools down, replenishes fluids, and seeks out the massage area. The first step of the post-event massage is to conduct a short interview to assess the athlete's post-race condition. The therapist should be aware of signs of hypo- or hyperthermia, cramps, spasms, or muscle strain. Questions that the therapist might ask of the athlete include:

- How do you feel?
- Have you had any water or fluids since the competition?
- Have you completed your cool-down practices?
- Do you have any problems or discomfort?
- How long ago did you finish your event?
- How did you perform in the competition?
- Did you have any problems during the race?
- Are there any areas on your body that you want me to concentrate on?
- As I work on you, let me know if what I do is uncomfortable.

It is advisable to observe the athlete closely during the interview for signs of exhaustion or depression. Have the athlete sit on the table and remove his shoes during the conversational interview. Be aware of any blisters, abrasions, contusions, spasms, or strains, and apply appropriate first aid or obtain the assistance of the attending medical personnel. It is a good idea to continue light conversation throughout the post-event massage.

The post-event massage concentrates on the muscle groups used during the exercise and the athlete's areas of concern. If time allows, include the rest of the body to enhance relaxation. The massage can be performed without lubricant and through the sports clothing if given on site or can include the use of some lubricant on the bare skin if private facilities are available.

The general procedure for each involved body area would include the following:

- Long effleurage strokes and kneading to flush out the area
- Light compressions to the entire area
- Jostling and traction shaking of the limb
- Range of motion and light stretching
- Repeat effleurage strokes
- Feather, nerve strokes from proximal to distal aspect of the area being massaged.

General Procedure for Pre- or Post-Event Massage

At a sporting event where pre- and post-event massage is given, it is wise to have a general routine prepared that you can then adapt to the sport and to any injuries or complications that an athlete has incurred. As you use these routines more, you will begin to find a pattern that is comfortable for you. More event experience will lead to a feel for which techniques are best for the athlete and when certain ones are not beneficial.

The following is a general event sports massage routine that can be used if you join a state sport massage team or are accepted as a team member to provide massage at a national or international event (e.g., Olympics/Paralympics or World Games). The sidebars list ideas for stretches as well as sports-specific common problems.

As you escort the athlete to the table, introduce yourself and conduct an interview. The following are sample questions and why they are important; they give some idea of the athlete's overall attitude, frame of mind, level of concentration, and focus. A triage person at the registration table can ask these questions also.

Pre-Event

- When and what is your event?
  Determines speed necessary and amount of time available for your session; enables your massage to be sports specific to the athlete's needs.
- Where are you in your in your warm-up routine?
  Helps to determine which techniques to use and how prepared the athlete is for the event.
- How did your training go? Are you feeling prepared?

Determines their frame of mind – whether the athlete is disappointed, ready, anxious, nervous, calm, focused, eager, or similar moods.

- Did you incorporate massage during your training?
  If yes and regularly – once a week, twice a month – the athlete can tell you what works for him, the pressure and techniques he is used to, and other personal preferences. If no, you know not to do deep or trigger-point work, which could affect his performance.
- Do you have any chronic or acute injuries?
  Makes you aware of sensitive areas and any specific work or treatments the athlete has received.
- What do you want me to focus on?
  Remember, the person on the table is the one living in his body – he might want you to focus on legs if he is running, or upper body if he is swimming — or relaxing if he is anxious. Listening is a key component when working with athletes.
- Let me know if my pressure is too deep or light or if something hurts.
  Initiates good communication and rapport.

Post-Event

- How long has it been since you finished your event?
  Gives you an idea whether the athlete has allowed himself time to cool down (physically and mentally).
- How are you feeling? Hot, warm, cold?
  Alerts the therapist to any conditions such as hyper- or hypothermia, heat exhaustion, spasms, or trauma that might require medical attention.
- Have you had something to eat or drink?
  Lets you know whether the athlete has replenished his body with nutrients and fluids.
- Have you cooled down, stretched, walked around?
  It is important to do this before massage; it allows the recovery process to begin.
- How do you feel about your performance?
  Determines the athlete's state of mind – disappointment, excitement, determination to continue to the next level, and ideas on what he needs to improve on.
- Did you have any problems (e.g., falls, cramping, injuries) during the event? If so, have you been to first aid/medical? How are you feeling now?
  Helps you to focus on problem areas immediately or determine whether the athlete needs to be referred to a medical professional.
- Where do you need work done? Where would you like me to focus?
  Allows you to meet the athlete's needs to help him to recover more quickly or address a weak or injured area, or complement his cool-down/recovery/relaxation process.
- Let me know when my pressure is too deep or light or if something hurts.
  Stresses communication and rapport.

Remember that pre-event massage should be done at a faster pace (with some exceptions) than post-event massage. Generally, in pre-event massage,

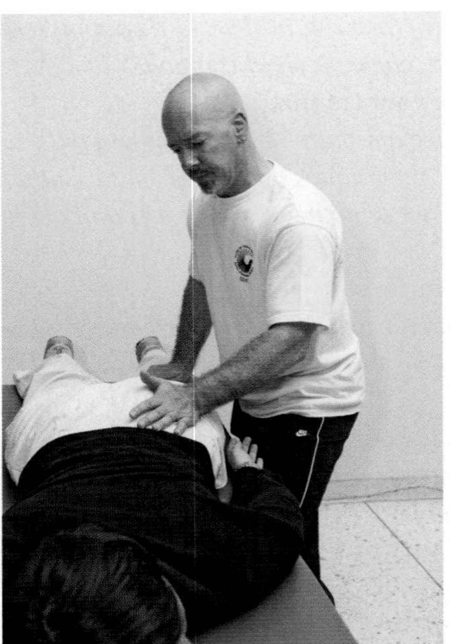

FIGURE 18-5 Begin with compressions to the gluteals and continue with rhythmic compression strokes all the way up the back.

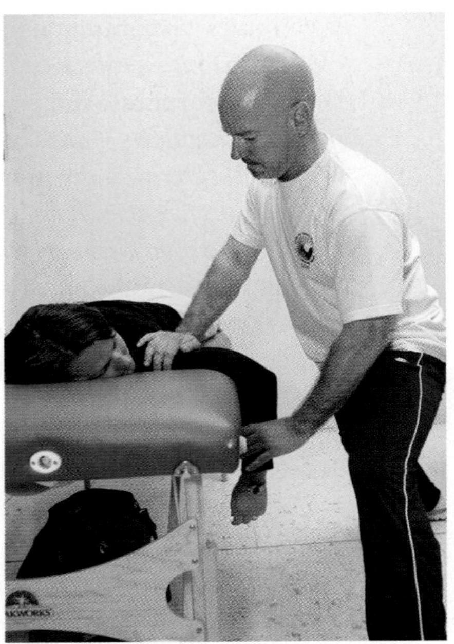

FIGURE 18-6 Apply compression and petrissage from the shoulder to the wrist.

conclude each area with tapotement and in post-event massage, conclude each area with effleurage and nerve strokes.

Have the athlete lie on the table (either supine or prone is fine to start). Make sure to use a bolster under the knees when supine to reduce strain on the low back, and under the ankles when prone (or have the feet hanging off the edge of the table) to reduce cramping in the calves. You may help him remove his shoes (if post-event, look for blisters he may not know about).

Prone – Back/Upper Body

- Begin with gentle rocking, starting with the back and then going down each leg. Use this time to assess the body, noting any tense or sensitive areas.
- Apply compressions on the gluteals, move up the erectors to the trapezius, rhomboids, and scapulas; continue the rocking motion (Figure 18-5).
- Apply petrissage to the same areas, paying attention to any areas of tension.
- On the next pass, apply circular friction to this same area using the heel of your hand or fingertips.
- Apply direct pressure to stress points, paying attention to the athlete's response.
- Apply petrissage and circular friction with the thumbs and fingers from the base of the neck to the occiput; then gently squeeze the neck.
- After compressions into the belly of the upper trapezius, a general kneading can be done.
- Apply compressions to the deltoids down through the triceps.

Scapula Release

Bring the arm above the head, apply traction for two to three seconds. Return the arm to the side of the body, and then place the athlete's hand on the low back (check for any shoulder injuries first, then the comfort level of this position). Place your bottom hand under the shoulder, top hand on the scapular with fingers wrapped around the medial board of the scapula, and apply a gentle traction (see Figure 18-7a-c).

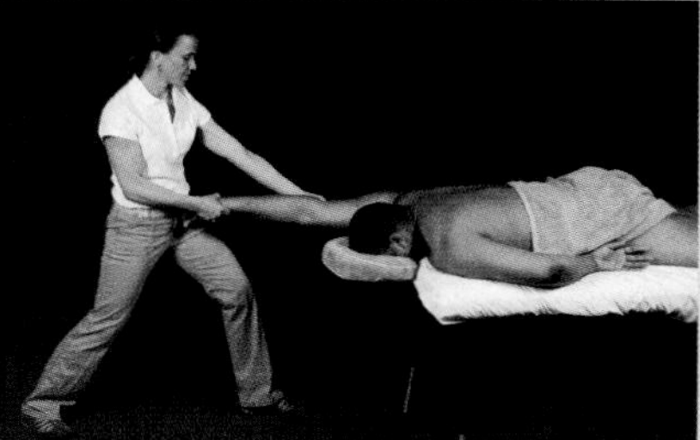

FIGURE 18-7A Bring the arm above the head, and apply traction for 2 to 3 seconds.

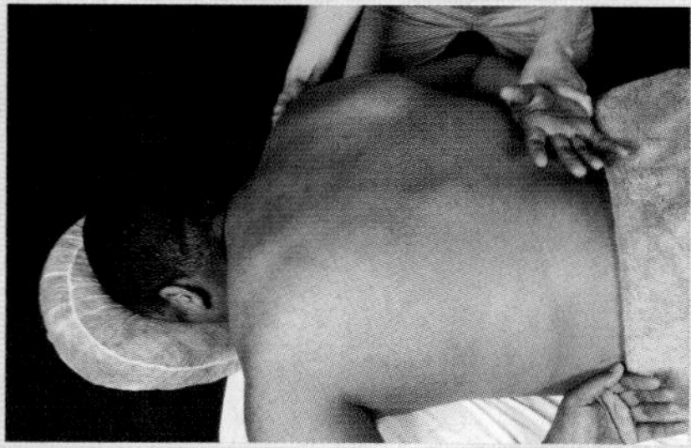

FIGURE 18-7B Return the arm to the side of the body, and then place the hand on the low back. Check for any shoulder injuries first; then check the comfort level of this position.

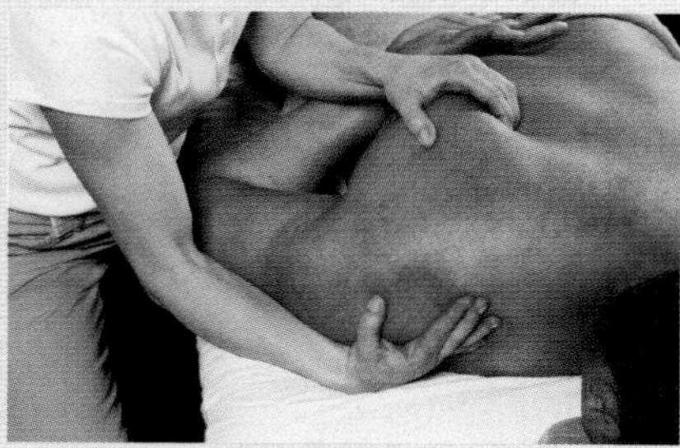

FIGURE 18-7C Place your bottom hand under the shoulder, top hand on the scapula with fingers wrapped around the medial border of the scapula, and apply a gentle traction.

- Let the arm hang off the side of the table. Grab it around the biceps/triceps with both hands and jostle. Return the arm to the table (see scapula release sidebar for stretch).
- Apply compression, petrissage, and friction to the forearm and palm of the hand (Figure 18-6).
- Light tapotement can be used for pre-event massage. Finish with long effleurage strokes during post-event massage.

Repeat the routine on the other side of the body.

Prone – Lower Body

- Bend the knee to 90 degrees, grasp the ankle with both hands, and lift the leg slightly off the table allowing the leg to abduct slightly; gently shake the leg. Extend the leg, returning the foot to the bolster.
- Apply compressions (Figure 18-8) on the gluteals and hamstrings (two to three passes).
- Jostle and then petrissage the hamstring.
- Spread hamstring muscles (see the accompanying Spreading the Hamstring sidebar and Figure 18-9 a and b for a description of this).
- Apply petrissage and compressions on the gastrocnemius.
- Grasp and lift the gastrocnemius with gentle shaking.
- Bend the knee to 90 degrees; use a wringing motion on the gastrocnemius from the knee to the Achilles tendon.
- Lift and shake the leg (as in Step 1).

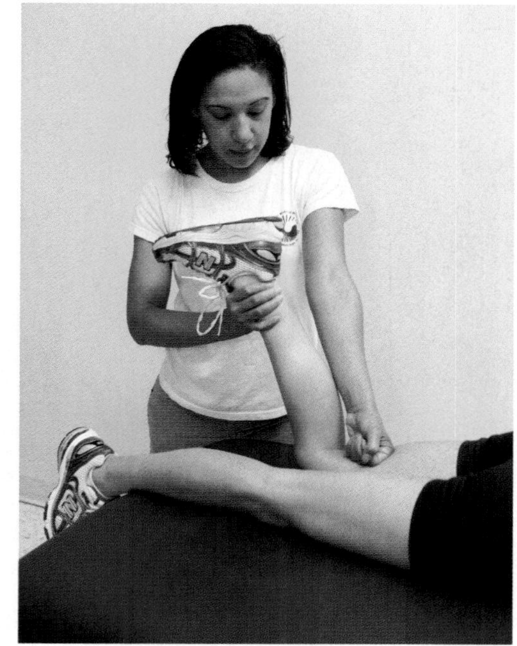

FIGURE 18-8 Compressions and petrissage increase circulation and warm the posterior thigh.

Spreading the Hamstring

With fists together on the hamstring, apply pressure and then slowly bring the fists apart, spreading the fibers apart (Figure 18-9a and b).

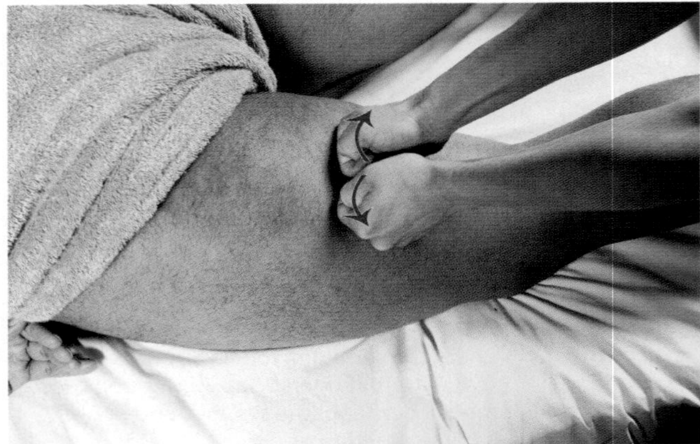

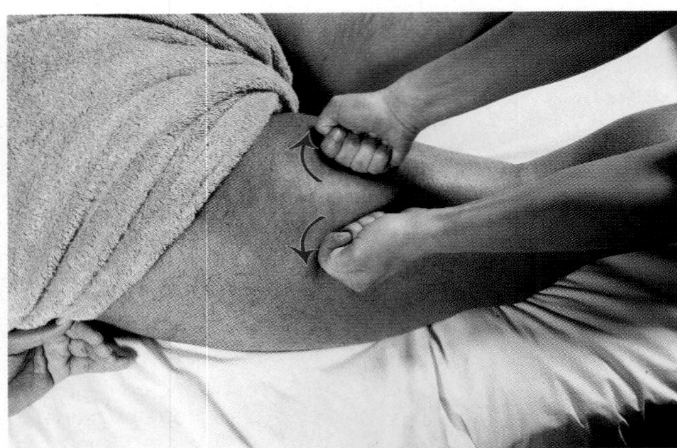

FIGURE 18-9A, B Spreading the hamstrings: with fists together on the hamstring, apply pressure, and then slowly bring the fists apart, spreading the fibers.

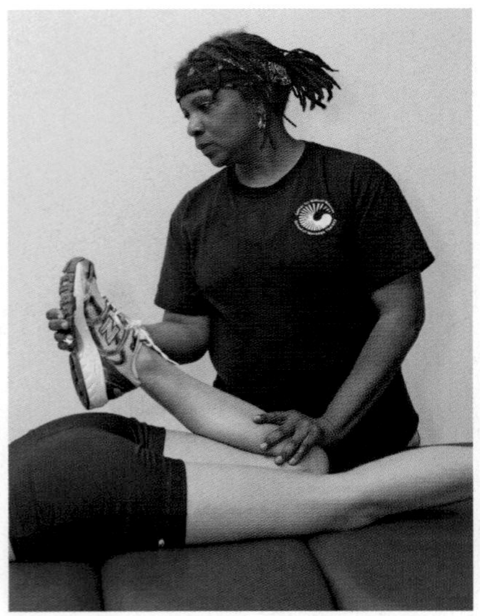

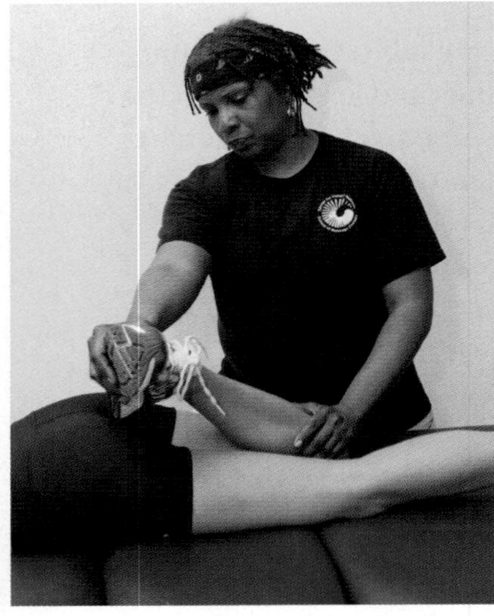

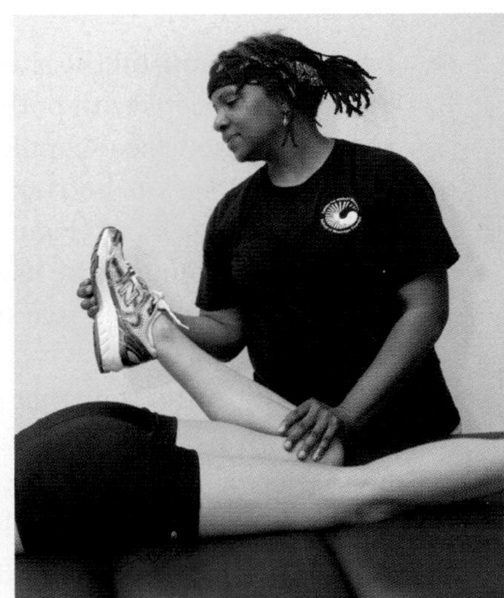

FIGURE 18-10A-C Move the athlete's heel toward the buttocks to stretch the quadriceps.

- Quadriceps stretch (Figure 18-10a-c): Heel toward buttocks to athlete's tolerance. Hold for two to three seconds, release, and repeat several times.
- External and internal hip rotation: With one hand on the buttocks, use the other hand on the ankle to rotate the leg externally, then internally for gluteal and piriformis stretch.
- With the knee still at 90 degrees, rotate the ankle clockwise and counterclockwise, then dorsiflex the ankle to stretch the gastrocnemius. Return the leg to extension.

- Foot (optional at events): Using fist, knuckles, or thumbs, apply compressions to the sole of the foot, then circular friction. You can end with tapotement (be aware of blisters or injury, especially post-event).
- Pre-event massage – complete with tapotement to the back of the leg and gluteals. Post-event – finish with long effleurage to the back of the legs.
- Repeat on the other leg.

Before asking the athlete to turn over, do some gentle rocking of the whole body to bring it together.

Supine – Lower Body

Quadriceps

- Standing at the end of the table, cup both ankles/heels in your hands and apply traction for a few seconds. Release and rock the legs. Repeat traction and rocking again.
- Apply compressions to the upper leg, proximal to distal, covering all quadriceps muscles (Figure 18-11).

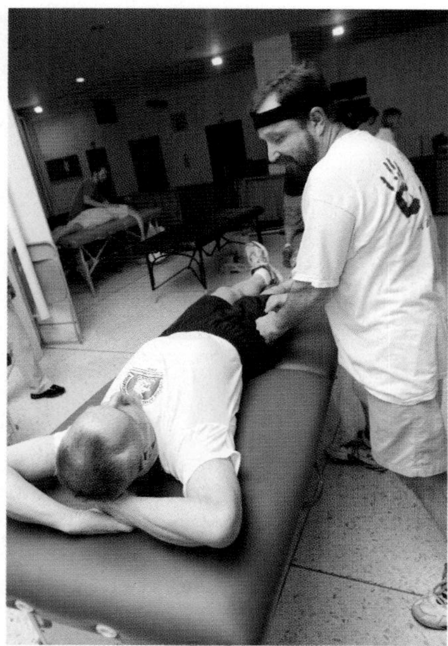

FIGURE 18-11 Compressions to the anterior thigh increase circulation.

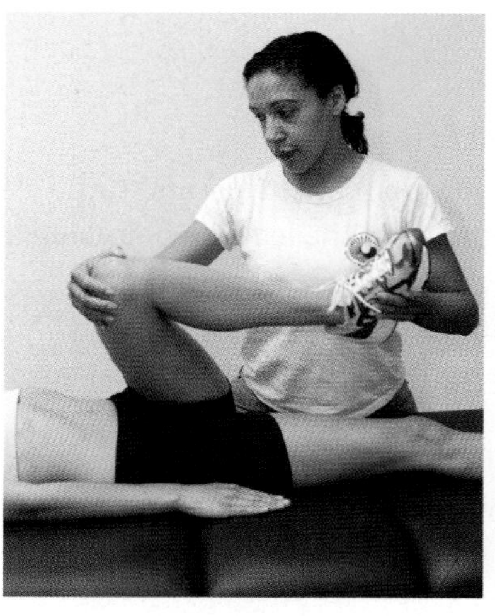

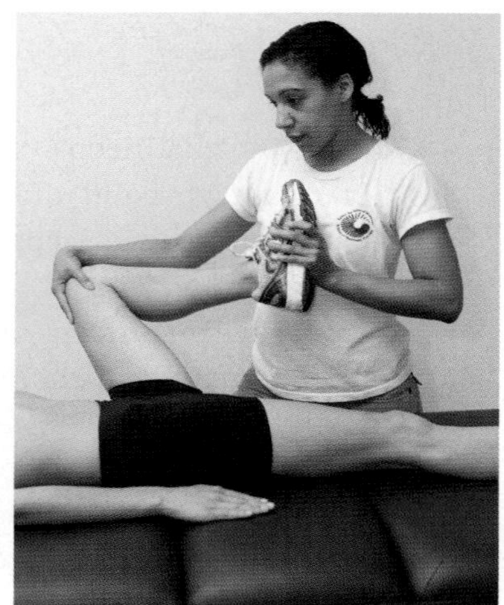

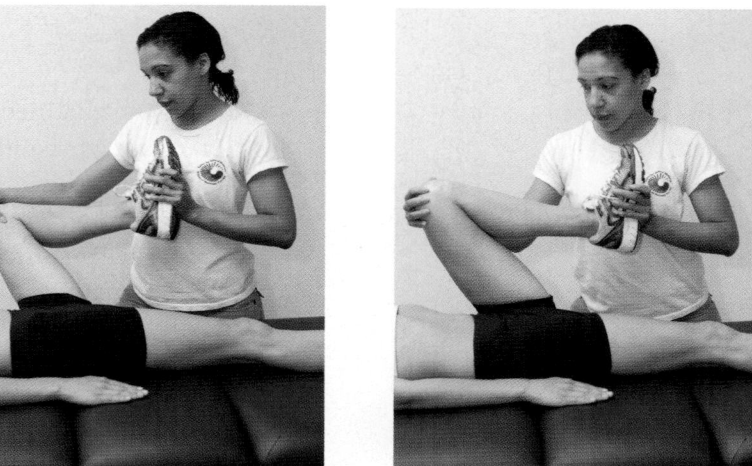

FIGURE 18-12A-C ROM of the hips helps to stretch and relax the athlete.

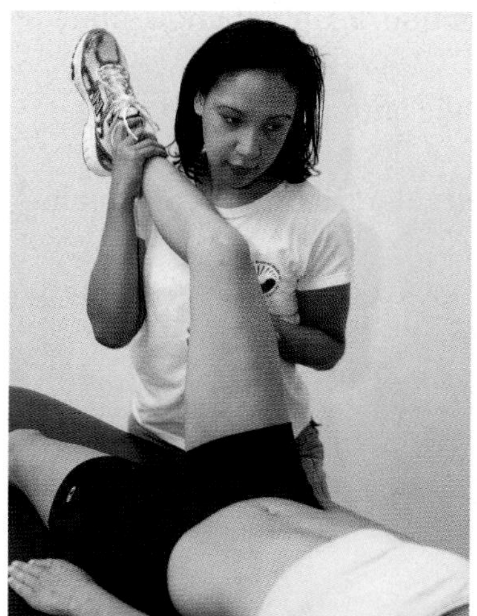

FIGURE 18-13 Flex the hip and extend the knee to stretch the hamstrings gently.

Quadriceps Stretch

Have the athlete lie on his side, keeping the spine straight. The lower leg should be bent at the knee and hip (knee to chest). The upper leg (parallel to the table at all times) should be bent at the knee, with the athlete's upper hand holding it at the ankle (a towel can be wrapped around the ankle if he cannot grab it). The hamstring should first engage to extend the leg, and then the athlete (or therapist, if assisting) should pull on the ankle to get a little more stretch in the quadriceps. Hold for two seconds, release to starting position, and repeat five or more times. The body should be in alignment at all times, not rolling back when the quad is in full stretch. The stretch should be felt at the top of the quadriceps (Figure 18-14 a and b).

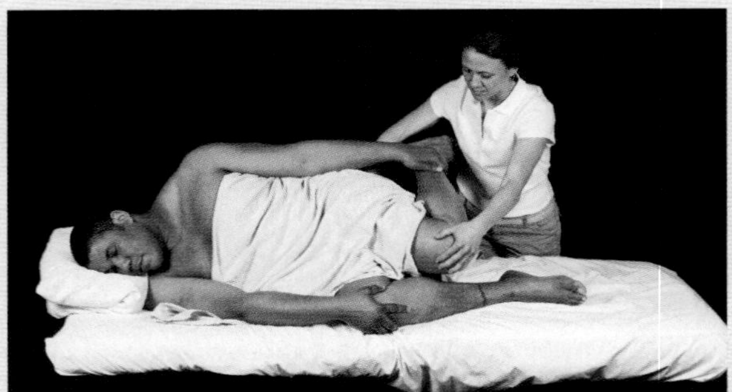

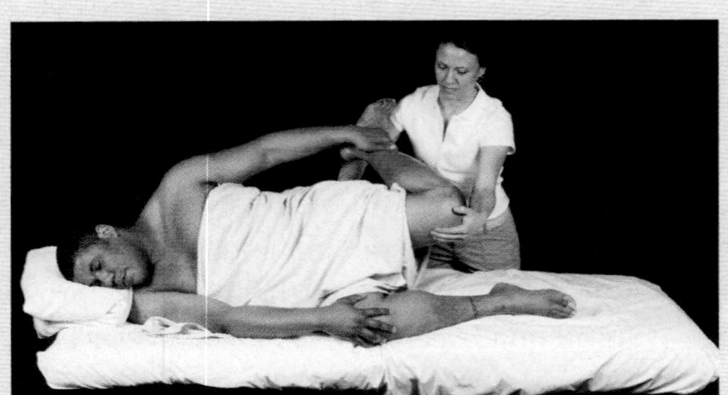

FIGURE 18-14A, B Quadriceps stretch.

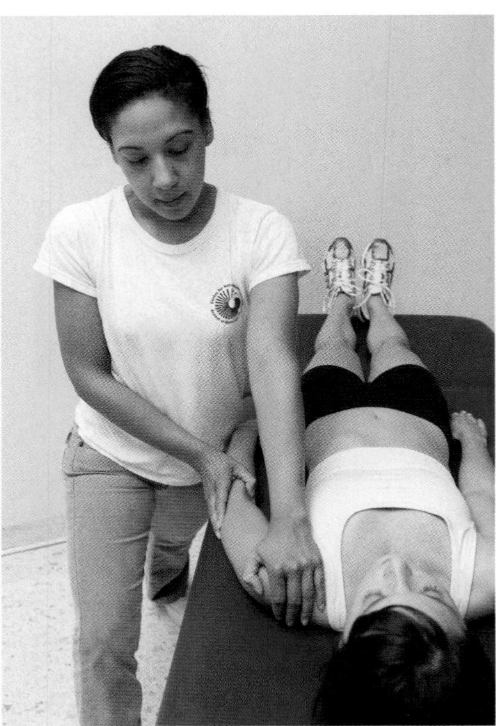

FIGURE 18-15 Apply compression strokes to the pectoralis, deltoids, and biceps.

- Jostle the quadriceps.
- Place outside hand under the leg (on hamstring) and top hand on the quadriceps. Lift and drop the leg, like bouncing a basketball.
- Petrissage quadriceps and adductors.
- Apply spreading technique as done on the hamstring.
- Jostle.
- Bend the knee to 90 degrees, flex at the hip to 90 degrees; take the knee to the chest and do ROM for the hip (Figure 18-12a-c). Extend the leg back to the table.

Knee and Lower Leg

- With opposing thumbs, effleurage around the patella OR use cross-fiber friction on patella tendon/ligament above and below patella.
- Apply compressions on the tibialis anterior and peroneus muscles.
- With thumbs or fingers, apply circular friction to the tibialis anterior.
- Dorsiflex the foot to stretch the gastrocnemius and soleus.
- Traction and shake the leg again.
- Pre-event – apply percussion to thigh. Post-event – apply effleurage to front of leg.
- Repeat on the other leg.

Upper Body

Chest and Arms

- Hold the hand and laterally raise the arm to the side of the table (shoulder height). With flexed elbow, shake the arm. Return it to the table.
- Apply compressions to the pectoralis, deltoids, biceps, and forearm (Figure 18-15).
- Petrissage the deltoids, biceps, and forearm.
- Use the tips of fingers to apply friction to the palm of the hand and around the wrists.
- Apply long effleurage strokes up the arm.
- Do ROM for the shoulder.
- End by shaking the arm.

Shoulders, Neck, and Head

- Stand or sit at the head of the table and apply petrissage and friction to the upper trapezius muscles of the shoulders and up the neck.
- Do gentle stretching of the neck (flex right and left, lift chin to chest).
- With your fingertips, apply circular friction to the scalp.
- To end, place your hands on the shoulders and apply pressure (pressing the shoulders down toward the feet).
- End with nerve strokes or gentle rocking.

Massage during Training

Training massage – also called *restorative, preventive*, and *maintenance massage* – is the most beneficial form of massage for the athlete. It is considered a regular and valuable part of the training regime and allows the athlete to train at a higher level of intensity, more consistently, with less chance of injury. Training massage increases blood and lymph circulation, which allows more efficient oxygen and nutrient supply to the cells as well as more efficient removal of metabolic waste. It helps to identify and address areas of tenderness and restriction. All of these benefits make more intense and frequent workouts possible, thereby improving overall performance. The initial strokes used during regular training sessions to warm up the tissue and increase circulation provides an opportunity to find stressed areas that might require specific attention. Contractures and constricted muscle tissue containing trigger points can be released. Massage reduces minor cross-fiber adhesions resulting from microtrauma, thereby increasing muscle response and flexibility. Massage also alleviates muscle-boundness (by breaking down muscle bundles) so that muscle contractions and relaxation are more efficient, allowing finer-tuned muscle response.

Another benefit of restorative massage is the breaking down of transverse adhesions that might be the result of previous injuries. This promotes muscle power, better circulation, less chance of reinjury, increased mobility, increased flexibility, and better performance. The athlete can achieve maximum effort sooner, more often, and maintain it longer with fewer, if any, ill effects.

The massage process systematically involves every part of the athlete's body, concentrating on those muscle groups and body parts specifically involved in the sport and including other areas that are indirectly involved. Training massage maintains muscles in the best possible state of nutrition, flexibility, and vitality.

Restorative Massage Techniques

Techniques of restorative massage vary according to specific application. The primary techniques in this aspect of athletic massage include all of the techniques of pre- and post-event massage, plus neuromuscular and myofascial techniques such as deep cross-fiber friction, trigger-point therapy, and active joint stretches to reduce soft tissue lesions and constrictions. Effleurage and petrissage are also used, but to a lesser degree. There are several therapist-assisted joint movements that are very effective in this stage of massage. They include MET, position release, and passive and active joint movements. (See Chapter 15 for more details about these techniques.)

Regular restorative massage sessions help to increase flexibility and ROM, which translates into increased power and better performance. Restorative massage provides the opportunity to locate and deactivate trigger points and stress points before they become problems.

There is no standard or set procedure for athletic massage owing to the variety of sports situations to which this technique is applicable. There is a process to follow in choosing an effective treatment plan, however. When interviewing the client, you should find out the following:

- The sport or sports in which the athlete is involved
- The location and extent of present areas of concern
- The location and extent of previous injuries and surgeries
- The workout schedule and upcoming competitions
- The extent to which the athletic massage is to be incorporated in the athlete's training

By learning the client's regular sports, the practitioner can give special consideration to related muscle areas. Trouble areas can point to particular muscle groups on which to concentrate.

Being aware of previous injuries can also target trouble areas. Often an injury occurs as a result of a muscle's not being flexible enough or being unable to let go. Trouble areas also indicate fascia that could be stuck or bound together. Injuries, especially when muscle spasm or tears exist, also point to synergistic, opposing, or compensating muscles as being primary or potential problems.

Workout schedules indicate how serious a person is about a particular sport and can also reveal injury-prone "weekend warriors." How much or how often the athlete wants to include massage in his training program helps the practitioner to determine the frequency and intensity of treatments. If the plan is to include only one or two sessions, the massage should be limited; however, if several regular sessions are planned, a thorough preliminary massage can be given. Work can then be done systematically on trouble areas or areas that receive continuous and intense use.

Goals for restorative massage vary according to the needs of the athlete but can include:

- Identifying and releasing hypertonic/spasmed muscle
- Identifying and releasing fascial constrictions caused by repetitive stress or previous injuries
- Enhancing or restoring flexibility or ROM

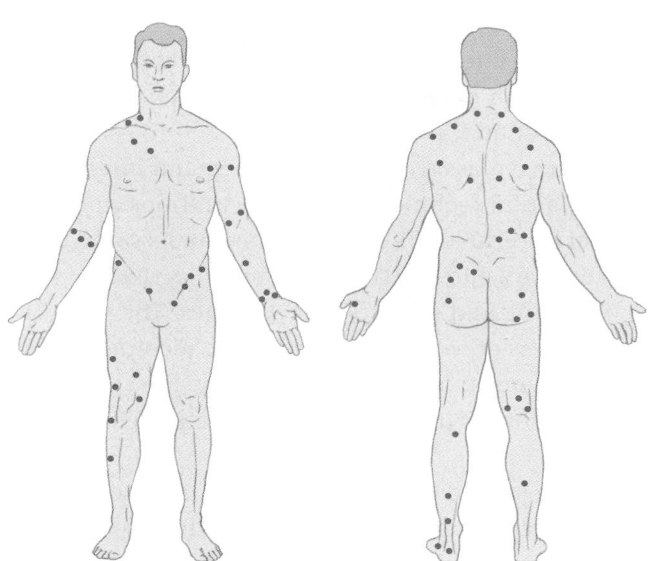

FIGURE 18-16 Major tender points of the body: (a) anterior and (b) posterior views.

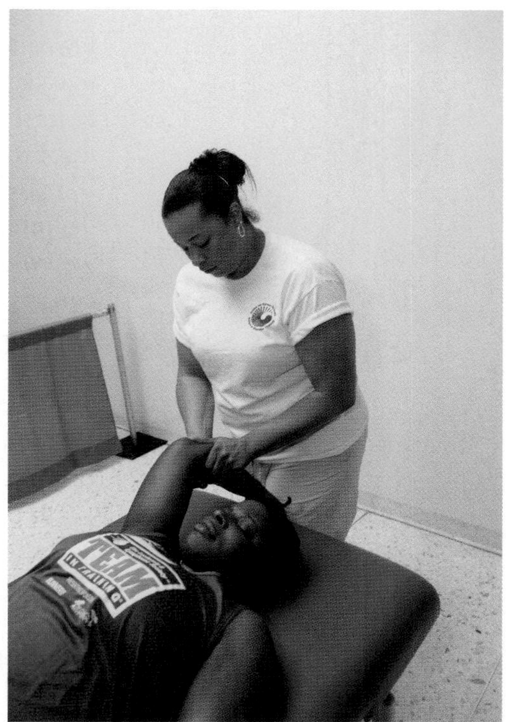

FIGURE 18-17A Cross-fiber friction on stress points helps to reduce adhesions and fibrosis.

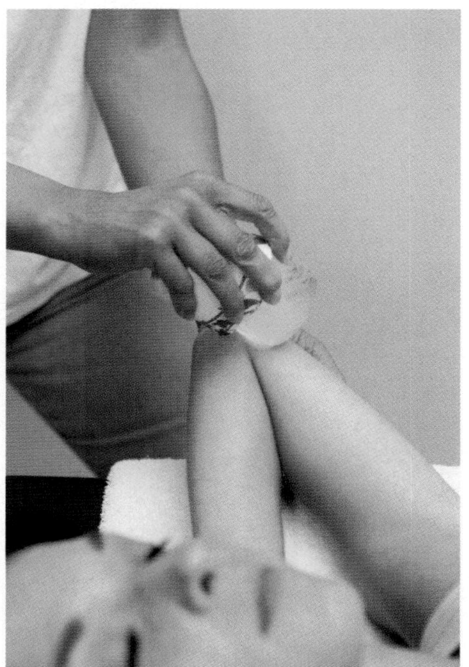

FIGURE 18-17B Following cross-fiber friction with ice massage helps to reduce or prevent local inflammation.

Restorative massage sessions are generally done in a clinical setting where the athlete disrobes and is draped as in a Swedish massage. Sessions are 30 to 90 minutes long and can be whole body or site specific. The first massage is primarily a hunt-and-search process using petrissage, compression, and deep stroking to seek out muscle bundles, spasms, and tender points as well as constrictions and areas of fibrosis. To the client, such trouble areas are generally painful when palpated.

Muscles often contain tender points that are located either in taut bands in the muscle body (trigger points) or where the muscle ends and joins the tendon or tendon sheath (stress points). The musculotendinous junction is where fascia and connective tissues are more prevalent. Because many muscle fibers terminate here, the area is vulnerable to strain, microtrauma, and the subsequent development of adhesions and fibrosis that become tender stress points. This is also where the ratio of blood vessels to tissue is less, and therefore where fatigue occurs first. Often when a muscle is headed for trouble, the first indication appears in these areas (Figure 18-16).

Deep pressure on tender points gives the first clue to future problems. Early treatment of the muscles associated with the tender points can stop an injury long before it begins to affect the athlete's performance adversely. Once the trouble areas have been identified, the procedure for working on them is to deactivate the trigger point and reduce the fibrosis and adhesions at the attachment stress points. Trigger points are located in taut bands of muscle and are treated with trigger-point pressure release or position release techniques, followed by METs to help to return the muscle to its normal resting length. Stress points at attachment sites are treated by compression and site-specific cross-fiber friction to reduce adhesions and

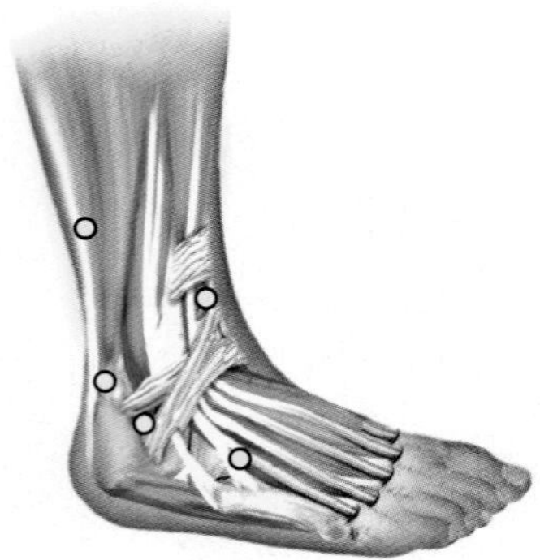

FIGURE 18-18 Common stress points of the foot and ankle.

fibrosis (Figure 18-17a). Extensive cross-fiber friction can be followed by ice massage (Figure 18-17b) to aid in reducing or preventing local inflammation. Fascial restrictions are addressed with myofascial techniques such as skin rolling, broad plane releases, stretches, and traction.

Some applications of restorative massage tend to be deep and intense, but deep techniques do not mean painful techniques. All interventions must stay well within the pain tolerance of the athlete. The athlete must understand that a certain amount of discomfort can be a part of a treatment and be willing to work with the therapist on deep breathing and relaxation techniques. The practitioner must not persist if in the process of working the muscle it becomes tighter. This could cause the condition to worsen or cause actual injury. The athlete and practitioner should work together for the improvement of the athlete's ability to train and condition his body.

If the restorative massage is deep and intense, it is like an intense workout and should be done on days when training is light or on days the athlete is not training. Intense restorative massage should not be given just before a competition. Allow at least a couple of practice days between a restorative massage and an event so that the athlete can adapt to changes in strength, speed, and timing.

General Problem Areas and Suggested Massage

The following are common trigger points and potential stress points that can be addressed during restorative massage.

The Foot and Ankle

The heels absorb a great deal of shock in sports such as jogging and running, and muscles can become painful to pressure (Figure 18-18).

Athletic Foot Massage: To apply general massage to the foot, have the athlete lie face down with feet over the edge of the table. (You can sit on a stool if you are more comfortable.) Use your thumbs to apply deep friction to the bottom of the foot. Apply cross-fiber friction to any tender points on the bottom of the foot, pause, then repeat the movement. (Note: Friction is contraindicated in the case of plantar fasciitis.) Flex and rotate the foot.

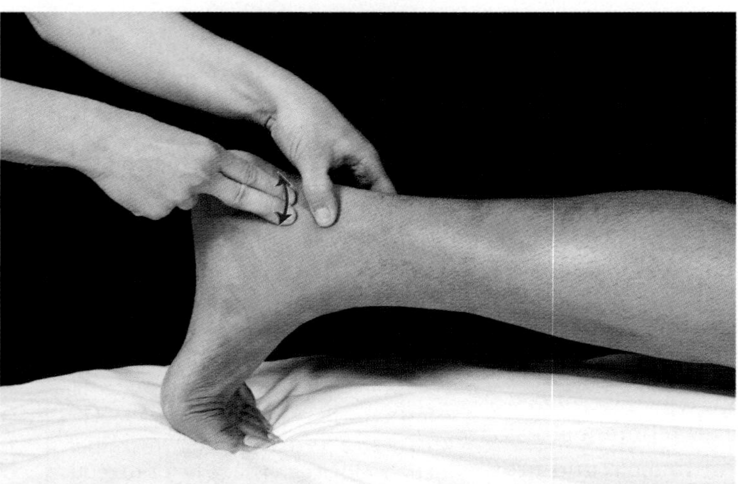

FIGURE 18-19 To apply transverse friction to a lesion on the Achilles tendon, stretch the tendon while friction is applied. The foot is flexed dorsally. The tendon is displaced to one side with the thumb of one hand. Transverse friction is applied with a braced finger directly to the site of the lesion.

Achilles Tendon

The Achilles tendon, which connects the soleus and gastrocnemius to the calcaneus, can become swollen and painful if the ankle has been strained or if the tendon has been pulled at its attachment to the heel. Stress points might have formed at the attachment to the heel, along the tendon, or at the musculotendinous junction of the calf muscle.

Massage: Caution: It is contraindicated to do deep strokes along a fibrous tendon like the Achilles tendon because this technique tends to aggravate abnormal conditions such as pulls and tears. Palpate the tendon from the attachment to the musculotendinous junction and note any tenderness. Stretch the tendon before applying cross-fiber friction. To do this, with the athlete lying prone, dorsally flex the ankle. With one thumb, move the tendon to the side and with a braced finger of the other hand apply transverse friction massage to the site of tendonosis (Figure 18-19). Search the calf muscle for related fibrosis or trigger points. Address any trigger points in the gastrocnemius or soleus muscles. If there are stress points at the musculotendinous junction, use your thumbs to apply repeated direct pressure movements, followed by cross-fiber friction. Repeat direct pressure, followed by compression with your hand. Finish with gliding strokes from the heel to the knee.

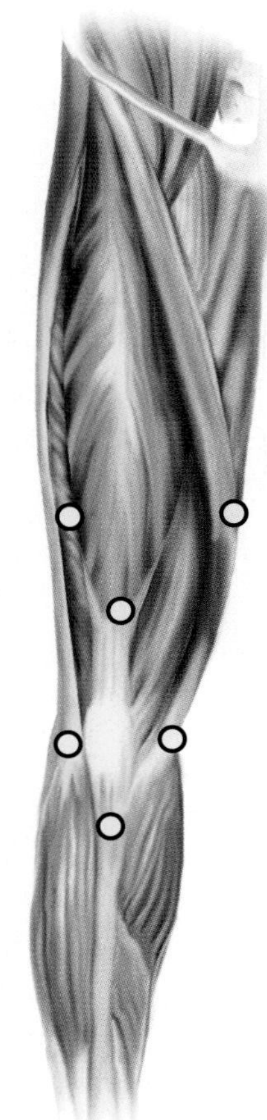

FIGURE 18-20 Common stress points of the anterior leg.

Ankle Strains and Twists

The feet and ankles play an important part in sports and, owing to the varied and stressful movements required of them, are prime targets for injury and fatigue.
Massage: Use your thumb and forefinger to apply pressure and cross-fiber friction to the stress points near the ankle bone. Release and repeat; this must be done gently, because the area might be painful. Apply friction to the instep, working gently and from the toes to the heel. Move to the stress point of the outer ankle, and apply direct pressure to any stress points followed by cross-fiber friction. Release and repeat the movement. Shake and rotate the foot, then gently stretch it in every direction.

Front of the Leg

Sports such as skiing, skating, ice hockey, surfing, horseback riding, and cycling all require quick reflexes and muscle power. Although the neck, shoulders, and back are under some stress in these sports, the muscles of the lower body also undergo stress and strain. Often, there is pain in the knee and thigh areas (Figure 18-20) after a day of heavy exertion.
Massage: With the athlete supine on the table, apply petrissage followed by compression on the quadriceps and adductors. Use your fingertips or thumbs to apply circular friction over and around the knee. Use the tips of your fingers to apply direct pressure to the stress points around the knee, and then follow with cross-fiber friction. Repeat the sequence several times. Using compression and deep gliding strokes, locate the stress areas in the thighs above the knee and in the groin and inguinal fold. Treat any trigger points located in taut bands using repeated direct pressure. Wherever fibrosis or fascial constrictions are found, use cross-fiber or other myofascial techniques. Apply compressions to the entire thigh, and use passive joint movements to the knee and hip to stretch the muscles gently. Finish the massage by applying deep strokes from knee to hip, shaking, jostling, and rolling the thigh.

Runner's Cramp

Runners often suffer from muscle cramps, spasms, or tightening of the calf muscle. Ice can be applied to the area in spasm. Have the athlete sit on the side of or lie down on the massage table. Hold the foot in a neutral position, and ask the athlete to tighten the antagonist muscle to the one in spasm by pulling his toes toward his knee for seven to ten seconds. Ask the athlete to relax, and as he

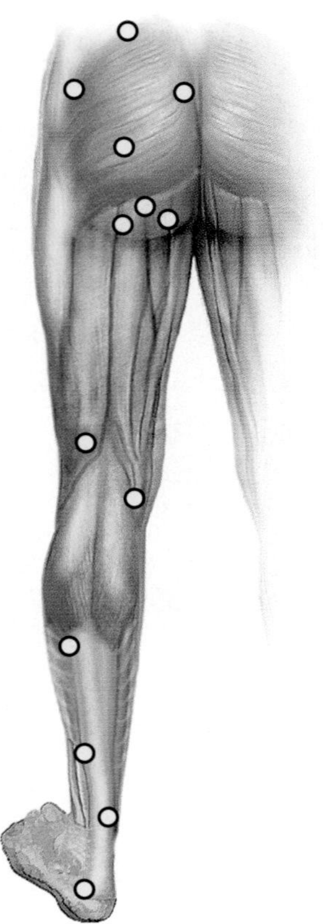

FIGURE 18-21 Common stress points of the posterior leg and buttock.

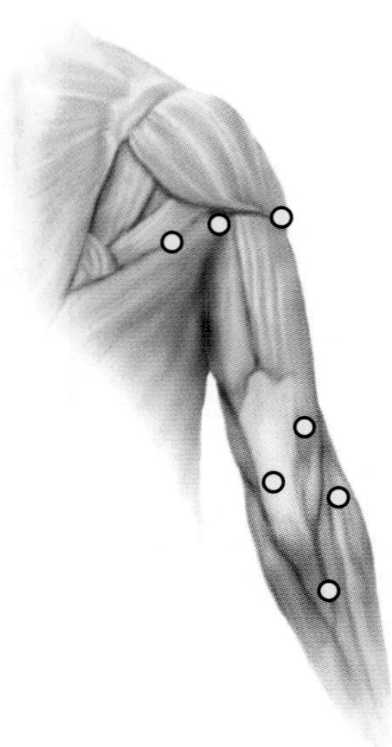

FIGURE 18-22 Common stress points of the elbow and arm.

does, gently stretch the spasmed muscle by dorsally flexing the ankle. Repeat the process several times (reciprocal inhibition).

Massage: To massage the leg, have the athlete lie face down on the table. After the spasm subsides, bend and flex the knee several times. Flex the ankle, and rotate it several times. Locate any trigger points in the calf muscles, and then with your thumb or finger, apply pressure for ten counts, release, and repeat the movements. Use MET/reciprocal inhibition to release tension further in the calf muscles. Apply steady, firm compression movements to the calf. Apply direct pressure to any stress points near the muscle attachments for ten counts, release, and follow with cross-fiber friction. Repeat the compression. Apply several deep strokes from heel to knee. Shake and jostle the calf muscle from knee to ankle and apply effleurage to the area.

Hip, Leg, and Buttocks

In the hip area, there are three main stress areas of concern to a therapist: the side of the hip, the back of the leg, and the buttocks (Figure 18-21).

Massage: Have the athlete lie facedown on the table. Apply petrissage and compression to the gluteal area. Use your thumb or a soft fist to apply deep pressure all over the gluteal area. Locate any taut bands, hypertonic areas, or tender points in the buttock. Apply pressure for ten counts, release, and repeat the movement several times. Controlled use of the elbow is very effective in this area. Apply cross-fiber friction for 20 counts. Release and repeat the movement. Find the tender points along the iliac crest, and apply direct pressure using the thumb or elbow. Apply for ten counts; release and repeat the movement. Apply cross-fiber friction for 10 counts to each affected area; release and repeat the movement. Repeat the cross-fiber friction, and finish with deep shaking and vibration movements.

Strain to Hamstrings

Sports requiring sustained leg tension for some time can lead to strain. Examples of such sports are dance and distance running. Generally, the strain will be in the back mid-thigh extending to the back of the knee.

Massage: Apply petrissage and compression movements to the back of the leg. Locate and treat any trigger points located in taut bands of muscle with repeated deep pressure, followed by MET/reciprocal inhibition. Use your thumb to locate the stress points behind the knee and in the gluteal crease at the ischial tuberosity. Apply direct pressure for 10 counts. Release and repeat. Apply cross-fiber friction for 10 counts. Release and repeat. Slightly flex the knee while supporting the ankle. Use the palm of your hand to apply compression over the entire back of the thigh from the buttock to the knee. Finish the massage with deep gliding strokes along the hamstring from knee to hip.

Calf

Tennis and similar games place stress on the muscles of the calves and ankles, often causing spasms.

Massage: Have the athlete lie face down. Apply petrissage and compression strokes from the knee to the ankle. Bend the knee and flex the ankle several times. Locate the stress points at the outside of the knee joint. Use the thumbs to apply direct pressure, holding for ten counts. Release and repeat the movement. Follow with cross-fiber friction on the stress points. Repeat the direct pressure and friction on the lower stress points of the ankle. Use the palm of your hand to apply deep compression all over the calf muscles. Apply cross-fiber friction along fibrous bands in the muscle and deep strokes from heel to knee, followed by shaking and jostling of the muscle and finally effleurage.

The Elbow and Arm

The muscles in the arm and shoulder can become strained by overuse from an activity such as tennis. Muscles can be stiff and sore. The extensor muscles of the forearm is usually affected (Figure 18-22).

Massage: Using the heel of the hand, apply compression to the wrist for ten counts. Apply petrissage and compression from the wrist, up to the elbow and the shoulder, and then back down to the wrist so that the entire arm is covered. Find the pressure point near the lateral epicondyle of the elbow, and with the thumb, apply direct pressure for about ten counts, followed by cross-fiber friction at the attachment site of the muscle. Release and repeat the cross-fiber friction three or more times. Using cross-fiber friction, move distally to the next tender point. Follow along the length of the muscle, repeating the cross-fiber friction where the muscle fibers seem stuck together. Follow this with several more compressions along the muscle. Apply deep stroking movements along the muscle from insertion to origin, and follow these with shaking and jostling movements. Repeat the same procedure to other stress points, and finish with general compression on the entire arm, gentle passive joint movements, stretching, and soothing effleurage. Ice massage can be applied to reduce any inflammation or residual soreness. Instruct the athlete to rest the arm, and repeat the treatment daily until all symptoms are gone.

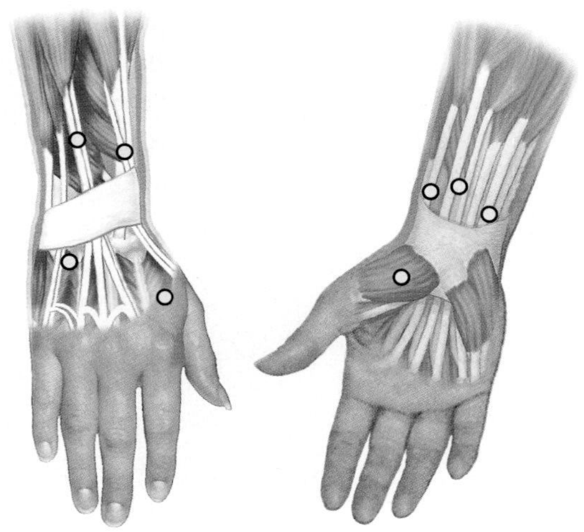

FIGURE 18-23 Common stress points of the wrist.

The Wrist

The ligament, tendons, and muscles of the wrist can be affected by tension caused by grasping and tensing for long periods (Figure 18-23). Examples include grasping the handlebars of a bicycle and lifting weights.

Massage: Find the stress points around the wrist. Use your fingertips or thumbs to apply direct pressure to the stress points, holding for ten counts. Release and then repeat the movements several times. Apply cross-fiber friction for ten counts; release and repeat. Use your thumb to apply cross-fiber friction all around the wrist. Follow with a series of compressions using the heel of the hand. Apply compression up the forearm from wrist to elbow, going all around the arm. Repeat these movements several times. Finish the massage by applying passive joint movements, gently stretching the wrist in all directions.

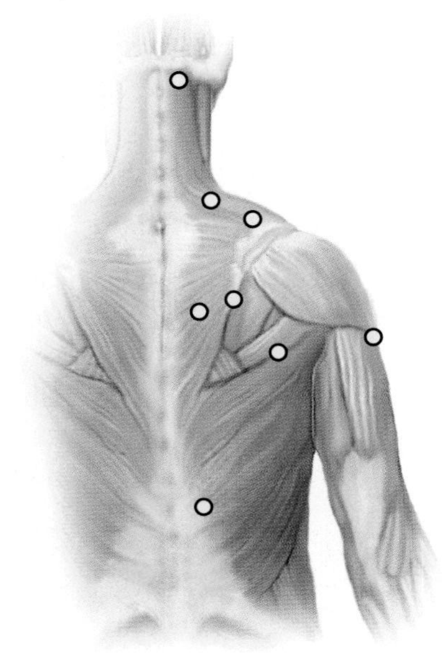

FIGURE 18-24 Common stress points of the back and shoulder.

Back, Shoulder, and Neck

The back and shoulder muscles are often strained during weightlifting, bowling, golf, and other sports. Shoulder joint injuries are due to such sports as baseball, bowling, basketball, and other sports requiring exertion of the arm and shoulder (Figure 18-24). These usually result in strain or injury to the rotator cuff or associated muscles.

Massage: Have the athlete lie face down on the table. Apply petrissage and compressions over entire back and sides of the neck. Apply deep gliding strokes to the side of the neck and downward on the shoulder. Repeat until the area has been covered. Use the thumb or elbow to apply deep pressure and cross-fiber friction at high-stress areas. Release and repeat the movement. Find the stress points on and around the shoulder blade. Apply direct pressure for ten counts; release and repeat the action. Apply cross-fiber friction for 10 counts; release and repeat the movement. Do this sequence several times, finishing the massage with compression done with the palm of the hand.

Triceps Strain

Triceps strain is a condition that usually occurs when the muscle is overused and stressed.

Massage: With the client lying prone on the table, begin with petrissage and compression over the triceps. Locate any stress points. Use the thumb or fingertip to apply direct pressure for ten counts. Release and repeat the movements. Apply cross-fiber friction for ten counts. Release and repeat the movements. Do this sequence (gently) several times. Apply deep strokes from elbow to shoulder; then shake and flush out the area.

Midback and Lower Back

Massage: Have the athlete lie on the table face down. Apply petrissage from the crest of the ileum to the rib cage on each side of the body. Apply skin rolling to the lumbar area. Find the stress points in the muscular bands along each side of the spine. With the thumb, apply direct pressure for ten counts. Release and repeat the movement all the way down the back. Do the sequence down the back several times, working with the client's breathing. Apply pressure on the exhale and release on the inhale. Apply cross-fiber friction with the thumb. Release and repeat the movement, moving an inch or so down the back. Use the palm of the hand to apply several compressions on the muscles along the spine. Use the thumb to apply cross-fiber friction on the outside of the muscle. Do this sequence several times. Apply deep strokes with the thumbs or the flat of the elbow from the top of the shoulders down to the tailbone, and then shake and vibrate the muscles back up to the shoulders. Apply compressions to the buttocks with your hand, and finish by flushing out the area with effleurage.

The Groin

The groin is more likely to be pulled in sports such as horseback riding, gymnastics, and soccer. This is a painful condition caused by overstretching of the gracilis and adductor muscles located high on the inner thigh.

Massage: Have the athlete lie on his side with the affected leg on the bottom. The knee of the top leg is bent, and the bottom leg remains fairly straight. Stand behind the athlete and apply compressions to the inner thigh with the palm of the hand. Search for any taut bands containing trigger points. Treat trigger points with repeated trigger-point pressure release. Locate any stress points at muscle attachments. Use the thumb to apply pressure and cross-fiber friction for 20 counts. Release and repeat the movement. Because this area will be quite tender, be gentle. Find any tension in the area and apply compression with a soft fist or the palm of the hand. Release and repeat the movement.

Massage During Rehabilitation

Rehabilitation massage focuses on the restoration of tissue function following injury. The best way to treat an injury is to prevent it. Massage during training is invaluable for locating potential trouble spots and relieving them before they progress into debilitating injuries. When injury does occur, however, massage can be an important part of the rehabilitation program. Treatment strategy varies, depending on the nature and stage of healing of the injury. Rehabilitation athletic massage accomplishes the following:

- Shortens the time it takes for an injury to heal
- Helps reduce swelling and edema
- Assists in forming strong, pliable scar tissue
- Maintains or increases ROM
- Eliminates splinting in associated muscle tissue
- Locates and deactivates trigger points that form as a result of the trauma
- Assists in getting the athlete back into training sooner with less chance of reinjury

Valuable therapeutic modalities used in rehabilitation massage include

- Lymph massage – to control reduce and swelling
- Neuromuscular techniques – to increase circulation, reduce muscle tension, and deactivate trigger points
- Myofascial techniques – to soften connective tissue and reduce adhesions and fascial constrictions
- Hydrotherapy – to reduce swelling and pain, or increase circulation and promote relaxation
- Swedish techniques – to promote circulation and relaxation and to reconnect and integrate the injury back into the whole

The massage therapist must have a thorough anatomic understanding of the structures involved and the nature of the injury, including the severity and the stage of healing. The application of proper techniques to the type of injury is important.

The massage practitioner should practice therapy at this level only after receiving proper training under the supervision of a qualified instructor who is familiar with sports injuries and the practice of therapeutic athletic massage. Before attempting rehabilitation massage, the therapist must be well trained in sound evaluation and treatment techniques. When skillfully applied, massage

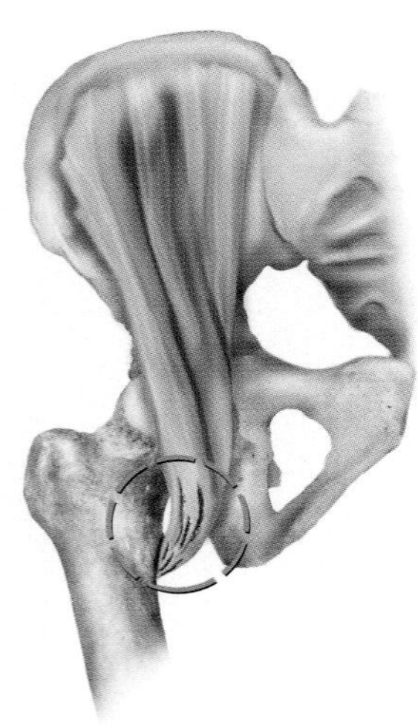

FIGURE 18-25A Grade I: Overstretched fibrous tissue with some microtrauma.

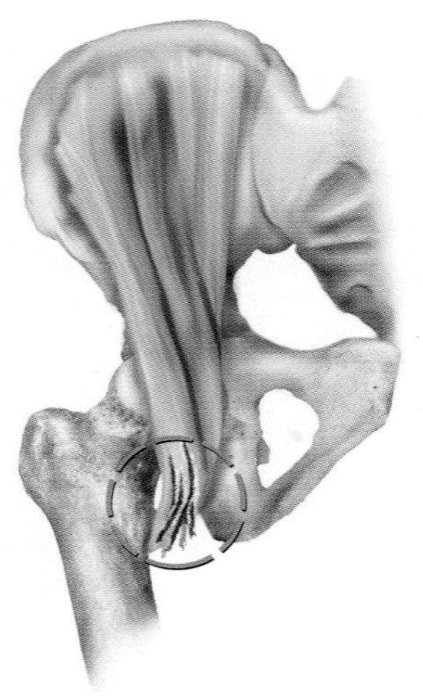

FIGURE 18-25B Grade II: Some tearing of the fibrous tissue.

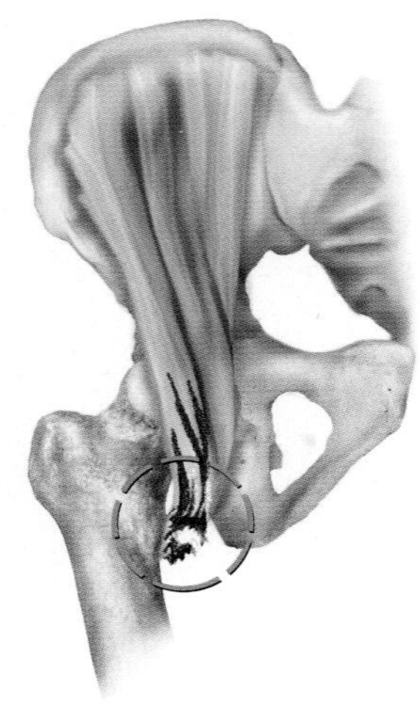

FIGURE 18-25C Grade III: Severe tearing of the fibrous tissue with loss of function.

can reduce the healing time, with return to full function; however, improper application of techniques can prolong healing time and result in more severe injury.

General rules for the application of rehabilitation massage are

- Do not massage directly on the site of an injury or trauma during the acute stage or when it is inflamed.
- Do not stretch muscle or fibrous tissue that is in the acute stage of injury.
- Never cause pain! Pain is the guide for proper application of all techniques. Less pain, more gain.
- Apply cross-fiber friction and stretching only after inflammation and swelling have subsided and the healing process is well established.
- When in doubt — don't.

The advantages of massage therapy are numerous. Prompt application of the appropriate therapy can reduce much of the swelling and pain caused by an injury. Proper therapy allows the injured tissues to remain proximal to each other so that healing progresses faster and with less need for the body to produce excess scar tissue. When massage is administered, the quality of healed tissue is far superior than if an injury were left to heal on its own.

Proper massage therapy improves circulation, enabling excess fluid and damaged tissue to be carried away. With improved circulation, more nutrients are brought to the rebuilding tissue so that it becomes strong, pliable, and heals more quickly. Research has also shown that with massage therapy, fibrosis caused by muscle injury is reduced and the presence of transverse adhesions is almost nonexistent.

Appropriate treatment and accelerated healing of injuries mean that the athlete's downtime is cut to a minimum. With continued treatment during the rehabilitation period, there will also be fewer ill effects on performance.

Therapy can be given at the rate of once or twice a day during the time the athlete is out of training and every other day or every third day until he is back to a full training schedule. Massage for new or fresh injuries should be given only by properly trained therapists in conjunction with a physician's approval.

Athletic Injuries

It is the nature of athletes to push their abilities to their limits and beyond to excel at their particular sports. Because of the rigorous training and participation in competition, athletes' bodies are continuously exposed to stress, strain, fatigue, and sometimes microtrauma or more serious injury. Maximal athletic effort is physical abuse.

Most athletic injuries are either the result of trauma (contact with another athlete or in a fall) or the result of excessive and/or repeated stress to an area of the body. Injuries of the traumatic sort are often in the form of broken bones, dislocated joints, and torn ligaments. Such injuries are generally accidental and cannot be prevented. Injuries of the second type are far more common and generally affect the soft tissue in the form of muscle strains, pulls, and tears, or inflammation of tendons and ligaments. These are usually the result of fatigue, overtraining, poor tissue integrity, muscular weakness, imbalance, or biomechanical deviation. Most of these injuries are preventable and treatable by massage and proper training.

Athletic injuries are categorized according to the onset and duration of the injury. Acute injuries have a sudden and definite onset and are usually of relatively short duration. Chronic injuries have an indefinite onset, can linger for several weeks or even months, and can be the result of repeated injuries in the same area. Examples of acute injuries include dislocations, sprains, strains, lacerations, fractures, and contusions. Strains and sprains and their side effects respond well to massage therapy. *Strains* involve the tearing of muscle tissue or tendons; *sprains* involve ligaments or joint capsules. The severity of strains and sprains is graded as follows (Figure 18-25 a-c):

Grade I: Mild pain
Severe overstretching of the fibrous tissue, with little or no damage
Full ROM and full strength available

Grade II: Moderate to severe pain
Swelling and possible discoloration
Some tearing of the fibrous tissue
Reduced ROM and strength

Grade III: Immediate pain
Severe or complete tissue rupture
Extensive swelling and tissue deformity
No strength or ROM

Soft tissue injuries progress through identifiable stages of healing. The acute or inflammatory stage is the generally the first 24 to 72 hours just after the incident, depending on the type and severity of the injury. The goal during the inflammatory stage is to control or reduce swelling and interrupt the pain cycle without further disrupting the injured tissue. The early subacute phase is also known as the *regenerative stage,* during which fibroblasts have migrated into the area to produce collagen fibers to begin to mend the damaged tissue. During the regenerative stage, treatment goals include continuing to reduce swelling and encourage the development of a pliable, functional scar. A later portion of the subacute phase is called the *remodeling* or *maturation* stage, when the healing tissue is well on its way to recovery. Goals during the maturation stage include reducing adhesions and fibrosis, improving flexibility and strength of the injured tissues, and addressing any conditions of associated or compensating structures.

Massage directly on acute injuries is contraindicated; however, prompt first aid greatly reduces secondary injury caused by swelling. First aid for acute soft tissue injuries, such as sprains, strains and contusions, involves PRICE (protect, rest, ice, compression, elevation) for the first 24 to 48 hours to help to reduce pain, swelling, and spasm. (Read more about PRICE in Chapter 13, Hydrotherapy.) Use caution when applying ice to avoid skin burn and nerve damage.

During the acute stage of a soft tissue injury, lymph massage can be applied proximal to the injury site. Lymph massage begins at the terminus at the base of the neck and progresses toward the injury site. Clear the nodes at the catchment site nearest the injury and continue with slow circles while approaching the injury. Do not massage directly over the injury or distal to the injury. Reverse the progression to encourage lymph circulation away from the injury toward the heart. (Read more about lymph massage in Chapter 16.)

After one or two days of rest, the injury enters the early subacute stage. Most of the swelling and inflammation has subsided, and the tissues are beginning the healing process. Lymph massage is valuable to reduce any residual swelling. Contrast hydrotherapy treatments can be used to increase circulation to help promote healing. Each series should end with cold. Massage treatments are begun to stimulate circulation to and away from the area. Gentle myofascial techniques help to mobilize the tissue so that as the tissue regenerates, strong, pliable, and flexible scar tissue forms. Gentle cross-fiber friction and pain-free passive and active ROM exercises help to encourage the development of strong, functional scar tissue. Neuromuscular techniques can be used on associated structures to reduce muscle tension and trigger points. Extreme caution must be used not to aggravate the injury or cause more damage to the tissues. Pain is the indicator to the athlete and therapist of the intensity of the techniques. As the tissues continue to mend and get stronger, the aggressiveness of the therapy increases until the athlete returns to full participation.

During the remodeling or maturation stage, the tissues continue to heal. Myofascial techniques at and around the injury site help to create a strong, flexible scar while minimizing adhesions and fibrosis in the neighboring tissues. Lymph massage is usually not necessary at this stage because most of the inflammation and swelling has subsided; however, ice packs or ice massage following deep work at the injury site minimizes local inflammation. Neuromuscular and myofascial techniques can be used on associated or compensating structures to relieve tension, trigger points, or fascial constrictions that might have developed as a result of the injury.

Chronic injuries have a gradual onset, tend to last for a long time, or recur often. Often they are the result of repetitive stressful activity and are sometimes labeled *overuse syndrome*. Repeated or extreme stresses cause microscopic lesions in the connective tissue of the tendons, muscles, or the musculotendinous or tenoperiosteal junction. This in turn causes local, low-grade inflammation, selected muscle spasms (taut bands), reduced circulation to the area, pain, and dysfunction. Examples of chronic injury include chronic muscle spasm, tennis elbow, shin splints, tendonosis, fasciitis, and iliotibial band syndrome.

Chronic conditions suggest a varied therapeutic response according to the structures involved and the nature of the injury. Myofascial techniques reduce adhesions and fascial restrictions. Cross-fiber friction breaks down adhesions and helps to realign fiber integrity at the injury site. Neuromuscular techniques help to identify and decrease the presence of trigger points and muscle tension. Hydrotherapy helps to soften connective tissues preceding treatment (hot packs or baths) and reduce local inflammation following deep treatment (ice massage or packs). Swedish techniques increase circulation, promote relaxation, and integrate injured and compensating structures into the whole body. Treatment includes work directly on the injury site and indirectly on areas of the body that are either associated with or compensating for the injured area. If there is still time after direct work on the injury and indirect work on the compensating structures, finishing with Swedish techniques leaves the athlete with a sense of relaxation, connectedness, and completion.

Soft Tissue Lesions and Injury

Connective tissues form a continuous netlike framework throughout the body. Connective tissue consists largely of a fluid matrix (ground substance) and collagen fibers that support, bind, and connect the wide range of body structures.

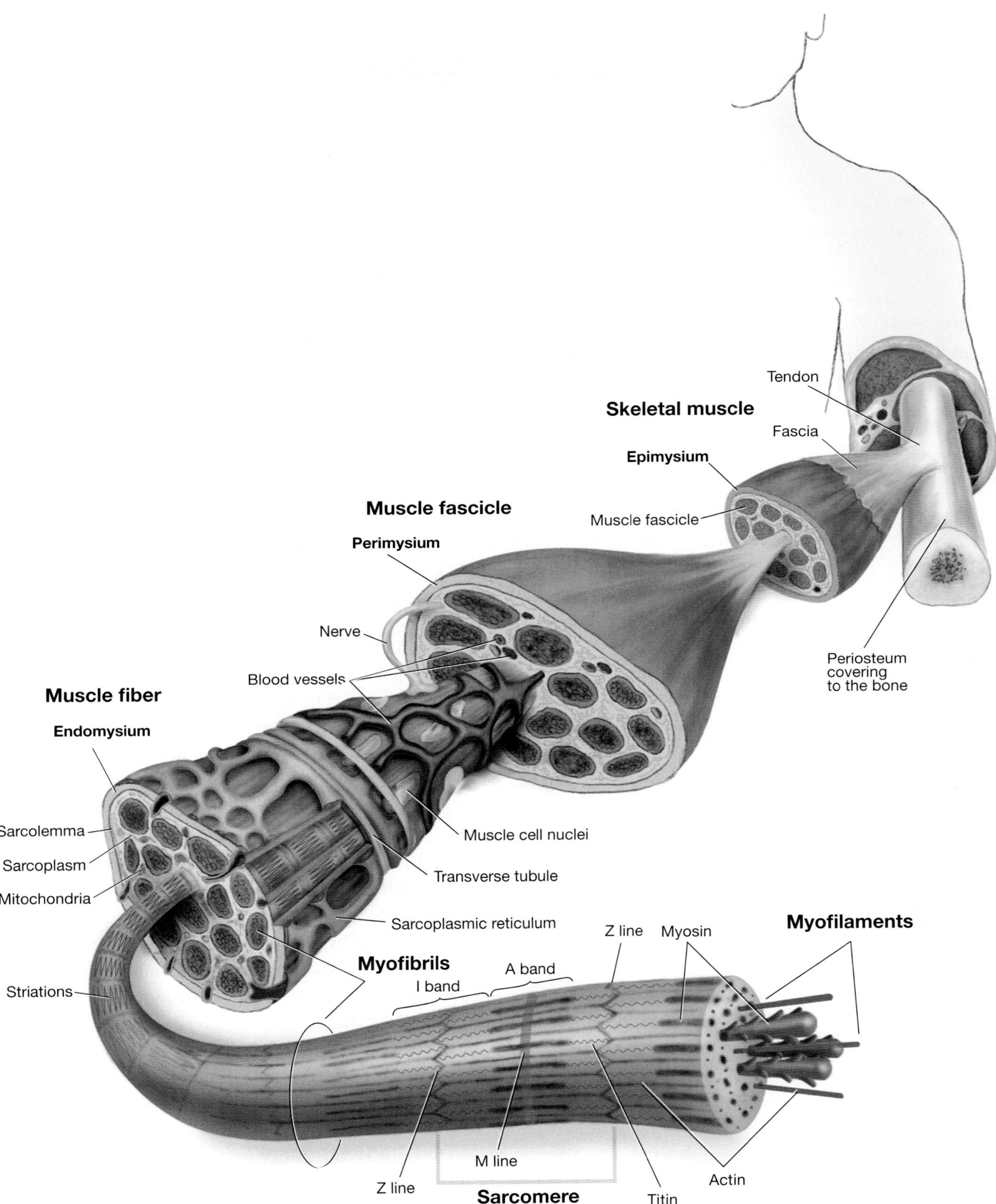

FIGURE 18-26 Muscles are contractile organs that are compartmentalized, organized, and supported by intricate layers of connective tissue or fascia.

epimysium

is the layer of connective tissue that closely covers an individual muscle.

perimysium

separates the muscle into bundles of muscle fibers.

fascicle

is a bundle of muscle fibers.

endomysium

is the delicate connective tissue covering of muscle fibers.

Collagen fibers provide the tensile strength in connective tissue. Depending on the consistency of the connective tissue and the varying proportions of fluid to fibers, a wide array of fibrous connective tissues are formed. Some examples are the fluid intercellular environment, superficial fascia that is just beneath the skin, and the fascia of the muscles, tendons, ligaments, and even bone.

The muscular system is a highly organized system of compartmentalized contractile fibrous tissues that work together to produce movement. The fibrous tissue is organized and supported by an intricate network of fascia. Fascia organizes muscles into functional groups, surrounds each individual muscle, extends inward throughout the muscle-creating muscle bundles, and eventually houses each muscle fiber. Fascia also creates the supporting structure for the intricate network of blood vessels and nerves. The connective tissue projects beyond the ends of the muscle to become tendons, which connect the muscles to the bones and other structures. Fascia supports the muscle fibers in such a way that when the fibers contract, a force is exerted on whichever structure the muscle is attached to, causing movement (Figure 18-26).

The layer of fascia that closely covers an individual muscle is the **epimysium** (ep-ih-**MIS**-ee-um). The **perimysium** (per-ih-**MIS**-ee-um) extends inward from the epimysium and separates the muscle into bundles of muscle fibers or **fascicles** (**FAS**-ih-kls). Within the fascicle, each muscle fiber is covered by a delicate connective tissue covering called the **endomysium** (en-do-**MIS**-ee-ium). The **sarcolemma** (cell wall) of the muscle cell and the endomysium are intimately connected and act as a unit, so that when the muscle fiber contracts and shortens, the fascia covering moves right along with it.

The connective tissue organizes the muscle fibers, connects the muscle to tendons, tendons to bones, and even bones to bone. Without this complicated system of connecting sheets, hinges, and ropes that transfer the action of the muscle fibers to the levers of the skeleton, motion and postural stability would not be possible.

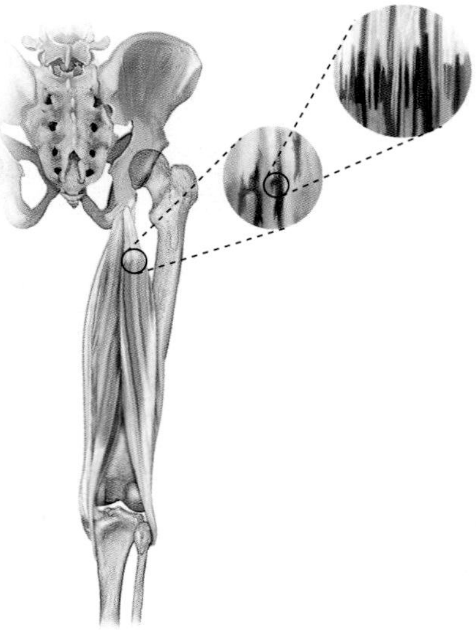

FIGURE 18-27 Soft tissue injuries occur when the tissue is pulled and stretched to the point that the integrity of the collagen fibers is broken.

Soft tissue injuries are the result of overstretching and eventual breaking of the collagen fibers in one or more layers of the fascia or connective tissue. Whether it is microtrauma in or between the muscle fibers, strained muscles, or torn ligaments, stresses to the connective tissue exceed their tensile strength, resulting in the tearing of collagen fibers in the connective tissue (Figure 18-27).

The healing process in all soft tissue injuries is essentially the same. The cell damage initiates an inflammatory response. Extra fluid is infused into the area (swelling). The positive effects of swelling are to immobilize the area and supply an environment rich in leukocytes and fibroblasts so that the natural healing process of the body can start to repair the injury. The negative effect is that the swelling creates pressure in the tissue, which causes further tissue damage and separates the ends of the injury and connective tissue layers, slowing healing. Inflammation and swelling are accompanied by pain.

The fluid carries an abundance of fibroblasts that within a couple of hours of the injury begin to lay down new collagen fibers to secure the injured tissue. Within two to three days, the early subacute or regenerative phase begins when collagen formation is at its maximum. Fibroblasts generate collagen fibers that extend in random directions, forming a cobweb-like network that adheres to any structure in the vicinity. Collagen formation that reconnects the injured tissue forms scar tissue. The crisscross formation of fibers that connect to structures other than the injured tissue forms undesirable adhesions between the layers of fascia that restrict mobility and flexibility in the healed tissues.

The swelling that takes place when tissue is injured also creates space between the various layers of fascia. Wherever swelling has separated tissues,

TABLE 18-1

REHABILITATION MASSAGE ACCORDING TO STAGE OF HEALING

STAGE OF HEALING	GOALS OF TREATMENT	TREATMENT MODALITY
Acute	Reduce swelling	PRICE
First 24 – 72 hours after injury	Reduce pain	PRICE
Inflammatory stage	Encourage edema uptake	Lymph massage proximal to injury
	Decrease spasm	Gentle position release or NMT –reciprocal inhibition using the antagonist to the injured tissue
Early subacute stage	Continued uptake of excess tissue exudate	Lymph massage proximal to and at injury site
Regeneration phase	Facilitate strong flexible scar formation	Cross-fiber friction after swelling is reduced and there is no discoloration around the injured tissue
Granulation tissue forms	Maintain ROM	Pain-free passive and active joint movements
	Minimize compensating structures	Neuromuscular techniques to reduce tension and trigger points in compensating muscles
	Minimize local inflammation after deep massage	Ice massage
Late subacute stage	Prepare the area, soften connective tissue	Hydrotherapy – heat packs
Remodeling or maturation phase	Facilitate strong scar formation	Cross-fiber techniques at the site of injury
	Reduce adhesions and fascial constrictions	Myofascial techniques – site-specific and broad plane to address neighboring and associated tissues
	Increase flexibility and strength	Neuromuscular techniques – reciprocal inhibition and postisometric relaxation, passive and active joint movements
	Minimize local inflammation of treatment	Ice massage
	Address compensating areas	NMT to relieve tension, trigger points, and stress points in compensating structures
	Integrate injury	Swedish massage techniques to reconnect injury to adjacent areas
Chronic injuries	Prepare the area, soften connective tissue	Hydrotherapy – heat packs
	Identify and release muscle tension in surrounding, associated tissues	Neuromuscular techniques to release trigger points, stress points, and tension in area
	Reduce adhesions and fibrosis at and around injury	Site-specific and broad cross-fiber friction
	Increase ROM	METs, stretching, active and passive joint movements
	Release fascial constrictions	Myofascial techniques – site-specific and broad plane releases
	Minimize local inflammation of treatment	Ice massage over injury site after deep cross-fiber work
	Integrate injury	Swedish massage techniques to reconnect injury to adjacent areas

collagen fibers form to adhere the separated tissue. The more extensive the swelling, the more extensive is the formation of fibrosis and adhesions. The more severe the injury and the greater the separation in the injured tissue, the more extensive is the formation of scar tissue. As swelling is reduced, the fibrosis left behind sticks or glues the adjoining layers of fascia together. This type of gluing can also be the result of stressed and confined muscle movement over a long period. The resulting fibrosis reduces mobility and flexibility, leaving a reduction of power and a greater chance of reinjury. Both of these conditions can be greatly reduced with proper first aid and athletic massage therapy.

Proper first aid, represented by the acronym PRICE (protect, rest, ice, compress, elevate), greatly reduces swelling and the accompanying secondary trauma. With reduced swelling, the space between the ends of the injured tissue and between associated connective tissue layers is minimized. This minimizes the formation of scar tissue, fibrosis, and adhesions.

As the tissue heals, proper therapy, including massage, encourages new fibers to form along appropriate lines of stress (Table 18-1). Properly applied transverse friction massage and gentle stretching helps to organize and align collagen fibers to produce strong, pliable tissue at the same time as it breaks down unwanted interfiber cross-links and adhesions.

CONTRAINDICATIONS

The athlete's physician (employed by the organization or school) takes case histories and is responsible for preseason evaluations and for advising the athlete on health care and care of injuries. The physician treats illnesses and injuries and is responsible for rehabilitation of the athlete. The massage practitioner or trainer works under the direction of the physician and follows her guidelines when massage is to be a part of treatment or rehabilitation of injuries.

The physician or practitioner avoids doing anything that might make her liable or subject to malpractice. *Negligence* is defined as imprudent action, failure to act properly, or failure to take reasonable precautions. Athletes understand that there are always some risks involved and that a physician or therapist is not held liable for poor judgment on the part of the athlete. Athletic massage is contraindicated in any abnormal condition, acute injury, illness, or disease except as advised by the athlete's physician.

There are times when an amateur or school athlete requests the services of the massage practitioner. The same contraindications for massage apply for this client as for the professional. The client must take responsibility for his own health and provide a physician's report if deemed necessary. Any heart condition, anemia, diabetes, thyroid disorders, liver, kidney and lung conditions, cancer, skin disease, varicose veins, hypertension, internal injuries, wounds, or similar conditions are contraindications for massage. In these cases, massage would be done only by an experienced massage therapist who has continued her education, by the recommendation of the client's physician, and at the request of the client.

SUMMARY

Athletic or sport massage is therapeutic massage specifically designed to address the concerns of athletes as they train and participate in their chosen athletic endeavors. An athletic massage therapist must have a thorough understanding of the structure and function of the human body as well as the physical demands of the athletic activities in which the client participates. There are three basic applications of athletic massage: event massage, restorative or training massage, and rehabilitative massage.

The three classifications of event massage include

- Pre-event massage – takes place before an event to assist in the athletes' warm-up and to prepare the major muscle groups used during the event to prepare for the exertion.
- Intra-event massage – massage between events to assist athlete to recover from one athletic activity and prepare for an upcoming event.
- Post-event massage – massage after an event to normalize the tissues and relax the athlete after competition.

Techniques used during event massage include effleurage, compression, jostling, and joint movements. Event massages are given at the site of the competition or event and are usually rather fast paced and short.

Restorative or training massage is usually done in a clinical setting, uses many of the same techniques of event massage plus techniques to identify and address conditions in the soft tissue that might be inhibiting performance or are potential injuries waiting to happen. Restorative massage allows the athlete to train harder with less chance of injury. Besides techniques used in event massage, restorative massage uses myofascial techniques such as cross-fiber and broad plane stretches, neuromuscular techniques such as stripping, trigger-point releases, and METs.

Rehabilitation massage focuses on the restoration of tissue function following injury. Therapeutic modalities used in rehabilitative massage include both hot and cold hydrotherapy, lymph massage, myofascial and neuromuscular techniques, and various Swedish massage techniques. Rehabilitative massage addresses the injury and related conditions so the athlete can return to action more quickly with fewer repercussions from the injury and less chance of reinjury.

QUESTIONS FOR DISCUSSION AND REVIEW

1. What is athletic/sports massage?
2. Define adaptive sports massage.
3. In addition to a thorough understanding of human anatomy and physiology, which four major body systems and their functions must the therapist know?
4. What is the overload principle?
5. What are negative effects of exercise?
6. What techniques are commonly used in athletic massage?
7. What is the primary goal of compression?
8. In athletic massage, what does the term *hyperemia* refer to?
9. In athletic massage, how is deep pressure used?

10. Who popularized the use of transverse friction massage for treating soft tissue lesions?
11. What is the objective of using cross-fiber friction in athletic massage?
12. What are the three basic applications for athletic massage?
13. What is the goal of each application of event athletic massage?
14. When is massage considered to be the most beneficial to the athlete?
15. What are stress points, and where are they generally located?
16. Why must the therapist be sure to apply proper techniques at all times?
17. What is the best way to treat an athletic injury?
18. What are some beneficial advantages of rehabilitation massage?
19. How does massage therapy affect the healing time of injuries?
20. Who is qualified to give athletic massage to new or fresh injuries?
21. What is PRICE?
22. Differentiate between acute and chronic injuries.
23. Which massage techniques should be used at the site of acute muscle injuries?
24. Differentiate between a strain and a sprain.
25. When is athletic massage contraindicated?

CHAPTER

19 Massage for Special Populations

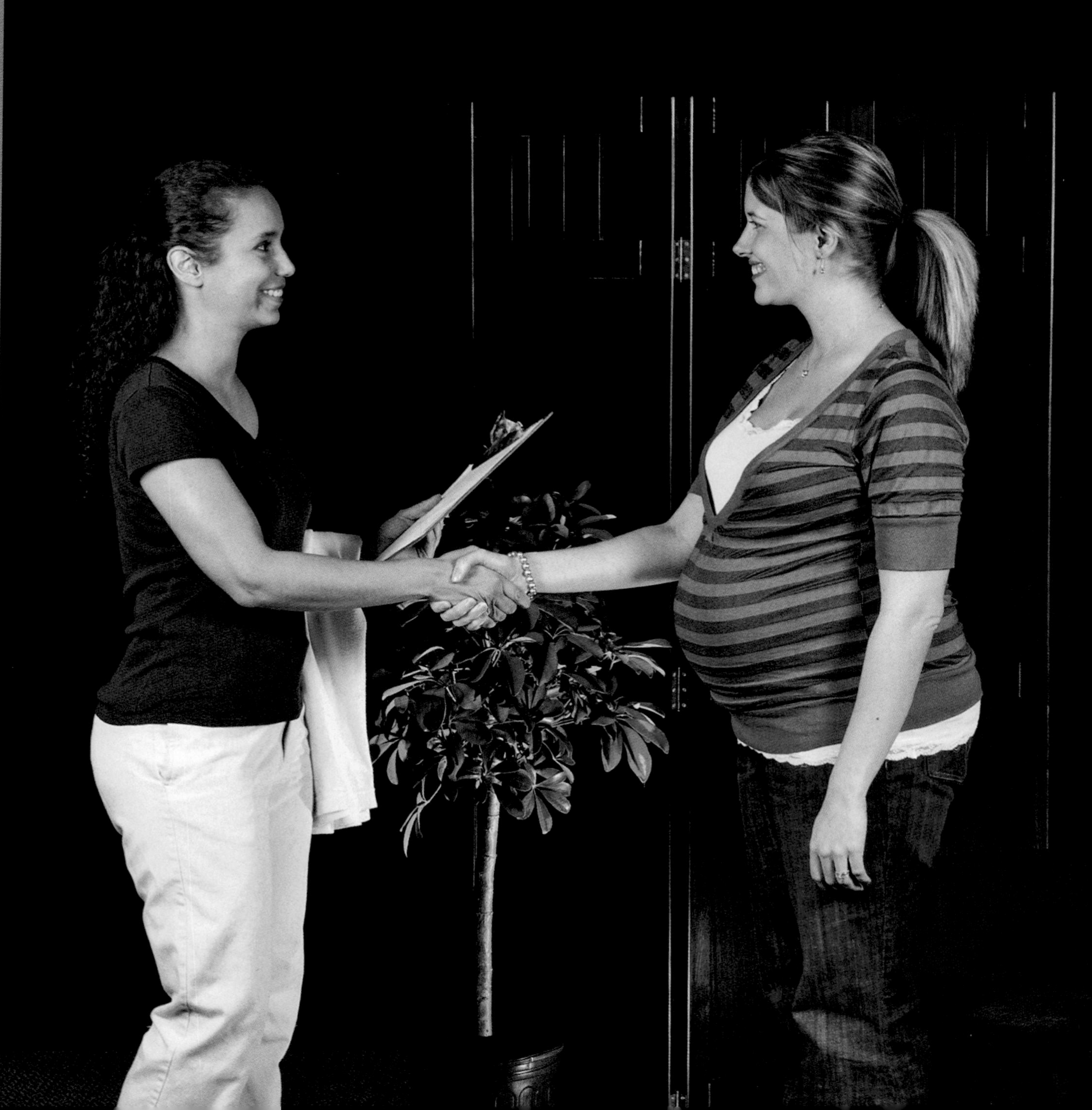

LEARNING OBJECTIVES

After you have mastered this chapter, you will be able to

1. **Explain the benefits of prenatal massage.**
2. **Explain the contraindications for prenatal massage.**
3. **Demonstrate proper positioning when massaging a pregnant woman during each trimester.**
4. **Describe various maternal concerns (by trimester) that are considerations for massage.**
5. **Describe the benefits of infant massage.**
6. **Explain special considerations for providing massage services to children.**
7. **Differentiate the considerations of working with older clients who are frail and those who are robust.**
8. **Explain the accommodations and considerations for providing massage to people with various disabilities.**
9. **Explain the major considerations when providing massage to people with critical illnesses such as HIV/AIDS or cancer.**

INTRODUCTION

Massage in some form is beneficial for nearly everyone, male or female, young or old, active athlete or sedentary businessman. This chapter focuses on certain populations that can benefit from special consideration when providing massage services. Because of unique physiologic needs or characteristics, certain segments of the population require or at least benefit from physical assistance, special positioning, and adaptation of massage technique to accommodate the particular conditions that a client might present. These groups include women who are pregnant, infants, children, older clients, people with disabilities, critically ill patients (including those infected with HIV), and those with cancer or in hospice care. These considerations are introduced in this chapter, but the student interested in providing therapeutic services to these populations as a part of her practice is encouraged to seek additional training from a qualified instructor.

PRENATAL MASSAGE

During pregnancy, a woman's body experiences many physical and hormonal changes to accommodate for the gestation and delivery of a baby. Physical changes include an enlarging abdomen and breasts and weight gain. Strain is increased on the lower back, hips, and lower extremities because of increasing weight. Hormones cause softening of ligaments and other connective tissue in preparation for delivery and can play a part in the emotional swings that some expectant mothers experience.

In normal, healthy pregnancies, massage has proved to be beneficial to both mother and unborn child. Properly applied massage can aid relaxation, benefit circulation, and soothe nerves. Prenatal massage is performed as any regular massage is, except for the following considerations.

Positioning

The client can assume any of several positions, depending on which is more comfortable. Early in the pregnancy, before the abdomen starts to protrude, the prone and supine positions can be used. When the fetus has grown enough to "show," special considerations to provide comfort to the mother and safety to the fetus must be made. If the client chooses a supine position, arrange pillows or a foam wedge under her back to support her in a semi-reclining (45-degree to 70-degree) position. Place a small pillow or folded towel under her head to support the head and neck, and place a pillow or a small bolster (6 or 8 inches) under the bend of her knees to take the strain off the lower back and abdominal muscles (Figure 19-1). During the second and third trimester of the pregnancy, use the supine position (with great caution or not at all) because the weight of the fetus can press on the descending aorta and impede the flow of blood to the placenta.

The mother might prefer a side-lying position and might find this more comfortable throughout the pregnancy. Plenty of pillows and bolsters are used to comfortably support the head, womb, upper leg, and arm (Figure 19-2).

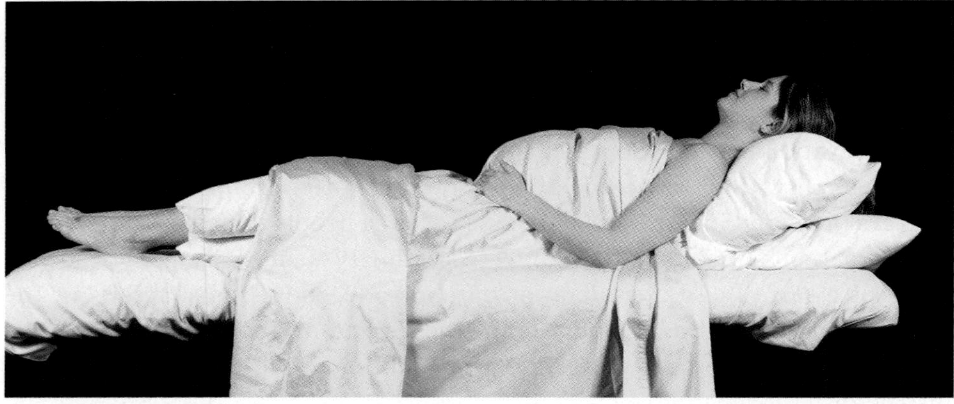

FIGURE 19-1 In the supine position, the pregnant client should be supported in a semi-reclining position to prevent pressure from the fetus on the major abdominal blood vessels.

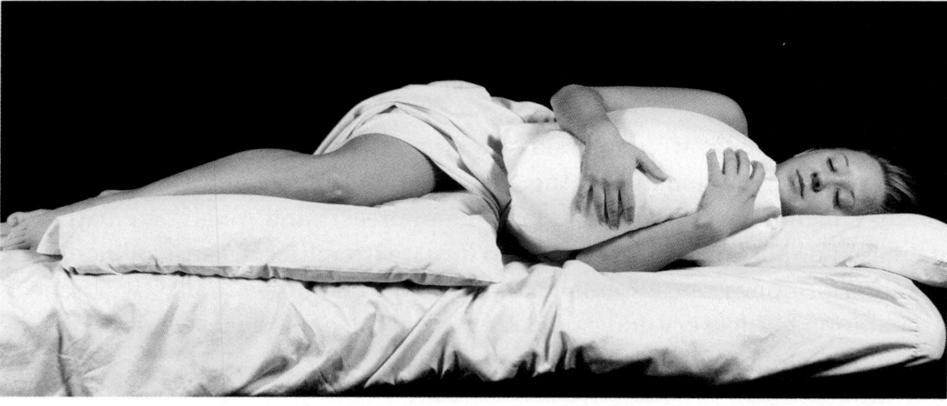

FIGURE 19-2 The side-lying position is a comfortable position to be used throughout pregnancy. When the client is on her side, pillows are placed under her head, abdomen, and upper knee, or between her legs. Another pillow for the upper arm to hug positions the woman in a comfortable fetal pose.

Ask the client to indicate if she becomes uncomfortable at any time during the treatment.

During the first two to three months of pregnancy, the prone position can be used, but only if it is comfortable to do so. Some women feel uncomfortable lying on their stomachs immediately. As the abdomen becomes larger, however, pillows placed underneath the client's head, chest, pelvis, and legs can add to her comfort. A soft rolled towel can also be placed under the collarbone to ease pressure on the chest (which can also be used for nursing mothers). During the second and third trimester, a Preg-pillow can be used for a safe and comfortable prone position for short periods. A Preg-pillow is a cushion, 6 to 8 inches thick, with space cut out for the enlarged abdomen and breasts. There are commercially available cushions and bolsters specifically designed for prenatal massage that safely and comfortably support the mother in side-lying and prone positions (Figure 19-3).

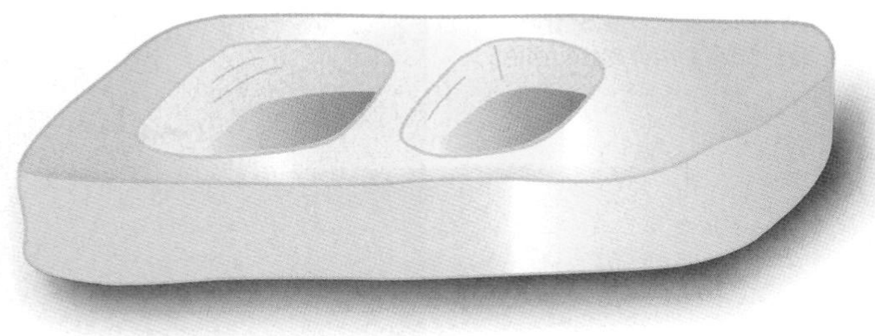

FIGURE 19-3 A Preg-pillow is a special supporting cushion with cutouts for the womb and breasts that can be used to allow even a full-term mother to lie safely and comfortably in the prone position.

Body Areas Subject to Discomfort

During pregnancy, the neck, upper and lower back, hips, legs, and feet appreciate special attention. The upper back and neck often feel strained because of the head-forward position that is common during pregnancy. Tension in this area can lead to tension headaches. The neck is most easily accessed, with the client in a semi-reclining or side-lying position (Figure 19-4).

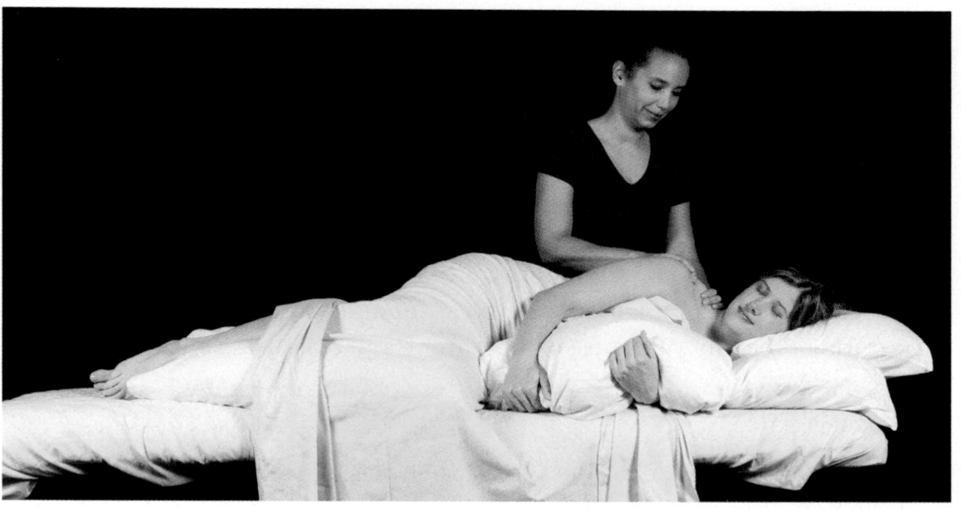

FIGURE 19-4 The upper back and shoulders are easily accessed while the pregnant mother is in the side-lying position.

The lower back experiences extra strain, especially in the later stages of pregnancy, owing to the extra weight of the protruding abdomen and the hormonal changes that soften the ligaments in preparation for delivery. Massage to the lower back can be applied in the side-lying position (Figure 19-5). Lateral and abdominal muscles are also under strain from carrying the extra weight and from stretching to accommodate the growing fetus. Light effleurage is soothing and helps to relieve the tension in the muscles. Any deep massage technique directly on the abdomen is contraindicated during pregnancy. Abdominal

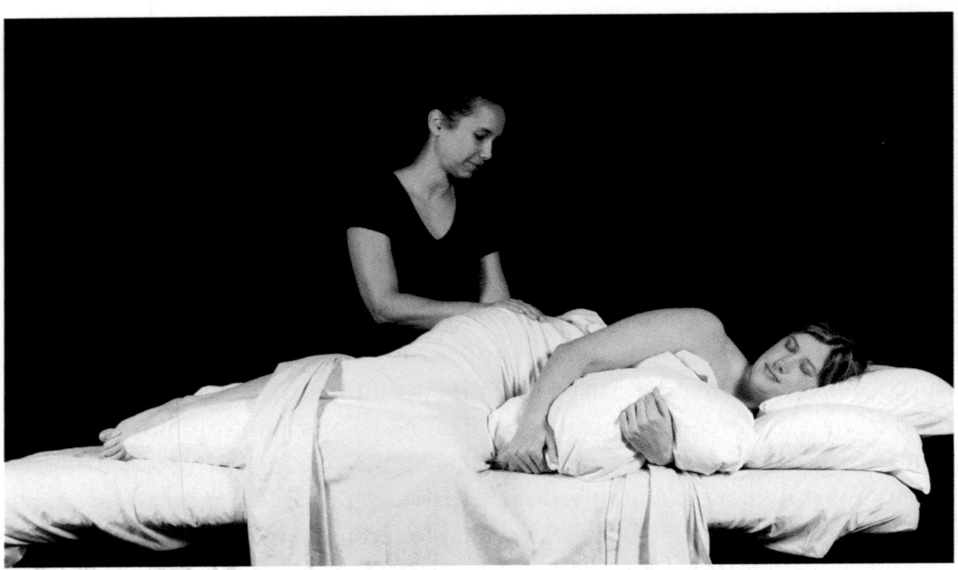

FIGURE 19-5 Massage of the lower back offers welcome relief.

massage is restricted to very light effleurage during the second and third trimester. Avoid all abdominal massage in the first trimester.

The added weight and reduced activity that accompany pregnancy often result in fatigue and minor swelling in the legs and feet. Regular, gentle massage of the feet and legs helps to reduce the fatigue and swelling. If edema is minimal, it is acceptable to massage (effleurage or lymph massage) the legs and arms. If the edema is serious, massage should not be done, and the client should be referred to her physician.

Be present to assist the client onto the table and into a comfortable position. A step stool is helpful for the client to get onto and off the table easily. Have lots of bolsters and pillows handy to provide comfortable positioning. A bathroom and robe should be easily accessible because the growing fetus tends to press on the mother's bladder, prompting frequent and urgent urination. Plan on a relatively short massage. Most pregnant women cannot remain comfortable lying down for more than 45 or 50 minutes, although some enjoy a 90-minute massage. Women often comment on how pleasant and soothing they find massage to be during pregnancy because of its calming and reassuring effects.

Contraindications for Prenatal Massage

There are some special considerations when performing massage on a pregnant woman. Pregnant women should receive permission from their doctors or maternity specialists before receiving prenatal massage. Before beginning a prenatal massage, ask the expectant mother whether there is any reason why massage would not be advisable. Massage is contraindicated when the woman is experiencing morning sickness, nausea, or diarrhea, or has any vaginal discharge or bleeding. High blood pressure, excessive swelling in the arms or legs, abdominal pain, or a decrease in fetal movement are contraindications for massage and warning signs for immediate referral to a physician. High blood pressure and excess edema are contraindications, and patients with these conditions should be referred to a physician. *Preeclampsia*, a type of toxemia, is a condition sometimes occurring in the latter half of pregnancy and is characterized by high blood pressure, edema (swelling of hands, feet, and face), and sodium retention. Indications of this condition include excessive weight gain or protein in the urine. The expectant mother sometimes suffers headaches and dizziness and, in serious cases, convulsions. When toxemia is suspected, the expectant mother should see her physician without delay.

Varicose veins are often a problem during pregnancy owing to the effects of progesterone and relaxin on the blood vessels and to the increased pressure on the main blood vessels that return blood from the legs. Light effleurage can be done around, but not on, affected areas.

Pregnancy increases the chance of deep vein thrombosis (DVT) especially in the legs, because of hormonal changes that increase blood **coagulability**. DVT in previous pregnancies increases the risk of their occurring again. DVT symptoms include pain and swelling at the blood clot's location. Blood clots also can cause redness and tenderness around the site. Owing to the possibility of DVT, deep or heavy massage on the legs is avoided during pregnancy. If signs of DVT are present, refer the client to the doctor.

coagulability

a measure of the bloods ability to coagulate.

If there are any other health concerns, obtain permission and a recommendation from the woman's maternity health care provider before providing massage services. During pregnancy, do not give massages when contraindications are present. Problems can occur during pregnancy, and the expectant mother should be under her physician's care regarding diet, exercise, and massage. Many physicians do recommend massage for its therapeutic effects during pregnancy, however.

Maternal Concerns by Trimester

The length of a normal human pregnancy is approximately 40 weeks. Physical changes that the mother experiences and the development of the fetus are continuous throughout the pregnancy; however, for the sake of discussion, the term of the pregnancy is divided into three trimesters, each being about 13 weeks in length. During each trimester, there are unique concerns for the mother and special considerations for providing massage.

First Trimester (Weeks 1–13)

Early in the first trimester, the woman might not know she is pregnant although hormonal changes are already happening. About a week after fertilization, the embryo embeds in the wall of the uterus. Hormonal changes cause the breasts to enlarge and become tender or sensitive. Often the woman experiences nausea (especially in the morning, but sometimes throughout the day), mood swings, fatigue, and sensitivity to certain tastes or smells.

During the first trimester, the mother is at a higher risk of having a miscarriage, which is a natural termination of the pregnancy before the fetus has reached viability. Because of this, many suggest that a woman should not receive massage during the first trimester. Generally, healthy women during a low-risk pregnancy enjoy and benefit from massage throughout the pregnancy. If there are conditions and factors that increase the risk of complications, massage should be postponed until written permission is obtained from the client's doctor or maternity specialist. High-risk factors include

- Mother's age under 20 and more than 35 years (some sources specify under 17 and more than 40 years)
- Complications in previous pregnancies
- Previous spontaneous abortions (miscarriages)
- Multiple gestation (twins or triplets)
- Maternal illnesses: diabetes mellitus; chronic hypertension; cardiac, renal, connective tissue, or liver disorders
- Rh-negative mother, or genetic problems, including diethylstilbestrol (DES) exposure, and other uterine abnormalities
- Fetal genetic disorders
- Drug or other hazardous materials exposure (Osbourne-Sheets, 1998, p. 50)

Massage Considerations for the First Trimester

Provide massage to a pregnant woman only after she has received permission from her doctor or midwife. Positioning considerations during the first trimester are minimal. Supine and prone positions are suitable as long as the client is comfortable. Sometimes a woman's breasts are too tender for her to be comfortable in a prone position, so make accommodations by using special bolsters with breast recesses or using a side-lying position. Avoid all abdominal massage or stimulation of any reflex points on the ankles, legs, or feet that relate to the uterus or reproductive organs. If the client is experiencing nausea or morning sickness, schedule the massage at a time of day when those symptoms are minimal, and avoid any rhythmic, rocking movements that might exacerbate the nausea. Focus on techniques to reduce stress and relieve fatigue and nausea. Areas to work on include the upper back, shoulders, lower back, and legs.

Second Trimester (Weeks 14–26)

In the second trimester, the fetus grows from about three inches long to about twelve inches, and the mother begins to "show" as her abdomen begins to protrude. By around week 20 to 22, the mother begins to feel the baby move. As the uterus grows, connective tissues are stretched to their limits or beyond, and stretch marks begin to appear. The growing uterus often puts pressure on the blood and lymph vessels in the abdomen, resulting in swelling (edema) in the legs and ankles. The body also starts to produce the hormone relaxin, which softens the connective tissues in the pelvis in preparation for the delivery of the baby. Relaxin also softens ligaments in other joints of the body, and so the massage therapist must use caution when performing range of motion (ROM) exercises to avoid overstretching the tissues. During the second trimester, as the fetus grows, the mother's body undergoes more changes, with weight gain and a shift in the center of gravity. As her abdomen grows, the mother can begin to experience back, pelvic, hip or leg pain and constipation and heartburn.

Massage Considerations for the Second Trimester

The continuing development of the fetus and the accompanying growth of the abdomen during the second trimester present some concerns for positioning and bolstering for the comfort of the client and the safety of the baby. During the early part of the second trimester, the supine position can be used; however, after about the 20th week, the uterus has grown large enough that it can put pressure on the major blood and lymph vessels in the abdomen, and use of the supine position should be limited to no more than 10 to 15 minutes. A safer supine alternative is to use a semi-reclining position, where pillows, a foam wedge, or a back jack is used so that the pregnant woman's head, shoulders, and torso are elevated at a 45- to 70-degree angle. Another bolster is placed under the knees.

Another option is to place the expectant mother in the *left lateral tilt position* by placing a small bolster under the right shoulder and hip. This allows the fetus to shift to the left enough so that the fetus does not press against the abdominal vena cava and aorta. This reduces the chance of cutting off circulation to the placenta while maintaining a comfortable position for the client in an adjusted supine position.

Because of her protruding abdomen and often very tender breasts, the prone position is not recommended during the second trimester, unless special bolstering such as a Preg-pillow or a Body Support System is used to remove pressure on the breasts and uterus. A well-bolstered side-lying position that provides good access to the neck, back, and legs without putting undue pressure on the breasts or uterus is preferred. Provide adequate support for the neck and head so that the cervical spine is aligned with the thorax and the lower shoulder is comfortable without excess pressure from the weight of the torso. Extend the bottom leg and provide enough pillows or bolsters under the bent upper leg to maintain a horizontal line between the hip, knee, and ankle. Provide a small pillow or bolster under the abdomen to support the uterus and another pillow for the client to hug to support the upper arm. This semi-fetal position is very comfortable for a pregnant woman at any stage of her pregnancy because it allows her to relax and talk while the therapist has easy access to most parts of her body.

During the second trimester, areas of the body to massage include the neck, shoulders, and upper back to relieve stress. The lower back and hips are beginning to feel the extra strain from the weight changes and benefit from massage. Light circulatory or lymphatic massage to the feet and legs is relaxing and helps to relieve some of the swelling that often accompanies pregnancy. Watch for varicose and spider veins, and avoid all but the lightest massage where they are present. Check for varicose veins before the client lies down because they are more visible during weight bearing. The presence of varicose veins increases the possibility of asymptomatic deep vein thrombosis (DVT) or blood clots in the legs. Because of the increased possibility of DVT during pregnancy, avoid any deep massage of the legs, especially on the medial side of the calf or thigh. Use only the lightest effleurage and never any deep techniques on the abdomen.

The Third Trimester (Weeks 27–40+, birth)

During the third and final trimester of pregnancy, the uterus continues to grow as the baby doubles in length to approximately 20 inches and triples in weight to an average of 7.5 lbs. As fetal growth continues, the mother's weight increases and shifts anteriorly, often resulting in discomfort from musculoskeletal strain through the back, pelvis, and legs as well as the neck and shoulders. The uterus can grow large enough to reach the rib cage and put pressure on several anatomic structures, resulting in a variety of discomforts:

- Pressure against the diaphragm causes shortness of breath and/or hyperventilation.
- Pressure on the stomach and intestines causes heartburn, constipation, and hemorrhoids.
- Pressure on the bladder causes frequent urination.
- Pressure on the deep lymph vessels increases edema in the legs.
- Pressure on the deep blood vessels increases the likelihood of varicose veins.
- Pressure on various nerves can cause burning, tingling, or numbness.
- Pressure against the abdominal muscles causes the connective tissue of the linea alba to separate (diastus recti) to allow more room for the fetus.
- Sometimes, owing to pressure from the fetus and the effects of the hormone relaxin, the symphysis pubis separates.

Late in the third trimester, the baby will "drop" head down into the pelvis in preparation for the birth. The mother probably begins to experience mild, irregular practice contractions (Braxton-Hicks) as the uterine muscles tense for short periods, signaling the imminent arrival of the newborn. Labor actually begins when the contractions become more regular, last for 30 seconds or longer, and continue long enough to push against and begin to dilate the cervix.

Massage Considerations during the Third Trimester

Positioning of the client during the third trimester of pregnancy requires consideration for the comfort of the mother and safety of the baby. Use of the supine position, even for a short while, creates a risk of reduced blood flow to the fetus and should be avoided. Likewise, avoid the prone position because it creates excess inter-uterine pressure on the developing fetus.

A semi-reclining position, with the head and shoulders elevated 40 to 70 degrees and a bolster under the knees, is safe and comfortable. Because many women assume this position during labor and delivery, it is helpful for her to become accustomed to being relaxed in this position. A well-bolstered side-lying position is preferred for the comfort of the client, safety of the fetus, and the ease of application of massage to most of the body.

Massage during the third trimester should focus on relaxation. The goal is to reduce anxiety and stress and relieve the strain on weight-bearing joints and muscles associated with increased weight. The lower back, hips, upper torso, shoulders, and neck benefit from the relief of tension. The arms, legs, and feet often experience increased fluid retention (edema) and benefit from circulatory and lymph massage. As explained earlier, when varicose veins are present, use only the lightest techniques to encourage circulation. Use only light circulatory and lymph massage on the medial legs or thighs as a precaution in case of the presence of DVTs. Avoid deep pressure on the acupressure points on the outside of the foot or inside the leg (three inches above the medial malleolus), which stimulate uterine activity. In the third trimester, the stretched muscles and skin of the abdomen can benefit from superficial effleurage. The baby might respond by moving or kicking. All deep massage to the abdomen and legs is contraindicated.

Massage During Labor

A physician might recommend light effleurage on the patient's abdomen and upper legs as a means of obtaining relief between contractions. Lower back pains can also be relieved by the application of firm continuous pressure. During a contraction, pressure can be applied to both sides of the spine in the area of the sacrum.

Massage Following Birth

Mothers request massage throughout pregnancy and after childbirth. As soon as the mother receives permission from her doctor or midwife following birth, a massage can be beneficial. In the first six to eight weeks after the birth, the new mother's body is going through many changes, and the emphasis of the massage should be on relaxation. Massage helps to relieve neck, shoulder, and lower back discomfort and is an aid in the relief of tension. When combined with proper exercise and diet, massage can be of value in regaining normal weight and firming slack muscles.

INFANT MASSAGE

Infant massage has been documented as a cultural activity in families, passed down from mother to daughter for centuries. From Bali to Nigeria, mothers have taught their daughters traditional massage routines that nourish infants throughout the world. In 1976, Fredrick Leboyer, author of *Birth Without Violence*, published *Loving Hands*, which documents the flowing rhythms of the traditional Indian art of baby massage, bringing this art and practice to a global awareness. He describes it as "a silent dialogue of love between a mother and her baby. Some kind of ritual or ballet-slowness, controlled strength, tenderness, and dignity."

As a young woman on a quest to India in 1973, Vimala Schneider McClure witnessed infant massage, but little did she know it would shape many years of her life. On returning to the United States, she developed a more active form of this massage, wrote a small booklet in the mid-1970s, and later authored *Infant Massage, A Handbook for Loving Parents*. She helped to initiate the formation of the International Association of Infant Massage Instructors, which co-owns Certified Infant Massage Instructor (CIMI).

After becoming a licensed massage therapist in 1976, Diana Moore started working with young families just as her grandmother, also a massage therapist, had done before her. She met McClure in 1980 and trained to instruct people in infant massage. As the first official director of the International Infant Massage Instructors Association, she helped to make infant massage more professional. In 1992, Diana incorporated the International Loving Touch Foundation, reaching out to train professionals internationally, including those in the orphanages of Romania, as caregivers who work with institutionalized children and infants. Now social workers, pediatric occupational therapists, pediatric physical therapists, child life specialists, pediatric nurses, and massage therapists are being trained to teach parents this simple and effective massage to add to their skill tool boxes for parenting and receive CIMI credentials. In 2007, the State of Oregon Health Addictions and Mental Health Division added infant massage as an evidence-based practice preventive program for parents and professionals, another step in establishing the benefits of infant massage.

Tiffany Field, PhD, is the undisputed master of touch research. In 1992, she received funds from Johnson & Johnson Company to establish the Touch Research Institute at the University of Miami. Ground-breaking research supporting massage of preterm neonates started substantiating the benefits of infant massage in 1995. Numerous studies at the Touch Research Institute and other venues from 1995 to the present have substantiated the value of infant massage for the infant and the caregiver. It was during one of the Touch Research Institutes studies that it was established that the pressure must be firm to effect the touch receptors, and that infants in the neonatal intensive care unit (NICU) nursery would actually gain weight and go home earlier because massage stimulated the vagus nerve and release of food absorption hormones.

Since the breakthrough by the pioneers in touch with infants in the 1970s, several other professionals have contributed to the development of infant massage. They are too numerous to mention; however, many children in this world have benefited from all who instruct caregivers in this simple and effective loving touch.

A debatable topic among infant massage instructors is who is best suited to actually administer infant massage. Generally speaking, massage students want to perform the massage; after all, what massage therapist would not want to massage an adorable newborn? With **bonding** being the most important benefit and being reciprocal for both the **primary caregiver** and the infant, however, the massage therapist must consider her own motives. Are you providing tools to primary caregivers to help aid in the daily care routines for the infant? Are there specialized techniques in which you are trained that must be done by the therapist alone? After reading *The Vital Touch* by developmental psychologist Sharon Heller, one will undoubtedly be convinced that the parent or primary caregiver should be the one sharing in the nourishing touch with the newborn. Only when advanced techniques are used or the parent is unavailable should those outside the family unit engage in the massage activity. The **skinship** that is formed between the newborn and the caregiver has the power of cementing the relationship not only a lifetime but also for generations. Some studies done by the Touch Research Institute trained volunteer senior citizens to administer the massage. Not only did the infants benefit, but the seniors were noted to suffer from less depression, drink less coffee, and also felt a connection to the infants.

Bonding

a unique relationship between two people that is specific and endures through time.

Primary caregiver

a person or persons whose responsibility is rearing the child. This might be a parent, grandparent, adoptive parent, or a nanny.

Skinship

the sensitivity to communicate through the skin. A parent who forms this might be aware of the infant's body tension, heart rate, and movement of the digestive system, which cues an awareness of hunger.

The International Loving Touch Foundation recommends that the massage instructor use a life-sized doll (typically close to the size of the infant; if the infant is premature, a 12- to 18-inch doll; for full-term infants, a 23-inch doll with a soft body) to demonstrate the strokes and have the parents follow along on their infants (Figure 19-6). The reasons for use of the demonstrative doll-teaching technique is to create confidence in parenting, and to monitor appropriate skills as well as the use of firm but gentle pressure.

Two massage routines are commonly taught, a simple routine for premature and the newborn infants, and a more active routine for 6- to 8-week old and older infants. Both of these routines can be taught to the primary caregiver by a certified instructor.

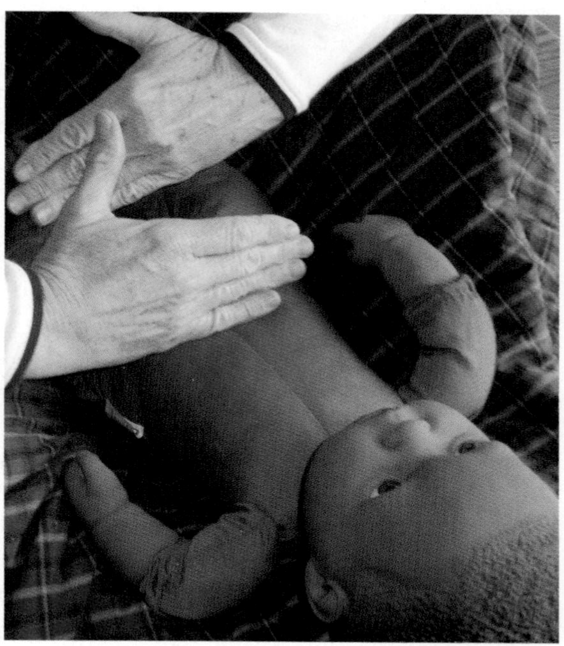

FIGURE 19-6 An infant-sized doll is used to demonstrate the massage while the mother follows along on her infant.

Benefits

- Bonding: creation of a close relationship that endures through time. A parent who is taught to touch in a loving caring way is less likely to touch abusively.
- Relief of tension and pain: Humans are one of the mammals that require total care as infants.
- Stimulation of several body systems such as circulation and the digestive system (specifically gas, constipation, colic), the immune system, and hormones.
- Relaxation.

Contraindications

The parent or caregiver should consult the infant's physician if there are any medical problems that raise any concerns. Instructors have an opportunity to see infants and should be familiar with normal infant development, referring the family to appropriate sources if developmental delays or other medical issues are observed. Massage is stimulation to the largest sensory organ of the body. Sometimes the baby can become easily overstimulated, and so the pace might need to be slowed down and stationary touch used. The baby's cues as to his willingness to engage in the massage must be honored. In most cases, the contraindications for infant massage are the same as for adult massage.

Communication

The baby must be willing to engage in the massage. This is not something done *to* an infant, but something done *with* them. We ask for permission. Get the infant's attention by gently cradling the head, making eye contact, and verbally asking permission to massage: "Would you like a massage?" Then look for signs of engagement.

- Signs of Engagement: Eye-to-eye contact, cooing, smiling, alert connection.

- Signs of Disengagement: Looking away (gaze aversion), frowning, fussing, crying, sleeping, coughing.

Choosing a Massage Lubricant

When choosing a massage lubricant for infant massage, keep it simple, one type of oil, no blends. Acceptable choices are sweet almond oil, grape seed oil, or olive oil. After the infant's hands or feet are massaged, they might end up in the baby's mouth, and so it is important to use an edible, food-grade oil. It is better not to use fragrances or scents, because infants and parents bond through smell. To test for an allergy to the oil, dab a small amount on infant's interior wrist and wait 15 minutes. If there is any reaction, choose a different lubricant.

Where to Massage

It is preferable to do the infant massage on a blanket on the floor, where infants are safe. Newborns usually do best in a nest of pillows, slightly elevating the head and torso. An infant might roll or fall off of a massage table. The room should be quiet and warm (75 °F) because infants chill quickly and do not have the ability to warm up easily.

Well Baby Active Massage Routine

Massage for babies six weeks and older can be an eclectic mix of Swedish, Asian, reflexology, and conditioned relaxation response (CRR). The Asian strokes initiate the routine to relax the baby's tense arms and legs, which have a tendency to curl into a fetal tuck. The Asian strokes are performed proximal to distal on the arms and legs to drain tension and stress from the body. Swedish strokes, including effleurage or gliding, petrissage, friction, and percussion, are also incorporated into the routine. Basic reflexology can be administered to the feet. A fun stroke that catches the baby's attention is a simple gliding stroke, called the *airplane runway*, that glides off of the body to end in the air. Typically, massage to each part of the body is completed with the Asian or the CRR to drain tension away from the body. In this playful routine, most parents learn the cute names given to strokes, helping create a joyful, playful interaction.

A full-body well-baby routine generally lasts about 20 minutes, or as long as the infant is willing to engage. The infant first must become accustomed to being touched. Typically, a baby can tolerate 5 to10 minutes, perhaps (if you are lucky) 20 minutes. Because an infant's nervous system can be sensitive, the massage should start slowly on the legs, which are usually less sensitive. Primary caregivers are encouraged to pick up their infants and attend to their needs

Conditioned Relaxation Response

Infants have a tendency to stay in a fetal tuck, in which their arms and legs are tucked into their body. Gently using jostling or tapping of the triceps helps to initiate relaxation of the arm. Verbal cuing by saying, "relax your arm" allows the baby to learn to relax at a young age. As they do relax, respond with positive reinforcement.

When Massage Does Not Work

Infants are unpredictable, and sometimes more active touch does not work. When all else fails, stationary touch provides warmth and comfort. Allow the hand to sink in, providing a comforting touch.

when appropriate. Unlike a mature adult, infants do not always participate in a full massage.

Simplified Routine

The simplified routine developed for preterm infants, as well as newborn to six-week-old babies is gentle, firm, and slow gliding with range of motion (ROM). The Touch Research Institute has developed a very basic routine that typically can be performed in 15 minutes at a very slow pace. It begins with the infant prone, working from the head down to the ankles. The baby is then turned face-up, and a slow-paced ROM of the legs and arms is performed. The infant is returned to the prone position and receives more slow-paced gliding strokes. This routine helps the infant to become accustomed to receiving touch so that, as they grow, they become more comfortable with a more active routine.

Well-baby Massage Routine

With the infant in a supine position, without lubricant, cradle the baby's head and ask for permission to begin the massage. When permission is given, proceed to rub your hands together with oil, and cue the baby that the massage is about to begin.

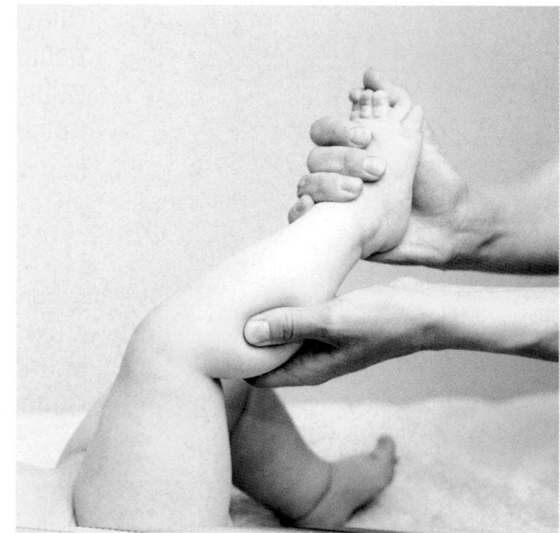

FIGURE 19-7 Gliding and friction on the leg from the hip to the ankle.

Lower Extremities: Supine Position

Typically apply three passes of the stroke or as tolerated.

1. Gliding-proximal from hip to ankle, alternating hands (Figure 19-7)
2. Wringing friction of leg
3. Circular friction in a fanning motion with thumbs on the plantar surface of foot
4. Digital petrissage to toes
5. Gliding on the plantar surface of the foot from heel to toes with visual airplane cues
6. ROM for ankle
7. Circular friction to dorsal surface of foot
8. Effleurage of leg, distal to proximal
9. Rolling friction of leg
10. Superficial gliding
11. Jostling friction with verbal CCR

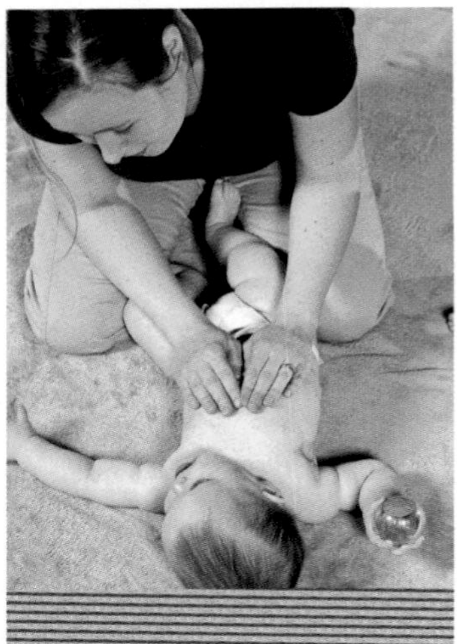

FIGURE 19-8 Gliding strokes from the rib cage to the pelvis.

Supine Torso

1. Joint movement and rocking of sacrum to reposition the infant and loosen abdominal muscles
2. Petrissage with paddling hands from under rib cage to pubic bone
3. Petrissage clockwise starting in lower left abdominal quadrant (hands of the clock), following the movement of the large intestine
4. Petrissage: "I Love You." This traces the descending colon, then the transverse/descending colon, then the U is formed with ascending/transverse/descending colon5. Digital fulling – using the pads of the fingers to walk across the abdomen left to right
6. Passive joint movement – knees to abdomen, hold three to five seconds
7. Stationary touch of abdomen, which can turn into gentle rocking (Figure 19-8)
8. Effleurage of chest midline to lateral, with palmer surface of the hands, changing into a heart-shaped stroke that encompasses the shoulders
9. Effleurage – hip to opposite shoulder, hands alternating in a slow rhythmic movement

Arms

1. Jostling friction on triceps with verbal CCR (allows arm to unfold from fetal tuck)
2. Circular friction – gently in armpit for lymph drainage
3. Gliding – proximal to distal with alternating hands
4. Wringing friction
5. Gliding of palmer surface of hand with verbal airplane runway cuing
6. Rolling petrissage of each digit
7. Gliding of dorsal hand to wrist
8. Effleurage of arm
9. Superficial effleurage of arm proximal to distal

Head and Face

Note that head and face can be sensitive. If the infant does not like it at first, go slowly, or use just stationary touch (no oil necessary).

1. Stationary touch by cradling head
2. Gliding on forehead following hairline, midline to temples

Colic/Gas/Constipation Routine

Repeat sequence three times; this can be done several times a day.

Petrissage paddling

Knee to abdomen passive joint movement

Petrissage clockwise (I-love-you stroke)

3. Gliding from inner canthi; tear ducts across eyelids
4. Circular friction of tear duct area
5. Glide midline from bridge of nose across cheeks to temples, and continue down below nose across cheeks
6. Glide, making a smile on the upper lip and lower lip
7. Circular friction with finger pads following above the jaw line then below the jaw line
8. Small circular friction of the ears then the scalp

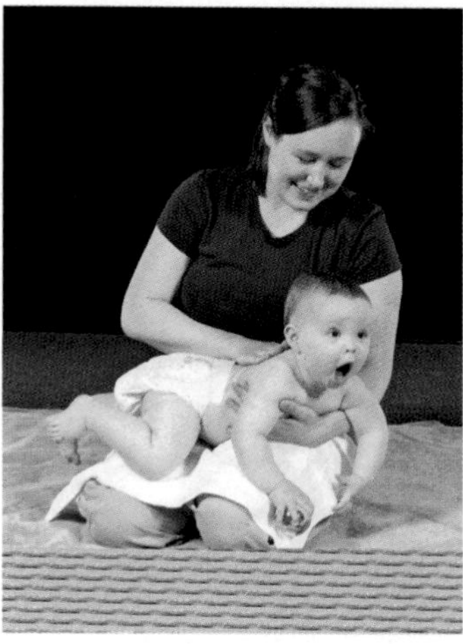

FIGURE 19-9 The baby lies across the lap for a soothing back massage.

Prone Position

Place the infant across the lap (Figure 19-9) or simply prone on the blanket.

Back

1. Effleurage from shoulders to buttocks
2. Wringing friction with alternating hands
3. Effleurage sweeping: Place one hand stationary on the lower buttocks for a gentle hold while the other hand sweeps from shoulder to buttocks
4. Circular friction of the erector spinae muscles
5. Petrissage of the larger muscles of the back
6. Effleurage superficial from head to toe. Hold the ankles in one hand while sweeping with the other
7. Vibration percussion of the back from shoulders to buttocks

Stretching

The baby is now dressed for this and supine.

1. Joint movement of arms – alternating arms across the chest with gentle traction

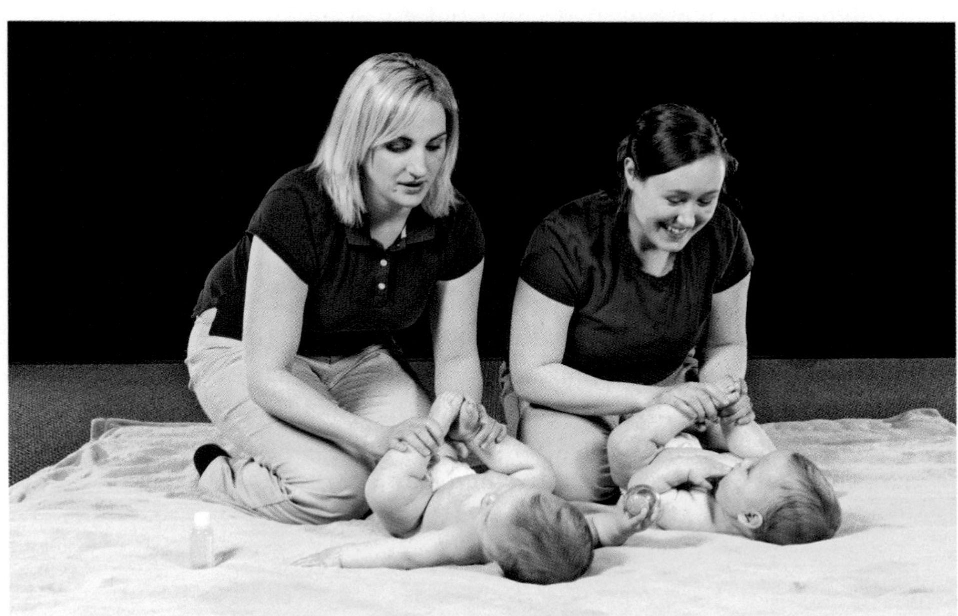

FIGURE 19-10 Passive joint movements of the knees to the chest can be done simultaneously or alternately.

2. Joint movement of appendages – opposite leg and arm stretching to midline to touch toes to hand
3. Passive joint movement, knees to abdomen; hold three to five seconds. This can turn into a run or walk movement of the legs (Figure 19-10)

Becoming an Instructor

Accredited continuing education classes for becoming a certified infant massage instructor (CIMI) are taught in a 2- to 4-day workshop format. Infant massage is a simple routine; however, working with parents and children takes a special background in communication, child development, and patience. It sounds easy to teach such a simple loving routine, but infants do not always cooperate, nor do they operate on a set schedule. The instructor must be adaptable to chaos and scheduling owing to the nature of the unpredictability of the new family. When investing your time, talent, and energy in any training, make sure that the trainer has a professional background in fields related to child development and touch therapies. The International Loving Touch Foundation offers 2- to 3-day workshops to become an instructor with a required take-home examination and teaching component to become a CIMI.

CHILDREN

Providing massage to children is not much different from providing it to adults. Most children enjoy physical touch. In fact, many parents massage their children to help them relax and fall asleep. Depending on the child's age and temperament, his attention span can be less than that of an adult. Typically, the younger they are, the shorter their attention span, although it does differ from child to child. The length of the massage should be adjusted accordingly. Children's bodies change quickly and drastically, and they are prone to growing pains. Their bone density is usually much lower, which allows fractures to occur more often. Children are fairly resilient but are prone to more illness as their immunity develops. Just as it is not appropriate to massage an adult with an illness such as a cold, it is equally so for children. Children often have higher fevers than adults, and fever is always a contraindication for massage. Because of the many changes and growth in children, sleep patterns are often associated with these changes. Regular massage can actually help with these sleep disturbances. Growth patterns during adolescence, especially during puberty, sometimes lead to discomfort with the body or a negative body image. Careful consideration in regard to this is highly important, and it might therefore be wise to massage some children through clothing. Another extremely important aspect in working with children is to notice any signs of abuse, such as bite marks, unusual scratches, burns, or bruises that might need to be addressed. (Reporting suspected child abuse to the proper authorities is required by law.) It is also important when working with children under the age of 18 years to always have a parent or guardian in the room while the massage is being performed (Figure 19-11) and to have a written consent to massage the child signed by the parent or guardian.

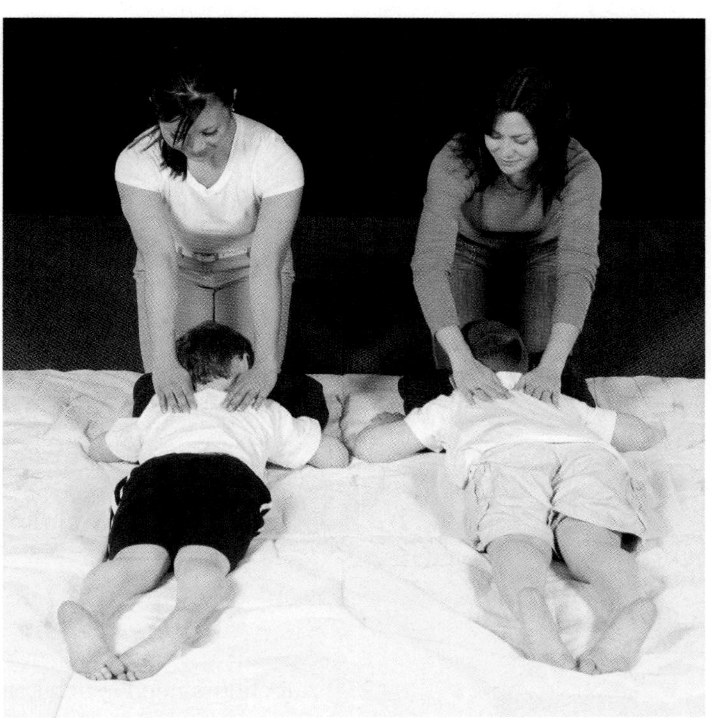

FIGURE 19-11 When a therapist is working with children, a parent or guardian must be present.

ELDERLY CLIENTS

In working with elderly clients (persons older than 65–70 years), it is important to determine if the client is robust (able to function normally and has a great deal of vitality) or frail (unable to function normally, has limited vitality, and often has age-associated illnesses). Sometimes older people are more robust than those who are younger. Chronological age may not be as good a determiner as physiologic age. Some 90-year-olds are in better health than some 70-year-olds.

Benefits to Massaging Elders

The benefits to working with elderly clients can be the same as with younger adults. Additionally massage can alleviate or partially alleviate age-related discomforts, assist in preventing illness from occurring, and possibly slow the aging process.

Some benefits of massage for older clients include:

- improving mobility, strength and flexibility
- improving the abilities to perform activities of daily living such as dressing, bathing, or climbing stairs
- increasing independence

Abdominal massage can help alleviate digestive problems such as indigestion and constipation. Massage helps to ease the anxiety associated with the aging process and helps to provide a social connection with others if loss of friends and family has occurred. As with any client, make sure an extensive client interview is done before performing the massage to ensure that there are no contraindications.

The Robust Older Client

There are fewer limitations and precautions for massaging older clients that are physiologically younger than massaging those who are frail; however, some precautions are still present and should be considered. Use extra pillows and bolsters to ensure the most comfort because lying on a massage table might be more uncomfortable. Limit the time that the client is face down to no longer than 15 to 20 minutes, because breathing can be a little more difficult. Clients might need help sitting up after the massage; make sure that the client is not lightheaded before leaving the massage room. You might not be able to work as deeply as with a younger client.

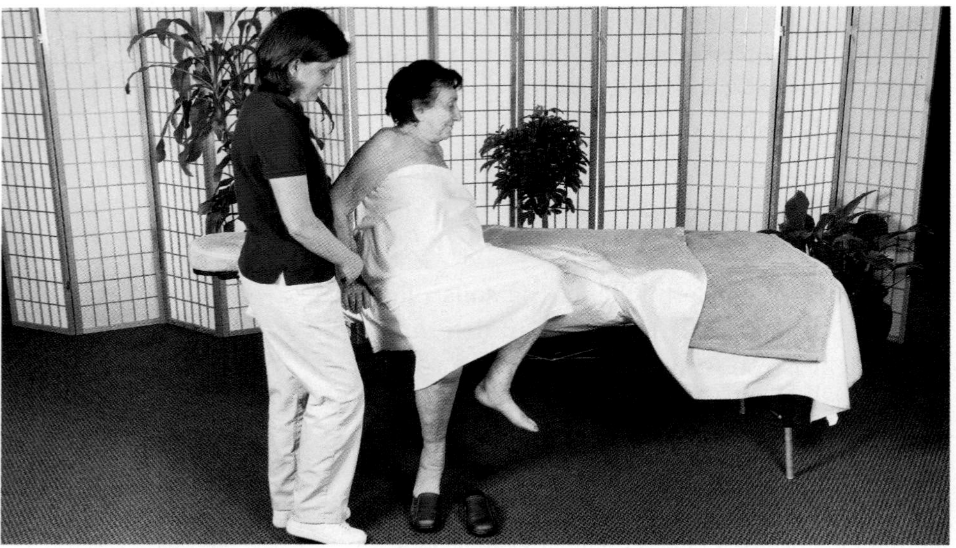

FIGURE 19-12 Working with elderly clients has many benefits for both the therapist and the client.

The Frail Older Client

Frail clients need special care and can be fragile to the touch. Their tissues can be more delicate and susceptible to bruising, and their skin can also be paper thin and more easily damaged. They might need assistance getting on and off the table (Figure 19-12) and with undressing and dressing. Be sure to ask if they need assistance. Some might simply need assistance fastening a bra or tying their shoes. They might need help turning over. Because often it is not wise to have older people lying face down, a side-lying position can be used for comfort and safety. You might need to massage an older client in his own bed (when doing home care) or work with him while he is seated in a chair. Use special care when doing ROM, and avoid excessive movements, especially if osteoporosis is present. Abbreviate the session to avoid fatiguing the client. Modifying the massage and using more stationary touch with light pressure instead of gliding strokes might be preferable (see www.comforttouch.com).

Most seniors with health concerns are under the care of one or more physicians and might be using several medications. Be sure to take a thorough medical history. The client may need assistance in filling out documents. Consider the medications that a client is using and any age-related conditions when choosing techniques, and check with the client's primary caregiver if in doubt. Remember, it is better to do too little than too to do much.

CLIENTS WITH DISABILITIES

There are special implications for working with clients who have varying types of disabilities. Some disabilities contribute to the client's ability to navigate the massage environment either from physical mobility limitations or from other impairments, such as blindness. In most cases, the actual massage is not so very different, but because of the disability, some accommodations should be made for the safety and comfort of the client. Some implications impede the ability to perform client intake or provide feedback during the massage. When working with people with disabilities, it is important to ask if they need assistance; do not just assume that they do. Different types of disabilities require different accommodations to provide the most effective massage therapy session.

Auditory Impairment

Clients can have complete or partial deafness that is either congenital or has developed from injury, illness, or the ageing process. Because the client might be able to read lips, speak slowly, face the client when speaking, and do not talk loudly unless they are partially deaf. It might also be a good idea to have paper and a writing utensil to communicate, especially during the client intake interview and during and after the massage session. If the client uses a hearing aid, avoid putting your hands too close to it during the massage as this can cause the device to squeal.

Massage considerations:

- Point to areas where clients can place clothing. Gesture how to get on the table and under the sheets.
- Be sure to read nonverbal cues, such as twitching, holding of breath, or moaning, and be ready to modify the massage. Asking the client about depth of pressure and other things might be difficult.
- To get a client's attention, tap him on the arm or shoulder.
- You might want to set up hand gestures with your client to reinforce communication before beginning the massage.
- Maintain contact throughout the massage (Ochsner, 2009).

Visual Impairment

Clients might have complete or partial blindness that is either congenital or has developed from injury or degenerative illness. Clients who are blind might have a service dog with them; therefore make sure that there is room to accommodate the dog. Companion dogs are working when in harness. Always ask the client for permission before interacting with the animal, so as not to distract it from its duty. If the blind client uses a cane, ask if you may guide them into the massage room. Offer the client an arm to rest her hand on as you lead her through the facility. Walk beside and slightly in front, while steering clear of any obstacles. Once the client is on the table, the massage can proceed normally, addressing stress or soft tissue conditions.

Massage Considerations:

- Help guide the client safely to the massage room.
- Be sure to help guide them up stairs or around doors and furniture.
- Help client fill out intake form and ask more detailed questions.
- Help client be aware of his surroundings, where he can place clothing, and where the table and linens are placed.
- Be sure to maintain contact during the massage (Ochsner, 2009).

Limited Mobility

Any number of factors can limit mobility, such as injury, illness, pain, paralysis, or weakness. The client might be using crutches, a walker, a cane, or a wheelchair and might need some assistance navigating the massage room and getting on and off of the massage table. Make sure that there is adequate wheelchair access or limited mobility access to your place of business. If the massage facility is not wheelchair accessible, it might be better to go to the client's home or a mutually agreed-on accessible establishment. Also make sure that the table is the appropriate height for a client who is paralyzed or has limited mobility so that he can safely (both to the client and the therapist) be helped on and off the massage table. Ask if any help is needed and how you can best provide any assistance they request. An electric or hydraulic lift table that lowers to chair height is a great advantage because it allows the client with mobility impairments to get onto the table easily. A person using a walker can simply sit down on the table, and a person using a wheelchair can more easily transfer onto the table. The table can then be raised to the proper height for the practitioner.

A person can experience limited mobility for a wide variety of reasons that can be explained more fully during the intake and medical history procedure. The massage can be designed to address conditions that are directly related to the impairment, such as circulatory or movement restrictions. Mobility aids such as crutches, walkers, and wheelchairs cause excessive stress and compensation patterns in the hands, arms, shoulders, and neck that can be addressed during the massage.

Massage Considerations:

- Carefully offer to help only when a client asks to be helped.
- Help the client to move on and off the table and when turning over, if requested.
- Make sure to have mobility aids nearby for easier access when your client needs them (Ochsner, 2009).

Paralysis

Paralysis is usually due to an injury or illness that adversely affects the nervous system. The extent of the paralysis and the part of the body affected vary, depending on the type of illness or the site of the injury. A stroke or cerebral vascular accident resulting in paralysis on one side of the body is known as *hemiplegia*. Spinal cord injury is another common cause of paralysis. The extent of the paralysis depends on the level of the spinal cord that was injured. The higher or closer to the head that the injury is located, the more extensive is the paralysis. Injury to the cervical spinal cord results in *quadriplegia*, when all four limbs (arms and legs) are affected. Injuries to the thoracic or lumbar spine result in *paraplegia*, or paralysis to the legs and lower body. Spinal cord injuries are classified as *complete*, when there is no nerve transmission through the injury site, and *incomplete*, when some amount of sensory or motor nerve activity exists and there is some sense of feeling or movement below the level of the injury.

Working with people with paralysis requires some special consideration. People with paralysis usually use some sort of mobility aid, such as crutches, manual or electric wheelchairs, or scooters, depending on their level of function. To provide services to this population, the massage facility must be wheelchair accessible. Otherwise, the therapist can choose to go to the client's home or other facility that is accessible.

A determination must be made whether to transfer the client onto the massage table, work with him while he remains in the wheelchair, perform the massage with the client in bed, or make some other accommodation. The client may need assistance with the transfer to the massage table. Ask the client if he requires assistance and then follow his instructions if they seem within your ability and safety considerations. It might be helpful to lower the table close to the height of the wheelchair seat. A hydraulic or electric adjustable table works well in these situations; the client can easily get on the table and then the table can be raised to the correct height for the therapist to perform the massage comfortably. Once the client is on the table, use plenty of bolsters to support him in a position of comfort.

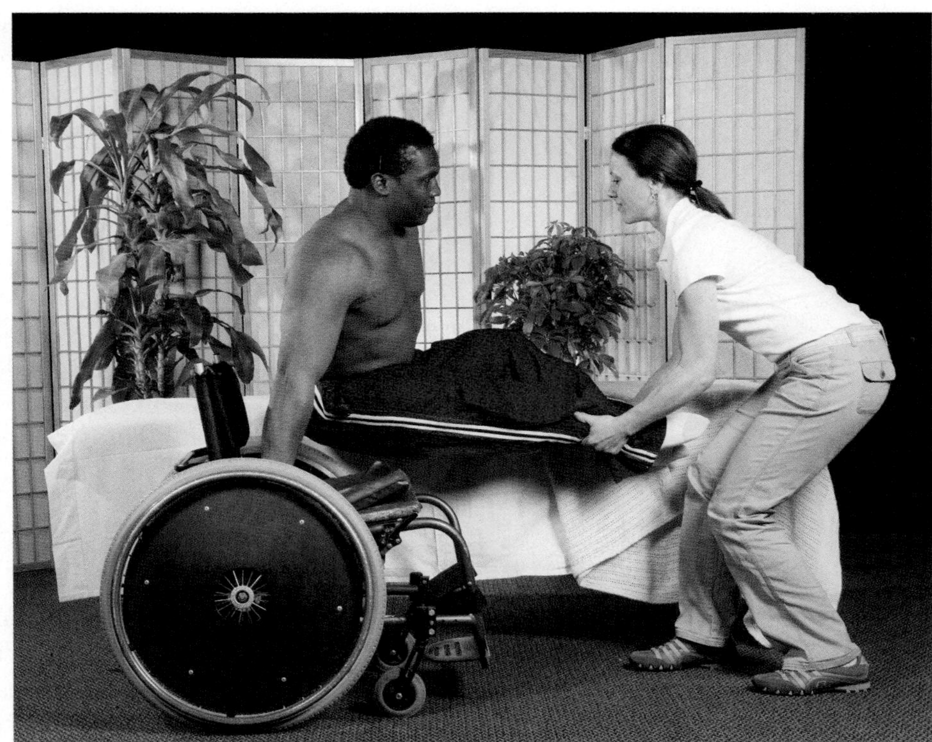

FIGURE 19-13 A client with paralysis might need assistance onto or off of the table. Ask the client if and how you may best assist them.

Massage for people with paralysis is very beneficial and deserves some special consideration. Paralysis usually affects only a portion of the body, limiting mobility and sensation. The rest of the body has relatively normal muscle and nerve activity, except that it can experience compensation patterns accompanied by tension or discomfort as a result of using mobility devises (wheelchairs or crutches) or adapting to life with paralysis. Because of compensating patterns from using mobility devices, a person with paralysis might have a sore back, shoulders, neck, and arms. Massage for the normal, nonparalyzed parts of the body is essentially the same as regular massage, concentrating on relaxation or addressing the tension created by the compensating movement patterns.

Massage to the paralyzed areas requires some caution. Paralysis is often accompanied by loss of sensation. Because the client cannot feel the paralyzed area, the therapist should avoid any deep techniques or excessive joint movements that might cause injury or pain.

Because of a lack of muscular activity and movement, circulation is compromised and connective tissue tends to stiffen, reducing flexibility. Long-term paralysis is often accompanied by muscle atrophy and joint stiffness, or even contractures. Gentle strokes that enhance lymphatic and venous circulation are beneficial. ROM techniques help to maintain flexibility but must be used with great caution.

Massage Considerations:

- Use care in helping client onto and off of the table (Figure 19-13) and turning over. Ask the client how best to assist them.
- If doing massage in the wheelchair, make sure that the wheel brakes are on.
- Be careful working on paralyzed extremities because of loss of feeling and delicate tissue.

- Do not perform massage if severe systemic symptoms are acute, especially respiratory failure or a compromised circulatory system.
- You might wish to do massage having the client in his own bed.
- Always work with client's physician.

Prosthetics or Amputees

A client might have lost a limb due to an injury or accident and might have been fitted with an artificial limb. The client might have been or is currently undergoing physical therapy. If so, working with their physical and/or occupational therapist can greatly enhance the client's ability and success with the prosthetic device. These clients can experience soreness at the prosthetic attachment or stump, might have sore muscles that have been compensating, or might have postural deviations.

Massage Considerations:

- Clients might (or might not) want to remove the prosthesis before or during massage.
- Ask permission if massage can be done to prosthetic attachment site (stump) and use care (it might be sore if recently fitted for a new prosthetic limb or might have limited sensation or numbness).
- Client might need help getting on and off the table and turning over.
- Client might have phantom pain that can be relieved through massage and can experience some reflex relief by working the **contralateral** limb (if it is present; Ochsner, 2009).

contralateral

referring to the body part on the opposite side of the body.

MASSAGE FOR THE CRITICALLY ILL

Massage is becoming a common part of preferred treatment with the critically ill patient. Many times, conditions are present that are normally contraindicated for massage; however, by making adjustments to the intent and delivery of the massage session, there literally are no contraindications for touch therapy. Depending on a person's condition, there are precautions and concerns as to how a massage should proceed.

Purpose

The intent of massage for the critically ill patient is to provide gentle and genuine caring touch therapy to bring comfort, pleasure, and relaxation to someone at a difficult time of life.

Benefits

- Helps to control discomfort and pain
- Improves mobility
- Helps reduce disorientation and confusion by bringing the person back to a more positive body awareness
- Reduces isolation and fear
- Helps to ease emotional and physical discomforts

- Allows the person to develop a more positive attitude about her situation or condition

Considerations and Precautions

As always, it is important for the practitioner to be conscious and aware of the client's needs. Conditions dictate how much can be done and which precautions should be used. When in doubt about how or whether to proceed because of a person's condition, always ask the client first. Generally, clients are very aware of any precautions concerning their condition. It is also important to communicate with the physician or the caregiver in charge. A critically ill person's physical and emotional condition is constantly changing. Continually assess the client visually, verbally, and tactually, and adjust the massage accordingly. The practitioner must be open to the needs of the person at that moment.

Techniques

Many of the common massage techniques are designed for the relatively healthy person. When working with the critically ill, it is essential to be aware of each individual person's needs and tolerances. Many massage techniques are made to stimulate circulation and stir up wastes and toxins. These might not be appropriate when massaging a person suffering from a critical illness. With the critically ill patient, the body might be having a hard time eliminating waste and might not tolerate more waste being pushed into the system.

Techniques should soothe and add comfort. Touch, slow and gentle stroking, and energy work are the most common choices for massaging the critically ill client. Depending on the tolerance of the client, the length of a session might be abbreviated. Rather than a full massage that lasts an hour or more, the situation might call for the back and shoulders or just the feet to be massaged for 15 minutes. This is a time to underdo rather than overdo, and it is a time to be supportive and calming. The touch session might involve simply holding the client's hand and responding to the person. Client feedback is often compromised in critical illness. The client might have difficulty moving, talking, or giving verbal cues, and if he is heavily medicated, he might be unable to let you know if you are hurting him. Pain medication can alter perception to touch, so it is best to keep the pressure light.

Any and all contact that is made is an integral part of the session. Your mere presence is as important as the manipulations that you use. Your actions, voice, breathing, and movements should all reflect the caring, nurturing, and compassion of the session. More often than not, persons who are critically ill are touch starved because family and friends may be too fearful or uncomfortable to touch those who are ill. In the words of Irene Smith, of Service Through Touch:

> We give massage primarily for relaxation and pleasure. The patient may be under a high level of stress due to fear, pain, and anxiety on the physical, emotional and spiritual levels. Slow, gentle, loving touch is used in order to offer the patient a time of peace and quiet. Peace and quiet and gentleness are three very valuable healing qualities.

PRECAUTIONS FOR WORKING WITH HIV-INFECTED CLIENTS

human immunodeficiency virus (HIV)

is a virus that can multiply and destroy a portion of the immune system.

acquired immune deficiency syndrome (AIDS)

is a condition caused by HIV infection whereby a portion of the immune system is destroyed, making it easy for the infected person to acquire life-threatening diseases.

The **human immunodeficiency virus (HIV)** is the causative agent for the **acquired immune deficiency syndrome (AIDS).** The only way to determine whether a person is HIV positive is through a simple blood test. Not everyone who is HIV positive develops AIDS, and being HIV positive is no longer a death sentence. Through medication, the progression of the disease can be slowed or stopped. Even more than other critically ill clients, those infected with HIV are even more touch starved because of people's fear in contracting the illness, even though massage can be of great benefit to those who have contracted HIV. The associated stigma of those who are HIV infected has even given rise to this disease's being a protected entity, ensuring the privacy of those who are infected.

Stages of HIV Infection

opportunistic infection

is caused by organisms commonly found in the environment and our bodies that become deadly when the body's immune system is weakened.

There is a continuum of stages of HIV infection. After being infected with the virus, a person might experience no symptoms for a long period. This period can be a matter of months, several years, or, with modern drug therapy, can continue indefinitely. When the immune system begins to weaken, mild symptoms appear. As the immune system continues to weaken, the symptoms become more severe. Symptoms continue to become more severe as the body loses its ability to fight off infections. When an HIV-infected person has a T-cell count of 200 or less and/or is diagnosed with an **opportunistic infection,** that person has AIDS.

Opportunistic infections are caused by organisms that are commonly found in the environment and that many of us already have in our bodies. Normally our immune system protects us against these bacteria, parasites, fungi, and viruses. With the immune system weakened by HIV, the uncontrolled organisms become deadly. Common opportunistic infections associated with AIDS include:

- *Pneumocystis carinii pneumonia (PCP).* PCP is caused by a protozoan commonly found in the lungs. When the immune system is weakened, as in AIDS, the organism multiplies and causes the disease. PCP is the most common opportunistic disease of persons with AIDS. Unless you have an immune deficiency, there is no concern about catching PCP.
- *Cryptococcal meningitis.* Cryptococcal meningitis is caused by the fungus Cryptococcus neoformans. This fungus is found in the environment and grows in pigeon droppings. Dust containing the fungus is inhaled, and it spreads to the meninges of the central nervous system, creating the symptoms of the disease.
- *Toxoplasmosis.* Toxoplasmosis comes from a protozoan that is usually acquired through eating raw or undercooked meat. If the immune system is weak, the infection can spread to the heart, lungs, or brain. In AIDS patients, the infection often affects the brain, resulting in lesions and neurologic complications.
- *Candida.* The fungus *Candida albicans* is normally found in the intestines, mouth, and vagina. When a person's resistance is reduced because of illness, immunosuppressive drugs, or broad-spectrum

antibiotics, Candida infections can occur. In people with AIDS, the Candida infection can appear in the mouth, where it is called *thrush*, or it can appear as a rash on the skin. Do not touch a Candida rash, because it can be very sensitive and also can spread from one part of the body to another.

- *Herpes.* There are three forms of the herpes virus, all of which are very contagious:
  Herpes simplex I causes fever blisters and cold sores on the face and mouth.
  Herpes simplex II causes painful sores around the genitals and anus and is sexually transmitted.
  Herpes varicella-zoster is also called *shingles* and causes painful blisters that tend to follow specific nerve pathways.
- *Kaposi's sarcoma (KS).* KS is a form of cancer of the cells that line certain blood vessels and produces lesions that can appear on the skin. The lesions are bluish to reddish purple and can be smooth or raised. They can be closed, in which case massaging over them is acceptable, or they can be open, in which case the same precautions as with blood products must be observed.
- *Other rashes.* The person with AIDS can have any number of rashes caused by fungi or reactions to medications. Most rashes are contraindicated to massage. Simply avoid the area where there is a rash and proceed to another area of the body.

Transmission of HIV

The virus that causes AIDS is transmitted from person to person only through the exchange of body fluid that contains the virus. The transmission of HIV requires three simultaneous conditions:

1. The virus requires a proper environment to survive. The virus is found in blood, semen, vaginal fluids, and mother's milk in high enough concentrations to be virulent. HIV has also been found in sweat, tears, and rarely in saliva.
2. The substance containing the virus must have a sufficiently large concentration of the virus to cause an HIV infection. There is no known case of HIV infection caused by contact with sweat, tears, or saliva.
3. The virus must have a port of entry; that is, there must be a way for the virus to enter the body. Some ways in which this can occur are engaging in unprotected sexual activity, sharing needles used for injecting drugs or applying tattoos, receiving transfusions with infected blood, transmitting in utero to an unborn child, or by nursing an infant when the mother is infected.

Precautions Against Infection

Understanding the stages of HIV infection and the factors necessary for transmission of HIV can help to guide the practitioner when determining which precautions to take.

Always be aware of standard infection precautions, or Universal precautions, when working with any client. These precautions are designed to prevent blood or any other body secretions from entering the practitioner's body through any opening such as open sores or cuts.

The client with AIDS is more at risk than the therapist, because they have a weakened immune system and are susceptible if the practitioner has any type of virus or contagious disease. If the practitioner has any kind of open sore or wound, it should not come in contact with the client, which is no different than any massage safety considerations on other clients. If the client with AIDS has an open sore, this should be covered, and be considered a local contraindication as with any other client. In other words, do not treat a client with AIDS any differently than anyone else.

The primary infection precaution is thorough hand washing. Thorough hand washing is accomplished by scrubbing the hands vigorously with a germicidal soap for at least 20 seconds before and after each massage session. When it is deemed necessary, the hands can be washed during the session. The hands are washed before the session to protect the client, who might be susceptible to infection. Thorough hand washing after the session protects the therapist and anyone with whom the therapist comes in contact after the session.

The Use of Gloves

The use of gloves is a secondary infection precaution and never replaces the need for thorough hand washing. Either vinyl or latex gloves can be used. When oil is used as a lubricant, latex gloves can break down or tear. Double gloving can be used when added protection is a concern. In situations in which the client is susceptible to infection, sterile latex gloves can be used.

A practitioner should use gloves:

- When handling blood, feces, or any other body fluids or secretions or linens soiled with them.
- When the practitioner has an open sore, cut, or broken cuticles on the hands.
- Whenever you as a practitioner do not feel comfortable without them. (Always explain to your client why you are wearing gloves and make sure that she agrees before proceeding.)
- When the client requests that you wear gloves.

Caring for Equipment

Tables and other surfaces that have been contaminated with blood or other bodily fluids can be cleaned and sanitized with a 10 percent solution of chlorine bleach. This can be made by mixing one part chlorine bleach with nine parts water. Alcohol can be used to disinfect surfaces contaminated by other body fluids and secretions.

Linens can be disinfected by washing them in hot water with detergent and one cup of bleach and drying them in a hot dryer.

Following these general infection precautions does minimize the risk to you and your clientele; however, it does not eliminate the fact that some risk is involved. If any questions or concerns arise as a result of working with a person who has an HIV infection or any other infectious disease, contact your local infection control center. There is an infection control center located at your local hospital or medical center.

(For more information about massage for HIV-infected persons or massage for the critically ill, contact www.everflowing.org [Service Through Touch].)

Massaging People with Cancer

Until recently, massage has been considered to be a contraindication when working with persons with cancer because of the effects it has on blood and lymph circulation and the fear that massage might actually spread the cancer. Pioneers such as Debra Curties, Gayle MacDonald, and others have examined the development of cancer and the mechanics of how it spreads and have concluded that when certain precautions are taken and guidelines followed, the risks of massaging persons with cancer are minimal when weighed against the many benefits provided by skilled touch. Two books recommended for anyone considering working with people with cancer are *Medicine Hands: Massage Therapy for People with Cancer* by Gayle MacDonald and *Massage Therapy and Cancer* by Debra Curties.

Certain types of massage or massage techniques are contraindicated for people with cancer or for those undergoing cancer treatment; however, many techniques provide support and relief to people with this devastating disease. With a clearer understanding of the disease, careful consideration, and some specific guidelines, massage can now be offered to a population that might find great benefit in their increased comfort and enhanced quality of life. In fact, massage is used in many cancer centers and hospitals as an integrated therapy for cancer patients.

People who receive a diagnosis of cancer suddenly face a life-threatening and life-changing situation that requires hard choices and the likelihood of invasive medical procedures. They are suddenly facing a fight against a disease that will deeply affect their mental, emotional, and physical well-being. The adverse physical effects of cancer can stem from the disease itself or from the rather aggressive treatment required to fight it. Common cancer therapies tend to be invasive, painful, stressful, and sometimes even disfiguring. Emotional side effects of cancer or its treatment include mood swings, depression, a sense of hopelessness, confusion, or decreased cognitive skills. Massage provides both physical and emotional support to people dealing with cancer.

Benefits of massage for persons with cancer include pain relief or control and relief from depression. Massage has been effective in reducing nausea, eliminating insomnia, promoting relaxation, reducing anxiety, increasing body awareness, and helping to restore a positive body image. Massage induces relief from muscle tension, spasms, and fatigue. Further effects of massage include improved lymph movement, reduced edema and swelling, better digestion and

Box 19.1

BENEFITS OF MASSAGE TO PERSONS WITH CANCER

Provides some pain relief or control
Reduces nausea
Improves digestion and elimination
Relieves stress
Promotes relaxation
Helps insomnia
Reduces anxiety
Provides some relief from depression
Provides some relief from muscle tension and spasm
Helps improve flexibility
Helps to restore ROM
Improves lymph movement and reduces edema
Increases body awareness
Restores positive body image
Enhances self-esteem
Improves outlook on life
Improves quality of life
Boosts the healing process
Promotes health
Feels good at a time when many things feel bad

elimination, better flexibility, an improved outlook on life, and enhanced self-esteem. Massage restores ROM and promotes health, and, simply put, it feels good. It imparts an improved quality of life and a boost to the healing process. The intention of providing massage to people with cancer is to relax, restore, and nurture. Massage provides comfort and support even though it is not necessarily intended to "fix" anything (see Box 19.1).

Massage that reduces stress levels has been found to reduce the levels of cortisol and glucocorticoids in the blood and therefore can inhibit the spread of the disease. Higher levels of these stress-related hormones have been linked to increased tumor proliferation.

It has been shown that people with cancer who receive massage can experience many benefits. In studies at the Touch Research Facility at the University of Miami, massage has been shown to increase certain immune factors in the bloodstream. Avoiding gentle, comfort-giving touch does not stop metastatic cells from breaking away from a primary tumor, moving through the bloodstream, and stopping in host tissues to form secondary tumors, but it can deny a population under myriad stressful conditions the many benefits of skilled touch.

Each situation is different, considering the type of cancer, the stage of the disease, the level of treatment or state of remission, the state of the immune system, the stamina and attitude of the person, and many other factors. The decision to do massage must be made on an individual basis.

Cancer Metastasis

There is limited knowledge as to why cancer strikes; however, there is more and clearer understanding of how it spreads. **Metastasis** is the manner in which cancer spreads. Metastasis, or proliferation of cancer cells, is a complex process that is still under investigation in the fight against this disease. Even though modern medical practices are very successful at eliminating the primary tumors associated with cancer, the fact that the cancer metastasizes to other locations is usually the cause of death. Usually by the time a palpable tumor is detected and diagnosed, metastasis has already started. It is estimated that in 30 to 50 percent of people with cancer, metastasis has begun before they receive their initial treatment.

Cancer spreads in four ways:

- direct invasion of nearby structures
- within body cavities
- through the bloodstream
- through the lymph system

Three stages of metastasis are of concern to the massage therapist (Figure 19-14a and b):

- cells breaking off of the primary tumor
- circulation through the blood and lymph vessels
- implantation of cancerous cells at secondary sites

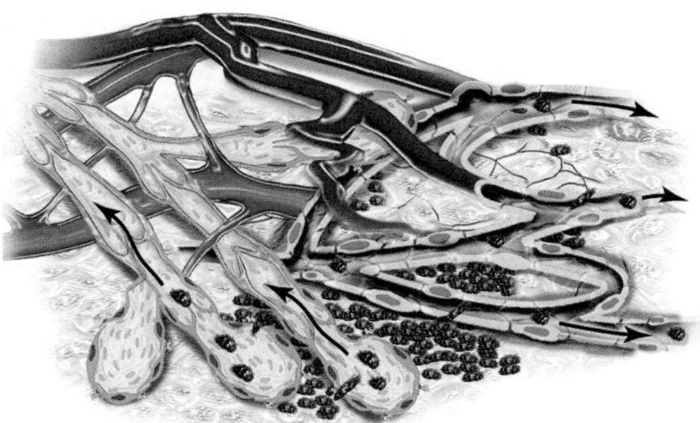
A. Cancer cells shedding

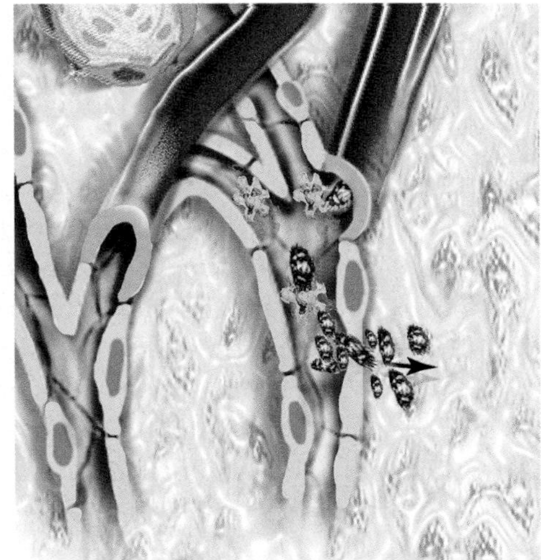

B. Cancer cells implanting

FIGURE 19-14 Cancer cells shed from the primary tumor, enter the bloodstream, and implant in a secondary site.

Cancers that metastasize through the bloodstream seem to be the most lethal. The means by which this happens is very complicated. Simply stated, cancerous cells from a tumor slough off and pass through the walls of the blood vessels that feed the tumor. Mechanical processes such as direct pressure or intense movement close to a tumor can enhance shedding of cells from a primary tumor. Therefore massage, stretching, or joint movements on or near the site of the tumor are contraindicated, especially if the tumor is in superficial tissues. When cancer cells enter the circulatory system, they enter into a very hostile environment in which far fewer than one percent of them survive. Factors that cause their destruction include the fact that cancer cells are unable to absorb nutrients while moving through the bloodstream, that the immune system is designed to seek and destroy abnormal cells, and that cancer cells are not built to withstand the turbulent forces of movement in the circulatory system. The longer cancer cells remain in circulation, the less likely they are to survive. Fewer than one percent of metastatic cells from a tumor survive in the bloodstream, and fewer than one percent of those cancer cells are able to initiate the metastatic process (Groenwald and Frogge, 1995; Curties, 1994). Cells can clump together to increase their chance at survival. Eventually the cells move into and lodge in a capillary bed, where they adhere to the wall of the

metastasis

is the spread of cancer from one site to another location in the body.

blood vessel. With the right conditions, they grow or penetrate the capillary wall, invading the interstitial space, and begin growth as a secondary tumor.

Cancerous cells can also enter the bloodstream by means of the lymph system. Cells shed from the primary tumor and into the interstitial spaces, where they are absorbed into lymph capillaries. They travel into lymph vessels and to regional nodes where they are either destroyed by the immune system or proliferate in the node. Malignant cells can enter the bloodstream through the nodal capillaries or pass on through infected lymph nodes to the thoracic or right lymphatic ducts and then into the bloodstream through the vena cava.

If the effects of massage increase the volume and speed of blood and lymph circulation and increase immune function, the agitated hostile environment would be more likely to suppress metastatic cell survival in the bloodstream than to support it. The long-held assumption that massage spreads cancer through the blood and lymph system is largely unfounded and without merit. As of the most current revision of this text, there has been no definitive study done examining whether massage affects the spread of cancer.

Implantation at a secondary site happens when viable malignant cells reach the capillary bed of a preferred host tissue. The cancerous cells adhere to the capillary walls, are able to penetrate the capillary wall, move into the new site, and establish themselves as a secondary site. Most cancers seek out and prefer certain host tissues or organs as secondary sites. These patterns of metastasis are clearly documented and must be considered when determining where and how to administer massage techniques. Secondary sites are often in deep, major organs where distal circulatory massage is of minor consequence.

The question is, does massage increase the chances of malignant cells' implanting in a secondary site? There is no available data one way or another, so it is prudent to take a precautionary approach. Depending on the site of the primary tumor, massage should be avoided in the area or areas of probable secondary sites, especially if those sites are in superficial tissues. There is no conclusive research regarding the risks of massage during the stages of metastasis; however, by observing certain precautions, the therapist can minimize the risks of spreading the cancer.

Classifications of Cancer

There are many types of cancer as well as different stages of the disease process. Cancer is defined by type, grade, site, and stage.

The *type* of cancer is determined by the kind of tissue in which the cancer cells begin to develop:

- carcinoma—originates in the epithelial tissue that lines organs and vessels
- myeloma—originates in bone marrow
- sarcoma—originates in the supportive and connective tissues such as muscles, cartilage, and bone
- lymphoma—originates in lymphatic tissue
- leukemia—originates in tissues that form blood cells

Grading involves the microscopic examination of tumor cells that have been harvested through biopsy. The degree of abnormality of the cells determines the grade of the cancer. Grade levels are from 0 to 4, in which 0 indicates normal cells and grade 4 indicates highly abnormal, undifferentiated, cancerous cells.

Site refers to the location of the primary tumor and is often reflected in the name describing the cancer. Cancer tumors are usually named after the part of the body where the cancer first began. Its name does not change even if the cancer spreads to another part of the body. For example, if breast cancer spreads (metastasizes) to the lung, it is still named and treated as breast cancer.

The *stages* of cancer refer to a system of quantifying the status of the primary tumor, the regional lymph node involvement, and the areas of metastasis that uses numerical values to express the extent of involvement of the disease. The treating physician, usually an oncologist, is the best source for obtaining information as to the location, type, and extent or probable sites of metastasis for the cancer.

Stage defines the growth of most cancers:

- *Stage I*: Cancer is still small and contained in the original tumor.
- *Stage II*: Cancer has grown and/or spread to nearby lymph nodes.
- *Stage III*: Cancerous cells have spread to regional lymph nodes and/or other tissues in the area.
- *Stage IV*: Cancer is well developed and has spread to other tissues or organs in the body.
- *Recurrent*: Cancer has returned after being treated. It might come back at the original site or another part of the body.

Another classification scheme of staging considers the cancer distribution in terms of primary tumor (T), regional lymph node involvement (N), and extent of metastasis (M). The T component indicates the size and invasiveness of the primary tumor. The N component indicates the absence or extent of invasion of cancer cells in the regional lymph nodes. The M component indicates whether the cancer has spread to other parts of the body.

- Tumor (T)
  - T0 No evidence of tumor
  - T1–4 Increasing tumor size and involvement
- Node (N)
  - NX Lymph node involvement cannot be assessed
  - N0 No evidence of lymph node involvement
  - N1–4 Increasing degrees of lymph node involvement
- Metastases (M)
  - M0 No evidence of distant metastases
  - M1 Evidence of distant metastases

Progression of the Disease

Cancer develops progressively from an alteration in certain cells to uncontrolled growth that invades tissues and organs. Clinically, a person with cancer goes through a succession of experiences as she learns of the disease, makes decisions for treatment, progresses through treatment, and deals with the outcome. Persons with cancer exhibit different conditions and have varying needs at each level.

Box 19.2

Important Considerations when considering massage for persons with cancer

The type and location of cancer
The stage of progression of the cancer
Possible secondary sites of metastasis
The treatment type and stage
The condition of the immune system
The stamina of the person
The attitude of the person
The belief and desire of the person regarding massage
The purpose of the massage
Therapist's intention and quality of touch

The five phases of progression are

1. onset
2. diagnosis/pretreatment
3. treatment—surgery, radiation, chemotherapy, alternative and complementary
4. remission/survivorship
5. advanced terminal/terminal

Choices for massage therapy must be made on a case-by-case basis. A thorough intake procedure, safe practice, and informed client consent become essential.

Intake Procedure for Persons with Cancer

During the intake consultation, a medical history is taken to gather information about the client, the type of cancer, stage of the cancer, the course of treatment (type and timing), the side effects, the names of the treating physicians, and the level of health, stamina, and emotional state of the client. Become as informed as possible. Learn about the kind of cancer, where it is located, primary secondary sites (areas where the particular cancer tends to metastasize to), type of treatment, side effects of the treatment, treatment schedule, symptoms of the cancer, and the treatment. Questions that cannot be answered by the client can be referred to the client's doctor. The Internet is also a rich source of information about different types of cancer and treatment (see Box 19.2).

Adjust the Massage to the Client's Health Status

A person's level of health can vary greatly depending on where the client is in the progression of the disease or treatment. Attitude, stamina, and health status influence the choice of massage treatment.

Adjust the Massage to the Cancer Site

Many cancers have a specific location where there is a tumor, whereas some, such as leukemia or lymphoma, have no specific location. By knowing the location of the cancer, the therapist can avoid circulatory massage or pressure to the local area of the cancer or its possible sites of metastasis. Massage that puts pressure on the site of a tumor is contraindicated owing to the concern of dislodging tumor cells. If there is a secondary site where the cancer is suspected to have spread, local and regional massage is contraindicated in that area as well.

Adjust the Massage to the Cancer Treatment

Cancer treatments are often quite invasive and have numerous side effects, many of which must be taken into consideration by the massage therapist. Side effects from cancer intervention can last for days, weeks, or even years after treatments are completed. Massage, when applied with knowledge and understanding, might provide relief for some of the unpleasant treatment side effects. These same treatments and their accompanying side effects are the reason for many massage modifications and contraindications.

Types of Cancer Treatment

After a person receives a diagnosis of cancer, a course of treatment is prescribed. The treatment depends on the type and stage of the cancer and can include one or a combination of the following modalities:

- Surgery
- Chemotherapy
- Radiation
- Bone marrow transplant
- Treatment with other drugs (e.g., steroids, narcotics, and antidepressants)
- Complementary and alternative therapies

Surgery

Surgery is often the first intervention in cancer treatment. Generally, the primary tumor and often the local or regional lymph nodes are surgically removed. Recent surgery increases the chance of a blood clot or thrombus forming in a blood vessel such as in a vein in the leg or in the area of the surgery. This is a serious consideration for the massage therapist, because circulatory massage could dislodge the clot and it would become a floating embolus in the bloodstream. The embolus would circulate back to the heart and then into the pulmonary arteries, where it would eventually lodge in one of the smaller arteries and become a pulmonary embolism, which is a life-threatening condition.

Because of the concern of thrombosis, massage on or around the incisions from surgery is contraindicated. Massage to the lower limbs is also contraindicated for postsurgical patients. Always consult the client's physician to determine when it is safe to massage the lower extremities or the incision after surgery, asking the physician specifically when the danger of thrombosis is past.

The site of the incision is a local contraindication unless the therapist has specific training in working with scar tissue and adhesions and has the physician's approval. Reasons for being a contraindication include the following:

- It is the site of a recent tumor.
- The tissue is actively healing.

- There may be clotting.
- It may still be inflamed or irritated.

Another postoperative concern is infection, either at the incision site or systemically. The postsurgical client is often in the hospital under close supervision so that any sign of infection is quickly treated. Any areas of infection or inflammation are contraindicated for massage, and the client should be referred to the treating physician immediately. A common side effect or symptom of cancer surgery or other treatment is fever. Whenever fever is present, massage is contraindicated.

Surgery often involves the removal of regional lymph nodes, which sometimes causes lymphedema in the limb distal to the missing nodes. Excess fluid fills the interstitial spaces of the limb distal to the affected lymph nodes owing to interference in the normal lymph channels. General massage or massage techniques that apply pressure to the affected areas are contraindicated because they can exacerbate the condition. Only light manual lymph drainage techniques can be employed, and only after consulting with the treating physician.

During the client intake, the therapist should be very thorough in determining the kind of surgery, when it was performed, the location and extent, if lymph nodes were removed, and how well the client recovered. When the therapist has formulated a treatment plan, she should check with the treating physician and obtain an informed consent from the client before proceeding with massage therapy.

Chemotherapy

Chemotherapy uses chemicals usually administered intravenously or orally to kill, sterilize, or weaken the cancer cells so that other chemical or radiation treatments will eradicate the cancer. Some types of chemotherapy can target specific cancer cells or specific properties of those cells; however, many types of therapies cannot differentiate, so many fast-growing normal cells are affected. Dosages are controlled to obtain the maximum effect on the cancer without overwhelming the normal tissues.

Many of the side effects from chemotherapy stem from the destruction of the fast-growing cells of the respiratory organs, digestive tract, and bone marrow. They include nausea, diarrhea, vomiting, mouth sores, constipation, skin rashes, weight loss, fever, hair loss, reduced white and red blood cell count, reduced platelet count, pain, fatigue, and nervous symptoms such as vertigo and peripheral neuropathy. Each of these side effects has implications for the massage therapist.

Effects from chemotherapy can range from mild to severe, with the most difficult time within the first 24 to 72 hours following treatment. General massage during this time can be too taxing, whereas short gentle touch sessions can help to reduce muscle tension, anxiety, and nausea.

Clients receiving chemotherapy may have an intravenous (IV) catheter located semipermanently on their body. Care must be taken not to disturb the catheter either by positioning or massage.

When white blood cell counts are low, the immune system is compromised and the client is more vulnerable to infection. Therapists should avoid contact if they or anyone in their close surroundings (family or colleagues) is ill.

If the treatment has reduced the client's platelet count, the client might be prone to bruising or bleeding because platelets control clotting. The therapist might need to adjust the massage to prevent bruising or damaging delicate tissues.

Reduced red blood cell counts cause anemia, which results in fatigue, intolerance to cold, occasional dizziness, and shortness of breath. The therapist should consider keeping the session brief and light to avert fatigue and keep extra blankets handy to avoid chilling the client. Be careful when helping the client up from the table in case of dizziness.

Hair loss or alopecia is sometimes accompanied by irritation of the scalp. This condition must be approached delicately because of the client's body image. It is important to ask the client about any scalp condition and any desire for touch. The client might choose to keep a wig or head covering on during the massage, or the client might want a thorough head massage. Stimulating the scalp with massage is usually well received in these cases. Care must be taken to not get lotion or oil on the head covering or hairpiece. Any scalp irritation is a contraindication for massage.

Digestive abnormalities are common with chemotherapy. Nausea and diarrhea contraindicate general circulation massage, especially joint movements and rocking, which can cause more queasiness. Light comforting touch or massage to specific areas of discomfort can be very helpful. The location of the nearest restroom should be pointed out to the client just in case they need to get there in a hurry.

Chemotherapy can cause skin rashes, dryness, and weeping or open lesions. It also can cause areas to become supersensitive. These conditions contraindicate local massage.

Weight loss (cachexia) is common owing to chemotherapy and the ravaging effects of later stages of the disease. The loss of adipose and muscle tissue, especially if the patient is confined to bed, increases the possibility of pressure sores. Massage can help to prevent pressure sores from forming but is contraindicated on or close to decubitus sores/ulcers. Muscle loss can result in stiff or hypermobile joints. If ROM is used, it must be done carefully and gently. Fatigue and a loss of stamina often accompany weight loss, and the massage must be adjusted to support and not tire the client.

Some forms of chemotherapy affect the central or peripheral nervous system, causing pain, burning, or tingling sensations. If your client has these symptoms, talk with the client's doctor to determine the cause and what you can do. Peripheral neuropathy, a common side effect, causes numbness, burning, tingling, or pain in the feet and hands. Gentle massage sometimes relieves symptoms; however, deep pressure or any methods that exacerbate the symptoms are contraindicated.

If a person is receiving chemotherapy, the preferred time to receive massage might be before this treatment. Massage given before the invasive treatment can help to relieve stress and lower anxiety levels, which can result in less severe reactions to the treatment. Massage may be resumed after the chemotherapy, when the side effects have subsided to the point that the client can easily tolerate touch. Family members can be shown slow-stroke back massage and neck and shoulder relaxation massage to assist their loved ones through this difficult time.

Persons with cancer, especially those in treatment, experience increased stress that can result in increased muscle tension accompanied by fatigue and pain. Massage works wonders, when applied within the client's safe practice limits, to alleviate muscle tension and associated symptoms.

Radiation

Radiation therapies usually beam radiation directly at a tumor site to either destroy the cancer cells and reduce the tumor size or more often to destroy cancer cells' capability to reproduce. The problem is that the cancer cells often cannot be singled out, and normal tissue cells in the irradiated area are also damaged. In some cases, a larger area or the whole body is irradiated. In these instances, only the patient is exposed to the radiation, and there is no concern of radiation exposure to the therapist or others. For some types of cancer treatment, an implant or radioactive iodine is used. In these instances, the patient is isolated until the danger of exposure to others is reduced to safe levels.

To help control or aim the radiation, spots are inked or tattooed on the patient's body. These spots are not to be tampered with while the patient is undergoing treatment.

Massage for Persons Receiving Radiation

There are no clear massage protocols while a person is undergoing radiation; each case must be considered on its own merits. The therapist should consult the treating physician regarding the advisability of working in the area being treated. After a radiation session, the client might experience fatigue and/or nausea, which preclude massage until those symptoms pass. The area being irradiated requires special consideration. The area that has recently been radiated might have some of the same symptoms as a burn; however, the burn is from the inside out and can appear pink or angry. The irradiated tissue is very fragile and can continue to degrade for a time after the actual treatment, much as a sunburn gets worse even after exposure has ceased. The patient is usually under doctor's orders regarding care of or using lubricants on the affected area. The massage therapist should regard these instructions carefully. Abide by all restrictions regarding touch or lubricants. Avoid working on the area for three to five days or until the burning effects completely subside. If there are any lesions, wait until they are completely healed. Remember, the damaged tissue is not only on the surface; there can be similar conditions at the exit site of the radiation. Local and regional massage is contraindicated for radiation sites. Affected areas of the skin can remain sensitive to heat and pressure long after treatment.

A locally radiated area does not preclude massage on other parts of the body, although the massage might need to be modified to accommodate for other side effects such as nausea or fatigue. In the case of fatigue, modify the massage session in consideration of the stamina of the client by using light, nonintrusive techniques in an abbreviated session. If the client is experiencing nausea, avoid joint movements, rocking, or passive movement techniques that might aggravate the nausea. If the radiation has destroyed any lymph nodes, lymphedema is often a concern. Follow the same guidelines discussed in the previous section on surgery.

Massage seems to be more effective before chemotherapy and radiation treatments because it seems to improve the client's outlook and reduces anxiety. As a result, recovery from the treatment is quicker, and many of the side effects, such as fatigue and nausea, seem less drastic.

Transplants

Bone marrow and stem cell transplant therapies are some of the most drastic treatments done. They involve whole-body irradiation followed by transplant surgery so that more rigorous chemotherapy can be done. The patient's health is extremely compromised. The patient's immune system is weakened, and he might be in isolation. Total-body irradiation can result in extensive skin burns. It is a time when the patient is debilitated and weak from repeated interventions in the attempt to fight the cancer.

Massaging Persons with Cancer

To provide safe and effective massage, the therapist must find out as much about the illness, treatment, and the client as possible. Most people in cancer treatment are very knowledgeable about their condition and will know of any restrictions. If the client is in the acute stage of the disease and in treatment, work closely with the medical team and the client when formulating a treatment plan. The treating physician might provide a massage recommendation or prescription and agree to inform the massage therapist of any changing conditions that could influence the choice of massage treatment.

In this difficult time, massage must be gentle, supportive, and compassionate. The massage session is one of the few times the patient experiences soothing, noninvasive, and pleasurable touch.

Adjust the massage session to the cancer, the treatment, and the client's level of health. Most special considerations have to do with site restrictions, positioning, pressure sensitivity, or stamina. If the client fatigues easily or has a low energy level, adjust the massage accordingly. This can be done by shortening the length of the session, lightening the pressure, and slowing the pace of the massage. How much adjustment is made in these areas depends on the client's condition and needs. Listen to the client, and be there for him. Careful questioning, observation, and intuition are key to determining a course of action. It is better to do too little than too much. This is not a time to fix anything or further deplete a client's energy, but to provide relaxation, comfort, and ease.

When a treatment plan is developed and discussed with the client, with the potential risks and benefits, the client should sign an informed consent form releasing the therapist from any liability as far as the proliferation of the disease. Massage, within safe parameters, can then proceed. The client makes the decision to proceed; nevertheless, it is wise to do less rather than more.

As people progress deeper into the disease and become more ill, the benefits they receive from massage increase. In hospice settings, where patients have a prognosis of less than six months to live, massage has been shown to improve the quality of a person's experience by reducing pain, muscle tension, and anxiety, and improving circulation, appetite, sleep, and general comfort. Skilled touch communicates a sense of caring, comfort, and acceptance.

This is a time for nurturing touch. When light Swedish techniques might even be too much, modalities such as Reiki, therapeutic touch, or mild polarity can be used. Persons with cancer are not the only ones to consider. Spouses and close family members are also under increased stress and can benefit from massage. Many times, family members who are part of the client's support group can be taught simple or specific massage techniques so that they can provide caring touch to the person with cancer on a more routine basis. This not only provides additional comfort to the client, it also empowers family members by giving them something positive that they can do to support their loved one.

There are many conditions during the course of cancer that warrant precautions regarding the application of massage; however, at any stage of the disease, some form of skilled touch provides many benefits that are welcomed by the person having the disease.

Guidelines for Massaging Persons with Cancer

- Before any massage is given to a new client, a complete medical history is taken.
- The physician/oncologist is consulted, and a recommendation for massage is obtained.
- A treatment plan is developed, and the client is fully informed about the effects of massage therapy before giving informed consent.
- When doing massage, use light to moderate pressure, shorter sessions, and positioning for comfort.
- Deep massage is contraindicated in that it overstresses the body.
- Massage or direct pressure in the local area of the tumor as well as the regional area where affected lymph nodes might reside is contraindicated.
- Avoid circulatory massage at probable secondary metastatic sites.
- Avoid massage treatment in the event of infection or fever.
- Adjust massage according to the current state of client's health:
  Know the stage of the disease and the client's stamina, attitude, and emotional state.
  Adjust the type of massage, depth, duration, and speed.
  Consult with client, caregiver, family, and physician.
- Adjust massage according to the treatment regime.
- Consult with medical personnel.
- Consider the client's state of fatigue, nausea, and well-being.
- Be aware of chemotherapy concerns—low blood counts, white cell, red cell, platelet; IV ports.
- Be aware of radiation concerns—skin rashes and burns, hair loss, tissue fragility, infection, fatigue.
- Be aware of surgery concerns—increased chance of blood clots, hemorrhage, thrombosis; avoid massage on the site of any incision; specialized scar massage can be started in four to six weeks, after approval from doctor.

- Be aware of a client's impaired awareness to pain or sensory loss—might be due to disease-related neurologic damage, pharmaceuticals, depression, surgery, or near-death withdrawal. Proceed with caution.
- Adjust your treatments to best serve the client—obtain client feedback from previous sessions as well as current needs to adapt the session to best serve the client's needs.

Hospice and End-of-Life Care

Many of the same precautions apply to caring for someone at the end of her life (i.e., one with a terminal illness that will not heal and who has no other medical treatment options for a cure) as treating someone who is critically ill. Terminal illnesses can be advanced stages of cancer, organ failure (e.g., congestive heart failure, chronic obstructive pulmonary disease, advanced diabetes, hepatitis or kidney failure), degenerative illnesses, severe trauma or injury, neurologic disorders (e.g., Parkinson's, amyotrophic lateral sclerosis, Huntington's, or stroke), complications from severe eating disorders or malnutrition, and any number of other life-threatening illnesses. People who have acquired the services of hospice (either at a hospice center or home hospice care) are at the very end of their lives. The goal at this point is not *quantity* of care but rather *quality* of care, in which the goal is to make the patient as comfortable (reducing pain) and as comforted (having someone to give empathy) as possible. Hospice professionals help to comfort family and friends and often helps the patient and loved ones deal with the transition and grief of accepting death.

Massage during Hospice and End-of-Life Care

Much of the massage care, which typically applies to avoiding massage because of contraindications, differs at this point. Although care and gentle work is imperative, it is the premise that quality of life (not quantity) governs which kind of massage performed. It is absolutely important to work with hospice caregivers and physicians. The involvement of family and friends is also important. This is not work for the faint at heart. Working with someone who is about to die takes much grounding and shielding as well as strength and compassion. Often, the patient is heavily medicated to cope with pain, and gentle care must be provided. Often the patient can tolerate at most only 15 to 20 minutes of touch. Only light compression, feather stroking, working on hands or simply holding the client's hand, or energy work is indicated. Maneuvering around IVs and working on the patient within the medical bed (e.g. at a hospital, hospice center, or even in the patient's home) is necessary. Sometimes the family might ask that they be left alone with the patient to die and this should be absolutely honored, especially to say goodbyes. Always ask if the time is appropriate. Sometimes working on the family and visitors can also be a good idea, but always ask first. Some types of energy work such as therapeutic touch and Reiki can actually help a dying patient to accept death as part of life and may provide solace and tranquility enough to pass on. Grief counselors available to the families and visitors are also there to help the caregivers (including massage and touch therapists) work through the very real grief often felt when a patient has passed.

SUMMARY

There are many styles, modalities, and modifications of massage that make it applicable to innumerable situations and conditions. This chapter introduces how massage can be modified and applied to a wide range of conditions, from prenatal and infant massage, to working with minors and elderly clients, to those with disabilities and critical illnesses like AIDS and cancer, to those in hospice care at the end of their lives. Throughout life, from the very earliest weeks to the final stages, massage effectively provides comfort and relaxation. By taking into consideration the current needs and condition of the person at the time that they are seeking massage, therapists can make accommodations, choose techniques, and make modifications to create a massage experience that is rewarding and beneficial.

QUESTIONS FOR DISCUSSION AND REVIEW

1. How does massage benefit a woman during a normal, healthy pregnancy?
2. Which consideration(s) should be made when positioning a woman in the second and third trimesters of pregnancy?
3. Which type of massage is applied to a woman's abdomen during the first trimester of pregnancy?
4. What are common contraindications for prenatal massage?
5. Who is best suited to perform infant massage?
6. List at least four benefits of infant massage.
7. Which considerations should be made when massaging minors?
8. Which accommodations should be made when providing massage to someone who is hearing impaired?
9. Which accommodations should be made when providing massage to someone whose vision is impaired or is blind?
10. When massaging a person with paralysis, which considerations should be observed?
11. How does massage benefit a person who is critically ill?
12. How is the HIV/AIDS virus transmitted from person to person?
13. Why is massage contraindicated for people with cancer?
14. What are some of the benefits of massage for people with cancer?
15. How can the practitioner reduce the chances of promoting metastasis when massaging people with cancer?
16. What are the stages of cancer?
17. What are the common treatments for cancer?
18. What are some important considerations when determining whether to massage a person with cancer?
19. When a person is receiving chemotherapy or radiation treatment, when is a good time for them to receive massage and why?
20. Which modifications can be made to massage for a client who tends to fatigue easily?

CHAPTER

20 Massage in Medicine

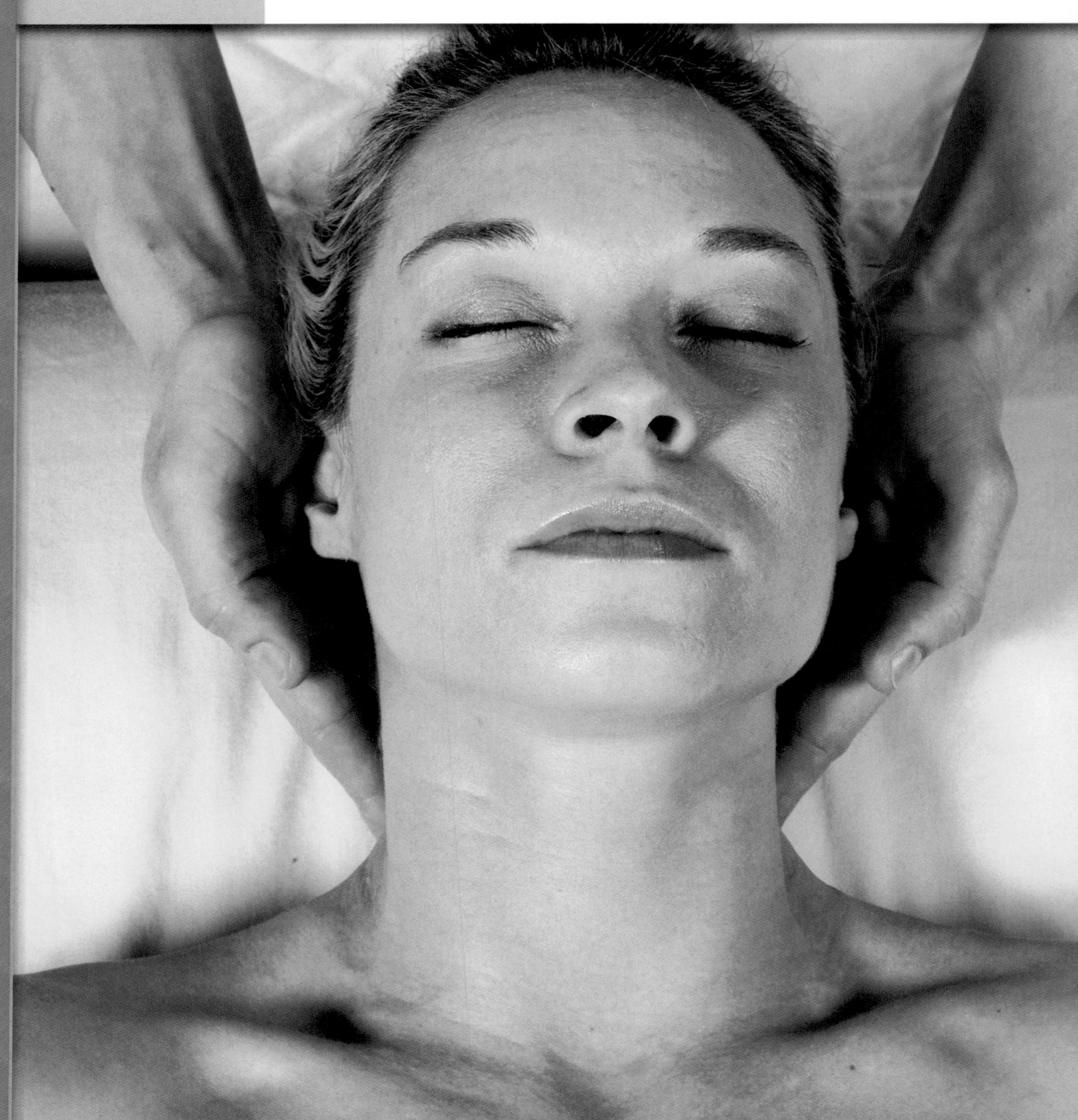

LEARNING OBJECTIVES

After you have mastered this chapter, you will be able to

1. **Explain the historical significance that massage has had in medicine.**
2. **Explain how massage reemerged in the United States as alternative medicine.**
3. **Differentiate among the terms *alternative, complementary,* and *integrative* medicine.**
4. **Explain the role of massage in integrative medicine.**
5. **Describe the role of the patient in integrative medicine.**
6. **Define CAM.**
7. **Explain how massage might fit into a hospital setting.**
8. **Define *medical massage*.**
9. **Demonstrate billing insurance for massage.**

MASSAGE IN MEDICINE THROUGHOUT HISTORY

Many massage techniques were developed and used as part of healing or medical practice. The earliest medical literature from Persia, Egypt, Japan, and China all make reference to various treatments that include the use of massage techniques, although the actual term *massage* did not appear in medical literature until the end of the nineteenth century. There is evidence that the Greeks in the times of Hippocrates and Asclepiades employed massage-like treatments for medical purposes. Exercise, diet, bathing, and massage were all important aspects of preserving health in Roman culture. The fall of the Roman Empire ushered in the Dark Ages (AD 470–1500), a time when few Western medical or historical books were written and much recorded history was lost. As the Roman Empire declined, the Arabic Empire flourished. In Persia, physicians such as Rhazes and Avicenna authored important texts on medical practices that included references to the use of exercise and rubbing for the treatment of disease and preservation of health.

In the West, by the sixteenth century, medical practitioners again began using mechanotherapy. French physician Ambrose Paré (1517–1590) wrote about the positive effects of friction treatments in the healing process. In 1569, Mercurialis of Italy published *De Arte Gymnastica,* which included the benefits of manual therapies when integrated with other treatments. The sixteenth, seventeenth, and eighteenth centuries saw literature from English, French, Italian, and German authors describing the use of massage-like treatments, exercises, and other physical treatments for the purpose of maintaining health and treating disease.

References to massage techniques are found in medical literature from the United States and Europe dating from the 1700s to the present day. Techniques were referred to as rubbing, frictions, gymnastics, medical movements, and medical rubbing.

Per Henrik Ling developed a system of movements that he called *medical gymnastics* and, in 1813, opened the Royal Swedish Central Institute of Gymnastics, where he taught the Ling System until his death in 1839. The popularity of what was to become known as the *Movement Cure* or the *Swedish Movements* spread throughout Europe. In 1858, Dr. Charles Fayette Taylor traveled to England to learn this cure and returned to New York to practice and teach the technique. At the same time, his brother, George Henry Taylor, attended the Sotherberg Institute in Stockholm and completed full training in the Movement Cure before returning to New York to join his brother Charles. Although their combined practice lasted only about a year, they both continued to practice, write about, and teach these techniques until their deaths in 1899.

In 1902, Douglas Graham, M.D., of Boston published *Manual Therapies, A Treatise on Massage,* which clearly described the effects of massage and helped massage to gain more credibility in the medical profession.

James Mennell (1880–1957) published *Physical Treatment by Movement, Manipulation and Massage* in 1920. He was a medical officer and lecturer of massage in England and was very influential in the early development of physical therapy.

Mary McMillan received her training and early experience in England. She moved to the United States to become the director of massage and medical gymnastics at Children's Hospital in Portland, Maine, and later took a position at Walter Reed Army Hospital. She was an instructor for reconstruction aides in physiotherapy during World War I and became director of physiotherapy at the Harvard Medical School from 1921 to 1925, where she wrote the definitive text *Massage and Therapeutic Exercise.*

Massage for treating orthopedic conditions continued to expand in the United States until approximately 1945. Massage as physiotherapy was used extensively in the rehabilitation of those wounded in World War I and World War II. Massage was also a common prescription for victims of the polio epidemic during the 1940s and 1950s.

The use of massage in physiotherapy declined between 1940 and 1950 owing to the fact that it was strenuous, time-consuming, and required extensive training. Physical therapy began relying more on exercise and the use of a variety of machines, medicines, and mechanical modalities for treatment. The use of massage in the medical field in the United States was nearly nonexistent after the early 1950s.

Even though the use of massage in medicine declined, exercise and massage continued to be popular for the maintenance and promotion of physical health. Swedish massage, which included Swedish movements, hydrotherapy, and sometimes colon irrigation and diathermy, remained popular with natural health enthusiasts. Swedish massage practitioners could find employment in health clubs or spas, sanatoriums, YMCAs, and resorts.

Manual therapies and massage-like procedures have been considered part of medical practice since ancient times. Massage practices of physical manipulations and applications have also flourished in nonconventional healing practices and folk medicine. After falling into obscurity in the 1950s, massage began to reemerge during the human potential movement of the 1960s and 1970s.

The reemergence of massage in the United States happened outside of **allopathic medicine.** Classic Swedish massage was joined by reflexology, shiatsu, acupressure, and other alternative practices. More therapeutic modalities began to emerge, each carrying the name of the person who devised it, such as Reichian therapy, Rolfing, Alexander technique, Feldenkrais, and Trager, among others. Cross-fiber techniques of James Cyriax and trigger-point therapies described by Simons and Travell gained acceptance and popularity. English osteopaths Stanley Lief and Boris Chaitow developed Neuromuscular Technique (NMT), which has been popularized in the United States by Judith Walker and Paul St. John. John Upledger developed Craniosacral Therapy. In the 1980s, massage gained popularity among athletes because of its ability to reduce the stress of intense workouts, enhance performance, and promote the healing of soft tissue injuries. Many techniques found to be effective when addressing soft tissue conditions in athletes also were effective for hypertonic or dysfunctional conditions in the general population.

allopathic medicine

treatment of disease or injury with the use of medications and surgery.

Massage had turned a corner from being simply relaxing and feeling good to being therapeutic and directed toward improving a person's physical condition. All of these modalities were developed outside of Western medical practices and were considered alternative practices. More and more people began to regularly seek out the services of these alternative practitioners to help to maintain and improve their health. Massage and massage-like practices were accompanied by a wide array of health and healing practices that were considered to be *alternative medicine.*

ALTERNATIVE AND COMPLEMENTARY MEDICINE

The term **alternative medicine** implies that people were seeking services of alternative health practitioners instead of going to allopathic physicians. In fact, many were using the services of conventional doctors and alternative practitioners for the same physical conditions. Many times, this was done without clients informing their medical doctors that they were visiting alternative practitioners at the same time. In the 1980s, the term **complementary medicine** emerged and began to gain popularity, implying that the alternative practices could work along with more conventional medicine for the benefit of the client. A change in terminology was accompanied with a change in attitude. Some alternative practices, massage among them, were becoming more acceptable socially and in the medical community.

alternative medicine

is a term that implies using services other than those usually received from allopathic physicians.

complementarymedicine

is the term that took the place of "alternative medicine" and implies that the alternative practices can work along with more conventional medicine for the benefit of clients.

The establishment of the National Center of Complementary and Alternative Medicine (NCCAM) as a part of the National Institutes of Health (NIH) generated increased research in CAM therapies (http://nccam.nih.gov). Senate bill 2440 established the NCCAM in the fall of 1998. On July 13, 2000, President Clinton, by executive order, appointed members and the chair for the White House Commission on CAM policy to develop administrative and legislative recommendations to increase benefits and protect the public by providing consistent and credible research. Results of clinical studies were published in the *Journal of the American Medical Association* and other prestigious scientific and medical journals.

Complementary and Alternative Medicine Defined

The Panel on Definition and Description, CAM Research Methodology Conference, Office of Alternative Medicine, NIH, Bethesda, Maryland, April 1995, defined *complementary and alternative medicine* as a broad domain of healing resources that encompasses all health systems, modalities, and practices and their accompanying theories and beliefs, other than those intrinsic to the politically dominant health system of a particular society or culture in a given historical period. CAM includes all such practices and ideas self-defined by their users as preventing or treating illness or promoting health and well-being. Boundaries within CAM and between the CAM domain and the domain of the dominant system are not always sharp or fixed.

Research continues at hospitals and academic institutions across the United States. Because of these reported findings, more medical doctors are supporting the use of various CAM therapies along with prescribed medical care. More doctors are using CAM therapies for their own health maintenance. Nearly one half of U.S. medical schools are offering some education on CAM.

Complementary and alternative medicine (CAM) encompasses several healing practices, philosophies, and therapies that conventional Western medicine does not include, study, accept, or generally offer (See Box 20.1).

Box 20.1

Cam Modalities

A wide variety of health or healing practices is included in CAM. Here is a partial list:

Acupuncture
Alexander technique
Aromatherapy
Asian bodywork (therapy)
Ayurveda
Biofeedback
Chelation therapy
Chinese herbal medicine
Chiropractic
Color therapy
Deep breathing exercises
Diet therapy
Folk medicine
Glandular therapy
Guided imagery
Herbal medicine
Homeopathy
Humor therapy
Hydrotherapy
Hypnosis
Light therapy
Massage
Meditation
Movement therapies
Music therapy
Naturopathy
Neurolinguistic programming
Nutrition counseling
Pet therapy
Prayer and spiritual healing
Progressive relaxation
Reiki
Shiatsu
Sound therapy
Visualization
Yoga

Alternative versus Complementary versus Holistic versus Integrative Medicine

Complementary and alternative medicine encompasses many therapies that have developed outside of the Western medical model and are not necessarily based on surgical or biochemical theories. The term *CAM* is well recognized, partially because of the creation in 1998 of the NCCAM at the NIH. Other terminology is often used interchangeably, such as *holistic medicine, body-mind therapies,* or *integrated medicine,* although each of these terms has special considerations.

Holistic means to look at the whole picture. When applied to health, holistic takes into account the whole person and not just the symptoms. All of the things affecting the health of the person—including spiritual, physical, mental, emotional, social, and environmental factors—are considered. Holistic treatment can include medical intervention combined with music in a conducive setting while the patient would also receive massage, acupuncture, Reiki, or hypnosis and participate in a support group. Holistic approaches also emphasize wellness, healthy lifestyle, and active participation by the person in her healing process. Diet, imagery, positive thinking, meditation, and motivational tools are commonly used together.

Mind-body medicine considers the power of the mind or thought processes and their effect on the physical. Techniques include positive attitude, hypnosis, and guided imagery, as well as meditation, relaxation techniques, tai chi, and yoga. Mind-body response is supported by studies in psychoneuroimmunology and is the source of healing from within, spontaneous healing, and the placebo effect.

Integrative medicine combines complementary and alternative medicine with allopathic medicine. In an integrated model, a health care team, including doctors, massage therapists, acupuncturists, nutritionists, other selected health providers, and the patient meet together and cooperate to create a plan to best benefit the health maintenance of the patient. Integrative medicine effectively combines high technology and high touch to provide the best overall support for the patient. Recognizing that mind, body, spirit, emotion, and environment all play a part in healing the whole person, in which no one system has all the answers, many resources can be combined to support health on many levels.

Integrative medicine combines complementary and alternative medicine with allopathic medicine.

According to Andrew Weil, *alternative* insinuates "instead of"; *complementary* indicates a nice add-on, fluff; *integration* is a true coming together and cross-acceptance of the medical models. It is the meeting of the minds, worlds,

Box 20.2

Complementary or Alternative?

In 2002, the Medical Subject Headings Section staff of the National Library of Medicine classified alternative medicine under the term *complementary therapies*. This is defined as therapeutic practices that are not currently considered an integral part of conventional allopathic medical practice. Therapies are termed as *complementary* when used in addition to conventional treatments and as *alternative* when used instead of conventional treatment.

and philosophies. In keeping with Weil's model, he is training physicians in the practice and implementation of integrative medicine. In this model, the physician is still the director and decides which course to take, whereas in a true integrative model, the patient would be the director. Innately, patients know what they need. If they are interested in their health, they can make choices when given the appropriate information.

In 1993, David Eisenberg, MD, published a study in the *New England Journal of Medicine* that surveyed people across the United States in 1990. It revealed startling use of unconventional therapies and CAM modalities for chronic or serious health problems. Thirty-four percent of the respondents reported using at least one unconventional therapy the previous year. The survey showed that 83 percent of those visiting alternative practitioners for serious medical conditions had also visited allopathic doctors in the same year for the same condition; however, 72 percent of those did not tell their conventional doctor that they had sought out or used alternative therapies.

In 1997, another study by Eisenberg indicated that 40 percent of all Americans and more than 50 percent of people between the ages of 30 and 55 years had used some form of alternative therapy. Indeed, in 1997, there were an estimated 629 million visits to alternative practitioners, compared with 386 million visits to primary care physicians. Both surveys indicated that an overwhelming majority of patients seeing alternative practitioners were also seeing allopathic physicians. The study also showed that in 1997, Americans spent more than $27 billion on alternative therapies, which exceeded the out-of-pocket spending for all U.S. hospitalizations.

Surveys conducted in 2002 and again in 2007 by the NIH also indicated that 38 percent of the adult population in the United States had used some CAM in the previous 12 months. This survey was based on over 23,000 interviews. Chiropractic and massage virtually tied as the most popular practitioner-delivered complementary modality used. The use of massage increased by nearly 60 percent from 2002 to 2007. The use of non-vitamin, non-mineral natural products was the most popular CAM modality, followed by deep breathing and meditation. According to the survey, conditions for which CAM was most frequently used included back, neck, and joint pain; arthritis; anxiety; headaches; and insomnia.

The surveys show that the American public continues to use and support the use of alternative therapies. Patients are choosing CAM with their pocketbooks.

INTEGRATIVE MEDICINE

Integrative medicine combines conventional allopathic medicine with appropriate complementary and alternative medicine (CAM) modalities to provide the highest benefit to the client. Integrative medicine programs focus on assisting patients in the creation of customized wellness plans for optimal health that are as responsive to patient's initial concerns as they are to patient's changing health needs, taking into consideration all aspects of well-being. These plans include recommendations from a wide range of appropriate therapeutic interventions from both conventional and complementary/alternative practices. An integrative program might include conventional medications and diagnostic medical screenings and examinations, herbal supplements, Oriental medicine, and acupuncture (Figure 20-1), physical therapy, nutritional therapy, movement, and exercise assessments. The plan might also include stress reduction and mind-body interventions such as biofeedback, massage, art and music therapy, yoga, and meditation. Above all, these plans are founded in mutual trust and respect between patient and practitioner, with the understanding that each person has a significant, innate capacity for healing that can be supported and enhanced.

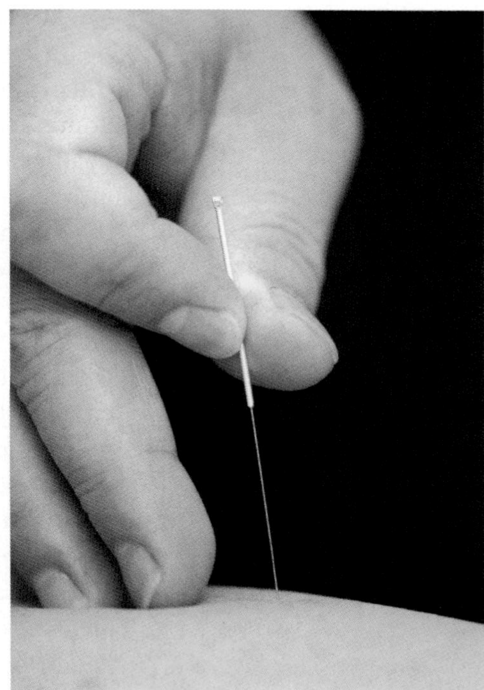

FIGURE 20-1 Integrative medicine recognizes that mind, body, spirit, emotion, and environment all play a part in healing the whole person.

By combining modalities to reduce symptoms, enhancing the ability to control pain and anxiety, and better managing stress and improving quality of life, integrative medicine is particularly successful at assisting patients who have chronic medical conditions. Patients with chronic health problems, ranging from arthritis to headaches to life-threatening illnesses such as heart disease and cancer, combine traditional medical care with integrative methods to ensure that their physical and emotional well-being is addressed. A close collaboration among the physician, integrative medicine team, and the patient helps to choose treatments and services that can be thoroughly integrated into the patient's overall medical care.

Integrative medicine is a health care program that is principled in science and tradition, in which the patient is treated as a whole person and respected as an individual being. The patient in an integrative medicine program is encouraged to participate fully in health care choices to attain optimal health. Patients are listened to and treated with respectful consideration as a partner in the development of their health plan. They are given recommendations founded in Western/conventional medicine combined with appropriate lifestyle recommendations such as diet and exercise, appropriate CAM treatment options such as herbal medicine, acupuncture, massage, biofeedback, yoga, and stress reduction techniques. A care plan is tailored to fit each patient's needs and to honor each patient's personal healing process. The patient is also given the help needed to sort through the myriad complexities within complementary, alternative, and conventional health options to customize a health plan that is right for that person.

Many health centers and hospital complexes around the United States have opened centers of integrative medicine. These centers offer a variety of alternative or complementary health services in conjunction with mainstream Western allopathic medical practices. Practitioners from a wide variety of CAM modalities are available to provide their services. Each practitioner is part of the health team, integrating services to support and enhance the health and well-being of the patient. Many of the integrative health services provide wellness services to hospital staff and outpatient services to people in the community. Many also provide services for hospital inpatients in certain circumstances and under the supervision of the medical staff.

Because integrative clinics are connected to hospitals, the CAM modalities used at those clinics are gaining acceptance and recognition by parts of the medical community and the community at large. Integrative medicine programs see themselves as agents of change, dedicated to the transformation of health care from a disease-oriented, physician- and technology-centered model into a wellness, patient-centered orientation that understands and empowers the integration of body, mind, spirit, and community in health care.

As the medical community gains a better understanding of the level of interventions available from different types of massage and other CAM therapies, patients will benefit by integrating CAM and conventional medical practices with their physician's referral, recommendation, or at least, knowledge and cooperation. Patients' reports of positive outcomes from the use of CAM modalities are part of what changes the attitudes and opinions of the medical community. Educating the medical community and the community at large is an ongoing function of the integrative clinic, the practitioners who practice there, and the participants who benefit from the services.

Massage is often the first choice, or at least on the top of the list, for patients using integrative medicine. Massage therapy might be the remedy for a specific condition, or massage therapy might be an adjunct therapy to complement a therapy regime. Massage therapy is one of the most effective CAM modalities for relieving stress and managing pain that is associated with so many pathologic conditions. Massage is one of the most popular and requested CAM modalities, and it is the most familiar. Massage therapy is the mainstay of many CAM and integrative clinics.

Just as there are numerous complementary and alternative practices in integrative medicine, there are also many different styles of massage and touch therapies used in integrative medicine clinics, according to the circumstances and needs of the patient/client. Some of the variations of somatic therapy found in integrative clinics include Swedish massage, NMT, trigger-point methods, craniosacral, Rolfing, manual lymph drainage technique, infant massage, pre- and postnatal massage, and energy modalities including Reiki, therapeutic touch, and shiatsu.

Classic Western or Swedish massage is very popular when the client is seeking respite from the rigors of more stressful conventional medical treatments. Circumstances might prompt special considerations, such as cancer treatment, AIDS, prenatal care, preoperative preparation, postsurgical recovery, or recovery from a traumatic accident. Massage increases relaxation, promotes well-being, and reduces anxiety in patients undergoing more invasive therapies. Massage is about touch and human contact. It is a key to wellness.

Lymph drainage therapy is offered in many integrative clinics to assist patients who experience lymphedema following the surgical removal of lymph nodes or other congestive conditions.

Massage services that are specific to the client's condition can also be requested. This might be the request of the patient, the suggestion of the integrative team coordinator, or a prescription from the client's physician. Specific massage might be orthopedic massage to reduce pain and increase range of motion (ROM) and function to a particular body area, or scar tissue massage to reduce the detrimental effects of excessive scar formation. If there is any consideration of submitting billing to insurance, a prescription from the client's physician is required. (More on insurance billing can be found later in this chapter.)

The experience of working in an integrative clinic helps the therapist to become more aware and knowledgeable about other therapies. A massage therapist who is knowledgeable about other CAM therapies is able to suggest other CAM modalities or refer clients to other therapists who might be able to support the client in her healing journey. Massage becomes a doorway to open clients to using other CAM therapies.

Working in an integrated system, especially a hospital-related program requires the massage therapist to follow set guidelines and protocols. Protocols are established for each CAM service offered. Protocols and procedures delineate the standard of care to the patient; define relationships and communication between practitioners, staff, and administration; reflect professional standards; and ensure that all practices are within the policies of the hospital and other legal entities. The Joint Commission on Accreditation of Healthcare Organizations (JCAHO) routinely reviews hospital operational policy and practices before providing accreditation for their continued operation. During these surveys, protocols, policies, and procedures must be clearly stated and meet professional standards before the hospital or the program is accredited.

If an integrative clinic is a hospital department or if massage therapists are employed by the hospital, therapists might need to meet certain competencies for the hospital to maintain its accreditation. Those competencies might be evaluated through written tests, hands-on demonstrations of competence, verbal examinations, or a combination of the three. If a massage therapist is working in a particular department, such as the birthing center, and is doing postpartum massage, she will be required to show that she has knowledge of positioning the patient, understands precautions about working with new mothers, and is knowledgeable about epidurals or cesarean sections. There might be competency examinations for each massage modality.

Record Keeping

Clear and accurate documentation is required when working in an integrative setting. When working in an integrative clinic, especially in a hospital setting, a massage therapist must follow hospital regulations regarding patient safety, record confidentiality, and patient information. Patient records provide communication from patient to provider and from provider to provider. Records must be accurate, stating what the practitioner saw and did. Accurate records become the communication tool among various modalities and the means by which the coordinator follows the patient's progress and counsels the patient regarding health care decisions.

Documentation of massage services is included in the patient's chart. Clear, concise language describes the services provided. Documentation of massage includes the assessment, type of massage given, effects of the treatment, any physical observations, and follow-up recommendations. Most hospitals use a central charting system in which all health care providers, doctors, nurses, physical therapists, and CAM practitioners document in the same chart. The SOAP charting system (see Chapter 9) of documentation is commonly used in the medical community and is well suited to CAM practices; however, many settings use a descriptive explanation of services. The practitioner should learn and follow the documentation procedure that the facility uses.

CHIROPRACTIC AND MASSAGE

Many massage therapists work in chiropractors' offices. The relationships between the chiropractic and massage practices vary between offices. Often, the massage therapist is an independent contractor who simply rents a space in the chiropractor's office. The massage therapist might be responsible for scheduling his own appointments and might work entirely independently from the chiropractor. On the other hand, the office receptionist might handle all scheduling and billing for services. Occasionally, the chiropractor might refer one or more of his patients for massage when soft tissue conditions need to be addressed. The chiropractor might suggest that the patient receive a short massage before the adjustment because it helps her to relax and prepares the tissues so that the chiropractor's manipulations are easier and more effective. Some patients prefer a massage after being adjusted by the chiropractor. They think that the effects of the combined treatment far exceed the effects of either treatment given by itself. The chiropractor might also diagnose a soft tissue condition and refer the patient to the massage therapist for several therapy sessions (Figure 20-2).

Massage and chiropractic therapies together can address structural alignment issues and the soft tissue conditions that so often accompany them. The massage therapist spends the time to work with the soft tissue to increase circulation, reduce spasms, deactivate trigger points, and increase ROM. The chiropractor is then easily able to adjust the spine and other joints to improve the overall structure and function of the client.

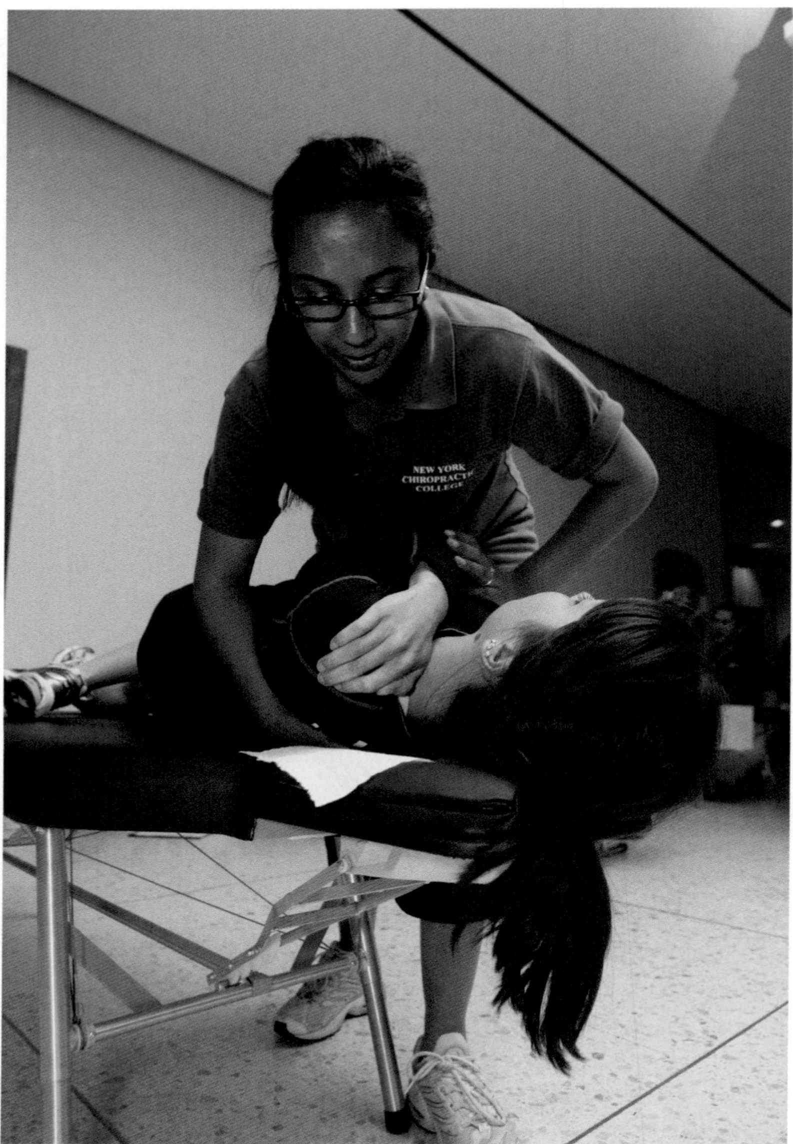

FIGURE 20-2 Chiropractors adjust spinal vertebrae to improve structural alignment.

HOSPITAL-BASED MASSAGE

Hospital-based massage, as its name suggests, takes place in a hospital environment. The therapist might be employed by the hospital, could be an independent contractor, or could even be a volunteer or work through an associated hospital program, such as an associated integrative clinic. Sometimes the therapist is associated with the physical therapy department. Therapist services can be available to hospital staff, patients, or patients' families. Benefits of massage to staff include decreased staff turnover, increased productivity, improved morale, decreased sick time, decreased worker compensation claims, and improved quality of patient care. Benefits of providing massage to patients include improved sleep, reduced need for pain medication, earlier discharge, and more satisfaction regarding patient care.

Providing massage services to patients requires a recommendation, referral, or prescription by the patient's doctor. Even without a prescription, the physician must provide a recommendation or release for the massage. A prescription is required before any third-party (insurance coverage) payment can be pursued. If the therapist is working as an employee of the hospital and has a prescription to provide massage, insurance reimbursement might be available through the hospital's patient billing services. Usually the patient requests the massage. Services are generally provided on a cash basis, whereby the patient pays the therapist directly. Services are usually performed with the patient in the hospital bed. The therapist might encounter a wide variety of medical conditions. Careful consideration must be given to medical equipment (e.g., catheters and monitors) that might be around the hospital bed and connected to the client. The massage therapist must have a clear understanding of related pathologies and indications and contraindications of each of the clients when working in a hospital environment.

Hospitals can seem impersonal and intimidating. Receiving a massage from a caring massage therapist helps to relieve the feeling of being institutionalized and improves the patient's overall sense of well-being (Figure 20-3). Studies have

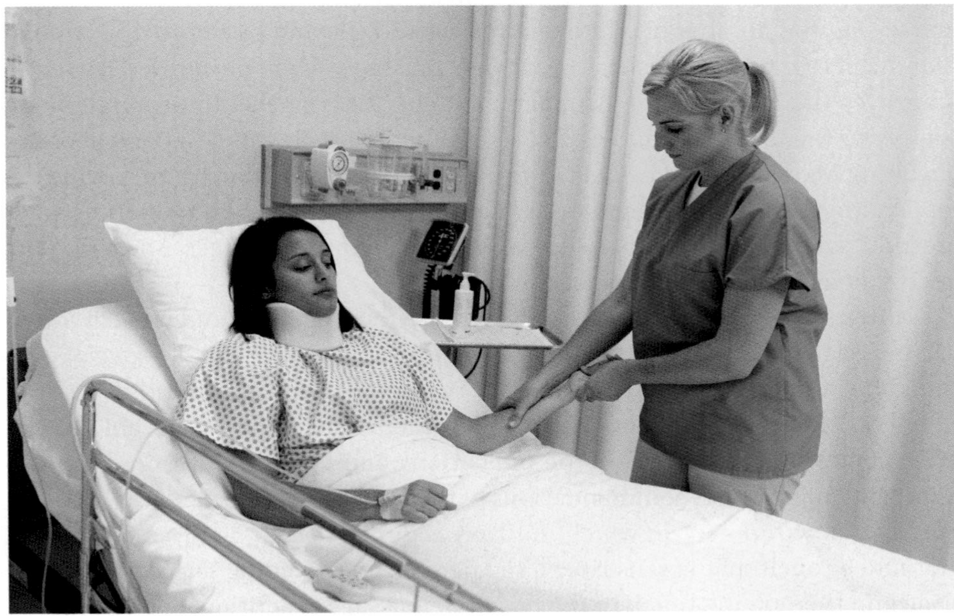

FIGURE 20-3 For patients staying in the hospital, massage from a caring massage therapist can reduce anxiety, improve sleep, and improve the overall sense of well-being.

found that massage reduces anxiety, improves sleep, and reduces requests for pain medication.

Some hospital areas in which massage is performed include prenatal, postnatal, preoperative, and cancer treatment areas. Massage before surgery helps to reduce a patient's anxiety and also seems to reduce the time spent in recovery.

Massage services have become a common addition to birthing centers. Massage helps to promote relaxation during the birthing process. It also helps to reduce the back pain often associated with labor. Acupressure can help to stimulate contractions and ease the process.

Massage during cancer treatment provides a service that feels good when most treatment feels bad. Given before invasive treatments such as radiation or surgery, massage can help to reduce anxiety. Massage has also been found to reduce pain. After surgery and the initial healing, massage can help to reduce scar tissue, relieve edema, and help the client to regain a better sense of self.

Massage is valuable after trauma, such as motor vehicle accidents, to help people to reintegrate their own bodies, which many times have gone through radical changes.

Massage is valuable in the treatment of injuries to soft tissues and joints and is prescribed in a wide range of conditions. Massage is used in some cases to treat nervous fatigue, insomnia, headache, tension, stress, and other disorders.

In a hospital setting, massage is used as part of the physiologic and psychological rehabilitation process. When a person becomes ill or is injured, it is common to feel a sense of apprehension, insecurity, and anxiety, which often leads to restlessness and insomnia. A good massage increases the patient's comfort, induces relaxation, and helps to relieve anxiety. When a patient is confined to bed for a period of convalescence, muscles lose their tone, joints become stiff, and skin develops sensitivity. Unless a patient is turned or can move, bedsores might develop. Massage helps to prevent these problems.

In addition to increasing the patient's comfort, massage aids healing by increasing the number of white and red blood cells and by improving circulation, which in turn nourishes the tissues. Massage, when performed correctly, improves the action of the lymphatic system. It also helps to promote blood supply to the brain and nerves so that the patient feels more in control of her faculties. Massage is used as an aid to preventing constipation by improving the peristaltic action of the small intestines and colon. There are numerous ways in which massage has been found to benefit patients of all ages. Many doctors recommend it as an aid to a speedier recovery.

Often the massage services provided are modifications of classical Swedish massage to help to soothe and reduce stress. There are usually special considerations and precautions because of the population receiving the massage services. It is essential that the massage therapist be knowledgeable of the pathologies present, aware of the indications and contraindications for massage, and follow the recommendations of the attending physician.

In an environment in which most procedures tend to be invasive, there is not much touch that is sensitive to the person. By providing services like massage and therapeutic touch in the hospital, massage practitioners can begin to bring compassionate touch back into health care.

Contraindications for Massage in Health Care

Unlike the practitioner who works with healthy clients, the massage therapist in a health care setting often works with people who are ill, injured, or recovering. The stage of the person's illness or injury often determines the extent to which a massage might be given beneficially, or whether it should be given at all. Massage must be approved by the patient's physician.

Massage brings more fluid, blood, nutrients, and oxygen to affected areas of the body, but sometimes massage must not be given to or near an affected part. The patient's physician will note deterioration of muscles or skin that could benefit from massage and will also note any contraindications for massage. The therapist does not apply massage in cases of illness or injury without the supervision or permission of the patient's physician.

The following is a general review of contraindications:

- Bleeding (internal or external)
- Skin problems such as rashes, growths, lesions
- Newly formed scar tissue, scabs, wounds, and burns
- Infections, swollen areas, pain, inflammation, heat in the area
- Nausea, vomiting, and fever
- Edema: Excessive lymph fluid often causes swelling in feet and legs, particularly in elderly people. Sometimes the physician recommends gentle effleurage or lymph drainage therapy in the direction of the lymphatic flow to help to relieve this condition.
- Varicose veins: Veins in the legs become dilated and lengthen owing to increased blood pressure. In mild cases, massage may be performed on nearby areas but not directly on the affected part.
- Inflamed joints such as arthritis and bursitis: massage is not performed on the area when it is painful and inflamed.
- Cancer: When any symptom of cancer is detected or if any condition is suspected to be cancerous, massage is avoided on or near the area.

The following are warning signs that are associated with cancer and are contraindications for massage. Clients who show any of these signs should be referred to a doctor:

- Any sore that has not healed normally
- A mole, skin tag, or wart that is changing in color or size
- Lumps underneath the arms or in the breasts
- Persistent hoarseness, coughing, or sore throat
- Abnormal functioning of any internal organ, such as changes in the bladder or bowels
- Discharge or bleeding from any part of the body
- Persistent indigestion or difficulty in swallowing

MASSAGE AS MEDICINE

Currently, massage and manual therapies are experiencing a resurgence in popularity within the medical profession. As research continues to verify the benefits of massage and patients continue to profess its value and request referrals

Box 20.3

A Case of Neck Pain

A prospective client comes for a massage for relief of headaches, neck and shoulder pain, and pain and tingling in her arm that has been intermittent but persistent since an automobile accident she was in several months ago. Before proceeding with any massage treatments, the therapist refers the client to her physician for a full examination and an accurate diagnosis. The client can also request a prescription from the physician for massage and provide for release of medical information so that the massage therapist may contact the physician. In so doing, the massage therapist protects the client and himself by making sure that there is an accurate diagnosis and that there are no hidden medical conditions. Having a prescription for massage also opens the possibility of obtaining insurance coverage for the massage services. This might increase the likelihood of more extensive and consistent massage services to achieve lasting relief for the client.

from their doctors for massage, more doctors are writing prescriptions for massage (Box 20.3). Some of these physician-prescribed massages take place in hospitals and integrative or medical centers; however, most of the time, medically prescribed massages occur in the office or studio of independent massage therapists. A massage to address a condition diagnosed by a physician can be considered a *medical massage* (Box 20.4).

medical massage

medically prescribed massage performed with the intention of improving pathologies diagnosed by a physician.

Medical massage is sometimes defined as medically prescribed massage performed with the intention of improving pathologies diagnosed by a physician. Medical massage is generally practiced on patients to bring about a medical goal for health improvement. Medical massage is part of the medical treatment.

Box 20.4

Conditions That Benefit from Medical Massage

Medical massage can be an effective treatment for several conditions, especially when stress or musculoskeletal issues are involved. Some diagnosed conditions that are referred for medical massage include

- Anxiety
- Athletic injuries
- Back pain
- Carpal tunnel syndrome
- Edema
- Emotional stress
- Fibromyalgia/fibrositis
- Headaches
- Insomnia
- Migraines
- Myofascial pain
- Neck pain
- Osteoarthritis
- Postinjury rehabilitation
- Repetitive strain injuries
- Sciatica
- Sprain/strain
- Temporomandibular joint dysfunction
- Tendonosis and other tendon injuries
- Thoracic outlet syndrome
- Whiplash

The goal of the massage therapist providing medical massage is to apply techniques that positively and directly affect the diagnosed condition. The therapist must be familiar with the pathologies involved and with therapeutic modalities that positively address the conditions. The therapist might use a variety or combination of modalities or procedures during the treatment, such as Swedish massage, NMT, craniosacral therapy, myofascial release, lymphatic drainage, massage for cancer patients, orthopedic massage, trigger-point therapy, soft tissue mobilization, or acupressure, depending on the condition and the skills of the therapist. Medical massage is specifically directed to resolve conditions that have been diagnosed by a physician and focuses treatment on the areas of the body related to the diagnosis and prescription.

Medical massage is directed toward a diagnosed medical condition or at least is given with the consideration of a medical condition being present. The massage might be directed toward a soft tissue condition to improve function, relieve tension, increase ROM, and/or relieve associated pain. Massage can also be prescribed to help to manage stress and anxiety related to pathologies or medical conditions that are otherwise unaffected by the massage.

Medical massage sessions follow a therapeutic procedure (see Chapter 17). The prospective client comes to the session with some condition or injury and seeks a massage to remedy or improve the medical condition. A physician or chiropractor has previously diagnosed the condition, and the client has a prescription or recommendation for massage. A concise health and client history helps the therapist to better understand the client's conditions and concerns. A thorough assessment at the beginning of the first session further determines the tissues involved. The therapist must have an acute awareness of indications and contraindications for the diagnosed conditions. Techniques are chosen, a care plan is created, and the treatments commence. The therapist continually assesses the tissues and responses of the client while performing appropriate techniques to address the condition. Massage services are directed toward the affected condition according to the doctor's diagnosis. Sessions of medical massage are usually shorter and more frequent. Full-body massages are generally not warranted. When the condition subsides or improves to a level where there is no further improvement, the goal for the treatments is accomplished, and further treatments are discontinued.

INSURANCE REIMBURSEMENT FOR MASSAGE

Massage therapists in many parts of the United States are experiencing the advantages and frustrations of obtaining reimbursement from insurance companies for the work they do on massage clients who have been injured and referred to them from a doctor or chiropractor. The decision to accept insurance cases into a massage practice requires some consideration of the pros and cons of working with the clientele and their insurance companies.

Working with the clients can be very rewarding as they find relief from their injuries with the soft tissue interventions of medical massage. With the doctor's recommendation and prescription, the regular massages are therapy that would otherwise be unavailable to the client.

The therapist, however, must be willing to provide services to the client and prepare the necessary paperwork to bill the insurance company, then patiently wait or battle for reimbursement while the insurance company processes the claim. Usually reimbursement payments are fairly prompt; however, the insurance company sometimes request more information or review a claim. Sometimes the waiting continues for months or even years, after which the therapist's fees for service might be reduced or even denied. Knowledge of proper billing practices reduces the frustration of resubmitting claims and increases the promptness and probability of being paid by the insurance companies. Proper billing requires close attention to detail when preparing claims, clear communication with the company agent, and accurate record keeping while documenting client progress and billing information.

There are a wide variety of types of insurance providers. Most do not reimburse massage therapists for the services provided. HMOs and PPOs will not cover the services of a massage therapist unless the therapist is listed as a provider in the group. Even then, massage services are usually available to the subscriber only at a reduced rate. Government health insurance (e.g., Medicare and Medicaid) does not cover massage services. Most major medical insurance policies do not cover massage therapy at this time. As massage becomes more recognized as a cost-effective alternative, however, this could change.

The types of insurance cases that are more likely to cover massage therapy are state worker's compensation, auto insurance, and some personal injury (PI) cases. In Washington state, legislation was passed in 1996 requiring insurance companies to reimburse licensed massage therapists for services performed on patients when prescribed by a doctor. The state of Florida also has legislation that requires insurance providers to reimburse massage therapists for certain types of services. When a therapist decides to accept insurance cases, it is a good idea to start slow, learn the ropes, and become comfortable with the process. Begin with one or two insurance claims. Learn the intricacies of correctly filling out and submitting the necessary paperwork and communicating with insurance agents. Proper filing of insurance claims requires considerable time. If the owner of a massage business decides to accept several insurance clients, she might want to consider contracting with a billing service to file claims, thereby leaving more time to see clients.

Filing a Claim

The process in which insurance billing is done is fairly standardized. Following a procedure when working with insurance cases and billing insurance companies can simplify the process and increase the chance of prompt payment from the insurance company. Organization, clear documentation, perseverance, patience, attention to detail, and promptness are required to reap the benefits of insurance reimbursement successfully.

For a claim for massage therapy to be considered by an insurance company, the massage treatments must be considered to be medically necessary. Medical necessity can be determined only by a doctor, chiropractor, or possibly a physical therapist and is documented by a letter of referral and/or a prescription. A referral to a massage therapist must include a statement of medical necessity and a prescription that includes a diagnosis of the condition, an order for services to be preformed, the frequency of treatments, and how long the treatments will continue until the patient will be reevaluated by the doctor. The billing to the insurance company must reflect massage services as they appear on the prescription.

If during the intake assessment the massage therapist recognizes conditions related to the client's injury beyond those indicated on the doctor's prescription, the therapist can request that the doctor rewrite the prescription to include the additional conditions so that they are included in the insurance claim. The client can return to the doctor and ask that the related condition be added to the diagnosis, or the therapist can call and inform the doctor of his observations, and ask whether the physician would consider amending the prescription. Otherwise, even if the therapist addresses the additional conditions during the therapy session, he may bill the insurance company only for the work done on the conditions listed on the prescription.

When making the first appointment with a new client, the therapist should determine whether it is an insurance case. If it is, the client is instructed to bring the necessary information to the first appointment, or better yet, the therapist collects the necessary preliminary information over the phone to obtain verification from the insurance carrier before the client arrives for the first appointment. The therapist must obtain verbal verification from the insurance company before providing any services to the client.

Verification or Authorization

Before beginning any massage on a new insurance client, the therapist must obtain verification over the telephone from the insurance adjuster that the massage services are covered on the client's policy. The therapist should have the following information before calling for verification:

- client name
- name of policyholder, if different from the client
- insurance company name
- adjuster's name and phone number
- insurance ID number (Social Security Number)
- claim number
- date of incident/injury

The therapist must also have a prescription and preferably a referral letter from a physician or chiropractor. The prescription should include a diagnosis and a treatment plan to include the number, frequency, and duration of the massage treatments to be given.

Obtain verification of the following: does the client have coverage for massage therapy services? Which **current procedural terminology (CPT) codes** are covered? Is there a limit on coverage either in number and frequency of treatments or monetary limit of benefits? What is left under the limit? Is there a deductible? How much and which portion has been met? When does the deductible renew? What percentage of fees does insurance reimburse? Is there a **co-pay**? What is it? If it is a worker's compensation claim, obtain an authorization to proceed.

Worker's compensation requires authorization before services are rendered. Any services provided before authorization is obtained do not have to be reimbursed by the insurance carrier. Rules for worker's compensation vary

current procedural terminology (CPT) codes

were developed and are maintained by the American Medical Association and categorize and quantify medical services and provide a common language and a base for communication between physicians, therapists, patients, and insurance companies.

co-pay

is the portion of the fee for service that the patient is responsible for at the time of service.

from state to state. Before accepting any claims, call the workers' compensation division of the department of employment in your state for information and ask for a fee-for-service manual. Workers' compensation is generally provided from an insurance company designated by the client's employer at the time of the injury. By the time the client comes for treatment, she should have a prescription from the physician, the name of the claims agent or case manager, the agent's phone number, and a claim number. The prescription must include the diagnosis, the prescribed treatment, the frequency of treatments, the duration of treatment, and the physician's license number and signature. The prescription

Box 20.5

Client Information Required for Insurance Verification

The following information is required to obtain verification or authorization from the insurance carrier that massage services are covered by the client's policy. The therapist should not expect to be paid for any services provided to the client before obtaining verification. Even getting verification does not guarantee payment for all the services that are submitted for reimbursement. The therapist needs the following information from the client to contact the insurance company for verification:

- A prescription or a doctor's referral that contains:
  Physician's name and license number
  Diagnosis (ICD-9 code)
  Prescribed treatment (CPT codes)*
- Insurance information
  Name of the insured person
  Name of the insurance company
  Adjuster's name and phone number
  Name of policyholder, if different than name of insured
  Policy number
  Claim number
  Date of injury
  When speaking to the adjuster, verify what will be covered by insurance.
- Will insurance cover the services of a massage therapist?
- Verify that the CPT codes for the prescribed treatment will be reimbursed.
- What is the amount of time allowed per treatment per diagnosis?
- What is the duration of treatments or number of sessions allowed?
- Ask about the deductible:
  How much is the deductible?
  Has the deductible been met?
  When does it renew?
- Ask about co-pay:
  Is there a per-visit co-pay?
  How much is it?
- Ask about percentage of coverage information.
  Remember that verification does not guarantee payment.

*ICD-9 and CPT codes are described on pages 767–768.

must prescribe "massage therapy" or include specific CPT codes that are within the massage therapist's scope of practice.

When communicating with an adjuster or insurance claims agent, it is essential to document the conversation. Record the date and time (to the minute), the name of the agent or agents, and exactly what was said. If an agent transfers the therapist to another party, get the name and the direct phone number of that person in case the transaction is disconnected.

The massage therapist should always obtain a verbal verification of a client's insurance coverage over the telephone before performing any services on that client. Telephone authorization or verification must be followed up with a confirmation letter restating what was verified during the telephone conversation. Fax or mail the confirmation letter to the insurance carrier, requesting a written confirmation of coverage.

Documentation for an Insurance Claim Client

During an initial interview, the client with an insurance claim completes several forms and a preliminary assessment. At the initial interview, the client completes and signs a Medical Information Release Form and an Agreement for Payment Form. The Intake Form and the doctor's prescription should have sufficient information to contact the insurance adjuster for verification of coverage. The Medical Information Release Form is required by law and allows the therapist to share information regarding the client's health (related to the injury) with the insurance company, other health practitioners related to the case, or lawyers or the

Box 20.6

Documentation for Insurance Clients

During the initial visit, the client is requested to fill out several documents, including

- *Client Intake Form*: This form is designed so that the information that it contains will transfer to the 1500 Health Insurance Claim Form.
- *Medical History Form*: May be part of the intake form or a separate document.
- *Medical Information Release Form* (Figure 20-4): This is required to share confidential information with insurance companies, physicians, or attorneys.
- *Agreement for Payment Form* (Figure 20-5): This states that the client is responsible for any fees not covered by insurance.
- *Assignment of Benefits Form* (Figure 20-6): This instructs the insurance carrier to pay the therapist directly for services billed.
- *Informed Consent Form*: This is a client's written authorization for professional services based on adequate information from the massage therapist about the massage, including expectations, potential benefits, possible undesirable effects, and professional and ethical responsibility.
- *Initial Assessment Form*: This will contain current findings related to the physician's diagnosis.

The preliminary visit of an insurance client requires extra time to fill out required documents and to perform an initial assessment. The insurance company might or might not reimburse for the extra time required for the initial assessment.

Medical Information Release Form

Client's Name ______________________________________

Address ____

I hereby authorize ________________________ to release to any physician, insurance company, or attorney directly involved in my case any medical records or other information necessary for the purpose of administration, evaluation, or payment of debt related to my illness/injury sustained on (date) __/__/____.

This authorization remains valid from the date it is signed until revoked by me, in writing to both this provider and the insurance company.

Signed _________________________________ Date _________________________

FIGURE 20-4 Medical Release Form.

Agreement for Payment Form

I understand that I am responsible for all fees charged for professional services rendered. All fees are due at the time of service unless other arrangement are made in advance. If insurance is billed for services, I understand that I am responsible for any charges not covered including co-payments, unpaid percentage of coverage, and deductibles. In the event of insurance nonpayment or denial, I also understand that I am responsible for all fees and will make whatever arrangements possible to make full payment.

I understand that your time is valuable and that 12 hours' notice is required for cancellations and I will be charged for missed appointments without giving proper notice.

Client's Name ______________________________________

Address ___________________________ City ____________ State ____ ZIP _______

Client Signature ____________________________ Date ______________________

FIGURE 20-5 Agreement for Payment Form.

Assignment of Benefits

I hereby direct my insurance provider ______________________ to assign and make direct payment to _________________________, my health care provider, all monies for medical claims submitted by them on my behalf for medically necessary treatment.

Client's Name ______________________________________

Address ___________________________________ Policy Number _______________

Client Signature ______________________________ Date ______________________

FIGURE 20-6 Assignment of Benefits Form.

courts involved with the case. Patient information is not shared or released without the patient's authorization, and then only necessary information is provided and only to those professionals involved or related to the case. The Agreement for Payment Form establishes the client's responsibility for any payment of fees for services that is not paid by the insurance company or in a court settlement. The client should also sign an Assignment of Benefits Form, a copy of which is sent to the insurance company with the first claim so that the carrier can send the claim benefits directly to the therapist for the services performed. Another copy is kept in the client's file so that when sending in future claims, and the client is not available to sign forms, the proper blank can be filled in with "signature on file."

Another important form when working with insurance companies is a receipt for services. The receipt should include all information necessary for the insurance company, the client, and the therapist regarding the session. The receipt should include the following information:

Date of service
Client's name
Charges for service
Payments and adjustments
Previous and current balance
ICD-9 (diagnosis) and CPT (procedural) codes
Therapist's name, address, phone number, and provider number, if there is one
Client's next appointment

During the initial evaluation, the therapist carefully documents any conditions relevant to the client's injury or complaint. The physician's prescription designates specific areas of the body to apply selected procedures. The tissues in the designated area(s) are assessed with palpation, and the condition of the specific muscles is documented on the preliminary assessment form. Tension, trigger points, hypertonicity or hypotonicity, inflammation, swelling, or any other conditions are indicated. Following the session, changes to these conditions are documented.

When performing medical massage or filing for insurance payment, every massage or therapy session must be clearly documented. Usually, this documentation is kept only in the client's files and is not included when filing a claim unless requested by the insurance company. A narrative SOAP note style of documentation is preferred (see later).

The therapist might be required to submit documentation to insurance companies or, if the case goes to court, to attorneys, and therefore it is imperative to keep clear, concise client records.

When performing massage for medical purposes, whether at the request of a physician or from the prescription, or when expecting reimbursement from insurance, it is essential to keep accurate documentation of each and every therapy session. Documentation includes forms completed during the intake procedure, individual session notes, and a receipt for services. Progress or session notes document each session and help the therapist and the client to follow the course and progress of the treatment. Documentation is required for communicating with others involved, such as medical personnel, insurance companies, and even lawyers or the courts. Clear session notes provide documentation that the session happened. They also show proof of progress, which is vitally important to insurance companies as they review and determine to continue payment of benefits.

Insurance companies pay only for services that are deemed medically necessary. The insurer determines medical necessity by reading documentation presented by the service providers. The client's medical history, especially related to the current injury or condition, the referral and prescription from the doctor, the initial assessment, and progress notes are essential documents with which the insurer determines whether to reimburse for the massage therapy services.

Most of the documentation remains in the client files, except the receipt for services, a copy of which is given to the client and a copy is kept in a file for bookkeeping. Copies of the client's medical history, initial assessment, physician's referral and/or prescription, session notes, and the assignment of benefits form will accompany the **1500 Health Insurance Claim Form** as attachments with the initial claim that is sent to the insurance company. It is very important to keep copies of everything that is sent to the carrier. Follow-up submissions of claims for the same incident might require only the 1500 Health Insurance Claim Form, unless the insurance company requests session/SOAP/progress notes and a copy of the prescription with each claim submission. The therapist should ask the claims adjuster during the initial verification to determine the particular company policy regarding which documentation accompanies submitted claims.

1500 Health Insurance Claim Form

is a standardized form created by the Health Care Financing Administration to be used by service providers when billing insurance for medical expenses.

Insurance companies usually prefer progress notes to be in a story form following a SOAP format. The use of abbreviations is discouraged. If abbreviations are used, include a key with every report. Session notes should be typed or written very clearly and easy to read and understand.

The initial SOAP documentation includes the name of the client, name of the physician, name of the therapist, the date of service, location, and type of visit (initial or the number in the series) in the header of the document.

- The **S** (subjective) portion contains the client's experience of the condition, including complaints and symptoms, when and how it started, what makes it better or worse, what has been done about it and the results, and the client's impression or response to the treatment.
- The **O** (objective) portion contains the therapist's observations of visual and palpatory findings, as well as results of any examinations and tests. Remember, when billing insurance, all objective and subjective findings must directly correspond to the diagnosis on the physician's prescription.
- The **A** (assessment) portion of the report contains the physician's findings or diagnosis as well as the functional outcome of the massage session.
- The **P** (plan) portion contains the treatment plan as directed by the physician, including the type, duration, and expected outcome or results.

SOAP documentation for follow-up sessions is somewhat briefer. The header contains the same information as the initial session document.

- The **S** portion contains the client's updated, current experience of her condition, including reactions or responses to the previous massage session.
- The **O** portion contains the therapist's visual and palpatory findings as well as the results of any examinations or assessments.
- The **A** portion reports any functional outcome that the therapist observes or the client reports as a result of the session.
- The **P** portion describes the procedure used and any suggested exercises.

1500 Health Insurance Claim Form

Insurance companies have adopted a standardized form for billing purposes. The 1500 form was created by the Health Care Financing Administration and is now used throughout the insurance industry, eliminating the confusion of different forms for every company. The Center for Medicare and Medicaid Services (CMS) uses an identical form for billing of Medicaid and Medicare Part B services.

The 1500 Health Insurance Claim form was designed to be read by optical character recognition (OCR) software, which is the reason that it is printed with specialized red ink. The form ideally should be filled out using a typewriter or a computer, using black ink. Handwritten forms cannot be read by computer and can result in a delay of payment. If the form is handwritten, use black ink and very legible handwriting. If using a computer, make sure the printer is aligned properly so that all entries are clearly readable. Use all uppercase (capital) letters and an easily read (Courier or Arial, 10 or 12 point) font. Do not copy, staple, paper clip, tape, or fold the form. There are a few software companies that have developed programs to assist in the preparation of the 1500 Health Insurance Claim Forms using client information from client intake and history documents.

The intake form can be designed so that it contains all the necessary information to transfer to the 1500 Health Insurance Claim Form.

The 1500 form also requires the use of procedural codes that refer to the services provided (CPT codes), diagnostic codes that refer to the doctor's diagnosis (ICD-9 codes), and place of service codes, indicating where service is provided.

ICD-9 codes are published by the U.S. Health Services and Health Care Financing Administration and specifically relate to the condition of the client as diagnosed by a physician. *ICD-9* is an acronym for International Classification of Disease, 9th Revision, Clinical Modification. The system was first created by the World Health Organization (WHO) and has been modified in the United States. Every health condition has an assigned decimal number that is used on insurance forms to aid in the uniform reporting of ailments. A medical diagnosis and corresponding ICD-9 codes can be provided only by the doctor. It is preferred that the doctor or the physician's office includes the ICD-9 codes on the prescription. If a prescription does not have an ICD-9 or CPT codes, the physician's office can be called to supply or verify the codes. Usually the doctor's office is very cooperative about supplying the proper codes. Remember, it is outside a massage therapist's scope of practice to diagnose or provide ICD-9 codes; however, it *is* the therapist's responsibility to enter the correct ICD-9 code for the client's condition on the 1500 Health Insurance Claim Forms.

ICD-9 codes

are a system of decimal numbers that correspond to medical conditions diagnosed by doctors. ICD-9 is an acronym for International Classification of Disease, 9th Revision, and is published annually by the U.S. Health Services and Health Care Financing Administration.

Current procedural terminology (CPT) codes were developed by the American Medical Association to categorize and quantify medical services accurately. The codes provide a common language and a base for communication among physicians, therapists, patients, and insurance companies. CPT codes also list the allowable fees for each listed procedure. It is necessary to verify with the insurance adjuster which codes are currently recognized and reimbursed. Worker's compensation claims also require the use of CPT codes; however, worker's compensation may update codes covered in their fee schedules only every several years; therefore contact the state worker's compensation office to obtain the most recent fee schedule.

CPT codes are arranged according to medical specialty, in which specified levels of medical training or certification are required to use particular codes. Massage therapy falls within the category of physical medicine. A therapist must have proper training for the codes that they bill for, even to the extent that they could explain the technique and reasons for using it in a court of law. As of the latest revision of this text, the following CPT codes are most commonly suggested to be used by massage therapists. The therapist should always verify with the insurance carrier which codes are considered for reimbursement.

97010 Application of a modality to one or more areas; for example, hot or cold packs

97124 Therapeutic procedure, one or more areas, each 15 minutes; massage, including effleurage, petrissage, and/or tapotement (stroking, compression, percussion)

97140 Manual therapy techniques (e.g., mobilization/manipulation, manual lymphatic drainage, manual traction); one or more regions, each 15 minutes

Note: This code replaces 97250 (deleted in 1999). Use this code for all therapeutic work. See 97124 for standard massage.

Codes change often. Because of the widening acceptance of massage and other complementary health practices, new codes are being considered to better describe the various therapies. Practitioners should stay informed of changes in the CPT codes. CPT codes are revised yearly with a new CPT manual published annually. Manuals are sold at most major booksellers or can be obtained through the American Medical Association or on their Web site, www.ama-assn.org. Rather than purchasing the code books, the therapist can determine the proper codes to use from the physician's office or the insurance carrier. Contact each claims adjuster when beginning a new case to verify which codes to use. Insurance might not pay for the evaluation done during the preliminary client visit. If the insurance company wants evaluations and will pay for them, ask the adjuster which code to use to cover this service.

Insurance usually pays for only one hour of "physical medicine" per date of service and for a maximum of four 15-minute procedures. Many carriers allow only two units or procedures on a specified area of the body. Each CPT procedure delineates a 15-minute increment; therefore four increments or units constitute one hour. When listing the procedures on 1500 Health Insurance Claim Form, put one unit on each line. It is the therapist's responsibility to know that the codes used are proper and within his scope of practice.

State worker's compensation determines the reimbursement scale for every procedure listed in the CPT codes that is covered by worker's compensation. It is necessary to obtain authorization for every worker's compensation claim. When calling for worker's compensation authorization, call the insurance adjuster of the company carrying the policy, *not* the state worker's compensation office. After authorization is received, the therapist agrees to accept the payment schedule from worker's compensation insurance and not charge the client anything above what is paid by the insurance company. The therapist can request a claim's guide or a fee-for-service manual from the state worker's compensation office that should include which procedures are covered and the fee allowed for each procedure.

Place of service codes on the 1500 Health Insurance Claim Form go in Box 24b. Codes that massage therapists might use are these:

11 office
12 home
21 inpatient hospital
22 outpatient hospital
34 hospice
61 inpatient rehabilitation facility
62 outpatient rehabilitation facility

The therapist completes the 1500 Health Insurance Claim Form, including services provided specific to the diagnosed conditions and the individual and total cost of those services. The therapist includes their tax ID number—either Social Security number or employer identification number—the address where services were provided, and business or billing address, and then signs and dates the document.

The completed 1500 Health Insurance Claim Form with the required supporting attachments is sent to the insurance adjuster. If it is an initial filing, a copy of the prescription, initial assessment, typed session progress notes, and the assignment of benefits form is included. Insurance companies pay only for medical care that is considered medically necessary. The company makes the determination of medical necessity according to the documentation, including physician's referral and prescription, the initial visit/history documents, and the individual session progress notes. These documents must be complete and clear. The insurance carrier might require progress notes from each session to be included with subsequent claim submissions. The treatment and documentation must coincide with the physician's prescription and diagnosis of the patient's complaints to be considered by the insurance company for reimbursement. Be prompt when submitting claims; file the first claim as soon as possible after the client's initial visit. It is preferred that no more than two or three visits be included on a single form. Smaller claims seem to be paid more quickly. Always retain a copy of everything that is sent to the adjuster.

Insurance companies are supposed to respond to claims within 30 days from when they were submitted. If the therapist does not receive any notification in six weeks (include time for mail delivery), they should contact the adjuster to inquire as to the status of the claim. Document the inquiry. If it is a phone call, document the date and time (to the minute), the person with whom the therapist spoke, what was said, and the tone in which it was said. The agent might say that the claim is under review or that they need more documentation. If denial or reduction of fees is part of the conversation, be sure to document any and all reasons. Be as diplomatic as possible when working with insurance adjusters; remember, it is better to have them as an ally than an adversary. If diplomacy fails, persistence and assertiveness might be required to move the process. If the insurance company continuously delays action or payment on a claim, the therapist might inform the client and have her or her attorney contact the company. Another avenue of recourse is to contact the state insurance commissioner to file any concerns. If all else fails and the claim is denied or fees reduced, contact the client, inform her of the decision, and remind her that according to the signed agreement, she as the client is now responsible for the balance due.

SUMMARY

Many of the techniques now referred to as massage were developed as health-promoting remedies or part of a medical treatment in the earliest development of these practices. The earliest medical literature from Persia, Egypt, Japan, and China all make reference to various treatments that include the use of massage-like techniques, although the actual term *massage* did not appear in medical literature until the end of the nineteenth century. Massage-like practices continued to be a part of healing and remedial practices in many cultures around the world throughout history. In Western cultures, references to massage techniques are found in medical literature from 1700 on to the present day.

During the first half of the twentieth century, massage continued to gain credibility and acceptance within the medical field in the form of physiotherapy. It was practiced in hospitals and rehabilitation sanatoriums as a part of the rehabilitation of wounded soldiers returning from World War I and World War II. Physiotherapy was also used for recovering victims of the polio virus. By the 1950s, the use of massage in physiotherapy declined because it was strenuous, time-consuming, and required extensive training. Physical therapy began relying more on exercise and the use of a variety of machines, medicines, and mechanical modalities for treatment. The use of massage in the medical field in the United States was nearly nonexistent after the early 1950s.

Swedish massage maintained a relationship in the natural health field and was practiced in health clubs or spas, sanatoriums, YMCAs, and resorts. Massage began to reemerge during the human potential movement of the 1960s and 1970s outside of allopathic medicine. Classic Swedish massage was joined by reflexology, shiatsu, acupressure, and other alternative practices. In the 1980s, massage gained popularity among athletes owing to its effects on reducing the stress of intense workouts and its effectiveness in promoting the healing of soft tissue injuries. Many of the techniques found to be effective when addressing soft tissue conditions in athletes also were effective for hypertonic, painful, or dysfunctional conditions in the general population. Clients sought the services of massage practitioners to remedy their aches and pains as an alternative to seeking medical treatment. Massage became classified as an alternative medicine along with practices such as acupuncture, nutritional therapy, herbal therapy, and other practices that are not considered an integral part of conventional allopathic medical practice. A study by David Eisenberg in 1991 indicated that an astonishing number of people were seeking the services of alternative practitioners. The study showed that there were more visits to alternative practitioners than to doctors and expenditures to alternative practitioners exceeded the out-of-pocket money paid to hospitals. In the 1980s, the term *complementary medicine* gained popularity, implying that the services of the alternative practitioner would complement those of allopathic medicine, rather than be an alternative to it. The National Center of Complementary and Alternative Medicine (NCCAM) was established in 1998 as a part of the NIH to develop administrative and legislative recommendations to increase benefits and protect the public by providing consistent and credible research. Research into the effects of massage and other complementary practices continues at hospitals, academic institutions, and in private clinics across the United States. Because of reported findings, more medical doctors now support the use of various CAM therapies along with prescribed medical care.

Integrative medicine combines complementary and alternative practices with allopathic medicine to create a care plan that is tailored to fit each patient's needs to honor each patient's personal healing process. It includes recommendations from a wide range of appropriate therapeutic interventions from both conventional and complementary/alternative practices to provide the highest benefit to the client. A patient can meet with an integrative team consisting of a medical doctor and a wide variety of alternative practitioners to develop a care plan to best serve her individual needs.

Integrative medicine is particularly successful at assisting patients who have chronic medical conditions by combining modalities to reduce symptoms, to enhance the ability to control pain and anxiety, and to better manage stress and improve quality of life. A close collaboration between the physician, integrative medicine team, and the patient enables a choice of treatments and services that are thoroughly integrated with the patient's overall medical care.

Integrative medical clinics are often associated with a hospital and offer a variety of alternative and complementary services to hospital patients and staff. A massage therapist working in a hospital-related program is required to follow set guidelines and protocols that delineate the standard of care to the patient; define relationships and communication between practitioners, staff, and administration; reflect professional standards; and ensure that all practices are within the policies of the hospital and other legal entities. Accurate documentation that follows hospital protocols is essential in that it is the communication tool between providers and the means by which the coordinator follows the patient's progress and counsels the patient regarding health care decisions.

Massage in the twenty-first century is reemerging as an integral part of people's health practices. Whether it is to manage stress or pain on a regular basis or as part of an integrated treatment plan for handling cancer or other illness, massage and bodywork are becoming a common choice for persons seeking better health. As research continues to verify the benefits of massage and patients continue to profess its value and request referrals from their doctors for massage, more doctors and patients are making massage a part of their medical treatment. Massage that is prescribed by a physician or chiropractor to address a diagnosed condition can be considered a medical massage and is part of a medical treatment. The therapist can use a variety of techniques with the intention of directly and positively addressing the diagnosed condition. Medical massage is especially effective for musculoskeletal and stress-related conditions.

A client seeking medical massage has seen a physician and has a prescription for massage. That prescription should contain a diagnosis and an order for massage therapy services to be performed, including the frequency of treatments, and how long the treatments will continue until the patient will be reevaluated by the doctor. The massage session should follow a therapeutic procedure with a thorough assessment, treatment plan, massage, and evaluation. Massage services are directed toward the affected condition according to the doctor's diagnosis. Sessions of medical massage are usually shorter and more frequent. When the condition subsides or improves to a level at which there is no further improvement, the goal for the treatments is accomplished and further treatments are discontinued.

Because medical massage is done according to a doctor's prescription, certain types of insurance reimbursement are available. There are pros and cons to working with a clientele and their insurance companies that the therapist must consider before accepting insurance cases. Working with the clients can be very rewarding; however, insurance billing requires extra paperwork, and sometimes dealing with the insurance companies can be time-consuming and frustrating. Whereas most major medical policies, HMOs, PPOs, and government insurance such as Medicare and Medicaid do not cover the services of a massage therapist, personal injury from auto insurance and workers' compensation claims are more likely to pay for massage therapy when prescribed by a doctor or chiropractor. Filing an insurance claim is a fairly standardized yet rather complicated process. Successful reimbursement requires close attention to detail when preparing claims, clear communication with the company agent, and accurate record keeping while documenting client progress and billing information. Medical necessity must be established. The client must have a prescription that contains a diagnosis, including ICD-9 codes and an order for massage, including CPT codes. The billing to the insurance company must reflect massage services as they appear on the prescription. Different insurance companies require different documentation when filing a claim; however, almost all companies use the standardized 1500 Health Insurance Claim Form accompanied by other documentation. It is necessary to contact the claims agent for the case to verify that services are covered and which documentation is required. Patience and persistence are necessary when depending on insurance companies to pay for services provided to clients, because it can take months or even years to be reimbursed, or in some cases, the claim is reduced or denied, in which case it is imperative that the client understands that she is responsible for payment for any services not reimbursed by insurance.

Historically, massage is closely associated with medical practices when working with musculoskeletal conditions and physical rehabilitation. In the mid-twentieth century in the United States, massage fell out of favor in the medical community, only to reemerge as a most popular form of complementary and alternative therapy in the beginning of the twenty-first century. Continuing research, better training, and patient demand are restoring massage therapy to be a viable and valuable component of the health care system.

QUESTIONS FOR DISCUSSION AND REVIEW

1. What did Charles Fayette Taylor and George Henry Taylor have in common?
2. Define CAM.
3. Differentiate between alternative medicine and complementary medicine.
4. What is integrative medicine?
5. What is the role of massage in integrative medicine?
6. What are some considerations for hospital-based massage?
7. What are the seven early warning signs for cancer?
8. Define medical massage.
9. Why should a massage therapist obtain verification before providing massage services for a client seeking insurance reimbursement?
10. What is a 1500 Health Insurance Claim Form?
11. What are ICD-9 codes?
12. What are CPT codes?
13. Which documents should be included in an initial insurance claim?

CHAPTER

21 Other Somatic Therapies

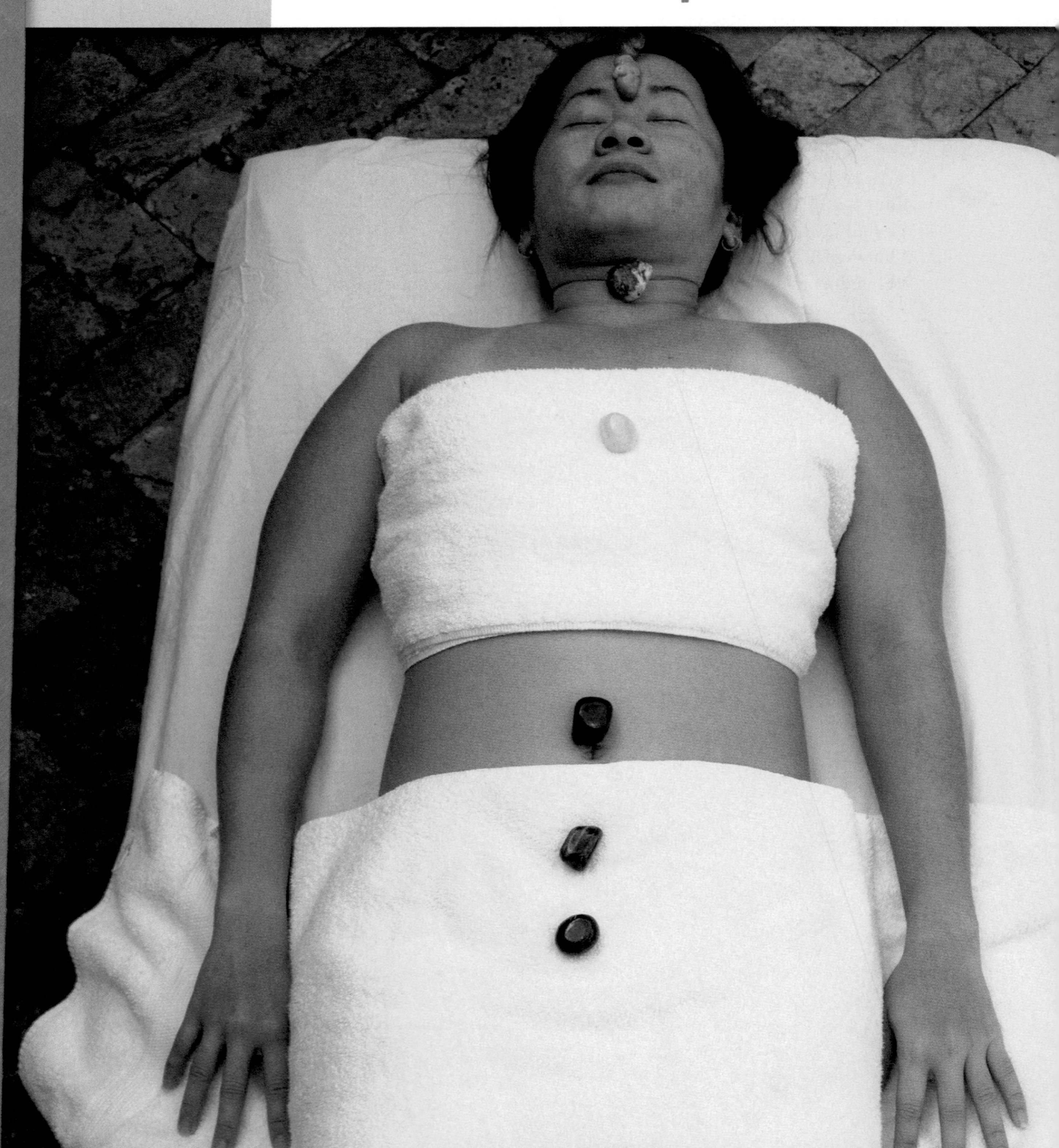

LEARNING OBJECTIVES

After you have mastered this chapter, you will be able to:

1. **Describe basic chair massage techniques and demonstrate a simple chair massage routine.**
2. **Define reflexology and be able to locate reflexology points on feet and hand maps and demonstrate a basic foot reflexology sequence.**
3. **Explain the basic philosophy of acupressure and acupuncture.**
4. **Describe shiatsu as related to pressure points of the body.**
5. **Describe the location of the seven chakras.**

INTRODUCTION

Recent years have seen a resurgence of interest in various touch therapies that relate to the maintenance of physical, mental, and emotional health. Many of these techniques have origins in the far Eastern philosophies of Japan, China, and India. The techniques discussed in this chapter are chair massage, reflexology, acupuncture, acupressure, shiatsu, and chakra energy healing techniques.

It is not within the scope of this book to cover in detail every therapy style; however, the serious student or practitioner is encouraged to continue her training by exploring various styles and sharpening her skills to serve her clientele better. Continuing education through advanced programs at schools or in workshops is necessary to stay current with new developments and techniques available to the massage professional. There is a wealth of reference material listed in this book's bibliography. The brief discussions in this chapter will acquaint the practitioner with the basic concepts of a variety of techniques. At the end of the chapter is a partial list of other popular somatic therapies that the serious student might want to explore.

CHAIR MASSAGE

Chair massage is a growing, highly visible branch of professional massage. In airports, shopping malls, convention centers, supermarkets, street corners, dentists' offices, the workplace, and other venues, chair massage practitioners are introducing thousands of people who ordinarily might not consider receiving table massage to the benefits of skilled touch.

History

The origins of chair massage can be traced to the earliest history of bodywork. Centuries-old Japanese block prints illustrate bathers, newly emerged from the tub, receiving massage while seated on a low stool. Indeed, many styles of East Asian table or floor massage traditionally perform a portion of each session (often at the beginning or end) with the client sitting up rather than lying down.

In the modern bodywork tradition, methodologies such as Rolfing, Feldenkrais, and Alexander techniques regularly work with clients in a seated position.

As a discrete segment of the contemporary profession, this style of bodywork was formulated and popularized by David Palmer, a former massage school owner. Palmer began experimenting with massaging seated clients in 1982 as a way of making it easier for his students to introduce their services to potential clients. In 1986, he developed the first specialized chair for seated massage and began training practitioners at other bodywork schools throughout the country.

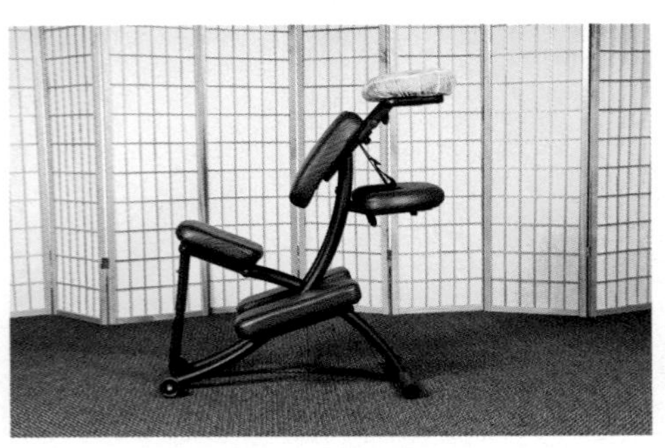

FIGURE 21-1 Massage chairs are available from several manufacturing companies.

Today, massage chairs are available from more than a dozen different manufacturers (Figure 21-1). Most bodywork schools include some form of chair massage in their core curriculum. Seated massage is widely available around the world and is considered an integral part of the massage profession.

Advantages of Chair Massage

Chair massage has made skilled touch physically, psychologically, and financially accessible to the general public. Because the client does not disrobe and no lubricants or lotions are used, a practitioner with a portable massage chair is no longer restricted to working in a private room behind closed doors. Chair massage has been performed on planes and trains, in gyms and beauty salons, at the beach and state fairs, in RV parks and flea markets, on movie sets, and in professional ballparks. On-site chair massage is offered in teacher's lounges and corporate offices, providing professional people with relaxing and rejuvenating breaks in their busy schedules. The variety of locations is limited only by the imagination of the practitioner.

For those who have a personal history of negative touch experiences, chair massage is a way to reintroduce positive touch into their lives. Shelters for battered women and programs assisting victims of physical, sexual, and emotional abuse or other forms of post-traumatic stress disorders often include chair massage among their services. Chair massage can be helpful in reconnecting clients with emotions that must be processed for successful recovery.

Finally, because a typical chair massage session lasts only 5 to 20 minutes, not only is it well-suited to the fast pace of urban living, but it also makes a massage significantly more affordable. Whereas relatively few people choose to spend $45 to $60 a week on a table massage, $5 to $15 a week is more manageable. The low cost of chair massage makes it the easiest way to experience massage for the first time and to integrate regular massage into a healthy lifestyle.

The Role of Chair Massage in a Bodywork Practice

Because the best way to learn massage is by doing massage, the versatility of chair massage makes it ideal for students and new practitioners. It is much easier to learn than table massage, and students can begin their practice massages sooner. Because chair massage is so user-friendly, more people are willing to offer their bodies for practice. If you are setting out on a massage career, chair massage is one of the best ways to introduce clients to your touch and market your table practice.

A regular chair massage clientele also provides good balance to a table practice by helping to prevent the "cabin fever" syndrome, which occurs when practitioners begin to tire of the same four walls day after day. Seated massage also allows bodyworkers to interact with their community in a broader, more spontaneous way, which some practitioners find helps to keep their practices, and their lives, fresh and exciting.

A growing number of practitioners now make chair massage their exclusive bodywork practice. Some prefer it for the same reason the general public does: the perceived safety and control that comes with not having to deal with modesty issues behind closed doors. Others see chair massage as the best way to accomplish the goal of introducing new markets to professional touch. For whatever reason they like it, chair massage is a valuable addition to every bodyworker's toolbox.

The Process

Because chair massage is done mostly through the clothing without lubrication and tends to be high volume (larger numbers of clients in a day than table massage), certain adjustments are necessary.

Gliding or effleurage movements are generally not possible through clothing. Without these "resting" strokes, kneading movements tend to tire the hands quickly. Consequently, superficial or deep touch, combined with friction, compression, percussive techniques, and perhaps some simple stretches are more commonly employed. Virtually all of the acupressure techniques of East Asian bodywork, traditionally done through clothing or a towel, are ideally suited for this style of bodywork.

The head, neck, shoulders, arms, back, and hips of a client seated in a massage chair are most readily accessible to the practitioner. In one newer method of chair massage, however, a lower leg and foot massage can be done by seating the client in a traditional chair or turned around backward in a massage chair.

The determining factors in the creation of a personal chair massage routine are the length of the massage and the special needs of the target market. For example, if you provide services to a large number of people in a short period, each session is necessarily shorter. If the client is wheelchair bound, the lower back might not be as accessible as in other clients, and that factor will dictate the kind of massage you can perform.

There are also a few special hygiene considerations. Because the chair is not draped with a sheet, particular care must be exercised in cleaning the vinyl surfaces that come in contact with clients' skin. The face cradle and armrest (also knee rest and chest pad if the client is wearing shorts or without a shirt) should be sanitized with an antimicrobial wipe or spray solution after each use. Likewise, without a sink nearby, practitioners should be prepared to sanitize their hands by using a similar procedure.

In addition, face cradle covers should always be used and changed with each client. Because the face cradle is typically tilted, try to pick covers that do not slide off the vinyl. Although cloth covers work well, if you are massaging 20 or more clients a day, laundering can become a major expense. A soft paper towel is a convenient alternative. A less labor-intensive choice is a set of disposable hair coverings with elastic bands around the edges (worn by nurses and food service workers). They are available from medical supply stores or massage chair manufacturers at a very low price.

As with table massage, every client must be screened before sitting in a massage chair. Although chair massage can be used as part of an overall remedial treatment plan, by far its most common uses are to provide relaxation, reduce stress, and promote health. An abbreviated version of a standard table screening probably suffices, with strong adherence to the rule "When in doubt, don't." Because time pressures often do not permit extended assessment, a conservative approach to screening is more appropriate for chair massage.

There is one special screening consideration: because the client is seated rather than prone, she might experience a sudden drop in blood pressure, possibly leading to symptoms of fainting. This rarely occurs when a client is lying on a table because gravity keeps blood (and thus oxygen) moving to the head. The most common reasons seated clients might faint or experience symptoms of fainting is because they missed a meal and their blood sugar is low, or because they have a history of fainting. If they have missed a meal, a quick snack—a muffin or a glass of juice—usually makes them feel more comfortable. If they have a history of fainting, ask them to let you know immediately if they feel any lightheadedness, nausea, sudden sweating, or clamminess. In addition, be alert during the massage for fidgeting, particularly if you see the client lift her head away from the face cradle. Stop the massage and ask if she feels all right. If not, immediately position her so that she can place her head between her knees or so that she is lying prone. Although fainting is not a common experience, the potential for it does exist, and a wise practitioner is prepared to handle it.

Sample Brief Chair Massage Routine:

After a brief consultation to determine if there are any contraindications or special considerations, introduce the client to the massage chair and explain how to sit in the chair (Figure 21-2a). Make any adjustments to the chair, such as the height of

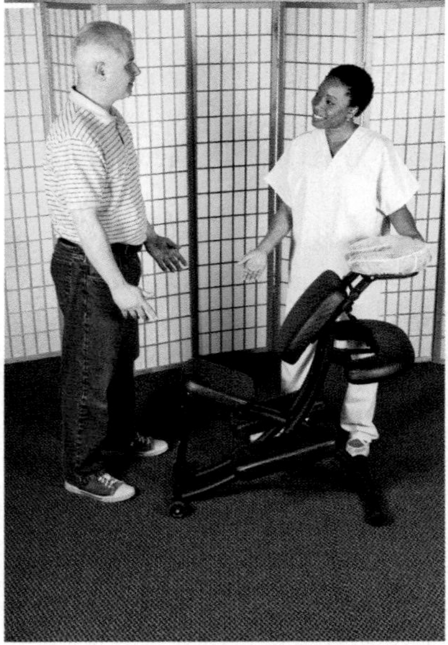

FIGURE 21-2A Explain to the client how to sit in the massage chair.

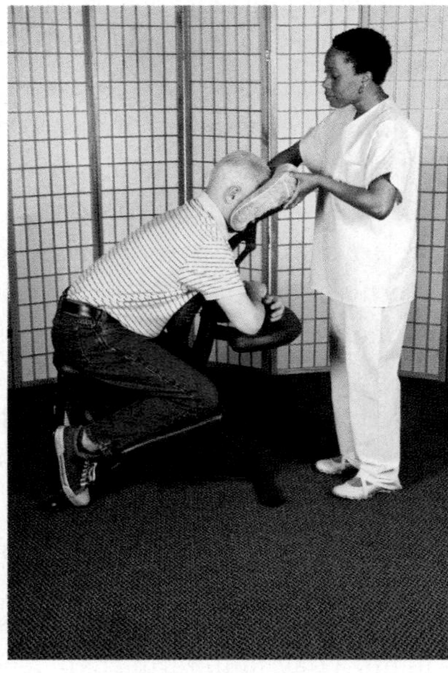

FIGURE 21-2B Adjust the chair to fit the client comfortably.

the chest pad and the height and angle of the face rest (Figure 21-2b). When the client is comfortably seated, begin by making contact with and performing compressions on the shoulders (Figure 21-3) and then work down the back along each side of the spine. Repeat this sequence a few times, going more deeply with each pass. Then using palms or fists in small circular motions, massage down either side of the spine. After a couple of passes, change to using the pads of the fingers to apply pressure along side of the spine and around the scapulae (Figure 21-4). Change to using the thumbs to apply pressure very close to the spine from the base of the neck to the top of the hips, making sure to change hand positions, keeping the wrists as straight as possible. Move down an inch at a time and repeat. Change to fists (instead of thumbs) once you get close to the lower back, and work until you reach the hip bone. Return to compressions with the hands, and then press the forearms onto the upper trapezius muscles, alternating pressure on each shoulder (Figure 21-5a). Then turn to face the client. Press palms of the hands down onto the shoulders, using a circular and pressing motion simultaneously, and alternating. Continue by using circular friction with the pads of the fingers on either side of the neck, making sure that you do not work too anteriorly. Repeat, alternating between pressing the shoulders and massaging the neck (Figure 21-5b). Use the

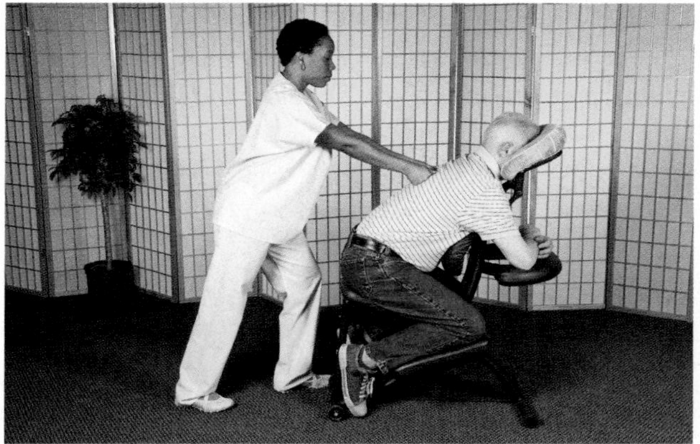

FIGURE 21-3 Apply compressions to the shoulders and down the back.

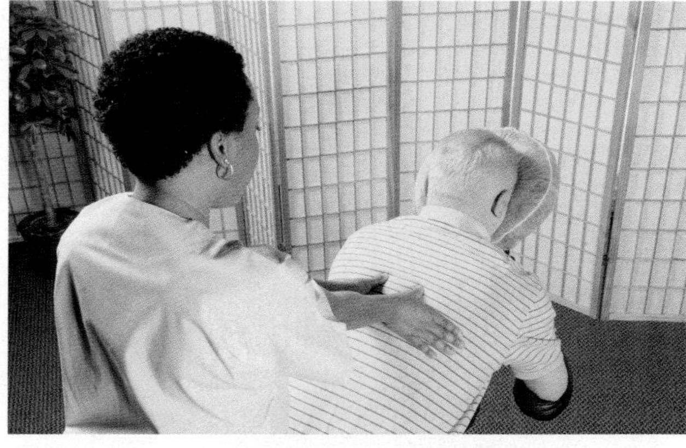

FIGURE 21-4 Use the thumbs, hands, and elbows to apply compressions around the scapula.

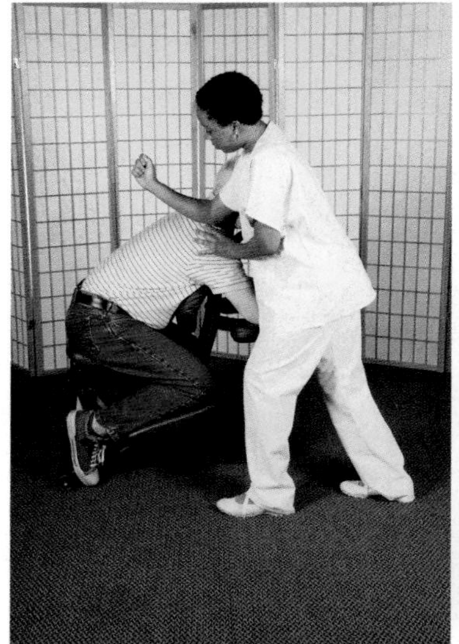

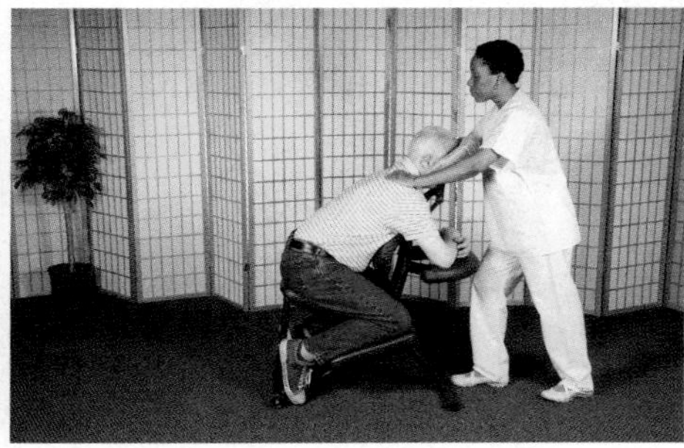

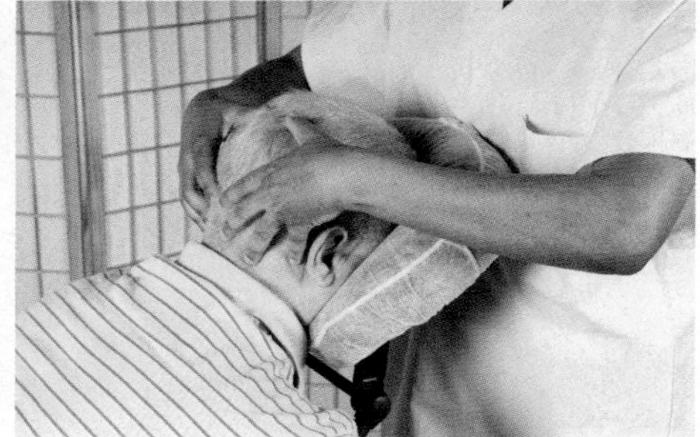

FIGURE 21-5 A-C Face the client, and apply compression and petrissage to the upper shoulders and up the sides of the neck to the back of the head.

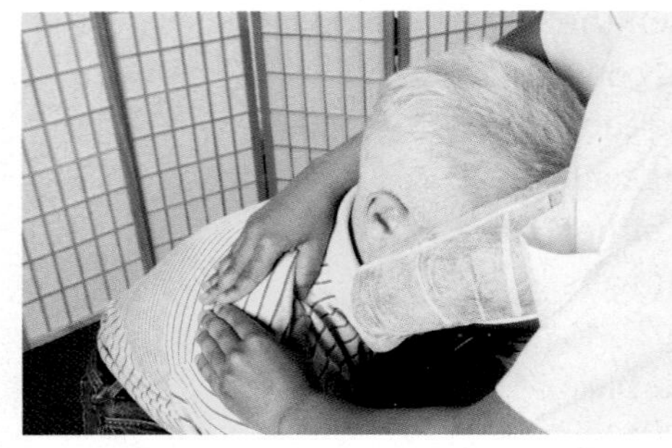

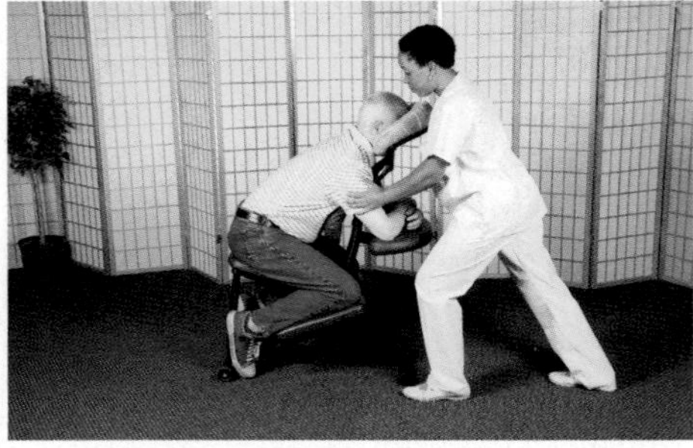

FIGURE 21-6 A AND B Move to the side of the chair and compress the shoulders from front to back. Then compress the arm from the shoulders to the wrist.

pads of fingers to apply circular friction from the tops of the shoulders up the sides and back of the neck toward the base of the skull (Figure 21-5c). Then hook fingertips under base of skull and pull gently, elongating the neck and holding that position for a few seconds.

Step to the client's side. Perform compressions with one palm in front and one palm in back of the shoulder, squeezing gently (Figure 21-6a). Then perform compressions down the arms (Figure 21-6b). With the client's palms facing up and resting on the armrest, massage the hands by working the entire palm and between the tendons on the back of the hand (Figures 21-7 a and b). Then massage each finger and thumb from the base to the tips, lightening the pressure as you move down to the nails. Next, place arm at the client's side and lightly shake the arm by placing hands on either side and move them back and forth (similar to starting a fire with a twig) and move down the arm to the hands (Figure 21-8). Return the hands and arms to the armrest. Repeat the entire sequence on the other shoulder, arm, and hand. Walk around to the client's back and work down the client's back, performing compressions as before (Figure 21-9). Then massage the scalp with fingertips (make sure to ask first. If you are in the workplace, many people do not want their hair mussed) by pressing down and moving the scalp and not the hair, so that minimal mussing occurs (Figure 21-10). Then perform light hacking and tapotement (percussion) on the shoulders and down along

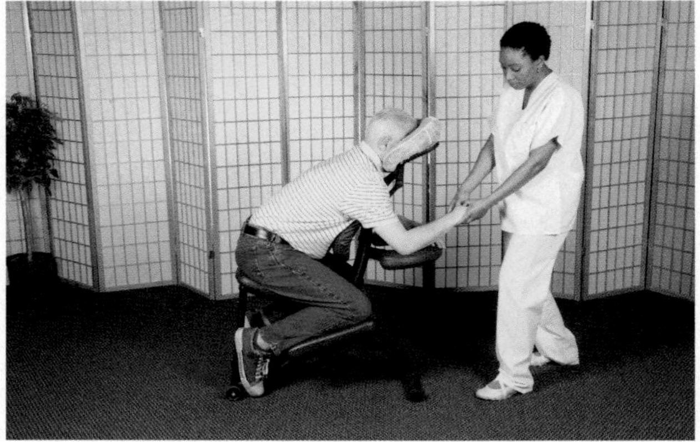

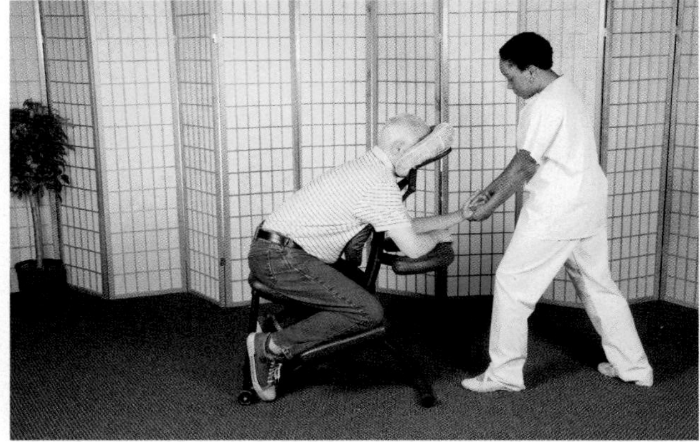

FIGURE 21-7 A AND B Massage the hand.

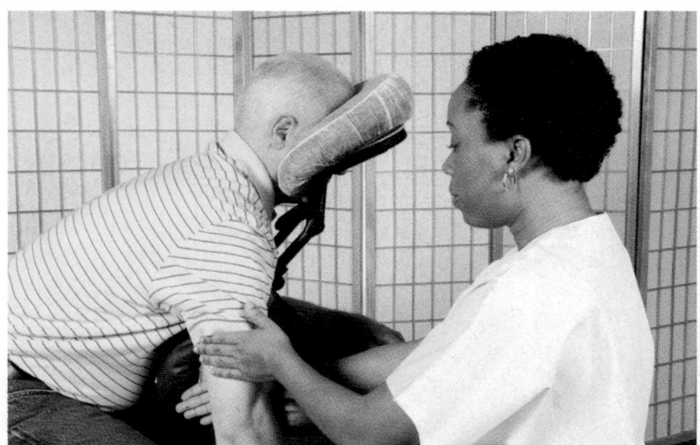

FIGURE 21-8 Let the hand and arm hang, and wring and roll the arm from the shoulder to the hand. Then put the hand back on the arm rest, and massage the other arm and hand.

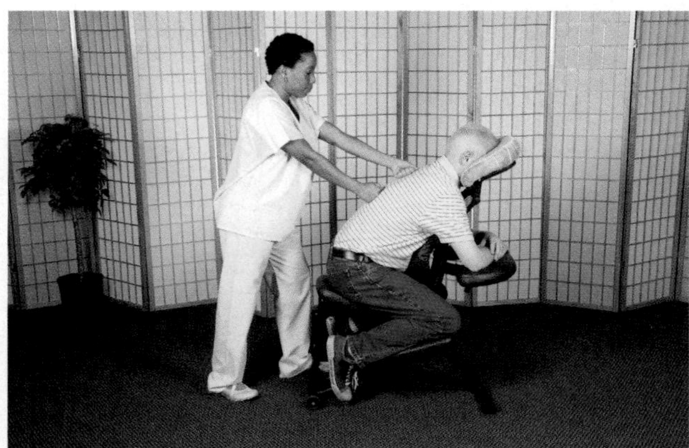

FIGURE 21-9 Walk around to the client's back and work down the client's back, performing compressions.

either side of the spine (Figure 21-11). End with light feather strokes (nerve strokes), starting with the top of the head and along the spine to the lower back. Repeat twice.

Variations can easily be added to elongate the session; this is merely a basic routine to get started.

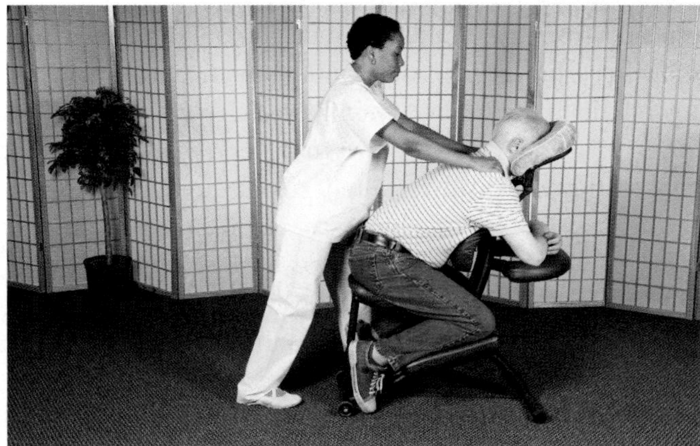

FIGURE 21-10 Return to the shoulders and up the neck with petrissage and friction. If appropriate and after asking the client if it is permissible, massage the scalp.

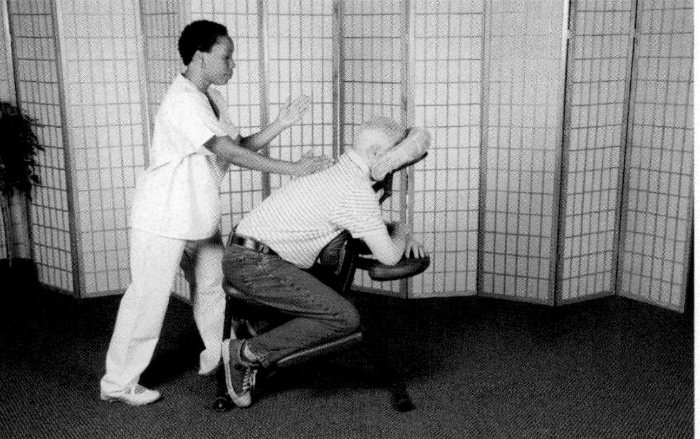

FIGURE 21-11 Perform light hacking and tapotement (percussion) on shoulders and down along either side of the spine. Finish with nerve strokes all the way down the back.

REFLEXOLOGY

Reflexology is the art and science of stimulating the body's own healing forces by locating and stimulating certain points on the body that affect organs or functions in distant parts of the body. It is a form of compression massage, using mainly the thumbs in a technique called *thumb walking*. Reflexology is based on the principles that reflex points in the hands and feet are related to every organ and area of the body.

History of Reflexology

The roots of reflexology have been dated as far back as more than 4,000 years ago with painted hieroglyphs in ancient Egypt. Reflexology as it is known in the West began as zone therapy. There are ten zones that run longitudinally from the top of the head to the hands and feet (Figure 21-12). The person that popularized zone therapy is Dr. William Fitzgerald, who later joined forces with Dr. Joe Riley to make others more aware of this practice. They later met Eunice Ingham, who eventually wrote two books that furthered the popularity of reflexology (i.e., *Stories the Feet Can Tell* and *Stories the Feet Have Told).* Eunice devoted her life to the practice and instruction of reflexology.

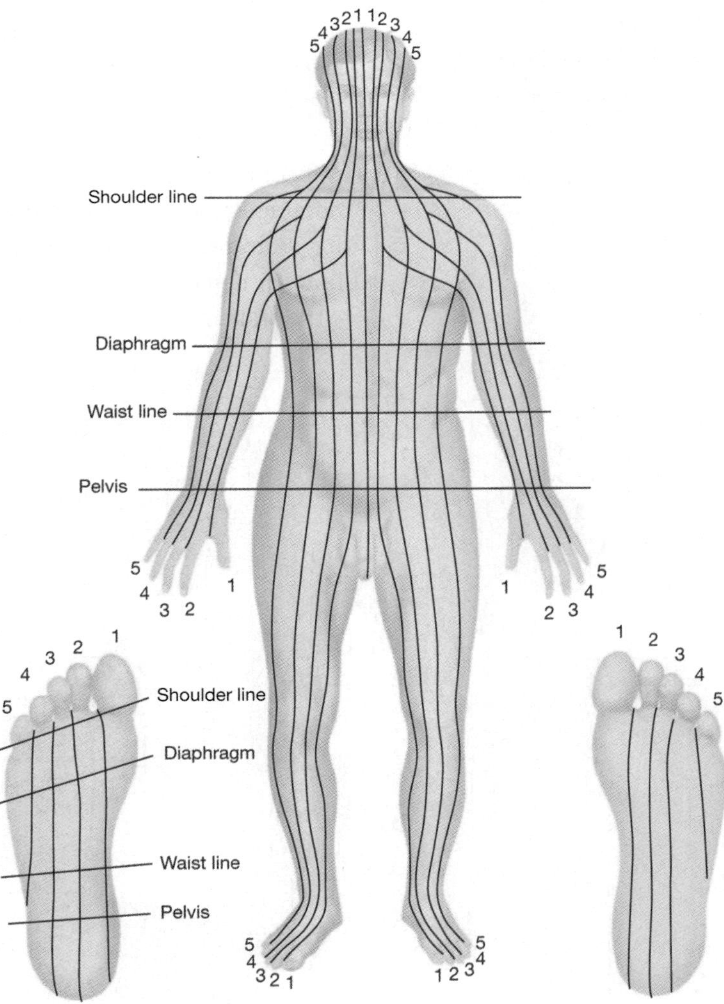

FIGURE 21-12 The body is divided into ten zones that reflect on the hands and feet.

STUDENT ACTIVITY

To learn the reflexology maps of the feet, put on white socks and draw the maps in different colored markers on the socks. It is more convenient to pair up with another person and draw on each other's feet. To learn the maps of the hands, put on white gloves or latex-free gloves and draw maps with colored markers on the hands. Hint: it is easier to draw one hand at a time instead of wearing gloves on both hands while drawing. You might also find it easier to draw on another's hand than on your own.

How Reflexology Works

By applying pressure to a reflex point, the practitioner can stimulate certain beneficial changes in a distant area of the body related to that point. For example, when reflex massage is given to certain points on the big toe, it is said to relieve headache and tension. Activating these links through stimulating reflex points can relieve tension, improve the blood supply to certain regions of the body, and help to normalize body functions. When an organ is distressed, it becomes inflamed or congested. That inflammation triggers the brain to send messages down to the corresponding reflex point, creating an inconsistent texture or sensitivity. A reflexologist feels for inconsistencies such as knots, harder areas, swelling, crunchiness, or an area that is sensitive. Maintaining good communication with your client is important, asking them to tell you if any point is sensitive. Usually areas of inconsistencies are sensitive, although sometimes an area is sensitive without any inconsistencies and sometimes there are inconsistencies without any sensitivity. When one of these areas is found, the practitioner applies pressure to that point repeatedly and then proceeds with the routine.

Reflexology Session

During a reflexology session, the practitioner works on each foot, feeling for these inconsistencies and sensitive areas, keeping in constant communication with the client. Learning the maps of the feet and hands is imperative to the practice of reflexology (Figures 21-13 a–d and 21-14). The basic routine varies from practitioner to practitioner but usually follows each zone from the heel to the toe. The routines can last anywhere from 20 minutes to 90 minutes, depending on the needs or desires of the client. The more time that is available, the more time that can be spent working each reflex area that indicates an imbalance. Reflexology is not a cure-all nor can it be used to diagnose. It merely detects imbalance, congestion, or inflammation and can send messages back to the brain to affect the areas by sending endorphins and more circulation to that area.

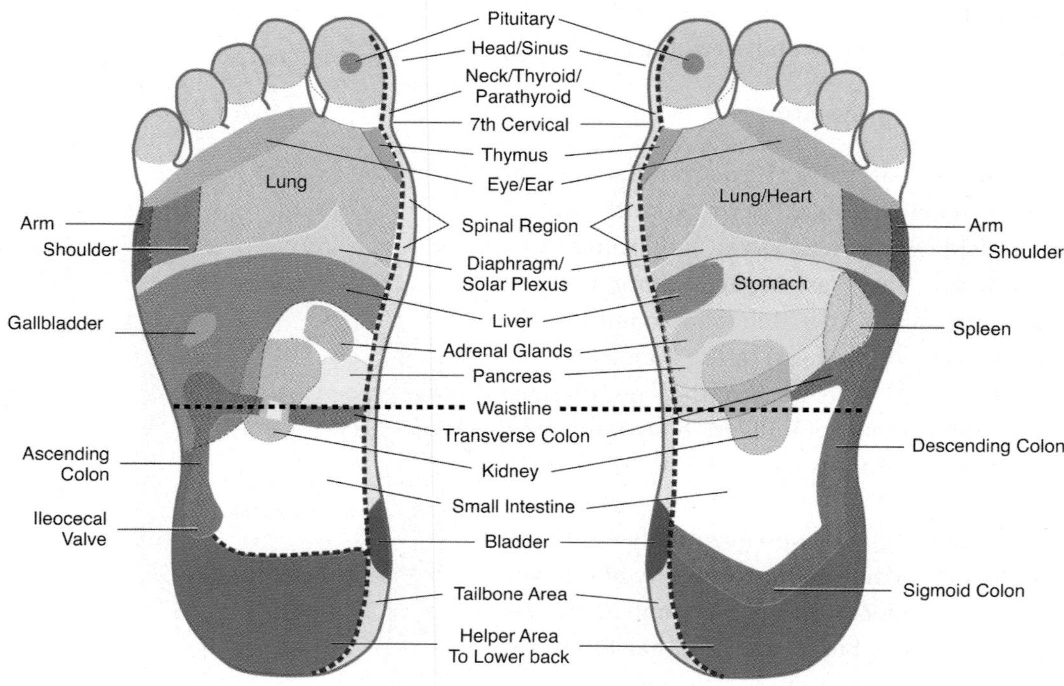

FIGURE 21-13A

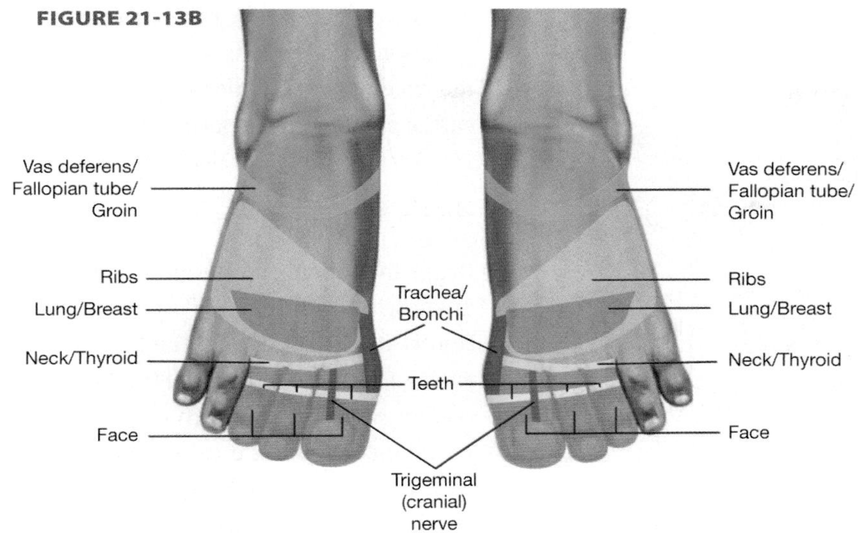

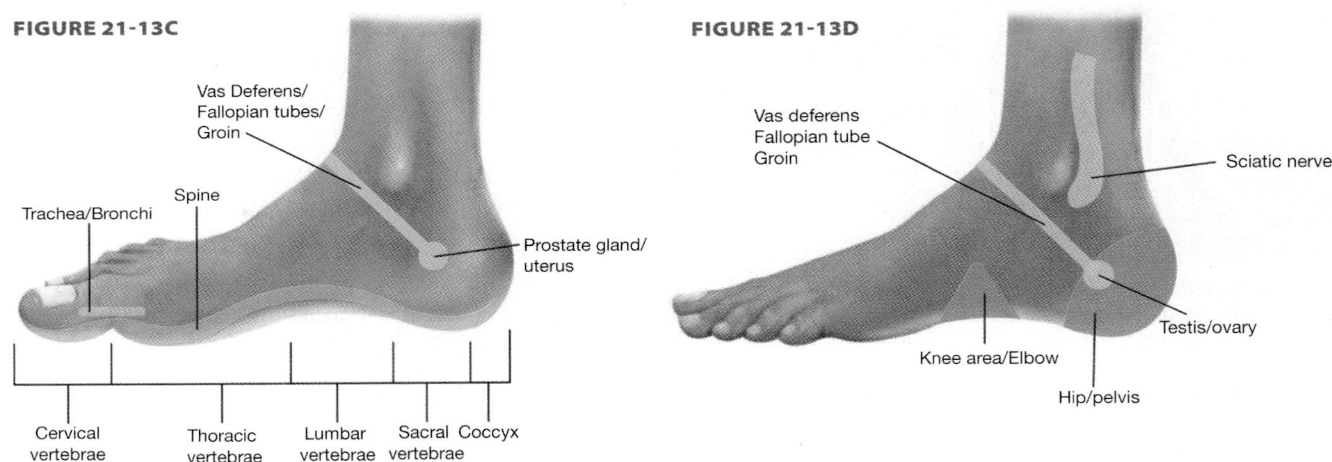

FIGURE 21-13 A-D The foot reflexology chart indicates points on the foot that reflexively correspond to other areas of the body. A) Bottom of the foot. B) Top of the foot. C) Medial side of foot. D) Lateral side of foot.

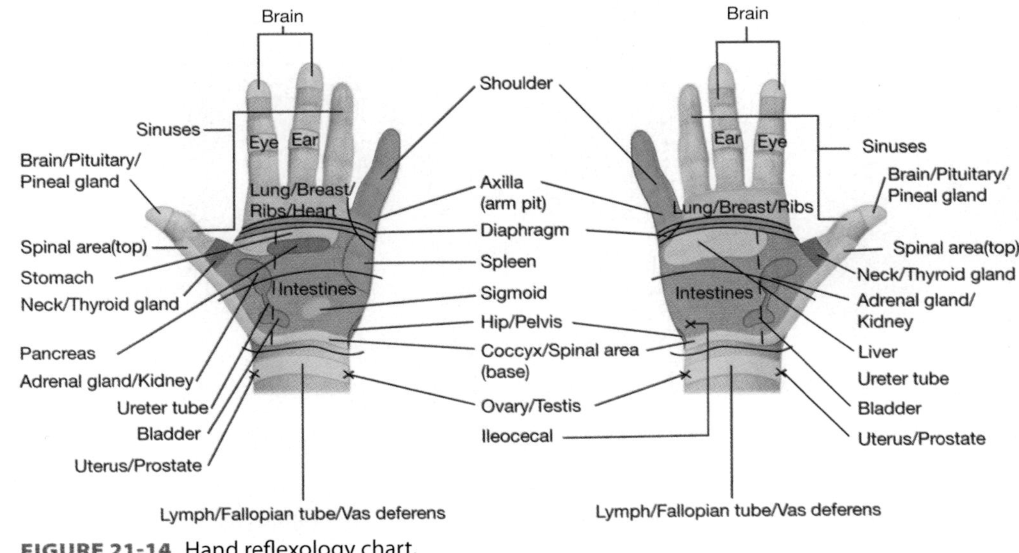

FIGURE 21-14 Hand reflexology chart.

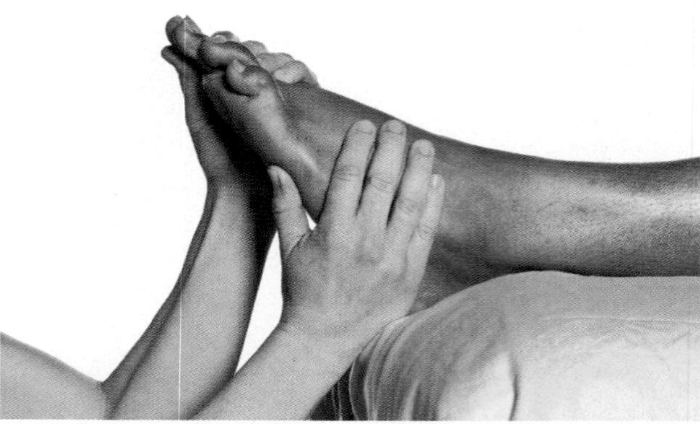

FIGURE 21-15A Thumb walking is initiated by holding the foot firmly with one hand and placing the flat of the tip of the thumb of the other hand on the sole of the foot.

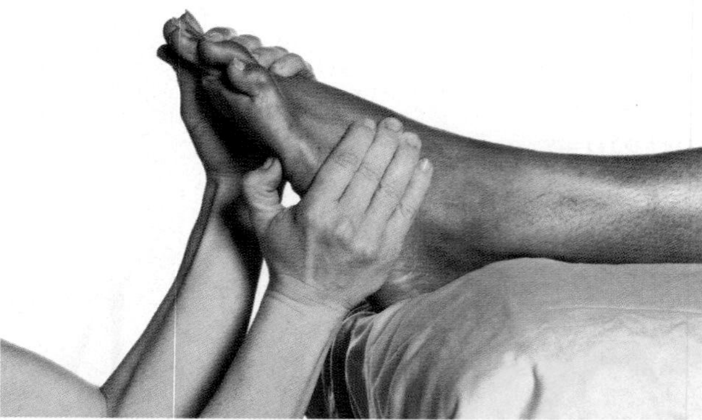

FIGURE 21-15B Bend the last joint of the thumb so the thumb tip is perpendicular to the surface of the foot, and apply pressure with the tip of the thumb. After a short time, roll off of the tip of the thumb to the initial position, move slightly to a new position, and repeat the process.

Integral to the practice of reflexology is the detection of slight variations and textures in the feet and hands and learning the reflexology maps. Reflexology can also be practiced on the ears, a practice called *auriculotherapy.*

Basic Routine

Begin by applying general compressions on one foot and ankle with both hands. Perform some light and brisk friction strokes to warm up the foot. Then methodically work each zone on the bottom of the foot, starting with the most medial zone using the thumb-walking technique, similar to the movement of a caterpillar or inchworm. Press down with the thumb; then let pressure up but not off the foot. Then "scoot" the thumb about a quarter to a half inch and press down again (Figure 21-15 a andb). To work each zone, start on the medial aspect of the bottom of the foot near the heel and thumb walk to the big toe. Starting again near the heel, thumb walk up more toward the middle of the foot to the second toe. Repeat on a line to the third toe, then the forth, and finally the little toe. Then do finger walking (same as thumb walking but with fingertips) on the dorsal (top) side of the foot, being careful not to put too much pressure on bony areas. Be sure to communicate freely and openly with the client, and be sure to apply sustained and repeated pressure to any areas that are sensitive or have evidence of congestion or inflammation (Figure 21-16 a andb). It might be necessary to switch hands throughout the routine so that the wrist can be held as straight as possible. Work the zones on the top of the foot, making sure to massage between the tendons instead of on them. Then finger walk across (horizontally) from the base of the toes on the plantar side, working toward the heels like the rungs of a ladder (about a half inch apart). Then finger walk diagonally, working the bottom of the foot just as before, making sure to go both directions like an X.

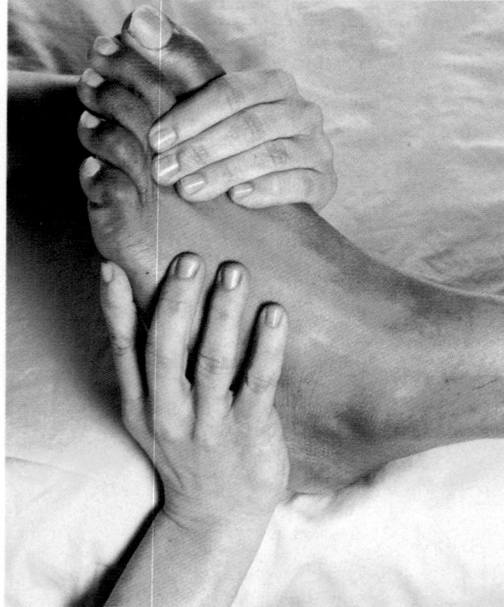

FIGURE 21-16A Finger walking is similar to thumb walking but is done with the index or second finger on the side or top of the foot.

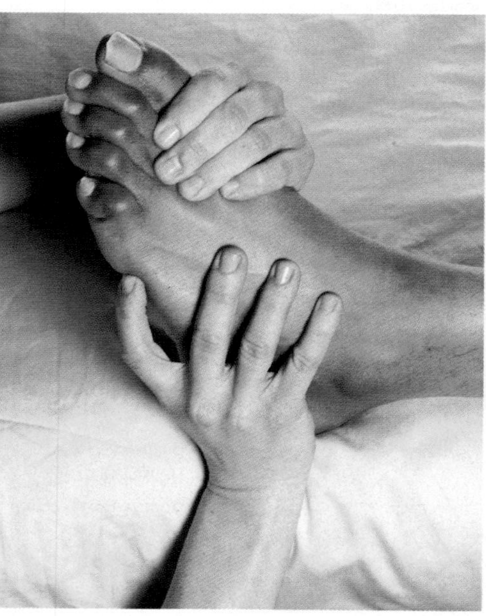

FIGURE 21-16B Apply pressure with the tip of the finger. Release, move to the next spot, and repeat the sequence.

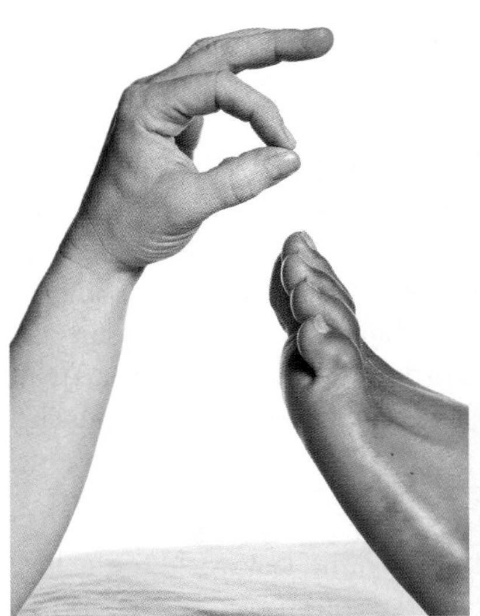

FIGURE 21-17A The pincher or tweezer grip is used on or between the fingers or toes.

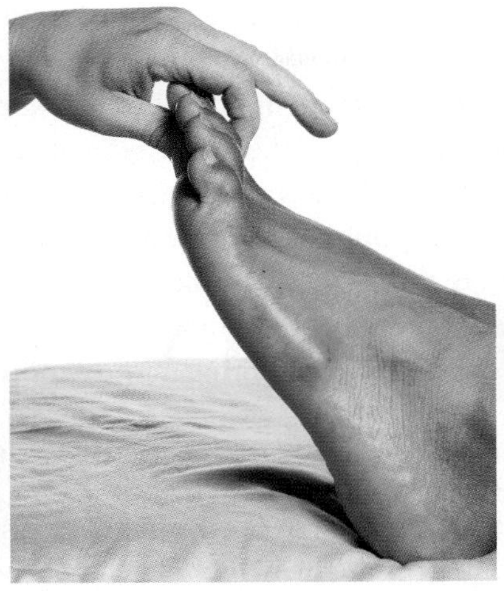

FIGURE 21-17B Massage the fingers or toes using the pincher grip.

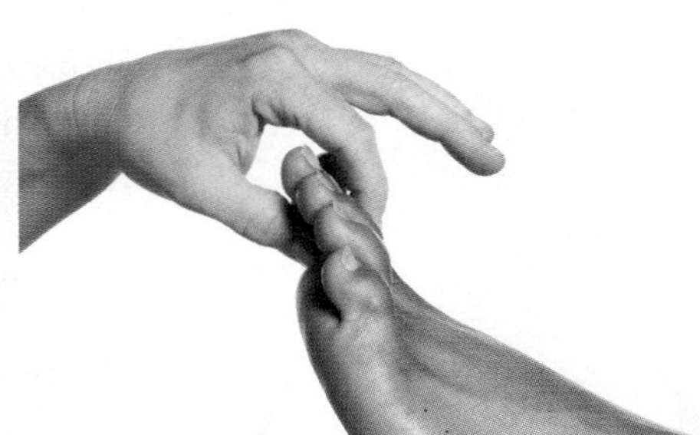

FIGURE 21-17C Grasp the skin between the toes or between the thumb and first finger with a pincher grip.

Repeat on the top of the foot with fingertips. Next, work the toes by pressing them between your thumb and finger, being careful and lessening the pressure on the nails (Figure 21-17 a–c). Work the areas around the ankle, working either side of the Achilles tendon by gently pinching and pulling. Next, finger walk across the top of the ankle where it meets the foot. Then lightly stretch the foot by squeezing the sides of the foot toward each other both toward the bottom and toward the top of the foot. Lightly stretch the foot and ankle by dorsiflexion and plantarflexion. Next, take the foot in both hands and tug gently to provide light traction. Then lightly jostle (shake) the foot by placing the palms of the hand on either side of the foot or hand and then moving them back and forth, shaking the foot (Figure 21-18). For each symptom or illness that a client might describe, apply sustained pressure on the reflex areas to each organ within that specific system of the body. For example, if someone has stomach ulcers, work the reflexes for each organ of the digestive system. To conclude, do a few nerve strokes (light feather stroke), and then repeat the series on the other foot.

There are many variations on this basic routine and certainly more complex routines, although all of them start or include the techniques described here.

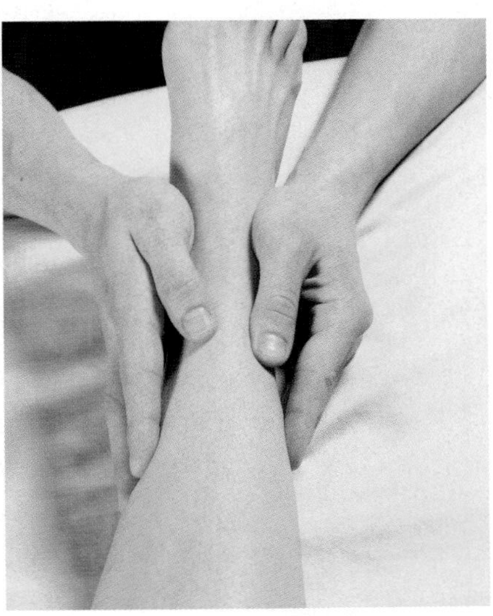

FIGURE 21-18 Jostle the foot by placing one hand on either side of the ankle and shaking it back and forth.

ENERGETIC MANIPULATION

The concept of energy is difficult to perceive through the lens of the modern world, because so much of today's view is based solely on what is visible. If it cannot be seen, it is difficult to accept as real. All through the ages, however, particularly in East Asia, another level of reality has been understood—one in which the whole of existence is intertwined with a vast web of invisible energy. From this perspective, every facet of creation is not only connected to everything else but also affects everything else.

Almost every culture in the world has a history of delving deeply into the study of energy, and this energy has been called by many names. To the followers of Islam, it was known as *baraka*. To the Hebrew nations, it was *ruach*. India has termed it *prana*, and the cultures of Asia have named it *qi* or *ki*. (Qi in China is pronounced "chee," and ki in Japan is pronounced “key.”) Even here in the West there has been an accumulating interest in this field, and we too have developed our own terminology—calling it *orgone* or describing it as human vitality or **bioenergy**.

bioenergy

is the vital life force in all living matter.

Most of the energetic healing arts being practiced today and the wide range of studies conducted in the field of energy come from China and India. Both of their systems have shared ideas and concepts, and the principles from which they operate permeate throughout both countries. Their central tenets can easily be seen in both cultures. From these cultures, practices have been developed not only to measure and gauge the energetic state of a human being but also to discover ways to affect and treat the body's energy system to bring it into a more balanced and healthful state of being.

The Energetic Manipulations of China

The most prevalent form of energy work practiced around the world today first originated in China. The origin of Chinese bodywork is often credited to the legendary Chinese Yellow Emperor, Huang Ti, who is thought to have lived over 5,000 years ago. Huang Ti is the author of the oldest written Chinese medical text, entitled *The Yellow Emperor's Classic of Internal Medicine*. The first written descriptions of massage therapy are found in this book.

Although their various methods of treatment were honed and crafted over time through the rigorous process of trial and observation, the core theories, principles, and understandings of Eastern medical knowledge were not created. Instead, they were “received” by the Taoist monks.

According to history, the ancient sages of China spent countless hours in meditation, delving into the inner landscape of human consciousness to understand the nature of existence. Through this process, the holy sages were said to have attained a state of being in which the workings of the entire universe came to be understood. From this place they saw that a human being was not an isolated entity but rather an integral and interconnected part of the many layers of creation.

They came to understand that human beings stood between heaven and earth, connected and nourished from both above and below. Chinese *ideograms*, written symbols that represent an idea or object directly rather than a particular word or speech sound, depict a human being's connection with heaven and earth by portraying the human body with roots spreading from a human's feet and branches reaching into the sky from the tips of the fingers. These ancient seers also understood that the very same laws and energies that limited and governed the entire universe were also contained within every person. Just as a drop of water from the ocean contains all the properties of that ocean, man was seen as reflecting the very same forces and energies that make up all of existence. From this perspective it was understood that man is not just a part of nature—he *is* nature in microcosmic form. Through these insights, a comprehensive system of health and well-being was eventually created and came to be known as traditional Chinese medicine (TCM).

Chinese knowledge of anatomy was limited to conjecture and speculation because it was considered inconceivable to show disrespect to one's ancestors by dissecting what was once the residence of the soul. This led to a system of medicine that developed its tools of diagnosis by physicians who were masters of energy development and movement and who carefully studied the patterns of disharmony that a patient exhibited. Signs and symptoms were considered against the landscape of the patient's home environment, while taking into consideration the patient's normal personal state to test for abnormal fluctuations. The physicians' diagnostic process, including examination of the tongue and pulses, evolved to such a high level of sensitivity that they became capable of sensing and distinguishing the subtlest fluctuations in the internal system of the body. Because these nuances could be detected only by subtle palpation, practitioners of acupuncture and oriental medicine were required to have mastery over bodywork as well.

Physicians were also trained in the martial arts, usually in several styles, so that they could master and develop the physical body and sensitivity to the energy system that is the basis of TCM. According to TCM, the vital force, or *qi*, of the universe infuses the human body and flows through it in a complex system of energy channels, some of which can be accessed through palpation and pressure in massage and through using needles on specific points in acupuncture. The mind, the body, and the emotions are all a part of and a manifestation of this energy system. It is the disturbance of this energy system that creates disease or "dis-ease," whereas the balancing of the energy system is the hallmark of health and well-being.

Although TCM has been practiced for thousands of years, it is only in the last 20 to 30 years that it has been gaining popularity outside the borders of Asia. The integration of TCM into the field of complementary and alternative medicine (CAM) has been a rather slow process, despite the fact that most people who have encountered TCM usually recognize its tremendous worth—even if they do not understand it. One of the major factors behind the strength of the recent growth of this minimally invasive form of medicine is its effectiveness in treating a broad range of conditions. This, coupled with a lack of side effects, produces a win-win situation that many people recognize immediately.

TCM is a complex subject and requires a serious commitment to its study and practice, especially if one aims to use it as the basis of assessment and treatment for one of the many forms of Asian bodywork therapy practiced today.

Qi: The Fundamental Substance of Existence

At the heart of TCM is the view that everything in existence, all matter, is composed of a fundamental substance known as *qi*. *Qi* is the all-important and underlying spark of life, without which there would be no movement or action. It gives the lungs the ability to breathe and the eyes the power to see. It gives the mind the ability to think and the heart the ability to feel. Because *qi* gives power to everything, without this current of energy, we cannot be alive. In all of the theories composing traditional Chinese medicine, this is perhaps the most critical, because it lays the foundation for understanding the interconnectedness of all things and gives explanation to the idea that this energy or *qi* underlies and enlivens the physical body. When all matter can be understood as a gradient of *qi*, it becomes easier to conceive of the interconnectedness and underlying unity among all things.

Yin and Yang

The traditional Chinese medical system is based on the primary concept of yin and yang. This is the concept that a polarity of forces exists throughout the universe, actively changing throughout the day, season, and lifetime, but that overall maintains a necessary balance (Figure 21-19). While *qi* describes the substance with which everything

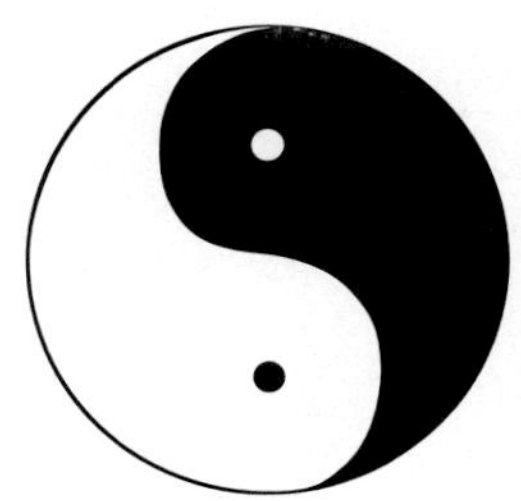

FIGURE 21-19 *Yin yang* symbol depicting balance and change.

is made, yin and yang describe one of the primary dynamics of that substance. When translated, *yin* refers to the shady side of a hill, whereas *yang* represents the sunny side. What is viewed as dark, passive, heavy, or slow is described as yin. What is seen as bright, active, light, or fast is described as yang. Yin represents the earth below and yang represents the heavens above. Yin is the feminine power of nurturing, soothing, and encompassing while yang is the driving, masculine force of action and movement. Personalities, too, can be understood through this principle, with yin describing the characteristics of introversion whereas yang expresses the qualities of the extrovert.

The concept of yin and yang is not applied to define and restrict something permanently as either yin or yang; rather, it is relative and used to understand the relationship between two parts of anything. Because of this, what was yin in one relationship can become yang in another and vice versa. For example the density of water is yin when compared with the fineness and freedom of mist, which is yang. When water is compared with ice, however, the flowing, active, always-in-motion substance of water becomes yang relative to the density and fixed nature of ice, which is yin. Yin and yang also represent constant change and movement—one of the central pillars of Chinese philosophy. These two complementary yet opposing forces give life and definition to all things, without which nothing could exist. Easy cannot exist without difficult, hard cannot exist without soft, and good cannot exist without evil.

Some Aspects of Yin and Yang:

YIN	YANG
dark	light
night	day
low	high
cold	hot
inside	outside
contracting	expanding
passive	active
deficient	excessive
weak	forceful

Yin and Yang in the Body:

YIN	YANG
front of the body	back of the body
inner body	outer body
lower body	upper body
underactive	overactive
coldness	hotness

Although yin and yang seem to be diametrically opposed, one has no meaning without the other. There is continuous and constant vying as one creates and transforms into the other while simultaneously holding the other in check. It is said that when yin and yang are in balance, there is harmony and well-being. The outcome of long-term disharmony is disease. If yang is too strong or excessive, yin will appear to be too weak. If yang is weak, yin will be overbearing. If the imbalance becomes too severe, yin and yang will separate, and the result is death of the organism. Breathing, digestion, metabolic rest and activity, and even the seasons are examples of this interaction. This relationship is considered to be the source of all change and movement.

The Five Elements

The deeper the energetic theory of traditional Chinese medicine is explored, the more detailed it becomes. In the next phase, energy or *qi* is further broken down into the Five Elements (Figure 21-20). Whereas the theory of yin and yang reveals broad strokes, finer details can be determined by applying the principle of the Five Elements. Five Element theory breaks everything down into five fundamental energies, substances, and qualities that constitute our existence—wood, fire, earth, metal, and water. Each element is host to myriad qualities and correspondences, ranging from physical organs to emotional states to the seasons of the year (Table 21.1). With this approach, even something as nebulous as imbalances in someone's psychology can be explained, understood, and treated by applying it to the Five Elements. As a result, the principle of the Five Elements can be used as another essential diagnostic tool for the Asian bodywork practitioner. There are very specific correspondences to each of the elements, which are clearly stated in the TCM literature, and these correspondences are the foundation of assessment.

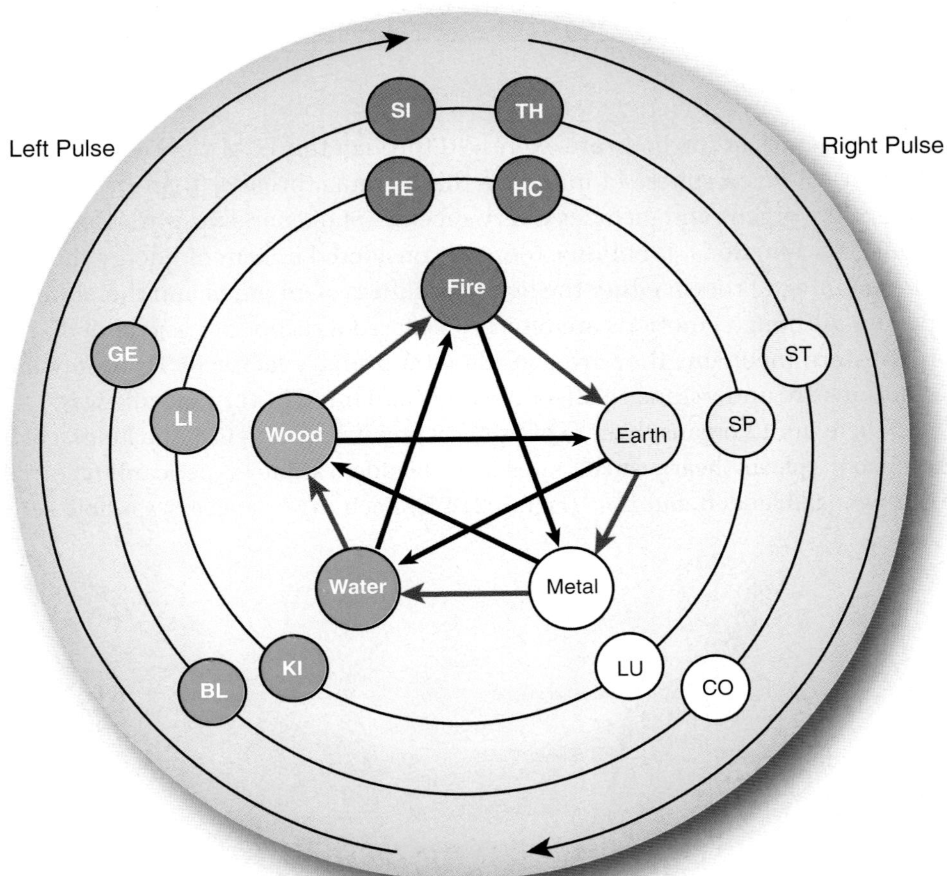

FIGURE 21-20 The relationships of the five elements to each other and their related organs are depicted in this diagram. The arrows in the center that look like a star depict the ko or control cycle: Wood controls earth by covering it or holding it in place with roots. Earth controls water by damming it or containing it. Water controls fire by dousing or extinguishing it. Fire controls metal by melting it. Metal controls wood by cutting it. The next arrows that form a pentagon depict the shen or creative cycle: Water engenders wood. Wood fuels fire. Fire creates earth (ashes). Earth engenders metal. Metal engenders water. The two rings indicate the solid (yin) and hollow (yang) organs that are associated with the elements. The outer circle (arrows) indicates the location of the pulse points that are used for diagnosis.

TABLE 21.1

SOME OF THE CORRESPONDENCES FOR THE FIVE ELEMENTS					
Element	Fire	Earth	Metal	Water	Wood
Color	Red	Yellow	White	Black/Blue	Green
Climate	Heat	Damp	Dry	Cold	Wind
Season	Summer	Late Summer	Fall	Winter	Spring
Yin Organ	Heart	Spleen	Lung	Kidney	Liver
Yang Bowel	Small Intestine	Stomach	Large Intestine	Bladder	Gallbladder
Taste	Bitter	Sweet	Spicy	Salty	Sour
Sense Organ	Tongue	Mouth	Nose	Ears	Eyes
Tissue	Blood Vessel	Muscle	Skin	Bone	Sinew
Emotion	Joy	Worry	Grief/Sadness	Fear	Anger

The Organs

Further details of the body are expressed through the TCM view of the organs. Each organ has a sphere of influence that is much broader than the Western view of the organs and includes a very specific set of energetic, physiologic, and emotional functions. Emotions, too, are considered a form of energy that can play an integral role in either the health or illness of an organ and therefore of a person. Although emotions are often considered a secondary aspect of disease in Western medicine, they are considered a primary factor in TCM, in which emotions are understood to affect the body and mind in very specific ways.

There are 12 organs that are of primary importance in TCM: the lungs, colon, stomach, spleen, heart, small intestines, bladder, kidneys, pericardium, triple warmer, gallbladder, and liver (Figure 21-21). Each organ conveys a whole set of

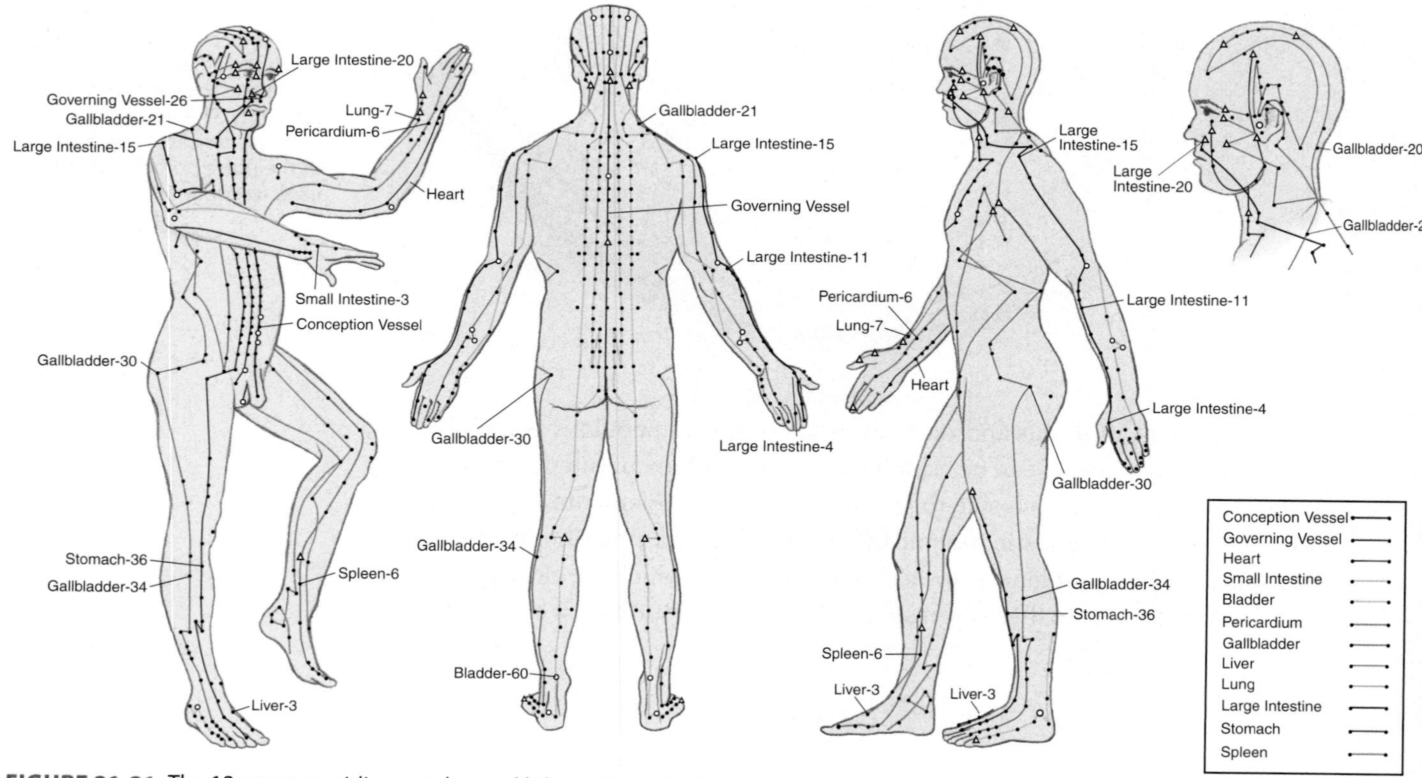

FIGURE 21-21 The 12 organ meridians are located bilaterally on the body.

functions and characteristics that represent their sphere of influence on the physical body. For example, the lungs not only regulate respiration but have other functions, such as the descending and dispersing of *qi* throughout the body, helping to create the *qi* that flows through the channels and regulating the opening and closing of the pores of the skin. The emotional state of grief is most often associated with the lungs.

The Channels and Points

Qi also refers to the energy that circulates in a network of meridians, channels, and collateral pathways in the body. These pathways are like rivers of *qi* (energy) that course along the extremities, into the body, and through related organs. They are what feed and enliven every muscle, tissue, and cell in the body, and it is these lines of energy that are the major focus of the many forms of Asian bodywork therapy. There are *twelve organ meridians,* or *channels.* They run bilaterally, are associated with organs, and are classified as being either yin or yang. Two of the organ meridians, the triple warmer and the pericardium are related to body functions more than to actual organs. In addition, there are two *extraordinary vessels* that are single channels, which also have points known as the *conception* and *governing vessels.* These two channels are considered part of the *eight extraordinary vessels,* another group of pathways, which store and release energy to the twelve organ meridians as needed for better regulation and harmonization of *qi.*

Along these meridians are small areas of high conductivity called *acupoints* (acupuncture points). There are 365 acupoints, located on the organ meridians where the *qi* (or *ki*) flows more superficially. Here they can most easily be influenced and affected by several modalities such as pressure, heat, electricity,

TABLE 21.2

ORGAN MERIDIANS			
ORGAN MERIDIAN	**YIN OR YANG**	**ELEMENT**	**LOCATION**
Lung	Yin	Metal	Chest to end of thumb
Large intestine	Yang	Metal	Index finger to face
Stomach	Yang	Earth	Face to front of body to end of second toe
Spleen	Yin	Earth	Medial side of large toe to inside of leg to chest
Heart	Yin	Fire	Chest, near axilla to inside of arm to end of little finger
Small intestine	Yang	Fire	Small finger to back of arm to side of face
Bladder	Yang	Water	Medial side of eye, over head, and down back and back of leg to little toe
Kidney	Yin	Water	Bottom of foot and along inside of leg to upper chest
Pericardium	Yin	Fire	Chest to end of middle finger
Triple warmer	Yang	Fire	End of ring finger back to side of head
Gallbladder	Yang	Wood	Side of head and body and alongside leg to fourth toe
Liver	Yin	Wood	Big toe and along inside of leg to the bottom of the rib cage
Governing vessel	Yang		Tip of tailbone, up midline of back, and over the head to upper lip
Conception vessel	Yin		Perineum and up the front of midline to bottom lip and chin
The Eight Extra Meridians Having a Regulatory Effect			
Conception vessel	Governing vessel		
Regulatory channel of *yin*	Regulatory channel of *yang*		
Connecting channel of *yin*	Connecting channel of *yang*		
Belt channel	Vital or penetrating channel		

needles, and touch. It is at these points that acupuncturists insert their needles or Asian bodywork therapists apply their hand techniques, manipulations, and pressure to stimulate, move, and balance the body's energy system.

These meridians have been mapped on the body very specifically in terms of location and direction of energy flow. Those seriously interested in pursuing mastery of the subject, and related massage and bodywork forms, must understand the direction of *qi* flow within each of the meridians, as well as learn the pathway of each meridian as it traverses the body and their most commonly used points. These points have a range of functions and indications, and their use is integrated within the course of an energetic manipulation treatment based on the practitioner's assessment. The specific manipulation of acupoints also can positively affect the immediate area where they are located, or can have positive influence and benefits that reach as far as the other end of the body, depending on the particular point and the channel treated. Although each of the twelve main channels has a deep and a superficial part, it is the superficial aspect of the channel that contains the acupoints, which are massaged and treated by the Asian bodywork therapist or acupuncturist.

Achieving the balance of yin and yang or removing blockages that impede the flow of *qi* within the body is the aim of most energy therapists. Imbalance in the body is recognized by several signs and symptoms. Various therapists have differing means of recognizing imbalances and offering techniques for affecting and regulating energy flow so that a more healthful condition can be achieved.

Methods of Energy Assessment

A great deal of information can be gathered about a person's energetic condition by closely assessing and analyzing the subtle signs and symptoms of the physical body. One of the main tools of assessment used in TCM is pulse diagnosis (Figure 21-22). The ability to read the manner in which energy flows through each wrist at different depths reveals different characteristics of a person's state of heath. From a TCM perspective, the pulse reflects more than the heart rate, which beats at a rate of 60 to 90 beats per minute in its normal state. An experienced practitioner can discern more than 25 varying qualities in the pulses. According to TCM, after much practice and experience in reading the pulses, properly detailed information on a client's state of internal health (including the organs, the weakness or strength of the *qi*, the channels, blood, and any deficiencies or excesses of yin and yang) can be revealed. It can also provide information about one's constitution.

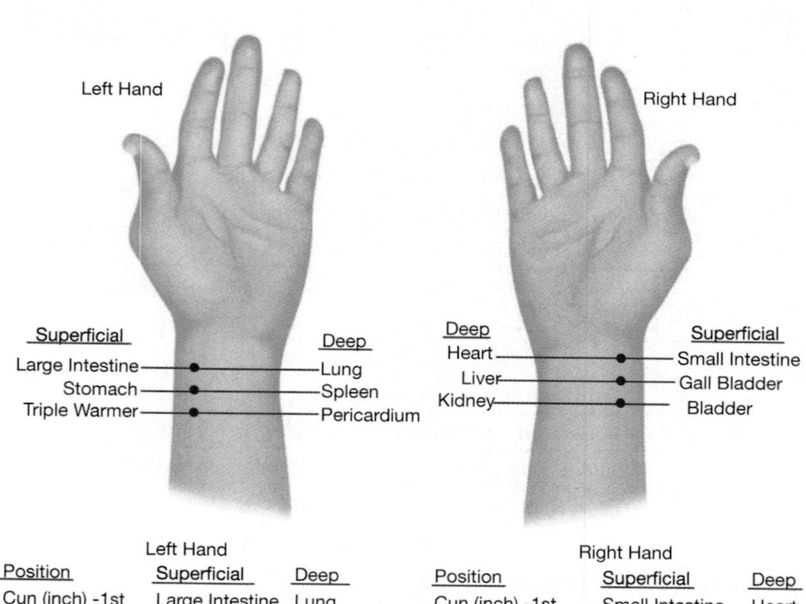

Left Hand

Position	Superficial	Deep
Cun (inch) -1st	Large Intestine	Lung
Guan (barr) -2nd	Stomach	Spleen
Chi (foot) -3rd	Triple Warmer	Pericardium

Right Hand

Position	Superficial	Deep
Cun (inch) -1st	Small Intestine	Heart
Guan (barr) -2nd	Gall Bladder	Liver
Chi (foot) -3rd	Bladder	Kidney

FIGURE 21-22 Pulse diagnosis is usually done on the radial artery at the wrist. The condition of the organ qi is indicated by the quality of the pulse.

There are three main pulse positions on each wrist, taken at the radial artery, and each position has both a superficial (yang) and deep (yin) location, accounting for all 12 of the major organs. At each position, the therapist gauges the pressure, speed, stability, and depth of each pulse to determine that organ's condition. For example, a strong, wiry pulse on the liver position that feels like a guitar string points to overactive liver energy, which can indicate stress, frustration, anger, high blood pressure, and other conditions. A pulse that seems to float closer to the surface of the skin at the lung pulse position, which can be felt as soon as the therapist touches the wrist but disappears when some pressure is applied, indicates that the immune system is fighting off a pathogen such as a cold or influenza.

Pulse diagnosis is usually coupled with the diagnosis of the tongue, where aspects like the color, shape, markings and coatings of the tongue all have very specific meaning and are used for assessment. If the tip of the tongue is a bright red, this indicates a buildup of heat in the chest, which is affecting the energies of the lungs or heart. A commonly seen marking called "scalloping," which occurs when the tongue is being pressed into the teeth, is a sign of deficiency in the energies of the spleen, which controls the digestive process in TCM and therefore has a whole set of implications for treatment.

These and other TCM methods of assessment, such as listening and smelling, in addition to palpation and looking are known as the *Four Traditional Methods of Assessment* and reflect back to the fundamental philosophy that underlies TCM, that a "man is a microcosm of the universe." For Chinese people, this idea is reflected in all aspects of life. Just as the qualities of a tree are contained within a single seed, the qualities of an entire human being can be found reflected into various parts of the body. Although the tongue and pulse diagnosis are the most frequently used forms of TCM assessment, the same signs and symptoms manifesting as energetic imbalances in a person can be read in other areas of the body, including the face, the abdomen (as used in Japanese *hara* diagnosis), the ear (used in auricular acupuncture), and the hand and foot (used in reflexology and acupuncture).

These methods can often seem strange and mysterious at first, but they reflect the traditional view of the human body seen as a holy vessel. Instead of physically cutting the body open and looking inside to understand the workings of its internal structure, physicians had to develop other ways of obtaining the necessary information, assessing its meaning, and treating the findings.

Methods of Treating Energy

In the thousands of years since the inception of the energy system, various means of treating it have been devised. One of the oldest, most widely practiced, and most documented of the energetic modalities used today is acupuncture. Acupuncture treatment dates back more than 5,000 years. Currently in China, physicians study not only Western medical course work but also acupuncture, bodywork, and herbs, and then specialize in either Eastern or Western medicine. Acupuncture, once ridiculed in the West as quackery, now has become mainstream in many countries. Clinical trials using Western research methods have demonstrated acupuncture's efficacy with regard to pain relief, addictions, nausea and vomiting, childbirth, infertility, and the treatment of many serious and chronic conditions. Many studies have shown the immune-boosting effects of acupuncture therapy. Acupuncture is a wonderful adjunct to massage, especially in the treatment of musculoskeletal problems. In acupuncture, very fine, sterile needles are inserted into the superficial layer of the skin and used to stimulate specific energy points (acupoints) that are chosen by the acupuncturist after the extensive process of assessment.

Various combinations of points can be used, depending on the goal of the treatment. The effect of the needles can be boosted by twirling them with the fingers, attaching metal leads that pulse with a therapeutic current of electricity, and applying an herb such as mugwort to the top of an acupuncture needle and burning it to add heat into the acupoints through the needle itself. This is known as *moxibustion*, which can take many other forms.

The purpose of acupuncture treatment is to balance the energy system and assist the body in self-healing. Although acupuncture is still considered a form of CAM in the West, it has been making its way more and more into the mainstream, including major hospitals. Many hospitals now offer acupuncture treatment as a complementary therapy. In the East, acupuncture is still one of the most prevalent forms of medicine practiced.

Today, various forms of energetic bodywork that have emerged and evolved from the original form of Chinese bodywork are often practiced in conjunction with acupuncture. In the past, the physicians of China were required to learn bodywork to build proficiency with their hands and develop the palpation skills necessary for the subtleties of the TCM diagnostic procedures, such as in reading the pulses. At one point, in the era of the Tang dynasty (618–907 CE), bodywork reached such a pinnacle that doctoral degrees were offered in its study at the Imperial College of Medicine (Sohn & Sohn, 1996).

Tuina

One of the Chinese forms of energetic bodywork commonly practiced today is *tuina*. *Tuina* is currently considered a serious medical art in China. Prior to this, massage in China was called *anmo*, and in Korea *amma*. Tuina is a form of healing grounded in the theory, principles, and assessment methods of TCM and with its own comprehensive system of techniques and treatments.

Tuina is a vigorous form of bodywork that uses robust techniques to move energy along the pathways or meridians. One of the main features of this modality is the sprawling array of techniques that are at the practitioner's disposal. Strokes can be fast and percussive or slow and penetrating. Muscles can be wrung, twisted, kneaded, and stretched, and joints can be vibrated, jostled, manipulated, and tractioned. Some techniques require lifting half of the patient's body to perform effectively. Because of the wide variety of "tools" at the therapist's disposal, practitioners must listen carefully and palpate and feel astutely for the patient's energetic imbalances and needs.

Acupressure

Today, acupressure can refer to any of several treatment systems that incorporate various manipulations of the acupoints. Its basic philosophy, theory, and principles are rooted in traditional Chinese medicine, however. Most Eastern cultures incorporate some form of point pressure in their traditional bodywork therapy.

Acupressure is often used to facilitate better circulation of blood and *qi* to an affected area and to relieve pain. Techniques usually include various pressures of touching, pressing, or rubbing one or more points, depending on what is to be achieved. Acupressure and many of the health practices of Asian origin are often used in conjunction with diet, herbs, exercise, and meditation. As always, the goal is to balance the physical and psychological aspects of a person's being by harmonizing and balancing the underlying energy system.

The Chinese method of acupressure can also be viewed as a close relative of some of the lineages and variants of Japanese shiatsu, particularly in the West, especially given the fact that China greatly influenced the development of the Japanese energetic healing arts. It is not uncommon to find the terms *shiatsu* and *acupressure* being used interchangeably to describe hybrid forms of Asian bodywork therapy. Today acupressure is also the foundation of other forms of bodywork, including the popular *Jin Shin Do* Bodymind Acupressure and some other forms of *shiatsu*.

Shiatsu

A style more meditative and less assertive than the work of *tuina* is a popular Japanese form of bodywork called *shiatsu*. Literally, the word *shiatsu* means "finger pressure," but the simplicity of this definition belies a rich undercurrent that is both sophisticated and comprehensive in its approach. The original seeds of this modality spread from China and carried overseas to Japan. This was during the height of bodywork in China, and at this time, Japan followed suit by requiring their physicians to learn bodywork to practice medicine.

The Japanese word **shiatsu** (composed of *shi* [finger], and *atsu* [pressure]), means pressure of the fingers or digits, although practitioners of the shiatsu technique can use the elbows, knees, and feet as well. In a sense, it is based on acupuncture theory but without the use of needles. The purpose of shiatsu is to increase circulation of *ki* (qi) and restore energy balances in the body. It is also an aid in soothing the nervous system and is said to be particularly effective in relieving headache, fatigue, insomnia, nervous tension, sore and stiff muscles, and disorders such as constipation and high blood pressure.

shiatsu

is similar to acupuncture but uses finger pressure instead of needles.

Like acupuncture, shiatsu recognizes strategic points (called *tsubo*) or energy pathways situated on the meridians. Instead of using needles, the shiatsu expert uses the ball of the thumb, the forearm, the palm, the heel of the hand, the elbow, the knee, or the foot to apply pressure. The treatment can be given to the entire body to restore complete harmony or according to specific needs. By applying pressure to the points, the natural recuperative powers of the body are generated; toxins are dispersed; muscles are relaxed; circulation of *ki*, blood, and lymph is improved; energy is released or balanced; and the entire body is revitalized.

To be effective, the practitioner must build strength and dexterity of the fingers, thumb, and entire hand. Pressure is applied with only the tips of the fingers or the thumb pointing straight into the point. One finger with another finger placed over it as a brace is also used (Figure 21-23a). The palm of the hand or other body parts are sometimes used to apply pressure over a larger area. Three fingers held together can

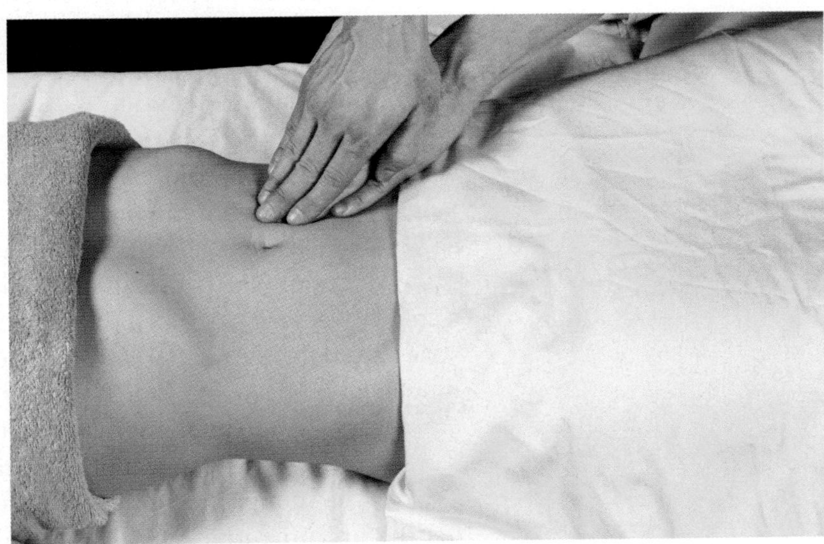

FIGURE 21-23A Braced fingers are used to apply pressure to the *tsubo*.

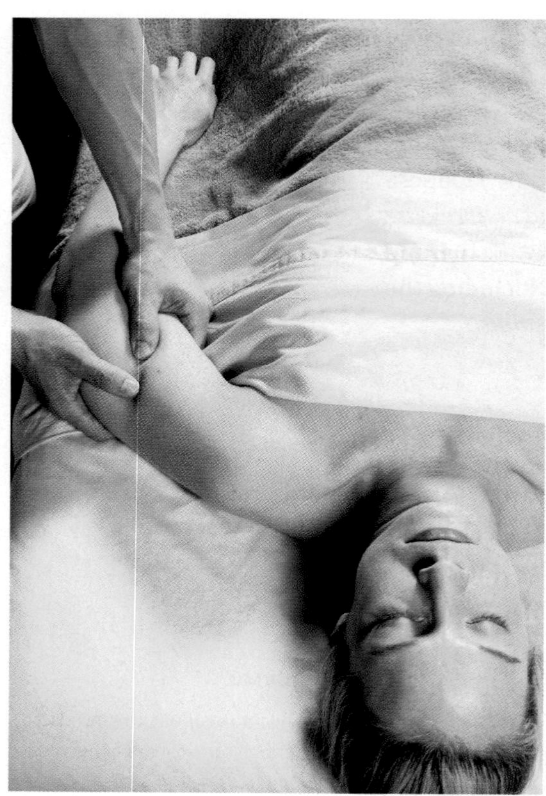

FIGURE 21-23B The thumbs are effective in the practice of shiatsu.

be used generally for the face, abdomen, and adjacent areas. The thumbs are used most often in shiatsu. Only the ball of the thumb is used to press straight down (no rubbing motions) on the pressure points (Figure 21-23b). Pressure is exerted perpendicularly to the surface of the skin with the pads of the fingers or thumb, for two to five seconds or more, depending on the area being treated.

Although traces of its Chinese lineage and TCM can easily be seen, shiatsu has grown and matured into its own distinct form and has also branched into colorful varieties. Some of the forms practiced today are Namikoshi Shiatsu, Five Elements Shiatsu, Ohashiatsu, Integrative Eclectic Shiatsu, and more. Today one of the most prevalent forms of shiatsu is Zen shiatsu.

Zen Shiatsu

Zen shiatsu still strongly follows the theories and principles of TCM, but its creator, Shizuto Masunaga, has made distinct modifications, altering the system of channels according to his personal experience with the movement of energy. In the traditional system of China, there are six channels along the arms and six channels on the legs. Masunaga thought that the meridian system of TCM was not sufficient to address the fact that the energy of each channel permeates the entire body, and so he developed what he thought was a more complete and integrated map of the energy channel system. His meridian system depicts the six channels on the legs also running on the arms and the six channels on the arms also running on the legs. In addition, all 12 channels travel through the organs of the abdomen (*hara*), where they can be palpated and used in the process of *hara* diagnosis.

The *hara* is considered both the physical center of gravity and the center of power. This area, like the tongue and pulse, can be palpated and studied to determine a person's energetic qualities. *Hara* diagnosis is the primary assessment technique of Zen shiatsu and is often used in the prescribing of herbs and acupuncture. *Hara* diagnosis consists of evaluating which energies are *kyo* (or empty) and which energies are *jitsu* (or full), to determine the right course of action in treatment

The distinctions between the work of practitioners in China and those of Japan can easily be seen as represented in their approaches to energy work. In acupuncture, the needles used in China are much bigger than the ones used in Japan, and the techniques applied by practitioners trained in the Chinese lineage are much more vigorous in their approach. In the Japanese model, the work is more contemplative. Greater levels of subtlety are valued and sometimes just a single needle can be used to treat the whole body. These same differences in styles are reflected in their styles of bodywork. A session of shiatsu moves at a much slower pace, and much greater importance is laid on moving with the correct breath and approaching the treatment with the correct frame of mind.

According to American Organization for Bodywork Therapies of Asia (AOBTA, a nonprofit professional membership organization representing instructors, practitioners, schools, and programs, and students of Asian Bodywork Therapy [ABT]), there are many forms of energetic Asian bodywork in practice today that consider the element of energy from the Eastern perspective.

These include but are not limited to acupressure, *Anma*, ANMA Therapy, *Chi Nei Tsang*, Five Element Shiatsu, Integrative Eclectic Shiatsu, Japanese Shiatsu, *Jin Shin Do* Bodymind Acupressure, *Jin Shou Tuina*, Macrobiotic Shiatsu, *Nuad Bo 'Rarn* (Traditional Thai Bodywork), Shiatsu, Shiatsu Anma Therapy, *Tuina*, Zen shiatsu, medical *Qigong*. For more information and brief definitions of each of these forms of Asian bodywork therapy, visit www.aobta.org.

OTHER RELATED ENERGETIC THERAPIES

The energetic therapies of India bear some resemblance to those of their neighbors. As in the founding of TCM, the depth of India's knowledge was said to have come not from the hands of man but through the grace of a higher source. In the same fashion as China, the ancient *Rishis* (holy seers) were said to have embarked on an inward journey, and after great time spent in devoted meditation, they were permitted to know the secrets of the universe. In this manner, the gifts of a unique insight and subtle way of understanding anatomy, physiology, psychology, astronomy, and spirituality came flooding in, eventually resulting in *Ayurvedic medicine*, also known as *Ayurveda*.

Ayurvedic medicine, one of the world's oldest medical systems, evolved in India over the course of thousands of years. Today in the United State it is considered its own system of CAM. Several therapies are used as part of treatment and include herbs, ayurvedic massage, and specialized diets. The key principles of this system of energetic medicine and treatment concern the idea of an underlying universal energetic interconnectedness, the body's constitution, and a triad of life forces known as the three *doshas*.

Marma-Point Therapy

Another one of the ancient energetic treatment modalities associated with Ayurvedic practice is *marma*-point therapy. Like the points of TCM, *marmas* are specific energy sites on the body that, when properly treated, have powerful functions of balancing, relaxing, and enhancing. The purpose of massaging the *marma* points is to move stagnant and blocked energies by either arousing or calming the *doshas*. There are 107 marmas around the body, with the major points corresponding to the 7 chakras. The 108th marma is considered to be the mind. Each point ranges in size from one to six inches in diameter, and they are approached with extreme subtlety. Much gentler than a regular massage, the strokes used to stimulate the *marmas* are lightly initiated and build with pressure as the treatment progresses. The points are manipulated and massaged in specific sequences of treatment. Practitioners of this form of energetic massage usually train with master practitioners of Ayurvedic medicine and their studies often include the use of different herbs and essential oils.

Thai Massage

Thai medicine consisted of four limbs : spiritual practices, nutritional guidelines, herbal medicine, and massage known as *Nuad Bo-Rarn* ("ancient massage"), or Thai massage as it is now known in the west. The fact that they called it "ancient massage" was a sure indication that it was considered sacred and had been handed down throughout the generations. As is typical of indigenous peoples, the Thai continued to develop their own form of massage by assimilating Buddhism, yoga, Ayurveda, and traditional Chinese medicine.

Ayurvedic medicine is also the foundation for the ancient practice of yoga, and the familial resemblance between Thai massage and yoga is immediately apparent. Whereas other forms of bodywork use massage techniques as their primary method of treatment, Thai massage utilizes yoga-like stretches as the major means to achieving the ends. For this reason, Thai massage has been playfully dubbed as "yoga for lazy people" and is also known as Thai yoga therapy. Thai massage also uses muscle compression, joint mobilization, and acupressure during treatment.

Reiki

Literally translated, *Reiki* is Japanese for "spiritually guided life energy." Practitioners of this form are said to be channels for an energy that comes from the wisdom of a higher source. This means that they are not exerting any of their own force, but that they are simply allowing themselves to be open to the universal pool of energy that exists all around us. Therapists use *mantras* (sounds, syllables, words, or groups of words that have special vibrational qualities and thought, capable of catalyzing healing and spiritual transformations), symbols, and the power of intention to open their circuits to allow the *qi* to flood into their pores. This energy is then routed through the minor chakras in the palms of the hands and poured into the body of the recipient. Receivers of Reiki can feel warmth or vibration coursing through them, and the effects of treatment can continue for days after the session. Because givers of Reiki are not siphoning from their own limited reservoir of energy, they are not drained at all after the treatment. In fact, they often report feeling more enlivened because the energy is passing through them as they pass it on to others.

In the previous modalities discussed, physical contact was a large component of the treatment process. Reiki, however, is an energetic form of bodywork that mostly does not use touch at all. In fact, in this energetic modality healing is even said to be possible over a distance.

Polarity Therapy

Polarity Therapy is an eclectic system of healing, created by Dr. Randolph Stone (1890–1981), that draws from a huge resource of knowledge. Stone was known to be a consummate explorer, and his prolific interrogation into the field of healing through energy brought him many admirers across a broad scope of professions. With a background in chiropractic, osteopathic, and naturopathic medicine, Stone began his developments in energy work with a firm foundation of the body's structure. His later explorations in the Eastern arts of energetics, including the Ayurvedic medicine of India, TCM, yoga, and reflexology, helped to create a form of bodywork that spans the range of different approaches from somatic to energetic.

His multifaceted approach gelled into a synthesis of traditional theories and modern scientific research. He studied deeply into the intricate pathways of energy and how they flowed through and around the human body. His research covered so much territory that today it is difficult to define his work concretely. Two practitioners of polarity therapy can be so different that it might appear that their work comes from two different spheres. One treatment might approach the client with the greatest of subtleties and barely a touch, whereas another client's session might be bold and assertive, with vigorous strokes and hearty amounts of force applied.

Therapeutic Touch

A popular form of energetic bodywork used by nurses is *Therapeutic Touch*. Its approach and theories are nowhere near as complex as the others, and befitting the goals of its creators, Dora Kunz and Delores Krieger, Ph.D., RN, *Therapeutic Touch* is a form of compassionate healing meant to be used by anyone without formal training.

Modalities like Reiki require the assistance of a master in the field to give what is called an "attunement" before a person can become an energetic conduit. In modalities such as acupuncture, years of schooling and intensive training are necessary to digest its teachings properly before being able to provide the correct course of treatment. In Therapeutic Touch, it is taught that the ability to heal is inherently ingrained in each person, and therefore one can be a vessel for this healing no matter what his age or education. Therapeutic Touch is a simple and direct form of energetic bodywork that is being practiced by nurses in hospitals all over the country. It seeks to balance the human energy field or aura by contacting and moving it with the hands held above and off the body. The practice of Therapeutic Touch, much like those of the traditional forms of Chinese massage therapy, is predicated on the underlying assumption that human beings are complex energy fields.

The term *Therapeutic Touch* is actually a misnomer, because its practice actually requires no physical contact, hence its alternative name Noncontact Therapeutic Touch (NCTT). The focus of treatment is on the underlying human energy field that extends beyond the limits of the physical body rather than the physical body itself, so that the hands actually do not touch the other person.

CHAKRA ENERGY WORK

The word *chakra* is derived from Sanskrit and means "wheel" or "disk." The first recorded information came from ancient Indian texts such as the Upanishads and Yoga Sutras, dating back to 1200 BC. Chakras are thought to be rotating energy vortices located along the central line of the body and are considered focal areas for the reabsorption and transmission of energy (Figure 21-24). There are seven major chakras

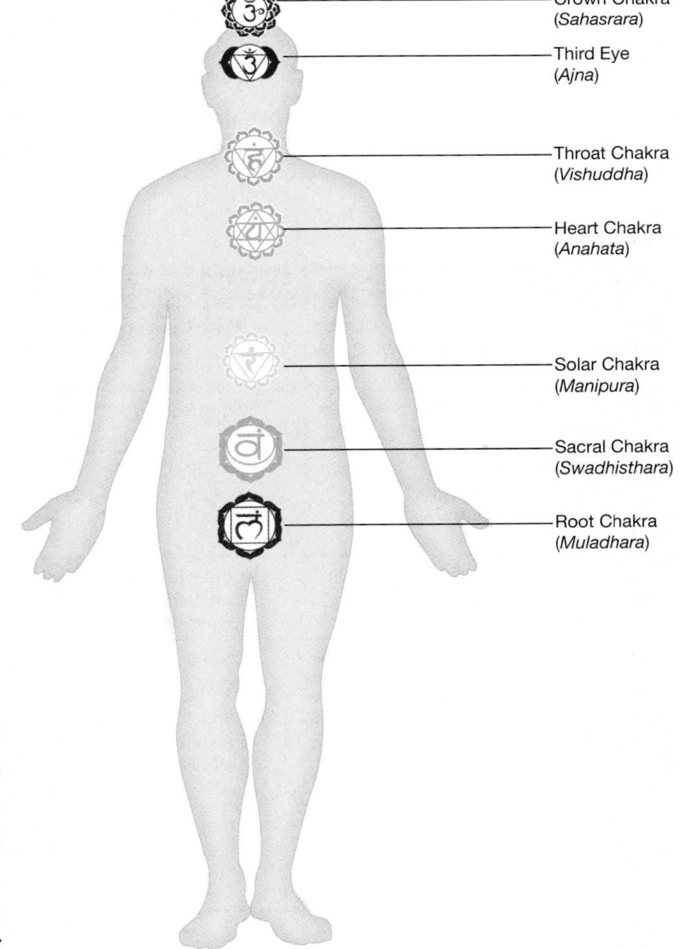

FIGURE 21-24 The location of the seven chakras in the body.

or energy centers that are located between the base of the spine and the top of the head. These energy centers are places where the energy (*qi*) often stagnates and becomes blocked. According to yogic philosophy, the chakras also reflect and represent psychological layers of the mind and levels of consciousness. It is thought that very concentrated and specific practices, including meditation, aimed at opening these energy centers leads to spiritual development and evolution for the person. The seven major chakras each relate to a specific gland, organ, color, emotion, tone, and various other traits (Table 21.3). Chakras that are blocked might have "stuck" energy and often cause physical, emotional or spiritual "dis-ease"; open chakras initiate health.

At the core of this kind of energy work is intent. When the intent of a practitioner is to heal and have only positive regard for their clients, then healing is facilitated in the client. Effective massage therapists use intent as a guiding force for any type of bodywork. Chakra work can easily be incorporated into any type of massage because it is based on intent.

There are numerous ways in which a client or practitioner can open or clear a chakra and help to balance the body's energy patterns. In addition to laying hands on or above these chakras, one can place crystals on them or use a pendulum to open and balance chakras. It is thought that if a chakra is open, the feelings, organs, and other systems related to that chakra function more healthily. Balance among the charkas promotes balance between the physical, mental, emotional, psychological, and spiritual health of the person.

A chakra chart with the different positions, organs that each governs, emotion, and sense is shown in Table 21.3.

TABLE 21.3

CHAKRA CHART

Chakra & Location	Sanskrit Name & Meaning	Color	Main Concern	Identity Intention	Body Part	Element	Endocrine gland	Sense	Tone
Crown (7th) Top of head	Sahasrara Thousandfold	Violet, gold, white	Spirituality	Universal Self-knowledge	Skin, brain energy	Thought/ cosmic	Pineal	Beyond Self	B
Third Eye (6th) Above and Between eye-brows	Ajna To perceive/ To know	Indigo	Intuition, Wisdom	Archetypal Self-reflection	Eyes	Light/ telepathic energy	Pituitary	Sixth sense	A
Throat (5th) Base of neck	Vishudda Purification	Blue	Communication, Self-expression	Creative Self-expression	Mouth, throat, ears	Ether	Thyroid	Hearing	G
Heart (4th)	Anahata	Green	Love & Relationships	Social Self-acceptance	Heart, chest, lungs, circulation	Air	Thymus	Touch	F
Solar Plexus (3rd) Above navel	Manipura Lustrous Gem	Yellow	Personal power, Self Will	Ego Self-definition	Digestive tract, muscles	Fire	Pancreas	Sight	E
Sacral or Belly (2nd) Below navel	Svadhisthana Sweetness	Orange	Emotional balance, Sexuality	Emotional Self-gratification	Sex organs, bladder, womb, prostate	Water	Sex glands	Taste	D
Root (1st) Pelvic floor	Muladhara Root or Support	Red	Survival, Physical needs	Physical Self-preservation	Bones, skeleton	Earth	Adrenals	Smell	C

Box 21.1

Sample Chakra Clearing Exercise

Clearing Chakras Using Pendulums

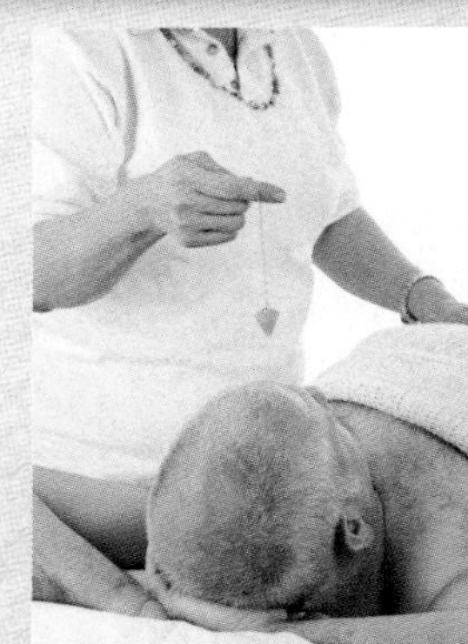

FIGURE 21-25 Hold the pendulum in the right hand, with the chain draped over the index finger.

Making pendulums: All that is needed to make a pendulum is some string or light chain and a washer or simple pendant. Make sure that the string or chain is at least a foot long. Place string or chain in right hand and clasp hand around the end with the string or chain draped over your index finger (Figure 21-25).

Let the pendulum hang straight down. After it stops moving, ask the pendulum out loud, "Show me a 'yes'." Observe the way that the pendulum begins to move. It might move in a circle, clockwise or counterclockwise, or it might just swing back and forth. Allow the pendulum to stop and ask it out loud, "Show me a 'no'." Observe how the pendulum swings that is different from the 'yes' movement. You now have a positive and negative indicator from the pendulum and are ready to proceed, using the pendulum as a tool to balance the chakras.

Have the client lie supine, with bolsters under the knees. They remain clothed for this.

Start with the root chakra. Hang the pendulum over their root chakra and ask "Is this _______'s (your client's name) root chakra?" If it says yes, continue. (It will indicate a positive, yes response with the same motion as you observed in the previous exercise.) If it says no, then move the pendulum slightly until the pendulum gives a yes indication that it is over that chakra. When it does indicate yes, ask the pendulum to move in the direction that the chakra is moving. Note: Clockwise is the natural flow of a chakra and is healthy. If it is counterclockwise or still, it is either blocked or healing.

- Ask the pendulum if the chakra is moving too fast.
- Ask the pendulum if the chakra is moving too slow.
- If the pendulum is moving counterclockwise, ask if the chakra must change direction. Sometimes it will say no and needs to keep moving that direction.
- If the pendulum says yes, that the chakra is moving too fast, too slow, or the wrong direction, ask the pendulum to correct the movement. (It will speed up, slow down, or change direction when it is corrected.)

Then move up to the next chakra (belly or sacral, depending on which terminology you use because it is stated as both in different texts) and repeat the sequence. Continue to balance each chakra in turn, up to the crown chakra. When the process has been repeated through each chakra, thank the pendulum, and the balancing is complete.

ADDITIONAL SOMATIC THERAPIES

Somatic therapies include many different applications of techniques that affect the well-being of the person. Most of these therapies are hands-on techniques; however, they can focus on various aspects of the body/mind. Many of these therapies can be classified according to their intent or the aspect of being to which they are directed. Some therapies are directed at the energetic aspect, others at movement, and others at physiologic tissue manipulation.

Listed here are some of the somatic therapies that are popular today. They are organized according to the broad classifications of energy, movement, or manipulative therapies. Using this type of classification is somewhat difficult, however, because several of the therapies fit into more than one classification—for example, shiatsu is a manipulative technique that affects the energy systems of the body.

Energy Techniques

Do-in
Five Element Shiatsu
Jin Shin Do
Jin Shin Jyutsu
Touch for Health
QiGong

Movement Techniques

Alexander Technique
Aston Patterning
Feldenkrais
Pilates
Tai Chi Chuan
Yoga

Manipulative Techniques

Anmo
Ayurvedic Massage
Bindegewebsmassage or connective tissue massage
Esalen Massage
Lomi Lomi
Pfrimmer Deep Muscle Therapy
Rolfing/Structural Integration/Hellerwork
Soft Tissue Release
SOMA Neuromuscular Integration
Trager Method
Watsu
Zero Balancing

Other Related Therapies Not Classified Above

Applied Kinesiology
Aromatherapy

SUMMARY

This chapter focuses on several bodywork methods prevalent in the field of somatic therapy. Although this is not an exhaustive list, it does provide a brief history and introduction to chair massage, reflexology, acupuncture, acupressure, shiatsu, and chakra balancing techniques. Elements of each of these techniques can easily be incorporated into a massage therapist's practice. Even though these modalities have been explained briefly, it is wise for a massage therapist to engage actively in continuing education to practice these types of bodywork.

QUESTIONS FOR DISCUSSION AND REVIEW

1. Where can chair massage be practiced?
2. What are some of the advantages to providing chair massage?
3. What is reflexology?
4. How does reflexology work?
5. Where is acupuncture said to have originated?
6. In Eastern thought, there are two parts that contrast or exist as opposites of the same phenomenon. What are these two parts called?
7. What are the three main techniques used in acupressure?
8. What is the meaning of the Japanese word shiatsu?
9. What are charkas, and where are they located?

PART 4

MASSAGE BUSINESS ADMINISTRATION

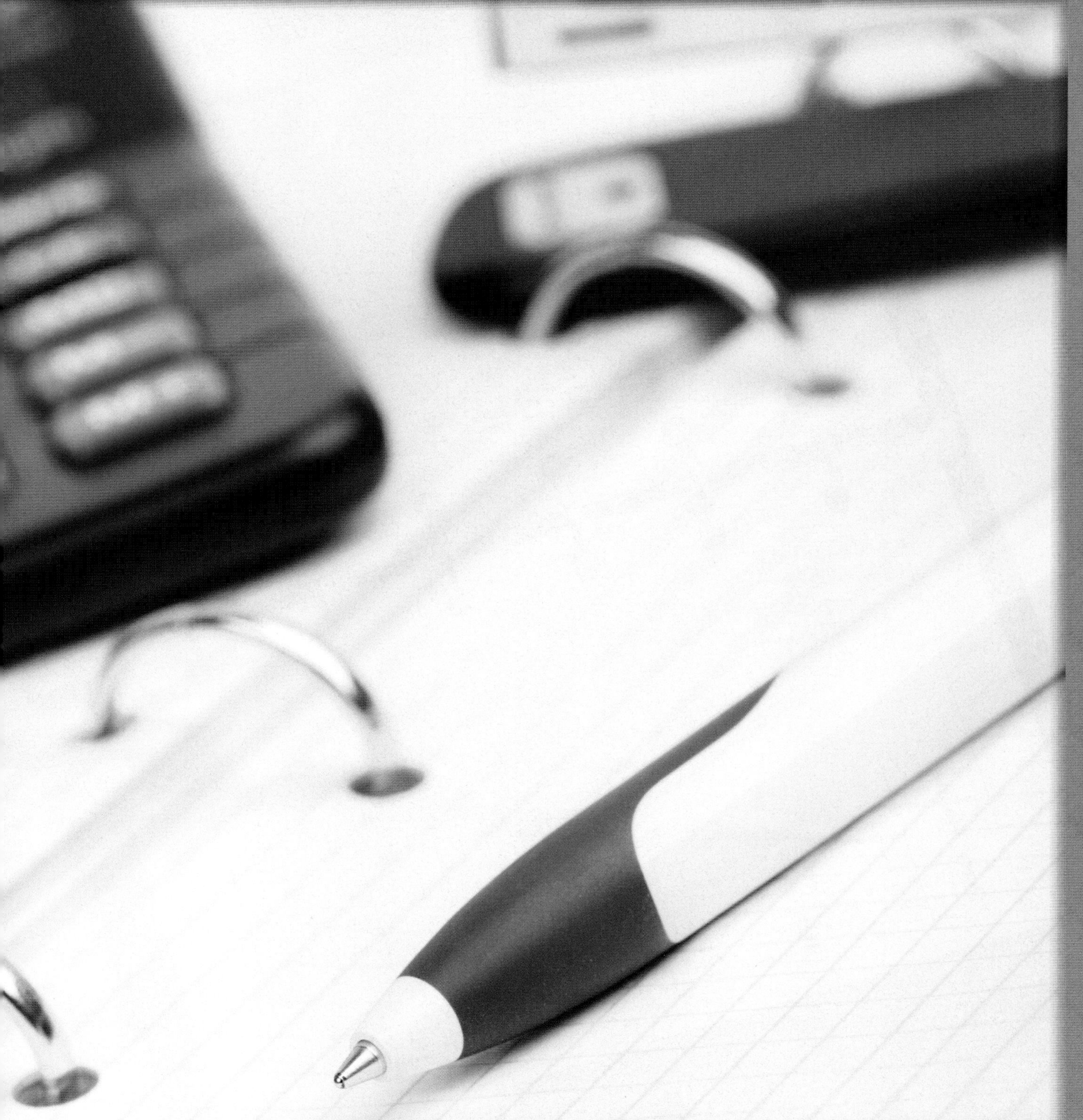

CHAPTER

22 Business Practices

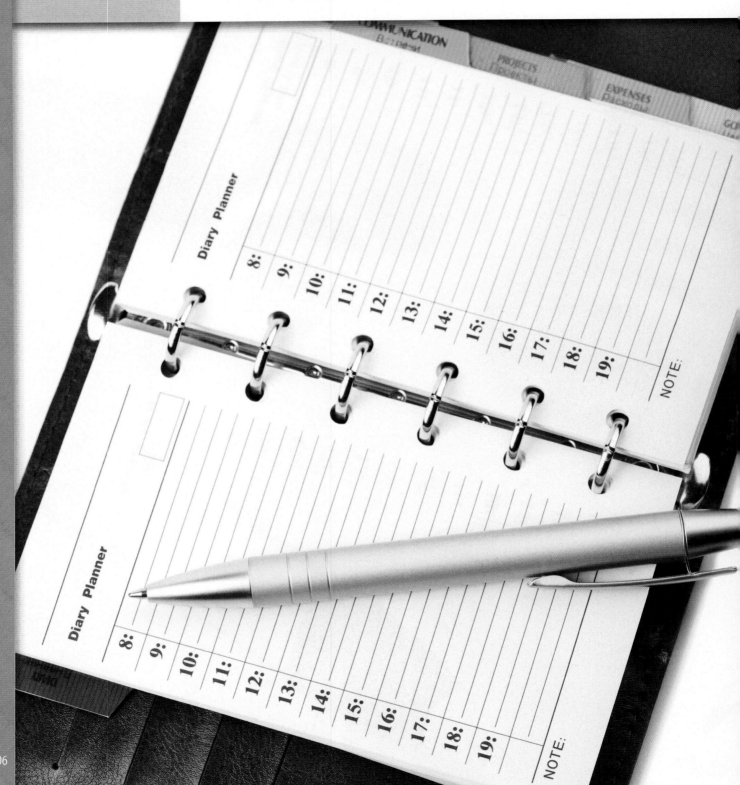

LEARNING OBJECTIVES

After you have mastered this chapter, you will be able to:

1. **Differentiate between being employed and self-employed.**
2. **Create a résumé and cover letter for a prospective employer.**
3. **Explain the relationships among attitude, self-image, and business success.**
4. **List the major expenses related to starting a massage business.**
5. **Explain the difference between a partnership, a corporation, and a sole proprietorship.**
6. **Explain the advantages and disadvantages of operating your own business.**
7. **List the various permits and licenses required to operate a massage business and where to obtain them.**
8. **List the types of insurance a massage business owner should carry to protect the business.**
9. **Describe a physical layout for a beginning business operation.**
10. **Explain the importance of business location to the success of a personal service business.**
11. **Explain why careful planning is important before opening a business.**
12. **Explain why keeping accurate records is necessary in a successful business.**
13. **List the major ingredients of a basic bookkeeping system.**
14. **Explain the importance of marketing to business success.**
15. **Define a target market.**
16. **Make a checklist of factors to consider before opening a business.**

INTRODUCTION

One of the greatest rewards of being a massage professional is seeing the relaxed smile on a client's face after a good massage. Most people who decide to become massage practitioners do so because they want to help people feel better. Of course, another objective of becoming a massage therapist is to produce an income. Research continues to show the positive effects of massage for relief from stress and painful conditions. Studies indicate that more people are turning to massage for relaxation, pain relief, and improvement of their overall health and wellness. As the emphasis on wellness and physical fitness continues to grow, there will be more employment opportunities for ethical and well-trained massage practitioners. According to the U.S. Department of Labor, employment opportunities for massage therapists are expected to increase by 20 percent between 2006 and 2016.

There are positive indications for increasing successful employment opportunities for energetic, enterprising massage therapists. However, because there are a limited number of massage positions available, many massage practitioners opt for self-employment. It is wonderful to have the independence of operating a business, but it is also comes with the responsibility of making sure that the business thrives and supports the therapist. The self-employed massage business person is owner, organizer, manager, bookkeeper, sales staff, and advertising executive as well as maintenance person and janitor. To be successful—to attain a desired level of practice and comfort—the self-employed person must develop some sense of business practice.

The practitioner who wishes to gain valuable experience can look for employment in a health club, at a resort hotel or spa, on a cruise ship, in conjunction with a medical facility, or as a freelance professional. An ambitious practitioner can choose to open her own business or occupy space within an established salon, clinic, or studio. Regardless of the environment in which the practitioner works, it is important to know something about business procedures. This includes keeping records, understanding laws and regulations, being familiar with insurance requirements, and much more. The practitioner who understands business procedures is more likely to succeed because she is more aware of the importance of good customer relations, more involved in the overall operation of the business, and more profit conscious. This chapter covers basic business skills that provide the basis for a successful massage practice.

Determining Whether to Be Self-Employed or Employed

As the popularity of massage continues to grow, there are more opportunities for the massage practitioner to find employment. Most of the opportunities, however, require the practitioner to be self-employed. Unless there are established massage businesses, spas, or medical facilities that employ massage therapists in the area, or there is the possibility to work for a concessionaire in a resort area or on a cruise ship, the chances are that the practitioner will need to create a place to practice.

One of the first steps in planning a massage practice is to consider which kind of massage business operation to work in or to have. Regardless of the

The advantages of being employed include

- being able to focus on giving massage
- coming to work at a regularly scheduled time
- equipment and supplies are provided
- providing massage or services as directed by the employer
- a regular take-home paycheck
- taxes and Social Security are automatically deducted from earnings
- the practitioner can learn from other practitioners at the facility or from training offered by the facility
- the owner or manager takes care of the business responsibilities

situation, there are both advantages and disadvantages. The following discussions explore some possible practice alternatives for the massage practitioner.

If the option is available, a practitioner can choose to be employed by an established massage practice or business. In an established business, the novice practitioner has the opportunity to gain valuable experience without the time and financial commitment of running a business. When working as an employee, a practitioner is paid by the hour or by commission, in which case they are paid a portion of the fees collected for the massages that they perform.

Besides the opportunity to gain valuable experience, advantages of being an employee include having facilities, supplies, scheduling, and reception services provided; receiving a steady paycheck with taxes withheld; and receiving any employee benefits, including vacation, sick days, and health insurance.

Some disadvantages are that the practitioner receives only a small portion of the money collected for massage services and works on someone else's schedule. In some cases, the practitioner must follow set session protocols, use specified products, and sign noncompete agreements so that they can not perform massages anywhere else while working at the establishment.

Deciding to work for someone else means that the practitioner must seek out an employer. Possible employment situations include the following:

- Alcohol or abuse treatment centers
- Athletic clubs
- Athletic teams
- Beauty salons
- Chiropractic clinics
- Cruise ships
- Dance companies or schools
- Day spas
- Destination spas
- Hospitals
- Hotels or resorts
- Integrative health centers
- Massage franchise businesses
- Physical therapy or medical clinics
- Ski resorts
- Sports medicine clinics
- Wellness centers

Seeking Employment

A practitioner can do several things to increase the chances of securing a rewarding and satisfying job. Make a list of clinics, spas, salons, athletic clubs, and chiropractic or medical offices that already have or would be interested in offering massage services. Check online and in the classified section of the local paper for massage employment ads. Contact the businesses either in person or over the phone to determine if they might be hiring and the qualifications that they require for a massage therapist.

Résumé and Cover Letters

Once there is a list of possible employment opportunities, prepare a résumé and a cover letter specific to each organization or business. A *résumé* is a document that you prepare to present to a prospective employer that lists your qualifications for employment, whereas the cover letter introduces you and indicates why you want to work for the company. The information on the *résumé* usually includes:

- Contact information – name, address, telephone information, and e-mail address. This is usually in boldface and can be the header of the résumé.
- A profile of the position being applied for, or
- A summary of who you are, including expertise, experience, and personal attributes that make you a good candidate for the position
- Qualifications, including credentials held such as licensure, national certification, insurance, and certifications for modalities that you are qualified to perform
- Education – a listing of schools and seminars that you have completed relevant to the position for which you are applying. You can include the number of hours and the main techniques learned.
- Employment history – List present and past employment, including the dates of employment (most recent first), name and address of employer, and a summary of your duties that might relate to the position that you are seeking.
- Affiliations, awards, and articles – Include any association memberships, awards you have received, articles or publications you are featured in, presentations you have given, or experience you have related to the position you are seeking.

Try to limit the résumé to one page. The résumé should reflect the depth of your experience and the knowledge that you have gained relative to the position for which you are applying (Figure 22-1).

The résumé should be accompanied by a cover letter that is addressed specifically to the prospective employer to whom you are applying. It serves as an introduction that tells the company who you are, the position to which you are applying, how you heard about the job, and why you should be hired. Tailor the letter to each prospective employer, because form letters are never as effective when you are trying to make a good impression. The cover letter has three basic sections—the introduction, the body, and the close. Begin by introducing yourself and stating the position in which you are interested. The body of the letter

Resume resource

Many word processing programs have résumé templates. Web sites such as www.careerbuilder.com, www.monster.com, and www.hotjobs.com have tools to assist in creating résumés and cover letters.

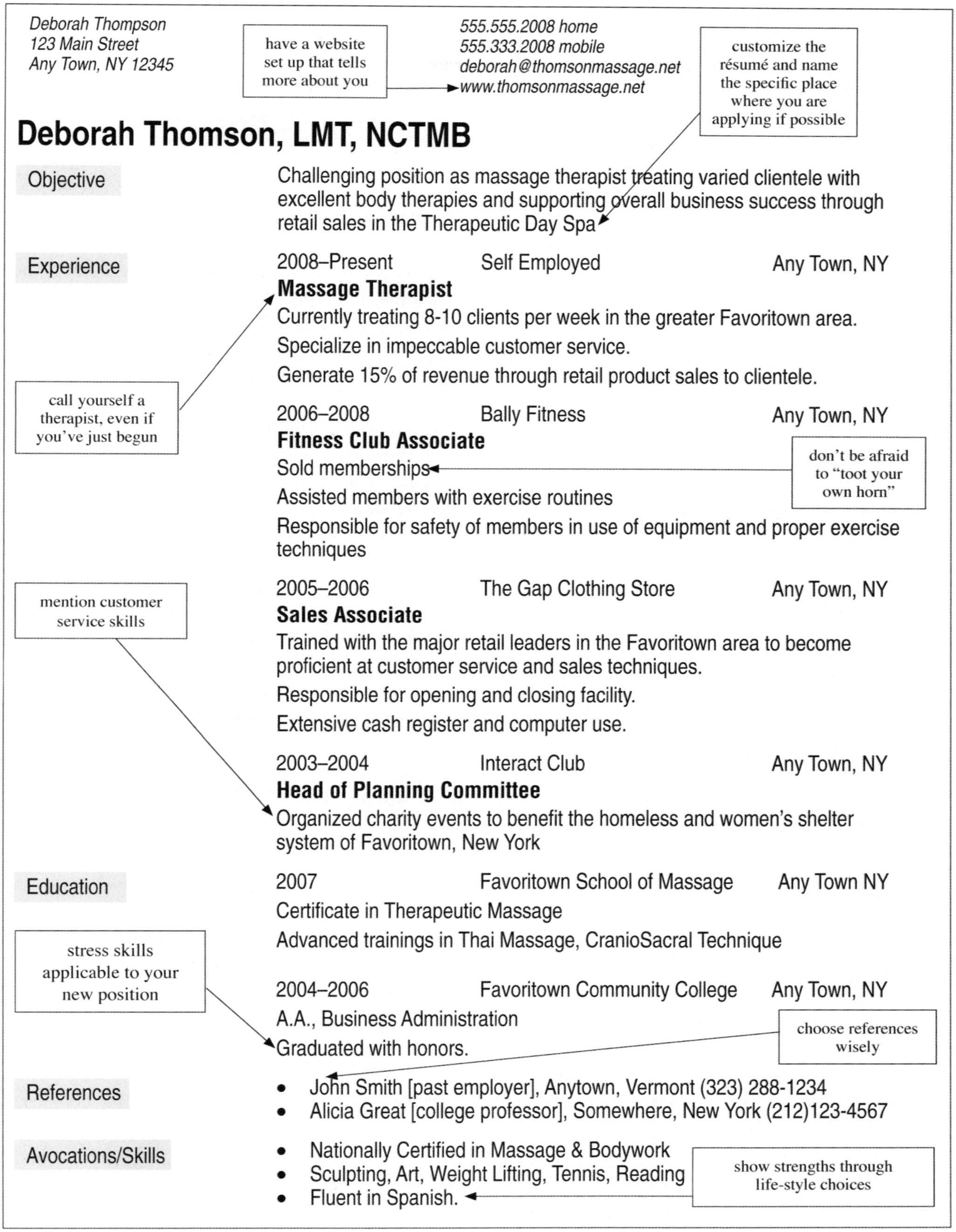

Deborah Thompson
123 Main Street
Any Town, NY 12345

have a website set up that tells more about you

555.555.2008 home
555.333.2008 mobile
deborah@thomsonmassage.net
www.thomsonmassage.net

customize the résumé and name the specific place where you are applying if possible

Deborah Thomson, LMT, NCTMB

Objective

Challenging position as massage therapist treating varied clientele with excellent body therapies and supporting overall business success through retail sales in the Therapeutic Day Spa

Experience

2008–Present Self Employed Any Town, NY
Massage Therapist
Currently treating 8-10 clients per week in the greater Favoritown area.
Specialize in impeccable customer service.
Generate 15% of revenue through retail product sales to clientele.

call yourself a therapist, even if you've just begun

2006–2008 Bally Fitness Any Town, NY
Fitness Club Associate
Sold memberships
Assisted members with exercise routines
Responsible for safety of members in use of equipment and proper exercise techniques

don't be afraid to "toot your own horn"

mention customer service skills

2005–2006 The Gap Clothing Store Any Town, NY
Sales Associate
Trained with the major retail leaders in the Favoritown area to become proficient at customer service and sales techniques.
Responsible for opening and closing facility.
Extensive cash register and computer use.

2003–2004 Interact Club Any Town, NY
Head of Planning Committee
Organized charity events to benefit the homeless and women's shelter system of Favoritown, New York

Education

2007 Favoritown School of Massage Any Town NY
Certificate in Therapeutic Massage
Advanced trainings in Thai Massage, CranioSacral Technique

stress skills applicable to your new position

2004–2006 Favoritown Community College Any Town, NY
A.A., Business Administration
Graduated with honors.

choose references wisely

References

- John Smith [past employer], Anytown, Vermont (323) 288-1234
- Alicia Great [college professor], Somewhere, New York (212)123-4567

Avocations/Skills

- Nationally Certified in Massage & Bodywork
- Sculpting, Art, Weight Lifting, Tennis, Reading
- Fluent in Spanish.

show strengths through life-style choices

FIGURE 22-1 Sample résumé.

describes how your skills are suited to the job and are of benefit to the business. In the closing, express your appreciation for their time and consideration. Indicate your interest in an interview or state that you will contact them in the near future to request an appointment for an interview. Make a note, and be sure to make the follow-up telephone call after a few days, allowing enough time for them to receive and examine your documents.

The Interview

After presenting the résumé and the cover letter to a prospective employer and before being hired, an interview will probably be scheduled, in which a representative for the employer meets with the job applicant to determine if they might be a good fit for the business. The representative might be the owner or manager of the business or part of the company human resources department. The interview is an opportunity for the employer to get to know the prospective employee and it is a chance for the applicant to find out more about the business and the position. This is the chance for prospective employees to impress on the employer that their personality, interests, and skills are such that they cannot only do the job, but that they will be an asset to the business.

Before meeting the potential employer, learn as much about the company and the position as possible. If possible, visit the business as a customer to see which services are offered and get a feeling for the way that the business operates. Candidly speak to an employee to obtain an idea of what it is like working there. Visit the employer's Web site, if they have one. Try to learn about the company history and who the prospective clientele is. This type of information helps when formulating questions that you might have for the interviewer.

Be prepared when you come to the interview. Be ready to answer questions about your career goals, what qualifies you for the position, and how you would benefit the company. Prepare a list of questions of your own to determine the job's responsibilities; which type of clientele are served, which kinds of massage are advertised or performed, and who is responsible for scheduling, for collecting fees, and which materials or equipment is provided.

Dress and act like a professional. Appearance is a first impression and is vital to a successful interview. Look as good as possible from head to toe:

- Clean, neat clothes appropriate to the business
- A well-groomed hairstyle
- Teeth brushed and fresh breath (no gum or candy)
- Minimal jewelry (no piercings or tattoos visible)
- Clean, trimmed fingernails (no polish)
- Clean, polished shoes

Be sure to bring any documentation you may need to the interview, including:

- A current massage license (if required in the location)
- Proof of liability insurance
- A picture ID
- Social Security number

Your confidence, professionalism, and personality are major factors that are just as important as education or massage skills. Maintain a positive attitude throughout the interview. Stay relaxed, smile, and make eye contact when answering or asking questions.

If you are being considered for hire, you probably will need to demonstrate a massage. This might happen during your initial interview, so be prepared. Bring your own lubricant, and if appropriate, a uniform to change into before the massage. You might be asked to massage the interviewer or someone else as the interviewer observes. Treat the demonstration as a regular massage. Include an intake interview. Listen for any concerns, complaints, or possible contraindications and administer the massage according to the client's feedback. Take into consideration the style of massage provided by the business. Ask for feedback concerning the recipient's comfort about the room temperature and the pressure you use. Practice impeccable draping, yet be smooth with your technique when transitioning from stroke to stroke and between body parts. Before completing the massage, ask if there is anything else the recipient would like to have done. Allow them to rest for a moment, and then be sure to assist them into a sitting position.

As the interview draws to a close, restate your interest in the position, including the strengths and skills that you can bring. Asking when a decision will be made and how and when you may contact the employer shows your consideration and also reinforces your desire for the position. Shake hands with the interviewer, thanking them for taking the time to meet with you, and let them know that you will be in touch. Leaving them with your business card is a professional gesture, giving them another easy means to contact you. Within 24 hours, send a thank-you letter or e-mail to the person who interviewed you. If you said that you would contact the interviewer in two to three days to find out their decision, be sure to make the phone call. Even if you did not get the job, thank them again for their time.

Use the interview as a learning experience. After the interview, perform a self-assessment. What went well? What did not go well? What can be done to improve your performance before the next interview? Remember to keep a positive attitude. The right opportunity is waiting for you.

ATTITUDE/SELF-IMAGE/PUBLIC IMAGE

As a massage therapist, you are not only a health care practitioner, but you are also a businessperson. Being a successful businessperson requires a positive self-image. A positive self-image means that you feel good about who you are and what you are doing. A good self-image is a positive attitude reflected in the enthusiasm and quality exhibited in your work and other activities. There is a sense of excitement about what you are doing. This is usually accompanied by a desire to be involved and to learn more. A positive attitude and an inner knowledge that "I will attain my goals" is a major advantage in being successful.

A good self-image and a positive attitude are the foundations for creating a good public image. Your public image is perceived through your appearance, the way you do business, and how you interact with your clients and associates. Your public image relates to your reputation and the degree of professionalism with which you operate. Success depends on an excellent reputation, a good public image, and a high degree of professionalism.

Which Kind of Massage Operation Do You Want?

Most massage practitioners are self-employed or will be at some time in their career. There are many opportunities for qualified and industrious practitioners to be successful entrepreneurs. The following is a list of possible self-employment situations. Add to this list other situations that occur to you. Make a list of pros and cons (advantages and disadvantages) for each situation.

Independent Contractor

There are numerous opportunities to work in conjunction with an established organization or business as an independent contractor. Working as an independent contractor can be very similar to being employed by someone else, except that as an independent contractor, you determine your own work schedule, provide your own supplies, get paid a flat fee, and are responsible for your own taxes (including self-employment tax). Many times as an independent contractor, you simply rent a space and operate your business within another business. An example might be providing massage services in a spa or full-service beauty salon. You might also be hired as an independent contractor to provide massage services for an organization such as a dance company, sports team, or corporation. There are subtle differences between being an employee and an independent contractor that the practitioner must be aware of when considering employment that can have serious ramifications regarding earnings and taxes.

The Internal Revenue Service (IRS) differentiates between independent contractors and employees by examining three general criteria:

- Behavioral control – The independent contractor sets her own hours and determines the tasks to be done without specific training or direction. The employee is directed as to the hours to work, which tasks are to be performed, and how the work is to be done, and receives periodic feedback on performance. Specific training and equipment are often supplied.
- Financial control – The independent contractor might pay a flat fee (rent) or a percentage of fees received (commission) and realize a profit or loss from the enterprise. The employee receives a wage, salary, or commission, is not directly affected by the company's profits or losses, and is sometimes restricted from working for others doing the same labor. The employee has taxes, including Social Security/Medicare deductions, withheld from their paycheck. The employer is responsible to contribute to Social Security and pay for workers' compensation insurance and unemployment insurance. The independent contractor is responsible for paying their own self-employment taxes.
- Relationship with the business – An employee might receive paid vacations, sick pay, paid holidays, personal days, and insurance benefits. An independent contractor is responsible for covering his own insurance, sick days, and vacation. The employee might be required to sign a noncompete agreement. The independent contractor has the freedom to work for other companies at the same time. The independent contractor usually provides services according to a written agreement or contract drawn up between the business and the contractor.

If questions arise about whether a worker is an employee or an independent contractor, consult a lawyer who is familiar with local labor laws or complete and submit the IRS form SS-8.

Working Out of the Home

Operating a massage business out of your own home can be an economical alternative to having a separate office if you have a suitable space in your home that you can dedicate to your massage business. Before considering opening a massage business in your home, however, be sure to check out the local zoning regulations. A special variance to have a business in a residential area might be necessary. It is important to have an easily accessible bathroom, a clear entryway, and a waiting area. A massage business in your home is not only economical but also has certain tax advantages. Check with your accountant for full details.

There are also disadvantages to a home business. Having people coming into your home restricts your privacy. You must keep your home/office clean and sanitary. You must also maintain a quiet, professional atmosphere. This setup generally does not work well if there are children or pets, or if the household has a lot of daily traffic.

Outcalls Only

Some massage practices are set up as portable offices. With a portable table and/or massage chair, the practitioner goes wherever the client is. The overhead of such an operation is minimal. The convenience to the client is high, but for the practitioner, it is low. The workspace is whatever the client has available. The practitioner must carry her equipment in, set it up, then tear it down and carry it out at the end of each appointment. When doing only a few appointments a day or a week, this might be an ideal setup, but going to several appointments every day can be exhausting.

Safety is also a factor. Carrying a portable table into awkward locations can result in strain and injury. Going into unknown situations alone might result in a threatening encounter. Practitioners who do outcalls should have a system to protect themselves from the potential risk. When doing outcalls in a questionable situation, ensure your safety by making a telephone call to a colleague when you arrive at the appointment, giving the name and address of the party and the approximate time you will be finished, and then making another call to let your colleague know that you have finished and are leaving. Your phone calls will dissuade the client from any wrongdoing.

Working Out of a Separate/Private Office

A popular option among massage therapists is to rent a small private office. Depending on the size of the business, the office can be just one room or a complex of rooms where several practitioners work as employees, independent contractors, or partners. For a one-person operation, it is helpful to have at least two rooms, one as a therapy room and the other as an entry/waiting area.

Renting a Space in a Larger Office Complex

Another popular option for a therapist is to rent a space in conjunction with another complementary business operation, such as any of the following:

- A full-service beauty salon
- A chiropractor's office
- An athletic gym
- A sports clinic
- A hospital
- An alternative health clinic
- A doctors' complex
- A spa

These arrangements have many advantages in that the massage business has ready access to clientele as well as receptionist and waiting room facilities.

There are several possible alternatives when working out of or renting space from another business regarding how the rent is paid and what is included. They range from renting/leasing raw space (you bear all costs of modifications, maintenance, support services, and supplies) to a turnkey situation (a landlord prepares the space, supplies all the needs, and all the therapist must do is tell him what you want and come in and go to work). The amount of rent depends on what is included. In some cases, the rent is a flat amount; in other cases, it is a percentage of your sales. (In most situations, this author recommends a fixed rent amount because a percentage can vary widely and could be extremely high when the practitioner gets busy.) It is essential that whatever the terms of the agreement, they be put in writing in the form of a lease agreement or a contract that is signed by both parties. It is highly recommended that a lawyer examine the agreement to ensure that all parties comply with the law and that each party is duly protected.

> ## *Mini-lab*
>
> These are only a few of the many options available to the enterprising massage entrepreneur. Every option has its advantages and disadvantages.
>
> - For each of the options given here, make a list of pros and cons.
> - Think of three other possible options for a massage practice.
> - What would be the ideal massage practice you would like to work in?

Co-op an Office with Other Therapists

Often massage therapists rent a facility together, sharing the expenses of rent, utilities, and a receptionist/bookkeeper. This option is a way to provide an attractive facility for several practitioners yet keep the overhead affordable. It also provides flexibility in scheduling so that practitioners can work hours that suit them and clients have the option of receiving services at their convenience.

BEGINNING IN BUSINESS

As a business owner and manager, you must have knowledge of your field, good business sense, a sense of diplomacy, and clear business goals. In addition, you must keep accurate records and understand all business procedures involved in your kind of business. You can hire tax consultants and bookkeepers to do some of the more extensive work, but it is you, the owner, who is responsible for the success of the business.

Most people who succeed in the personal service business gain experience by learning while working for someone else. They learn efficient management, motivating employees, promoting good customer relations, and numerous other business procedures. After a practitioner has gained experience and knowledge, she might then decide to start a business or look for an established business to buy or manage.

If you are beginning a new business, consider several things. Which type of a business operation will it be? How will you finance the costs of equipment and other start-up costs before you can begin to generate income? Other considerations in starting a business are choosing a location, acquiring permits and licenses, and selecting adequate insurance coverage.

The Small Business Association (SBA) has a multitude of tools and services to assist the entrepreneur in the creation and development of a new business. (www.sba.gov, 1-800-8ask-sba.) One of those resources is SCORE—Councilors to America's Small Businesses. SCORE is a mentoring program in which volunteers, including working or retired business owners, executives, and corporate leaders, share their wisdom, offering free and confidential small business advice for entrepreneurs (www.score.org).

BUSINESS PLANNING

Business planning starts when a business is first conceived and continues throughout the life of the business. Planning is the first step in setting the stage for the development of the business. Planning involves clarifying your purpose, stating a mission, setting goals, and determining priorities.

A **mission statement** is a short general statement of the main focus of the business. Developing a mission statement requires careful consideration. The mission statement expresses the values and intent of the business and can be used on promotional material as a reflection of the business's public image.

mission statement

is a short, general statement of the main focus of the business.

A **purpose** is a theme that is derived from your dreams and ideals. You might have several purposes for doing business. Clarifying those purposes allows you to direct your energies toward those purposes.

purpose

is the business theme that is derived from the owner's dreams and ideals.

Some examples of a purpose might be:

- To provide a pleasant, environmentally friendly working environment
- To make a positive difference for my clientele
- To prosper and enjoy what I do

Goals are specific, attainable, measurable things or accomplishments that you decide on and make a commitment to achieve. The business goals that you set support your mission and reinforce your purpose. Setting goals clarifies your

goals

are specific, attainable, measurable accomplishments that you set and make a commitment to achieve.

intentions and directs your creative energy toward realizing your dreams, and ultimately toward success.

Goals can be short term or long term. You can have lifelong goals, 5-year goals, 1-year goals, 6-month goals, goals for next week, goals for tomorrow, or goals for today. Although it is helpful to include a deadline with a goal, it is not necessary. Keep your goals personalized and in the present tense. Make your goals realistic and attainable, but do not hesitate to think big. The more specific that your goals are, the better.

The following are some examples of goals:

- I will see 20 clients per week.
- I will attend the next national convention.
- I will spend at least three evenings per week at home with my family.
- I will increase my income by 20 percent this year.

Develop a Strategic Plan

It is helpful to write your goals down. Refer to them often to see how you are progressing. Setting goals is only a clarification of where you are heading. Once you set goals, it takes planning and commitment to realize them. Some goals are simple: "I will maintain my client files daily." Others are more complicated and have many subgoals contained within them. "I will increase my income by 20 percent this year." To accomplish the larger goal, it helps to break it into doable chunks, examine them, and develop a course of action.

List the benefits of attaining the goal. Brainstorm possible steps needed to reach the goal. Note potential obstacles or conflicts and solutions to those problems. Then develop a step-by-step plan of how to reach the goal. Include in the plan resources and timetables of what actions to take. After the plan is formulated, *do it!*

TYPES OF BUSINESS OPERATIONS

A business can be organized as a sole proprietorship, a partnership, or a corporation. Each type has advantages and disadvantages.

sole proprietor

is an individual business owner responsible for all expenses, obligations, liabilities, and assets.

As a **sole proprietor,** you are an individual owner and carry all expenses, obligations, liabilities, and assets. You receive all profits from your business and are responsible for all losses. Business obligations and debts are the owner's personal responsibility. Legally as a sole proprietor, you and the business are one and the same in the eyes of the law. If the business gets too far into debt, or in legal trouble, you as an individual are liable. There is the potential for numerous tax advantages, but you must comply with all tax responsibilities, including self-employment taxes. Many people prefer being a sole proprietor if they can handle the financial and personal responsibilities involved.

Most massage therapists are self-employed and are sole proprietors. If the business is run under a different name than that of the proprietor, the owner must register that name according to local statutes to protect the name and be sure that no other local business is already using it. This registration is referred to as *doing business as* (DBA) and can be done at a local county clerk's office. Being self-employed means being your own boss and setting your own schedule.

It also means that you are responsible for the success or failure of your business. Being self-employed requires you to be self-motivated and disciplined. You are solely responsible not only for working with clients but also for all promotional and operational activities.

A **partnership** might be the answer if you know someone who wants to invest and who is qualified to share the responsibility. The combined ability and experience of two or more people can make a business easier to operate. Although a partnership can relieve a sole proprietor of the pressures of doing everything herself, there are some drawbacks. A partnership is a relationship wrought with all the bonuses and misunderstandings of any interpersonal association.

partnership

is a business model in which two or more partners share responsibility and benefits of running the business.

One key to a good working partnership is a clear partnership agreement. Although it is not a legal requirement, a written partnership agreement can clarify the rights and responsibilities of each partner and strengthen the relationship. A partnership agreement should include the business goals, what each partner will contribute (i.e., money, material, and time), how the profits will be divided, and how the business will continue should one partner want out.

Legally, in a partnership, each partner is a co-owner and carries the same responsibilities as a sole proprietor in the case of debt and liability. There are also certain tax regulations specific to partnerships. Profits and losses are reported to the IRS on Form 1065. An accountant and a lawyer can be helpful if you are considering setting up a partnership.

A corporation is a legal entity with assets and liabilities separate from its owners. A **corporation** has advantages and disadvantages. It is subject to regulation and taxation by the state, and a charter must be obtained from the state in which the business operates. Management of the corporation is in the hands of a board of directors, the members of which determine policies and make decisions in accordance with the charter. Stockholders share in profits but are not legally responsible for the actions of the corporation. Stockholders and corporate owners are not directly liable for lawsuits and debts against the corporation. As a professional person, the corporation will not shield you from the liability of actions of gross negligence that result in a malpractice suit. If you are considering incorporating, consult with knowledgeable legal and financial authorities to determine whether it is worth the time, money, and effort that it takes.

corporation

is a business setup subject to state regulation and taxation. A charter must be obtained from the state in which the corporation operates.

Limited liability companies (LLCs) are a form of legal entity that is something between a partnership and a corporation. LLCs offer many of the benefits of a corporation with much less paperwork and other complications. Most states require an LLC to have at least two owners or members and to file an IRS Form 1065. The owners in an LLC are a separate entity from the business and are shielded from some of the personal liability of the business. Profits and losses from the business are divided among the owners and recorded on their individual income tax returns.

limited liability companies

are a form of legal entity, something between a partnership and a corporation.

If you are considering setting up a partnership, corporation, or an LLC, consult with a lawyer familiar with business law to determine the best type of business structure for your particular needs. Your local SBA office is a great resource for free business advice (www.sba.gov).

START-UP COSTS AND NEEDS

The start-up costs for beginning a business include all the expenses incurred before any revenues are collected. Those costs vary according to the size and complexity of the operation. Start-up costs are out-of-pocket expenses that must be considered during the planning stage and recovered before a profit is realized.

The two main reasons that small businesses fail are undercapitalization and poor management. Most massage practitioners are self-employed. They work out of their home, a small office space, a space shared with another practitioner, or in conjunction with another health care provider (e.g., doctor, chiropractor, or other professional person). Regardless of where you locate your practice, there are certain expenses in setting up the practice.

Start-up expenses include:

- Rent or lease: Can include first and last month's rent and a cleaning/damage deposit
- Utilities: Hook-up charges and deposits for electric, gas, telephone, telephone answering service, Internet access
- Equipment and supplies: Table, bolsters, therapy equipment, linens, massage oils, and laundry
- Furniture: Desks, chairs, supply cabinets, music system, file cabinet, and lighting
- Decorating supplies: Paint, curtains, plants, other items
- Office supplies: Calculator, printer, computer, pens, staple gun, writing paper, filing supplies, and appointment and receipt books
- Advertising expense: Ads and announcements, Web site
- Printing expense: Business cards, stationery, information forms, brochures
- Licenses and permits: Professional license, business license, professional membership, sales tax license
- Insurance: Professional liability, personal liability; premises, health, and disability insurance
- Initial operating expense: Opening business checking account with enough capital to cover miscellaneous expenses until the business is up and running
- Professional fees: Attorney, accountant, graphic artist, Web designer, business coach

When planning a business operation, it is important to establish good credit and banking relations. Many businesspeople rely on getting business loans when necessary to have sufficient working capital. It usually takes time to build clientele, and so money must be available to take care of necessary expenses. Always know where your money is being spent, and operate with sufficient cash flow. A major cause of small business failure is the owner's inexperience in judging overhead expenses and having inadequate capital to carry the business through slow periods. As income and profits grow, the budget can be increased for expansion of facilities, advertising, and other areas of growth.

BUSINESS LOCATION

One of the most important decisions that you can make concerning the success or failure of your business is where it is going to be located. Depending on how you structure the business, possible locations can vary. Massage businesses can be operated out of the practitioner's home, in a rented space in another business, or out of a freestanding office.

There are many factors to consider when renting or leasing a space for a massage business. The building in which a personal service business is located should be in good condition and in a fairly prosperous location. Choose a site that can accommodate your business needs, is pleasing to your clients, fits your image, and is properly zoned and within your budget. It must be easy to locate, with the address clearly visible from the street. It should be easily accessible and relatively quiet. An ideal space has one or more massage rooms, a reception/waiting area, an office, and bathroom facilities with a shower. The first impression that clients will have of you is the one they get when they walk into your place of business. Ask yourself, "Does this facility represent the quality with which I want to be associated?"

If a business is large enough to support a consistent advertising program, it can be located in an out-of-the-way, prestigious location. A smaller, less affluent business should be located near other active places of business to attract the attention of potential clients. Being near public transportation and having adequate parking facilities are important considerations.

After you have determined space requirements, have a clear price range in mind, an idea of the kind of location you want, and check the resources in your area. Realtors and the chamber of commerce can be good leads. If you want to work within another business, check out the local business directory or the Yellow Pages for businesses of the type with which you want to associate.

Before signing a rental agreement or lease, make certain that the space fits your needs. If remodeling is necessary or if the building must be "brought up to code," the costs can be overwhelming. Some questions to ask are:

- Does the massage area have individual heating and air-conditioning controls, and is it well ventilated?
- Will the massage rooms be quiet?
- Is the facility accessible to people with disabilities?
- Is the lighting appropriate, and are there sufficient outlets?
- Is there sufficient storage?
- How are the maintenance and utilities handled?
- Who is responsible for what, and how much can I expect to pay?

If you plan to lease a location or business, be sure that you insert into the lease agreement any options for removing or replacing fixtures, making repairs, changing specific structures, or installing equipment, plumbing, and electrical work.

When you are satisfied with the location and all provisions, it is important to get the lease agreement in writing. Do not necessarily sign the first lease that the landlord offers. Read the lease carefully to make sure that all provisions are clearly explained. All negotiations must be made and documented before the lease is signed. It is usually a good idea to review a business lease with an attorney before signing.

Many therapists choose to work independently out of their homes. This is an inexpensive alternative but sometimes does require a special use permit because of local zoning regulations. The portion of the home that is used for an office must be kept clean and neat if you choose this option. A clean bathroom, preferably with a shower, should be available for clients. There are certain tax deductions that can be claimed for having an office in the home (check with a tax accountant).

BUYING AN ESTABLISHED BUSINESS

You might have an opportunity to buy an established business, in which case you must weigh the advantages or disadvantages. Be sure the business has a good reputation, that it is worth the price being asked, and that it has an established clientele. It is a good idea to question customers as well as other business owners in the vicinity about the reputation of the business. Of course, you want to know why the present owner is selling. Obviously, it is no advantage to buy a business that is being sold because it is failing. Generally, the owner is moving, retiring, or changing occupations.

The price of buying an existing practice depends on several factors:

- the facility – rented, leased, or owned
- equipment fixtures and furniture
- reputation of the business
  - in the community
  - with local businesses
  - with suppliers and creditors
  - with other health care practitioners
  - with insurance providers
- projected income and expenses – Examining business records for the previous four or five years provides a good indication of expenses and income
- likelihood of client retention and loyalty

To enhance the likelihood of a smooth transition, it might be a good idea to arrange to work together with the seller of the business for a period of time to maintain relationships with existing suppliers, clients, local businesses, and referring agencies, if the seller is willing. This is also an opportunity for the seller to introduce the buyer to loyal customers, professional associates, and business networks.

It is important to consult a lawyer who can handle all legal aspects of the transaction to the satisfaction of everyone involved. A written purchase and sale agreement is needed. Also needed is a complete inventory of all fixtures, equipment, supplies, and materials as well as the value of each article that is to be part of the agreement. To avoid future misunderstandings, it is advisable to take photographs of furnishings and equipment. This will help to ensure that you receive the exact items listed. It is also necessary to examine all records to understand the assets and liabilities of the business that you are buying. An investigation should be made to determine any outstanding debts or obligations that might be held against the business.

LICENSES AND PERMITS

There are local, state, and federal regulations that must be considered when beginning, locating, or relocating a business. It is to the advantage of the business owner to be aware of and comply with all regulations in the process of organizing the business rather than to be surprised after the fact and have to pay heavy penalties or restructure or relocate the business. The following is a partial list of permits and licenses that might be required and who to contact to determine how to comply.

Planning and zoning permits: Required to ensure that the operation and location of the business complies with local zoning requirements. This might especially affect those who operate a business out of their home. *Contact:* County or city planning and zoning board.

Building safety permit: Might be required to obtain a business or professional license. Might be issued after the place of business has been inspected and found to be free of conditions that could pose a hazard to you or your clients and comply with building and fire codes. *Contact:* Local fire department.

Business license: Might be required to operate a business in the city, county, or state. *Contact:* City or county government, business licensing department.

Massage license: Can be a city, county, or state requirement to perform massage services for a fee. *Contact:* County/city licensing bureau or the state agency in charge of occupational or massage licensing.

Fictitious name statement (DBA): Required if the business name is different from the owner's name. A fictitious name statement, also called DBA (Doing Business As), is filed with the county to ensure that no other business uses the same name when doing business. *Contact:* County clerk's office.

Employer's identification number (EIN): This is the federal tax identification number issued to businesses and is used on all tax-related forms. An EIN is required of partnerships and businesses that hire employees. Sole proprietors can use an EIN or Social Security number. *Contact:* Internal Revenue Service.

Sales tax permit: Required if you sell products or if services are taxed. Provides information and materials to collect and file sales tax. *Contact:* State department of revenue.

Provider's number: This is an identification number issued to licensed health care providers. It is used and required when submitting claims to and receiving payment from medical insurance companies for services rendered. Massage practitioners in most states are not eligible to hold a provider's number but do receive third-party payments (insurance payments) by contracting with, billing through, or being an employee of a licensed provider (i.e., doctor, chiropractor, physical therapist).

PROTECTING YOUR BUSINESS

Adequate insurance against fire, theft, and liability is necessary to protect the business. To determine the specific types and amounts of coverage to cover your business and yourself, consult with one or more insurance agents. If you work out of your home, review your homeowner's policy concerning the liability of operating a business out of your home. If you lease an office, check the lease to determine which liability responsibilities are yours and which are the landlord's.

The following is a list of some types of insurance you may want to obtain.

Liability insurance covers costs of injuries and litigation resulting from injuries sustained on your property. This is usually a part of a homeowner's policy but might not cover business-related occurrences. Check with your insurance agent. A special rider to your homeowner's policy might be necessary, or you might need to purchase a separate policy.

Professional liability insurance, also called malpractice insurance, protects the therapist from lawsuits filed by a client because of injury or loss resulting from alleged negligence or substandard performance of a professional skill. Professional liability insurance can be purchased reasonably through some professional organizations such as the American Massage Therapy Association and the Associated Bodywork and Massage Professionals.

Automobile insurance: full coverage provides medical and liability insurance to the driver and any passengers, and covers the vehicle and its contents regardless of who is at fault.

Property insurance or fire and theft insurance covers fixtures, furniture, equipment, products, and supplies. If you rent or lease an office, the landlord might carry this insurance. Make sure that it is adequate. *Renter's insurance* is available through most major insurance companies for a relatively small premium that covers the loss of furniture and equipment in the case of theft, vandalism, fire, or other natural disasters. If you have an office in the home, be sure that your homeowner's policy is adequate to cover your office.

Medical/health insurance helps cover the cost of medical bills, especially hospitalization, serious injury, or illness.

Disability insurance protects the person from loss of income when she is unable to work because of long-term illness or injury.

Worker's compensation insurance is required if you have employees. It covers the medical costs for employees if they are injured on the job.

PLANNING THE PHYSICAL LAYOUT OF A BUSINESS

The layout of a business takes careful planning to achieve efficiency and economy of operation. After the building or space within a building has been decided, the interior must be designed to be a clean and safe environment for the comfort and privacy of the client. An efficient salon, studio, or clinic offering massage should have the following:

1. Air-conditioning and heating systems to provide warmth and comfort to clients.
2. Appropriate plumbing for showers and restrooms.
3. Adequate and appropriate lighting for the entire operation, including indirect lighting in the massage rooms.

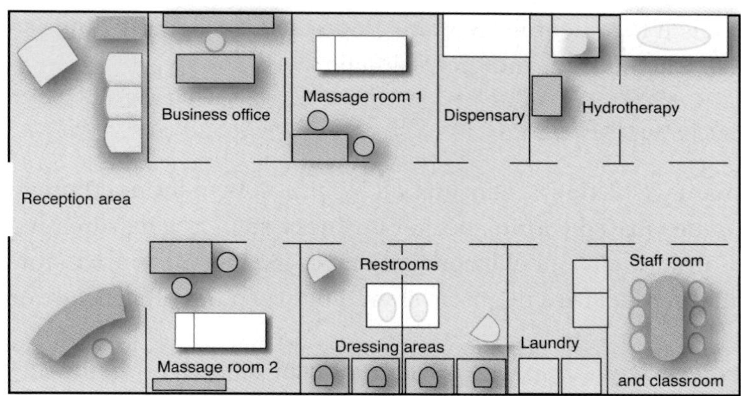

FIGURE 22-2 Floor plan A–ideal space, 28′ × 50′.

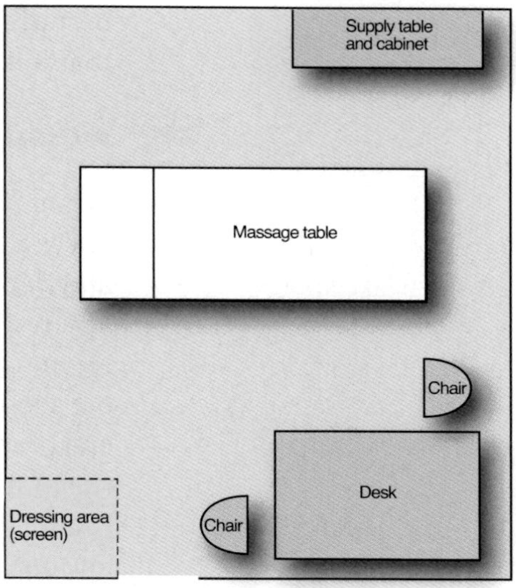

FIGURE 22-3 Floor plan B–basic space, 10′ × 12′.

4. A private massage room with adequate space for a massage table, maneuvering space around the table, a supply cabinet, possibly a dressing area, and, if consultations will take place in the room, a desk with two chairs.
5. Proper equipment and adequate space for its use.
6. Accessibility to all business areas for those who may have mobility impairments .
7. Furniture that is appropriate, attractive, durable, and in keeping with the dignity of the business.
8. An attractive and comfortable private consultation area.
9. An attractive and comfortable reception area.
10. An area suitable to carry out business practices such as maintaining client files, correspondence, making telephone calls, and scheduling appointments.

Clients form either a positive or negative first impression of a business operation by the appearance of the office facility. The decor and appointments need not cost a fortune but should give the impression that the business and the people employed there are highly professional. Your office can be one of your

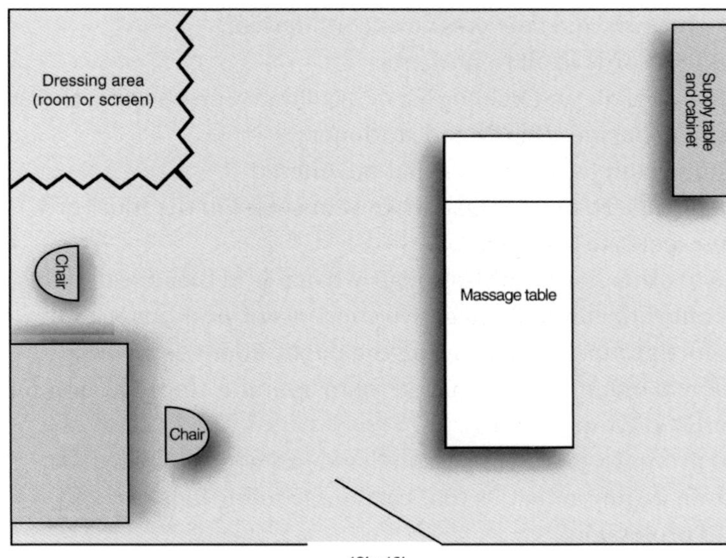

FIGURE 22-4 Floor plan C–functional space, 12′ × 16′.

best promotional tools if the client is favorably impressed. Design the office so that it is comfortable, uncluttered, and professional.

Massage Business Floor Plans

When planning a massage business, consider all facilities. As mentioned previously, a business can be located within another business, such as a hairdressing and skin care salon, athletic club, or chiropractic office. The reception area, storage, restrooms, and other facilities might be shared between the office, club, or salon.

Floor plan A shows adequate space for a larger business with room for several practitioners (Figure 22-2). The basic floor plan B (Figure 22-3) and the functional floor plan C (Figure 22-4) show only essential furnishings of a massage room. This is often the ideal plan for the beginning practitioner, to maintain a low operational cost.

BUSINESS ETHICS FOR THE MASSAGE PRACTITIONER

A massage practitioner must always practice according to a professional code of ethics. *Ethics* are standards of acceptable and professional behavior by which a person or business conducts business. Chapter 3 discusses ethics for the massage practitioner. Good business ethics provide guidelines for professional conduct when doing business. The following guidelines reflect ethical behavior for the massage business owner:

1. Always present a professional appearance.
2. Maintain a sense of dignity and professionalism in your work.
3. Project a pleasant, optimistic personality.
4. Treat each client with courtesy.
5. Maintain good health habits.
6. Keep surroundings neat, clean, and attractive.
7. Follow a systematic plan and organize your work properly.
8. Space appointments so that sufficient time is allowed.
9. Keep clients' records and conversations confidential.
10. Keep accurate records of all treatments.
11. Keep an active card file and mailing list of regular and prospective clients.
12. Use professional business cards and stationery.
13. Make periodic mailings of services that are offered.
14. Be sure that all advertising represents your business in the most professional and accurate manner.
15. Refer clients to other health professionals when it is in their best interest.
16. Make every effort to eliminate negative concepts of your business by speaking before groups and educating the public about your work.
17. Join professional organizations that strive to upgrade, improve, and set high standards for your business.
18. Continue to promote your own personal and professional growth.
19. Work to eliminate any activities that cast unfavorable light on your business and profession.
20. Be responsible in keeping your word and meeting your obligations.

21. Obey all laws and legal requirements regulating the practice of massage and your business operation.
22. Charge a fair price for services rendered.
23. Continue to build a good reputation by your own work and conduct.
24. Recommend massage treatments only as the client requires and desires them.
25. Be loyal to your employers, associates, and clients.
26. Keep your professional and private lives separate by maintaining professional boundaries and not discussing your personal problems with your clients.

SETTING YOUR FEES

As a businessperson offering a personal service, your income depends on the fees that you charge for your services. In determining your fee structure, consider several factors. There are various strategies you can use to set your fees.

You are a professional massage therapist selling a valuable service; therefore, set a fee that compensates you fairly and reflects your credibility. Consider the market and your competition. A little research can tell you which services are offered by other practitioners in the area and what they charge for those services. Set your fees in accordance with others in your area.

If you offer a unique service in high demand, your fee can be higher. If you are just beginning and want to attract more of the market, you might choose to set a lower fee or offer special introductory rates.

If you are self-employed and massage is your sole source of income, you must consider all of the costs of operating your business and determine how many sessions you must do at which rates to earn a living. If you are working for someone else, you might work for an hourly wage or for a percentage of each massage that you perform. You must determine what you are willing to receive for each massage that you perform. The percentage you receive might depend on who furnishes the equipment, supplies, and services such as telephone, receptionist, and advertising.

YOUR BUSINESS TELEPHONE

The business telephone is a powerful business tool. It is your contact with potential and steady clients. Anyone placing or receiving calls must know and use proper telephone techniques and courtesies. Your telephone number should accompany your business ads in telephone directories or newspapers and should be printed on your business cards. Therefore, the person answering the telephone should know how to do the following:

- Answer the phone professionally and in a courteous, friendly manner.
- Give accurate information and encourage a potential client to make an appointment.
- Make or change appointments for clients when necessary.
- Take messages accurately.
- Return all calls promptly.

- Place orders for supplies and other items when needed.
- Handle any complaints tactfully.
- Remind clients of appointments or needed services.
- Give accurate directions to the massage office from anywhere in the area.
- Build goodwill and new business.
- Screen calls.

In addition to the abovementioned, your business telephone serves as a security instrument in calling for help in case of emergency. For the protection of your employees and clients, the following phone numbers should be displayed near your business telephone:

- Nearest fire station.
- Nearest ambulance service and hospital emergency service.
- Police, local and state.
- Taxi service.
- Companies that provide needed services such as telephone and utilities.
- Names and telephone numbers of owners, managers, custodians, and employees.
- Names, addresses, and telephone numbers of all clients, which are kept in a private file but available in case of emergency.

If you work out of your home and use your personal telephone for business purposes, there are a few special considerations. Anyone who answers the phone must do it in a courteous, professional manner. Assume that every call is a business call. When the phone rings, put on a smile and answer by saying your name or the name of the business. Greet the caller by name. Ask, "What can I do for you today?" and then listen. Have a pen and paper ready to take notes. Respond to any questions professionally, or if you need more clarity, ask another question. When their questions have been answered, move them toward an action, preferably making an appointment.

When you are unavailable to answer the phone, an answering machine or voice mail can be used so that important calls are not missed. The outgoing message should be short and professional. It should contain a greeting, your name or business name, a request for information from the caller, and an indication when you will return the call. Messages should be responded to promptly, always within 24 hours if possible.

Business telephone expenses are tax deductible. If you use your home telephone for business purposes, the portion of your home telephone bill that is business related (i.e., long-distance business phone calls) is tax deductible if you maintain a telephone log book with the date, destination, and purpose for the call. (The base charges for your personal home phone are not deductible.) If you use your home phone number on your business cards and other advertising, it is considered a business phone and is subject to higher business telephone rates. If your phone is a business telephone (you pay business rates), the entire bill is tax deductible.

BASICS OF BOOKKEEPING

A good recordkeeping system is essential to the success of a business. You need to keep client records as well as records of income from both services and sales of products. Receipts, canceled checks, and invoices should be kept in appropriate files for tax purposes. Even though businesses hire accountants, it is still important for the self-employed practitioner, business manager, or owner to understand the basics of the system. It is more difficult to manage a business if you do not understand the principles of sound business administration and management. It is a plus for an inexperienced person to have some training in business administration before opening a business.

Without a proper bookkeeping system and accurate records, the owner or manager of a business would be unable to determine the progress of the business, especially the cost of doing business in relation to income. Business records are necessary to meet the requirements of local, state, and federal laws pertaining to taxes and employees. The manager of the business should see that records are kept properly for Social Security and taxes (i.e., state, local, and federal). If employees are involved, the manager should also be aware of recording payroll, wage and hour laws, workers' compensation, and any other laws or regulations that apply to hiring (or firing) employees.

A bookkeeping system should be only as complicated as the business requires. For a self-employed person, a simple system that records income and disbursements is sufficient. Once a good system is set up and kept current, it reduces the year-end tax preparation drudgery and offers an accurate accounting of the business's financial position. Consulting an accountant is helpful when setting up a bookkeeping system and advisable when preparing taxes. A good accountant knows the changing tax laws and can often find many deductions you might otherwise miss.

Accounting packages have been designed specifically for the massage therapist. They are usually advertised in one of the massage industry's journals or magazines. Make sure that they are updated and meet your needs.

A Word or Two about Using Computers

Computers have become an integral part of many business operations, streamlining various business activities and reducing paper usage. If you have a computer and are somewhat comfortable using it, the right software can make the process of bookkeeping much easier. There are several programs that enable the user to enter information and create reports easily. In programs such as Quicken and Quickbooks, by entering the information from your checkbook register (or writing your checks with the computer), you can generate a wide variety of reports and graphs. When recording checks, you enter the payee, the category, and the amount of the expenditure. Another feature allows you to break down your deposits into various income categories. With a couple of key strokes, you can create cash flow charts, income statements, accounts payable, accounts receivable, balance sheets, and several other reports. If you will be using an accountant to prepare taxes, ask them which software they recommend.

Other computer accounting programs allow even more functions, such as writing invoices and inventory control. There are a growing number of computer software packages that have been designed specifically for the massage business to manage client files, including appointments, SOAP notes, insurance, and financial files. Some of these programs include business accounting. Obtain the computer software that does what you require. Make sure that the software and hardware are reliable, and *always* back up your work.

If you do not have a computer and are unfamiliar with how to operate one, this might not the best time to start. You have enough on your hands getting your new business off the ground and most likely do not have a lot of capital in the bank to invest in the hardware and software that are required.

There are several ingredients to a workable bookkeeping system. The following section describes some of the basics.

Business Checking Account

A business checking account enables you to separate personal and business expenses. Open a separate account under the name of the business, and deposit all business income into the account. This will provide a record of your earnings. Use it whenever making cash disbursements. Pay all business bills by check, or a debit/credit card that provides a record of your expenditures. Write checks out of the business account to pay yourself. Then cash those checks or deposit them into your personal account to pay personal bills. This is called *personal draw* or *owner's expense*. Do not use the business account to pay personal or non-business expenses.

When a check is written, be sure to record clearly in the check register the check number, the date that the check was written, to whom the check was written, what the check was written for (the category or type of expense), and the amount of the check. All of this information must be recorded in the disbursement journal. If any of it is missing, it makes bookkeeping more difficult. An updated checkbook ledger is a good way to register disbursements and income; more complete ledgers are necessary to track a business's financial standing.

Petty Cash Account

petty cash fund is maintained to pay small disbursements for incidentals.

A **petty cash fund** can be maintained to pay small disbursements for incidentals such as parking fees, stamps, or copies. Receipts should be kept for each transaction, which should be properly recorded in the ledger. Occasionally, a check should be written from the business checking account to bring the petty cash fund back to a desired level.

Bank Statements and Reconciliations

Each month, the bank sends a bank statement listing the deposits that were made for the month, the checks that have been processed through the account, any bank charges or interest payments, and the balance left in the account. All of these figures should be compared with your records to make sure that neither you nor the bank has made any mistakes and that you agree on the balance in your account. On the back of most bank statements is a worksheet that can be used to reconcile your account. Be prompt in reconciling the statement with your checkbook. Note any errors, omissions, or miscalculations. Correct any mistakes and notify the bank immediately of any problems. Keep all bank statements, reconciliations, and canceled checks in your files a minimum of seven years as proof of expenditures.

Credit Cards

You might consider acquiring a credit or debit card to use solely for business purposes. Credit cards are wonderful if you are going to do any business traveling. You can use them to reserve and pay for hotels, plane tickets, or restaurant tabs. They are convenient, and all expenditures are listed on the credit card billing statements, which simplifies your bookkeeping. You must, however, still retain cash receipts for your tax records.

Just as checking accounts have a variety of charges and benefits, credit cards have different cost and amenities. They vary in the annual fee, the interest charged on the balance in the account, and the grace period allowed after a purchase is made before interest is charged on the balance. Your credit line also might vary, from $1,000 to $100,000 or more. Some credit cards have added benefits such as free travel insurance, discounts on car rentals, or no-fee travelers' checks. Several credit card companies offer a rewards program in which each dollar spent earns points toward airline travel, hotel stays, merchandise, or even cash back. By shopping around, you might be able to save long term. Regardless of the credit card that you decide on, if you pay off the balance promptly every month and keep the balance at zero, you will avoid paying exorbitant finance and interest charges.

Income Records

There are two basic steps to recording business income. The first step takes place when the income is first received and an invoice or sales slip is filled out. The second step is when the invoices are totaled, summarized, and recorded in an income ledger.

Writing out an invoice or a cash receipt every time money is taken in is a convenient way to keep track of how much money has been brought in and specifically for what. Invoices should be written in duplicate. The original goes to the client for his records, and the copy goes into the cash box or daily records. At the end of the day, week, or whichever recording period you choose, the invoices are tallied and recorded on the income ledger.

For a business that does only massage, a simple invoice that indicates how much the massage service costs is sufficient. If the business offers a variety of services and products, the invoice might be more complex. In states that have a sales tax, the invoice should have space for non-taxable services (or items), taxed items (retail sales), amount of sales tax, and the total. If you offer credit, it is a federal law that the terms of credit and finance charges are clearly disclosed on the invoice.

The invoice should include the following information:

- Your business name, address, and phone number.

- The invoice date.
- The client's name (and address).
- Date of the service or sales of goods.
- A description of services given.
- Amount charged for services.
- A description of goods sold.
- Amount charged for the goods sold.
- Amount of sales tax.
- The total.
- A space to indicate the date paid.
- A statement of appreciation for the client's business.

If you extend credit, you must include on the invoice all credit terms and finance charges. Keep a copy of the invoice for your records, and give a copy to the client.

The income ledger is a summary of all cash receipts or invoices. The information from sales invoices is tallied and posted on the income ledger. It is one of the most important business documents that you have. It shows you where your money is coming from and when it is or is not flowing. It is a primary source for preparing cash flow summaries, sales tax reports, and income taxes. It is also helpful when planning advertising, expenditures, and vacations.

How frequently the information is posted in the income ledger depends on the volume of business. The information that you need to note on a ledger sheet depends on the nature of your massage business. If all of your income is strictly from doing massage in your studio, the income ledger could be very simple. If your business sells any products or offers a variety of services, your income ledger will be more sophisticated, to reflect the different sources of incoming funds.

If your sales volume is quite large, daily posting might be appropriate. In most individual massage practices, however, weekly posting is sufficient. A word to the wise: don't let the paperwork pile up! Be prompt and do the book work regularly, because it really becomes a headache when you get behind. Each time you tally up your receipts to deposit your incoming funds in the bank, record your totals onto your income ledger, and your book work is done.

The income ledger should have a sufficient number of columns to list the classifications and sources of money coming into your business. Provide a column for income from massage services. If your business provides a variety of massage services that you want to track, you might want to include a separate column for each of those services. Examples might be outcalls, seated massage, hydrotherapy, or tanning booths. If your business sells massage-related products, include a column for retail or taxable sales and another column for sales tax. The sales tax column greatly simplifies filing quarterly sales tax documents. If you have any non-taxed income such as wholesale, out-of-state sales, or freight, include another column for non-taxed income. The last column on the ledger should record your total sales.

The sample ledger in Figure 22-5a has columns for the date, massage income, gift certificate income, non-taxed retail, taxable income, and sales tax. There is also a column for other income with a space for description of the income

Daily Income Ledger for Month of ________________ 20_____

Date	Massage Income	Gift Certificates	Other Income	Nontaxable Retail	Taxable Retail	Sales Tax	Total Income
Total							
YTD							

FIGURE 22-5A Sample income ledger.

Yearly Summary Income Ledger for 20_____

Month	Massage Income	Gift Certificates	Other Income	Nontaxable Retail	Taxable Retail	Sales Tax	Total Income
January							
February							
March							
1st Quarter							
April							
May							
June							
2nd Quarter							
July							
August							
September							
3rd Quarter							
October							
November							
December							
4th Quarter							
Yearly Total							

FIGURE 22-5B Sample yearly income summary ledger.

source. This might include freight, reimbursement for travel, or royalties. Finally, there is a column for the total. The amount in the total column should equal the sum of the other columns and be the amount that is recorded on the bank deposit slip.

Regardless of how often you post information in your books, keep the months separate and run monthly totals. This will become important information when planning specials, advertising, expenditures, and vacations. You can record monthly totals on a summary sheet like the one in Figure 22-5b to better track your business activity. It also simplifies quarterly and year-end taxes.

File all sales invoices and keep them for a minimum of seven years. Every month, bundle all the invoices together for that month and store them in a file. They are documents that support your records and tax returns, and you might need them if you are ever audited by the Internal Revenue Service (IRS).

Disbursement Record

The disbursement ledger is your record of all of the expenditures that the business pays out, including bills, loan payments, payroll, and the money that you pay yourself (personal draws). Some of these expenditures are tax deductible, and some are not. A huge advantage of being self-employed is that much of what you do or buy can be considered business related and is therefore tax deductible. Obtain and keep receipts for all expenditures and record them in the disbursement ledger. The function of the disbursement ledger is to separate and classify business expenditures both for tax purposes and so that you can easily identify where your money is going. You are thereby able to plan and budget better.

Nearly all of the information that goes into the disbursement ledger comes from the checkbook register or credit card statement. If for some reason there are any cash outlays or payments made with money orders, those should be posted in the disbursement ledger as soon as possible. Try to make *all* business expenditures from the checkbook or credit card. Even though information on the disbursement ledger comes from the checkbook register, it is still necessary to maintain both. The information that each document furnishes is different and important. The checkbook allows you to keep a running balance of the account and also provides a space for marking off canceled checks and posting deposits. The disbursement ledger includes expenditures paid by check, credit card, cash or money order and categorizes expenditures so that you can easily see how much you have spent on what.

Ideally, every entry on the disbursement ledger can be validated by a receipt. When you pay bills, pay them by check, put the check number on the receipt from the billing, and file that receipt. It is a good idea to bundle the receipts together each month, put them in an envelope, label it with the month and year, and keep it in a file. Keep all receipts a minimum of seven years in case of an audit.

The disbursement ledger (Figure 22-6) is divided into several columns. The first four columns contain the date of the expenditure, the check number (or whether the payment was made with cash or money order), the payee, and the amount of the check or payment. The rest of the columns represent the category of the expenditure. There are literally dozens of possible categories. (A list of 36 categories that are common in a massage practice follows later in this chapter.) A separate column for every category is impractical. The example disbursement ledger in this chapter has nine columns, most of which actually have two categories. One column is a catch-all *miscellaneous* column.

Most disbursements are tax deductible; however, some pay-outs, such as loan payments and owner's expenses, are not. Be sure to allow a separate column for nondeductible expenses. The last column is for the owner's draw, or the money that you pay to yourself. At the bottom of the ledger is a space to

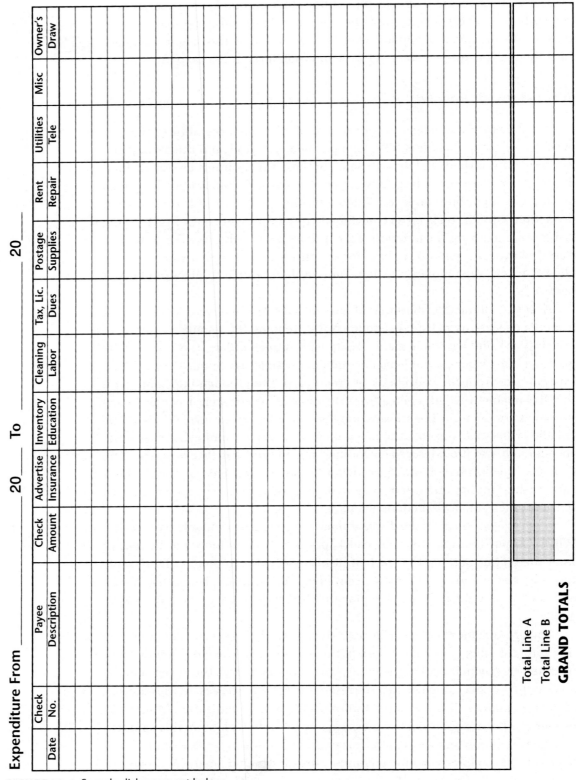

Expenditure From ______________ 20___ To ______________ 20___

Date	Check No.	Payee Description	Check Amount	Advertise Insurance	Inventory Education	Cleaning Labor	Tax, Lic. Dues	Postage Supplies	Rent Repair	Utilities Tele	Misc	Owner's Draw
		Total Line A										
		Total Line B										
		GRAND TOTALS										

FIGURE 22-6 Sample disbursement ledger.

total the figures in each column. The total of the category columns should equal the total in the *check amount* column. If it does not, recheck all figures and find your mistake.

It is a good idea to total all the columns of the disbursement ledger every month and record those totals on a summary sheet. This is a good way to keep track of your expenses and adjust your expenditures.

List of Business Expenses

Business expenses are partially or totally deductible from the business income when the profit or loss of the business is determined. These categories can be used when writing checks and on the disbursement ledger.

The following are possible expenses:

- Accounting expense
- Advertising
- Automobile expense
  - Fuel
  - Maintenance
  - Payments
  - License fees

(Another option is to keep track of mileage. Keep a record of the miles driven, date, and destination. An allowance per mile is used as a tax deduction.)

- Bad debts
- Bank fees
- Cleaning and janitorial
- Contract labor
- Convention and meeting costs
- Cost of products to be sold
- Depreciation of major business equipment expenditures
- Donations to charity
- Dues to business and professional associations
- Education expense
  - Seminars, professional journals, books, and other materials
- Entertainment
- Equipment expense
- Furnishings and fixtures
- Insurance premiums
  - Auto, liability, malpractice, health, fire, theft
- Interest paid on loans
- License and permit fees
- Office supplies
- Payroll, wages, and withholdings
- Postage, freight, and shipping
- Professional, legal, or consulting fees
- Refunds for services or products
- Rent
- Repair and maintenance
- Supplies

THE MASSAGE CLINIC

PROFIT and LOSS

January through December 2010

01/15/2011

Income		
Massage		36660.00
Gift Certificates		790.00
Total Massage		37450.00
Retail Sales		
Taxable	1380.65	
Non-taxable	776.60	
Total sales		2157.25
Other		1354.75
Total Income		**40,962.00**
Expense		
Accounting		150.00
Advertising		785.75
Conventions		395.00
Cost of products sold		950.29
Depreciation		0.00
Donations to charity		300.00
Dues		395.00
Education expense		850.00
Equipment		1295.95
Insurance		265.65
License and permits		125.00

Office supplies		632.35
Postage/shipping		78.50
Professional/legal		300.00
Rent		8100.00
Repair/maintenance		165.55
Taxes		
Property	196.65	
Sales	110.40	
Federal/state	3280.00	
Total taxes		3586.95
Telephone		777.60
Travel		
Auto/airfare	695.95	
Lodging	885.55	
Meals	156.69	
Travel/other	88.55	
Total travel		1826.74
Utilities		2645.45
Total Expense		**23,675.78**
Net Income/Loss		**17,336.22**

FIGURE 22-7 Profit and loss statement.

- Taxes
  Sales, property, state, federal
- Telephone, cell phone, Internet
- Travel, business-related
- Utilities

An expenditure that is not considered an expense is the owner's expense or salary paid to yourself.

Profit and Loss or Income Statement

An income statement or a profit and loss statement (P&L) is a summary of the income (revenue) and disbursement registers for a particular period, such as monthly, quarterly, or annually. The P&L is valuable for showing the profit that a business realized over a particular period and comparing it with other periods to determine if the business is meeting its financial goals. Income statements are also useful when preparing quarterly and annual tax documents.

To prepare a P&L statement, first list all sources of income or revenue and the amount collected from each source. Add the amounts to determine the total revenues. Next, list all expense categories and the amount spent for each category. Add those amounts to determine the total expense. Subtract the total expense from the total revenue to determine the net profit or loss for the particular period (Figure 22-7).

Note: If you use a computer, many software companies have accounting programs that include checking, income, and disbursement functions as well as profit and loss statements and other reports.

Business-related Receipts

Keep all receipts for every purchase or expenditure related in any way to the business. After recording transactions, file the receipts. Each month, create a new file so that the receipts are separated to reflect and support the entries in the monthly disbursement ledger. For tax reasons, keep all receipts for a minimum of seven years.

Accounts Receivable

Accounts receivable is a record of moneys owed to you by other persons or businesses. If you extend credit and bill your clients, you need to keep an ongoing record of each transaction. Record each charge and payment, including the date of the transaction and current balance. This does complicate the bookkeeping process considerably. To keep it simple, require cash payments at the time of service for everything except gift certificates, advance payments, insurance billings, and credit card payments (i.e., Visa and MasterCard).

Accounts Payable

Accounts payable records the money that you owe to other persons or businesses. If you buy supplies or services on credit, keep a file for each account or business that extends credit to your business. File statements and purchase orders so that you have an accurate record when it is time to pay the bills. Trades and barters should be recorded on a separate record.

Assets and Depreciation Records

Items and equipment purchased to be used in the business for an extended time (more than a year) are considered *business assets*. Supplies and inventory are not considered assets. Maintain a current record of business assets that includes an item description, date of purchase, and purchase price. Add new items when purchased and remove items when they are sold or retired from use.

Depending on the purchase price of a durable item and the business's financial situation, you can choose to declare it, for tax purposes, as a one-time business expense, or you can depreciate its cost over several years. Methods and schedules for depreciating different items vary according to the length of the useful life of the item. It is not within the scope of this book to discuss depreciation methods. Consult your accountant or refer to *The Tax Guide for Small Business,* published by the IRS, for detailed instructions. Maintain a depreciation record for all depreciable assets.

Keep a file for all major items and equipment, including purchase records, instruction manuals, service records, warranties, and guarantees.

Inventory

A good inventory system helps to ensure that you do not run out of supplies or are overstocked on items that do not move well. Supplies to be used are classified as *consumption supplies,* and those to be sold are classified as *retail supplies.* You might need to keep records of sales tax on supplies sold.

If you sell products as part of your business, you are required to take an inventory at the end of the year to determine the cost of goods sold for the year. The *cost of goods sold* is a business expense. The inventory still on hand at the end of the year is considered an asset and is not considered as cost of goods sold until the time it is sold:

To determine cost of goods sold:

  Determine cost of inventory as of January 1 of the tax year
+ Inventory purchased during the year
= Total inventory available for sale
- Cost of inventory as of December 31 of the tax year
= Cost of goods sold for the year

Mileage Log

All business-related travel should be recorded for tax purposes. Expenses for operating a vehicle for business are deductible from taxable income. This does not include travel from home to the place of business. If you travel from your home or office to do an outcall, however, the mileage to and from that destination is deductible. There are two ways of determining this deduction: the standard mileage allowance or actual automobile expense.

When an automobile is used in the course of the business, keep a mileage log and record all business travel. For each trip, record the destination, beginning and ending odometer readings, total miles traveled, and purpose of the trip. According to 2009 tax laws, a deduction of 55¢ per mile could be taken for business-related automobile use. (This figure does vary from year to year. Check with an accountant or the IRS for the current rate.)

If you deduct the actual auto expense, keep an itemized record of all expenses (e.g., fuel, service, insurance, license fees, parking, and depreciation records of actual purchase price). The auto expense is prorated between business use and personal use. For example, if you drove the vehicle 12,000 miles in a year and 4,000 miles was business related, you would deduct 33.3 percent of the total auto expenses from the business income.

Massage Clinic
Client Information Form

Name____________________ Birth Date ____________________

Address ____________________ Telephone ____________________

____________________ Business Phone ____________________

City/State/Zip ____________________ Social Security # ____________________

Occupation ____________________ Other Activities____________________

General Health Condition____________________ Blood Pressure ____________________

Have you had any serious or chronic illness, operations, chronic virus infections, or traumatic accidents? ____________________

Are you in recovery for addictions or abuse?____________________

Are you under a doctor's, chiropractor's, or other health practitioner's care? __________

If so, for what condition(s)? ____________________

Are you on any medication?_______ If so, what? ____________________

Do I have permission to contact your doctor/therapist?____________________

Names of doctors, chiropractors, or health practitioners:

Name____________________ Name ____________________

Address ____________________ Address ____________________

Telephone ____________________ Telephone ____________________

Why did you come for our services? (relaxation, pain, therapy, etc.)____________________

____

What results would you like to achieve with our work? ____________________

Have you had any massage therapy before?______If so, by whom? ____________________

How did you find out about our services? ____________________

Were you referred to this office?__________By whom? ____________________

In case of emergency notify: Name____________________Phone ____________________

I have completed this information form to the best of my knowledge. I understand the massage services are designed to be a health aid and are in no way to take the place of a doctor's care when it is indicated. Information exchanged during any massage session is educational in nature and is intended to help me become more familiar and conscious of my own health status and is to be used at my own discretion.

Our time together is precious, and I agree to cancel 24 hours in advance. Unless there is an emergency, if I miss an appointment, I agree to pay the full appointment fee.

Date____________________ Signature ____

FIGURE 22-8A Sample intake form.

Client Name ______________________________ Date 1st Session ____________

Address ____________________ City____________ St_______ ZIP_________

Phone (h)________________ (w)________________ Insurance ____________

Date	Service	Products	Tax	Charges	Credits	Balance	Comments

REFERRAL RECORD

Client Referred By ______________________________ Date ____________

New Clients Referred by This Client

Name	Date 1st Session	Acknowledged

FIGURE 22-8B Sample payment record.

Updated Client Files

The client file is the mechanism that practitioners use to record pertinent client information and document the work they have done with clients. The information that a practitioner keeps in the client files varies as much as the massage routines of different practitioners. Updated client files help the practitioner to render prompt and efficient service, ensure access to current information about the client, and provide some amount of legal protection for the practitioner in cases of litigation. Information that is often found in a client file includes intake information (Figure 22-8a), a treatment plan, informed consent, session documentation, and a record of payment (Figure 22-8b). Intake information includes name, address, phone, medical information, and history. A *treatment plan* provides a kind of a blueprint for the sessions that is updated periodically. Each session is documented with the type of service provided, the date given, the products used, and the results obtained. If a client is a physician referral or filing an insurance claim, documents include insurance information, a signed release of medical information document, assignment of benefits, financial responsibility, and consent-of-care forms. A payment record lists the amount charged and received for each item and service. Keeping accurate and updated records is a tedious but essential part of a professional operation. (See Chapters 9 and 17 for more information on client files.)

Appointment Book

The appointment book is possibly the most important document for organizing a successful and prosperous business, and it is an important tool in time management. A well-kept appointment book ensures that appointments are not missed and are scheduled so that you can be prompt and on time. There is nothing more embarrassing than to have two people show up for a massage at the same time. Keep the appointment book handy and always up to date. If you carry an appointment book with you, it can become a portable file to record mileage, important phone numbers, and business expenses, as well as appointments. It is still advisable to maintain a client appointment book at your office as well. Be sure to transfer information from your portable appointment book to your office book to avoid double bookings.

The appointment book should have enough space to record each client's appointment time, name, phone number (address and directions if it is an outcall), and possibly the amount that you receive from each client. All client information recorded in the appointment book is considered confidential and should be kept so that it is not in public view.

Many therapists now maintain their appointment calendars in electronic form on a computer, a personal digital assistant (PDA), or on an Internet website. The same information is recorded in the computerized appointment calendars as in the appointment book. Regardless of whether a paper-based or electronic appointment book is used, however, it is important to keep it updated, avoid double booking, and maintain the confidentiality of your clients' information.

Some clients prefer to book the same time on a regular basis. These regular customers are the mainstay of many businesses because they can be counted on for a certain amount of regular income.

Bookkeeping Tips

Record keeping is an essential part of maintaining a successful business. Once a filing and bookkeeping system is established, be persistent by continually updating the files. Here are a few tips that can simplify the task:

- Keep all records current.
- Review client files before each session, and document each session promptly after the session.
- When writing checks, record the amount and expenditure category in the check register.
- Keep and file all business-related receipts.
- Update income and disbursement ledgers regularly.
- Reconcile bank statements promptly.
- Keep all tax-related records:

Receipts	(keep at least seven years)
Ledgers, canceled checks, and so on	(keep at least seven years)
Tax returns	(keep indefinitely)
Real estate and business contracts	(keep indefinitely)

Preparation of Federal and State Taxes

If you have a net annual income of more that $600, you must file federal income tax forms. If you are a self-employed massage therapist, you are required to include a Schedule C (Sole Proprietorship Business or Profession Profit or Loss Form) and a Schedule SE (Social Security Self-Employment Tax Form) along with your federal income tax form. If you had any subcontractors to whom you paid more than $600 during the year, you must also file 1099s and the accompanying 1096 forms. Taxes must be filed each year before the April 15 deadline. If you are self-employed, you can expect to pay estimated state and federal taxes quarterly. The estimated tax is approximately one fourth of the previous year's income tax, and payments are due by the 15th of April, June, September, and January, respectively.

If you have been diligent in keeping your books, tax preparation is much simpler. Most of the information you need for tax forms comes right off your income and disbursement ledgers and summaries or can be retrieved as reports from your computer software program. Your disbursement ledger lists the amount and description of most of your business expenses. The exceptions are bad debts, automobile expenses, and business use of the home (if you work out of your home).

There are innumerable tax laws (including new ones almost every year), and unless you have a natural disposition toward preparing taxes, it is usually a good idea to seek the help of an accountant or a tax preparation professional. A competent tax preparer is well worth the expense and can usually save you money by pointing out deductions that you would otherwise miss and by making sure that all the proper forms are prepared correctly, thereby saving you mistakes and possible penalties. Even if you do use a tax preparer, however, you are ultimately responsible for your taxes. Being familiar with tax requirements can affect your bookkeeping, your business profits, and your relationship with your tax accountant. Besides, it can result in tax savings that your tax preparer fails to recommend. A good publication that provides up-to-date tax information is the *Tax Guide for Small Business,* prepared by the Internal Revenue Service and available at your local IRS office or online at www.irs.gov.

MARKETING

Marketing is the business activity done to promote and increase a business. It is anything that you do to make your business visible and bring it to the attention of the prospective client. Some marketing activities include advertising, promotion, public relations, referrals, and client retention. Marketing is an educational process of getting yourself and your services known. It is the enticement that encourages someone to seek your services. Marketing is an ongoing activity in business. The goal of marketing is to create and maintain a thriving practice. When developing marketing materials and practices in the field of massage, be certain that they reflect the image that you wish to portray.

Assess Marketing Needs

Your particular marketing needs are determined by several factors, including the amount of time or money that you can afford, your target market, and the size of your practice. If you are starting out in your practice, you may not have a large clientele and therefore have a lot of time but not a lot of money. More time can be spent on making contacts, giving presentations, writing articles, and making personal appearances. Concentrate on activities that are low-cost but more time-consuming. Actively educate the public about what you do and how it can benefit them.

If you have a fairly busy practice already, time is more limited, but you have a larger advertising budget. You might concentrate more on client retention, developing referrals, direct mail, and targeted advertising to announce special services.

Mini-lab

- Select two target markets that interest you.
- List the benefits of your services to this target.
- Which clubs or organizations cater to that target?
- List three ways of getting information about your services to this target market.

There are many marketing techniques to choose from that can be selected and designed to best suit a therapist's personal marketing needs.

Analyze Target Markets

Massage is a service that tends to appeal to specific segments of the population. Target groups are various segments of the population that have similar characteristics. Your target market consists of those target groups that you prefer to attract to your services. Selecting a target market enables you to modify your advertising and promotional activities to appeal to the specific group.

The parameters of target groups are innumerable. They can be very broad (i.e., women, athletes, elderly people, or professional persons). They can be highly specific (i.e., low-birth-weight infants, female runners, accountants, or abuse survivors). Several attributes that depict groups are age, gender, income, occupation, interests, and location.

There are at least two ways to determine your particular target market. One is to consider which type of clientele that you want to attract. When you have made your choices, contact clubs and organizations in your area that cater to persons from that group. Offer to be a speaker or perform a demonstration. Create brochures highlighting the benefits of massage for the specific conditions common to that group. Place ads and articles in magazines and newsletters specific to your target population. Make personal contact with people and participate in activities common to your target market.

Another way to determine your target market is to assess your client files to determine who is presently using your services and what they have in common. Then design promotional activities that reach that segment of the population.

It is wise to have more than one or even several target markets. The number depends on preference, expertise, and the size of your practice.

Business Promotion

The objective of promotion is to become known, to be visible to those in the community that might seek your service. It is also to create the desire in potential clients to use your services. Promotional activities, especially in a service industry such as massage, are largely educational in nature. Their objective is to let the target population know who you are, what you do, and how your services can benefit them.

Common methods of business promotion include public speaking and appearances, articles in professional magazines and newsletters, and booths at health fairs and other public functions. These provide excellent opportunities to educate prospective client groups. An excellent promotional tool to familiarize the public with the experience of touch and the benefits of massage is the *massage chair*. Chair massage has provided a means of bringing massage out of the private studio and into more public awareness. A massage chair can be set up essentially anywhere and provides the wider public the opportunity to experience the relaxing benefits of massage in a safe, nonthreatening environment without the need to disrobe. Many times, a chair massage leads a potential client to make an appointment for full-body massages.

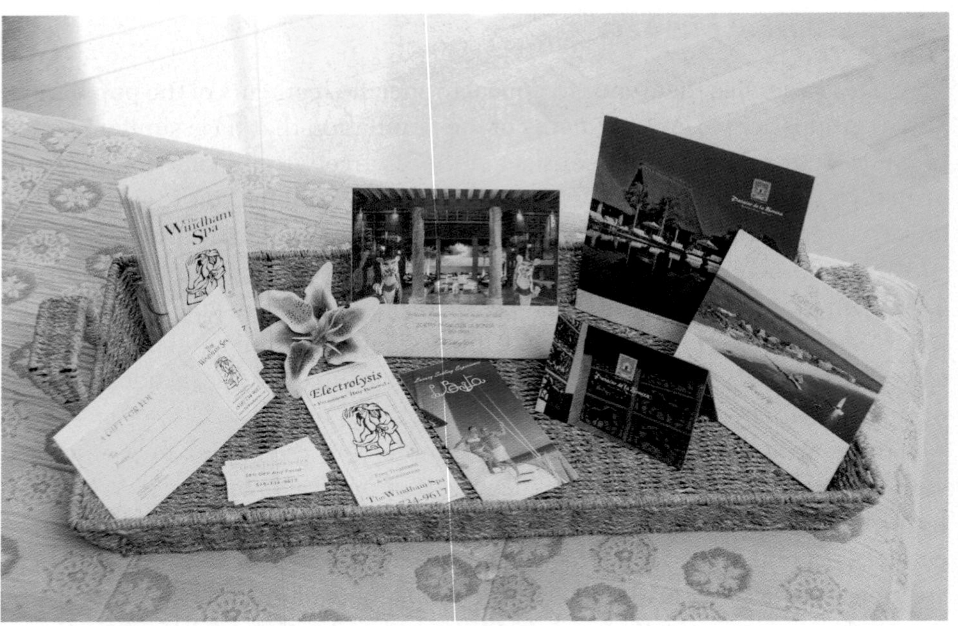

FIGURE 22-9 Effective advertising.

Developing Promotional Material

An important part of promotional activity is having appropriate printed materials to distribute when you meet potential customers. Printed materials include business cards, brochures, stationery, and newsletters. Your printed material should appeal to your target market and reflect your professionalism. Always include your name, business address, phone number, e-mail and/or website on every piece of promotional material.

One of the most important marketing tools is your business card. It serves as a reminder for prospective clients of who you are and how to contact you. Essential information to include on a business card is your name, title, and contact information. Your photo or a logo that illustrates who you are can also be added. Contact information includes the business phone number, possibly a cell phone number and e-mail address, and, if you have one, a Web address. If you have a business name and address, they can also be included. An effective business card reflects the image that you want to portray to your ideal clientele. The quality of paper, graphics, font selection, color, white space, and design are all chosen to reflect your professional image.

Whenever you speak to a group or one person about your services, be sure to leave a card or brochure. Even though you generally do not get a new client directly from your printed material, it serves as a reminder and contains information about how to contact you. (Figure 22-9).

Internet Marketing

As you know if you have a computer with Internet access, the Internet has created a new marketing possibility called the *Web site.* A Web site is an efficient and cost-effective way for the massage practitioner or business owner to communicate with clients or to market to new clients. The Web site can be used to advertise the business; provide educational information; describe services; list policies, procedures, and prices for services; and even book appointments. The Web site can contain articles on wellness, describe or show catalog products that are for sale, or contain links to other sites that might be of interest. The Web site can be used as a contact page for clients to download forms, ask questions, or make comments about services that they receive and make or cancel appointments. The Web site may be a simple one-page site with all the necessary information for a client to contact your business, or it can contain several pages filled with interesting and vital information. When you hand out your card at a networking event, you can refer the recipient to the Web site address printed on the card for more information about you and your business.

Building a Web site requires some skill. There are products available that simplify the process, so that it is possible for anyone with sufficient computer skills to build and maintain a site. To save time and possible frustration, however, hiring or trading for the services of an experienced Web designer and explaining which features that you want to include might be the wiser thing to do.

The practitioner might also stay in contact with clients or send out occasional promotional offers via e-mail. Social networking provides another marketing option associated with the Internet. Sites such as Facebook, MySpace, and Twitter are providing new opportunities for businesses and individual people to network with a selected or diverse audience about what they are doing. The fact that most households in the United States now are connected to the Internet and use it to gain information and communicate makes it an important and effective means of marketing and communication.

Advertising

Advertising is generally marketing activity that is done in return for direct payment. This includes magazine and newspaper ads and listings, signs, embossed pens and calendars, and similar materials.

Advertising is important to business success because it notifies the public about your services and how to contact you. When giving personal services such as massage, it is particularly important that your advertising not be misunderstood and that it creates a favorable impression to the public. Advertising should always reflect your professional status and the quality of your services. Keeping

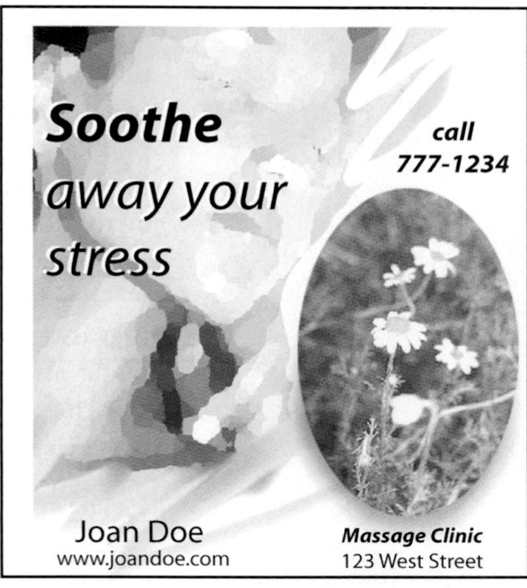

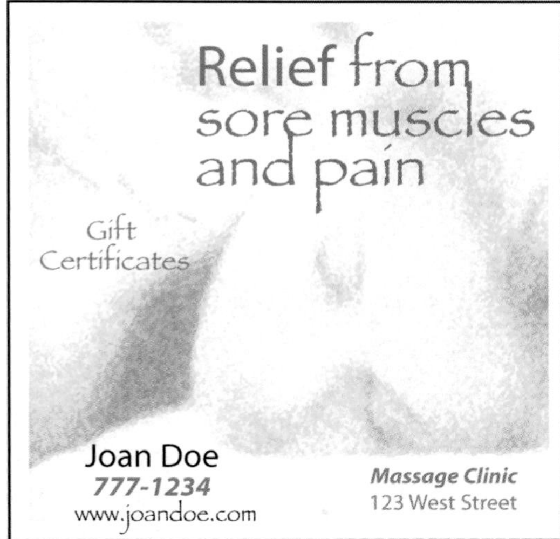

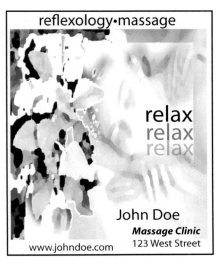

FIGURE 22-10 Effective advertising.

your name before the public is important to building your business and reminding clients to use your services.

Plan your advertising budget. You must try to obtain the most effective media for the amount of money that you have budgeted for advertising purposes. Newspaper advertising is generally an economical way to reach a large population when opening a new business. By placing your ad in a specific section of the newspaper, such as the health or sports section, you can target the ad to the market you want to reach. The people in the advertising department of the paper can help you to determine the cost, size, and style of your ad.

Placing a display ad or listing in local specialty magazines and newsletters that cater to your target market is another way to advertise your business. It might also be possible to submit an article to some of these publications that describe the benefits of massage for the targeted group.

A classified ad in the Yellow Pages of your local telephone directory is a fairly inexpensive and effective method of advertising for personal service businesses. Make sure to list your service under Massage–Therapeutic, with your credentials and association affiliations.

Direct mail is effective advertising for certain target markets. You might want to obtain a mailing list from a company that sells specifically targeted consumer lists.

Advertising consultants are expensive, but if you have a flexible advertising budget, you might find that a professional consultant can save you both time and money. A good consultant can help with creative ideas for logos, letterheads, and advertising that gets your message across in the most professional, tasteful, but dramatic way (Figure 22-10).

Public Relations

Some of the best advertising you can get is free. A feature article in a local newspaper is an excellent way to gain recognition in your community. News releases that announce classes that you offer or awards and certifications that you have received are also ways of promoting your business.

Offer to make personal appearances to give talks and demonstrations to various groups. You can offer to speak at social meetings, health clubs, sports events, schools, or as a guest on a radio or television talk show. You could act as guest instructor at a school or health facility where your type of personal services could be taught. Volunteer massage services at community events or races. Provide a booth at health fairs. Set up a massage chair at any conceivable venue where people gather or frequent such as malls, art fairs, or community or sporting events. Write articles for your own or other professional newsletters. Distribute brochures about massage or your business at events that prospective clients might attend. The possibilities are endless and limited only by your creative thinking.

An essential aspect in developing good public relations is networking. *Networking* is developing personal and professional contacts for the purpose of giving and receiving support and sharing resources and information. Become involved in networking groups such as the local Chamber of Commerce, Rotary, AARP, or other business groups. Participate in seminars or functions to meet others with whom you can develop networking relationships. Always keep business cards handy when attending these functions and distribute them freely. It is a good practice to give two or three cards at a time so that the recipient can pass one along to someone else. When you receive a business card from someone, make a note on the card as to what that person might provide for you. Keep a professional card file or a Rolodex™ with those cards, or an updated address book on your computer and refer to it when needs arise or when you are mailing out information.

Encouraging Referrals

One of the most effective and inexpensive methods of creating new business is through referrals. The two main sources of referrals are current clients and other health care professionals.

Satisfied customers are one of your most effective means of advertising. Remember, word-of-mouth advertising is the best advertising that there is, and the most important mouth is yours. Encourage referrals. Let your clients know that you not only appreciate their business but also that if they appreciate what you do, please tell others. Give them extra business cards and encourage them to tell their friends and associates about your services. Extend a special discount or even an occasional extra no-charge product or service to clients who make multiple referrals.

To promote referrals from other professionals, make yourself and what you do known to them. Explain how your services would benefit them and their clients. Write letters, and then follow up the letter with a telephone call. Set up a personal meeting or take them to lunch. Give them a treatment so that they can experience firsthand what you have to offer. Always present yourself in a professional manner. When other health care professionals send referrals, confer with them to determine their reasons and goals for sending the client to you. Report back to them about the client's progress as a result of massage. A good working relationship between health care professionals generates more referrals. It also initiates more holistic client care by promoting interdisciplinary treatment plans. Remember, it is necessary to have written permission from the client before sharing any confidential information with other health care professionals.

Whenever a new client comes in who has been referred by someone else, be sure to acknowledge the person who referred him with a thank-you note. When you do get referrals from someone, return the courtesy by referring people back or using that person's services yourself.

Remember the three Rs of referrals: request, reward, and reciprocate. *Request* referrals from satisfied clients and professionals. *Reward* those who send you referrals with prompt thank-you cards or personal telephone calls. *Reciprocate* by sending referrals or using the services of those who send you referrals.

Client Retention

Your clients are your most valuable asset. Clients who return on a regular basis are the mainstay of your practice. According to Cherie Sohnen-Moe *(Business Mastery,* 1997*)*, "On the average it costs six times as much money and takes three times the effort getting new clients as retaining current ones." Encourage clients to return for regular appointments. A weekly massage is a healthy investment. Before a client leaves your office, be sure that he has scheduled the next appointment.

Treat your clients with courtesy and respect. Give them service for which they not only want to return but will also want to refer others for. It requires more than just being a skilled massage technician to retain clients. Besides giving a good massage, make sure that your client feels cared for and appreciated. Document each session, paying attention to the client's personal interests, likes, and dislikes. Refer to your records before each visit to remind you of their idiosyncrasies. Avoid their dislikes, discuss their interests, and do those special little things they like. Always thank them for coming in.

Follow-up especially intense sessions with a telephone call to ask how the client is. Send cards for important occasions such as birthdays and holidays. Always send thank-you notes when a client sends a referral. If a client is deserving, send a certificate for a free massage. Many personal service businesses offer gift certificates or special prices to loyal customers.

Keep your clientele on a mailing list, send them newsletters, periodic flyers, birthday or holiday greetings, or offer special discounts during slow times.

Remember, the clients are your reason for practicing, they are the source of your income, and they deserve the best service that you can give.

BUSINESS LAW

In conducting business and employing help, it is necessary to comply with local, state, and federal laws and regulations. Federal laws cover Social Security, unemployment compensation or insurance, and tax payments on income, as well as several other taxes. Income tax laws are covered by both the state and federal governments. State laws cover sales taxes, licenses, workers' compensation, employment regulations, and the like. Business owners and managers may hire a lawyer or a tax accountant, but they should also be familiar with these laws and regulations.

HIRING EMPLOYEES

Hiring employees increases your potential to provide services to more people, but it also increases the employer's responsibility for record-keeping and tax regulations. An employer is required to maintain separate payroll records for each employee, withhold state and federal taxes, Social Security and Medicare deductions, prepare quarterly payroll tax returns, pay the employer's portion of social security and unemployment taxes, and purchase worker's compensation insurance.

Many businesses want to hire massage therapists as *contract labor*. When doing so, a person is an *independent contractor* and is hired on as her own boss for a per-client fee or a percentage without taxes, workers' compensation, or Social Security/Medicare being deducted from wages. An independent contractor is self-employed and is responsible for her own taxes. If you hire an independent contractor and pay her more than $600 in the course of a year, you are required to file tax forms 1099 and 1096. There are federal IRS guidelines that must be followed closely when using contract labor. Be sure to check with the state employment office or the IRS (www.irs.gov) for a copy of these guidelines before hiring contract labor.

If you are an employer, you are expected to be fair and honorable in handling employees, and you have a right to expect the same consideration from those you hire. Employees can make the difference between the success or failure of a personal service business. Clients often return to a place of business because they like the people who serve them as much as, if not more than, the products and services. The following are important considerations when hiring someone to represent your place of business. The potential employee should:

1. Have the necessary licenses or other credentials required by law.
2. Set a good example by having clean, healthy personal habits.
3. Be profit conscious and willing to work hard to achieve business goals.
4. Be courteous and professional when dealing with all clients.
5. Obey all rules, regulations, and laws pertaining to the business.
6. Be willing to learn new techniques and to grow both personally and professionally.
7. Be self-motivated and industrious.
8. Be honest and ethical.

CHECKLIST

In summary, there is more to being successful in a massage business than being able to perform a good massage. A positive attitude, clear goals, and some understanding of business practices are essential for success.

The following is a checklist of important basics to consider before opening a business of your own. Use this checklist as a guide to important factors before opening a business.

- Capital
  - Amount available
  - Amount required
- Organization
  - Sole proprietor, partnership, corporation
- Banking
  - Opening a business account
  - Deposits, drawing checks
  - Monthly statements
  - Establishing credit
  - Business loans
- Selecting a location
  - Population
  - Transportation facilities
  - Quiet enough to induce relaxation
  - Space required
  - Zoning ordinances
  - Parking
  - Accessibility
  - Adequate signage
  - Surrounding neighborhood

- Decorating and floor plan
  - Interior decorating
  - Installing telephones and Internet connection
  - Exterior decorating
- Bookkeeping system
  - Record of appointments
  - Receipts and disbursements
  - Petty cash
  - Profit and loss
  - Inventory
  - Client files
- Cost of operation
  - Supplies, depreciation
  - Rent, lights, utilities
  - Cleaning service, laundry
  - Salaries
  - Products for services
  - Telephone, Internet
  - Taxes, insurance
- Management
  - Methods of building goodwill
  - Client courtesies, gifts
  - Addressing complaints
  - Personnel relations
  - Public relations
  - Selling merchandise
- Equipment and supplies
  - Selecting equipment
  - Installation of equipment
- Marketing and public relations
  - Planning
  - Business cards and brochures
  - Direct mail
  - Internet
  - Newspaper
  - Newsletters and other print
  - Radio
  - Personal appearances
- Legal
  - Lease, contracts
  - Compliance with state, local, and government laws
  - Licensing of business
  - Licensing of managers and practitioners
- Ethics and professional growth
  - Setting goals
  - Courtesy
  - Observation of professional practices
  - Interaction with professional groups

- Insurance
  - Public liability and malpractice
  - Compensation, unemployment
  - Automobile
  - Fire and theft
- Methods of payment
  - Cash
  - In advance
  - Open account
  - Time payments
  - Charge cards

QUESTIONS FOR DISCUSSION AND REVIEW

1. How do attitude and self-image relate to business success?
2. Explain the difference between a partnership, a corporation, and a sole proprietorship.
3. Which start-up costs can you expect when beginning a massage business?
4. List five important considerations when choosing a location for a massage business.
5. List the various permits and licenses that might be required to operate a massage business.
6. List the types of insurance that a massage business owner should carry to protect the business.
7. Why is keeping accurate records necessary in a successful business?
8. List the major ingredients of a basic bookkeeping system.
9. What is marketing?
10. What are the main marketing techniques used in the massage industry?
11. Define target market.
12. What are the three Rs of referrals?

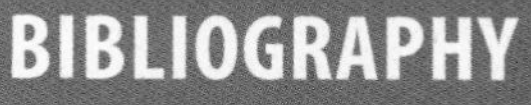

BIBLIOGRAPHY

Aaland, Mikkel. *Sweat: The Illustrated History and Description of the Finnish Sauna, Russian Bania, Islamic Hammam, Japanese Mushi-Buro, Mexican Temescal, and American Sweat Lodge.* Santa Barbara, CA: Capra Press, 1978.

American Massage Therapy Association. *The Business of Massage: The Complete Guide to Establishing Your Massage Career.* Evanston, IL: AMTA, 2009.

Andrade, Carla-Krystin; Clifford, Paul. *Outcome-Based Massage.* Philadelphia, PA: Lippincott Williams & Wilkins, 2001.

Archer, Pat. *Therapeutic Massage in Athletics.* Philadelphia, PA: Lippincott Williams & Wilkins, 2007.

Baby's First Touch. Portland, OR: International Loving Touch Foundation, 2005.

Barnes, John F. *Myofascial Release: The Search for Excellence.* Paoli, PA: John Barnes Rehabilitation Services, 1990.

Barnes, P.; Powell-Griner, E.; McFann, K.; Nahin, R. CDC Advance Data Report #343. *Complementary and Alternative Medicine Use Among Adults: United States, 2002.* May 27, 2004.

Barnes, P. M.; Bloom, B.; Nahin, R. CDC National Health Statistics Report #12. *Complementary and Alternative Medicine Use Among Adults and Children: United States, 2007.* December 10, 2008.

Barstow, Cedar. *Right Use of Power.* Boulder, CO: Many Realms Publishing, 2003.

Benjamin, Ben E.; Sohnen-Moe, Cherie. *The Ethics of Touch.* Tucson, AZ: Sohnen-Moe Associates, 2003.

Benjamin, Patricia J. *Professional Foundations for Massage Therapists.* Upper Saddle River, NJ: Pearson, 2009.

Biel, Andrew. *Trail Guide to the Body: How to Locate Muscles, Bones and More,* 3rd ed. Boulder, CO: Books of Discovery, 2005.

Born, Bryan A. *The Essential Massage Companion.* Berkley, MI: Concepts Born, 2005.

Bowman, Michelle; Lawlis, G. Frank. *Complementary and Alternative Medicine Management.* Gaithersburg, MD: Aspen Publishers, 2001.

Braun, Mary Beth; Simonson, Stephanie. *Introduction to Massage Therapy.* Philadelphia, PA: Lippincott Williams & Wilkins, 2008.

Callahan, Margery; Luther, David W. *The Medical Massage Office Manual,* 2nd ed. Steamboat Springs, CO: Author, 1999.

Calvert, Robert N. *The History of Massage.* Rochester, VT: Healing Arts Press, 2002.

Cantu, Robert I.; Grodin, Alan J. *Myofascial Manipulation: Theory and Clinical Application.* Gaithersburg, MD: Aspen Publishers, 1992.

Chaitow, Leon. *Positional Release Techniques,* 2nd ed. London: Churchill Livingston, 2002.

Chaitow, Leon. *Muscle Energy Techniques.* London: Churchill Livingston, 1996.

Chaitow, Leon. *Soft Tissue Manipulation.* Rochester, VT: Healing Arts Press, 1988.

Chaitow, Leon; Walker Delany, Judith. *Clinical Application of Neuromuscular Techniques, Vol. 1.* London: Churchill Livingston, 2000, 2008.

Chaitow, Leon; Walker Delany, Judith. *Clinical Application of Neuromuscular Techniques, Vol. 2.* London: Churchill Livingston, 2002.

Chapman, Cheryl; Kennedy, Eileen. Mastectomy Massage. *Massage Therapy Journal* 39(3), 91–99, Fall 2000.

Chilky, Bruno. *Silent Waves, Theory and Practice of Lymph Drainage Massage.* Scottsdale, AZ: International Health & Healing, 2002.

Clay, James H.; Pounds, David M. *Basic Clinical Massage Therapy,* 2nd ed. Baltimore, MD: Lippincott Williams & Wilkins, 2008.

Clemente, Carmine D. *Anatomy, A Regional Atlas of the Human Body,* 3rd ed. Baltimore, MD: Urban & Schwarzenberg, 1987.

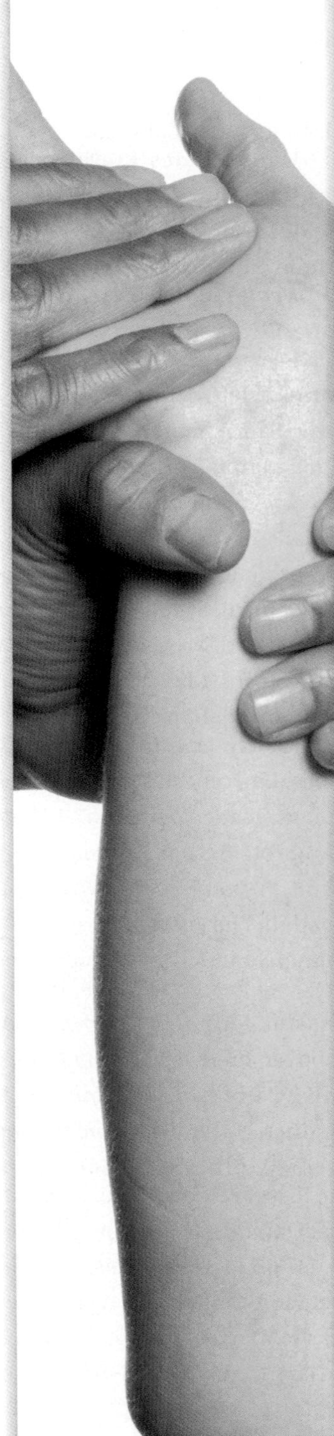

Consumer & Spa Trends Report. Presentation at 2004 Spa & Resort Expo and Conference by Spa Finder's, (212) 924-6800.

Curties, Debra. Cancer Treatments. *Massage Therapy Journal* 39(4), 80–85, Winter 2001.

Curties, Debra. Could Massage Therapy Promote Cancer Metastasis? *Massage Therapy Journal* 39(3), 83–88, Fall 2000.

Curties, Debra. *Massage Therapy and Cancer.* Moncton, New Brunswick, Canada: Curties-Overzet Publications, 1999.

Curties, Debra. Could Massage Therapy Promote Cancer Metastasis? *Journal of Soft Tissue Manipulation* 3–5, April/May 1994.

D'Ambrogio, K.; Roth, G. *Positional Release Therapy.* St. Louis, MO: Mosby, 1997.

Denning, Ed. *The Medical Code Manual for Massage Practitioners.* Clinton, OH: Massage Therapy Associates, 2001.

Devereux, Charla. *The Aromatherapy Kit.* London: Eddison Sadd Editions, 1993.

Dixon, Marian Wolfe. *Myofascial Massage.* Philadelphia, PA: Lippincott Williams & Wilkins, 2007.

Eisenberg, D. M.; Davis, R. B.; Etner, S. L.; Apple, S.; Wilke, S.; Van Rompey, M.; Kessler, R. C. Trends in Alternative Medicine Prevalence and Costs 1990–1997: Results of a Follow-Up National Survey. *Journal of the American Medical Association* 280, 1569–1575, 1998.

Eisenberg, D. M.; Kessler, R. C.; Foster, C.; Norwalk, N. E.; Calkins, D. R.; Delbanco, T. L. Unconventional Medicine in the United States: Prevalence, Costs and Patterns of Use. *New England Journal of Medicine* 328(4), 246–253, 1993.

Field, Tiffany. *The Amazing Infant.* New York: Blackwell Publishers, 2006.

Field, Tiffany, *Touch.* Cambridge, MA: MIT Press, 2001.

Findley, Thomas W.; Schleip, Robert. *Fascia Research Basic Science and Implications for Conventional and Complementary Health Care.* Munich, Germany: Elsevier GmbH, 2007.

Fong, Elizabeth; Ferris, Elvira B.; Skelley, Esther G. *Body Structures & Function,* 11th ed. Clifton Park, NY: Delmar, Cengage Learning, 1989.

Forman, Jeffrey. *Managing Physical Stress with Therapeutic Massage.* Clifton Park, NY: Cengage Learning, 2007.

Fritz, Sandy. *Fundamentals of Therapeutic Massage,* 4th ed. St. Louis, MO: Mosby, 1995, 2000, 2009.

Hart, Marcia. *Structural/Muscular Balancing.* Carson City, NV: Thoth, 1992.

Heath, A.; Bainbridge, N. *Baby Massage: The Calming Power of Touch.* New York: DK Publishing, 2000.

Heller, Sharon. *The Vital Touch.* New York: Henry Holt & Co., 1997.

Hess, Shelley. *Professional Reflexology Handbook.* Albany, NY: Milady, 1997.

Hoppenfeld, Stanley. *Physical Examination of the Spine and Extremities.* New York: Appleton-Century-Crofts, 1976.

Hungerford, Myk. *Beyond Sports Medicine.* Costa Mesa, CA: Sports Massage Training Institute, 1991.

Hungerford, Myk. *The Professional's Guide to Massage Therapy.* Costa Mesa, CA: Sports Massage Training Institute, 1988.

International Spa Association (ISPA) 2007 Spa Industry Study. Prepared by Association Resource Centre, Inc. (Contact ISPA in Lexington, Kentucky, at (888) 651-4772 for copies.)

Jones, Lawrence. *Strain and Counterstrain.* Colorado Springs, CO: American Academy of Osteopathy, 1981.

Juhan, Deane. *Job's Body: A Handbook for Bodyworkers.* Barrington, NY: Station Hill Press, 1987.

Kamoroff, Bernard. *Small Time Operator.* Laytonville, CA: Bell Springs, 1987.

Kapit, Wynn; Elson, Lawrence. *The Anatomy Coloring Book.* New York: Harper & Row, 1977.

Kendall, Florence; McCreary, Elizabeth. *Muscles: Testing and Function,* 3rd ed. Baltimore, MD: Williams & Wilkins, 1983.

Knapp, Joan E.; Antonucci, Eileen J. *A National Study of the Profession of Massage Therapy and Bodywork.* Princeton, NJ: Knapp & Associates, 1990.

Knaster, Mirka. *Discovering The Body's Wisdom.* New York: Bantam, 1996.

Leboyer, Fredrick. *Loving Hands.* New York: Alfred A. Knopf, 1976.

Lillis, Carol A. *Brady's Introduction to Medical Terminology.* Bowie, MD: Robert J. Brady, 1983.

Lindner, Harold H. *Clinical Anatomy.* Norwalk, CT: Appleton & Lange, 1989.

Lowe, Whitney. *Functional Assessment for Massage Therapists,* 3rd ed. Bend, OR: Orthopedic Massage Education and Research Institute, 1997.

MacDonald, Gayle. How Cancer Spreads. *Massage Therapy Journal* 39(4), 74–78, Winter 2001.

MacDonald, Gayle. *Medicine Hands: Massage Therapy for People with Cancer.* Findhorn, Scotland: Findhorn Press, 1999.

Madison-Mahoney, Vivian. *Comprehensive Guide to Insurance Billing.* Gatlinburg, TN: Author, 2002.

Magee, David. *Orthopedic Physical Assessment.* Philadelphia, PA: W. B. Saunders, 1987.

Malloy, Janice. Do the Benefits of Massage Outweigh the Risks? *Massage Therapy Journal* 39(4), 60–73, Winter 2001.

Manheim, Carol. *The Myofascial Release Manual.* Thorofare, NJ: Slack Incorporated, 2001.

McClure Schneider, Vimala. *Infant Massage: A Handbook for Loving Parents.* New York: Bantam, 1982.

McIntosh, Nina. *The Educated Heart.* Memphis, TN: Decatur Bainbridge Press, 1999.

Memmler, Ruth L.; Wood, Dena Lin. *The Human Body in Health and Disease,* 5th ed. Philadelphia, PA: J. B. Lippincott, 1983.

Meredith, S. *Your Happy Baby; Massage, Yoga, Aromatherapy and Other Gentle Ways to Blissful Babyhood.* New York: Ryland, Peters and Small, 2006.

Michlovitz, Susan L.; Wolf, Steven L. *Thermal Agents in Rehabilitation.* Philadelphia, PA: F. A. Davis Company, 1986.

Moody-French, Ramona. *Guide to Lymph Drainage Massage.* Clifton Park, NY: Milady, Cengage Learning, 2004.

Moor, Fred B.; Peterson, Stella C.; Manwell, Ethel M.; Noble, Mary C.; Meunch, Gertrude. *Manual of Hydrotherapy and Massage.* Oshawa, Ontario, Canada: Pacific Press Publishing, 1964.

Mulvihill, Mary Lou. *Human Diseases: A Systematic Approach,* 2nd ed. Norwalk, CT: Appleton & Lange, 1987.

Muscolino, Joseph E. *Kinesiology: The Skeletal System and Muscle Function.* St. Louis, MO: Mosby, 2006.

Osborne-Sheets, Carole. *Pre- and Perinatal Massage Therapy.* San Diego, CA: Body Therapy Associates. 1998.

Platzer, Werner. *Color Atlas and Textbook of Human Anatomy,* 3rd ed. Stuttgart, Germany: Georg Thieme Verlag, 1986.

Prudden, Bonnie. *Pain Erasure.* New York: M. Evans & Co., 1980.

Rattray, Fiona; Ludwig, Linda. *Clinical Massage Therapy.* Elora, Ontario, Canada: Talus Inc. 2000.

Salvo, Susan. *Massage Therapy Principles and Practice,* 3rd ed. Philadelphia, PA: W. B. Saunders, 1999, 2007.

Scheumann, Donald W. *The Balanced Body: A Guide to Deep Tissue and Neuromuscular Therapy.* Philadelphia, PA: Lippincott Williams & Wilkins, 2007.

Sieg, Kay M.; Adams, Sandra P. *Illustrated Essentials of Musculoskeletal Anatomy.* Gainesville, FL: Megabooks, 1985.

Sinclair, Marybeth. *Modern Hydrotherapy for the Massage Therapist.* Philadelphia, PA: Lippincott Williams & Wilkins, 2008.

Sinclair, Marybeth. *Pediatric Massage Therapy.* Philadelphia, PA: Lippincott Williams & Wilkins, 2005.

Smith, Genevieve Love; Davis, Phyllis E. *Medical Terminology,* 4th ed. New York: John Wiley & Sons, 1981.

Smith, Irene. *Guidelines for the Massage of AIDS Patients.* San Francisco: Service Through Touch, 1992.

Snyder, Daniel; Conner, LeAnne M.; Lorenz, Gregory F. *Kinesiology Foundations for OTAs and PTAs.* Clifton Park, NY: Delmar, Cengage Learning, 2005.

Sohnen-Moe, Cherie. *Business Mastery,* 3rd ed. Tucson, AZ: Sohnen-Moe Associates, 1997.

St. John, Paul. *St. John Neuromuscular Therapy Seminars, Manuals 1 & 4.* Largo, FL: Author, 1990.

Stamm, J. *Bright from the Start.* New York: Gotham Books, 2007.

Tappan, Frances M. *Healing Massage Technique: Holistic, Classical and Emerging Methods.* Norwalk, CT: Appleton & Lange, 1988.

Tappan, Frances M.; Benjamin, Patricia J. *Tappan's Handbook of Healing Massage Techniques.* Stanford, CT: Appleton & Lange, 1998, 2005.

Taylor, Kylea. *The Ethics of Caring.* Santa Cruz, CA: Hartford Mead, 1995.

Thompson, A.; Skinner, A.; Piercy, J. *Tidy's Physiotherapy,* 12th ed. Oxford, England: Butterworth & Heinemann, 1990.

Thompson, Diana L. *Hands Heal: Documentation for Massage Therapy.* Seattle, WA: Howling Moon Press, 1993.

Travell, Janet G.; Simons, David G. *Myofascial Pain and Dysfunction, The Trigger Point Manual.* Baltimore, MD: Williams & Wilkins, 1983.

Turchaninov, Ross; Cox, Connie. *Medical Massage.* Scottsdale, AZ: Stress Less Publishing, 1998.

Van Why, Richard. *The Bodywork Knowledgebase: Lectures on the History of Massage.* New York: Author, 1991.

Verklan, T.; Walden, M. (eds.). *Core Curriculum for Neonatal Intensive Care,* 3rd ed. Philadelphia, PA: Elsevier, 2004.

Voss, Dorothy E.; Ionta, Marjorie K.; Myers, Beverly J. *Proprioceptive Neuromuscular Facilitation.* Philadelphia, PA: Harper & Row, 1985.

Walton, Tracy. Clinical Thinking and Cancer. *Massage Therapy Journal* 39(3), 66–80, Fall 2000.

Williams, Donna. Touching Cancer Patients, Guidelines for Massage Therapists. *Massage Magazine* 84, 74–79, March/April 2000.

Williams, Ruth E. *The Road to Radiant Health.* College Place, WA: Color Press, 1977.

Wilson, Jacob. *Muscle Fibers—An In-Depth Analysis.* http://www.abcbodybuilding.com, 2004.

Wood, Elizabeth; Becker, Paul. *Beard's Massage,* 3rd ed. Philadelphia, PA: W. B. Saunders, 1981.

Yardley-Nohr, Terrie. *Ethics for Massage Therapists*. Philadelphia, PA: Lippincott Williams & Wilkins, 2007.

Yates, John. *A Physician's Guide to Therapeutic Massage*. Vancouver, British Columbia, Canada: Massage Therapists' Association of British Columbia, 1990.

Ylinen, Jari; Cash, Mel. *Sports Massage*. London: Stanley Paul, 1988.

APPENDIX 1

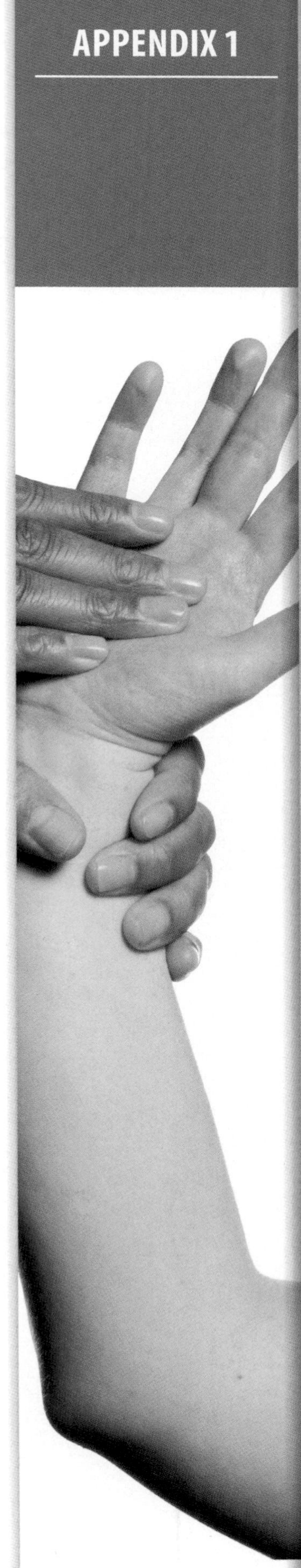

BASIC PHARMACOLOGY FOR MASSAGE THERAPISTS

by Faye N. Schenkman

Massage therapists frequently see clients who are taking prescription medications, vitamins, minerals, nutraceuticals, or herbal remedies. Often a client's complaints are not the result of a disease process but a reflection of the side effects of medications, or the interactions between different medications or between medications and supplements, which clearly can affect the progress of treatments. For example, if a client comes for treatment complaining of muscle aches and pains in the legs, and the massage therapist does not recognize that they are caused by the client's medication(s), the therapist might find that the treatments are ineffective because the symptoms will continue unabated as long as the client continues taking the medication(s). Conversely, massage therapists might find that because of the physiologic effects of massage on the body, their treatments can enhance the effects of certain medications, sometimes not only by improving the circulation of the medication but also its absorption. For example, if a client is taking an antihypertensive medication, the massage treatment can potentiate the medication's effects through improved circulation and muscle relaxation. This is a demonstration of how massage therapy can act as an adjunct to allopathic medicine, and how it can sometimes assist clients in lowering the dosage of their medication, or in some cases, eliminating the need for drug therapy altogether. Of course, such changes in medications must be conducted under the supervision of the clients' physician, because this is not within the scope of the massage therapist's practice. It should be noted, however, that massage can be practiced on many different levels. Clearly, the skill of the massage therapist is paramount in these cases. Practitioners of Asian bodywork therapies, who practice on an energetic as well as a physical level, can also find that they can help a client to minimize a drug's side effects and in some cases reduce its dosage by balancing that client's energy system.

A responsible therapist asks clients which medications, supplements, or herbs are being taken so that the therapist can look up information about them. Although it is unlikely that massage will cause any negative effects, it is still imperative that the massage therapist be familiar with the drugs and/or supplements that the client is taking and their potential side effects. The therapist should check if the client's complaints are related to the medications and whether the client needs to consult with the physician or other health care practitioner. In addition, the therapist must be aware that physical signs, such as bruising, can be caused by medication and must therefore be cognizant of when to refer clients to a doctor or other health care practitioner for further evaluation before continuing with treatments. The more informed that the therapist is about pharmacology, the better the therapist can help clients and ensure a happy outcome for all. Many laypeople are completely ignorant of their medications' effects on the body and are often unaware that the symptoms that they might be experiencing are the direct result of those medications. Clients are frequently embarrassed or afraid to question their physicians about the drugs that they have been prescribed or are afraid to tell physicians that they are taking supplements and herbs or seeing an alternative practitioner. Often clients feel more comfortable discussing their concerns with other health care providers, such as the massage therapist. Physicians often do not have the time to address their clients' questions, whereas massage therapists can provide a nurturing environment in which clients feel free to talk about their concerns. The ability of the massage therapist to discuss these issues intelligently and knowledgeably with the client is a great asset to both the client and the therapist's practice. A well-educated therapist can become a valuable resource of drug information for family and friends as well and can refer clients as needed.

Because of the myriad drugs on the market, many physicians are also unaware of the side effects of the drugs that they prescribe and are even more ignorant of the interactions of their drugs with those prescribed by other physicians. It is not uncommon for a client, particularly an elderly one, to be placed on numerous medications prescribed by a retinue of physicians, with no one overseeing the interactions of all the medications. Sometimes a client can experience lesser-known side effects, adverse reactions that are considered rarer for a particular medication, and therefore the client's complaints are not investigated properly. An informed massage therapist can recognize adverse effects and point out to clients the need to discuss medications with their physicians or encourage them to do so, in some instances acting as an advocate on their behalf.

As discussed earlier in this text, when a new client presents for treatment, the therapist should have the client fill out a patient intake form. This form should include questions concerning drug use, dosage, frequency of use, and duration. A sample of such a form is shown in Figure A-1.

With some clients, such a list might prove to be quite extensive. The massage therapist must do the necessary homework, checking out each and every

LIST ALL MEDICATIONS, VITAMINS, MINERALS, SUPPLEMENTS, AND HERBS.			
Name	Dosage-Strength (# per day)	Reason for Taking	Duration

FIGURE A-1 Sample Patient Intake Form.

entry for possible side effects that might influence the client's complaints and symptoms or that might affect the course of the massage treatment. Every therapist should purchase a text that gives necessary reference information. (See the Suggested Readings list at the end of this appendix for helpful information sources.) Therapists should also have a network of health care professionals to whom they can refer clients, if needed, for further evaluation.

The purpose of this appendix is to provide massage therapists with the basic and necessary information on pharmacology and to give them a framework within which to better assess and treat their clients. Although it is certainly not within the scope of their practice to prescribe any drug or supplement, massage therapists should be totally aware of their clients' conditions to be better able to treat them and help them to achieve an optimal state of wellness.

There are many different types of massage therapy. Within Asian bodywork alone there are numerous forms or styles, each one having its own variation of assessment and treatment, although all are rooted in the concept of an energy-based system. In Western massage, there are also many different methods and levels of treating. This appendix certainly cannot address all of the different ways and levels that various forms of massage can affect the body. Each therapist must hone palpatory skills, develop an awareness of the client as a "whole"—as a physical, emotional, mental, and energetic being. Therapists must be observant of clients' skin, musculature, posture, and such, and ask appropriate questions, always checking to see that their techniques are not causing more harm than good and using wisdom in deciding how much pressure can and should be applied. As long as therapists treat with the correct intention and take the time to assess clients properly, a favorable outcome will most often result.

WHAT IS PHARMACOLOGY?

Pharmacology is a science that studies the effects that substances have on living organisms, the nature of their chemical structure, how they act within the body, and how the body responds to them. The word *pharmacology* is derived from the Greek word *pharmakon,* which translates as "drug," and also involves its mechanism of action. Knowledge of pharmacology is essential for all health care practitioners who are involved in the treatment of disease in humans or animals.

Pharmacology
a science that studies the effects that substances have on living organisms, the nature of their chemical structure, how they act within the body, and how the body responds to them.

WHAT IS A DRUG?

Since time immemorial, humans have used plants, minerals, animals, insects, and other substances found in nature to treat disease. In modern times, drugs can be bioengineered or developed from gene therapy. According to the World Health Organization (WHO), 80 percent of the world's population continues to use herbs and other natural substances as their first line of defense against disease. In modern societies, however, synthetically produced chemicals are most often developed into drugs that are used in the treatment, prevention, cure, alleviation, or diagnosis of illness. This avenue is the most actively pursued by major drug companies today because natural substances cannot be patented. Research is therefore focused on artificially developed compounds in the competitive and lucrative world of the pharmaceutical industry.

Using a very broad definition, the term *drug* can also include common over-the-counter (OTC) substances such as nicotine, alcohol, and caffeine; illegal drugs such as cocaine, heroin, and marijuana; cosmetic substances; and even food additives or any substance that has an effect on the body.

Chemicals developed as drugs are often a double-edged sword. Although intended to have a selective action in the body, these drugs often fall short of that goal, producing instead several adverse effects, sometimes mimicking the very symptoms they are intended to relieve. Whenever more than one medication is taken, it is very possible that the combination of drugs might affect the expected response of each individual drug. One medication can affect another to increase, decrease, or cancel out the effects of the other, or to cause a different effect altogether.

All drugs, no matter what their origin, have one feature in common: they affect the body in some way, and they cause cellular changes to take place, which in turn cause an effect on the body's physiology. Some drugs affect the entire body; this is called a *systemic* effect. Other drugs are for local use only, limited to one area or aspect of the body.

Another factor that must be considered with medications is the client's age. For example, the geriatric population's ability to metabolize and excrete medications is much slower. Most drugs are eliminated through the kidneys; therefore if the drug is not excreted sufficiently and the client continues to take it, the drug can accumulate and build up in the body to toxic levels, which can become life threatening. This is particularly true in older clients. Elderly people also are often subjected to multiple physicians and multiple medications. In such cases, it is helpful to refer clients to someone such as a physician who specializes in geriatric or iatrogenic medicine or a nurse practitioner, who has an overview of all of these clients' pathologies and medications.

Children are an example of another population in which age influences the dosage of medications. Children react to medications differently from adults. They require smaller amounts of medication and need to be frequently monitored. Because many drugs have not been adequately tested on children, the effects of a medication can often be unpredictable.

Weight is also a factor in drug administration—heavier people usually need larger doses of medication than thinner people. Often the dosages of drugs are prescribed based on how much a client weighs. Certain people might be particularly sensitive regardless of their weight, however.

Women, men, people of different races, or persons in a diseased state do not always respond the same way to the same medications, owing to differences in hormone levels and body metabolism. Drugs are generally contraindicated if a woman is pregnant or nursing.

HOW ARE DRUGS NAMED AND CLASSIFIED?

Unfortunately, there is no uniform method for naming and classifying drugs. There are no international standards in pharmacology; therefore, the same medication can have multiple names, depending on the manufacturer and the country where it is being sold. In addition, individual drugs can belong to several different classifications.

Generic names are the common names of drugs. They contain prefixes and suffixes that indicate the drug classification and provide some clues as to its use and functions. When a company creates a new drug for market, it gives that drug a generic name. Once the drug is approved by the Food and Drug Administration (FDA), the pharmaceutical company gives it a trade name, usually something catchy that the public can remember easily. Generic names are usually recognized by their lowercase spelling; that is, the initial letter of the name is never capitalized.

Trade names are copyrighted brand names that often do not reflect the actions of the medication but rather are chosen because they are easy to recognize and remember. The initial letter of the name is always capitalized, and the name is sometimes followed with the symbol®, indicating that the name is a registered trademark. After 17 years, however, the pharmaceutical company loses the exclusive rights to that drug. Once the patent has expired, other companies may start to market the same drug, giving it their own trade name. Although the same medication can have multiple names from multiple manufacturers, the generic name remains the same.

The chemical name of a medication is based on the molecular construction of the compound. It is usually a long, complicated, and difficult name and of little consequence to the massage therapist.

The official name of the drug is the name as it appears in the official government reference book, the *United States Pharmacopeia/National Formulary* (USP/NF). This is usually the generic name.

For example, note the different names of the following drug:

Trade Name	Darvon
Drug Company	Eli Lilly
Generic Name	propoxyphene hydrochloride
Chemical Name	alpha-4 dimethylamino-3-methyl-1-2,2-diphenyl-2 butanol, proprionate hydrochloride

The naming of drugs is often based not only on chemical composition but also on marketing and the drugs' effects in the body. The massage therapist therefore should be acquainted with the different names of the same medication. In the same way that facial tissues can be referred to as Kleenex, Scott's, or Puffs, antihyperlipidemic agents such as atorvastatin calcium, fluvastatin sodium, lovastatin, pravastatin sodium, and simvastatin are known respectively by their trade names Lipitor, Lescol, Altocor or Mevacor, Pravachol, and Zocor. This appendix uses the trade names as examples for each category, because these are the names that are advertised to the public and are most recognizable to both the layperson and the massage therapist.

There are many different ways to classify drugs, because drugs having multiple therapeutic actions can be found under more than one classification. For example, aspirin can act as an analgesic (relieve pain), an antipyretic (reduce fevers), and as an anti-inflammatory (reduce inflammation). It therefore can be found under three classifications.

In addition, different systems of drug classification can be confusing because they are not standardized. Generally, drugs are classified based on their therapeutic effect, their pharmacologic actions, their actions at the molecular level, their origin (i.e., chemical, botanical, or animal), or their generic names.

HOW DO I LOOK UP A DRUG?

A valuable reference guide for the massage therapist is the *PDR Nurse's Drug Handbook*. This book provides an easy format for understanding individual **drug monographs.** The therapist can learn how to read and interpret the information for a multitude of commonly prescribed medications, including the generic names, their proper pronunciation, the trade name, the classification, whether a drug is a controlled substance, a drug's approved therapeutic uses,

drug monograph

a statement that specifies the ingredients a drug or class of drugs may contain, the directions for the drug's use, the conditions in which it may be used, and the contraindications to its use.

the contraindications, the special concerns, the side effects, the interactions with other medications or herbs, how the drugs are supplied, and the appropriate dosages.

The *Physicians' Desk Reference* (PDR) is also a valuable tool, but it is not as easy to navigate for the novice practitioner. There are also several good websites where practitioners can look up drugs and obtain all the necessary information. For example, www.drugs.com and www.webmd.com are two of the more common sites that offer accurate information on pharmaceuticals. There are also sites that will give you the different interactions between two or more medications. Those are very valuable for helping the practitioner to sort out client symptoms when multiple drugs are being taken. For example, www.drugs.com and www.medscape.com offer excellent information on drug interactions.

WHAT ARE SOME COMMON DRUG GROUPINGS?

The following are some common categories of drugs, the conditions that they treat, some of their side effects and contraindications (conditions or circumstances that indicate that a drug should not be given), and significant information that pertains specifically to the massage therapist. This list is by no means exhaustive but rather a general summary (Table A.1).

TABLE A.1

DRUG INDEX			
NAME	GROUP	MEDICATION FOR	PAGE #
A + D ointment	*Emollients*	Skin	876
Abelcet	*Antifungals*	Antibiotic	907
Abilify	*Antimanic Medication*	Antidepressant	913
Accolate	*Asthma Prophylaxis*	Respiratory	885
Accupril	*ACE Inhibitor*	Cardiovascular	890
Aciphex	*Proton Pump Inhibitor*	Gastrointestinal	881
Acromycin	*Tetracyline*	Antibiotic	906
ACTH	*Pituitaary Hormones*	Endocrine	898
Acthar	*Pituitary Hormone*	Endocrine	898
Acticin	*Scabicides and Pediculicides*	Skin	876
Actos	*Antidiabetic Drug*	Endocrine	900
Acyclovir	*Antiviral*	Antibiotic	907
Adapin	*Tricyclic*	Antidepressant	912
Adderall	*CNS Stimulant*	CNS	911
Advil	*NSAID*	Musculoskeletal	879
AeroBid	*Corticosteroids*	Respiratory	884
Afrin	*Decongestants*	Respiratory	886
Akne-Mycin	*Antibacterials*	Skin	877
Albuterol	*Bronchodilators*	Respiratory	884
Aldactone	*Diuretics*	Urinary	893
Aldomet	*Antihypertensives*	Cardiovascular	889
Aleve	*NSAIDs*	Musculoskeletal	879
Allegra	*Antihistamines*	Respiratory	886
Allerest	*Decongestants*	Respiratory	886
Allopurinol	*Gout Medications*	Urinary	893
Alupent	*Bronchodilators*	Respiratory	884
Alvesco	*Corticosteroids*	Respiratory	884
Amantadine	*Antiviral*	Antibiotic	907, 914

TABLE A.1 (CONTINUED)

DRUG INDEX			
NAME	GROUP	MEDICATION FOR	PAGE #
Amaryl	*Antidiabetic Drugs*	Endocrine	900
Ambien	*Nonbarbiturate*	Hypnotic	910
Amoxil	*Penicillins*	Antibiotics	905
Amphojel	*Antacids*	Gastrointestinal	881
Ampicillin	*Penicillins*	Antibiotics	905
Anafranil	*Tricyclic*	Antidepressant	912
Android	*Male Hormones*	Reproductive	901
Antagon	*Fertility Medication*	Reproductive	903
Antivert	*Bronchodilators*	Respiratory	883
Apidra	*Antidiabetic Drugs*	Endocrine	900
Apresoline	*Antihypertensives*	Cardiovascular	889
Apriso	*Anti-inflammatory*	Gastrointestinal	882
Aptivus	*Drugs to Treat AIDS*	Antiretrovirals	908
Aristocort	*Corticosteroids*	Skin, Musculoskeletal	876, 880, 899
Astepro	*Antihistamines*	Respiratory	886
Atarax	*Anxiolytic*	Antianxiety	913
Ativan	*Anxiolytic*	Antianxiety	913
Atrovent	*Corticosteroids*	Respiratory	884
Axid	*GERD, H2 Blockers*	Gastrointestinal	881
Azo-Standard	*Analgesics*	Urinary	894
Azulfidine	*Anti-inflammatory*	Gastrointestinal	882
Azulfidine	*Sulfonamides*	Antibiotic	906
Bacitracin	*Antibacterials*	Skin	877
Bactrim	*Sulfonamides*	Antibiotic	906
Beconase	*Corticosteroids*	Respiratory	884
Benadryl	*Antipruritics*	Skin	876
Benadryl	*Antihistamines*	Respiratory	886
Benemid	*Gout Medications*	Urinary	894
Betadine	*Anti-infectives*	Skin	877
Biaxin	*Macrolides*	Antibiotics	905
Bleomycin	*Antitumor antibiotics*	Antineoplastic	896
Bonine	*Antiemetics*	Gastrointestinal	883
Bumex	*Diuretics*	Urinary	893
BuSpar	*Anxiolytic*	Antianxiety	913
Bicillin	*Penicillins*	Antibiotics	905
Byetta	*Antidiabetic Drugs*	Endocrine	900
Cafcit	*CNS Stimulant*	CNS	911
Cancidas	*Antifungals*	Antibiotic	907
Captopril	*ACE Inhibitors*	Cardiovascular	890
Cardioquin	*Antiarrhythmic Drugs*	Cardiovascular	888
Cardizem	*Antihypertensives*	Cardiovascular	889
Cardura	*Alpha Blockers*	Urinary	895
Carmustine	*Alkylating drugs*	Antineoplastic	896
Ceclor	*Cephalosporins*	Antibiotic	905
Ceftin	*Cephalosporins*	Antibiotic	905

TABLE A.1 (CONTINUED)

DRUG INDEX			
NAME	GROUP	MEDICATION FOR	PAGE #
Celexa	*Serotonin Reuptake Inhibitor*	Antidepressant	912
Chlor-Trimeton	*Antihistamines*	Respiratory	886
Cialis	*Impotency Drugs*	Reproductive	901
Cipro	*Quinolones*	Antibiotics	906
Cisplatin	*Alkylating drugs*	Antineoplastic	896
Claritin	*Antihistamines*	Respiratory	886
Clearasil	*Keratolytics*	Skin	876
Climara	*Contraceptives*	Reproductive	902
Clomid	*Fertility Medication*	Reproductive	903
Codeine	*Antitussives*	Respiratory	885, 908, 909
Colace	*Laxatives*	Gastrointestinal	883
Colchicine	*Gout Agent*	Musculoskeletal	879, 880, 894
Combivir	*Drugs to Treat AIDS*	Antiretrovirals	908
Compazine	*Antiemetics*	Gastrointestinal	883, 914
Concerta	*CNS Stimulant*	CNS	911
Cordarone	*Antiarrhythmic Drugs*	Cardiovascular	888
Coreg	*Antihypertensives*	Cardiovascular	889
Corgard	*Antihypertensives*	Cardiovascular	889
Cortaid	*Antipruritics, Corticosteroids*	Skin	876
Cortisone	*Corticosteroids*	Musculoskeletal	880
Cortone	*Corticosteroids*	Endocrine	899
Coumadin	*Anticoagulant*	Cardiovascular	891, 892
Cozaar	*Angiotensin Blockers*	Cardiovascular	890
Crestor	*Antilipemic Drugs*	Cardiovascular	891
Crixivan	*Drugs to Treat AIDS*	Antiretrovirals	908
Cromolyn	*Asthma Prophylaxis*	Respiratory	884, 885
Cycrin	*Progesterone*	Reproductive	902
Cymbalta	*Serotonin Reuptake Inhibitor*	Antidepressant	912
Cystospaz	*Antispasmodics*	Gastrointestinal, Urinary	882, 894
Cytarabine	*Antimetabolite*	Antineoplastic	896
Cytotec	*Gastric secretion blocker*	Gastrointestinal	881
Dactinomycin	*Antitumor antibiotics*	Antineoplastic	896
Dalmane	*Nonbarbiturate*	Hypnotic	910
Danocrine	*Male Hormones*	Reproductive	901
Dapakene	*Anticonvulsant*	CNS	914
Darvon	*Opioid Analgesics*	Analgesic	865, 908, 909
Decadron	*Corticosteroids*	Musculoskeletal	880, 899
Deca-Durabolin	*Male Hormones*	Reproductive	901
Deltasone	*Corticosteroids*	Musculoskeletal	880, 899
Demadex	*Diuretics*	Urinary	893
Demerol	*Opioid Analgesics*	Analgesic	908, 909
Depakote	*Anticonvulsant*	CNS	913, 914
Depo-Estradiol	*Estrogens*	Reproductive	902
Depo-Provera	*Progesterone*	Reproductive	902
Depo-Provera	*Contraceptives*	Reproductive	902

TABLE A.1 (CONTINUED)

DRUG INDEX			
NAME	GROUP	MEDICATION FOR	PAGE #
Depo-Testosterone	*Male Hormones*	Reproductive	901
Desitin	*Emollients*	Skin	876
Desyrel	*Heterocyclic Antidepressant*	Antidepressant	913
Detrol	*Antispasmodics*	Urinary	894
Dexedrine	*CNS Stimulant*	CNS	911
Diabeta	*Antidiabetic Drugs*	Endocrine	900
Diflucan	*Antifungals*	Antibiotic	907
Digitalis	*Cardiac Glycosides*	Cardiovascular	888
Dilantin	*Anticonvulsant*	CNS	909, 914
Dilaudid	*Opioid Analgesics*	Analgesic	909
Dimetapp	*Antihistamines*	Respiratory	886
Diovan	*Angiotensin Blockers*	Cardiovascular	890
Ditropan	*Antispasmodics*	Urinary	894
Dulcolax	*Laxatives*	Gastrointestinal	883
Dyrenium	*Diuretics*	Urinary	893
Edecrin	*Diuretics*	Urinary	893
EES	*Macrolides*	Antibiotics	905
Effexor	*Serotonin Reuptake Inhibitor*	Antidepressant	912
Elavil	*Tricyclic*	Antidepressant	909, 912
Eldepryl	*Antiparkinsonian Medication*	CNS	914
Elidel	*Immunomodulators*	Skin	878
E-Mycin	*Macrolides*	Antibiotics	905
Enalapril	*ACE Inhibitors*	Cardiovascular	890
Epivir	*Drugs to Treat AIDS*	Antiretrovirals	908
ERYC	*Macrolides*	Antibiotics	905
Erygel	*Antibacterials*	Skin	877
Erythromycin	*Macrolides*	Antibiotics	905
Esidrex	*Diuretics*	Urinary	893
Estrace	*Estrogens*	Reproductive	902
Estraderm	*Estrogens*	Reproductive	902
Estratab	*Estrogens*	Reproductive	902
Estratest	*Male Hormones*	Reproductive	901
Exforge	*Angiotensin Blockers*	Cardiovascular	890
Factrel	*Fertility Medication*	Reproductive	903
Flexeril	*Muscle Relaxants*	Musculoskeletal	879
Flomax	*Alpha Blockers*	Urinary	895
Flo-Pred	*Corticosteroids*	Respiratory	884
Florinef	*Corticosteroids*	Adrenal	880, 899
Flovent	*Corticosteroids*	Respiratory	884
Fluorouracil	*Antimetabolite*	Antineoplastic	896
Follistim	*Fertility Medication*	Reproductive	903
Fortovase	*Drugs to Treat AIDS*	Antiretrovirals	908
Garamycin	*Aminoglycosides*	Antibiotic	904
Gelusil	*Antacids*	Gastrointestinal	881
Genapap ES	*Nonopioid Analgesic*	Analgesic	909

TABLE A.1 (CONTINUED)

DRUG INDEX			
NAME	GROUP	MEDICATION FOR	PAGE #
Glucophage	*Antidiabetic Drugs*	Endocrine	900
Glucotrol	*Antidiabetic Drugs*	Endocrine	900
Glynase	*Antidiabetic Drugs*	Endocrine	900
Glyset	*Antidiabetic Drugs*	Endocrine	900
Grifulvin	*Antifungals*	Antibiotic	907
Halcion	*Nonbarbiturate*	Hypnotic	910
Haldol	*Antipsychotic Medication*	Tranquilizer	914
Heparin	*Antithrombolyitic*	Cardiovascular	891, 892
Hibiclens	*Anti-infectives*	Skin	877
Histussin	*Antitussives*	Respiratory	885
Humibid	*Expectorants*	Respiratory	885
HydroDIURIL	*Diuretics*	Urinary	893
Hytrin	*Alpha Blockers*	Urinary	895
Ilosone	*Macrolides*	Antibiotics	905
Imodium, Imodium A-D	*Antidiarrhea*	Gastrointestinal	882
Inderal	*Antiarrhythmic Drugs*	Cardiovascular	888, 889
Interferon	*Antiviral*	Antibiotic	896, 907
Iophen	*Expectorants*	Respiratory	885
Isoptin	*Antiarrhythmic Drugs*	Cardiovascular	888
Isordil	*Coronary Vasodilators*	Cardiovascular	891
Kaletra	*Drugs to Treat AIDS*	Antiretrovirals	908
Kaopectate	*Antidiarrhea*	Gastrointestinal	882
Keflex	*Cephalosporins*	Antibiotic	905
Kenalog	*Corticosteroids*	Adrenal	899
Klonopin	*Anticonvulsant*	CNS	914
L-A	*Penicillins*	Antibiotics	905
Lamisil	*Antifungals*	Antibiotic	877, 907
Lanoxin	*Cardiac Glycosides*	Cardiovascular	887, 888
Lasix	*Diuretics*	Urinary	893
Levaquin	*Quinolones*	Antibiotics	906
Levitra	*Impotency Drugs*	Reproductive	901
Levothyroid	*Thyroid Medications*	Endocrine	899
Levoxyl	*Thyroid Medications*	Endocrine	899
Levsin, Levsinex	*Antispasmodics*	Gastrointestinal	882
Librium	*Anxiolytic*	Antianxiety	913
Lindane	*Scabicides and Pediculicides*	Skin	876
Lipitor	*Antilipemic Drugs*	Cardiovascular	891
Lithium	*Antimanic Medication*	Antidepressant	913
Lithobid	*Antimanic Medication*	Antidepressant	913
Loestrin	*Contraceptives*	Reproductive	902
Lomotil	*Antidiarrhea*	Gastrointestinal	882
Lopid	*Antilipemic Drugs*	Cardiovascular	891
Lorcet	*Antitussives*	Respiratory	885
Lovenox	*Antithrombolyitic*	Cardiovascular	892
Lozol	*Diuretics*	Urinary	893

TABLE A.1 (CONTINUED)

DRUG INDEX			
NAME	GROUP	MEDICATION FOR	PAGE #
Luminal	*Barbiturate*	Sedatives	910
Lunesta	*Nonbarbiturate*	Hypnotic	910
Lupron	*Fertility Medication*	Reproductive	896, 902–903
Maalox	*Antacids*	Gastrointestinal	881
Macrobid	*Antiurinary Drugs*	Antibiotic	908
Macrodantin	*Antiurinary Drugs*	Antibiotic	908
Marplan	*MAO Inhibitor*	Antidepressant	912
Maxaquin	*Quinolones*	Antibiotics	906
Maxipime	*Cephalosporins*	Antibiotic	905
Medrol	*Corticosteroids*	Musculoskeletal	880, 899
Megace	*Progesterone*	Reproductive	902
Metamucil	*Laxatives*	Gastrointestinal	883
Methotrexate	*Antimetabolite*	Antineoplastic	896
Mevacor	*Antilipemic Drugs*	Cardiovascular	891
Micronase	*Antidiabetic Drugs*	Endocrine	900
Milk of Magnesia	*Laxatives*	Gastrointestinal	883
Mitomycin	*Antitumor antibiotics*	Antineoplastic	896
Monopril	*ACE Inhibitors*	Cardiovascular	890
Morphine	*Opioid Analgesics*	Analgesic	908, 909
Motrin	*NSAIDs*	Musculoskeletal	879
Mucomyst	*Expectorants*	Respiratory	885
Myambutol	*Antituberculosis Drugs*	Antibiotic	907
Myciguent	*Antibacterials*	Skin	877
Mylanta	*Antacids*	Gastrointestinal	881
Nardil	*MAO Inhibitor*	Antidepressant	912
Nasacort	*Corticosteroids*	Respiratory	884
Nasonex	*Corticosteroids*	Respiratory	884
Nebcin	*Aminoglycosides*	Antibiotic	904
Neosporin	*Antibacterials*	Skin	877
Neo-Synephrine	*Decongestants*	Respiratory	886
Neurontin	*Anticonvulsant*	CNS	914
Nexium	*Proton Pump Inhibitor*	Gastrointestinal	881
Nicobid	*Antilipemic Drugs*	Cardiovascular	891
Nicoderm patch	*Smoking Cessation*	Respiratory	886
Nicorette gum	*Smoking Cessation*	Respiratory	886
Nicotrol inhaler	*Smoking Cessation*	Respiratory	886
Nitroglycerin	*Coronary Vasodilators*	Cardiovascular	890–891
Norinyl	*Contraceptives*	Reproductive	902
Noroxin	*Quinolones*	Antibiotics	906
Norpace	*Antiarrhythmic Drugs*	Cardiovascular	888
Norpramin	*Tricyclic*	Amtidepressant	912
Nortrel	*Contraceptives*	Reproductive	902
Norvir	*Drugs to Treat AIDS*	Antiretrovirals	908
No-stril	*Decongestants*	Respiratory	886
Novarel	*Fertility Medication*	Reproductive	903

TABLE A.1 (CONTINUED)

DRUG INDEX			
NAME	GROUP	MEDICATION FOR	PAGE #
Nuprin	*NSAIDs*	Musculoskeletal	879
Nystatin	*Antifungals*	Antibiotic	907
Omnipen	*Penicillins*	Antibiotics	905
Ortho-Novum	*Contraceptives*	Reproductive	902
Osmitrol	*Osmotic Drugs*	Urinary	893
Ovcon	*Contraceptives*	Reproductive	902
Ovral	*Contraceptives*	Reproductive	902
OxyContin	*Opioid Analgesics*	Analgesic	909
Pamelor	*Tricyclic*	Antidepressant	909, 912
Panadol	*Nonopioid Analgesic*	Analgesic	909
Paragard	*Contraceptives*	Reproductive	902
Parnate	*MAO Inhibitor*	Antidepressant	912
Patanase	*Antihistamines*	Respiratory	886
Paxil	*Serotonin Reuptake Inhibitor*	Antidepressant	912
Pepcid	*GERD, H2 Blockers*	Gastrointestinal	881
Percocet	*Opioid Analgesics*	Analgesic	909
Pergonal	*Fertility Medication*	Reproductive	903
Phenergan	*Antiemetics*	Gastrointestinal	883
Phenobarbital	*Barbiturate*	Sedatives	910
Pima Syrup	*Expectorants*	Respiratory	885
Plavix	*Platelet Inhibitors*	Cardiovascular	892
Polysporin	*Antibacterials*	Skin	877
Prandimet	*Antidiabetic Drugs*	Endocrine	900
Prandin	*Antidiabetic Drugs*	Endocrine	900
Pravachol	*Antilipemic Drugs*	Cardiovascular	891
Precose	*Antidiabetic Drugs*	Endocrine	900
Prednisone	*Corticosteroids*	Musculoskeletal	880, 896, 899
Premarin	*Estrogens*	Reproductive	902
Prevacid	*Proton Pump Inhibitor*	Gastrointestinal	881
Prilosec	*Proton Pump Inhibitor*	Gastrointestinal	881
Primatene	*Bronchodilators*	Respiratory	884
Prinivil	*ACE Inhibitors*	Cardiovascular	890
Pro-Banthine	*Antispasmodics*	Urinary	894
Procardia	*Antihypertensives*	Cardiovascular	889
Proscar	*Antiandrogens*	Urinary	895
Protopic	*Immunomodulators*	Skin	878
Proventil	*Bronchodilators*	Respiratory	884
Provera	*Progesterone*	Reproductive	902
Provera	*Contraceptives*	Reproductive	902
Prozac	*Serotonin Reuptake Inhibitor*	Antidepressant	912
Pulmicort	*Corticosteroids*	Respiratory	884
Pyridium	*Analgesics*	Urinary	894
Questran	*Antilipemic Drugs*	Cardiovascular	891
Rapaflo	*Alpha Blockers*	Urinary	895
Relafen	*NSAIDs*	Musculoskeletal	879

TABLE A.1 (CONTINUED)

DRUG INDEX			
NAME	GROUP	MEDICATION FOR	PAGE #
Relenza	*Antiviral*	Antibiotic	907
Remeron	*Heterocyclic Antidepressant*	Antidepressant	913
Restoril	*Nonbarbiturate*	Hypnotic	910
Retrovir	*Drugs to Treat AIDS*	Antiretrovirals	908
Rhinocort	*Corticosteroids*	Respiratory	884
Ribavirin	*Antiviral*	Antibiotic	907
Rifadin	*Antituberculosis Drugs*	Antibiotic	907
Risperdal	*Antipsychotic Medication*	Tranquilizer	914
Ritalin	*CNS Stimulant*	CNS	911
Robaxin	*Muscle Relaxants*	Musculoskeletal	879
Robitussin	*Expectorants*	Respiratory	885
Robitussin A-C	*Antitussives*	Respiratory	885
Rocephin	*Cephalosporins*	Antibiotic	905
Septra	*Sulfonamides*	Antibiotic	906
Serequel	*Antimanic Medication*	Antidepressant	913
Serophene	*Fertility Medication*	Reproductive	903
Seroquel	*Antipsychotic Medication*	Tranquilizer	914
Serzone	*Heterocyclic Antidepressant*	Antidepressant	913
Simcor	*Antilipemic Drugs*	Cardiovascular	891
Simethicone	*Antiflatulents*	Gastrointestinal	882
Sinemet	*Antiparkinsonian Medication*	CNS	914
Singulair	*Asthma Prophylaxis*	Respiratory	885
Solarcaine	*Antipruritics*	Skin	876
Soma	*Muscle Relaxants*	Musculoskeletal	879
Sonata	*Nonbarbiturate*	Hypnotic	910
Sorbitrate	*Coronary Vasodilators*	Cardiovascular	891
Stavzor	*Antimanic Medication*	Antidepressant	913
Streptomycin	*Antituberculosis Drugs*	Antibiotic	907
Sudafed	*Decongestants*	Respiratory	886
Sumycin	*Tetracyclines*	Antibiotic	906
Suprax	*Cephalosporins*	Antibiotic	905
Sustiva	*Drugs to Treat AIDS*	Antiretrovirals	908
Symmetrel	*Antiviral*	Antibiotic	907, 914, 915
Synthroid	*Thyroid Medications*	Endocrine	899
Tagamet	*GERD, H2 Blockers*	Gastrointestinal	881
Tamiflu	*Antiviral*	Antibiotic	907
Tapazole	*Antithyroid Medications*	Endocrine	899
Tapentadol	*Opioid Analgesics*	Analgesic	909
Tegretol	*Antimanic Medication*	Antidepressant	913
Tegretol	*Anticonvulsant*	CNS	909, 914
Tegrin	*Keratolytics*	Skin	876
Tekturna HCT	*Antihypertensives*	Cardiovascular	889
Tenormin	*Antiarrhythmic Drugs*	Cardiovascular	888, 889
Tessalon Perles	*Antitussives*	Respiratory	885
Theo-Dur	*Bronchodilators*	Respiratory	884

TABLE A.1 (CONTINUED)

DRUG INDEX			
NAME	GROUP	MEDICATION FOR	PAGE #
Thiotepa	*Alkylating drugs*	Antineoplastic	896
Thorazine	*Antipsychotic Medication*	Tranquilizer	914
Ticlid	*Platelet Inhibitors*	Cardiovascular	892
Tigan	*Antiemetics*	Gastrointestinal	883
Tofranil	*Tricyclic*	Antidepressant	909, 912
Tonocard	*Antiarrhythmic Drugs*	Cardiovascular	888
Torecan	*Antiemetics*	Gastrointestinal	883
Toviaz	*Antispasmodics*	Urinary	894
Tramadol	*Nonopioid Analgesic*	Analgesic	909
Trilipix	*Antilipemic Drugs*	Cardiovascular	891
Trimpex	*Antiurinary Drugs*	Antibiotic	908
Tri-Norinyl	*Contraceptives*	Reproductive	902
Tums	*Antacids*	Gastrointestinal	881
Tylenol	*Nonopioid Analgesic*	Analgesic	909
Tylenol with Codeine	*Opioid Analgesics*	Analgesic	909
Ureaphil	*Osmotic Drugs*	Urinary	893
Urecholine	*Cholinergics*	Urinary	894
Valisone	*Corticosteroids*	Skin	876
Valium	*Muscle Relaxants*	Musculoskeletal	879
Valium	*Anxiolytic*	Antianxiety	913
Valtrex	*Antiviral*	Antibiotic	907
Vanceril	*Corticosteroids*	Respiratory	884
Ventolin	*Bronchodilators*	Respiratory	884
Verelan	*Antihypertensives*	Cardiovascular	889
Viagra	*Impotency Drugs*	Reproductive	901
Vibramycin	*Tetracyclines*	Antibiotic	906
Vicodin	*Opioid Analgesics*	Analgesic	909
Videx	*Drugs to Treat AIDS*	Antiretrovirals	908
Vimpat	*Anticonvulsant*	CNS	914
Vinblastine	*Plant alkaloids*	Antineoplastic	896
Vincristine	*Plant alkaloids*	Antineoplastic	896
Viracept	*Drugs to Treat AIDS*	Antiretrovirals	908
Virazole	*Antiviral*	Antibiotic	907
Vivelle	*Estrogens*	Reproductive	902
Voltaren	*NSAIDs*	Musculoskeletal	879
Wellbutrin	*Heterocyclic Antidepressant*	Antidepressant	913
Xanax	*Anxiolytic*	Antianxiety	913
Xylocaine	*Antiarrhythmic Drugs*	Cardiovascular	888
Zantac	*GERD, H2 Blockers*	Gastrointestinal	881
Zarontin	*Anticonvulsant*	CNS	914
Zaroxolyn	*Diuretics*	Urinary	893
Zerit	*Drugs to Treat AIDS*	Antiretrovirals	908
Zestril	*ACE Inhibitors*	Cardiovascular	890
Zithromax	*Macrolides*	Antibiotics	905
Zmax	*Macrolides*	Antibiotics	905

TABLE A.1 (CONTINUED)

DRUG INDEX			
NAME	GROUP	MEDICATION FOR	PAGE #
Zocar	*Antilipemic Drugs*	Cardiovascular	891
Zofran	*Antiemetics*	Gastrointestinal	883
Zoloft	*Serotonin Reuptake Inhibitor*	Antidepressant	912
Zovirax	*Antivirals*	Skin	877, 907
Zyprexa	*Antipsychotic Medication*	Tranquilizer	914
Zyrtec	*Antihistamines*	Respiratory	866

It should also be noted that new drugs are continually being approved whereas others are being removed because of unwanted and serious side effects that were not apparent when the drug was first approved. By the time that this text is in print, most likely some of the information contained here will be outdated. The massage therapist must use additional sources of information, such as texts and the Internet, when researching a medication and also in determining whether massage is indicated or contraindicated.

DRUGS TO TREAT THE SKIN

The skin is an area of particular interest to the massage therapist. The massage therapist must always be aware of conditions that might be a contraindication for massage or for the therapist's own safety when touching other people who might have areas of concern.

Relevance for the Massage Therapist

Fungi, bacteria, and viruses can easily be transmitted through open cuts or broken skin. Universal precautions should always be observed. Any massage techniques that can irritate inflamed skin should be avoided. Universal precautions are infection control guidelines designed to protect health care practitioners and their clients from exposure to diseases spread by blood and certain body fluids. They stress that all clients should be assumed infectious for bloodborne diseases such as AIDS and hepatitis B.

Treatment for skin problems is usually topical; however, some conditions are systemic and require oral medication. It should be noted that many persons with skin conditions self-medicate without proper instructions or precautions. The FDA feels that over-the-counter (OTC) drugs are safe enough to use without a physician's supervision. Clients should be advised to discuss these problems with their physicians and, as with any medication, to read the instructions completely before embarking on a drug therapy.

Categories of Skin Medications

Antipruritics

These drugs are used to relieve allergic reactions that cause rashes and itching. They can contain local anesthetics, drying agents, or anti-inflammatory agents, such as corticosteroids and antihistamines.

Side Effects: Skin irritation, rashes, stinging and burning, allergic reactions, or sedation if antihistamines are included.

Contraindications or Cautions: Open wounds or prolonged use of corticosteroids.

Examples: Benadryl, Solarcaine, and Cortaid.

Corticosteroids

These drugs can be used locally or systemically to treat allergic skin reactions and inflammation. They are also used topically to treat eczema, psoriasis, and dermatitis.

Side Effects: Thinning of the skin with increased wounds and infections, increased fragility of blood vessels, irritations, ulcerations, slow healing, bruising, water retention, or edema.

Contraindications or Cautions: Bacterial, fungal, or systemic viral infections; open wounds; immunocompromised persons; children; pregnant or nursing women; acne.

Examples: Cortaid, Valisone, and Aristocort.

Emollients and Demulcents

These topicals are used to soothe or protect the skin.

Side Effects: Generally, there are no side effects, although the potential for an allergic reaction always exists.

Contraindications or Cautions: Known allergies to ingredients.

Examples: Desitin and A + D ointment.

Keratolytics

These drugs are used to treat abnormal flaking of the skin such as dandruff and psoriasis, or to catalyze peeling of the skin in conditions such as acne, calluses, and corns. Many keratolytics contain salicylic acid.

Side Effects: Skin irritations, burning, photosensitivity, or systemic effects in highly allergic persons.

Contraindications or Cautions: Open wounds, children, pregnant and nursing women. Keratolytics should not be used for any lengthy periods.

Examples: Tegrin, Neutrogena, and Clearasil.

Scabicides and Pediculicides

These drugs are used to treat scabies and lice, respectively. The infestation can be either on the head or body. The name of the infestation depends on where it occurs. Both organisms can be easily transmitted from one person to another through direct contact or through contact with contaminated clothing.

Side Effects: Irritations or rashes.

Contraindications or Cautions: Open, raw, or oozing skin; caution in the use of Lindane, which can be absorbed into the body, includes avoiding its use during pregnancy and lactation, and with children and older people.

Examples: Lindane, Acticin, and Nix.

Antifungals

These drugs are used in the treatment of candidiasis (vaginal, intestinal, systemic), aphtha (thrush), ringworm, or athlete's foot.

Side Effects: Skin irritation, itching, and burning.

Contraindications or Cautions: Some oral preparations can cause serious side effects and should be used only under a physician's supervision.

Examples: Lamisil, Lotrimin, Mycostatin, Monistat, Gyne-Lotrimin, and Tinactin.

Antivirals

These drugs are used in the treatment of herpes simplex (cold sores, genital herpes), herpes zoster (shingles), or varicella zoster (chickenpox). Treatments can be topical or oral.

Side Effects: Skin irritations.

Contraindications or Cautions: Hypersensitivity to formulation; use of the cream in the nose, eyes, or mouth.

Example: Zovirax (generally effective only on the first outbreak).

Anti-infectives

These drugs include antiseptics, used to inhibit the growth of bacteria, usually on the skin. The two major antiseptics currently used are Hibiclens (chlorhexidene) and Betadine (povidone-iodine).

Side Effects for Chlorhexidene: Skin irritation, allergic reactions, or photosensivity.

Side Effects for Povidone-Iodine: Skin irritations, allergic reactions, or temporary discoloring of the skin.

Contraindications or Cautions: Open wounds, eyes, ears, pregnant or lactating women. Hands must be washed thoroughly after use.

Examples: Hibiclens and Betadine.

Antibacterials

There are three OTC topical antibacterial medications. Those having a systemic effect and the potential for serious side effects are available only by prescription. Therapists should look up these medications for more information.

Side Effects: Inflammation, itching, rashes, superinfections, or pruritus.

Contraindications or Cautions: Known allergic sensitivity, use of topical products in or around the eyes, contact dermatitis, or conditions in which systemic absorption is possible.

Examples: Neosporin, Bacitracin, Polysporin, Myciguent, Akne-Mycin, and Erygel.

In 2008, the FDA approved the use of Acanya for patients 12 years old and older. This is a topical gel for the treatment of acne that is both an antibacterial and antibiotic combination. Acanya is a combination of benzoyl peroxide and clindamycin phosphate. This product can cause hypersensitivity to the sun and should not be used by people with a history of colitis or chronic diarrhea.

Immunomodulators

Immunomodulators affect the immune system and are used in the treatment of eczema and atopic dermatitis when other treatments have failed because of concerns about side effects. These medications are by prescription only, for children over the age of two years and adults.

Side Effects: Increased risk for skin cancer and lymphoma.

Contraindications or Cautions: The FDA has issued an alert that the topical eczema drugs Elidel (pimecrolimus) and Protopic (tacrolimus) could increase the risk of skin cancer and lymphoma and now must carry a black-box warning, the most serious alert. The new labeling states that these drugs should be used only if eczema has not responded to topical corticosteroids, which are the first choice for treatment.

Examples: Elidel, Protopic.

MUSCULOSKELETAL AND ANTI-INFLAMMATORY DRUGS

Generally, prescription drugs that are used to treat these problems fall into three categories: muscle relaxants, nonsteroidal anti-inflammatory drugs (NSAIDs), and corticosteroids. There are also several OTC medications that clients might fail to mention; therefore, they should be asked specifically about any self-medicating. It should be noted that in many cases OTC medications are prescription agents in a lower dose.

Relevance for the Massage Therapist

Musculoskeletal conditions are among the most commonly seen by the massage therapist. Neck and back pain are common complaints, and just as frequently, clients take some type of medication to ease their spasms, pain, and inflammation. Massage is excellent for helping clients to overcome these problems, but care should be taken not to use any techniques that might exacerbate inflammation or bruise the body. Because these medications are either anti-inflammatory or painkillers, they change the tissue response, in some cases dulling the sensations that the client feels. The client might show a false tolerance for pressure, and so the massage therapist should exercise great caution when applying pressure techniques. The therapist should communicate with the client so that, if possible, the client receives treatment when they are at the end of their dosage regimen rather than at the beginning or in the middle. In this way, the information gleaned is more accurate, and the therapist knows how much pressure and which techniques should be used.

Massage therapy can be of great benefit in helping clients to reduce the amount of medication that they need. Many of the prescription medications have serious side effects, which the therapist should be aware of when reviewing the clients' symptoms and complaints.

Categories of Musculoskeletal Medications

Skeletal Muscle Relaxants

These drugs are used to treat pain, spasms, muscle contractions, and restricted range of motion. Generally, acute back and neck problems are treated medically with a combination of muscle relaxants, bed rest, physical therapy, massage therapy, and analgesics. Muscle relaxants are for short-term use, until the pain subsides, and other adjunctive therapies such as massage and exercise can take over to strengthen and relax the muscles.

Side Effects: Dizziness, drowsiness, tremor, headaches, nausea, vomiting, diarrhea or constipation, urinary problems, liver toxicity, difficulty breathing, or confusion.

Contraindications or Cautions: Muscular dystrophy, myasthenia gravis, pregnant and nursing women, and children younger than age 12. These drugs can enhance the effects of alcohol, analgesics, psychotropic medications, and antihistamines.

Examples: Soma, Flexeril, Valium, and Robaxin.

Nonsteroidal Anti-inflammatory Drugs (NSAIDs)

These medications are used to treat inflammatory conditions such as arthritis, bursitis, gout, muscle strains and sprains, and spondylitis. Symptoms include inflammation, pain, swelling, heat, or limited range of motion (ROM). Often these drugs are used for prolonged periods in low doses as maintenance therapy, in contrast to the steroids, which should be used only for acute disorders. NSAIDs work by inhibiting the synthesis of prostaglandins, chemicals that create much of the inflammation and pain associated with conditions such as rheumatism, aches and pains, and sprains. Note that elderly people are particularly sensitive to the side effects from these drugs, which often cause stomach irritation and diarrhea. They should be advised to call their physician immediately if any of the negative symptoms are present.

COX-2 inhibitors are a newer class of NSAIDs that are supposed to pose less of a risk for gastrointestinal (GI) bleeding; however, recent studies have shown that they pose more of a risk for heart disease and stroke. Because of this, many of them have been recalled from the market by the FDA and drug manufacturers.

Side Effects: GI bleeding and ulceration, which is sometimes preceded by warning signs or symptoms; epigastric pain, nausea, heartburn, gastroesophageal reflux disease (GERD), constipation, tinnitus, headaches, dizziness, visual disturbances, hypersensitivity reactions, bronchospasm, or liver toxicity.

Contraindications or Cautions: Asthma, cardiovascular disease, kidney disease, liver disease, history of ulcers or inflammatory bowel disease, clotting disorders, thyroid disease, GERD, elderly patients, pregnant and nursing women, and children with viral infections.

Examples: Voltaren, Motrin, Advil, Nuprin, Aleve, and Relafen.

Gout Agents

Colchicine is a medication used to treat gout. Gout is caused by a buildup of uric acid crystals in different joints, especially the big toe, ankle, knee, and elbow.

Side Effects: Rashes, GI problems, diarrhea, and blood disorders.

Contraindications or Cautions: Blood dyscrasias; serious GI problems; hepatic, cardiac, or renal disorders; lactation; children, and elderly patients.

Example: Colchicine.

Adrenal Corticosteroids

Corticosteroids are secreted by the adrenal glands, which are located next to and on top of the kidneys. Corticosteroids act on the immune system to suppress the body's response to infection or trauma. Corticosteroids relieve inflammation, reduce swelling, and suppress symptoms in acute conditions. Corticosteroids also function as replacement therapy when the adrenal glands or pituitary glands are deficient or for their anti-inflammatory and immunosuppressant qualities. Corticosteroids are not meant to cure a disease but rather are used as adjunctive therapy in conjunction with other medications. They are used to treat conditions such as acute asthma attacks, acute skin conditions, acute rheumatism or arthritis attacks, acute attacks of colitis, and cancer treatments. Because their side effects are potentially very serious, they should be given for a short time only and locally whenever possible.

Side Effects: Nausea, vomiting, diarrhea, constipation, gastric ulceration or hemorrhage, headaches, vertigo, insomnia, psychosis, anxiety, easy bruising, skin thinning and tearing, fluid and electrolyte imbalance, edema, hypertension, congestive heart failure, increased chance of infections, delayed wound healing, or adrenocortical insufficiency.

Contraindications or Cautions: Long-term use, viral or bacterial infections, fungal infections, hypertension, congestive heart failure, psychosis or emotional instability, diabetes, children, pregnant or nursing women, history of seizures or immunosuppression, hypothyroidism, and cirrhosis.

Examples: Cortisone, Prednisone, Deltasone, Florinef, Decadron, Medrol, and Aristocort.

GASTROINTESTINAL MEDICATIONS

Gastrointestinal (GI) medications can be grouped into 11 categories based on their various actions in the body. Disturbances of the GI system are among the most common complaints of clients and one of the main areas where clients self-medicate. GI side effects are the most common among all medications. If the client complains of GI problems, one of the first areas to be considered should be the client's medications.

Relevance for the Massage Therapist

Many of the GI complaints are rooted in response to stress. Massage is most beneficial for helping clients to relax and as supportive therapy in the treatment of constipation or diarrhea. One of the positive results of regular massage treatment can be the reduction in the need for medication once the client can achieve deepening levels of relaxation.

Categories of Gastrointestinal Medication

Antacids

Antacids neutralize gastric hydrochloric acid and are among the most widely purchased OTC medications used to treat indigestion, heartburn, and sour stomach. They can also help in the treatment of gastric and duodenal ulcers. Because they interact with almost all other medications and have an impact on the effectiveness of other drugs, they should not be taken within two hours of other medications.

Side Effects: Constipation, diarrhea, electrolyte imbalance, urinary stones, osteoporosis, or flatulence.

Contraindications or Cautions: Kidney disease, liver cirrhosis, electrolyte imbalance, and congestive heart failure.

Examples: Tums, Maalox, Gelusil, Mylanta, and Amphojel.

Drugs to Treat Ulcers and Gastroesophageal Reflux Disease (GERD) (H2 Blockers)

Some of these drugs reduce gastric acid secretion by acting as histamine 2-receptor antagonists. They treat duodenal and gastric ulcers and give short-term relief from GERD.

Side Effects: Diarrhea, dizziness, rash, or headaches.

Contraindications or Cautions: Kidney disease, liver disease, children, and pregnant and nursing women.

Examples: Tagamet, Zantac, Pepcid, Axid (the last two are better tolerated in elderly patients with fewer adverse reactions).

Cytotec (misoprostol)

This is a synthetic drug used to block gastric acid secretion and to protect the mucosa from the effects of other drugs such as NSAIDs. It is not used for the treatment of ulcers.

Side Effects: Diarrhea, nausea, abdominal pain, menstrual problems, or spontaneous abortion.

Contraindications or Cautions: Women of childbearing age, pregnant women, and children younger than age 12.

Example: Cytotec.

Proton Pump Inhibitors

These drugs prevent gastric secretions. They are meant for short-term use in the treatment of GERD, ulcers, and erosive esophagitis.

Side Effects: Diarrhea, constipation, nausea, vomiting, abdominal pain, headaches, or dizziness.

Contraindications or Cautions: Lactating women, elderly clients, and children.

Examples: Prilosec, Prevacid, Nexium (now approved for children ages 1–11 years of age), Aciphex (approved for adolescents), and Protonix.

Carafate (Sucralfate)

This is a medication that inhibits pepsin, and it is used to treat ulcers in a local, rather than a systemic, way by forming a paste with hydrochloric acid that then covers the ulcer site, protecting it from further irritation.

Side Effects: Constipation (most common), diarrhea, indigestion, flatulence, dry mouth, gastric discomfort, urticaria, rash, insomnia, vertigo, angioedema, or facial swelling.

Contraindications or Cautions: Safety for use in children and during lactation has not been fully established.

Example: Carafate.

Antispasmodics/Anticholinergics

These medications work by decreasing motility in the GI tract.

Side Effects: Urinary retention, constipation, confusion, dry mouth, or blurry vision.

Contraindications or Cautions: Glaucoma, cardiovascular disease, myasthenia gravis, pregnancy, lactation, and obstructive GI disease.

Examples: Cystospaz, Levsin, and Levsinex.

Drugs for Inflammatory Bowel Disease

These drugs act as anti-inflammatory agents in the GI tract and are used to treat ulcerative colitis.

Side Effects: Nausea, vomiting, anorexia, headaches, dizziness, pruritis, or fever.

Contraindications or Cautions: Use with caution during lactation, in persons with known drug hypersensitivity or related drug hypersensitivity, and children younger than 2 years of age.

Example: Azulfidine, Apriso

Antidiarrhea Drugs

These medications have various modes of action in diminishing loose stools. Some act as adsorbents, whereas others slow intestinal motility.

Side Effects: Constipation, nausea, vomiting, abdominal distention, or confusion.

Contraindications or Cautions: Infants, elderly patients (unless under medical supervision), and ulcerative colitis.

Examples: Kaopectate, Lomotil (a controlled substance), Imodium, and Imodium A-D.

Antiflatulents

These drugs help to break up gas in the GI tract.

Side Effects: None.

Contraindications or Cautions: None.

Example: Simethicone.

Laxatives and Cathartics

These drugs help to stimulate evacuation of the intestines. Laxatives have a more gentle action than cathartics or purgatives, which promote a rapid evacuation. There are numerous subdivisions of laxatives, such as bulk-forming laxatives, stool softeners, mineral oil, saline laxatives, stimulant laxatives, and hyperosmotic laxatives. Each division should be investigated separately for more specific contraindications. Many clients self-medicate in this area. Massage can be very helpful in stimulating the movement of clients' colonic contents.

Side Effects: Generally rare but include diarrhea, anal irritation, or electrolyte imbalance.

Contraindications or Cautions: Acute abdominal pain, partial bowel obstruction, young children, debilitated persons, prolonged use, and congestive heart failure.

Examples: Metamucil, Colace, Milk of Magnesia, Dulcolax, and glycerin suppositories.

Antiemetics

These medications are used to treat nausea, vomiting, and motion sickness. There are many different drugs on the market, with different actions and means of administration.

Side Effects: Confusion, anxiety, drowsiness, vertigo, depression, blurry vision, or weakness.

Contraindications or Cautions: Children, pregnant and lactating women, geriatric or debilitated persons, seizures, and cardiac arrhythmias.

Examples: Torecan, Compazine, Tigan, Phenergan, Zofran, Antivert, and Bonine.

Biologic Agents

These are a relatively new class of medications, which are antibodies that block the action of tumor necrosis factor (TNF). TNF is a proinflammatory chemical that plays a major role in several inflammatory diseases such as Crohn's disease, ulcerative colitis, rheumatoid arthritis, and psoriasis. These medications are used when more traditional medications have failed.

Side Effects: Headaches, upper respiratory tract infections, abdominal pain, infections at the injection site, nausea.

Contraindications or Cautions: Increased risk for serious infections and potentially death because they affect the immune system and lower the body's ability to fight infections. Can cause lymphomas and other malignancies.

Examples: Cimzia, Remicade, Humira.

RESPIRATORY SYSTEM MEDICATIONS AND ANTIHISTAMINES

The main classifications of respiratory system drugs are bronchodilators, corticosteroids, mycolytics, expectorants, and antitussives.

Relevance for the Massage Therapist

Massage can be very beneficial for relaxing the muscles of the chest and upper back, thereby helping the client to take in more oxygen and breathe easier. Some respiratory medications can induce drowsiness, however, and relaxing massage techniques can exacerbate this symptom. The massage therapist therefore must be aware of any medications that the client is taking. Conversely, some medications can induce anxiety states, and the client might be unable to relax on the table no matter which efforts the therapist tries. Because many of these drugs can cause dizziness, the therapist should check to see if the client becomes dizzy when sitting up at the end of the treatment. If the client is dizzy, the therapist can press an acupuncture point directly under the client's nose in the center of the philtrum. The therapist can press the point with the tip of the index finger or instruct the client to do so. This is a very helpful technique for ameliorating dizziness. Because decreased sweating is sometimes a side effect of these medications, and the body's temperature can increase with the use of hydrocollators or other heat therapies, they should be avoided in these cases.

Many clients self-medicate in this area with OTC medications, and it is important to obtain a complete list of all drugs that clients are taking before beginning treatment.

Bronchodilators

These drugs act by alleviating bronchospasms and increasing the capacity of the lungs. These medications are used to treat acute respiratory conditions such as asthma and chronic obstructive pulmonary disease (COPD). There are three types of bronchodilators: sympathomimetics (adrenergics), parasympatholytics (anticholinergics), and xanthine derivatives. The therapist must research each category for more specific information regarding actions, side effects, and contraindications. General information is listed here.

Side Effects: GI effects such as nausea, vomiting, nervousness, tremors, dizziness, cardiac irregularities, hypertension, drowsiness, dizziness, confusion, agitation, seizures, or palpitations.

Contraindications or Cautions: Cardiovascular, kidney, pulmonary, or liver dysfunction; diabetes; children; elderly patients; and pregnant and lactating women.

Examples: Ventolin, Proventil, Primatene, Adrenalin, Alupent, Atrovent Albuterol, and Theo-Dur.

Corticosteroids

These drugs are discussed under Musculoskeletal Problems. For respiratory problems, corticosteroids can be administered orally, intravenously, or by inhaler or aerosol. Corticosteroids that are inhaled have less systemic effects than those that are taken orally or intravenously.

Side Effects: Coughing, fungal infections, sore throat, or dry mouth.

Contraindications or Cautions: Viral, bacterial, or fungal infections; hypertension; cardiac disease; diabetes; and kidney disease.

Examples: Vanceril, Beconase, Pulmicort, Rhinocort, Flovent, AeroBid, Nasonex, Nasacort, Flo-Pred and Alvesco.

Asthma Prophylaxis

These medications are used to prevent asthma attacks in clients who suffer from chronic asthma. They include antileukotrienes and cromolyn, which is usually listed separately because its action is different. Cromolyn can also be used in the prevention of exercise-induced asthma.

Side Effects: Headaches, dizziness, nausea, pain, fatigue, or infections.

Contraindications or Cautions: Liver toxicity, pregnant and lactating women, and children younger than age 12.

Examples: Accolate, Singulair, and Cromolyn.

Mucolytics and Expectorants

Mucolytics are drugs that liquefy pulmonary secretions, whereas expectorants increase secretions, reduce viscosity, and help to expel sputum. Expectorants are often combined in cough syrups to help with coughs caused by upper respiratory infections, bronchitis, and postnasal drip. A chronic cough can indicate a serious problem; however, any cough that lasts for more than a week or that recurs frequently needs the attention of a physician.

Side Effects: Drowsiness, nausea, vomiting, runny nose, or stomach upset.

Contraindications or Cautions: Cardiovascular disease, diabetes, pregnant and lactating women, and some clients with asthma.

Examples: Mucomyst, Humibid, Robitussin, Iophen, and Pima Syrup.

Antitussives

These are drugs used to prevent coughing in patients who have a nonproductive cough. Dry, persistent coughs can produce fatigue, prevent sleep, and sometimes cause pulled or strained muscles. Massage can help to relieve the pain of muscle strain and sprain, although narcotic antitussives are sometimes also used. Codeine is often used but can become addictive with long-term use if not monitored properly by a physician. There are several OTC cough syrups that combine several drugs—antitussives, expectorants, antihistamines, and decongestants. Clients should be encouraged to consult with their physicians, pharmacists, nurse practitioners, or medical assistants, because some of these ingredients are contraindicated with specific medical conditions. For example, decongestants can produce negative effects in persons with cardiovascular disease or thyroid conditions.

Side Effects of Narcotic Antitussives: Constipation, urinary retention, drowsiness, dizziness, nausea, vomiting, or respiratory depression. Non-narcotic antitussives do not depress respiration or cause addiction and have few side effects.

Contraindications or Cautions: Clients prone to addictions, asthma, and COPD.

Examples of Narcotic Antitussives: Codeine, Robitussin A-C, Histussin, and Lorcet.

Examples of Non-narcotic Antitussives: Robitussin and Tessalon Perles.

Antihistamines

These drugs provide relief from the symptoms of allergic reactions caused by histamine responses, such as inflammation, itching, and edema. They are also used to assist in treatment of anaphylactic shock after the acute stage has been treated with epinephrine and corticosteroids. Antihistamines are often used to treat the symptoms of allergic rhinitis, although when they are used to reduce nasal secretions in persons suffering from the common cold, the subsequent thickening of bronchial secretions can result in further airway obstruction, especially in those with COPD and asthma. Some antihistamines are also used to treat motion sickness and vertigo.

Side Effects: Dry eyes, ears, nose, and throat; drowsiness; dizziness; low blood pressure especially in elderly people; muscular weakness; urinary retention; constipation; visual disorders; insomnia; tremors; nausea; vomiting; anorexia.

Contraindications or Cautions: COPD, asthma, operating machinery or driving a car, elderly patients, cardiovascular disease, infants, pregnant and lactating women, seizure disorders, and benign prostatic hypertrophy (BPH).

Examples: Zyrtec, Dimetapp, Chlor-Trimeton, Benadryl, Claritin, Allegra, Astepro, and Patanase (nasal sprays).

Decongestants

Decongestants constrict the blood vessels in the respiratory tract, helping to shrink swollen mucous membranes, and open the nasal and sinus pathways. Also known as *adrenergic drugs*, these medications can be administered orally or nasally but should be used only on a short-term basis because they cause rebound congestion after a few days. Many decongestants, often sold OTC, are combined with antihistamines, analgesics, caffeine, or antitussives. Because of these combinations, the potential for negative side effects increases. Oral decongestants in particular, such as pseudoephedrine, can raise blood pressure; therefore, clients who already have high blood pressure should consult with their physician.

Effects: Anxiety, nervousness, tremor, seizures, palpitations, hypertension, headaches, or electrolyte imbalance. Rhinitis medicamentosa may occur if a patient has taken Afrin for 3 continuous days. This is called a *rebound effect.*

Contraindications or Cautions: Cardiovascular disease, diabetes, hyperthyroidism, elderly people, and pregnant and lactating women.

Examples: Afrin, Allerest, Neo-Synephrine, No-stril, and Sudafed.

Smoking Cessation Aids

These drugs are used in conjunction with behavior modification programs to help people stop smoking. Sometimes Zyban is also prescribed in smoking cessation.

Side Effects: Lightheadedness, nausea, vomiting, throat and mouth irritation, or cardiac irritability.

Contraindications or Cautions: Overdosage, pregnant and lactating women, and history of drug abuse or overdependence.

Examples: Nicorette gum, Nicoderm patch, and Nicotrol inhaler.

CARDIOVASCULAR MEDICATIONS

These include drugs that affect the heart and vascular system, and anticoagulants. There are seven subcategories of medications; however, some of the drugs have multiple uses and overlap categories.

Relevance for the Massage Therapist

Experts agree that cardiovascular disease is a leading cause of death in the United States. It is estimated that one in three Americans suffers from high blood pressure; therefore, massage therapists are likely to treat clients who are taking cardiovascular medications. Massage therapy can help to promote blood and lymph circulation through its vasodilatory effects and can augment the actions of certain medications. In addition, through the effects of massage on lowering blood pressure, clients might find that the dosages of their medications can be lowered. Many of these drugs work to lesson the sympathetic response and produce a parasympathetic response, and therefore therapists should always be mindful that clients, whether on medication or not, might get dizzy when they sit up at the end of the treatment. The client should be encouraged to wait before getting off the table. Gently pressing an acupuncture point directly under the nose in the philtrum can alleviate the dizziness. Therapists should do the following:

- Monitor the client's heart rate as well as be on the lookout for any unusual responses.
- Have their clients contact their physicians if they think there is cause for concern.
- Note that clients who are on diuretics might experience muscle cramps owing to loss of electrolytes and might need to discuss this with their physicians.

It is important to be aware that clients who are on blood-thinning medication can be particularly sensitive to pressure. Massage therapists must use a light touch, avoid any techniques that have the potential for bruising, and be on the lookout for any bruising or irritations from treatment. If bruising should occur despite the therapist's best efforts to use only very light techniques, the client should be informed and the treatment should be terminated.

Cardiac Glycosides

These medications are also called *cardiotonics* because of their ability to strengthen the heartbeat. They are used mostly in the treatment of congestive heart failure, in which the heart fails to pump properly and increases in size to compensate. In congestive heart failure, these medications increase the force of cardiac contractions without increasing oxygen consumption. Because the heart works more efficiently, it beats more slowly and decreases from its increased size, and the diuretic action decreases edema as well. Sometimes cardiac glycosides are also used with antiarrhythmic drugs to slow the heart rate in tachycardia, atrial fibrillation, or flutter. Lanoxin (digoxin) is the most commonly used drug in this category. Because there is a fine line between appropriate dosage and dangerous levels of toxicity, clients should be told to see their physician immediately if there are any side effects.

Side Effects: Anorexia, nausea, vomiting, diarrhea, abdominal bloating or cramping, headaches, fatigue, muscle weakness, vertigo, restlessness, irritability, tremors, seizures, blurry vision, cardiac arrhythmias, electrolyte imbalance, insomnia, and confusion, especially in elderly persons. A symptom of toxicity is seeing a yellow-greenish-bluish halo.

Contraindications or Cautions: Elderly clients, pregnant and lactating women, hypothyroidism, pulmonary disease, acute heart disease, and kidney disease.

Examples: Digitalis and Lanoxin (digoxin).

Antiarrhythmic Drugs

These medications are used to treat atrial or ventricular tachycardia, atrial fibrillation or flutter, and arrhythmias that are the result of digitalis toxicity. Most of these medications can lower blood pressure and slow the heartbeat, which, if not monitored properly, could lead to hypotension, bradycardia, and cardiac arrest. These drugs have the potential to make existing arrhythmias worse or cause new ones, and they can also cause negative effects when they interact with other medications.

There are several groups of antiarrhythmic drugs that function with different mechanisms of action. For example, beta-adrenergic blockers such as Inderal work by inhibiting adrenergic (sympathetic) nerve receptors; calcium channel blockers such as Isoptin work by suppressing the action of calcium in contraction of the heart muscle; Norpace decreases myocardial excitability and inhibits conduction; lidocaine is an anesthetic that stabilizes membranes; Pronestyl is used mostly as prophylactic therapy; and Quinaglute and Cardioquin decrease myocardial excitability. Extra caution in all of these categories must be exercised in elderly clients. Therapists should check each drug for more specific side effects and contraindications.

Side Effects: Hypotension, bradycardia, dizziness, confusion, insomnia, weakness, fatigue, nausea, vomiting, diarrhea or constipation, or edema.

Contraindications or Cautions: Diabetes, kidney disease, asthma, bradycardia, heart failure, pregnant and lactating women, children, and liver disease.

Examples: Tenormin, Inderal, Isoptin, Xylocaine, Cordarone, Tonocard, Cardioquin, and Norpace.

Antihypertensives

These medications are also called *hypotensives.* There are numerous drugs in this category that lower blood pressure. Clients who suffer from mild hypertension can often regulate their pressure with a program that includes dietary changes (e.g., reducing their salt intake), consistent massage therapy treatments, and appropriate exercise (e.g., walking, tai chi chuan). Nutritional counseling can also be of benefit. Therapists might want to network with a nutritionist and help their clients to establish a more wellness-oriented lifestyle. Note that antihypertensives do not cure high blood pressure; they simply manage the symptoms. Clients should never simply stop their medication on their own, because abruptly stopping can cause rebound hypertension. They should discuss their medication and concerns with their physician.

Hypertension is usually viewed as mild, moderate, or severe, and there are different drugs for each class. In addition, their actions vary. Patient history is also a factor in determining which medication is chosen. It is often difficult to choose the right drug initially, and clients often have their dosages and medications changed or combined, causing different kinds of side effects. Thiazide diuretics are sometimes used by themselves to treat mild hypertension but are more frequently combined with other hypotensive medications to lower high blood pressure. The types of antihypertensives are listed in the next sections.

Beta-Adrenergic and Calcium Channel Blockers

Examples: Inderal, Tenormin, Cardizem, Procardia, Coreg, Corgard, and Verelan (previously discussed under "Antiarrhythmic Drugs").

Aldomet (methyldopa)

This drug treats moderate to severe hypertension and is usually given with a diuretic. It can be used in pregnancy because it is safe for the fetus, but it is rarely used.

Side Effects: Low blood pressure, drowsiness, anemia, nausea, vomiting, diarrhea, constipation, a sore tongue, sexual dysfunction, liver problems, or nasal congestion.

Contraindications or Cautions: Liver disease, dialysis, and elderly clients.

Example: Aldomet.

Tekturna HCT

This drug has two FDA prescription medications in one tablet. Tekturna targets an enzyme in the body called *renin*, which can contribute to high blood pressure. Renin is produced in the kidneys and starts a process that leads to narrowing of the blood vessels. Hydrochlorothiazide is a diuretic. Diuretics cause sodium and water to move out of the body through urination, which reduces blood volume and blood pressure. This medication is not the first choice for treatment of hypertension.

Side Effects: Diarrhea, dizziness, flulike symptoms, allergic reactions causing swelling of the face, lips, mouth and tongue, which can cause difficulty in swallowing or breathing.

Contraindications or Cautions: Pregnancy, liver problems, lupus, kidney problems.

Example: Tekturna HCT.

Apresoline (hydralazine)

This drug is a peripheral vasodilator used in the treatment of moderate-to-severe hypertension, especially in clients with congestive heart failure. It is often administered with a diuretic and another hypotensive agent (e.g., a beta blocker), but it is very rarely used today.

Side Effects: Tachycardia, palpitations, headache, flushing, orthostatic hypotension, nausea, vomiting, diarrhea and constipation, blood abnormalities, or allergic reactions.

Contraindications or Cautions: Kidney disease, coronary artery disease, pregnant women, and lupus patients.

Example: Apresoline.

ACE Inhibitors

These drugs are called angiotensin-converting enzymes (ACE), which work to lower mild-to-moderate blood pressure and also treat congestive heart failure by decreasing vasoconstriction. They can be used alone or with a diuretic. ACE inhibitors can interact negatively with several other medications, and the client should be aware of the potential side effects from the interactions of these medications with other drugs.

Side Effects: Rash, photosensitivity, loss of taste, blood dyscrasias, renal disease, severe hypotension, cough, nasal congestion, or hyperkalemia.

Contraindications or Cautions: Renal disease, lupus, scleroderma, heart failure, pregnant and lactating women, and children.

Examples: Captopril, Enalapril, Accupril, Monopril, Zestril, and Prinivil.

Angiotensin Receptor Blockers

These drugs are generally used for clients who cannot tolerate ACE inhibitors.

Side Effects: Lower chance of taste loss, rashes, or cough than those caused by ACE inhibitors.

Contraindications or Cautions: Renal disease, lupus, scleroderma, heart failure, pregnant and lactating women, and children.

Examples: Cozaar and Diovan.

Note: A new medication was approved called Exforge, a combination of amiodipine, a calcium channel blocker (CCB), and valsartan, an antiotensin receptor blocker (ARB), in a single pill. Exforge was approved as a first-line treatment for high blood pressure.

Coronary Vasodilators

These medications are used to treat angina. Angina pectoris is pain in the chest as a result of ischemia, or decreased blood supply, to the heart muscle. When the coronary arteries are constricted or blocked, pain results. Coronary vasodilators are used to dilate the blood vessels and stop an attack of angina pectoris, or they can be used preventively to stop further attacks or at least reduce their frequency. The three subcategories of coronary vasodilators are nitrates, beta blockers, and calcium channel blockers.

Nitrates

Nitroglycerin comes in several different forms. These are administered for an acute attack, and if the attack is not halted after the first dose, additional doses can be given every 5 minutes, not to exceed three doses in 15 minutes. If three doses should fail to bring relief, a physician must be called immediately to avoid a myocardial infarction. Nitroglycerin is also available in timed-release capsules and tablets as well as in an intravenous (IV) solution. Persons using nitroglycerin preventively over the long term often use a transdermal ointment or a patch—the location must be only on the upper arm or body and must be rotated to avoid irritating the skin. Therapists should avoid any areas of skin irritation or raw areas as well as the area of the patch itself.

Side Effects: Headaches, postural hypotension including dizziness, flushing, blurry vision, dry mouth, nausea, vomiting, diarrhea, cold sweats, tachycardia, or syncope.

Contraindications or Cautions: Glaucoma, anemia, and frequent bowel movements. Note that alcohol interacts with nitrates and exacerbates their effects.

Examples: Nitroglycerin, Isordil, and Sorbitrate.

Beta Blockers and Calcium Channel Blockers

These drugs are discussed under Antiarrhythmic Drugs.

Antilipemic Drugs

These medications are among the most frequently prescribed drugs and are used to lower serum cholesterol and low-density lipoprotein (LDL), the "bad" cholesterol. Clients who have high cholesterol and high LDL (>130) are at a greater risk for myocardial infarction and atherosclerotic coronary disease. Dietary changes that include a low-fat and low-cholesterol diet as well as appropriate exercise, stopping smoking, and weight loss are all significant factors in lowering cholesterol; however, medications are frequently added in this effort. It should be noted that there are fairly new tests available that often provide better indications of coronary disease, such as C-reactive protein and homocystine tests. Clients should be advised to discuss these additional tests with their physicians before ingesting hyperlipidemia agents. All hyperlipidemia medications have potentially serious side effects, and sometimes two or three of them are combined. Types of hyperlipidemia agents include statins, niacin, and bile acid sequestrant.

Side Effects: GI upset, GI bleeding, bleeding gums, constipation, flushing, liver damage, muscle cramps, muscle weakness, renal failure, eye problems, cataracts (with long-term use), headaches, dizziness, insomnia, or fatigue, rhabdomyolysis.

Contraindications or Cautions: Liver, kidney, or gallbladder disease; diabetes, gout, allergies, alcoholism, ulcers, low blood pressure, pregnant and lactating women, and women of childbearing age.

Examples: Questran, Nicobid, Mevacor, Lipitor, Zocar, Lopid, Crestor, and Pravachol. Simcor is a new type of medication that combines a statin with niacin, whereas Trilipix is the first and only fibrate to be approved in combination with a statin to help to lower triglycerides and LDL cholesterol and to raise HDL cholesterol.

Anticoagulants and Antithrombolytics

These two classes of drugs include coumarin medications and heparins. Their mode of action is different—anticoagulants, such as Coumadin, prevent the blood from clotting and are referred to as blood thinners, whereas antithrombolytics, such as heparin, dissolve clots that have already been formed to prevent a cerebrovascular accident. They are also used with postsurgery clients such as those who have had a coronary bypass or hip or knee replacement. Particular caution must be exercised with elderly clients who are at higher risk for internal bleeding. Coumarin derivatives (warfarin) interact negatively with many drugs and herbal supplements. Some drugs increase the blood-thinning effect and greatly increase the potential for internal bleeding. These include aspirin and other NSAIDS.

Contaminated heparin, made in China, was responsible for several deaths in the United States. This has led to major concerns among scientists and lawmakers that America is too dependent on medications produced abroad and that the FDA lacks sufficient funds and manpower to oversee pharmaceutical factories overseas. This is clearly an issue that needs urgent government attention and intervention.

Side Effects: Major hemorrhage, minor bleeding, blood in the urine (hematuria) or stools (melena), or gums bleeding easily on brushing.

Contraindications or Cautions: GI problems, ulcers, liver or kidney disease, blood dyscrasias, pregnant women (heparin can be used with caution because it does not cross the placenta), and post-stroke.

Examples of Anticoagulants: Coumadin and aspirin.

Examples of Antithrombolytics: Heparin and Lovenox.

Platelet Inhibitors

These medications are used prophylactically to decrease platelet clumping in clients having a history of recent stroke, recent myocardial infarction, or peripheral vascular disease.

Side Effects: Headache, dizziness, weakness, nausea, vomiting, diarrhea, flushing, rash, or bleeding.

Contraindications or Cautions: Elderly clients.

Examples: Aspirin, Plavix, and Ticlid.

URINARY SYSTEM MEDICATIONS

The most frequently used drugs in this category are *diuretics*, which are drugs that increase the excretion of urine.

Relevance for the Massage Therapist

Massage can help to move fluids through the body and reduce edema, making these medications work more effectively. The therapist should be cognizant that the client might need to urinate midway through the treatment.

Diuretics

There are four classes of diuretics, depending on their actions: thiazides, loop diuretics, potassium-sparing diuretics, and osmotic agents. The condition being treated determines which type is used. These drugs also interact with several other medications and can have serious side effects. Because many of these drugs deplete potassium, potassium supplementation is often recommended.

Thiazides

These drugs are the most commonly used diuretic. They increase the excretion of water, sodium, chloride, and potassium. They are used to treat edema and hypertension and prevent stone formation in persons with hypercalciuria (too much calcium in the urine) and those suffering from electrolyte imbalance because of kidney disease.

Side Effects: Potassium deficiency, which can lead to cardiac arrhythmias; chloride deficiency, which can lead to alkalosis; muscle weakness or spasms; nausea, vomiting, or diarrhea; cramping; low blood pressure; vertigo; headaches; fatigue; skin conditions; hyperglycemia; or increased uric acid.

Contraindications or Cautions: Diabetes, gout, kidney disease, liver disease, long-term use, and elderly clients.

Examples: Lozol, Esidrex, HydroDIURIL, and Zaroxolyn.

Loop Diuretics

These drugs act directly on the loop of Henle in the kidneys, and although not classified as thiazides, they have a similar action in that they increase the secretion of water, sodium, chloride, and potassium. Their action is quicker than that of thiazides. They are used to treat edema from pulmonary, renal, or hepatic disease, as well as congestive heart failure, ascites, and hypertension.

Side Effects: Chest pain; electrolyte imbalance; potassium deficiency; vertigo; low blood pressure; GI effects including anorexia, nausea, vomiting, diarrhea, and abdominal pain; hyperglycemia; increased uric acid; blood dyscrasias; tinnitus; skin conditions; allergic reactions; headaches; muscle cramps; mental confusion; and dizziness.

Contraindications or Cautions: Liver disease, kidney disease, diabetes, gout, pregnant and lactating women, and children.

Examples: Edecrin, Lasix, Bumex, and Demadex.

Potassium-sparing Diuretics

These are used when deficiency of potassium has reached a dangerous level.

Side Effects: Excess potassium that can lead to cardiac arrhythmias, dehydration, weakness; GI symptoms, including nausea, vomiting, and diarrhea; fatigue; weight loss; and low blood pressure.

Contraindications or Cautions: Kidney disease, liver disease, and pregnant and lactating women.

Examples: Aldactone and Dyrenium.

Osmotic Drugs

These medications are most often used to reduce intracranial or intraocular pressure.

Side Effects: Fluid and electrolyte imbalance, headache, vertigo, mental confusion, nausea, tachycardia, hypertension, hypotension, allergic reactions, or severe pulmonary edema.

Contraindications or Cautions: Kidney and cardiovascular disease.

Examples: Osmitrol and Ureaphil.

Gout Medications

These drugs include uricosuric agents, which help with the urinary excretion of uric acid and which are used for chronic gout and gouty arthritis. The other type of medication used is allopurinol, which lowers uric acid levels. These drugs are not used in the treatment of acute gout attacks because they have no anti-inflammatory action nor do they relieve pain. Acute attacks are treated with medications in which colchicine, an anti-inflammatory, has been added.

Side Effects: Headaches, nausea and vomiting, kidney stones, rash, low blood pressure.

Contraindications or Cautions: History of kidney stones, history of peptic ulcer, nausea, vomiting, diarrhea, kidney disease, liver disease, and pregnant and lactating women.

Examples: Benemid and Allopurinol.

Antispasmodics

These drugs are anticholinergic, meaning that they block parasympathetic nerve impulses, which in turn reduce spasms in the urinary bladder.

Side Effects: Dryness, dizziness, drowsiness, headaches, urinary retention, constipation, blurry vision, mental confusion (especially in elderly clients), tachycardia, palpitations, nausea, vomiting, or skin reactions.

Contraindications or Cautions: Elderly clients, kidney or liver disease, GI obstruction, cardiovascular disease, prostatic hypertrophy, glaucoma, pregnant or nursing women, and children younger than 5 years of age.

Examples: Pro-Banthine, Detrol, Ditropan, and Cystospaz. Toviaz is a new medication indicated for the treatment of overactive bladder.

Cholinergics

In this case, cholinergics stimulate the parasympathetic nerves to help the urinary bladder to contract.

Side Effects: Nausea, diarrhea, vomiting, sweating, headache, bronchial constriction, or urinary urgency.

Contraindications or Cautions: Obstruction of the urinary tract, hyperthyroidism, peptic ulcer, asthma, cardiovascular disease, parkinsonism, and pregnant and lactating women.

Example: Urecholine.

Analgesics

The main analgesic used is Pyridium. It is used in the treatment of the burning, pain, and urgency of cystitis, procedures that irritate the lower urinary tract, or trauma. It is not to be taken for more than 2 days. Pyridium treats only the symptoms and not the cause of the condition. Anti-infective drugs are necessary to treat urinary tract infections.

Side Effects: Headaches, vertigo, mild GI disturbances, or orange-red urine.

Contraindications or Cautions: Kidney dysfunction and hepatitis.

Examples: Pyridium and Azo-Standard.

Drugs to Treat Benign Prostatic Hypertrophy

There are two classes of drugs to treat *benign prostatic hypertrophy* (BPH): antiandrogens and alpha blockers.

Antiandrogens

The main drug is Proscar, which is used to reduce the size of the prostate and the symptoms of BPH: urgency, nocturia, and urinary hesitancy. This medication does not cure BPH; it only suppresses the symptoms, which return once the medication is stopped.

Side Effects: Impotence, decreased libido or decreased volume of ejaculate, breast enlargement. Proscar can increase hair growth.

Contraindications or Cautions: Infections, liver disease, prostate cancer, urinary tract disease, and any allergies. The drug can be absorbed through the skin. If the film coating of the tablet has been broken or the tablet crushed, it should not be handled by a woman who is pregnant or planning to become pregnant. Any contact with Proscar by a developing male fetus could result in abnormalities of the external sex organs. Proscar should not be used in women or children.

Example: Proscar.

Alpha Blockers

The main drug was Flomax, which relaxes the smooth muscles of the bladder mouth and prostate, thus increasing the flow of urine and decreasing the symptoms of BPH. Rapaflo is a new drug, an alpha adrenoreceptor antagonist for the treatment of the signs and symptoms associated with BPH. Other drugs such as Hytrin and Cardura treat hypertension as well as BPH.

Side Effects: Dizziness, headaches, palpitations, or hypotension.

Contraindications or Cautions: Hypertension and concurrent use with warfarin.

Examples: Cardura, Flomax, Rapaflo, Hytrin.

ANTINEOPLASTIC DRUGS

Tumors are considered to be neoplastic ("new growth") cells. There are both benign and malignant tumors. Tumors that are considered to be benign do not metastasize (spread) from their original location. Tumors that are malignant, also known as cancers, metastasize by one of three means: extending or spreading into the adjacent tissues, spreading through the lymphatic system, or spreading via the blood. The growth of a tumor or cancer is called *carcinogenesis* or *tumorigenesis.* Cancer cells follow the path of least resistance. Some cancers have a strong genetic link, that is, mutations in the DNA. Other cancers can develop from environmental exposure to chemicals, toxins, viruses, stress, and other causes. Antineoplastic drugs stop the growth and spread of malignant cells. Generally, cancer is most successfully treated with combinations of therapies such as surgery, radiation, chemotherapy, medications, nutrition, and holistic therapies such as acupuncture, bodywork, imagery therapy, herbs, and supplements.

Chemotherapy involves using drugs, often in combination, to relieve the symptoms of cancer while attempting to kill the cancer cells. These drugs are called *cytotoxic,* meaning that they destroy cells. They are aimed at the cells that are metastasizing or spreading rapidly; however, because they are so toxic, they affect "good" cells as well, destroying healthy tissue and creating many negative side effects. Many of these medications also function to suppress the immune system, because cancer is considered to be an autoimmune disease. By decreasing the production of antibodies and phagocytes, the "defenders" of immunity, clients become more susceptible to infections, which can become in and of themselves life threatening.

Antineoplastic drugs are often given in very high doses on an intermittent schedule. After several weeks of chemotherapy, for example, a client may have a rest period before resuming treatments. The hope is that during this rest period, the client's good cells, tissues, and organs have a chance to recover from the chemotherapy. These medications are so toxic that they require special handling by health care personnel. Direct skin contact can result in absorption of these toxic chemicals. Pregnant women, those who are breastfeeding, or those who are trying to conceive should not care for clients receiving chemotherapy.

Relevance to the Massage Therapist

Massage can be very beneficial to patients undergoing chemotherapy, radiation, or both, as well as drug therapies. Many clients with cancer suffer from extreme stress and anxiety, and massage can help to alleviate these symptoms. In addition, massage can help the medications to circulate within the body and be more effective as well as help to alleviate some of the other symptoms such as constipation, weakness, fatigue, nausea, and vomiting. Treatments should be gentle and consistent. Care should be taken that the client does not get a chill or draft and that the client is not exposed to anyone with an infection. Certain tests that the client may be undergoing (e.g., PET scans) involve the injection of radioactive substances into the client. Clients should not receive a massage on the day that they have such tests.

There are seven classes of neoplastic drugs:

- Antimetabolites: Methotrexate is the most famous drug in this class. It is also used in the treatment of rheumatoid arthritis, psoriatic arthritis, and lupus. Other drugs in this category are fluorouracil and cytarabine.
- Alkylating drugs: Some examples of alkylating drugs are carmustine, cisplatin, and thiotepa.
- Plant alkaloids: Vinblastine and vincristine are examples of plant alkaloids.
- Paclitaxel (Taxol): Paclitaxel comes from the bark of the Pacific yew. It is often used as adjunct therapy in patients with metastatic breast or ovarian cancer.
- Antitumor antibiotics: Some examples include bleomycin, dactinomycin, and mitomycin.
- Hormone therapy: Hormone therapy consists of corticosteroids such as prednisone, antiestrogen drugs such as tamoxifen, and antiandrogen drugs such as Lupron Depot.
- Biologic response modifiers: Interferon is the most commonly used drug in this category. It also has an antiviral action.

All of these classes of drugs have a multitude of side effects. The most commonly experienced side effects are nausea, vomiting, diarrhea, rash, alopecia, loss of the ability to reproduce, neurotoxicity (including numbness, tingling, ataxia, and footdrop), visual disturbances, pain in the jaw, severe constipation, oral or GI ulceration, peripheral neuropathy, bone marrow depression, pulmonary disease, fatigue, weakness, osteoporosis, hot flashes, and so on.

Another type of drug administered in cancer therapy is the radioactive isotope. Sometimes radioactive material is planted inside the body in the form of capsules, needles, or seeds. Clients receiving such treatment should not be massaged until they are no longer a danger to others around them as certified by their physician.

Gardasil is a new vaccine given by injection and is used to prevent genital warts and cervical/vaginal cancers caused by certain types of human papillomavirus (HPV) in girls and young women. HPV can cause genital warts, cancer of the cervix, and various cancers of the vulva or vagina.

DRUGS THAT TREAT THE ENDOCRINE SYSTEM

The endocrine system regulates many important activities of the body. The term *endocrine* is a reference to a hormone, an internal secretion, which is produced by a ductless gland that secretes directly into the bloodstream. Hormones can be natural or synthetically produced. The four classes discussed here are pituitary hormones, adrenal corticosteroids, thyroid medications, and antidiabetic drugs. Hormones that affect the reproductive system are discussed under that category.

Relevance for the Massage Therapist

Treatment for clients taking hormones varies, depending on the type of hormone therapy they are undergoing. Hormones can affect the entire body. Generally speaking, the massage therapist should be aware of thin skin and easy bruising and adjust pressure as needed, using gentler techniques. For example, poor circulation and slow healing are some symptoms of type 2 diabetes; other symptoms include excessive weight gain, excessive thirst and urination, weakness, and vision problems. Massage therapists should be aware of these symptoms and refer clients to their physicians for approval of treatment if they have not already consulted with them. Massage can be very helpful to diabetic clients, improving their circulation and helping them to cope with stress more effectively. In addition, massage can help to lower blood glucose. This in turn might help the patient to lower the dosage of any medications, under a physician's supervision, of course. The therapist must also be aware of the signs and symptoms of hyperglycemia and hypoglycemia. Therapists should have some juice available should the patient experience a hypoglycemic attack during or after the treatment. To avoid major disruptions to the client's blood sugar, the therapist should treat the patient in the middle of their medication's dose, rather than at the beginning or the end. Therapists must also be aware if the patient has an insulin pump and avoid that area during treatment. The therapist must also pay particular attention to the level of pressure used or the use of heat therapies, because many diabetic clients not only bruise easily but also have decreased sensation owing to neuropathies.

Clients who are taking steroids sometimes find that their skin is easily irritated or inflamed. Therapists should be careful to avoid any techniques that might exacerbate these symptoms and be careful not to pull and tear any tissue.

Clients who are taking estrogen, birth control pills, or who are on hormone replacement therapy can develop problems with blood clots. Therapists should be mindful of the signs and symptoms of blood clots and refer these clients to a physician immediately if they suspect that a clot is present or if they notice excessive or unusual edema. Symptoms of a blood clot in the leg, when a clot obstructs blood flow and causes inflammation, include swelling, gradual onset of pain, redness, warmth to the touch, worsening leg pain when bending the foot, leg cramps (especially at night), and a bluish or whitish discoloration of the skin.

In general, massage can help to reduce stress and help balance the entire system, improving circulation and helping medications to move more freely through the system, as well as reducing any stagnation of fluids and swellings.

The classes of hormones are discussed in the next sections.

Pituitary Hormones

The pituitary is called the *master gland* of the body, because it regulates the functions of the other glands. It secretes four hormones: somatotropin, adrenocorticotropic hormone (ACTH), thyroid-stimulating hormone (TSH), and gonadotropic hormones (follicle-stimulating hormone [FSH], luteinizing hormone [LH], luteotropic hormone [LTH]). Abnormalities are treated by an endocrinologist. Two examples of medications used are Acthar and ACTH.

Adrenal Corticosteroids

Adrenal corticosteroids are secreted by the adrenal glands, which are located next to the kidneys. Their job is to suppress the body's response to infections or trauma. They are used for acute symptoms of inflammation, swelling, and when symptoms need to be suppressed. They are also used when secretions of the pituitary or adrenal glands are deficient. Corticosteroid therapy should be used on a short-term basis, and it can be used to treat conditions such as allergic reactions with rash or hives, flare-ups of rheumatoid arthritis, psoriasis, asthma, sarcoidosis, cancers, organ transplants, and ulcerative colitis. Long-term use of corticosteroids can suppress the pituitary gland and create atrophy, making the body unable to produce its own hormones. Steroids should therefore be used on a short-term basis only, and withdrawal should always be gradual.

Side Effects: Adrenocortical insufficiency, delayed wound healing and increased susceptibility to infections, muscle pain or weakness, osteoporosis, stunting of growth in children, cataracts, nausea, vomiting or diarrhea, hemorrhage, or easy bruising.

Contraindications or Cautions: Long-term use, viral or bacterial infections, fungal infections, cirrhosis, hypothyroidism, hypertension, diabetes, glaucoma, children, pregnant and lactating women, and history of seizures.

Examples: Cortone, Decadron, Florinef, Medrol, prednisone, Deltasone, Aristocort, and Kenalog.

Thyroid Medications

These medications can be natural or synthetic. They are used as replacement therapy for hypothyroidism caused by deficient thyroid function. Hypothyroidism causes the metabolism to slow, with symptoms of fatigue, dry skin, weight gain, sensitivity to cold, and irregular menstruation. This condition is diagnosed by blood tests, and periodic lab monitoring is necessary to maintain the correct dosage.

Side Effects: Usually caused by overdosage and can include palpitations, tachycardia, cardiac arrhythmias, increased blood pressure, nervousness, tremors, headache, insomnia, weight loss, diarrhea, intolerance to heat, or menstrual irregularities.

Contraindications or Cautions: Cardiovascular disease, elderly clients, and diabetes.

Examples: Synthroid, Levothyroid, and Levoxyl.

Antithyroid Medications

These drugs are used to treat hyperthyroidism.

Side Effects: Rash, urticaria, pruritis, or blood dyscrasias.

Contraindications or Cautions: Long-term therapy, patients older than 40 years, pregnant and lactating women, and liver disease.

Examples: Tapazole and PTU.

Antidiabetic Drugs

These drugs are used to lower blood glucose levels in persons with impaired metabolism of carbohydrates, fats, and proteins. There are two main types of diabetes: type 1, or insulin-dependent (IDDM), and type 2, or non–insulin-dependent (NIDDM). Type 2 has also been called *adult onset* because in the past it was usually found in adults more than 40 years old. In recent years, however, it has been discovered frequently in children and young adults because of the increase in obesity in children. Diabetes that occurs in pregnancy is called *gestational diabetes.*

Insulin is used for type 1 diabetes when there is insufficient insulin production from the islets of Langerhans in the pancreas. It is also given to clients with type 2 diabetes who cannot balance their blood glucose levels with diet and oral drugs. Traditionally, insulin was prepared from either beef or pork pancreas. Pork insulins are still used, but other forms, such as biosynthetic insulin (Humulin) and semisynthetic insulins (Iletin II purified), are available.

Hyperglycemia or elevated blood glucose can result from undiagnosed diabetes, not enough insulin, infections, emotional stress, trauma, pregnancy, or other endocrine disorders. Symptoms include excessive thirst, dehydration, anorexia, unexplained weight loss, frequent urination, weakness, or vision problems.

Hypoglycemia or lowered blood glucose can result from an overdose of insulin, not eating enough (e.g., dieting), excessive exercise, or change in the type of insulin. Symptoms include increased perspiration, irritability, confusion, tremors, headaches, tingling in the fingers, or blurry vision.

Persons who have type 2 diabetes sometimes are treated with dietary changes alone or with a combination of dietary changes and oral antidiabetic drugs. There are several classes of these drugs with differing modes of action, and often they are combined in treatment. They are called first-generation sulfonylureas, second-generation sulfonylureas, alpha-glucosidase inhibitors, biguanides, benzoic acid derivatives, and thiazolidinediones. It should be noted that many of these medications interact negatively with many other medications such as beta blockers, alcohol, NSAIDS, thyroid hormones, diuretics, steroids, oral contraceptives, and others.

Side Effects: GI distress, skin reactions, liver dysfunction, weakness, fatigue, headaches, or hypoglycemia.

Contraindications or Cautions: Liver and kidney dysfunction, severe infections, debilitated or malnourished persons, pregnant and lactating women, and children.

Examples: Amaryl, Glucotrol, Diabeta, Micronase, Glynase, Precose, Glyset, Glucophage, Prandin, Prandimet, Actos, Byetta and Avandia.

The FDA has approved a rapid-acting insulin called Apidra for treatment of children with diabetes.

REPRODUCTIVE SYSTEM MEDICATIONS

There are four main classes of hormones that regulate the functions of the reproductive system: gonadotropic, androgens, estrogens, and progestins. The gonadotropic hormones include FSH, which catalyzes the development of ovarian follicles in women and the production of sperm in the male testes; LH, which works with FSH to facilitate secretion of estrogen, ovulation, and development of the corpus luteum; and LTH, which stimulates the production of progesterone by the corpus luteum and secretion of milk by the mammary glands.

Relevance for the Massage Therapist

Therapists should be aware that blood clots are a potential side effect of estrogen therapy. Therapists should be on the lookout for easy bruising and use more gentle techniques as needed. They should also know the signs of blood clotting. Clients should be referred to their physicians immediately if the therapist suspects the presence of blood clots. Increased fluid retention is also possible when a client is taking estrogens and progestins. Massage improves the movement of blood and fluids throughout the system and helps to reduce edema. Any highly unusual signs should be noted and the client referred to a physician. Hormones can certainly affect emotions as well, and massage can be of great benefit in helping clients manage stress, balance the emotional states, and maintain a greater sense of wellness.

When treating clients on thyroid medication, remember that the thyroid is greatly affected by increasing stress, which, in turn, can affect how much medication a person needs to take. Massage can help to maintain emotional wellbeing, thus potentially reducing the need for higher dosages of medication.

Androgens—Male Hormones

Androgens stimulate the development of male characteristics and include testosterone and androsterone. Although these hormones are used in male subjects who show deficiency symptoms such as impotency, they are also used in women with advanced breast cancer, endometriosis, or fibrocystic breast disease. Use of anabolic steroids by athletes, especially teenagers, to build muscles and physique is illegal and potentially very dangerous. In addition to the side effects listed here, such drugs can produce psychosis, paranoia, depression, mania, and aggressive and violent behavior.

Side Effects: Edema, acne, deficient sperm production, increased or decreased libido, anxiety, depression, or headache.

Contraindications or Cautions: Cardiac, renal or hepatic disease; elderly men (can stimulate cancer), boys who have not yet reached puberty, and diabetic clients.

Examples: Danocrine, Android, Deca-Durabolin, Depo-Testosterone, and Estratest.

Drugs for Impotency

The most popular drug in this category is Viagra, which treats male erectile dysfunction.

Side Effects: Headaches, flushing, abnormal vision, dizziness, nasal congestion, dyspepsia, urinary tract infection, diarrhea, rash, angina, palpitations, or low blood pressure.

Contraindications or Cautions: Cardiovascular disease, kidney or liver disease, pregnant and lactating women, or use in children. These drugs should not be taken by people taking nitrates. **Examples:** Viagra, Cialis, and Levitra.

Estrogens

Estrogens are the female sex hormones produced mainly by the ovaries and secondarily by the adrenal glands. These hormones produce female sexual characteristics such as breast size, and during the menstrual cycle they produce the proper environment for the fertilization, implantation, and growth of the embryo. They also affect the secretions of the hormones FSH and LH from the anterior pituitary gland, which can prevent lactation and stop ovulation. At one time, estrogen therapy was extremely common for women entering menopause; however, recent studies have shown that the health risks are increased for women using these medications. The WHO now classifies estrogen as a known carcinogen.

Estrogen therapy is used in contraceptives, to treat menstrual problems, to treat menopausal symptoms, to prevent osteoporosis in postmenopausal women, to treat vaginal dryness, to inhibit lactation in nursing mothers, and in treatment for men with advanced prostate cancer.

Side Effects: Increased risk of stroke; myocardial infarction; thromboembolic problems; GI effects including vomiting, diarrhea, or constipation; weight gain; edema; skin discolorations; increased triglyceride levels; folic acid deficiency; liver disease; breakthrough vaginal bleeding;

increased risk of cervical erosion and candidiasis; headaches; migraines; depression; visual problems; gallbladder disease; cancer of the uterus; endometrial cancer; or breast cancer.

Contraindications or Cautions: Thromboembolus, stroke, myocardial infarction, liver disease, gallbladder disease, cancer, migraines, shortness of breath, seizures, asthma, kidney disease, and pregnant women.

Examples: Estrace, Estraderm, Depo-Estradiol, Premarin, Estratab, Climara, Vivelle and newly approved Premarin vaginal cream to treat moderate to severe post-menopausal dyspareunia (painful sexual intercourse).

Progesterone

Progesterone is a hormone secreted by the corpus luteum and adrenal glands. It is responsible for changes in the uterine endometrium in the second half of the menstrual cycle and is used to treat amenorrhea, abnormal uterine bleeding, and contraception. It is also used in postmenopausal therapy and as adjunctive therapy in the treatment of advanced endometrial or breast cancer. Synthetically produced progesterone drugs are called *progestins.*

Side Effects: Menstrual problems, breakthrough bleeding, spotting, edema, weight gain, nausea, breast tenderness, rash, headaches, depression, thromboembolic disorders, or decrease in bone density.

Contraindications or Cautions: History of depression, thromboembolic disorders, cardiovascular disease, liver disease, pregnant women, and cardiac or renal dysfunction.

Examples: Provera, Depo-Provera, Megace, and Cycrin.

Contraceptives

Contraceptives can be either estrogen-progestin combinations or progestin-only contraceptives. They are used to prevent pregnancy and to treat endometriosis, painful periods, heavy periods, irregular periods, acne, ovarian cysts, pelvic inflammatory disease, benign breast disease, and ectopic pregnancy.

Side Effects: Nausea, edema, weight gain or loss, breakthrough bleeding, mood changes, libido changes, migraine headaches, severe depression, blurry vision, or loss of vision.

Contraindications or Cautions: Thrombophlebitis or thromboembolic disorders, history of cerebrovascular accident, breast cancer or estrogen-dependent malignancy, pregnant and lactating women, liver disease, smoking, hypertension, diabetes, and gallbladder disease. They should not be prescribed to female clients older than age 35.

Examples: Ovral, Ovcon, Norinyl, Loestrin, Ortho-Novum, Tri-Norinyl, Depo-Provera, Nortrel and Paragard.

Lupron and Depot

These are used as antineoplastic drugs to stop the growth of hormone-dependent tumors. They are used in the treatment of prostate and breast cancers. Sometimes they are combined with tamoxifen for the treatment of breast cancer.

Side Effects: Hot flashes, headaches, insomnia, mood swings, nasal congestion, or weight gain or loss.

Contraindications or Cautions: Not to be used as a contraceptive or during pregnancy or lactation.

Examples: Lupron and Lupron Depot.

Fertility Medication

Clomid is a drug used for treatment of infertility. If Clomid on its own is unsuccessful, then injectable hormones to stimulate ovulation are sometimes recommended.

Side Effects: Nausea, vomiting, nervousness, insomnia, or multiple pregnancies.

Contraindications or Cautions: Ovarian cysts, endometrial cancer; liver, thyroid, adrenal disease.

Example: Clomid, Serophene, Novarel, Follistim, Pergonal, Factrel, Lupron, Antagon.

ANTI-INFECTIVE DRUGS

The most important first step in the treatment of infections is to identify the pathogen and then the specific medication to which it is sensitive. Often the physician orders a broad-spectrum antibiotic while waiting for the results of culture and sensitivity tests. This can sometimes cause additional problems if the organism is resistant to the antibiotic, or if it turns out that the pathogen is not bacterial but viral. Because antibiotics do not discriminate between good and bad bacteria, taking antibiotics when the infection is really viral can often compromise the immune system and inhibit the client's ability to heal from the organism. In addition, certain bacteria that are immune to specific antibiotics can pass that immunity to other types of bacteria. The result is that the antibiotics that are ineffective for one type of infection (e.g., respiratory) can prove to be ineffective for another type of infection, such as a urinary tract infection.

Relevance to the Massage Therapist

Persons taking anti-infective agents have a compromised immune system. Care must be taken by the massage therapist when treating immunocompromised clients so that they are not exposed to any infections, colds, or drafts. If the therapist is sick with a cold, no clients should be treated. Conversely, if the client is ill, it might be advisable to reschedule the appointment if the client is in the contagious stage of the disease, rather than expose the therapist and other clients to the pathogens. If there is inclement weather, the client should be instructed to reschedule rather than be exposed to conditions that can exacerbate the illness. GI distress is a common side effect of these medications. Massage can be very helpful for treating constipation or diarrhea, nausea, and abdominal bloating, as well as calming the client.

Of course, universal precautions should always be followed, especially when treating anyone suffering from pathogens.

Antibiotics

A major problem that has resulted from the overuse of antibiotics is the emergence of resistant strains of bacteria such as methicillin-resistant *Staphylococcus aureus* (MRSA) and *Clostridium difficile* (known colloquially as *C-dif)*, a bacteria that causes violent diarrhea and which has to be treated with vancomycin or metronidazole. This infection happens when a person takes antibiotics that kill off the healthy flora of the colon. Many antibiotics that at one time were in the forefront of the treatment of bacterial infections are no longer effective against these pathogens. Researchers are scrambling to discover new drugs so that organisms such as tuberculosis and *Staphylococcus aureus* can be kept under control. That is why antibiotics should never be used to treat the common cold, which is generally caused by a virus, even though patients, in their ignorance, often demand antibiotics from their physician.

Although there are numerous antibiotics, the side effects are generally of three types:

1. Allergic reactions, resulting in rashes, hives, or low fevers. In such cases, medication should be terminated. Sometimes a severe reaction, such as anaphylaxis, can follow a mild reaction and can be life threatening. *Anaphylaxis* is an allergic hypersensitivity reaction of the body to a foreign protein or drug. It can lead to anaphylactic shock, which can sometimes result in unconsciousness and death.
2. Tissue damage, hearing loss, kidney damage, liver damage, or blood dyscrasias (abnormalities in blood components). Sometimes the damage is permanent or can be reversed when the medication is discontinued.
3. Superinfections—new infections caused by resistant bacteria or fungi, as a result of killing off the normal bacteria in the intestines or mucous membranes, particularly when broad-spectrum antibiotics are used. It is helpful to eat yogurt or take a broad-spectrum probiotic supplement to replenish the gut continually with good bacteria.

Other common side effects can include headaches, diarrhea, constipation, nausea, vomiting, or blurry vision.

Contraindications and cautions especially apply to elderly clients, pregnant and lactating women, and anyone with a history of kidney or liver disease. Quinolones should not be prescribed to those younger than 18 years, and tetracyclines should never be given to children under the age of 9.

The most common groupings of antibiotics are discussed in the next sections.

Aminoglycosides

These drugs are used to treat infections caused by gram-negative bacteria such as *Escherichia coli, Pseudomonas,* and *Salmonella,* as well as gram-positive bacteria such as *Staphylococcus aureus.* Aminoglycosides are used for short-term treatment of serious infections only when other, less-toxic, antibiotics have failed. These antibiotics are generally administered intravenously because they do not absorb well in the GI tract.

Side Effects: Kidney disease, hearing loss, vertigo, headaches, tremors, numbness, seizures, blurry vision, or rash.

Contraindications or Cautions: Tinnitus, vertigo, hearing loss, kidney dysfunction, pregnant or nursing women, infants, or elderly people.

Examples: Garamycin, and Nebcin.

Cephalosporins

These drugs are semisynthetic antibiotics that are produced by a fungus. They are related to penicillin; therefore, clients who are allergic to penicillin can also be allergic to cephalosporins. They are broad spectrum and are active against many gram-positive and gram-negative bacteria.

Side Effects: Hypersensitivity, rash, edema, anaphylaxis (especially in those allergic to penicillin), blood dyscrasias, kidney disease, liver disease, nausea, vomiting, diarrhea, seizures, or respiratory distress.

Contraindications or Cautions: Renal disease, known allergies to penicillin, prolonged use leading to superinfections, severe colitis, pregnant or nursing women, and children.

Examples: Keflex, Ceftin, Suprax, Maxipime, Ceclor, and Rocephin.

Macrolides

These drugs are used to treat infections of the respiratory tract, skin (e.g., acne), and some sexually transmitted infections when the client is allergic to penicillin. Erythromycins are the best known antibiotics in this class and are considered to be the least toxic of all the antibiotics. They are chosen first if they are effective against an organism, rather than using more toxic antibiotics and running the risk of serious side effects. Pregnant women and children, for example, are good candidates for macrolides, if necessary. Unfortunately, there are now many erythromycin-resistant strains of bacteria. Erythromycin also has another use unrelated to its antibacterial activity—it is used in certain motility disorders of the GI tract because it stimulates gastric emptying.

Side Effects: Anorexia, nausea, vomiting, diarrhea, cramps, urticaria, and rash; superinfections.

Contraindications or Cautions: Liver dysfunction and alcoholism.

Examples: Biaxin, Zithromax, Zmax, Erythromycin, EES, E-Mycin, Eryc, and Ilosone.

Penicillins

These drugs are created by a particular species of fungus and treat many strains of streptococci, staphylococcus, and meningococcal infections, including respiratory and intestinal infections. Penicillins are the preferred antibiotic for treating gonorrhea and syphilis. Amoxicillin has been used to treat *Helicobacter pylori* infections in ulcer disease. Some semisynthetic penicillins have a broad spectrum of activity and are called *extended-spectrum penicillins.* Augmentin and Timentin are examples. A growing number of pathogens have become resistant to many forms of penicillin.

Side Effects: Hypersensitivity reactions range from rash to anaphylaxis, superinfections, nausea, vomiting, diarrhea, blood dyscrasias, kidney and liver disease, confusion, anxiety, or seizures.

Contraindications or Cautions: History of allergy to any drugs, kidney dysfunction, and electrolyte imbalance.

Examples: Amoxil, Omnipen, Bicillin L-A, and ampicillin.

Quinolones

Drugs such as Cipro (ciprofloxacin) or Levaquin are used to treat infections of the urinary tract, respiratory tract, GI tract, skin, bones, and joints. These medications have potentially severe side effects, especially in children and elderly patients. Unfortunately, some pathogens have already demonstrated resistance to the quinolones; therefore, these drugs should be used only when other antibiotics have failed or the client is allergic to other antibiotics. These medications should not be used in children younger than 18.

Side Effects: Nausea, vomiting, diarrhea, abdominal pain, colitis, headaches, dizziness, confusion, irritability, seizures, anxiety, superinfections, rash, or phototoxicity. Can cause injury to tendons.

Contraindications or Cautions: Elderly clients, children, adolescents, pregnant and lactating women, severe kidney disease, seizure disorders, and cardiac disease.

Examples: Cipro, Levaquin, Noroxin, and Maxaquin.

Tetracyclines

Tetracyclines are broad-spectrum antibiotics used to treat infections caused by rickettsia, Chlamydia, or uncommon bacteria. Severe cases of acne, Rocky Mountain spotted fever, Lyme disease, and atypical pneumonia are treated with tetracycline. Unfortunately, the number of organisms resistant to tetracyclines is growing, and therefore they should be used only after other antibiotics have failed.

Side Effects: Nausea, vomiting, diarrhea, superinfections, photosensitivity, discolored teeth in the fetus or children, or vertigo.

Contraindications or Cautions: Pregnant and lactating women, children younger than age 8, clients exposed to direct sunlight, liver or kidney disease, esophageal obstruction or dysfunction.

Examples: Sumycin, Vibramycin (doxycycline), and Acromycin.

Sulfonamides

These are some of the oldest anti-infective drugs. Because of increasing resistance to them, they are now used mostly in combination with other medications.

Side Effects: Rash, dermatitis, nausea, vomiting, diarrhea, high fever, headaches, stomatitis, conjunctivitis, blood dyscrasias, liver toxicity, kidney damage, or hypersensitivity reactions that can be fatal.

Contraindications or Cautions: Impaired liver or kidney function, urinary obstruction, blood dyscrasias, severe allergies, asthma, and pregnant or lactating women.

Examples: Azulfidine, Septra, and Bactrim.

Other Anti-infective Drugs

These include clindamycin (Cleocin), which is used to treat severe respiratory tract infections, severe pelvic infections, and certain bacteria associated with AIDS. Flagyl is a synthetic combination antibacterial and antiprotozoal drug useful in treating Crohn's disease and rosacea. Vancomycin (Vancocin) is the drug of last resort, which is used in the treatment of life-threatening infections when all other medications have failed. For example, it is the drug of choice for MRSA. Strains of pathogens are becoming increasingly resistant to this drug, however.

Antifungals

Antifungals are used to treat specific fungi, such as Candida or tinea. The medications used are very different in their actions. Some are administered intravenously for severe infections. Others are given orally, and some are used topically. Common side effects are headaches, fatigue, nausea, vomiting, diarrhea, and rash.

Side Effects: Headaches, chills, fever, hypotension, malaise, muscle and joint pain, weakness, anorexia, nausea, vomiting, cramps, anemia, or hypokalemia, which can lead to congestive heart failure.

Contraindications or Cautions: Children, pregnant and nursing women, and kidney or liver disease.

Examples: Diflucan, Cancidas, Lamisil, Grifulvin V, Abelcet, and Nystatin.

Antituberculosis Drugs

These drugs are used to treat tuberculosis (TB) if someone has been exposed to the disease, even though the person might not have symptoms, or if the TB test result is positive, and of course if someone has an active case of TB.

Side Effects: Nausea, vomiting, diarrhea, dizziness, blurry vision, headaches, fatigue, numbness, weakness, liver disease, or hypersensitivity reactions.

Contraindications or Cautions: Chronic liver disease, alcoholism, gout, kidney dysfunction, diabetes, ocular defects, pregnant and lactating women, and children.

Examples: INH, Myambutol, Rifadin, and Streptomycin.

Antivirals

Antivirals are used to treat a range of viruses and they share common side effects.

- Acyclovir (Zovirax, Valtrex) is used to treat initial outbreaks of herpes simplex, herpes zoster (shingles), and chickenpox infections.
- Amantadine (Symmetrel) is used to treat influenza A virus strains.
- Neuraminidase inhibitors (Tamiflu, Relenza) are a newer group of antivirals used to treat influenza A and B virus strains.
- Ribavirin (Virazole) is used to treat severe lower respiratory tract infections in children and in adults, hantavirus and hepatitis C.
- Interferons are used to treat AIDS-related Kaposi's sarcoma, chronic hepatitis B, and some cancers.

Side Effects: Nausea, vomiting, abdominal pain, diarrhea, rash, fatigue, or headaches.

Contraindications or Cautions: Children, pregnant women, and lactating women.

Drugs to Treat AIDS

These medications are called *antiretrovirals* and are classified by their mechanism of action. They include protease inhibitors, nucleoside reverse transcriptase inhibitors (NRTIs), and non-nucleoside reverse transcriptase inhibitors (NNRTIs). AIDS is often treated through a combination of drugs; this treatment is called *cocktail therapy*. Treatment does not eradicate the disease; instead it is aimed at attacking the virus at different stages in its evolution. All of these drugs potentially have the standard GI effects—nausea, vomiting, abdominal pain, and diarrhea, and can have much more severe adverse reactions, some having a high mortality rate.

Side Effects: Nausea, vomiting, diarrhea, hyperglycemia, exacerbation of existing diabetes, spontaneous bleeding, kidney stones, liver dysfunction, bone marrow suppression, pancreatitis, hypersensitivity reactions that can be fatal, severe rashes, dizziness, insomnia, confusion, hallucinations, or amnesia.

Contraindications or Cautions: Pregnant and lactating women, and children.

Examples: Viracept, Retrovir, Sustiva, Epivir, Videx, Combivir, Crixivan, Zerit, Aptivus, Kaletra, Norvir, and Fortovase.

Antiurinary Drugs

Most of these drugs prevent the growth of bacteria rather than kill them. They are usually used for recurrent urinary tract infections.

Side Effects: Nausea, vomiting, diarrhea, numbness, weakness, headaches, dizziness, weak muscles, or anemia.

Contraindications or Cautions: Liver or kidney impairment, anemia, diabetes, electrolyte abnormalities, asthma, pregnant and lactating women, and infants younger than 1 month old.

Examples: Macrodantin, Trimpex, and Macrobid.

ANALGESICS, SEDATIVES, AND HYPNOTICS

The purpose of analgesics is to relieve pain, that of sedatives is to calm, and hypnotics are to help the person to sleep.

Relevance to the Massage Therapist

Massage therapy can be very helpful for pain reduction and also for relaxation and calming patients. With consistent massage therapy treatments, a client might be able to reduce the dosage of medications. Massage therapists should work in conjunction with the client's physician in such matters. Some analgesics such as aspirin thin the blood and create the potential for bleeding and easy bruising. Therapists must be aware of such potential and adjust their pressure accordingly. In addition, the client's ability to discern pressure is sometimes impaired owing to the effects of the medication. Therapists must therefore be mindful that the client might not be aware enough to know whether the pressure is too much. Therefore, therapists should avoid using deep pressure techniques unless they are certain that they are not mistakenly injuring the client. Many of these drugs are also constipating, and massage can certainly help with this problem.

Analgesics

Analgesics can be classified as opioid (narcotics), nonopioid (non-narcotics), and adjuvant.

Opioid Analgesics

Opioid analgesics are a controlled substance and include natural opium alkaloids such as morphine and codeine as well as the synthetics such as Demerol and Darvon. Opioids tend to cause tolerance and dependence and can cause severe withdrawal symptoms if the drug is abruptly discontinued. For clients with bona-fide pain, the likelihood of dependence is extremely slim. A massage therapist must have a clear understanding of dependence, tolerance, and addiction.

Side Effects: Confusion, euphoria, restlessness, headaches, dizziness, nausea, vomiting, diarrhea, or physical and emotional dependence.

Contraindications or Cautions: CNS depression, liver and kidney disease, hypothyroidism, COPD, addiction-prone personalities, elderly clients, and pregnant and lactating women.

Examples: Demerol, Darvon, Dilaudid, OxyContin, Morphine, Percocet, Tylenol with codeine, Vicodin, and Tapentadol, a new drug that is a centrally acting oral analgesic. It is a unique drug with two mechanisms of action, combining mu-opioid receptor agonism and norepinephrine reuptake inhibition in a single molecule.

Nonopioid Analgesics

Many nonopioid analgesics are available OTC and are heavily advertised and very popular. Nonopioids are used to relieve mild-to-moderate pain, fever, and inflammatory conditions such as arthritis. They are also used with opioids to manage severe, acute, or chronic pain. The salicylates (e.g., aspirin, salsalate, choline magnesium trisalicylate) are used mostly for their analgesic, anti-inflammatory, and antipyretic qualities. Ibuprofen is also used as an analgesic. (NSAIDs are discussed elsewhere in this appendix.) Acetaminophen (Tylenol) has analgesic and antipyretic properties but has almost no effect on inflammation. Aspirin and acetaminophen are frequently combined to treat migraine headaches (Excedrin) and are combined with opioids for severe pain.

Side Effects of Salicylates: Bleeding, frequent bruising, tinnitus, drowsiness, dizziness, depression, or rash.

Contraindications or Cautions: GI bleeding, liver disease, asthma, kidney disease, pregnant and lactating women, and Hodgkin's disease.

Side Effects of Acetaminophen: Severe liver toxicity, rash, renal insufficiency.

Examples: Tylenol, Panadol, and Genapap Extra Strength.

Tramadol (Ultram)

Tramadol is a synthetic analgesic the effect of which is similar to that of opioids; however, it is a nonopioid and it is not a controlled substance.

Side Effects: Dizziness, headache, lethargy, nausea, constipation, anxiety, confusion, or rash.

Contraindications or Cautions: Head injury, liver and kidney disease, seizures, pregnant or nursing women, and children younger than 16.

Example: Tramadol.

Adjuvant Analgesics

These medications enhance the analgesic effect when used in conjunction with opioids and nonopioids. The two main classes of these drugs are anticonvulsants and tricyclic antidepressants. Anticonvulsants such as Dilantin and Tegretol are often used for the management of nerve pain from neuralgia, herpes, and cancer. Tricyclic antidepressants such as Elavil, Pamelor and Tofranil are used in the treatment of herpes, arthritis, diabetes, cancer, migraine or tension headaches, insomnia, and depression. Side effects of antidepressants include dry mouth, urinary retention, constipation, sedation, and arrhythmias. Side effects from anticonvulsants can also include dizziness, confusion, rash, nausea, vomiting, and diarrhea.

Sedatives and Hypnotics

These are controlled substances used in small doses to calm the client, and in larger doses to help the client to sleep. There are two classes of sedative-hypnotics: barbiturates and nonbarbiturates. These drugs can foster psychological and physical dependence, so they should not be used for long periods except in the treatment of epilepsy. Prolonged use produces a severe rebound effect, resulting in nightmares and hallucinations. Gradual reduction of dosage is essential to avoid rebound insomnia.

Barbiturates

Barbiturates are sedatives that can be very dangerous. Many suicides and fatalities from accidental overdose have been reported, especially when combined with central nervous system (CNS) depressants or alcohol. Children or elderly persons can manifest opposite behavior with these medications, such as hyperactivity, confusion, or hallucinations. Because of slower metabolism, barbiturates remain in the system longer and pose a greater threat to the elderly or weakened patient.

Side Effects: Depression, headache, fatigue, nausea, vomiting, constipation, rash, confusion, coma, or fatal overdoses.

Contraindications or Cautions: Elderly or debilitated clients; pregnant and lactating women; children; liver or kidney disease; depressed, mentally unstable, or suicidal persons; and those with addictive personalities.

Example: Luminal (phenobarbital—also used for seizures).

Nonbarbiturates

Even though these drugs are supposed to be safer than barbiturates, they have also been misused and have resulted in fatalities.

Side Effects: Nausea, vomiting, diarrhea, rash, or dizziness.

Contraindications or Cautions: Hypersensitivity; severe liver or renal impairment; elderly, debilitated, addiction-prone, depressed or mentally unstable people or those with suicidal tendencies; pregnant and lactating women; children; clients with COPD or sleep apnea.

Examples: Dalmane, Restoril, Lunesta, Halcion (rarely used), Ambien, and Sonata.

PSYCHOTROPIC MEDICATIONS, ALCOHOL, AND DRUG ABUSE

Psychotropic drugs are medications that have a therapeutic effect on a person's mind, emotions, and actions. There are several medications that have psychotropic effects that are secondary to their main functions. For example, many analgesics and sedatives can affect mental and emotional behavior.

Relevance for the Massage Therapist

Massage therapy treatments can help clients to relax and handle stress more productively and can also affect the dosage of medication being used. The therapist should be able to communicate with the client's psychiatrist or psychologist so that the client's best interests are served. If the massage therapist's clientele consists of clients who suffer from mental and emotional disorders, the therapist should take additional courses in psychology and study pharmacology further to understand what clients are experiencing and find ways to make the massage treatments better serve them. The mind, body, and emotions are intricately connected in one bioenergy system, and the positive effects of massage therapy and regular treatments can assist clients in moving toward greater well-being. Massage can help energize a depressed client or calm an agitated one. The therapist must assess each client individually and adjust treatment based on the findings. As with all clients, records that chart each session and the effects of the massage treatment should be kept.

The four classes of medications are CNS stimulants, antidepressants, anxiolytics, and antipsychotics.

CNS Stimulants

CNS stimulants are medications that affect the functioning of the CNS. One well-known drug in this class is caffeine citrate. Long-term use with high intake of caffeine in any form can result in tolerance, habituation, and psychological dependence. If caffeine is stopped suddenly, symptoms such as nervousness, anxiety, headaches, and dizziness can result. Because caffeine can cross the placenta and also be present in the milk of nursing mothers, it is generally recommended that pregnant and nursing mothers do not ingest foods and beverages or any drugs, including OTC medications that contain caffeine.

Other CNS stimulants include amphetamines such as Adderall, Ritalin, Concerta, and Dexedrine, all of which are used to treat attention deficit disorder (ADD) syndrome in children older than 6 years and narcolepsy. Prolonged use of CNS stimulants in children with ADD has been reported to suppress normal weight and height patterns temporarily and also to produce or exacerbate motor and vocal tics. Children must be observed very carefully for adverse effects. The use of amphetamines to lose weight is not advised, because tolerance develops very rapidly and a person can develop physical or psychological dependence quickly.

Side Effects: Nervousness, insomnia, irritability, seizures, psychosis, tachycardia, palpitations, hypertension, cardiac arrhythmias, dizziness, headaches, blurry vision, or GI distress.

Contraindications or Cautions: Treatment for obesity; patients suffering from anxiety; history of drug dependence, alcoholism, or eating disorders; hyperthyroidism; pregnant or nursing women; and abrupt withdrawal.

Examples: Cafcit, Adderall, Dexedrine, Ritalin, and Concerta.

Antidepressants

Antidepressants are also known as *mood elevators* and are used primarily to treat clients suffering from depression. Persons who are depressed can have a shortage of the neurotransmitters dopamine, serotonin, or norepinephrine. These substances, which are supposed to travel across the synapse between two neurons, sometimes fail to cross the synapse and instead get reabsorbed by one nerve ending; thus they are unable to perform their function. Clients who have this problem are said to suffer from a chemical imbalance that medication seeks to rectify.

There are four classes of antidepressants: tricyclics, monamine oxidase inhibitors (MAOIs), selective serotonin reuptake inhibitors (SSRIs), and heterocyclic antidepressants. (A new type of antidepressant was recently approved, Pristiq, a serotonin-norepinephrine reuptake inhibitor (SNRI) for adult patients with major depressive disorders.)

Tricyclics

Tricyclics take between two and four weeks to reach maximal effect. They have a mild sedative action and are generally taken many times during the day. Tricyclics generally have many side effects. They are also used as adjuncts in pain control. Tricyclics can interact with other medications, producing more severe side effects.

Side Effects: Dry mouth, increased appetite and weight gain, dizziness, drowsiness, constipation, urinary retention, palpitations, confusion, cardiac arrhythmias, or blurry vision.

Contraindications or Cautions: Cardiac, liver, kidney, and GI disease; elderly patients; glaucoma; obesity; seizures; pregnant and lactating women; use with MAOIs.

Examples: Elavil, Norpramin, Adapin, Tofranil, Pamelor, and Anafranil.

Monoamine Oxidase Inhibitors

MAOIs are used rarely because of potential serious side effects and negative interactions with food and other drugs. Persons stopping tricyclics must wait two weeks before starting MAOIs. These drugs are generally used for atypical depression, panic disorders, or phobias.

Side Effects: Nervousness, agitation, insomnia, headaches, stiff neck, hypertension, tachycardia, palpitations, chest pain, nausea, vomiting, diarrhea, or blurry vision. Interactions of the MAOIs with some drugs and food can cause a hypertensive crisis that can be fatal. Foods containing tyramine, tryptamine, or tryptophan such as yogurt, sour cream, all cheeses, turkey, liver, figs, bananas, and wines must be avoided.

Contraindications or Cautions: Clients with cerebrovascular and liver disease.

Examples: Marplan, Nardil, and Parnate.

Selective Serotonin Reuptake Inhibitors (SSRIs)

These are the first choice of drugs in the treatment of depression. They have fewer side effects and greater safety. Sometimes the client must be on the drug for two to four weeks before effects are seen. These drugs also can interact negatively with other medications such as anticoagulants and beta blockers, as well as other CNS drugs.

Side Effects: Sexual dysfunction, nausea, anorexia, diarrhea, constipation, sweating, insomnia, anxiety, nervousness, tremors, fatigue, dizziness, or headaches.

Contraindications or Cautions: Liver or kidney disease, suicidal history, diabetes, bipolar disorders, eating disorders, pregnant and lactating women. Should never be taken with MAOIs.

Examples: Prozac, Paxil, Zoloft, Celexa, Cymbalta, and Effexor.

Heterocyclic Antidepressants

These drugs are useful in treating severe depression and also in helping with smoking cessation. Some are used to treat clients suffering from both anxiety and depression and also help with the treatment of fibromyalgia. Others are useful for treating the agitation that elderly clients with dementia can experience. Heterocyclic antidepressants should never be taken with MAOIs.

Side Effects: Sleepiness, insomnia, restlessness, agitation, anxiety, dry mouth, dizziness, confusion, or weight gain.

Contraindications or Cautions: Suicidal history, seizures, and cardiac or liver disease.

Examples: Wellbutrin, Remeron, Serzone, and Desyrel (should not be taken by young men).

Antimanic Medications

These drugs are used to treat bipolar (manic-depressive) disorders. Clients must be monitored carefully for signs of toxicity.

Side Effects: GI distress, cardiac arrhythmias, low blood pressure, tremors, thyroid problems, coma, or muscle weakness.

Contraindications or Cautions: Seizure disorders, parkinsonism, cardiovascular and kidney disease, elderly clients, or thyroid disease. Blood levels of clients taking lithium must be monitored.

Examples: Lithobid (lithium), Tegretol, Serequel, Depakote, Stavzor, and Abilify, also used to treat both pediatric and adolescent patients with bipolar disorder and schizophrenia in adolescents.

Anxiolytics

These are medications that treat anxiety and act as minor tranquilizers. They are used for short-term treatment of anxiety, neurosis, some psychosomatic disorders, insomnia, and nausea and vomiting. When given in small doses, these drugs can reduce anxiety without causing drowsiness. Larger doses at bedtime are used for insomnia. These drugs are for short-term use only because persons can become physically and psychologically dependent on them. Withdrawal must be gradual, otherwise severe side effects, such as seizures and psychosis, can develop. Many of the anxiolytics are controlled substances.

Side Effects: Depression, hallucinations, confusion, agitation, bizarre behavior, amnesia, drowsiness, lethargy, headache, rash, or itching.

Contraindications or Cautions: Mental depression, suicidal history, pregnant and lactating women, children, liver and kidney disease, elderly clients, and persons operating machinery.

Examples: Xanax, Librium, Valium, Ativan, BuSpar, and Atarax.

Antipsychotic Medications

These drugs are major tranquilizers and are also called *neuroleptics*. They are used to treat psychoses and severe neuroses, relieve nausea and vomiting, and are used as adjunctive therapy with analgesics. These drugs can interact negatively with several medications such as antihypertensives and anticonvulsants.

Side Effects: Insomnia, agitation, depression, headaches, seizures, dry mouth, blurry vision, fever, jaundice, rash, confusion, drowsiness, weakness, constipation, or anorexia; parkinsonian symptoms such as tremors, drooling; involuntary and often irreversible movements (tardive dyskinesia) such as tics; dystonic reactions (spasms of the head, neck or tongue—more common in children).

Contraindications or Cautions: Seizure disorders, Parkinson's disease, severe depression, and pregnant women.

Examples: Thorazine, Haldol, Compazine, Risperdal, Zyprexa, and Seroquel.

Anticonvulsants

These drugs are used to reduce the severity and frequency of seizures in persons suffering from epilepsy. Although the cause of epilepsy is often unknown, seizures can be associated with disorders such as head trauma, brain tumors, chemical imbalances, cerebrovascular disease, or high fever. Medications should never be stopped abruptly. Drugs can be used to treat petit mal, also known as *absence epilepsy*—a momentary loss of consciousness without falling—or grand mal seizures. Grand mal seizures and temporal lobe seizures are generally treated with Dilantin, which can be combined with other drugs. Another drug, Tegretol, is used mainly for partial seizures. Preventive treatment is difficult because the medications must be adjusted to prevent seizures without sedating the client too much.

Side Effects of Drugs for Petit Mal Seizures: Drowsiness, dizziness, irritability, anorexia, nausea, vomiting, diarrhea, rash, or leukopenia.

Contraindications or Cautions: Liver and kidney disease, and pregnant and lactating women.

Examples: Zarontin, Klonopin, Dapakene, Depakote, Vimpat, and Neurontin.

Side Effects of Drugs for Grand Mal and Partial Seizures: Sedation, dizziness, headaches, blurry vision, GI distress, or rash.

Contraindications or Cautions: Liver disease, kidney disease, diabetes, low blood pressure, blood diseases, and congestive heart failure.

Examples: Dilantin and Tegretol.

Antiparkinsonian Medications

These drugs are used to treat Parkinson's disease, a neurologic disease with symptoms of muscle tremors, rigidity, and weakness of muscles. Medications are aimed at relieving symptoms. Sinemet is the main drug used for long-term treatment. Eldepryl is another drug used to treat Parkinson's disease. It is never used alone but is added to Sinemet when Sinemet becomes less potent or less effective. The dosage of Sinemet can be reduced to lessen the side effects. Use of Eldepryl is contraindicated with certain drugs when severe side effects can result, including death. A new drug for Parkinson's is Stalevo, which is a combination of three drugs: carbidopa, levodopa, and entacapone to provide longer-lasting relief from symptoms.

Side Effects: These are numerous and generally serious. They include anorexia, nausea, vomiting, anxiety, confusion, depression, psychosis, agitation, dizziness, syncope, low blood pressure, or involuntary movements.

Contraindications or Cautions: Bronchial asthma, emphysema, heart disease, low blood pressure, diabetes, kidney or liver disease, glaucoma, psychoses, and pregnant and lactating women. Clients must be weaned off the medication.

Examples: Sinemet and Eldepryl.

Anticholinergic Drugs

These drugs can help with mild forms of the disease and for symptoms induced by drugs. They include Cogentin, Artane, and Symmetrel (amantadine).

Side Effects: Dizziness, drowsiness, constipation, confusion, depression, nausea, tachycardia, dry mouth, urinary retention, headache, or insomnia.

Contraindications or Cautions: Elderly clients and benign prostatic disease.

Examples: Cogentin, Artane, and Symmetrel.

Drugs to Treat Alzheimer's Disease

These medications do not cure the disease but are aimed at slowing its progress. They include Cognex, Aricept, and Exelon. All of these drugs produce GI distress (e.g., nausea, vomiting, anorexia) and other side effects that can be severe.

Alcohol

Alcohol is perhaps the biggest drug problem in the United States today. Alcohol can be considered both a psychotropic drug and a CNS depressant. It is pharmacologically similar to ether and is rapidly absorbed from the GI tract into the bloodstream, causing excitement, sedation, and, finally, anesthesia. It decreases a person's ability to make decisions and impairs memory as well as mental and emotional functioning. Prolonged use affects most organs of the body, causing liver and pancreatic damage, malnutrition, cardiovascular effects, GI damage, and permanent CNS damage.

Side Effects of Chronic Alcoholism: Frequent falls and accidents, blackouts, memory loss, neuritis, muscular weakness, tremors, irritability, gastroenteritis, or neglect of personal appearance and responsibilities.

Drug Abuse

Drug abuse is the use of drugs for recreation or for purposes other than therapeutic reasons, for example, for weight loss or to improve athletic performance. Drug addiction means that the person has psychological dependence, physical dependence, tolerance, and withdrawal reactions with physiologic effects. Sometimes clients can become addicted to medications, especially when pain relief is being sought. Some of the major drugs that are abused are discussed in the next section.

Amphetamines

These are known as "uppers" and are sometimes illegally used for weight loss. Symptoms of chronic abuse are anorexia, mental confusion, social withdrawal, paranoia, or continuous teeth grinding.

Marijuana

This drug has euphoriant, sedative, CNS depressant, and hallucinogenic properties. Marijuana as a medication, however, can be very helpful for nausea induced by chemotherapy, for treatment of glaucoma, and as an appetite stimulant for persons suffering from cancer or AIDS. It has also been reported to have beneficial effects for persons suffering from multiple sclerosis, muscle spasms, and chronic pain. Cannabis seeds have been used traditionally in Chinese herbal medicine, in conjunction with other herbs, for the treatment of constipation. Despite its potential benefits, the U.S. government considers marijuana illegal to possess; however, several states including Oregon, Hawaii, Colorado, and California allow marijuana use for medical reasons.

Side Effects: Short-term memory loss, slowed reflexes, apathy, increased heart rate, or lung irritation.

Cocaine

Cocaine is a CNS stimulant that produces euphoria. Its only approved medical use is for topical application as a local anesthetic. Cocaine is highly addictive and a growing health problem in the United States. It can be sniffed or snorted, which can damage the mucous membranes of the nose. Intravenous use can be fatal, and smoking "crack" causes the most rapid addiction, sometimes after only one use. Withdrawal is very difficult, lengthy, and can lead to severe depression.

Side Effects: Euphoria, agitation, excitation, cardiac arrhythmias or failure, tremors and seizures, hallucinations, or possible psychosis.

Hallucinogens

Lysergic acid (LSD) and phencyclidine (PCP) are hallucinogens that can produce bizarre behaviors and distortion of perceptions.

Side Effects: Elevated blood pressure, increased heart rate and pulse, panic, paranoia, or psychotic episodes.

ANTICONVULSANT DRUGS, ANTIPARKINSONIAN DRUGS, AND DRUGS TO TREAT ALZHEIMER'S DISEASE

These drugs are becoming more common as the general population ages and lives longer than previous generations. Nervous system disorders can be helped by massage therapy.

Relevance for the Massage Therapist

Massage can potentiate or decrease the effects of medications; therefore, dosages of medications might need to be adjusted with consistent treatments. Therapists should observe their clients carefully during and after treatment to ascertain the effects of treatment with the medication and work together with the clients' physician as part of a total wellness program.

VITAMINS AND MINERALS

In 1912, the term *vitamin* was created by Casimir Funk, a Polish biochemist who theorized that inherent in foods were "vita-amines," compounds that were vital to life. Even though most vitamins were discovered in the early 1900s, 1920s, and 1930s, most medical doctors have held a rather dogmatic view that supplements are unnecessary if one ingests a balanced and healthy diet. The reality is that most people do not eat a highly varied, well-balanced diet that follows the government's guidelines on eating. Most people, however, do not choose foods that are very nutritious. On the contrary, obesity and diabetes have reached alarming rates, and at the same time, many people in this country are in fact undernourished. The average diet in the United States contains too much fat and not enough fruits and vegetables, whole grains, fiber, nuts and seeds, and legumes. People do not eat the same foods that their ancestors ate. Those born before World War II were not exposed to pesticides, herbicides, fungicides, preservatives, artificial ingredients, and toxic chemicals that now infest our food supply. In addition, modern fruits and vegetables are generally picked before they ripen, and so those foods are lacking in vital nutrients. If we take a loaf of bread, for example, we can see the dramatic difference in the way bread is prepared. A hundred years ago, bread was made using flour, water, butter, yeast, and sugar to help the yeast rise. Today more than 100 ingredients can be used to create a loaf of bread, many of them artificial chemical compounds that are added to the food, as well as the chemicals that leach into the food from manufacturing and packaging.

According to the U.S. Department of Agriculture (USDA), the nutrients in our soil have been severely depleted over the past six decades owing to chemical fertilization. As an example, USDA tests show that in 1948, a cup of spinach contained 158 mg of iron per 100 grams. Today, the content of iron per 100 g is about 2.7 mg. You would have to eat approximately 60 portions of spinach to receive the same amount of iron that you would have received from 1 cup in 1948.

In recent years, there have been numerous clinical studies demonstrating the benefits of nutritional supplements. Although skeptics might continue to claim that nutritional supplements pose a health risk, the facts are that 150,000 people die yearly from prescription medications, compared with the rare incidence of overdose of a nutritional supplement.

Linus Pauling, a two-time Nobel Prize winner and the founder of orthomolecular medicine (i.e., the use of vitamins and nutrients to treat disease), concluded that supplementation should be based not on deficiency of nutrients but on optimal intake. According to him, what should be emphasized is not the minimal requirements of nutrients but rather optimal nutrition, giving the body's cells the levels of vitamins, minerals, and supplements that help them to perform at their best. Currently, the Recommended Dietary Allowances (RDA) are established by the National Academy of Sciences and the National Research Council of the Food and Nutrition Board. These recommendations are considered by many researchers to be overly conservative and antiquated. They do not address the nutritional needs of people who are eating chemically laden foods, denatured foods, or people who are ill or sick. In addition, biochemical individuality exists in each person and, while everyone needs nutrients, the amounts from one person to the next vary. For example, one person might need 100 mg of vitamin C and another might need 1,000 mg. Stereotyped RDA values do not provide good nutrient guidelines.

Currently, a major project is under way to replace the RDA with Dietary Reference Intakes (DRI). The **Dietary Reference Intake** (or DRI) is a system of nutritional recommendations from the Institute of Medicine (IOM) of the United States National Academy of Sciences. The DRI system is used by both the United States and Canada and is intended for use by the general public as well as health professionals. In 1997, the DRI was created to expand the existing guidelines of the RDAs. RDA values still stand as the guideline for nutrient values, however. It remains to be seen whether the DRI will ultimately replace and be a significant improvement over the RDA.

Massage therapists have many clients who use vitamins daily. Most supplements are considered to be safe. A good multivitamin with minerals can provide health protection for about 10 cents a day. Multivitamins can help to protect against certain kinds of cancers, lower the risk of cardiovascular disease, strengthen the eyes against degenerative conditions such as cataracts and macular degeneration, and lower the incidence of birth defects. They also help to strengthen the immune system, reduce the number of sick days, and help aging people to strengthen their bones, reducing the risk of osteoporosis.

In addition, vitamins can help people who are nutrient deficient, for example, persons suffering from anorexia, alcoholism, or illness; persons suffering from GI diseases that result in leaky gut syndrome and loss of nutrients; pregnant and lactating women who require increased nutrients; children, adolescents, and menopausal women; and people who are nutrient deficient from medications, for example, deficiency of potassium from use of diuretics or deficiency of vitamin B1 from taking loop diuretics. New studies are emerging constantly that point to the importance of adequate vitamin intake. For example, current studies, such as those done at the University of Rochester Medical Center oncology center in 2008, have shown a link between adequate levels of vitamin D and breast cancer, and there might be links to other cancers as well. Other studies have demonstrated the importance of vitamin K2 in providing protection from osteoporosis, cardiovascular blockages, and pathologic calcification.

If clients are taking numerous vitamins on their own, they should be referred to a health practitioner or nutritionist who is skilled in assessing their condition and who can make the proper recommendations for supplementation. Many massage therapists further their studies in nutrition and enhance their practice in this way. In either case, each person should be under the care of a knowledgeable health care practitioner who can assist in choosing the right supplements for that person's health and well-being. Although there have been no studies on any possible interactions between massage therapy and vitamins and minerals, suffice to say that the massage therapist must be aware of all of the supplements and medications that a client is taking. In addition to referring the client to the appropriate health care practitioner, the massage therapist must always be vigilant for any potential interactions between treatments and what each client is taking.

Tables A.2 and A.3 provide a summary of the food sources, functions, and illnesses caused by deficiency or excess of the major vitamins and minerals.

TABLE A.2.

SUMMARY OF WATER AND FAT-SOLUBLE VITAMINS			
NAME	FOOD SOURCES	FUNCTIONS	DEFICIENCY/ TOXICITY
Vitamin A (retinol, beta carotene)	Animal Oily saltwater fish Whole milk, cream Butter, cheese Egg yolk Fish liver oils Plants Dark-green leafy vegetables Deep yellow or orange fruit and vegetables Fortified margarine	Dim light vision Maintenance of mucous membranes Growth of development of bones Healing of wounds Resistance to infection Beta carotene is an antioxidant.	Deficiency Retarded growth Faulty bone and tooth development Night blindness Decreased ability to resist infection—poor immune function Zinc deficiency Fat malabsorption Abnormal function of GI, genitourinary, and respiratory tracts owing to altered epithelial membrane Shriveled, thickened skin Xerophthalmia Toxicity Irritability, lethargy, headache Joint pain, myalgia Stunted growth, fetal malformations Jaundice, nausea, diarrhea Dry skin and hair

TABLE A.2. (continued)

SUMMARY OF WATER AND FAT-SOLUBLE VITAMINS			
NAME	FOOD SOURCES	FUNCTIONS	DEFICIENCY/ TOXICITY
Vitamin D3 (cholecalciferol)	Animal Fish oils Salmon, herring, mackerel, sardines Eggs, butter, milk Plants Fortified cereals	Healthy bones and teeth Muscle function Enables absorption of calcium	Deficiency Rickets (in children) Osteomalacia (in adults) Poorly developed teeth Osteoporosis Cancer (breast, prostate, colon) Fibromyalgia, Diabetes Depression Neurodegenerative Diseases Muscle spasms Toxicity Hypercalcemia Kidney stones, kidney damage Muscle/bone pain Nausea, anorexia
Vitamin E (tocopherol)	Plants Vegetable oils Seeds, nuts Wheat germ, cereals	Antioxidant	Deficiency Destruction of RBCs, muscle weakness Toxicity Prolonged bleeding time
Vitamin K (phytonadione)	Animal Egg yolk, cheese Liver Plants Vegetable oil Green leafy vegetables Cabbage, broccoli	Blood clotting	Deficiency Prolonged blood clotting Time Fractures Cancer Toxicity Jaundice in infants
Vitamin B1 (thiamine)	Animal Pork, beef, liver Oysters Plants Yeast Whole and enriched grains, wheat germ Legumes, collard greens, nuts, asparagus Oranges	Coenzyme carbohydrate metabolism Normal nervous and cardiovascular systems	Deficiency GI upset Neuritis, mental disturbance Cardiovascular problems Muscle weakness, fatigue Toxicity None known
Vitamin B2 (riboflavin)	Animal Milk Meat, liver Plants Green vegetables Cereals Enriched bread Yeast	Aids in energy metabolism of glucose, fats, and amino acids	Deficiency Cheilosis Glossitis Photophobia, vision problems, itching eyes Dermatitis, rough skin Toxicity None
Vitamin B6 (pyridoxine)	Animal Pork, beef, chicken, tuna, salmon Plants Whole grain cereals, wheat germ Legumes, peanuts, soybeans Bananas	Synthesis of amino acids Antibody production Maintenance of blood glucose level	Deficiency Anorexia, nausea, vomiting Dermatitis Neuritis, depression Elevated homocystine Increased heart disease risk Toxicity Seizures in newborn 120 mg—Neuropathy

TABLE A.2. (continued)

SUMMARY OF WATER AND FAT-SOLUBLE VITAMINS			
NAME	FOOD SOURCES	FUNCTIONS	DEFICIENCY/ TOXICITY
Vitamin B12 (cyanocobalamin) Niacin (nicotinic acid) Folacin (folic acid)	Animal Seafood/shellfish Meat, poultry, liver Eggs Milk, cheese Plants None Animal Milk Eggs Fish Poultry Plants Legumes, nuts Animal Organ meats Plants Green leafy vegetables Avocado, beets Broccoli, kidney beans Orange juice	Synthesis of RBCs Maintenance of nervous system Lipid metabolism Nerve functioning Synthesis of RBCs, leukocytes, DNA and RNA Needed for normal growth and reproduction	Deficiency Nerve, muscle, mental problems Pernicious anemia Fatigue Weakness Constipation Numbness and tingling in the hands and feet, dementia Toxicity None Deficiency Pellagra Anxiety Fatigue Elevated cholesterol Toxicity Vasodilation of blood Vessels Deficiency Increased risk of neural tube defects Macrocytic anemia Irritability, behavior disorders Toxicity None
Vitamin C (ascorbic acid)	Fruits All citrus, cantaloupe Plants Broccoli Tomatoes brussels sprouts Cabbage Green peppers	Prevention of scurvy Formation of Collagen Healing of wounds Absorption of iron Antioxidant	Deficiency Scurvy Poor healing Muscle cramps/weakness Ulcerated gums/mouth Capillary fragility Oxidative stress Toxicity Raise uric acid level GI distress Kidney stones Rebound scurvy in Neonates

TABLE A.3.

SUMMARY OF MAJOR MINERALS			
NAME	FOOD SOURCES	FUNCTIONS	DEFICIENCY/ TOXICITY
Calcium (Ca)	Milk, cheese Sardines Salmon Green vegetables except spinach	Development of bones and teeth Permeability of cell membranes Transmission of nerve impulses Blood clotting	Deficiency Osteoporosis Osteomalacia Rickets (in children) Toxicity None known
Potassium (K)	Oranges, bananas Dried fruits Tomatoes	Contraction of muscles Transmission of nerve impulses Carbohydrate and protein Metabolism Maintaining water balance	Deficiency Hypokalemia Toxicity Hyperkalemia
Sodium (Na)	Table salt Beef, eggs Milk, cheese	Maintaining fluid balance in blood Transmission of nerve impulses	Deficiency Hyponatremia Toxicity Increase in blood pressure
Chlorine (Cl)	Table salt	Gastric acidity Regulation of osmotic pressure Activation of salivary amylase	Deficiency Imbalance in gastric acidity Imbalance in blood pH Toxicity Diarrhea

TABLE A.3. (continued)

SUMMARY OF MAJOR MINERALS			
NAME	FOOD SOURCES	FUNCTIONS	DEFICIENCY/ TOXICITY
Magnesium (Mg) (DRI 320–420 mg)	Green vegetables Whole grains	Synthesis of ATP (adenosine triphosphate) Transmission of nerve impulses Relaxation of skeletal muscles	Deficiency (seldom) Imbalance Weakness Toxicity Diarrhea
Iron (Fe)	Meat Liver Eggs Poultry Spinach Dried fruits Dried beans Prune juice	Hemoglobin formation Resistance to infection	Deficiency (anemia) Pale Weak Lethargy Vertigo Air hunger Toxicity Vomiting Diarrhea Erosion of GI tract
Iodine (I)	Freshwater shellfish and seafood Iodized salt	Major component of thyroid hormones Regulating rate of metabolism Growth, reproduction Nerve and muscle function Protein synthesis Skin and hair growth	Deficiency Goiter Hypothyroidism Toxicity "Iodine goiter" Hyperactive, enlarged goiter
Zinc (Zn)	Meat Liver Oysters Poultry Fish Whole-grain bread and cereal	Wound healing Mineralization of bone Insulin glucose regulation Normal taste Antioxidant	Deficiency Poor wound healing Reduced taste perception Alcohol/glucose intolerance Toxicity GI distress Copper deficiency with extended use of high levels of zinc

HERBS AND SUPPLEMENTS

Herbalism is one of the oldest healing arts, with extensive roots in many cultures: Native American, Chinese, and Indian, just to name a few. Herbs are defined in different ways, depending on the discipline in which they are used. To a gardener, herbs are plants that help to decorate and beautify the land, whereas to a chef, herbs are used for culinary purposes. To a medical herbalist, however, herbs are defined as any plant material that can be used in medicine for healing. All of the parts of plants can be used in treatment—flowers, seeds, roots, stems, and fruit as well as nonflowering plants such as mosses, seaweed, ferns, and lichen. Chinese herbal medicine also includes nonbotanical substances such as minerals and entomologic and zoologic substances.

Throughout the world, the use of botanicals to treat disease far exceeds the use of conventional synthetic drugs. According to the WHO, 80 percent of the world's population uses herbal therapy as their first line of defense against illness. In many European countries (e.g., Germany), herbal medicine, called *phytotherapy*, is not considered alternative but mainstream, and physicians prescribe herbs more frequently than they do prescription drugs.

Most people do not realize that herbs form the foundation for much of modern medicine. Many years of scientific research resulted in the extraction of the active ingredients of plants and the creation of potent drugs. For example, aspirin came from willow bark, digoxin for heart failure from the foxglove, and steroids from the wild yam. Currently, about 25 percent of all prescription drugs are derived from botanical sources, whereas the other 75 percent of drugs are synthetically produced.

The United States has a long tradition of herbal medicine use, employing primarily native American plants and plants brought to U.S. shores by early settlers. Back in the 1700s and 1800s, the *U.S. Pharmacopeia,* our official compendium of medicinal substances, primarily contained entries of natural substances, including herbal extracts and whole herbs. Herbs were traditionally prepared as teas, tinctures, liniments, ointments, tablets, washes, douches, and poultices, and many modern herbalists still concoct their herbal remedies in myriad ways, depending on the needs of the client.

Today, the *U.S. Pharmacopeia* contains far fewer herbal medicines and a far greater number of synthetic drugs. This change in the makeup of the compendium took place over a period of years, beginning with the introduction of reductionism and the scientific analysis of herbs, the discovery of antibiotics, and the subsequent growth of the pharmaceutical industry. This shift continued, resulting in a complete departure from our natural herbal tradition as the active compounds of herbs were isolated, extracted, and concentrated.

Pharmacognosy is the study of natural drugs and their constituents and plays a major role in modern drug development. Because a plant cannot be patented, plants are researched for their active constituents, which are then isolated. In the United States, if the constituent is powerful enough, the drug company begins the process of obtaining FDA approval. Because it typically takes 10 to 18 years at a cost of hundreds of millions of dollars to obtain approval, and also because of the lack of patent protection for natural plants, the American pharmaceutical industry has done very little research on plant extracts as medicinal agents.

In contrast, European governments have made it economically possible for companies to research and develop herbs as drugs. In Germany, herbal products can be sold with drug claims if they have been proved to be safe and effective. The legal requirements for herbal products are the same for medications; therefore, whether the herbal product is given by prescription or sold OTC, it has met the requirements for safety and efficacy of use.

In Germany, a special expert commission called the German Commission E has developed a series of several hundred *monographs* (i.e., a treatise or detailed research article) on herbal products. This commission is composed of physicians, pharmacists, pharmacologists, toxicologists, representatives of the pharmaceutical industry, and laypersons. Its conclusions are independent of the German Federal Health Agency, the German counterpart of the FDA. Unlike the FDA, which relies on drug data compiled by the pharmaceutical manufacturers, the Commission E checks independent data from clinical trials, field studies, scientific literature, and traditional usage, including information from standard reference texts, and the expertise of medical persons. After completing its work, the commission issues a monograph with a positive or negative recommendation regarding medicinal use. Several reputable American herbal companies use the monographs from the German Commission E in the preparation of their herbal supplements and follow the recommendations of the commission regarding dosage and potency.

The supplement industry continues to grow dramatically worldwide as more and more consumers seek natural methods of managing their health. In this country, many studies have shown that consumers buy dietary supplements for many reasons—to prevent disease, as therapeutic agents for the treatment of diseases, to maintain health, and as adjunctive therapy for persons also receiving allopathic treatment.

In 1994, because of public demand, Congress passed the Dietary Supplement Health and Education Act (DSHEA), which recognizes herbs or other botanicals, vitamins, and supplements as dietary supplements distinct from drugs. According to the DSHEA, manufacturers cannot make statements that these substances cure or treat a disease, but they can make "statements of nutritional support" or "structure and function" claims. For example, a company cannot say that glucosamine sulfate treats or cures arthritis, but it can say that it helps to build and support joint cartilage. To make these claims, manufacturers must document and substantiate their statements. They must also state that their supplements are not drugs; their labels must say that they are "dietary supplements" and have a "supplement facts" panel on them.

The term *supplement* can cover a broad range of substances, including herbs and other botanicals, vitamins, minerals, antioxidants, enzymes, amino acids, metabolites, concentrates, constituents, extracts of natural substances, or combinations of these substances. The term *nutraceutical* is commonly used to describe supplements that combine several of these substances together in a formulation. For example, a supplement for cardiovascular support might include

Hawthorn berry—botanical
Ginger—botanical
Garlic—botanical
CoQ10—antioxidant
Vitamin C
L-Carnitine—amino acid
Magnesium—mineral
Potassium—mineral

Consumers must be educated about supplements and quality control, and they should be wary of fraudulent products. Products that are significantly cheaper than others; products that are not made by known, reputable companies; products that make claims of "cure" or "miracle"; or products the claims for which are not backed by scientific studies should be avoided. Consumers who wish to use the growing market of supplementation would be wise to consult with a certified herbalist, nutritionist, or other health care provider who is knowledgeable in the field of supplementation. Special warnings should be given to clients who have diabetes or who are taking cardiac drugs, particularly anticoagulants, because of the increased risk of serious interactions and side effects. Knowledge of the interactions between dietary supplements and medications is in its infancy. Clients therefore should consult not only with their physicians, who have limited information in this area, but also with qualified herbalists and nutritionists. Massage therapists should have such people involved as part of their network of health care professionals so that they can refer their clients to the best health care practitioner for their specific needs.

There are numerous herbal and nutraceutical remedies on the market today, and they are clearly beyond the scope of this appendix. Table A.4 lists some of the more popular ones with some information about their uses, cautions, and known interactions. Check the suggested reading list at the end of this appendix for additional sources of information.

TABLE A.4.

USES AND SIDE EFFECTS OF SOME HERBS AND SUPPLEMENTS		
HERBS OR SUPPLEMENTS	POSSIBLE USES	POSSIBLE SIDE EFFECTS/ACTIONS
Aloe Vera	Topical use for minor burns, minor wounds, sunburn, psoriasis, seborrhea, diabetes; internally as a laxative; antiulcer effects on the GI tract; immune enhancing and antiviral (used in treatment of HIV)	Not to be used for puncture wounds
Black Cohosh	Phytoestrogen for premenstrual syndrome (PMS), painful menses, menopausal symptoms, HBP	High doses can cause frontal headaches.
Cayenne	Topical pain relief, anti-inflammatory for arthritis; internally protective against gastroduodenal injury	Topically local burning sensation that usually fades with time; internally excessive doses can cause severe irritation of mucus membranes.
Chamomile	Anti-inflammatory, antispasmodic, inflammatory conditions of the GI tract, mild sedative, antiulcer	Persons with a known sensitivity to members of the Compositae family of plants (e.g., ragweed, daisies, chrysanthemums) might be allergic.
Coenzyme Q10	Improves blood circulation; increases tolerance to exercise; protects heart tissue from free-radical damage, congestive heart failure, hypertension, cardiomyopathy; periodontal disease; Parkinson's disease	Very safe, no serious side effects. Numerous drugs impair the synthesis of CoQ10 in the body (e.g., beta blockers, tricyclic antidepressants); therefore clients taking these drugs will find it useful to supplement with CoQ10.
Echinacea	Enhances resistance to infections, especially of the upper respiratory tract; assists in recovery from chemotherapy; anti-inflammatory	Side effects are rare; those allergic to the Compositae family of plants might be allergic. There are no data to suggest that long-term use of echinacea is harmful to immune function.
Evening Primrose Oil	Anti-inflammatory disorders, including rheumatoid arthritis, ulcerative colitis; diabetic neuropathy; hypotensive; PMS; source of gamma-linolenic acid (GLA)	Headaches, mild nausea; use caution in persons with a history of epilepsy.
Feverfew	Migraine headaches, tension headaches, arthritis	Has very few side effects; those allergic to the Compositae family might be allergic. Possible allergic dermatitis
Garlic	Lowers blood pressure, lowers cholesterol; antimicrobial against many types of bacteria, viruses, worms, and fungi; strengthens the immune system	Use with caution in patients on anticoagulants; can cause allergic contact dermatitis; irritation to the digestive tract
Ginger	Nausea, motion sickness, anti-inflammatory, antiplatelet, carminative; relaxes the intestinal tract; migraine headaches, arthritis	Contraindicated in persons with gallstones; not more than a daily dose of 1 g should be taken during pregnancy; possible heartburn at high doses
Gingko	Improves memory and cognitive function for ordinary memory loss, dementia, Alzheimer's; increases blood flow to the brain; tissue oxygenation and nutrition; improves peripheral circulation	Extremely small incidence of side effects; use with caution in clients on anticoagulants or antiplatelets
Panax Ginseng (Chinese, Korean)	Adaptogenic; tonic; cardiotonic, cancer preventive; improves performance and well-being; antifatigue	Contraindicated in acute illness, hypertension, insomnia, diarrhea, signs of heat; avoid concurrent use of stimulants
Glucosamine	Anti-inflammatory for osteoarthritis	Can increase insulin resistance in diabetes; mild GI distress
Green Tea	Cancer protective; decreased heart disease and cancer risk	Generally very safe—does contain some caffeine so it can cause nervousness or insomnia.
Hawthorn	Atherosclerosis, cardiac arrhythmia, congestive heart failure, angina, protects against myocardial damage; peripheral vascular disease, hypertension	No contraindications; can act with hypotensive drugs and increase their actions; modification of drug dosage can be necessary.
Licorice	Healing of peptic ulcers (deglycyrrhizinated licorice [DGL]); anti-inflammatory; antitussive; expectorant; menopausal symptoms	High doses can cause signs of pseudo-hyperaldosteronism—sodium retention and high blood pressure, which can be offset by following a high-potassium, low-sodium diet.
Melatonin	Insomnia, jet lag, cancer treatment—prevents some of the side effects of chemotherapy; helps to inhibit the growth of breast cancer cells; immune disorders, depression, seasonal affective disorder (SAD)	Can cause sedation and affect balance

TABLE A.4. (continued)

USES AND SIDE EFFECTS OF SOME HERBS AND SUPPLEMENTS		
HERBS OR SUPPLEMENTS	POSSIBLE USES	POSSIBLE SIDE EFFECTS/ACTIONS
Milk Thistle	Enhances liver function; alcoholic liver disease; cirrhosis; viral hepatitis; protects against hepatotoxic chemicals; prevents cholelithiasis—increases bile flow	Very safe, no adverse effects even with long-term use and high-dose administration; safe in pregnancy and lactation; can lower blood sugar.
Probiotics	Inflammatory bowel disease; antibiotic diarrhea; irritable bowel syndrome; eczema; vaginal candidiasis, traveler's diarrhea; acute infectious diarrhea in children—both prevention and treatment; prevents respiratory infection in children; prevents otitis media	No side effects or safety issues; no known drug interactions
Saw Palmetto	For treatment of benign prostatic hypertrophy (BPH); improves urinary tract symptoms in men	Very safe and well-tolerated

SUGGESTED READINGS

Bratman, S., and A. Girman (Eds.). *Mosby's Handbook of Herbs and Supplements and their Therapeutic Uses.* St. Louis, MO: Elsevier Science, 2003.

Harkness, R., and S. Bratman. *Mosby's Handbook of Drug-herb and Drug-supplement Interactions.* St. Louis, MO: Elsevier Science, 2003.

Hoffman, D. *Medical Herbalism.* Rochester, VT: Healing Arts Press, 2003.

Mills, S., and K. Bone. *Principles and Practice of Phytotherapy: Modern Herbal Medicine.* London: Churchill Livingstone, 2003.

Ottariano, S. G. *Medicinal Herbal Therapy: A Pharmacist's Viewpoint.* Portsmouth, NH: Nicolin Fields, 1999.

Spratto, G. R., and A. L. Woods. *PDR Nurse's Drug Handbook.* Clifton Park, NY: Delmar, Cengage Learning, 2005.

Woodrow, R. *Essentials of Pharmacology for Health Occupations* (4th ed.). Clifton Park, NY: Delmar, Cengage Learning, 2003.

APPENDIX 2

ANSWERS TO QUESTIONS FOR DISCUSSION AND REVIEW

Chapter 1: Historical Overview of Massage

1. Massage is the manual (use of hands) or mechanical (use of machines or apparatus) manipulation of a part of the body by rubbing, kneading, pressing, rolling, slapping, and similar movements for the purpose of improving circulation of the blood, relaxation of muscles, and other benefits to body systems.
2. Various artifacts show evidence that ancient civilizations used massage and exercise in their social, personal, and religious practices.
3. Massage is said to be the most effective and most natural means of obtaining relief from pain or discomfort, because a person can use both hands to rub, touch, or exercise a part of the body to obtain immediate relief.
4. The Chinese called their massage system *anmo* or *amma*. This method grew from various pressing and rubbing of parts of the body to produce therapeutic effects.
5. The Greeks and Romans were health and beauty conscious. Both men and women believed that exercise improved the body and the mind. Exercise and massage were used in the training and rehabilitation of gladiators. Both Greek and Roman physicians prescribed various kinds of exercise and massage movements as aids to the healing of diseases and wounds.
6. Hippocrates, the Greek physician, became known as the father of medicine and originator of the Hippocratic oath, which is still used as the ethical guide to the medical professions. The Hippocratic oath can be found in its entirety in most modern dictionaries.
7. The Middle Ages were called the Dark Ages because the arts and sciences were allowed to deteriorate, leading to the decline of learning.
8. As the Greco-Roman culture fell into the decay of the Middle Ages, many of the important teachings of the great physicians and philosophers were carried on by the Persians of the Arabic Empire. The Islamic Persian philosophers/physicians, Rhazes (or Razi) and Avicenna, who followed the teachings of Hippocrates and Galen, authored important books that eventually returned to the West by way of trade and conquest and paved the way for the Renaissance.
9. The Renaissance, meaning "rebirth," revived interest in the arts and sciences and renewed interest in health and personal hygiene practices.
10. The invention of the printing press in the latter part of the fifteenth century led to the publishing of more writings in the arts and sciences. This improved circulation of educational materials led to a better understanding of the value of massage and exercise as therapeutic aids.
11. Per Henrik Ling based the Swedish Movement Cure on the developing science of physiology applied to the treatment of disease. The system's primary focus was on gymnastics, which consisted of movements classified as active, duplicated, and passive.

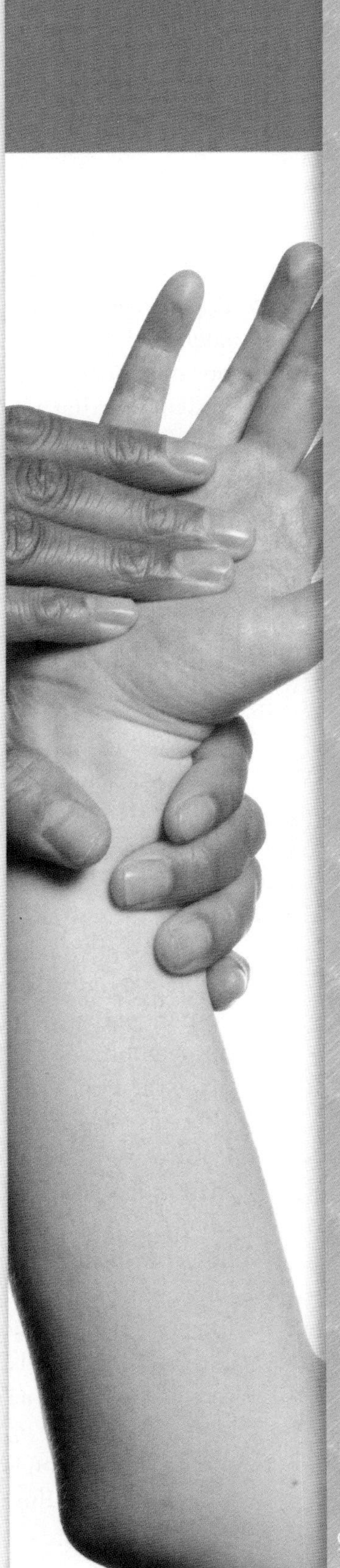

12. In 1858, the brothers Charles Fayette Taylor and George Henry Taylor started an orthopedic practice in New York. They specialized in the Swedish movements.
13. There were several reasons for the decline of the scientific and medical use of massage at the turn of the twentieth century. In 1894, an inquiry by the British Medical Association revealed numerous abuses in the education and practice of massage practitioners, including unscrupulous recruitment practices, inadequate training, deceptive advertising, and false certification. Technical innovations, such as the invention of electricity and various electrical apparatuses (e.g., the vibrator) and intellectual advances in medicine that led to new treatment strategies based more on pharmacology and surgical procedures, also had a detrimental effect on massage.
14. Because there were more diseases and injuries during wartime, physicians employed therapeutic massage and exercise more often. The good results led to wider acceptance of massage and exercise as aids to healing.
15. Manual massage became a secondary treatment following World War II because new mechanical and electrical devices were designed to take over some of the manipulative movements.
16. The increased awareness of physical and mental fitness, as well as the increasing cost of traditional medicine, opened the way for viable alternatives in health care. The development of the wellness model, which placed more emphasis on prevention and recognized the importance of controlling stress, has caused a renewed interest in massage.
17. Passive exercise of muscles incorporates massage and is done by the practitioner on the client. Active exercise of muscles is movement done by the person, as in sports or gymnastics.
18. The Japanese use a system called shiatsu (*shi,* fingers; *atsu,* pressure). It is the finger pressure method based on the Oriental concept that the body has a series of energy points. When pressure is properly applied to these points, circulation is improved and nerves are stimulated. This system is said to improve body metabolism and to relieve many physical disorders.
19. Athletes often have injuries and sore muscles that can be relieved by massage. Massage and proper exercise also help to prevent fatigue and contribute to the maintenance of optimal fitness.
20. A person contemplating a career in any important field should have some understanding of problems of the past and the progress that has been made over time. Understanding the past helps us to measure our own progress in the development of the art and practice of therapeutic body massage.
21. The Swedish massage system is still the most widely used and is most frequently incorporated into other systems.
22. The points of stimulation in Japanese massage *(tsubo)* are much the same as points used in Chinese traditional medicine.
23. Sports massage is used in sports medicine as an aid to treating injuries that have occurred during sports activities. It is also used as a means of keeping the athlete's muscles supple and strong.

Chapter 2: Requirements for the Practice of Therapeutic Massage

1. The practitioner must be concerned about the laws, rules, regulations, and obligations concerning the practice of therapeutic body massage, because the practitioner has a responsibility to the public and to individual clients. Massage is a personal, health-related service, and as such, strict rules must be observed.
2. The scope of practice defines the rights and activities legally acceptable according to the licenses of a particular practice or profession. *Scope of practice* is defined legally and determines the educational focus and requirements that become the national standards of a given profession.
3. Laws governing the practice of massage often differ because there are no national standards and some states have fewer complaints or problems, whereas others have found it necessary to establish state boards and

stringent guidelines for licensing practitioners, schools, and establishments.

4. Being licensed in one locality does not guarantee that the same license is valid or recognized in another locality. Because laws and regulations vary greatly from state to state and city to city, a practitioner who has a license and wishes to practice in another city or state should contact the proper agency in the area where the practitioner wishes to practice, provide proof of ability to meet any requirements, and make any applications that are required.
5. The general educational requirements to practice massage vary depending on discipline or techniques and the licensing requirements of the city or state where the practice is located. Because there is no national standard for massage therapy, licensing laws can contain no educational requirement or might require as much as 1,000 hours of training. Of the states that license massage at the time of publication of this text, the educational requirements vary from 500 to 1,000 hours of training.
6. A person might receive a certificate in recognition of an accomplishment or achieving or maintaining some kind of standard. Certificates are awarded by schools and institutions to show the successful completion of a course of study and by professional organizations to indicate that the recipient has met the qualifications to become a member or in recognition of achievements in the recipient's chosen profession.
7. The grounds on which the practitioner's license may be revoked, canceled, or suspended are the following:
   a. Practicing fraud or deceit in obtaining a license
   b. Being convicted of a felony
   c. Being engaged in any act of prostitution
   d. Practicing under a false or assumed name
   e. Being addicted to drugs, alcohol, or the like
   f. Being willfully negligent of the health of a client
   g. Prescribing drugs or medicine
   h. Being guilty of fraudulent or deceptive advertising
   i. Ethical or sexual misconduct with a client
   j. Practicing beyond the scope permitted by law or performing professional responsibilities that the licensee knows they are not competent to perform

Chapter 3: Professional Ethics for Massage Practitioners

1. It is important to have a code of ethics for your business to protect the public and your reputation.
2. A satisfied client is your best means of advertising, because that person will recommend you, your business, and your services.
3. Successful business managers know that employees who practice sound personal and professional ethics will help them to build their business and keep their customers.
4. Boundaries are the basis of ethics. By honoring personal and professional boundaries, a therapist can avoid ethical dilemmas.
5. Personal boundaries define a person's comfort zone and are either innate or developed beginning at a very early age. Professional boundaries are the basis for operating a professional practice that protects the safety of the client and practitioner, and they should be outlined in policy and procedure statements.
6. Some major areas to consider when establishing professional boundaries are location of service, interpersonal space, appearance, self-disclosure, language, touch, time, money, and sexual intimacy.
7. The power differential favors the person in the position of authority, usually the practitioner or therapist.
8. When a boundary is crossed, there is a feeling of discomfort.
9. The practitioner can reduce the risk of crossing a client's boundary by asking the client to articulate or speak up any time the practitioner says or does anything that causes any discomfort to the client.
10. *Transference* is the unconscious tendency for the client to project onto the practitioner

attributes of someone from a former relationship. *Counter-transference* is when the practitioner personalizes the relationship with the client.

11. It is always the responsibility of the practitioner to manage transference, counter-transference, and boundary issues.
12. A dual relationship is any situation that combines the therapeutic relationship with a secondary relationship that extends beyond the massage practitioner/client relationship. Examples might be when someone you know becomes a client, when services are bartered, or when a therapeutic relationship becomes a romantic relationship.
13. The appropriate response to sexual arousal depends on the circumstance. If there is discomfort on the part of either the client or the practitioner, immediate steps should be taken, such as massaging a less-sensitive area of the client's body, opening a dialogue with the client, or having the client turn over or change position. It is the practitioner's responsibility to act in a nonsexual manner, clarify to the client that there is no sexual intent or involvement in the relationship, and maintain the appropriate boundary.
14. Supervision means meeting with a professional or peer group to discuss questionable or uncomfortable situations that might occur during professional interactions such as transference, counter-transference, or sexual issues.
15. It is necessary for the massage practitioner to be concerned with personal hygiene and health habits because one's own good health inspires confidence on the part of clients. Good health is also a form of protection for the practitioner and the client.
16. Professional projection in attitude and appearance means that the practitioner acts, speaks, and dresses to project a professional image.
17. The term *human relations* is defined as the art of being able to work successfully with others and to give excellent service.
18. The practice of good human relations is important because it helps the practitioner to interact successfully with different personalities.
19. When building your business image, pay attention to the use of appropriate wording in your business name and in advertising so that potential clients receive the right message.

Chapter 4: Human Anatomy and Physiology Overview

1. *Anatomy* is defined as the study of the gross structure or morphology of the body or the study of an organism and the interrelations of its parts.
2. *Physiology* is the science and study of the vital processes, mechanisms, and functions performed by the various systems of the body.
3. *Kinesiology* is the scientific study of muscular activity and mechanics of body movement.
4. *Pathology* is the study of the structural and functional changes caused by disease.
5. Disease is an abnormal and unhealthy state of all or part of the body wherein it is incapable of carrying on its normal function.
6. A *symptom* is caused by the disease and is perceived by the person, such as dizziness, chills, nausea, or pain. A symptom is a clear message to the person that something is wrong. *Signs* of a disease are observable indications such as abnormal pulse rate, fever, abnormal skin color, or physical irregularities.
7. Regardless of the source or nature of stress, the physiologic reaction of the body is essentially the same. When we encounter high levels of stress, our bodies respond with the "fight-or-flight" reactions. The adrenal secretions, adrenaline and cortisol, give us a physical and mental boost that heightens senses, sharpens reflexes, and strengthens muscles.
8. There are two responses to pain: psychological and physical. The physical response to pain is very similar to the body's response to stress. Blood pressure and pulse increase, blood flow is shifted from the intestines and brain to the muscles, and mental alertness intensifies, readying the body for a fight or flight. The physical experience also informs us of the location, intensity, and duration of the pain.
9. The pain-spasm-pain cycle is associated with muscle spasms. The natural reflex reaction

to the tissue damage and pain is a contraction of the muscles that surround the injury. Contracted muscles pinch the blood vessel and capillaries in the muscles, restricting blood flow and causing ischemia. Metabolic activity of the muscles increases as oxygen and nutrients are burned, producing increased amounts of metabolic wastes. Lactic acid and other toxins collect in the tissues, and soon ischemic pain appears. Reflex reactions to the ischemic pain mirror and perpetuate the reaction to the original injury to become a vicious cycle.

10. In the case of the pain-spasm-pain cycle wherein pain is intensified because of ischemia, skillfully applied massage therapy diverts some attention away from the acute intensity of the pain and gives the client a chance to relax and disassociate from the noxious stimulus, possibly long enough to shut down the fight-or-flight reaction. Massaging the contracted ischemic tissues relieves the chronic spasms and restores circulation. As oxygen and nutrients flood the area and lactic acid and other irritants are removed, the pain disappears and mobility is restored.
11. *Infection* is the result of the invasion of the body by disease-producing microorganisms such as bacteria, viruses, fungi, or protozoa. If microorganisms enter the body in sufficient numbers to multiply and become harmful and are capable of destroying healthy tissue, the body reacts by developing an infection. Inflammation is a protective and healing response that happens when tissue is damaged. Blood vessels in the area of the damaged tissues dilate, increasing blood flow to the area; capillary walls become more permeable, allowing large quantities of blood plasma and white blood cells to enter the tissue spaces; and leukocytes flood the area to engulf and digest the invading organisms and the damaged tissue debris.
12. The four principal signs and symptoms of inflammation are swelling, redness, heat, and pain.
13. *Fever* is a warning sign that usually accompanies infectious diseases or infected burns and cuts. A disturbance of the body's heat-regulating system causes an elevated body temperature.
14. Extreme or prolonged fever can be dangerous or even fatal. Prolonged fever causes dehydration, and therefore fluids must be replaced. Fevers above 106° to 108°F may cause damage to the tissues of the kidneys, liver, or other organs or may cause irreparable brain damage, possibly resulting in death.
15. Medical terms are usually compound words constructed of root words, or stems, prefixes, and suffixes. Anatomic terms often include more than one word. Generally the first word acts as an adjective and indicates the region or location of the structure. The second word is the noun and names the structure.
16. The stem, or root word, generally indicates the body part or structure involved. A prefix is added in front of the stem to further its meaning. Suffixes often denote a diagnosis, symptom, or surgical procedure or identify a word as a noun or adjective.

Chapter 5: Human Anatomy and Physiology

1. All living matter consists of various cells.
2. Nucleus, cytoplasm, and the cell membrane or wall.
3. The nucleus and the centrosome control cell reproduction.
4. As long as the cell receives an adequate supply of food, oxygen, and water, eliminates waste products, and is surrounded by a favorable environment (i.e., proper temperature and the absence of waste products, toxins, and pressure), it will continue to grow and function. When these requirements are not provided, the cell stops growing and will eventually die.
5. Cell reproduction in human tissue occurs by the process called *mitosis*, the indirect division of cells.
6. The five phases of mitosis are interphase, prophase, metaphase, anaphase, and telophase.
7. Catabolism and anabolism.

8. *Anabolism* is the process of building up larger molecules from smaller ones.
9. *Catabolism* is the process of breaking down larger molecules into smaller ones.
10. Enzymes are protein substances that act as organic catalysts to initiate, accelerate, or control specific chemical reactions in the metabolic process, while they themselves remain unchanged.
11. All tissues are composed of specialized cells.
12. The four main categories of tissues are epithelial, connective, muscular, and nervous tissue.
13. The endoderm, mesoderm, and ectoderm are the cell layers of the embryo that form the primary germ layers, which in turn form all of the tissues and organs of the body.
14. Epithelial tissues cover all surfaces of the body, both inside and out, and function in the process of absorption, excretion, secretion, and protection.
15. The two main types of membranes are epithelial and connective.
16. The three types of muscle tissue are skeletal, smooth, and cardiac muscle tissue.
17. Striated muscle tissue is made of cylindrical fibers, is found in voluntary muscles, and appears striated if observed under a microscope. Smooth muscle tissue fibers are not striated and are found in involuntary muscles.
18. Cardiac muscle tissue is found only in the heart.
19. The main function of nervous tissue proper is to initiate, control, and coordinate the body's adaptations to its surroundings and environment.
20. Liquid tissue is found in blood and lymph.
21. The main function of connective tissue is to bind structures, to create a framework, and to provide support.
22. The main function of areolar (loose) tissue is to bind the skin to underlying tissues and to fill spaces between the muscles.
23. Adipose tissue is areolar tissue with an abundance of fat-containing cells.
24. The three types of cartilage are fibrous, hyaline, and elastic.
25. Bone tissue is made hard by mineral salts, calcium phosphate, and calcium carbonate.

The Anatomic Position of the Body

1. Anatomic position shows a person from the front standing upright with the palms of the hands facing forward.
2. The three imaginary planes are called the *sagittal* (vertical), the *coronal* (frontal), and the *transverse* (horizontal) planes.
3. When studying anatomy, you should know the anatomic position and the regions and planes of the human body to describe the position of a structure or to locate one structure in relation to another. Once you know the body planes, you can understand the location of body cavities and which organs are located in a particular cavity.
4. The subdivisions of the ventral cavity are the thoracic cavity, containing the heart and lungs; the abdominal cavity, containing the liver, stomach, spleen, pancreas, small and large intestines; and the pelvic cavity, containing the bladder, rectum, and some of the reproductive organs. The dorsal cavity is divided into the cranial cavity, containing the brain, and the spinal or vertebral cavity, containing the spinal cord.
5. The four main anatomic parts of the body are the head, consisting of the cranium and the face; the spine, including the vertebrae and the sacrum; the trunk, including the chest or thorax and the abdomen and the organs that they contain; and the extremities-the upper extremities, including the shoulders, arms, and hands-and the lower extremities, including the hips, legs, and feet.
6. The ten most important systems of the body are the integumentary (skin), skeletal, muscular, nervous, endocrine, circulatory (blood and lymph-vascular), digestive, excretory, respiratory, and reproductive systems.

Answers to Matching I

1. g; 2. j; 3. i; 4. k; 5. h; 6. e; 7. c; 8. b; 9. d; 10. a; 11. f

Answers to Matching II

1. f; 2. c; 3. i; 4. g; 5. a; 6. d; 7. j; 8. b; 9. e; 10. h

System 1: The Integumentary System—The Skin

1. The integumentary system, also called the skin, is the external covering and largest organ of the body.
2. The skin protects the parts of the body situated beneath its surface, regulates body temperature, and functions as an organ of secretion and excretion, absorption, and respiration.
3. The two main layers of the skin are the epidermis and the dermis.
4. The layers of the epidermis are the stratum corneum, lucidum, granulosum, spinosum (also called stratum mucosum), and germinativum.
5. Keratin is both hard and soft. Soft keratin is found in the skin, and hard keratin is found in hair and nails.
6. Subcutaneous tissue is a layer of fatty tissue found below the dermis. It contains a network of arteries and a superficial and deep layer of lymphatics.
7. The color of the skin depends partly on the blood supply but more on melanin, the pigment or coloring matter deposited in the deepest layer of the epidermis and the superficial layer of the dermis.
8. The layers of the dermis are the papillary and the reticular layers.
9. A *gland* is an organ of either excretion or secretion, taking materials from the blood and forming new substances.
10. The two major glands in the skin are the sudoriferous glands, which excrete sweat, and the sebaceous glands, which secrete sebum.
11. *Sebum* is an oily substance of the sebaceous glands. A *duct* is a passage or canal for fluids.
12. Appendages of the skin include hair and nails. In addition, the oil and sweat glands are appendages.
13. A *lesion* is a structural change in tissues caused by injury or disease.
14. Contact dermatitis is a skin condition or reaction caused by some substance or exterior agent that causes a rash or irritation on contact with the skin.
15. The practitioner observes the client's skin condition for possible contraindications for massage or to observe and bring to the client's attention conditions they may not be aware of.

System 2: The Skeletal System

1. The skeletal system is composed of bones, cartilage, and ligaments.
2. The functions of the skeletal system are:
   a. To offer a framework that supports body structures and gives shape to the body
   b. To protect delicate internal organs and tissues
   c. To provide attachments for muscles and act as levers in conjunction with muscles to produce movement
   d. To manufacture blood cells in the red bone marrow
   e. To store minerals such as calcium phosphate, calcium carbonate, magnesium, and sodium
3. Organic matter of bones consists of bone cells, blood vessels, connective tissue, and marrow. Inorganic matter consists of calcium phosphate and calcium carbonate.
4. Two types of bone tissue are cancellous (spongy) tissue and dense (compact) tissue. Dense bone tissue is found on the outer portion of the bone just under the periosteum. Cancellous tissue is found on the interior of flat bones and in the ends of long bones.
5. The periosteum covers and protects bone.
6. Bones receive their nourishment through blood vessels that enter through the periosteum into the interior of the bone. Bone marrow also aids in the nutrition of the bone.
7. Flat bones, such as the skull; long bones, such as the legs; short bones, such as the fingers; and irregular bones, such as the vertebrae of the spine.
8. Yellow bone marrow is found in the medullary cavity of the long bones. Red bone marrow is located in the ends of the long

bones and in flat bones. In infants and young children, red marrow also occupies the cavities of long bones.

9. Red bone marrow is the site of blood cell synthesis.
10. The main parts of the skeleton are the axial skeleton and the appendicular skeleton.
11. The three classifications of joints are synarthrotic joints such as those in the skull, which are immovable; amphiarthrotic joints, which have limited motion; and diarthrotic joints, which are freely movable.
12. Articular cartilage cushions bones at the joints.
13. Bones are supported at the joints by ligaments.
14. Joints are lubricated by synovial fluid or synovium.
15. There are approximately 206 bones in the adult human body.
16. The form or outline of the bones must be carefully followed and the limitations of the range of movements be considered when practicing massage therapy. Knowing the names of bones serves as a guide in recalling the names of related structures connected with the body part being massaged.
17. Pivot joints, as in the neck between the atlas and the axis. Hinge joints include the elbow, knees, and two distal joints of the fingers. Ball-and-socket joints are in the hips and shoulders. Gliding joints, as in the spine or hand. Saddle joints, as in the wrist, thumb, and ankle.
18. A *fracture* is a break or rupture of a bone.
19. A *sprain* is an injury to a joint that results in the stretching or tearing of the ligaments. In a class I sprain, there is a stretch in the ligament, some discomfort, and minimal loss of function. In a class II sprain, the ligament is torn, with some loss of function. In a class III sprain, the ligaments are torn, and there is internal bleeding and severe loss of function.
20. *Arthritis* is an inflammatory condition of the joints often accompanied by pain and changes of bone structure. The three most common types of arthritis are rheumatoid arthritis, osteoarthritis, and gouty arthritis.
21. *Osteoporosis* literally means porous bones and is a condition in which minerals are drawn out of the bones, leaving them brittle and weak. When massaging a person with osteoporosis, the therapist must not use heavy pressure or forceful joint movements, either of which could fracture the weakened bones.
22. Three abnormal curves of the spine are as follows: *kyphosis* is an exaggerated convex curve usually associated with the thoracic spine. *Lordosis* is an exaggerated concave curve usually associated with the lumbar spine. *Scoliosis* is an abnormal lateral curve of the spine.

Answers to Matching I

1. i; 2. g; 3. b; 4. e; 5. h; 6. f; 7. j; 8. c; 9. a; 10. d

Answers to True or False Test

1. F; 2. T; 3. T; 4. F; 5. F; 6. T; 7. T; 8. T; 9. T; 10. F

Answers to Matching II

1. c; 2. e; 3. h; 4. j; 5. b; 6. a; 7. d; 8. i; 9. f; 10. g

System 3: The Muscular System

1. Muscles are contractile fibrous tissue that produces various movements of the body.
2. There are approximately 600 muscles in the human body.
3. Voluntary (striated) muscle is found in the muscles that attach to the skeleton; involuntary (nonstriated) muscle is found in the hollow muscular organs such as the stomach, intestines, bladder, and blood vessels; heart (cardiac) muscle is found only in the heart.
4. Voluntary muscles can be controlled by the will; involuntary muscles are not controlled by the will and receive nerve stimulation from the autonomic nervous system.
5. The characteristics that enable muscles to produce movement are irritability, contractility, and elasticity.
6. Skeletal muscles are striated muscles attached to the bones of the skeleton.
7. The functional unit of skeletal muscle is the muscle cell or muscle fiber.

8. The striated appearance of voluntary muscle is due to the arrangement of the actin and myosin in the myofibrils.
9. Beside the muscle fibers, muscle contains a variety of connective tissue, blood and other fluids, blood and lymph vessels, and nerves.
10. Muscles are attached to bones, cartilage, ligaments, tendons, skin, and sometimes to each other.
11. The *origin* of a muscle refers to the more fixed attachments, such as muscles attached to bones, that act as anchors for movements.
12. The *insertion* of a muscle refers to the attachments that perform the action, such as muscles attached to skin, other muscles, or the more distal and movable attachment.
13. Tendon or sinew attaches muscles to the bone.
14. The function of fibrous connective tissue is to organize and support muscle tissue, blood vessels, and nerves. Connective tissue anchors the muscle fibers and connects them to the structures that they act on.
15. Fascia is connective tissue that organizes muscles into functional groups, surrounds each individual muscle, extends inward throughout the muscle creating muscle bundles, and eventually surrounds each muscle fiber. The fascia projects beyond the ends of the muscle to become tendons or flat tendinous sheaths (aponeuroses) that connect the muscles to other structures. The *superficial fascia* is situated just below the skin and covers the entire muscular system.
16. The three layers of connective muscle are the epimysium, which covers the muscle, the perimysium, which separates the muscle bundles, and the endomysium, which surrounds each muscle cell.
17. A *motor unit* is all of the muscle fibers that are controlled by a single motor neuron.
18. Acetylcholine is a chemical neurotransmitter found at the myoneural junction. When a nerve impulse travels to the end of a motor neuron, acetylcholine is released and travels across the gap to excite the muscle cell to contract.
19. Muscles receive energy from the breaking down of adenosine triphosphate (ATP) into adenosine diphosphate (ADP).
20. Oxygen debt results from the muscles expending energy faster than the body can supply the oxygen needed to produce the energy. When oxygen debt becomes extreme, the muscles stop functioning in a condition known as *muscle fatigue*.
21. The term *myofascial* was coined to refer to the combination of muscle tissue and its related connective tissue or fascia.
22. Type I, slow twitch fibers, have a relatively slower contraction time and a high resistance to fatigue. They contain a high number of mitochondria, large amounts of myoglobin, and have an ample capillary supply, giving them a rich, red color. Type IIb, fast twitch fibers, produce powerful, high-velocity contractions for short periods. They contain few mitochondria, low myoglobin content, and few capillaries, which give them a lighter, whitish color.
23. When massage practitioners understand how muscles function, they are better able to apply massage techniques that can relax tense muscles and rejuvenate tired muscles.
24. *Extensibility* is the ability of muscle fibers to lengthen and stretch.
25. An *isometric* muscle contraction is a static contraction wherein the distance between the ends of the muscle does not change, and so there is no movement. With an isotonic muscle contraction, the distance between the ends of the muscle changes, and there is movement.
26. Eccentric and concentric muscle contractions are both isotonic contractions. In a concentric contraction, the ends of the contracting muscle are coming closer. In an eccentric contraction, the ends of the contracting muscle are moving farther apart.
27. *Prime mover* and *agonist* both refer to the primary muscle that is responsible for a specific movement.
28. When the elbow is flexed, the triceps become the antagonist.
29. The three components of motion are flexion/extension, adduction/abduction, and rotation.
30. Diarthrotic joints are freely movable.
31. There are three degrees or grades of muscle strain. Grade I is an overstretching of a few of the muscle fibers with a minimal tearing

of the fibers. Grade II involves a partial tear of between 10 and 50 percent of the muscle fibers. Grade III is the most severe injury, with between 50 and 100 percent muscle tearing.
32. *Muscle atrophy* is a degenerative process caused by muscle disuse. The muscle fibers reduce in size, blood supply is reduced, and the muscle weakens.
33. Ampiarthrotic joints have limited motion.
34. Synarthrotic joints, as in the skull, are functionally immovable.

Matching Test I

1. c; 2. e; 3. a; 4. b; 5. d

True or False Test I

1. F; 2. F; 3. T; 4. T; 5. F

Matching Test II

1. c; 2. d; 3. b; 4. e; 5. a

True or False Test II

1. T; 2. F; 3. F; 4. T; 5. T

Matching Test III

1. b; 2. c; 3. d; 4. e; 5. a

True or False Test III

1. T; 2. F; 3. T; 4. F; 5. T

Matching Test IV

1. e; 2. a; 3. d; 4. c; 5. b

True or False Test IV

1. F; 2. F; 3. T; 4. T; 5. T

Matching Test V

1. b; 2. c; 3. d; 4. e; 5. a

True or False Test V

1. T; 2. T; 3. F; 4. T; 5. F

System 4: The Circulatory System

1. The heart, blood vessels (i.e., arteries, veins, and capillaries), lymph vessels, and the fluids that circulate through them are the main parts of the circulatory system.
2. The two divisions of the circulatory system are the blood-vascular system and the lymph-vascular system.
3. The heart is an efficient pump that keeps the blood moving in a steady stream through a closed system of blood vessels.
4. The pericardium is a protective sac surrounding and supporting the heart in position and at the same time allowing it to move frictionlessly as it continually pulsates.
5. The chambers of the heart are the right atrium (or auricle), the right ventricle, the left atrium, and the left ventricle.
6. Two sets of nerves, the vagus and sympathetic nerves, regulate the heartbeat.
7. The arteries carry blood away from the heart to the capillaries.
8. An *arteriole* is the microscopic final division of the arteries before the capillaries.
9. Movements of the arterial walls are controlled by vasomotor nerves from the autonomic nervous system consisting of the vasoconstrictor nerves and the vasodilator nerves.
10. The capillaries connect the smaller arteries with the veins. The permeable walls of the capillaries allow a two-way diffusion of substances between the blood and the tissue fluid, thereby bringing nourishment to the cells and removing waste products.
11. The veins carry blood from the various capillaries back toward the heart. Veins of general circulation carry waste-laden, oxygen-poor blood from the body, whereas pulmonary veins carry freshly oxygenated blood from the lungs.
12. A *venule* is the smallest vessel of the venous system that collects blood from the capillaries.
13. The purpose of the venous pump is to assist in moving the blood through the veins and toward the heart.
14. The main artery is the aorta.
15. Two portions of the blood-vascular system are the pulmonary circulatory system and the general or systemic circulatory system.
16. The pulmonary veins carry freshly oxygenated blood.
17. The constituents of blood include plasma, red corpuscles, white corpuscles, and platelets.

18. The red blood cells primarily carry oxygen from the lungs to the cells and carbon dioxide from the cells to the lungs.
19. The primary function of white blood cells is to protect the body against disease by combating different infectious and toxic agents that can invade the body.
20. Blood carries water, oxygen, food, and secretions to the body cells.
21. Blood carries carbon dioxide gas and metabolic waste products away from the body cells.
22. The blood protects the body against extreme heat or cold, harmful bacteria, and the excessive loss of blood by forming an external clot.
23. Normal body temperature is 98.6(F (37(C).
24. The lymph system includes the lymph, lymphatics, lymph ducts, lymph nodes, glands, and lacteals. Also considered a part of the lymph system are the tonsils, the spleen, and the thymus gland.
25. The function of the lymph-vascular system is to collect excess tissue fluid, invading microorganisms, damaged cells, and protein molecules. The lymphoid tissue also produces lymphocytes, a white blood cell that is an important element of the body's immune system.
26. The lymph nodes filter harmful bacteria and toxic matter from the lymph and are the site of production of lymphocytes.
27. The parts of the body containing lymph nodes are the back of the head, around the neck muscles, under the armpit, under the pectoral muscles, along the blood vessels of the abdomen and pelvis, the back of the knees, and the groin.
28. Lymph is derived from interstitial or extracellular fluid.
29. Lymph returns to venous blood through the brachiocephalic veins near the junction of the jugular vein.
30. Lymph drainage is draining of lymph fluids from various areas of the body.
31. The lacteals are lymphatic vessels that carry chyle from the small intestine to the thoracic duct.
32. Massage increases flow of lymph and prevents stagnation.
33. Lymphatics are named according to their location in the body.
34. The lymphatic pump is similar to the venous pump. A system of valves in the lymph vessels operates so that external pressure on the walls of the vessel force the movement of lymph through the vessel in one direction.
35. Tissue fluid becomes lymph when it enters through the wall of a lymph capillary. From there, lymph flows into larger lymphatics and into the first of possibly several lymph nodes. Eventually, the lymph flows out of the nodes, through another lymph vessel, and into either the right or thoracic lymph duct. From the lymph duct, lymph flows into the brachiocephalic vein.

Matching Test I

1. b; 2. c; 3. d; 4. e; 5. a

True or False Test I

1. T; 2. F; 3. T; 4. F; 5. T

Matching Test II

1. d; 2. a; 3. e; 4. c; 5. b

True or False Test II

1. T; 2. F; 3. T; 4. F; 5. F

System 5: The Nervous System

1. The nervous system controls and coordinates the functions of other systems of the body so that they work harmoniously and efficiently. The primary function of the nervous system is to collect a multitude of sensory information; process, interpret, and integrate that information; and initiate appropriate responses throughout the body.
2. The main parts of the nervous system include the brain, spinal cord, and the peripheral nerves.
3. A nerve cell is called a *neuron* and consists of a cell body, a single axon, and numerous dendrites.
4. Neurons have the ability to react to certain stimuli (irritability) and to transmit an

impulse generated by that stimulus over a distance or to another neuron (conductibility).

5. A *synapse* is the junction between two nerve cells where a nerve impulse is transmitted from one nerve cell to another.
6. A sensory neuron or afferent neuron carries impulses from the sense organs in the periphery of the body toward the central nervous system (CNS). A motor or efferent neuron carries impulses away from the CNS to the muscles or glands that they control. Interneurons, located in the spinal cord or brain, transmit impulses from one nerve cell to another.
7. A nerve is a bundle of nerve fibers held together by connective tissue that extends from the CNS to the tissue that the neurons innervate.
8. An efferent nerve or motor nerve is composed of motor neurons that carry impulses from the CNS to the tissues they innervate.
9. An afferent nerve or sensory nerve is composed of sensory neurons that carry impulses from the body toward the CNS.
10. A mixed nerve is composed of both sensory and motor nerves. Most nerves in the body are mixed nerves.
11. The two divisions of the nervous system are the CNS and the peripheral nervous system.
12. The CNS consists of the brain, which is located in the cranium, and the spinal cord, which is located in the vertebral canal of the spine.
13. The *meninges* form a fibrous connective tissue covering of the CNS, consisting of the dura mater, the arachnoid mater, and the pia mater.
14. Cerebrospinal fluid is a clear fluid derived from the blood and secreted into the inner cavities or ventricles of the brain. Cerebrospinal fluid carries some nutrients to the nerve tissue and carries wastes away; however, its main function is to protect the CNS by acting as a shock absorber for the delicate tissue.
15. The main parts of the brain are the cerebrum, the cerebellum, and the brain stem, consisting of the midbrain, the pons, and the medulla oblongata.
16. The peripheral nervous system consists of all the nerves that connect the CNS to the rest of the body and therefore is located throughout all the innervated tissues of the body.
17. The two divisions of the peripheral nervous system are the somatic nervous system and the autonomic nervous system.
18. There are 12 pairs of cranial nerves.
19. The 12 cranial nerves are the I olfactory nerve, II optic nerve, III oculomotor nerve, IV trochlear nerve, V trigeminal or trifacial nerve, VI abducent nerve, VII facial nerve, VIII acoustic or auditory nerve, IX glossopharyngeal nerve, X vagus or pneumogastric nerve, XI spinal accessory nerve, and XII hypoglossal nerve.
20. There are 31 pairs of spinal nerves.
21. The spinal nerves are numbered according to the vertebral level where they exit the spinal column. They are numbered as follows: cervical nerves—C1 through 8; thoracic nerves—T1 through 12; Lumbar nerves—L1 through 5; sacral nerves-S1 through 5; and one pair of coccygeal nerves.
22. A nerve plexus is a network or gathering of nerves located outside of the CNS.
23. The important nerve plexuses are the cervical plexus, formed by the spinal nerves C 1–4, serving the structures in the region of the neck; the brachial plexus, formed by the spinal nerves C5–T1, serving the shoulder, arm, and part of the chest; the lumbar plexus, formed by the spinal nerves T12–L4, serving the muscles and organs of the abdomen, hip, and upper leg; the sacral plexus, formed by the spinal nerves L4–S4, creating the sciatic nerve and serving the legs; the coccygeal plexus, formed by part of S4 and S5, serving the area around the coccyx.
24. The autonomic nervous system regulates the action of glands, smooth muscles, and the heart.
25. The parasympathetic and sympathetic are the two divisions of the autonomic nervous system. The activity of the sympathetic system is primarily to prepare the organism for energy-expending, stressful, or emergency situations. Stimulation of the sympathetic nerves can bring about rapid responses, such as increased respiration, dilated pupils, and increased heart rate and cardiac output. Blood vessels dilate, the skin constricts, and

the liver increases conversion of glycogen to glucose for more energy. There is increased mental activity and production of adrenal hormones. The parasympathetic nervous system balances the action of the sympathetic system. The general function of the parasympathetic division is to conserve energy and reverse the action of the sympathetic division.

26. The involuntary muscles, heart, lungs, stomach, intestines, and blood vessels are supplied by the sympathetic nervous system, as are the adrenal and salivary glands, the bladder, and reproductive organs.
27. *Reflex action* is the involuntary response of a muscle to a stimulus.
28. Proprioception is a system of sensory and motor nerve activity that provides information as to the position and rate of movement of different body parts to the CNS. Proprioception provides information as to the state of contraction and position of the muscles.
29. Two categories of proprioceptors are spindle cells and Golgi tendon organs. Spindle cells, located mostly in the belly of the muscle, record changes in the length and stretch of the muscle as well as how far and fast the muscle is moving. The Golgi tendon organs are located in the tendon near its connection to the muscle and record the amount of tension produced in muscle cells that occurs as a result of the muscle stretching and contracting and the amount of force pulling on the bone to which the tendon attaches.

Matching Test I

1. c; 2. d; 3. e; 4. b; 5. a

True or False Test I

1. F; 2. T; 3. F; 4. T; 5. T

Matching Test II

1. e; 2. d; 3. a; 4. c; 5. b

True or False Test II

1. F; 2. T; 3. T; 4. F; 5. T

Matching Test III

1. b; 2. e; 3. a; 4. c; 5. d

True or False Test III

1. T; 2. F; 3. F; 4. T; 5. T

Matching Test IV

1. b; 2. e; 3. d; 4. c; 5. a

True or False Test IV

1. F; 2. T; 3. T; 4. F; 5. T

Matching Test V

1. e; 2. c; 3. b; 4. a; 5. d

True or False Test V

1. T; 2. F; 3. T; 4. F; 5. T

System 6: The Endocrine System

1. The endocrine system is composed of a group of glands the functions of which are vital to the maintenance of health.
2. The major function of the endocrine system is to assist the nervous system in regulating body processes.
3. A duct gland possesses a duct or canal that carries its secretions to their destination, whereas a ductless gland has no duct and therefore must depend on the circulatory system to carry its secretions to various affected tissues.
4. The blood supplies the raw materials that glands use to produce secretions. The nerves control many of the functional activities of the glands.
5. Sebaceous glands are duct glands that provide sebum (oil) to lubricate the skin.
6. A ductless or endocrine gland has no duct but delivers its secretion directly into the bloodstream, affecting the growth, development, sexual activity, and health of the entire body, depending on the gland's target organs and the quality and quantity of its secretions.
7. The pancreas and sex glands (gonads) function as both duct and ductless glands.
8. The ductless or endocrine glands produce hormones.
9. Hormones are specialized to act on specific tissues (target organs) or influence certain processes in the body. Some have a profound effect on physical or sexual development. Others regulate metabolism or body chemistry. Some hormones stimulate or restrain the activity of another gland. The endocrine glands operate cooperatively with one another and the nervous system to maintain a state of homeostasis within the organism.
10. The important endocrine glands are the pituitary gland, thyroid gland, parathyroid glands, adrenal glands, sex glands (gonads),

and pancreas. Other organs that have hormone-producing tissue include the pineal gland, the hypothalamus, the kidneys, the placenta, and intestinal mucosa.

11. Most diseases or dysfunctions of the endocrine system are the result of overactivity or underactivity of one or more glands. Overactive or hyperactive glands oversecrete hormones owing to lack of regulation or glandular tumors. Underactive or hypoactive glands secrete insufficient amounts of their respective hormones.
12. The pituitary gland is often called the *master gland* because many of the hormones it secretes stimulate or regulate other endocrine glands.
13. The hormone-producing parts of the adrenal glands are the adrenal cortex and the medulla.
14. The male sex glands produce testosterone, and the female sex glands produce estrogen and progesterone.

Answers to Matching I

1. a; 2. f; 3. g; 4. a; 5. b; 6. i; 7. a; 8. e; 9. h; 10. e; 11. a; 12. g; 13. f; 14. c; 15. a

Answers to Matching II

1. j; 2. a; 3. h; 4. d; 5. g; 6. f; 7. b; 8. i; 9. e; 10. c

System 7: The Respiratory System

1. The major respiratory organs include the nose, nasal cavity, pharynx, larynx, trachea, bronchial tubes, and the lungs.
2. The respiratory system is responsible for the vital exchange of oxygen and carbon dioxide.
3. The lungs are two sacs composed of spongy tissue, blood vessels, connective tissue, and microscopic air sacs called alveoli.
4. The three levels of respiration are external, internal, and cellular, or oxidation. External respiration takes place in the lungs. Internal respiration takes place between the bloodstream and the cells of the body. Cellular respiration or oxidation takes place within the cells.
5. The alveoli are microscopic air sacs at the terminal ends of the bronchioles, which are surrounded by the pulmonary capillaries, where the exchange of carbon dioxide for oxygen takes place.
6. Breathing or ventilation is the process of inhaling and exhaling air.
7. The natural rate of breathing is 14 to 20 breaths per minute.
8. The *diaphragm* is a muscular sheet separating the thorax from the abdominal cavity and is the major muscle used in breathing.

System 8: The Digestive System

1. Structures of the digestive system include the alimentary canal and accessory digestive organs. The alimentary canal consists of the mouth, pharynx, esophagus, stomach, small intestine, and large intestine. The accessory organs include the teeth, tongue, salivary glands, pancreas, liver, and gallbladder.
2. The main functions of the digestive system are digestion and absorption. Digestion is the process of converting food into substances capable of being used by the cells for nourishment.
3. Absorption is the process in which the digested nutrients are transferred from the intestines to the blood or lymph vessels so that they can be transported to the cells.
4. The physical process of digestion involves the teeth, which tear and grind the food, and the action of the muscles, which churn and mix the food as well as push it through the digestive tract.
5. Enzymes aid digestion.
6. In the mouth, food is chewed and mixed with saliva, and carbohydrates begin to be digested to the sugar stage.
7. The *alimentary canal* is a muscular tube about 30 feet long that extends from the mouth to the anus. The wall of the alimentary canal consists of four distinct layers: the mucosa or mucous membrane is made up of epithelial cells, connective tissue, and a variety of digestive glands. This layer protects the underlying tissues and carries on secretion and absorption. The submucosa consists of connective tissue, nerves, and blood and lymph vessels that serve to nour-

ish the surrounding tissues and carry away the absorbed material. The muscular layer has two layers of smooth muscle that churn the contents and propel it through the canal. The serous layer is the outer covering of the tube.

8. *Peristaltic action* is a rhythmic, wavelike muscular action of the smooth muscles of the alimentary canal that propels and churns the food throughout the length of the canal.
9. In the stomach, food is mixed with gastric juice and protein digestion begins.
10. The parts of the small intestine are the duodenum, the jejunum, and the ileum.
11. Digestive secretions in the small intestines are supplied by the liver, pancreas, and glands in the small intestine.
12. In the small intestine, food is completely digested.
13. The blood vessels and lacteals in the villi in the walls of the small intestine absorb the end products of digestion.
14. The rectum of the large intestine eliminates undigested food waste from the body.

System 9: The Excretory System

1. The organs that compose the excretory system are the lungs, kidneys, skin, liver, and large intestine.
2. The body will become poisoned by its own waste products.
3. The excretory system eliminates metabolic waste and undigested foods from the body.
4. The urinary system includes two kidneys, two ureters, the bladder, and a urethra.
5. The functional unit of the kidney is the *nephron*.
6. A urinalysis indicates the presence of white blood cells, blood, glucose, or other chemicals in the urine that can be an indication of metabolic imbalance, infection, or numerous other conditions.
7. A change in the color of the urine, such as cloudiness or a reddish or brownish color, can indicate infection or other health problems.
8. The liver secretes bile.
9. The main excretory function of the liver is the production of urea, which is returned to the blood to be excreted by the kidneys. The liver also excretes bile into the small intestines.

System 10: The Human Reproductive System

1. The reproductive system is the generative apparatus necessary for organisms to reproduce organisms of the same kind or species.
2. Asexual reproduction, as in some one-celled organisms, means that no partner is needed to reproduce. In humans and animals, reproduction is sexual and requires a male and female to reproduce.
3. A *gonad* is a sex gland-the ovary in the female and the testes in the male.
4. A *zygote* is the fertilized ovum, the cell formed by the union of a spermatozoon (sperm) with the ovum (egg).
5. The reproductive system in males includes two testes, two vas deferens, two seminal vesicles, a prostate gland, the bulbourethral glands (Cowper's glands), and the penis.
6. The functions of the male reproductive system are the production of sperm, the production of the male hormones, and the performance of the sex act.
7. The reproductive system in women includes two ovaries, two fallopian tubes (oviducts), a uterus, a vagina, and the vulva or external genitalia.
8. The functions of the female reproductive system are to produce the ovum and female hormones, to receive the sperm during the sex act, and to carry the growing fetus during pregnancy.
9. From the beginning of conception until approximately the third month of pregnancy, the developing child is called an *embryo*. After that time, it is called a *fetus*.
10. Ovulation is the discharge of a mature egg cell from the follicle of the ovary.
11. Pregnancy lasts approximately 40 weeks, or 280 days.

Chapter 6: Effects, Benefits, Indications, and Contraindications of Massage

1. The main physiologic benefits of massage are stimulation of the muscular, vascular, and glandular activities of the body. Circulation is increased, and soreness and stiffness of the muscles relieved.
2. The psychological benefits of massage result from the reduction of tension and relief from stress and anxiety. Massage can also promote a sense of renewed energy and well-being. Massage helps the client to feel healthier, more invigorated, and more energetic.
3. Massage has direct mechanical effects and indirect reflex effects on the body.
4. Massage is beneficial to all body systems, including the circulatory, nervous, skeletal, muscular, digestive, glandular, integumentary (skin), respiratory, and excretory systems.
5. Massage benefits the development of the muscular system by way of stimulation of its circulation, nerve supply, and cell activity. Massage is also an effective means of relaxing tense muscles and releasing muscle spasms. Massage prevents and relieves stiffness and soreness of muscles. Muscle tissue that has suffered injury heals more quickly and with less connective tissue buildup and scarring when therapeutic massage is applied appropriately and regularly.
6. Nearly all massage movements enhance circulation; however, stroking, kneading, and compression most effectively promote circulation.
7. Massage relieves stiff, sore muscles by improving circulation of the blood through the body part. It helps in the removal of waste products and supplies the cells with oxygen and nourishment.
8. Cross-fiber friction and compression movements prevent the formation of adhesions and fibrosis in muscles.
9. The immediate effects of massage on the skin include increased circulation of the blood, which nourishes the skin, improves tone, and helps to normalize the functioning of the sebaceous (oil) glands.
10. Depending on the type of massage movement applied, the nervous system can be stimulated or soothed.
11. Friction, vibration, and light percussion movements produce a stimulating effect on the nervous system.
12. Gentle stroking, light friction, and petrissage produce a sedative effect on the nervous system.
13. Massage affects the quality and rate of blood flowing through the circulatory system. Direct and reflex effects of massage increase circulation and stimulate the production of red and white blood cells.
14. Massage movements are directed toward the heart to facilitate the flow of blood and lymph back toward the heart.
15. Light or deep stroking, light percussion, friction, petrissage, and compression are all useful in increasing the flow of blood and lymph.
16. Massage improves the circulation of the blood, which in turn supplies beneficial nutrients to the skin.
17. When the client has a condition that appears to be a contraindication to massage, massage should be avoided.
18. *Contraindication* means the expected treatment or process is inadvisable. In massage it refers to any condition in which massage is inadvisable because it would not be beneficial or could be dangerous.
19. It is important to take a client's medical history to help to determine potential indications and contraindications for the massage.
20. The practitioner should have a thermometer to take a client's temperature if a fever is suspected. Massage is not recommended when the client's temperature is abnormally high. An abnormally high temperature is an indication of illness, infection, or other health problems.
21. Massage should be avoided when there is a contraindication, such as a physical or mental condition that needs medical attention or when there is doubt of its benefits. The therapist should refer the client to an appropriate health professional in this case.
22. The signs of inflammation are heat, swelling, pain, and redness.

23. In the case of local inflammation, massage must be avoided on the inflamed area and applied to the area of the body proximal to the inflammation to promote circulation toward and away from the area.
24. The practitioner can recognize varicose veins as bluish, protruding, thick, bulbous, distended superficial veins usually found in the lower legs.
25. A *hematoma* is a mass of blood trapped in some tissue or cavity of the body and is the result of internal bleeding. When the hematoma is in the acute phase, massage is contraindicated because of the risk of reinjuring the tissue. Once the bruise has changed colors, light massage can enhance circulation to the area and actually assists the healing.
26. Certain areas of the body are sites of possible endangerment because relatively unprotected anatomic structures could be injured by certain massage manipulations, such as major nerves, blood vessels, or vital organs that might be vulnerable to deep manipulations.

Chapter 7: Equipment and Products

1. The massage practitioner should project a professional image of relaxed confidence.
2. A massage space should be comfortable, clean, and free of distractions and safety hazards. It should be of an adequate size, well ventilated and a comfortably warm temperature.
3. A room that is 10 feet by 12 feet allows ample space for a massage table, desk, dressing area, and other equipment and supplies necessary to perform massage.
4. Equipment should be checked for safety and sanitation. Supplies must be checked to ensure an adequate supply and to see that they are clean and stored properly.
5. Preparation is essential to good service, and it shows that the therapist is a professional.
6. Lubricants, creams, and powders are products used for body massage.
7. The massage room is usually most comfortable for clients when the temperature is 72° to 75°F.
8. The height of the massage table should be adjusted to give the practitioner more leverage to do the massage efficiently. Correct height also allows for good body mechanics and prevents the practitioner from becoming fatigued.
9. Soft, natural, indirect lighting is best in the massage room.
10. Some people find music distracting and prefer absolute quiet.

Chapter 8: Sanitary and Safety Practices

1. All states have laws pertaining to sanitation for the protection of the public. These laws protect both clients and practitioners.
2. As a practitioner, you should practice the rules of sanitation because you are responsible for safeguarding the client's health as well as your own health.
3. The practitioner should have some knowledge of bacteria to understand the importance of preventing the spread of disease.
4. Pathogenic bacteria are harmful, whereas nonpathogenic bacteria are harmless and sometimes helpful.
5. The body produces antibodies to inhibit or destroy invading harmful bacteria.
6. Three forms of pathogenic (harmful) bacteria are cocci, bacilli, and spirilla.
7. The strict practice of sanitation is the best prevention against the spread of harmful bacteria.
8. Universal precautions is a system of infection control that is to be employed whenever there is a chance of exposure to or possible contact with human blood or other bodily fluids.
9. Before using any disinfectant or antiseptic product, read the manufacturer's instructions and follow them.
10. Disinfectants are used in the practice of massage to keep all equipment and the premises in a clean, sanitary condition.
11. The best method for keeping the hands and nails clean is to scrub them with antibacterial soap and warm water for a minimum of 15 seconds. The hands are then rinsed thoroughly and dried with a clean towel. The towel is then used to turn off the water

so that the hand is not recontaminated by touching the faucet.

12. Suitable strengths for cresol and Lysol used to clean floors, sinks, and restrooms are 1 to 5 percent.
13. *Sterilization* is the procedure for making an object germ-free by destroying bacteria, both the harmful and harmless kinds.
14. Safety is an attitude put into practice that is concerned with the prevention of situations and elimination of conditions that might lead to injury of the massage practitioner or client.
15. Safety considerations in a massage practice need to focus on (1) the facility, (2) the equipment, (3) the massage practitioner, and (4) the client.

Chapter 9: Consultation and Documentation

1. The consultation is important to obtain certain data regarding the client's conditions and to determine the most effective treatments.
2. An assessment includes taking the client's medical history, observing the client's actions, and performing verbal and manipulative tests that might indicate the client's conditions.
3. A preliminary assessment is advisable when performing massage therapy because it clarifies the client's conditions, reveals indications and contraindications, determines whether referral to another health professional is advisable, and indicates which therapeutic techniques to use.
4. The treatment plan is an outline that is created from the information gained during the assessment that the practitioner can follow when giving massage treatments.
5. The treatment plan is formulated using information from the intake and medical history forms, the interview, and preliminary assessment to formulate session goals and choose massage techniques.
6. *Informed consent* is an educational and informative process that ensures that the client has received and understands the nature and extent of the massage services before giving consent to proceed.
7. The practitioner discloses adequate information regarding the practitioner's credentials, the services offered, and the policies and procedures used during the sessions and describes the massage techniques to be employed as well as projected effects and outcomes, including benefits and possible side effects.
8. Accurate records are important to both the practitioner and client because special information might be needed for reference. Well-kept records also help the practitioner to determine and render the most effective treatments.
9. Information that is often found in a client file includes intake contact information (i.e., name, address, telephone numbers), medical information and history, treatment plan and recorded notes, and financial and billing information.
10. The client might not understand why premassage procedures are necessary or might feel uneasy and not know what is expected.
11. Being able to anticipate and answer questions that the client might ask gives the practitioner more credibility.

Chapter 10: Classical Massage Movements

1. The six basic classifications of movements are touch, stroking, kneading, friction, percussion, and joint movements.
2. The practitioner should regulate the intensity of pressure, direction of movement, and duration of each type of manipulation to meet the client's needs.
3. Light movements should be applied over thin tissues and bony parts.
4. Heavier movements should be applied over thick tissues and muscular parts.
5. Massage is generally applied in a centripetal direction, or toward the heart.
6. Massage strokes directed away from the heart should be light enough that they do not affect fluid flow.
7. The approximate duration of a full-body massage is about one hour.

8. In massage technique, touch is the stationary contact of the practitioner's hand and the client's body.
9. Light or superficial touch is purposeful contact in which the natural and evenly distributed weight of the practitioner's finger, fingers, or hand is applied on a given area of the client's body. The main objective of light touch is to soothe and to provide a comforting connection that is calming and allows the powerful healing mechanisms of the body to function. Touch is effective in the reduction of pain, lowering of blood pressure, control of nervous irritability, or reassurance for a nervous, tense client.
10. Deep touch is performed with one finger, thumb, several fingers, or the entire hand. The heel of the hand, knuckles, or elbow can be used according to desired results. Deep touch is used when calming, anesthetizing, or stimulating effects are desired. Deep pressure is useful in soothing muscle spasms and relieving pain at reflex areas, stress points in tendons, and trigger points in muscle.
11. Aura stroking is done with long, smooth strokes, where the practitioner's hands glide the length of the client's entire body or body part, coming very close to but not actually touching the body surface.
12. Another name for feather stroking is nerve strokes. These are usually used as the final stroke to the individual areas of the body.
13. *Effleurage* is a succession of strokes applied by gliding the hand over a somewhat extended portion of the body.
14. Superficial stroking is a kind of effleurage that requires the lightest possible touch.
15. Deep gliding strokes require firm pressure.
16. Superficial gliding strokes produce soothing effects and overcome tiredness or restlessness.
17. Deep gliding strokes have a stretching and broadening effect on muscle tissue and fascia. They also enhance and stimulate the venous blood flow.
18. Kneading movements are applied by grasping muscular tissue with one or both hands and then squeezing, rolling, or pinching with a firm pressure.
19. Kneading enhances the fluid movement in the superficial as well as the deeper tissues.
20. The classical term that means the same as kneading is *petrissage*.
21. Fulling is recommended for the muscular areas of the arms and legs.
22. Friction movements are applied to the body by moving more superficial layers of flesh against the deeper tissues to flatten, broaden, or stretch the tissue.
23. Heat created during friction movements affects the connective tissues surrounding the muscles, making them more pliable so that they function more efficiently.
24. Cross-fiber friction uses short, deep strokes transverse to the direction of muscle, tendon, or ligament fibers. The fingers do not move over the skin but move the skin and superficial tissues across the target tissue.
25. Compression movements are rhythmic pressing movements directed into muscle tissue perpendicular to the body part by either the hand or fingers.
26. Compression movement invigorates the body, stimulates the flow of blood and lymph, and prevents muscular stiffness following exercise. Compression movements cause increased circulation and a lasting hyperemia in the tissue.
27. Vibratory movements are applied with a continuous shaking or trembling movement by means of the practitioner's hands or an electrical vibrator.
28. Vibration is safe at a rate of 5 to 10 times per second by hand, 10 to 100 times per second by electrical vibrators.
29. The practitioner can control the effects of vibratory movements by controlling the rate of vibration, intensity of pressure, and duration of treatment.
30. Excessive vibration produces a numbing effect.
31. Percussion movements are applied with quick striking movements performed with both hands simultaneously or alternately.
32. Percussion movements are slapping, beating, hacking, cupping, and tapping.
33. Percussion movements tone the muscles and stimulate the nervous and circulatory systems.

34. Joint movements can be used to manipulate any joint in the body, including joints of the toes, knees, hips, arms, the vertebrae, or even the less movable joints of the pelvis and cranium.
35. Two types of joint movements are active joint movements and passive joint movements.
36. During an active assistive joint movement, the client is instructed to perform a motion at the same time the practitioner assists the movement. During an active resistive movement, the client is instructed to make a motion while the limb is held to resist movement.
37. Range of motion (ROM) is the movement of a joint from one extreme of the articulation to the other.
38. *End feel* is the change in the quality of the feeling the therapist senses as the end of a joint movement is approached.
39. Pressure is regulated during a massage according to the technique used and according to the intended outcome. The rule is to begin with a light and sensitive touch, increase the pressure as you work into an area, and then gradually reduce pressure as you leave the area.
40. A person's pain threshold is the amount of discomfort or pain that can be tolerated without adverse reactions. When the pain threshold is violated, the client tenses up and the massage work becomes less effective or can even be counterproductive.

Chapter 11: Application of Massage Technique

1. The massage practitioner must develop strong, flexible hands to deliver massage movements to the body over an extended period and to control the pressure and rhythm while working over the contours of the body.
2. Body mechanics is the observation of body postures in relation to safe and efficient movement in daily living activities.
3. Using good body mechanics increases the strength and power available in a movement while at the same time reducing the risk of potential injury to the person performing the massage.
4. To increase the power and strength in a movement and at the same time conserve energy, the practitioner must use the muscles in the legs and the movement of the whole body to deliver the strokes. Keeping the hands in good alignment and close to the practitioner's body and moving the whole body conserves energy and increases the power and strength when performing massage.
5. Correct posture and stances aid balance; allow the delivery of firmer, more powerful massage strokes; conserve strength; and sustain energy when it is necessary to perform multiple massages.

Chapter 12: Procedures for Complete Body Massages

1. The practitioner should wash hands before and after each treatment.
2. For reasons of safety and liability, it is advisable that the practitioner assist the client onto the table at the beginning of a massage and into a sitting position and off of the table at the end of the massage.
3. Chilling of the client's body can be prevented by keeping the room warm and by using proper draping.
4. Two common methods of draping are the top cover method, which uses a table covering and a separate sheet or towel to cover the client, and full sheet draping, which uses a double-sized sheet to cover the table and wrap the client.
5. Besides draping, the therapist can ensure the client's warmth by keeping the room at a comfortable temperature or using an electric mattress pad or supplying extra coverings.
6. The practitioner can avoid scratching the client by filing the fingernails short and smooth and removing jewelry.
7. Heavy pressure, rapid movement, or jarring contact cause fear and should be avoided.
8. It is better for the client to receive a massage before eating a meal.

9. The average duration of a massage is about an hour.
10. Massage should never be applied to an area where there is injury or abrasion of the skin, fever, inflammation of joints or veins, or when other contraindications are present.
11. Before a body massage, check facilities for readiness, obtain and arrange supplies, and check self for readiness. Obtain necessary information about client's needs and wishes, advise the client regarding preparation procedures, and assist as necessary.
12. The position that the client assumes first for a massage depends on the treatment to be given and the preference of the therapist and the client; however, generally the massage begins with the client in supine (face up) position.
13. The order of massage movements is determined by the purpose of the massage and the preference of the therapist. Movements should follow a logical sequence, such as
    a. Begin with the hands and arms, right then left
    b. Proceed to front of the legs and feet, left then right
    c. Continue movements over chest, neck, and abdomen
    d. The client then turns over to assume a prone (face down) position
    e. Begin with the back of the legs, right then left
    f. Finish the massage with the back of the body
14. The final considerations of massage involve completing the client's record card, suggesting supplementary services, placing supplies in their proper places, discarding refuse, and arranging the massage table and bath for the next client.
15. Undesirable aftereffects can include a slight headache, upset stomach and nausea, or the feeling that comes with the onset of a cold. Such reactions are due to an increase in metabolic waste material in the circulatory system. This waste material puts an extra burden on the excretory system. If this waste is not flushed out of the system, it will be reabsorbed into the tissues. The particular symptom that the client experiences depends on the organs that are being overtaxed.
16. The client should drink plenty of water to keep the system flushed out following a massage.

Chapter 13: Hydrotherapy

1. Hydrotherapy is the application of water in any of its three forms (i.e., ice, water, vapor) to the body for therapeutic purposes.
2. The qualities of water that make it an effective therapeutic tool are that it is readily available, is relatively inexpensive to use, has the ability to absorb and conduct heat, provides buoyancy, and is a solvent.
3. The three classifications of the effects of hydrotherapy on the body are thermal, mechanical, and chemical.
4. Water treatments that involve hot or cold applications should not be given when the client has cardiac impairment, diabetes, lung disease, kidney infection, extremely high or low blood pressure, an infectious skin condition, or the inability to feel hot or cold. Treatments that tend to raise the body's core temperature are contraindicated during pregnancy and for those with multiple sclerosis.
5. Cryotherapy is the application of ice for therapeutic purposes.
6. The local application of ice acts as an analgesic to reduce pain and causes vasoconstriction to limit swelling. It is beneficial on painful, inflamed, and swollen areas.
7. In the acronym PRICE, P = protect, R= rest, I= ice, C= compression, and E= elevation. PRICE is the standard first-aid treatment when a soft tissue injury such as a sprain or strain occurs. It reduces swelling, pain, and the secondary tissue damage that results from excessive swelling.
8. CBAN is the acronym for cold, burning, aching and numbness. These describe the series of sensations that result from applying ice to an area of the body.
9. Cold applications are beneficial because they improve circulation, stimulate nerves, and increase the activity of body cells. Cold applications help reduce swelling and pain.

10. Cold applications are undesirable over prolonged periods because they can produce a depressing effect. If after a cold bath or shower the client comes out chilly, shivering, blue-lipped, or goosefleshed, it indicates that the client's body reaction is not good.
11. Four convenient ways to apply cryotherapy are cold compresses, ice packs, ice massage, and immersion baths.
12. Thermotherapy is the application of heat to the body for therapeutic purposes.
13. Hot water applications improve skin functions by promoting perspiration and by increasing the circulation of blood to the surface of the skin.
14. The skin can tolerate 110°F of hot water for short periods and approximately 130°F of steam vapor. Water above 104°F over a prolonged period can cause hyperthermia, a potentially dangerous condition.
15. Two objectives of baths are external cleanliness and stimulation of bodily functions.
16. A warm bath is 95° to 100°F, equal to 35° to 37.7°C. A hot bath is 100° to 104°F, equal to 37.7° to 40°C.
17. The average duration of a cold bath, shower, or sitz bath is approximately three to five minutes.
18. The duration of a hot saline or sitz bath is approximately 5 to 10 minutes.
19. The purpose of a cabinet bath is to induce perspiration that contributes to a weight reduction and to induce relaxation. It is also considered to be a cleansing procedure.
20. Safety precautions to observe during the operation of a bath cabinet include following the manufacturer's instructions for use of the cabinet and observing the client's general reactions, state of health, and tolerance to temperature.
21. The main benefits of a whirlpool bath are increased blood circulation, the soothing of nerves, and relaxing of the muscles.
22. Contrast therapy is the alternating application of hot and cold applications to a portion of the body.
23. Contrast therapy is one of the most effective methods of increasing local circulation by causing an alternating vasodilation and vasoconstriction of the blood vessels in an area.

Chapter 14: Massage in the Spa Setting

1. The origins of the word *spa* come from a Latin acronym for *sanitas per aqua,* or "health through water." The term might also have derived from the Latin verb *spagere,* which means to sprinkle or flow, like a fountain or spring.
2. In Rome, early spas or baths were called *thermae.* In Turkey they were called *hammam,* and in Japan they were called *Onsen.*
3. In 2007, the U.S. spa market was a $9.4 billion industry with 14,600 locations and 111 million guest visits.
4. The major categories of spas are destination spas, hotel/resort spas, day spas, club spas, medical/dental spas, and mineral spring spas.
5. Some of the spa modalities in addition to massage that therapists might be required to perform include body wraps, body scrubs, foot treatments, back treatments, scalp treatments, face treatments, cellulite treatments, aromatherapy, parafango, clay/mud/seaweed treatments, specialized rituals and exotic services such as Ayurvedic and Indonesian treatments, herbal detoxification treatments, and hydrotherapy baths and showers.
6. The most important points to keep in mind while practicing massage in a spa setting are: scope of practice, intake procedures, optimal number of massages per day, timing of services, guest greetings, preparation, and cleanup.
7. The major challenges to consistently giving high-quality therapeutic massage in the spa setting are low expectations, time constraints, and inexperienced clients. To overcome them, therapists should pay special attention to the timing, transitions, and uniqueness of each massage.
8. No. The rules and laws vary widely state to state regarding what a massage therapist can and cannot do in the spa setting. In some states, the law requires massage therapists to perform body wraps and exfoliation treat-

ments; in others, the law allows untrained spa technicians to perform these treatments.

9. A spa cellulite treatment features vigorous massage, wrapping, and special products (usually seaweed-based) to promote an improved appearance to affected areas. It often includes underwater massage in a hydrotherapy tub.
10. A spa parafango treatment uses a blend of paraffin wax and fango (mud from a volcanic source) that is smoothed onto a part of or the whole body while warm and then is wrapped.
11. In the spa industry, *aromatherapy* can be defined as the use of essential oils processed from herbs, flowers, fruits, spices, stems, bark, and roots in massage, inhalation, or other modalities to affect mood and improve health and well-being.
12. Some carrier oils commonly used for aromatherapy massage include apricot kernel, avocado, grapeseed, jojoba, sesame, sweet almond, and wheat germ.
13. Some distinctions that make an aromatherapy massage different from a Swedish massage include the following: therapists should check for guests' sensitivity to aromas and explain therapeutic outcomes prior to treatment. During the treatment, strokes are predominantly light and flowing, and time is allowed for the client to experience the aromas. Blankets and/or an infrared heating lamp should be in place if necessary to keep the client warm.
14. Spas offer body wraps for heating the body; detoxification; to relax and improve mood and well-being; to nourish, cleanse, and improve the superficial contour the skin; for purging and drawing impurities out through the pores, softening the skin, improving joint elasticity, remineralizing the skin and entire body; and less frequently for weight-loss or inch-loss.
15. The main benefits of exfoliation are that it assists the skin's own regenerative processes, aids in the absorption of spa products applied afterward, thoroughly cleanses and promotes overall hygiene, and creates a healthy glow and radiant shine to the skin.
16. The principle maneuver for all exfoliation techniques is a circular scrubbing action. This is to avoid stretching the delicate connective tissues of the skin too far in any one direction.
17. A spa's company policies cover time concerns, appearance, attitude, professional development, and physical attributes.
18. As a part of professional career management, the spa, in exchange for a percentage of the price of each treatment, offers therapists many benefits, including built-in clientele, marketing, advertising, appointment booking, billing, payroll, supplies, equipment, training, support staff, and a clean facility.
19. A *Vichy shower* is a multihead inline shower extending out over a treatment table, under which clients recline on a wet table to receive spa services. It is primarily used for body wraps and exfoliation services, but it can also be used during specialty massages.
20. A *wet table* is a specially constructed waterproof treatment table with built-in drainage used in spas for exfoliation and body wrap services.
21. Customer service can be defined as the ability of an organization or individual to take care of the needs, wishes, questions, requests, and complaints of its clientele. Excellent customer service consists of doing these things consistently, to a very high standard of satisfaction, and in a largely transparent manner.
22. Most spas depend on retail profits to keep the business operational. Without these profits, many spas would close, and many therapists would be out of work. It is therefore in spa therapists' best interests to help with retail sales, as long as these sales are executed with integrity, honesty, and skill.
23. The main teamwork skills required to work successfully in a spa are being able to follow direction, anticipate others' needs, present a united front, and pitch in toward a common goal, regardless of whether a particular task is in the therapist's job description.
24. Therapists should come to spa job interviews prepared to talk about how they chose massage as a career, past work situations, attitude toward clients, and how they would

deal with problems on the job. In addition, they should have some knowledge of the spa where they are applying and be able to explain why they want to work at that particular facility.

25. Therapists considering opening a spa should start out slowly, honestly assess their own limitations, enlist valuable allies, and keep learning information from diverse fields such as bookkeeping, management, retail, housekeeping, human resources, equipment maintenance, customer relations, and, of course, hands-on skill.

Chapter 15: Clinical Massage Techniques

1. Neurophysiologic therapies recognize the importance of neurologic feedback between the CNS and the musculoskeletal system in maintaining proper tone and function. Alterations or disturbances in the neuromuscular relationship often result in dysfunction and pain. Neurophysiologic therapies use methods of assessing tissues and soft tissue manipulative techniques to normalize the tissues and reprogram the neurologic loop to reduce pain and improve function.
2. Neuromuscular therapy was developed in England in the 1930s by Dr. Stanley Lief. It has been popularized in the United States through the teachings of Paul St. John, Leon Chaitow, and Judith DeLany.
3. Abnormal tissue signs that indicate neuromuscular lesions include
   - Congestion in the tissues
   - Contracted tissue or taut, fibrous bands
   - Nodules or lumps
   - Trigger points
   - Restrictions between the skin and underlying tissues
   - Variations in temperature (warmer or cooler than surrounding tissues)
   - Swelling or edema
   - General tenderness

   Neuromuscular lesions are always hypersensitive to pressure and often associated with trigger points.
4. The four-step protocol for addressing neuromuscular dysfunction is as follows: a. Decrease ischemia and trigger points in soft tissue. b. Restore flexibility with joint mobilization and stretching. c. Rebuild strength with exercise and weight training. d. Restore endurance with conditioning exercises.
5. The primary treatment techniques used in neuromuscular therapy include gliding, ischemic compression, and stretching.
6. A trigger point is a hyperirritable spot that is painful when compressed. When stimulated, active trigger points refer pain and tenderness to another area of the body. Latent trigger points exhibit pain only when compressed and do not refer pain.
7. Myofascial trigger points are found in muscle tissue or its associated fascia. They are located in a taut band of muscle fibers.
8. Central trigger points are located near the middle of the muscle body and are thought to be associated with the motor end plate of the motor nerve. Attachment trigger points are located either at the myotendinous junction or the osseous attachment of a muscle and are thought to be caused by the continuous tension of the taut band caused by the central trigger point.
9. The criteria for recognizing active trigger points are the following: a. A palpable, taut band in the muscle. b. An exquisitely tender nodule in located in the taut band. c. Pressure applied to the nodule provokes pain, numbness, or tingling in a referred area. d. There is a reduced ROM in the tissue housing the suspected trigger point.
10. Procedures for deactivating trigger points include injections, stretch and spray, active stretching, and ischemic compression. Trigger-point pressure release, position release, and muscle energy techniques (METs) are modalities available to massage therapists to reduce trigger-point activity.
11. The two basic inhibitory reflexes produced during MET manipulations are postisometric relaxation and reciprocal inhibition.
12. The three active joint movements used in MET are contract-relax or agonist-contract,

antagonist-contract, and contract-relax-antagonist-contract.

13. Passive positioning techniques are perhaps the gentlest of soft tissue manipulations, wherein joints associated with constricted muscles are passively placed into their preferred position of greatest comfort.
14. Three important considerations of passive positioning techniques are
    a. Gently moving a joint into its position of maximal comfort
    b. Holding that position for an adequate period
    c. Slowly and passively returning the joint to its neutral position
15. Strain-counterstrain was developed by Dr. Lawrence Jones.
16. In strain-counterstrain, the preferred position is determined by palpating and monitoring the sensitivity of the associated tender points while positioning the joint. When the client indicates that the pain in the point is reduced and there is a noticeable "letting go" in the palpated tissues, when the pain or discomfort in the joint is also reduced, and when the client is in a comfortable position, the correct position has been established.
17. The primary techniques used in structural muscular balancing include precision muscle testing, passive positioning, directional massage, and deep pressure.
18. Preferred position pertains to moving the body or a body part in a manner that is away from pain, toward ease and the body's preference. Movements are away from bind and restrictive barriers and toward comfort.
19. *Myofascia* refers to skeletal muscle tissue and all of the connective tissue associated with it, including tendons, ligaments, and the attachments of muscles to bones and other structures. The myofascial system also includes neuromuscular connections and related superficial fascia.
20. Superficial is located just below the skin and is continuous over the entire body, connecting the skin to the deeper fascia.
21. Three techniques for assessing myofascial restrictions include postural assessment, skin rolling, tissue excursion or fascial glide, and positional testing or ROM.
22. Hands-on techniques for myofascial massage include skin rolling, cross-handed stretch, and traction. Cross-fiber techniques and J-strokes are direct connective tissue techniques.
23. The craniosacral system is a semi-closed hydraulic system composed of the meninges, the cerebrospinal fluid, the physiologic structures that control the fluid's input and output, and related cranial and spinal bones.
24. *Deep tissue massage* refers to various regimens or massage styles that affect the deeper tissue structures of the body. Deep tissue massage techniques affect the various layers of fascia that support muscle tissues and loosen bonds between the layers of connective tissues.
25. Structural integration attempts to bring the physical structure of the body into balance and alignment around a central axis.

Chapter 16: Lymph Massage

1. Three people who have had a major influence on the development of lymph massage are Dr. Emil Vodder, Dr. Johannas Asdonk, and Dr. Bruno Chikly.
2. Lymph circulation begins when interstitial fluid enters the initial lymphatics or lymph capillaries. Lymph continues from the capillaries into the pre-collectors and then into the larger lymph collectors on its way to the lymph nodes. It flows from the nodes into larger vessels and on into either the thoracic or right lymphatic ducts before it re-enters the venous system in the subclavian vein at the angulus venosus.
3. The four functions of lymph nodes include the following: a. The filtration of toxins and other elements from the lymph. b. The breakdown or destruction of harmful substances by the action of lymphocytes and phagocytes. c. Concentration of lymph by reabsorbing fluid back into the venous system. d. Production of monocytes and lymphocytes.

4. Lymphocytes (leukocytes) are white corpuscles found in lymphatic tissue, blood, and lymph. They are active in the immune responses of the body and play a major part in healing wounds and fighting infections.
5. Lymph is the portion of the interstitial fluid that is absorbed into the lymph capillaries. It consists of water, proteins, cellular debris, bacteria, viruses, and other inorganic materials.
6. Correct lymph massage helps to stimulate the flow of lymph, which rids the body of toxins and waste materials. Lymph massage promotes the balance of the body's internal chemistry, purifies and regenerates tissues, and helps to normalize the functions of all body organs and the immune system.
7. The sequence of movements generally begins and ends at the site of the collecting lymph nodes that drain the area being massaged. The lymph massage sequence begins proximally to clear out the lymph channels and works distally and then again from distal to proximal, finishing by once again helping to clear the area of the lymph nodes.

Chapter 17: Therapeutic Procedure

1. The four steps of the therapeutic procedure are assessment, planning, performance, and evaluation.
2. The purpose of assessment is to review any information available at the onset of the process to best understand the present conditions. During the planning stage, the information gained from the assessment is used to determine strategies and select therapeutic techniques to address specific conditions found during the assessment. The performance is the actual application of the selected techniques. The evaluation examines the outcome of the session in regard to the effectiveness of the selected procedure for the condition.
3. The therapeutic process can be implemented for long-range goal setting, covering several sessions; short-range planning, covering a single session; and during an actual massage session.
4. Five parts of the assessment are taking a client history, client interview, observation, palpation, and examination.
5. The pain scale is a subjective tool with which clients can describe the relative pain or discomfort they are experiencing on a scale of 1 to 10, where 1 is no pain and 10 is excruciating, unbearable pain. Clients are able to express the level of pain that they are experiencing at the beginning of the session and again at the end to indicate any improvement. The therapist is able to determine the amount of pressure to use in certain interventions by asking for the client's feedback using the pain scale.
6. When ROM is being tested, passive movement, active movement, and restricted movement are examined.
7. Soft tissue barriers represent the limits within which tissues are manipulated. The resistive barrier marks the first sense of tissue stretch. The physiologic barrier represents the extent of tissue stretch and easy, painless movement. The anatomic barrier represents the anatomic limit of a particular tissue. To move beyond the anatomic limit would result in tissue damage.
8. Soft tissues that can be palpated from superficial to deep include just above the surface of the skin, the skin surface, the superficial fascia including lymph nodes and blood vessels, muscles and related structures and textures, the musculotendinous junction, tendons, bones, ligaments, and joints.
9. According to Dr. James Cyriax, contractile tissues are the fibrous tissues that have tensions placed on them during muscular contractions and include muscle tissue, tendons, and the muscle attachments. Inert tissues are the tissues that are not contractile, such as bone, ligament, bursae, blood vessels, nerves, nerve coverings, and cartilage. *End feel* refers to the quality of the sensation that the therapist feels while passively moving a joint to the full extent of its possible range.
10. Three classifications of normal end feel are hard, soft, and springy.

11. Abnormal end feel is similar to normal end feel except that there is reduced movement or associated pain.
12. *Acute* and *chronic* are terms used to describe a condition, pain, or illness. Acute refers to a condition with a sudden onset and relatively short duration. Chronic refers to a lingering or ongoing condition.
13. The appropriate intervention in the initial stage of an acute soft tissue injury is protect the area, rest, ice, compression, and elevation (PRICE).
14. Information from the medical history, intake form, interview, observation, movement assessments, palpation, and the client's needs and concerns are used to develop a treatment or care plan.
15. Assessment findings and treatment plans are discussed with the client so that the client can actively participate in the therapy, better understand the condition and treatment, and give informed consent to proceed with the session.
16. A therapeutic massage is like an intense conversation in that the therapist listens, observes, and examines the client to get an idea of the condition. Then the therapist's hands listen to the client's body and respond with manipulative touch. The body listens to the manipulations and responds. Hearing and feeling these responses, the therapist chooses the next delivery, and so on.
17. Postural muscles respond to stress by shortening and becoming hypertonic, whereas phasic muscles fatigue and weaken in response to stress.
18. The evaluation is important because
    - The client and therapist can gauge the effectiveness of the selected course of therapy according to the success in attaining the goals.
    - It provides a rationale for applying similar therapies for similar conditions in the future.
    - It is the grounds for altering portions or all of the process to achieve desired results more effectively.
    - It helps to determine whether goals have been met and whether referral to another professional is warranted.

Chapter 18: Athletic/Sports Massage

1. *Athletic massage*, also called *sports massage*, is the application of massage techniques that combine sound anatomic and physiologic knowledge, an understanding of strength training and conditioning, and specific massage skills to enhance athletic performance.
2. *Adaptive sports massage* is sports massage for athletes with physical or mental disabilities, given with special consideration for the specific disability that the athlete might have.
3. The therapist must know the functions of the circulatory, skeletal, muscular, and nervous systems of the body.
4. The overload principle in conditioning refers to the necessity of applying stresses to the body greater than it is accustomed to increase strength or endurance.
5. Negative effects of exercise include
    - Increased metabolic waste buildup in the tissues
    - Strains in the muscle or connective tissue, which can range from microscopic microtrauma to major injury
    - Inflammation and associated fibrosis
    - Spasms and pain that restrict movement
6. Techniques commonly used in sports massage include those of Swedish massage plus compression, cross-fiber friction, deep pressure, and active joint movements.
7. The primary goal of compression is to create hyperemia in the muscle tissue.
8. In athletic massage, *hyperemia* refers to the increased amount of blood and other fluids in and moving through the muscle tissue.
9. In athletic massage, deep pressure is used to relieve stress points and deactivate trigger points.
10. Transverse friction massage was popularized by the British osteopath, Dr. James Cyriax.
11. The objective of using cross-fiber friction in athletic massage is to reduce fibrosis, encourage the formation of strong, pliable

scar tissue at the site of healing injuries, and prevent or soften adhesions in fibrous tissue.

12. The three basic applications for athletic massage are event massage, restorative massage during training, and massage during injury rehabilitation.
13. The goal of pre-event massage is to increase circulation and flexibility in the areas of the body about to be used. The goal of intra-event massage is to encourage a quick recovery from the previous activity, address any areas of tension or concern that might have developed during the activity, and help the tissues to prepare for the upcoming event. The goal of post-event massage is to increase circulation to clear out metabolic wastes, reduce muscle tension and spasm, and quiet the nervous system.
14. Massage is considered to be most beneficial to the athlete when it is a regular part of scheduled training.
15. Stress points are areas of chronic stress or the site of microtrauma that are generally located at the ends of muscles or in taut bands of muscle tissue.
16. The therapist must be sure to apply proper techniques to avoid aggravating a condition or causing permanent damage to the area.
17. The best way to treat an athletic injury is to prevent it.
18. Beneficial advantages of rehabilitative massage include
    - Shortens the time it takes for an injury to heal
    - Maintains or increases ROM
    - Helps to reduce swelling and edema
    - Helps to form strong, pliable scar tissue
    - Eliminates splinting in associated muscle tissue
    - Locates and deactivates trigger points that form as a result of the trauma
    - Helps get the athlete back into training sooner with less chance of reinjury
19. Proper massage therapy improves circulation, enabling damaged tissue to be carried away while making rebuilding nutrients available so that healing time is reduced.
20. Massage for new or fresh injuries should be given only by properly trained therapists in conjunction with a physician's approval.
21. PRICE is an acronym for protect, rest, ice, compression, and elevation. This represents proper first aid for soft tissue injuries.
22. Acute injuries have a sudden and definite onset and are usually of relatively short duration. Chronic injuries have a gradual onset, tend to last for a long time, or recur often.
23. Massage is contraindicated at the site of fresh acute muscle injuries.
24. Strains involve the tearing of muscle tissue or tendons. Sprains involve ligaments or joint capsules.
25. Athletic massage is contraindicated in any abnormal condition, injury, illness, or disease, except as advised by the athlete's physician.

Chapter 19: Massage for Special Populations

1. Massage benefits a woman during a normal, healthy pregnancy by promoting relaxation, soothing nerves, relieving strained back and leg muscles, and instilling a sense of well-being.
2. During the second and third trimesters, the supine position should be used for short periods only and the prone position should not be used at all, unless special bolsters are used to take all pressure off of the uterus. A semi-reclining or side-lying position is more appropriate for the comfort of the mother and the safety of the fetus.
3. All massage to the abdomen is contraindicated during the first trimester of pregnancy.
4. Contraindications for prenatal massage include morning sickness, nausea, or diarrhea, or any vaginal discharge or bleeding. High blood pressure, excessive swelling in the arms or legs, abdominal pain, or a decrease in fetal movement, preeclampsia, and toxemia also contraindicate prenatal massage.
5. The person or persons best suited to provide infant massage are the parent or primary care giver of the infant.
6. Four benefits of infant massage are

a. Bonding: creation of a close relationship that endures through time
b. Relief of tension and pain
c. Stimulation of several body systems, such as circulation and the digestive system, the immune system, and hormones
d. Relaxation

7. Children generally have shorter attention spans, and therefore the massage should be shorter. A guardian or adult should be present in the massage room during the massage and must sign a written consent form.
8. When working with someone with a hearing impairment, if they read lips or wear hearing aids, face them when you speak. Do not put your hands too close to the hearing aids when doing massage. Have a piece of paper and pencil handy to communicate if necessary. Use hand gestures to clarify communication, and tap the client to get the person's attention.
9. When providing massage services for someone who is blind, offer them an arm to lead them into the facility. If the client has a guide dog, make a space for the dog to stay in the room and do not interact with it without first asking permission from the owner. Assist the client in filling out all forms. Help the client to become aware of where to place clothing, where the table is, and how to get on the table and under the drapes. Once the client is on the table, the massage can proceed normally.
10. When providing massage to a person who is partially paralyzed, if the paralysis is accompanied by a loss of sensation, the therapist should avoid any deep techniques or excessive joint movements that might cause injury or pain. Massage on the nonparalyzed areas can be as if on a regular client and focused on tension caused by compensating patterns.
11. Massage for the critically ill helps to control discomfort and pain; improves mobility; helps reduce disorientation and confusion by bringing the person back to a more positive body awareness; reduces isolation and fear; and helps to ease the emotional and physical discomfort of the ill person.
12. The virus that causes AIDS is transmitted from person to person only through the exchange of body fluid that contains the virus.
13. Massage has been considered to be a contraindication when working with persons with cancer because of the effects it has on blood and lymph circulation and the fear that massage might actually spread the cancer.
14. Some benefits of massage for people with cancer include the following: pain relief or control; reduced nausea; better digestion and elimination; stress relief; relaxation; help for insomnia; reduced anxiety; relief from depression; relief from muscle tension and spasm; better flexibility; restored ROM; improved lymph movement; reduced edema; increased body awareness; restored positive body image; enhanced self-esteem; improved outlook on life; improved quality of life; boosts to the healing process; health promotion; and feeling good at a time where many things feel bad.
15. The practitioner can reduce promoting metastasis when massaging people with cancer by not massaging or putting pressure on the primary site of the cancer, avoiding infected lymph nodes, and not performing circulatory massage on possible secondary sites.
16. The stages of cancer are a classification of the growth or progress of the disease: stage 1: Cancer is still small and contained in the original tumor; stage 2: Cancer has grown and/or spread to nearby lymph nodes; stage 3: Cancerous cells have spread to regional lymph nodes and/or other tissues in the area; stage 4: Cancer is well developed and has spread to other tissues or organs in the body; Recurrent: Cancer has returned after being treated. It might recur at the original site or in another part of the body.
17. The common treatments for cancer are surgery; chemotherapy; radiation therapy; bone marrow transplant; treatment with other drugs such as steroids, narcotics, and antidepressants; and complementary and alternative therapies.
18. Important considerations when performing massage on people with cancer include the type and location of cancer; the stage of

progression of the cancer; possible secondary sites of metastasis; the treatment type and stage; the condition of the immune system; the stamina and attitude of the person; the belief and desire of the person regarding massage; and the purpose of the massage. Always work under the supervision of the client's physician.

19. Massage seems to be more effective before chemotherapy and radiation treatments because it seems to improve the client's outlook and reduces anxiety. As a result, recovery from the treatment is quicker, and many of the side effects such as fatigue and nausea seem less drastic.
20. If the client fatigues easily or has a low energy level, adjust the massage by shortening the length of the session, lightening the pressure, and slowing the pace of the massage. How much adjustment is made in these areas depends on the client's condition and needs. It is better to do too little than to do too much.

Chapter 20: Massage in Medicine

1. Charles Fayette Taylor and George Henry Taylor were brothers who both traveled to Europe, one to Sweden and the other to England, to study the Swedish Movement Cure. They both returned to New York, where they practiced, taught, and wrote about the cure until their deaths in 1899.
2. CAM is an acronym for complementary and alternative medicine.
3. The term *alternative* medicine insinuates using unconventional medical practices instead of conventional allopathic medical practices. The term *complementary* medicine insinuates using conventional allopathic methods along with unconventional practices to address a medical condition.
4. Integrative medicine combines conventional allopathic medicine with appropriate alternative and complementary practices to provide the best possible health benefits to the client/patient.
5. Massage is the most requested integrative medicine (IM) modality and the mainstay of many integrative medicine clinics. Several massage modalities are practiced in IM clinics, including classical Swedish for stress and pain relief, NMT, trigger-point, manual lymph drainage, pre- and postnatal massage, and energy modalities to serve a variety of patient conditions.
6. For hospital-based massage, the patient must have a referral, prescription, or at least a release from the attending physician for massage. The massage will probably take place in the patient's hospital bed, so the therapist must make certain adjustments, such as working around medical equipment. The therapist must be aware of the client's condition, special precautions, contraindications, and indications, and work according to the physician's recommendations.
7. Warning signs of cancer include the following:
   - Any sore that has not healed normally
   - A mole, skin tag, or wart that is changing in color or size
   - Lumps underneath the arms or in the breasts
   - Persistent hoarseness, coughing, or sore throat
   - Abnormal functioning of any internal organ, such as changes in the bladder or bowels
   - Discharge or bleeding from any part of the body
   - Persistent indigestion or difficulty in swallowing
8. *Medical massage* can be defined as medically necessary massage performed with the intent of improving pathologies or conditions diagnosed by a physician.
9. A massage therapist should obtain verification from the insurance company to determine whether and to which extent massage services are covered by the client's insurance policy. The therapist can also inquire about the correct CPT codes to use; if there is a deductible and has the deductible been met; and if there is a co-pay and how much it is.
10. The 1500 Health Insurance Claim form is a standardized form created by the Health Care Financing Administration that is used

throughout the health care and insurance industry for billing purposes.

11. ICD-9 codes are diagnostic codes used by doctors to aid in the uniform reporting of ailments. ICD-9 is an acronym for the document International Classification of Disease, 9th Edition, in which every human health condition is assigned a decimal number.
12. CPT is an acronym for current procedural terminology codes, which were developed by the American Medical Association to categorize and quantify medical services and create a common base of communication between physicians, therapists, patients, and insurance companies.
13. Documents that should be included in an initial insurance claim include the 1500 Health Insurance Claim form, the physician's prescription and/or referral, the client history, initial assessment, preliminary session notes, and the assignment of benefits form.

Chapter 21: Other Somatic Therapies

1. Chair massage can be practiced in airports, shopping malls, convention centers, supermarkets, street corners, dentists' offices, the workplace, and any other venues where there is room to set up a massage chair. Chair massage has been performed on planes and trains, in gyms and beauty salons, at the beach and state fairs, in RV parks and flea markets, on movie sets, and in professional ballparks. The variety of locations is limited only by the imagination of the practitioner.
2. Chair massage has made skilled touch physically, psychologically, and financially accessible to the general public. Because the client does not disrobe and no lubricants or lotions are used, a practitioner with a portable massage chair is no longer restricted to working in a private room behind closed doors. For those who have a personal history of negative touch experiences, chair massage is a way to reintroduce positive touch into their lives. The low cost of chair massage makes it the easiest way to experience massage for the first time and on an ongoing basis.
3. Reflexology is used to stimulate the body's own healing forces through the stimulation of reflex points on the hands, feet, or other areas of the body.
4. By applying pressure to a reflex point, the practitioner can stimulate certain beneficial changes in a distant area of the body related to the point. Activating these links through reflex massage can relieve tension, improve the blood supply to certain regions of the body, and help to normalize body functions.
5. Acupuncture is said to have originated in China more than 5,000 years ago.
6. Yin and yang are the two parts that contrast or exist as opposites of the same phenomenon.
7. Acupressure techniques include rubbing, touching, and pressing of pressure points.
8. The Japanese word shiatsu (*shi,* finger; and *atsu,* pressure) means pressure of the fingers.
9. Chakras are thought to be rotating energy vortices located along the central line of the body from the base of the spine to the crown of the head and are considered focal areas for the reabsorption and transmission of energy.

Chapter 22: Business Practices

1. A positive attitude and good self-image are reflected in the enthusiasm and quality exhibited in your work. They are the foundation for creating a good public image. A good public image and good business practices breed success.
2. A sole proprietorship is a business owned and operated by a single person. In a partnership, two or more people combine resources to operate a business. In both a sole proprietorship and a partnership, the owners are responsible for the obligations and liabilities of the business and take the profits. A corporation is managed by a board of directors, the owners are not directly liable, and the profits are shared by the stockholders.
3. Start-up costs of a massage business can include rent or lease, equipment, supplies, furniture and decorating costs, printing and advertising, license, insurance, and other miscellaneous expenses.

4. The location for a massage business should accommodate your business needs, be pleasing to clients, fit your image, be properly zoned, and be within your budget. The office location must be easy to locate, with the address clearly visible from the street. It should be easily accessible and relatively quiet. An ideal space would have one or more massage rooms, a reception/waiting area, an office, and bathroom facilities with a shower.
5. Permits and licenses necessary to operate a massage business might include fictitious name statement; business license; massage license, sales tax permit; planning and zoning permits; building safety permit; and employer's identification number (EIN).
6. The types of insurance that a massage business owner should carry to protect the business include liability insurance, malpractice liability insurance, automobile insurance, fire and theft insurance, medical health insurance, and workers' compensation insurance.
7. Keeping accurate records is necessary in a successful business in that it records the progress of the business, especially the cost of doing business in relation to income. Business records are also necessary to meet the requirements of local, state, and federal laws pertaining to taxes and employees.
8. The major ingredients of a basic bookkeeping system are a checking account with an updated ledger, income and disbursement ledgers, accounts receivable and accounts payable files, bank statements and reconciliations, filed business receipts, an inventory system, an assets and depreciation file, and a mileage log.
9. Marketing is the business activity done to promote and increase a business. Marketing is an educational process of getting yourself and what you do known. It is the enticement that encourages people to seek your services.
10. Marketing activities commonly used in the massage industry include advertising, promotion, public relations, referrals, and client retention.
11. A *target market* is a segment of the population with certain characteristics that make them good prospective consumers of a particular product or service.
12. The three Rs of referrals are
    a. Request: Request the referral.
    b. Reward: Acknowledge and reward the person who sends the referral.
    c. Reciprocate: Use the services of or send referrals back to those who send you referrals.

GLOSSARY

Absorption: The process in which the digested nutrients are transferred from the intestines to the blood or cell lymph vessels.

Accessory Digestive Organs: Consist of the teeth, tongue, salivary glands, pancreas, liver, and gallbladder.

Acquired Immune Deficiency Syndrome (AIDS): A condi thattion caused by HIV infection whereby a portion of the immune system is destroyed, making it easy for the infected person to acquire life-threatening diseases.

Acquired Immunity: Results from an encounter with a new substance, which triggers events that induce an immune response specific to that particular substance.

Actin: A protein in muscle tissue that forms filaments that interact with myosin filaments to cause muscle contractions.

Active Joint Movements: Movements in which the client actively participates by contracting the muscles involved in the movement.

Active Range of Motion: The client moves the limb or the joint without any intervention from the practitioner to assess any Alimitation in the joint movement.

Acute: A condition with a sudden onset and relatively short duration.

Adenosine Triphosphate: A molecule that stores energy in the body and releases it when it breaks down into ADP.

Adipose Tissue: Areolar tissue with an abundance of fat cells.

Adrenal Glands: Situated on the top of each kidney, produce epinephrine, norepinephrine, and corticosteroids.

Aerobic Cellular Respiration: Makes energy for reconstituting ADP in cell mitochondrion.

Afferent Nerves: Carry impulses toward the spinal cord and brain.

Agonist: A muscle that is the prime mover.

Alimentary Canal: Consists of the mouth, pharynx, esophagus, stomach, and small and large intestines.

Allergen: Antigen that can cause an allergic response in some people.

Allopathic Medicine: Treatment of disease or injury with the use of medications and surgery.

Alternative Medicine: A term that implies using health supportive services other than those usually received from allopathic physicians.

Amitosis: A process of cell division in which the nucleus and cytoplasm split in two.

Anabolism: The process of building up of larger molecules from smaller ones.

Anaerobic Respiration: A process in which glucose is broken down in the absence of oxygen.

Anatomic Barrier: Refers to the anatomic limit of motion of particular tissue. To move beyond the anatomic barrier would cause injury and disruption of tissues and supportive structures.

Anatomic Position: Standing with feet shoulder-width apart, arms at the side, with the palms of the hands facing forward.

Anatomy: The study of the gross structure of the body and the interrelations of its parts.

Anatripsis: The art of rubbing a body part upward.

Aneurysm: A local distention or ballooning of an artery due to a weakening wall.

Angulus Venosus: The juncture of the jugular and subclavian veins.

Antagonist: The muscle that performs the opposite movement portionof the agonist.

Antibodies: A class of proteins produced in the body in response to contact with antigens that immunize the body.

Antigen: Anything that can trigger an immune response.

Aorta: The main artery of the body.

Aortic Semilunar Valve: Part of the heart that permits the blood to be pumped from the left ventricle into the aorta.

Appendicular Skeleton: Made up of bones of the shoulder, upper extremities, hips, and lower extremities.

Arachnoid Mater: The middle space of the meninges.

Areolar Tissue: Loose connective tissue that binds the skin to the underlying tissues and fills the spaces between the muscles that makes up fascia.

Aromatherapy: The use of essential oils processed from herbs, flowers, fruits, stems, spices, and roots in massage, inhalation, or other modalities to affect mood and improve health and well-being.

Arteries: Thick-walled muscular and elastic vessels that transport oxygenated blood from the heart.

Arterioles: Small blood vessels between the arteries and the capillaries.

Articular Cartilage: A layer of hyaline cartilage covering the end surface of the epiphysis.

Atherosclerosis: Characterized by an accumulation of fatty deposits on the inner walls of the arteries.

Atoms: Consist of subatomic particles that all substances are composed of.

Autoimmune Disease: Occurs when the immune system mistakes self for nonself and attacks itself.

Autonomic Nervous System: Regulates the action of glands, smooth muscles, and the heart.

Axial Skeleton: Made up of bones of the skull, thorax, vertebral column, and the hyoid bone.

Axon: Conducts impulses away from the nerve cell body.

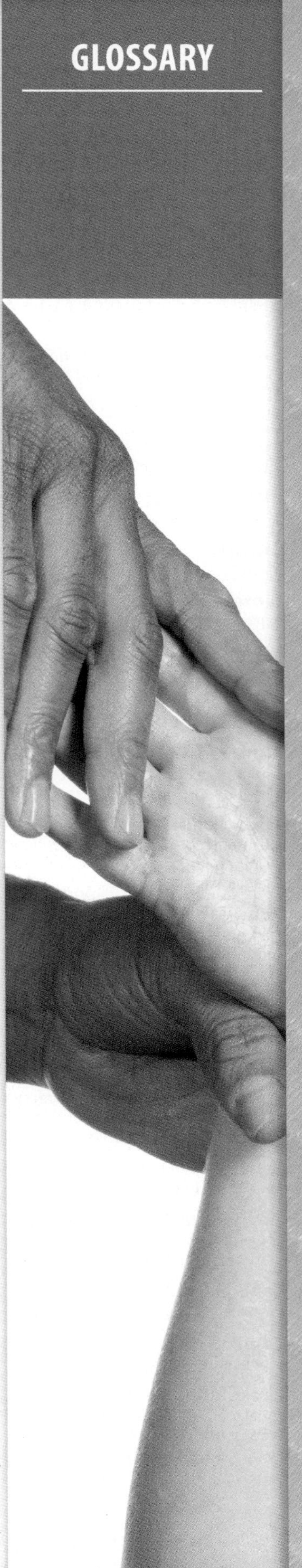

Ayurveda: An ancient system of Indian medicine and healing; it has been modified in recent years for use in spa treatments such as body scrubs, face treatments, and massages.

Bacteria: Minute, unicellular organisms exhibiting both plant and animal characteristics and are classified as either harmless or harmful.

Bania: A Russian-style communal steam bath.

Basal Cell Carcinoma: A type of skin cancer.

Beating: The heaviest and deepest form of percussion and is done over the denser areas of the body.

Bicuspid (Mitral) Valve: Part of the heart that allows blood to flow from the left atrium into the left ventricl bye.

Bile: A bitter, alkaline, yellowish-brown fluid secreted by the liver that aids in fat digestion.

Bioenergy: The vital life force in all living matter.

Bioforce: The vital life force in all living matter.

Bladder: An organ where the urine is stored.

Blood Platelets: Or thrombocytes, are colorless, irregular bodies, much smaller than red corpuscles.

Bonding: A unique relationship between two people that is specific and endures through time.

Bone Tissue: Connective tissue in which the intercellular substance is rendered hard by mineral salts, chiefly calcium carbonate and calcium phosphate.

Boundaries: Personal comfort zones that help a person to maintain a sense of comfort and safety. They can be professional, personal, physical, emotional, intellectual, and sexual.

Brachial Plexus: Composed of four lower cervical nerves and the first pair of thoracic nerves that control arm movements.

Bursae: Fibrous sacks lined with synovial membrane and lubricated with synovial fluid, functioning as a cushion in areas of pressure.

Calcitonin: A hormone that controls the level of calcium in the blood.

Cancellous Bone: Located inside long bones and flat bones, consists of irregularly shaped spaces defined by thin, bony plates.

Cancer: The uncontrolled growth and spread of abnormal cells in the body.

Capillaries: The smallest blood vessels and connect arterioles with the venules.

Capsular Pattern: Refers to the proportional limitation of any joint that is controlled by muscular contractions.

Cardiac Muscle Tissue: Occurs only in the heart and is responsible for pumping blood through the heart into the blood vessels.

Cardiovascular System: A network of structures including the heart, blood vessels, and blood that pumps and carries blood throughout the body.

Carrier Oil: Massage lubricant into which essential oils are blended for aromatherapy applications.

Cartilaginous Joints: Joints held together with cartilage with no joint cavity.

Catabolism: The breaking down of larger substances into smaller ones.

Cell Membrane: The wall or outer border of a cell that permits soluble substances to enter and leave the protoplasm.

Cells: Basic functional units of all living matter.

Centering: A visualization practice based on the concept that you have a geographical center in your body about two inches below the navel.

Central Nervous System: Consists of the brain and spinal cord.

Centripetal: Referring to a direction, toward the center (heart).

Cerebrospinal Fluid: Flows through and around the brain and spinal cord to nourish and protect them.

Cerebrovascular Accident: Or stroke, is caused by a blood clot or ruptured blood vessel in or around the brain that subsequently destroys nerve tissue.

Cervical Plexus: Consists of the four upper cervical nerves that supply the skin and control the movement of the head, neck, and shoulders.

Chair Massage: Takes place in a chair, which is a better choice for people unable to or not amenable to receiving full-body massage on a table.

Chirugy: Healing with the hands.

Chronic: A lingering or ongoing condition.

Chucking: A friction massage movement that involves the flesh being grasped firmly in one or both hands and moved up and down along the bone.

Chyle: A cloudy liquid, consisting mostly of fats, that passes from the small intestines, through the lacteals, and into the lymph system.

Circular Friction: A massage movement in which the fingers or palm of the hand move the superficial tissues in a circular pattern over the deeper tissues.

Coagulability: A measure of the blood's ability to coagulate.

Coccygeal Plexus: Formed from a portion of the fourth sacral nerves, the fifth sacral nerve, and the coccygeal nerve.

Code of Ethics: A set of guiding moral principles that governs a person's choice of action.

Compact Bone Tissue: Forms the hard bone found in the shafts of long bones and along the outside of flat bones.

Complementary Medicine: The term that took the place of "alternative medicine" and implies that the alternative practices can work along with more conventional medicine for the benefit of clients.

Compression: Rhythmic pressing movements directed into muscle tissue by either the hand or fingers.

Congenital: A condition or disease that is present from the time of birth.

Connective Tissue Massage: Massage directed toward the subcutaneous connective tissue, believed to affect vascular and visceral reflexes related to a variety of pathologies and disabilities.

Contractile Tissues: The fibrous tissues that have tensions placed on them during muscular contractions.

Contractility: The ability of a muscle to contract or shorten and thereby exert force.

Contract-relax Technique: A Muscle Energy technique that incorporates postisometric relaxation theory, which states that as soon as an isometric muscle contraction releases, the muscle relaxes.

Contraindication: Any physical, mental, or emotional condition a client may have that may cause a particular intervention or treatment to be detrimental or unsafe.

Contralateral: The body part on the opposite side of the body.

Contrast Therapy: The alternating application of heat and cold for therapeutic purposes.

Contusion: A common type of hematoma that is generally not too serious (also called, bruise).

Co-pay: The portion of the fee for service that the patient is responsible for at the time of service.

Coronal Plane: Divides the body into the front and back.

Corporation: A business setup subject to state regulation and taxation. A charter must be obtained from the state in which the corporation operates.

Countertransference: When a therapist or practitioner personalizes a therapeutic relationship by unconsciously projecting characteristics of someone from a former relationship onto a client. This is almost always detrimental to a therapeutic relationship.

Cranial Nerves: Twelve pairs of nerves that emerge from the brain through openings in the base of the cranium.

Craniosacral Therapy: A gentle, hands-on method of evaluating and enhancing the functioning of the craniosacral system.

Cretinism: Caused by a lack of thyroxin during fetal development and results in a dwarfed stature and mental retardation.

Cross-fiber Friction: A massage technique that is applied in a transverse direction across the muscle, tendon, or ligament.

Cryotherapy: The application of cold agents for therapeutic purposes.

Cupping: A massage percussion technique used by respiratory therapists to help break up lung congestion.

Current Procedural Terminology (CPT) Codes: Developed and are maintained by the American Medical Association that categorize and quantify medical services and provide a common language and a base for communication between physicians, therapists, patients, and insurance companies.

Cushing's Syndrome: Results from excess glucocorticoid production and is characterized by obesity, muscle weakness, elevated blood sugar, and hypertension.

Cytoplasm: All of the substance within the cell wall other than the nucleus.

Cytoplasmic Organelles: Discrete structures within a cell, having specialized functions, identifying molecular structures, and a distinctive chemical composition.

Décolletage: The area of the upper chest above the breasts and onto the front of the neck.

Decubitus Ulcers: Bedsores.

Deep Fascia: Refers to fibrous tissue sheaths that penetrate deep into the body, separating muscle groups.

Deep Gliding: Indicates that the effleurage technique uses enough pressure to have a mechanical effect.

Deep Tissue Massage: Refers to various regimens or massage styles that are directed toward the deeper tissue structures of the muscle and fascia.

Deep Transverse Friction Massage: Massage that broadens the fibrous tissues of muscles, tendons, or ligaments, breaking down unwanted adhesions and restoring mobility to muscles.

Dendrite: A nerve cell appendage that connects with other neurons to receive information.

Dermatome: An area of the skin supplied by nerve fibers originating from a single spinal nerve root.

Dermis: The deeper layer of the skin that extends to form the subcutaneous tissue.

Diabetes Mellitus: Caused by decreased output of insulin by the pancreas.

Diaphysis: The bone shaft between the epiphyses.

Diathermy: The application of oscillating electromagnetic fields to the tissue.

Differentiation: The repeated division of the ovum during early developmental stages, resulting in specialized cells that differ from one another.

Diffusers: Devices using fans, heat, or steam dispersion to release the aromas of essential oils into a room for therapeutic and/or esthetic purposes.

Diffusion: A process in which substances move from an area of higher concentration to an area of lower concentration.

Digestion: The process of converting food into substances capable of being used by the cells for nourishment.

Disease: An abnormal and unhealthy state of all or part of the body wherein it is incapable of carrying on its normal function.

Disinfection: A medium level of decontamination, nearly as effective as sterilization, but it does not kill bacterial spores.

Dopamine: A neurotransmitter that controls fine movement, emotional response, and the ability to experience pleasure and pain.

Draping: The process of using linens to keep a client covered while receiving a massage.

Drug Monograph: A statement that specifies the ingredients a drug or class of drugs may contain, the directions for the drug's use, the conditions in which it may be used, and the contraindications to its use.

Dr. Vodder's Manual Lymph Drainage: A method of gentle, rhythmic massage along the superficial lymphatics that aids in lymphatic system functioning and treats chronic lymphedema.

Dry Room: A massage room used for spa treatments performed without the use of showers and baths.

Dura Mater: The outer layer of the meninges.

Eccentric Contraction: Occurs when a muscle contracts while the ends of the muscle move farther apart.

Ectoderm: The outermost layer of cells of the zygote.

Edema: A condition of excess fluid in the interstitial spaces.

Effleurage: A succession of strokes applied by gliding the hand over an extended portion of the body.

Elasticity: The tissue's ability to return to normal resting length when a stress that has been placed on it is removed.

Embolus: A piece of a clot that loosens and floats in the blood.

Empty End Feel: An abrupt restriction to a joint movement caused by pain.

Emulsion: A uniform mixture of two or more liquids, such as an essential oil and a massage lotion.

End feel: The change in the quality of the feeling a practitioner senses as they move a client's limb through a ROM and the end of a movement is approached.

Endocardium: The thin, innermost layer of the heart.

Endocrine glands: Are ductless glands that depend on the blood and lymph to carry their secretions to various affected tissues.

Endoderm: The innermost layer of cells of the zygote.

Endomysium: The delicate connective tissue covering muscle fibers.

Endurance: The act, quality, or power of withstanding hardship or stress.

Enzymes: Proteins that act as catalysts for chemical reactions in metabolism while remaining unchanged themselves.

Epicardium: The protective outer layer of the heart.

Epidermis: The outermost layer of the skin.

Epilepsy: A neurologic condition in which there is an abnormal electrical activity in the CNS without apparent tissue abnormalities.

Epimysium: The layer of connect tissueive fascia that closely covers an individual muscle.

Epinephrine: "Fight-or-flight" hormone that prepares the body to respond to emergencies.

Epiphysis: An enlarged area on the ends of long bones that articulates with other bones.

Epithelial Tissue: A protective surface layer that functions in the processes of absorption, excretion, secretion, and protection.

Esalen Massage: A style of massage developed at Esalen Institute in northern California that features long, flowing strokes that connect all parts of the body into a whole.

Estrogen: A female hormone responsible for development of secondary sexual characteristics.

Exfoliation: Any of several spa treatments the primary purpose of which is to cleanse the body of dead skin cells, thus softening the skin, helping the body to eliminate better through the skin, preparing it for better absorption of other therapeutic products.

Exocrine glands: Are duct glands that possess tubes or ducts leading from the gland to a particular part of the body.

Extensibility: The ability of a muscle to stretch.

Exteroceptors: Nerve ends that record conscious sensations such as heat, cold, pain, and pressure throughout the body.

Fascia: Fibrous connective tissue that forms a network throughout the body, surrounding every structure to support, separate, and give shape to the body.

Fascicle: A bundle of muscle fibers.

Feather Stroking: massage technique that requires very light pressure of the fingertips or hands with long flowing strokes.

Fetus: The developing child from the third month of pregnancy until birth.

Fever: An elevated body temperature.

Fibrocartilage: Dense connective tissue found between the vertebrae and pubic symphysis.

Fibrous Connective Tissue: Composed of collagen and elastin fibers that are closely arranged to form tendons and ligaments.

Fibrous Joints: Have no space and are held together by fibrous connective tissue.

Filtration: A process in which blood pressure pushes fluids and substances through the capillary wall and into the tissue spaces.

Fixator: Muscles that act to stabilize a body part so that another muscle can act on an adjacent limb or body part.

Flat Palpation: Done with the fingertips or thumb either in line with or perpendicularly across the fibers of the muscle tissue.

Fomite: An object or material that is likely to carry infection, such as clothing, dirty linens, or used hypodermic needles.

Freely Flexible Range of Movement: The pliable and easily movable range of the tissue.

Fungus, *pl.* fungi: A diverse group of organisms, potentially capable of causing disease, that thrive or grow in wet or damp areas and live by absorbing nutrients from organic matter.

Gait: A pattern or manner of walking.

Gait Assessment: Observing the manner in which a person walks to determine constrictions or related conditions.

Gate Control Theory: The positive effects of relaxing massage interrupts the transmission of pain sensations of affected nociceptors from entering the central nervous system by stimulating other cutaneous receptors.

General (Systemic) Circulation: The blood circulation from the left side of the heart throughout the body and back again to the heart.

Gestation: The physiologic condition that occurs from the time an ovum is fertilized until childbirth.

Gliding: The massage technique of gliding the hand smoothly over some portion of the client's body with varying amounts of pressure.

Goals: Specific, attainable, measurable accomplishments that you set and make a commitment to achieve.

Golgi Tendon Organs: Multibranched sensory nerve endings located in tendons.

Gonorrhea: A venereal disease characterized by a discharge and burning sensation when urinating.

Grounding: Based on the concept that you have a connection with the earth and with the client and that you function as a grounding apparatus in helping the client to release tension.

Gymnasium: A center where exercise and massage are combined to treat disease and promote health.

Hacking: A massage percussion technique that consists of rapid striking movements that can be done with one or both hands.

Hammam: A Turkish steam bath with elaborate cleansing, exfoliation, and massage rituals passed down for centuries, played an important role in Ottoman culture.

Hard End Feel: A bone-against-bone feeling.

Hematoma: A mass of blood trapped in some tissue or cavity of the body and is the result of internal bleeding.

Hemiplegia: Unilateral paralysis caused by a stroke.

Hemoglobin: An iron-protein compound in red blood cells capable of carrying oxygen from the lungs to the cells and carbon dioxide from the cells.

Herniated Disk: A weakening of the intervertebral disk resulting in a protrusion into the vertebral canal, potentially compressing the spinal cord.

Herpes: A virus that affects the mouth, skin, and other facial parts, commonly called cold sores and fever blisters.

High Blood Pressure: An elevated pressure of the blood against the artery walls.

Hippocratic Oath: A code of ethics for physicians.

Homeostasis: The internal balance of the body.

Hospitality Industry: The combined hotel, resort, restaurant, and entertainment industries that rely especially on customer service and professional hospitality for their success.

Human Immunodeficiency Virus (HIV): A virus that can multiply and destroy a portion of the immune system and is the causitive agent of aquired immunedeficiency syndrome (AIDS).

Hydrocollator: An electrical appliance used to heat and store moist hot packs.

Hydrotherapy: The application of water in any of its three forms to the body for therapeutic purposes.

Hyperactive Glands: Oversecrete hormones owing to lack of regulation or glandular tumors.

Hyperemia: Hyper = increased or excessive; -emia = blood; increased blood in an area of the body.

Hypoallergenic: Relatively unlikely to cause an allergic reaction.

ICD-9 Codes: A system of decimal numbers that correspond to medical conditions diagnosed by doctors. ICD-9 is an acronym for International Classification of Disease, 9th Revision, and is published annually by the U.S. Health Services and Health Care Financing Administration.

Ice Massage: A local application of cold achieved by massaging a cube of ice over a small area such as a bursa, tendon, or small muscle.

Immune System: Helps to protect the body and keep it safe from pathogens and diseases.

Inert Tissues: The tissues that are not contractile such as bone, ligament, or nerves.

Inflammation: A protective tissue response characterized by swelling, redness, heat, and pain.

Inflammatory Response: A natural process of healing and repair when soft tissue is injured.

Informed Consent: A client's written authorization for professional services based on adequate information from the massage therapist about the massage, including expectations, potential benefits, possible undesirable effects, and professional and ethical responsibility.

Innate Immunity: Immunity that is passed on from the mother and is present from birth.

Insertion of a Muscle: The more mobile attachment of a muscle to bone.

Intake Specialists: Also known as hospitality coordinators, spa concierges, and other titles, are spa employees who focus on pairing guests with appropriate treatments, therapists, services, and lifestyle choices during their stay at the spa.

Integrative Medicine: Combines complementary and alternative medicine with allopathic medicine.

Integumentary System: Composed of the skin, hair, and nails.

International Spa Association (ISPA): A professional organization consisting of member spas, owners, directors, technicians, consultants, writers, marketers, and suppliers of products and equipment who meet at conventions and roundtables to create standards, share information, and chart directions for the development of the spa industry worldwide.

Interneuron: Carries impulses from one neuron to another.

Irritability: Or excitability, is the capacity of muscles to receive and react to stimuli.

Ischemia: Localized tissue anemia caused by obstruction of the inflow of blood.

Ischemic Compression: Is a massage and neuromuscular technique that involves digital pressure directly into a trigger point.

Islets of Langerhans: Found in the pancreas, produce insulin and glucagon.

Isometric Contraction: Occurs when a muscle contracts and the ends of the muscle do not move.

Isotonic Contraction: Occurs when a muscle contracts and the distance between the ends of the muscle changes.

Jostling: Is a friction massage technique that ivolves grasping the entire muscle, lifting it slightly away from its position, and shaking it quickly across its axis.

Kidneys: Bean-shaped glands that filter the blood.

Kinesiology: The scientific study of muscular activity and the anatomy, physiology, and mechanics of body movement.

Kiva: An underground chamber used by the Pueblo tribe of Indians for ceremonial sweats and other rituals.

Lacteals: Lymphatic capillaries located in the villi of the small intestine.

Ligaments: Bands of fibrous tissue that connect bones to bones.

Limited Liability Companies: A form of legal entity, something between a partnership and a corporation.

Liquid Tissue: Connective tissue represented by blood and lymph.

Local Infection: Invading organisms confined to a small area of the body.

Lumbar Plexus: Formed from the first four lumbar nerves.

Lymphatics: Small, intermediate lymph vessels.

Lymphedema: An accumulation of interstitial fluid, or swelling, in the soft tissues caused by inflammation, blockage, or removal of the lymph channels.

Malignant Melanoma: The most serious form of skin cancer.

Marrow: The connective tissue filling in the cavities of bones that forms red and white blood cells.

Massage: The systematic manual or mechanical manipulations of the soft tissues of the body for therapeutic purposes.

Medical Gymnastics: Gymnastics applied to the treatment of disease, consisting of active, duplicated, and passive movements.

Medical Massage: Medically prescribed massage performed with the intention of improving pathologies diagnosed by a physician.

Medullary Cavity: A hollow chamber formed in the shaft of long bones that is filled with yellow bone marrow.

Meiosis: Cell division that takes place in the sex organs of animals to produce the egg and sperm required for fertilization, and in which the resultant cells have only one half of the hereditary chromosomes as the parent cell.

Meningitis: An acute inflammation of the pia mater and arachnoid mater around the brain and spinal cord.

Menopause: The physiologic cessation of the menstrual cycle.

Menstruation: The cyclic, physiologic uterine bleeding that occurs at about four-week intervals during the reproductive period of the female.

Mesoderm: The middle layer of cells of the zygote.

Metabolic Wastes: Products formed from cell metabolism.

Metabolism: The process taking place in living organisms whereby the cells are nourished and carry out their activities.

Metastasis: The spread of cancer from one site to another location in the body.

Mission Statement: A short, general statement of the main focus of the business.

Mitosis: The process of cell division in which a cell divides into two cells identical to the parent cell.

Mitral Valve: Part of the heart that allows blood to flow from the left atrium into the left ventricle.

Molecules: Specific arrangements of atoms.

Morphology: The science or study of the structure of an organism or body.

Motor (Efferent) Neuron: Nerve cells that carries nerve impulses from the brain to the effectors.

Motor Unit: Consists of a motor neuron and all of the muscle fibers it controls.

Multiple Sclerosis: Occurs in young adults and results from the breakdown of the myelin sheath.

Muscle Energy Technique: MET, or PNF stretching, uses neurophysiologic muscle reflexes to improve functional mobility of the joints.

Muscle Fatigue: A condition in which the muscle ceases to respond because of oxygen debt from rapid or prolonged muscle contractions.

Muscle Spindle Cells: Sensory organs in muscle that detect the rate of stretch in muscles.

Muscle Tone: A type of muscle contraction present in healthy muscles even when at rest.

Myocardium: The cardiac muscle.

Myofascial: The combination of muscle tissue and its related connective tissue or fascia.

Myoneural Junction: The connection point of the motor nerve and the muscle cell.

Myosin: A protein that forms filaments that make up nearly 50 percent of muscle tissue and are involved in muscle contraction.

Neat: Refers to the application of an essential oil at its full, undiluted strength.

Nephron: The functional unit of the kidney.

Nerve Cell: The structural unit of the nervous system.

Nerve Fibers: Projections from the body of the nerve cell that carry nervous impulses.

Nerves: Bundles of fibers held together by connective tissue that originate in the brain and spinal cord and distribute branches all over the body.

Nervous System: Controls and coordinates all the body systems and includes the nerves, spinal cord, and brain.

Nervous Tissue: Composed of neurons; it initiates, controls, and coordinates the body's adaptation to its surroundings.

Neurologic Pathway: The route that a nerve impulse travels through the nervous system.

Neuromuscular Techniques: A group of techniques that assess and address soft tissue dysfunction by affecting the neurologic mechanisms that control the muscle.

Neuron: Or nerve cell, is the structural unit of the nervous system.

Neurotransmitter: A chemical that communicates a nerve signal across a synapse.

Nonverbal Communication: Also known as body language, is how a person's posturing, gestures, and facial expressions provide information about his mental, emotional, or physical condition.

Norepinephrine: "Fight-or-flight" hormone that prepares the body to respond to emergencies.

Nucleus: The main central body of living cells that contains the genetic information for continuing life.

Onsen: Japanese hot springs at the site of natural volcanic spring water, usually with massage and other relaxing therapies available.

Opportunistic Infection: Caused by organisms commonly found in the environment and our bodies that become deadly when the body's immune system is weakened.

Oral Cavity: Or mouth, prepares food for entrance into the stomach.

Organ Systems: Several organs working together to perform a bodily function.

Organs: Combination of tissues and cells that form a complex structure to perform a certain function within the system.

Origin of a Muscle: The point where the end of a muscle is anchored to an immovable section of the skeleton.

Ortho-bionomy: A healing system created by Dr. Arthur Pauls based on the body's self-correcting reflexes.

Ovaries: Glandular organs in the female pelvis that produce the ovum and female sex hormones.

Overload: The principle of applying stresses that are greater than what the body is accustomed to forcing it to adapt to the heavier load by increasing strength or endurance.

Ovulation: The discharge of a mature ovum from the follicle of the ovary.

Pain: Is a primarily protective function in that it warns of tissue damage or destruction somewhere in the body. It is the result of stimulation of specialized nerve endings in the body.

Palpation: A skill and an art developed by the therapist that is a primary assessment tool allowing the therapist to listen to the client's body through the therapist's hands.

Parafango: A combination of paraffin wax and fango mud used in spa wraps and localized applications to soften, moisten, and purify the skin while warming and relaxing the muscles.

Paraplegia: Paralysis of the lower extremities; does not affect the arms or hands.

Parasite: An organism that can potentially cause disease that exists and functions at the expense of a host organism without contributing to the survival of the host.

Parasympathetic Nervous System: Functions to conserve energy and reverse the action of the sympathetic division.

Parathormone: A hormone from the parathyroid glands that regulates the blood level of calcium.

Parkinson's Disease: Occurs as a result of the degeneration of certain nerve tissues that regulate body movements.

Partnership: A business setup in which two or more partners share responsibility and benefits of running the business.

Passive Joint Movements: A massage technique where the therapist moves a body part to stretch the fibrous tissue and move the joint through its range of motion without assistance of the client.

Pathology: The study of the structural and functional changes caused by disease.

Pericardium: A double-layered membrane that encloses the heart.

Perichondrium: The membrane covering cartilage.

Perimysium: Connective tissue or fascia that separates the muscle into bundles of muscle fibers.

Periosteum: A fibrous membrane that functions to protect the bone and serves as an attachment of tendons and ligaments.

Peripheral Nervous System: Consists of all the nerves that connect the CNS to the rest of the body.

Peristalsis: The wavelike muscular action of the alimentary canal.

Petrissage: A massage technique that lifts, squeezes, and presses the tissues.

Petty Cash Fund: Maintained to pay small disbursements for incidentals.

Phagocytes: Blood cells that are able to engulf and digest cellular debris and foreign bodies in the tissues.

Phagocytosis: A process in which leukocytes engulf and digest harmful bacteria and other cellular debris.

Pharmacology: A science that studies the effects that substances have on living organisms, the nature of their chemical structure, how they act within the body, and how the body responds to them.

Phlebitis: An inflammation of a vein accompanied by pain and swelling.

Physiologic Barrier: Represents the extent of easy movement allowed during passive or active movements.

Physiology: The science and study of the vital processes, mechanisms, and functions of an organ or system.

Physiopathologic Reflex Arc: A self-perpetuating dysfunctional neurologic circuit.

Pia Mater: The innermost layer of the meninges.

Pincer Palpation: Employed in areas where the muscle tissue can be picked up between the thumb and fingers of the same hand (e.g., sternocleidomastoid muscle) where the belly of the muscle is rolled between the thumb and fingers.

Pituitary Gland: A small gland, often called the master gland, because the hormones it secretes stimulate or regulate other glands.

Plastic Body Wrap: A thin, transparent, disposable plastic sheet used to wrap directly around the client's skin during mud, clay, and seaweed body wraps.

Polarity Therapy: Uses massage manipulations derived from Eastern and Western practices developed Dr. Randolph Stone.

Position Release: A method of passively moving the body or body part toward the body's preference and away from pain, seeking the tissue's preferred position. Movements are toward ease and away from bind, away from any restrictive barrier and toward comfort.

Postisometric Relaxation: Means that following an isometric contraction, there is a period of relaxation during which muscle impulses are inhibited.

Pregnancy: The physiologic condition that occurs from the time an ovum is fertilized until childbirth.

Primary Caregiver: Person or persons whose responsibility is rearing the child. This might be a parent, grandparent, adoptive parent, or a nanny.

Prime Mover: The primary muscle responsible for a specific movement. Also called the agonist.

Progesterone: A female hormone that prepares the uterine lining for implantation, aids maintaining pregnancy, and stimulates development of mammary glands for nursing.

Proprioceptors: Sensory nerve endings located in muscles or fascia that sense where the body is and how it moves.

Protoplasm: A colorless, jelly-like substance contained within the cellular membrane in which food elements, such as protein, fats, carbohydrates, mineral salts, and water, are present.

Pulmonary Circulation: The blood circulation from the heart to the lungs and back again to the heart.

Pulmonary Semilunar Valve: Part of the heart that directs blood from the right ventricle into the pulmonary arteries.

Purpose: The business theme that is derived from the owner's dreams and ideals.

Quadriplegia: Paralysis of the arms and legs caused by a stroke or spinal cord injury.

Range of Motion: The movement of a joint from one extreme of the articulation to the other.

Reciprocal Inhibition: Occurs when a muscle acting on a joint contracts and the opposing muscle is reflexively inhibited.

Red Corpuscles: Or erythrocytes are blood cells that carry oxygen from the lungs to the body cells and transport carbon dioxide from the cells to the lungs.

Reflex: The simplest form of nervous activity, which includes a sensory and motor nerve.

Reflex Arc: The nerve pathway of a reflex.

Reflexology: A massage technique that stimulates particular points on the surface of the body, which in turn affects other areas or organs of the body.

Resistive Barrier: Also known as the pathologic barrier, is the first sign of resistance to a movement as tissue is moved and manipulated through its range of motion.

Reticular Tissue: Composed of fibers that form the framework of the liver and lymphoid organs.

Rocking: A push-and-release movement applied to the client's body in either a side-to-side or an up-and-down direction.

Rolfing: A bodywork system developed by Dr. Ida Rolf that aligns the major body segments through manipulation of the fascia or the connective tissue.

Rolling: A rapid back-and-forth movement with the hands, in which the flesh is shaken and rolled around the axis of the body part.

Sacral Plexus: Formed from the fourth and fifth lumbar nerves, and the first four sacral nerves.

Sagittal Plane: Divides the body into left and right parts.

Saliva: A fluiid produced by the salivary glands of the mouth contains enzymes that begin to digest carbohydrates.

Sanitation: The third level of decontamination practiced in the massage studio and is done with soaps or detergents and water.

Sarcolemma: The cell wall of the muscle cell.

Sarcomere: The smallest functional unit of the muscle cell containing the actin and myosin filaments.

Sarcoplasmic Reticulum: A network of membranous channels within the muscle cell that release calcium ions, causing muscle contraction.

Scar: A dense fibrous tissue that forms as an injury, wound, burn, or sore heals.

Sciatic Nerve: The largest and longest nerve in the body.

Scope of Practice: Defines the rights and activities legally acceptable according to the licenses of a particular occupation or profession.

Sensory Neuron: Carries impulses from sense organs to the brain.

Septum: The wall that separates the heart's chambers.

Sequence: The pattern or design of a massage.

Serotonin: A neurotransmitter that helps regulate nerve impulses and influences mood, behavior, appetite, blood pressure, temperature regulation, memory, and learning ability.

Sexually Transmitted Diseases: Associated with the sexual organs and are characterized by sores and rashes on the skin.

Shaking: A massage technique that allows the release of tension by gently shaking a relaxed body part so that the flesh flops around the bone.

Shiatsu: A massage technique from Japan in which points of stimulation are pressed to effect the circulation of fluids and ki (life force energy).

Shingles: An acute inflammation of a nerve trunk by the herpes varicella-zoster virus, or a short, repeated gliding stroke using alternating hands.

Sign (of Disease): An observable indication of disease or bodily disorder.

Skeletal Membrane: Covers bone and cartilage.

Skeletal Muscles: Attached to bone by tendons and are responsible for moving the limbs, facial expression, speaking, and other voluntary movements.

Skin Brushing: A light, brisk brushing using a dry vegetable bristle bath brush.

Skinship: The sensitivity to communicate through the skin. A parent who forms this might be aware of the infant's body tension, heart rate, and movement of the digestive system, which cues an awareness of hunger.

Slapping: A percussion massage technique that uses a rhythmic, glancing contact of the flat surface of the hand with the body.

Smooth Muscle Tissue: Muscle tissue of mmany organs that lacks striations and cannot be stimulated to contract by conscious effort.

Soft End Feel: A cushioned limitation in which soft tissue prevents further movement, such as knee flexion.

Soft Tissue Barriers: Notable physiologic changes in the quality of movement in soft tissue that represent the limits within which the tissues can be effectively manipulated.

Sole Proprietor: An individual business owner responsible for all expenses, obligations, liabilities, and assets.

Somatic Nervous System: Consists of the nerves that connect the central nervous system to the voluntary muscles and skin

Spa Massage: Any massage given by a therapist within the structure and limitations of the spa setting, usually referring to the spa's basic Swedish massage, but also applicable to advanced modalities given in the spa.

Spindle Cells: Proprioceptive nerve ends located in the belly of muscle, alert the CNS as to the length, stretch, and speed of muscle contractions.

Spondylosis: A degenerative arthritic condition affecting the vertebrae.

Spongy Bone: Located inside long bones, consists of irregularly shaped spaces defined by thin, bony plates.

Sports Massage: A method of massage designed to enhance an athlete's performance.

Sprain: An injury to a joint resulting in stretching or tearing of the ligaments.

Sterilization: The most complete process of removing pathogens; this destroys all living organisms, including bacterial spores.

Stress: Any psychological or physical situation or condition that causes tension or strain.

Stretching: Passive and active stretching of muscle and connective tissue to achieve normal resting length.

Strigil: A curved, usually metallic, instrument used in ancient Greece and Rome to scrape dead skin cells, oil, and dirt from bathers' skin.

Subcutaneous Tissue: Regarded as a continuation of the dermis, also called superficial fascia.

Superficial Fascia: The connecting layer between the skin and those structures underlying the skin.

Superficial Gl Swedish massage etechniqu where the practitioner's hand conforms to the client's body contours so that light pressure is applied to the body from every part of the haend as th hand lightly slides ofer an extended of the client's body.

Sweat Lodge: A Native American enclosure for sweating, cleansing, and purification, in which participants pour water ceremonially over heated stones to create heat while praying and chanting.

Sympathetic Nervous System: Supplies the glands, involuntary muscles of internal organs, and walls of blood vessels with nerves.

Symptom: Subjective evidence of disease or bodily disorder.

Synapse: The junction where nerve signals jump from one nerve to another.

Synergists: Muscles that assist the agonist.

Synovial Joints: Freely movable joints with a joint cavity surrounded by an articular capsule.

Synovial Membrane: A connective tissue membrane lining cavities and capsules in and around joints that produce synovial fluid.

Syphilis: A serious disease that is transmitted by sexual contact with an infected person.

Systemic Circulation: The blood circulation from the left side of the heart throughout the body and back again to the heart.

Systemic Infection: Invading organisms that have spread throughout the body.

Tapotement: Percussion massage movements include tapping, slapping, hacking, cupping, and beating.

Tapping: The lightest, most superficial of the percussion techniques performed with the finger tips.

Tendons: Fibrous connective tissue bands that attach muscle to bone.

Testes: Two small, egg-shaped glands that produce the spermatozoa.

Testosterone: A male hormone responsible for development of secondary sexual characteristics.

Tetany: A sustained muscle contraction that usually affects the hands and feet.

Therapeutic Procedure: The process of acquiring a concise medical history, assessment procedures to determine constricted and painful conditions, developing treatment plans, performing appropriate treatment practices to address the conditions more specifically, and evaluating the results.

Thermae: Hot springs or baths, especially the baths of ancient Rome.

Thermal Blanket: Thin polyethylene and metallic-coated sheet that retains heat during spa body wraps and aromatherapy. Also known as a space blanket.

Thoracic Duct: The largest lymph vessel that collects lymph from both legs and the left side of the rest of the body just before lymph reenters the venous blood stream.

Thrombophlebitis: The inflammation of veins from blood clots.

Thyroxin: A thyroid hormone that stimulates the metabolic rate of the body.

Tissues: Collections of similar cells that carry out specific bodily functions.

Touch for Health: A simplified form of applied kinesiology that involves techniques having both Eastern and Western origins.

Touching: Is a massage technique that refers to the stationary contact of the practitioner's hand and the client's body.

Transference: When a client personalizes, either negatively or positively, a therapeutic relationship by unconsciously projecting characteristics of someone from a former relationship onto a therapist or practitioner.

Transverse Plane: Divides the body horizontally into an upper and lower portion.

Transverse Tubules: A system of channels within the muscle cell containing extracellular fluid that helps transmit nerve impulses throughout the cell.

Tricuspid Valve: Part of the heart that allows blood to flow from the right atrium into the right ventricle.

Trigger Point: A hyperirritable nodule associated with dysfunctional contractile tissue that illicits a pain response when digital pressure is applied.

Triiodothyronine: A thyroid hormone (T3) that stimulates the metabolic rate of the body.

Tschanpua: A Hindu technique of massage in the bath.

Tsubo: Points on the body that are sensitive to pressure applied during shiatsu.

Tumor: An abnormal growth of swollen tissue that can be located on any part of the body.

Universal Precautions: A system of infection control that protects persons from exposure to blood and bloody body fluids.

Uterus: A pear-shaped, muscular organ of the female reproductive system that expands during pregnancy to accommodate the fetus.

Vaccine: Contains microorganisms that are either dead, or weakened or altered forms of a live infectious organism that stimulates an immune response without causing an illness.

Vagina: A muscular tube leading from the vulva to the cervix and is the lower part of the birth canal.

Vasoconstriction: The contraction of the arterial walls.

Vasodilation: The relaxation and enlargement of the arterial walls.

Veins: Thinner-walled blood vessels that carry deoxygenated blood and waste-laden blood from capillaries back to the heart.

Venereal Diseases: Known as sexually transmitted disease (STD) are associated with the sexual organs and are characterized by sores and rashes on the skin.

Venules: Microscopic vessels that continue from the capillaries and merge to form veins.

Vibration: A massage technique involving the continuous trembling or shaking movement delivered either by the practitioner or an electrical apparatus.

Vichy Shower: A multihead inline shower extending out over a treatment table, under which clients recline on a wet table to receive spa services.

Virus: A class of submicroscopic pathogenic agents that transmit disease.

Voluntary Muscles: Skeletal muscles that can be activated by conscious effort.

Watershed: The separation of flow of lymph into different drainage territories.

Wellness: Behaviors and habits that have a positive influence on health.

Wet Room: A tiled treatment room with plumbing that contains one or more of the following: wet table, shower, Vichy shower, hydrotherapy tub, Swiss shower.

Wet Sanitizer: Any receptacle large enough to hold a disinfectant solution in which the objects to be sanitized can be completely immersed.

Wet Table: A specially constructed waterproof treatment table with built-in drainage used in spas for exfoliation and body wrap services.

White Corpuscles: Or leukocytes, protect the body against disease by combating infections and toxins that invade the body.

Wringing: A massage technique consisting of a back-and-forth movement in which both hands are placed a short distance apart on either side of the limb and work in opposing directions.

INDEX

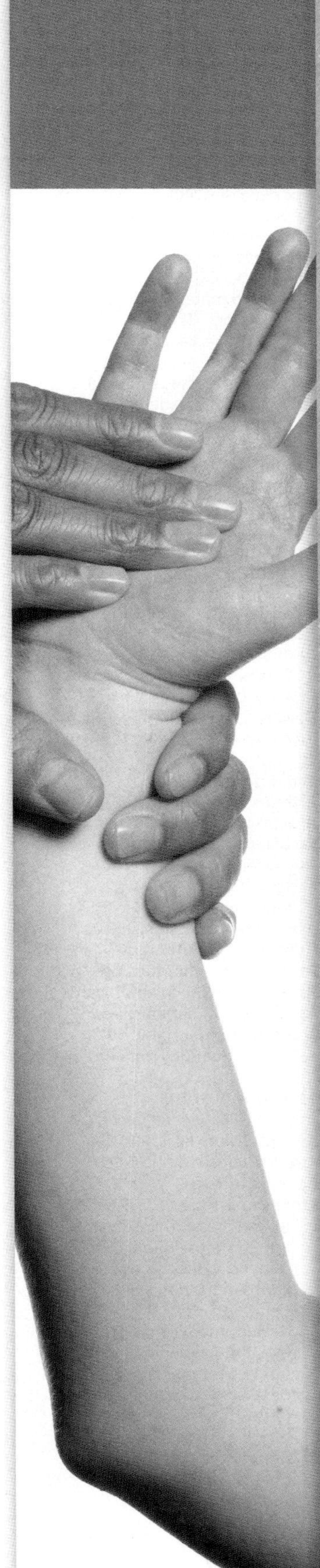

A

B

E

F

J

K

L

N

U

V

U

V

W

Y

Z